EIGHTH EDITION

8

FRANK H. NETTER, MD

Netter's Atlas of HUMAN ANATOMY

Classic Regional Approach

with LATIN TERMINOLOGY

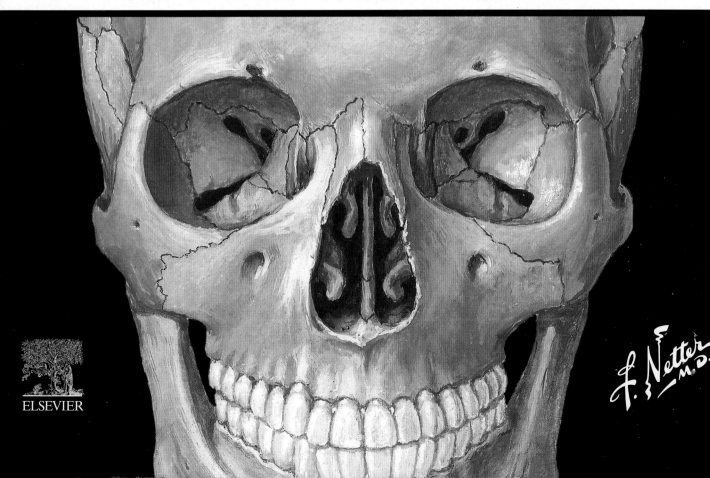

ELSEVIER

ELSEVIER
1600 John F. Kennedy Blvd.
Ste. 1600
Philadelphia, PA 19103-2899

ATLAS OF HUMAN ANATOMY: CLASSIC REGIONAL APPROACH
WITH LATIN TERMINOLOGY, EIGHTH EDITION

978-0-323-76023-2

Notices

Knowledge and best practice in this field are constantly changing. As new research and experience broaden our understanding, changes in research methods, professional practices, or medical treatment may become necessary.

Practitioners and researchers must always rely on their own experience and knowledge in evaluating and using any information, methods, compounds, or experiments described herein. In using such information or methods they should be mindful of their own safety and the safety of others, including parties for whom they have a professional responsibility.

With respect to any drug or pharmaceutical products identified, readers are advised to check the most current information provided (i) on procedures featured or (ii) by the manufacturer of each product to be administered, to verify the recommended dose or formula, the method and duration of administration, and contraindications. It is the responsibility of practitioners, relying on their own experience and knowledge of their patients, to make diagnoses, to determine dosages and the best treatment for each individual patient, and to take all appropriate safety precautions.

To the fullest extent of the law, neither the Publisher nor the authors, contributors, or editors, assume any liability for any injury and/or damage to persons or property as a matter of products liability, negligence or otherwise, or from any use or operation of any methods, products, instructions, or ideas contained in the material herein.

International Standard Book Number: 978-0-323-76023-2

Publisher: Elyse O'Grady
Senior Content Strategist: Marybeth Thiel
Publishing Services Manager: Catherine Jackson
Senior Project Manager/Specialist: Carrie Stetz
Book Design: Renee Duenow

Printed in India

9 8 7 6 5 4 3

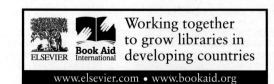

Working together
to grow libraries in
developing countries

www.elsevier.com • www.bookaid.org

CONSULTING EDITORS

Chief Contributing Illustrator and Art Lead Editor

Carlos A. G. Machado, MD

Terminology Content Lead Editors

Paul E. Neumann, MD
Professor, Department of Medical Neuroscience
Faculty of Medicine
Dalhousie University
Halifax, Nova Scotia
Canada

R. Shane Tubbs, MS, PA-C, PhD
Professor of Neurosurgery, Neurology, Surgery, and
    Structural and Cellular Biology
Director of Surgical Anatomy, Tulane University School
    of Medicine
Program Director of Anatomical Research, Clinical
    Neuroscience Research Center, Center for Clinical
    Neurosciences
Departments of Neurosurgery, Neurology, and Structural
    and Cellular Biology, Tulane University School
    of Medicine, New Orleans, Louisiana
Professor, Department of Neurosurgery and Ochsner
    Neuroscience Institute, Ochsner Health System, New
    Orleans, Louisiana
Professor of Anatomy, Department of Anatomical
    Sciences, St. George's University, Grenada
Honorary Professor, University of Queensland, Brisbane,
    Australia
Faculty, National Skull Base Center of California,
    Thousand Oakes, California

Electronic Content Lead Editors

Brion Benninger, MD, MBChB, MSc
Professor of Medical Innovation, Technology, &
    Research; Professor of Clinical Anatomy
Executive Director, Medical Anatomy Center
Department of Medical Anatomical Sciences
Faculty College of Dentistry
Western University of Health Sciences
Lebanon Oregon;
Faculty, Sports Medicine, Orthopaedic & General Surgery
    Residencies, Samaritan Health Services, Corvallis,
    Oregon;
Faculty, Surgery, Orthopedics & Rehabilitation, and
    Oral Maxillofacial Surgery, Oregon Health & Science
    University, Portland, Oregon;
Visiting Professor of Medical Innovation and Clinical
    Anatomy, School of Basic Medicine, Peking Union
    Medical College, Beijing, China;
Professor of Medical Innovation and Clinical Anatomy
    Post Graduate Diploma Surgical Anatomy, Otago
    University, Dunedin, New Zealand

Todd M. Hoagland, PhD
Clinical Professor of Biomedical Sciences and
    Occupational Therapy
Marquette University College of Health Sciences
Milwaukee, Wisconsin

Educational Content Lead Editors

Jennifer K. Brueckner-Collins, PhD
Distinguished Teaching Professor
Vice Chair for Educational Programs
Department of Anatomical Sciences and Neurobiology
University of Louisville School of Medicine
Louisville, Kentucky

Martha Johnson Gdowski, PhD
Associate Professor and Associate Chair of Medical
    Education, Department of Neuroscience
University of Rochester School of Medicine and Dentistry
Rochester, NY

Virginia T. Lyons, PhD
Associate Professor of Medical Education
Associate Dean for Preclinical Education
Geisel School of Medicine at Dartmouth
Hanover, New Hampshire

Peter J. Ward, PhD
Professor
Department of Biomedical Sciences
West Virginia School of Osteopathic Medicine
Lewisburg, West Virginia

Emeritus Editor

John T. Hansen, PhD
Professor Emeritus of Neuroscience and former Schmitt
    Chair of Neurobiology and Anatomy and Associate Dean
    for Admissions University of Rochester Medical Center
Rochester, New York

Latin Lead Editor

Paul E. Neumann, MD
Professor, Department of Medical Neuroscience
Faculty of Medicine
Dalhousie University
Halifax, Nova Scotia
Canada

EDITORS OF PREVIOUS EDITIONS

First Edition
Sharon Colacino, PhD

Second Edition
Arthur F. Dalley II, PhD

Third Edition
Carlos A. G. Machado, MD
John T. Hansen, PhD

Fourth Edition
Carlos A. G. Machado, MD
John T. Hansen, PhD
Jennifer K. Brueckner, PhD
Stephen W. Carmichael, PhD, DSc
Thomas R. Gest, PhD
Noelle A. Granger, PhD
Anil H. Waljii, MD, PhD

Fifth Edition
Carlos A. G. Machado, MD
John T. Hansen, PhD
Brion Benninger, MD, MS
Jennifer K. Brueckner, PhD
Stephen W. Carmichael, PhD, DSc
Noelle A. Granger, PhD
R. Shane Tubbs, MS, PA-C, PhD

Sixth Edition
Carlos A. G. Machado, MD
John T. Hansen, PhD
Brion Benninger, MD, MS
Jennifer Brueckner-Collins, PhD
Todd M. Hoagland, PhD
R. Shane Tubbs, MS, PA-C, PhD

Seventh Edition
Carlos A. G. Machado, MD
John T. Hansen, PhD
Brion Benninger, MD, MS
Jennifer Brueckner-Collins, PhD
Todd M. Hoagland, PhD
R. Shane Tubbs, MS, PA-C, PhD

OTHER CONTRIBUTING ILLUSTRATORS

Rob Duckwall, MA (DragonFly Media Group)
Kristen Wienandt Marzejon, MS, MFA
Tiffany S. DaVanzo, MA, CMI
James A. Perkins, MS, MFA

INTERNATIONAL ADVISORY BOARD

PREFACE

The illustrations comprising the *Netter Atlas of Human Anatomy* were painted by physician-artists, Frank H. Netter, MD, and Carlos Machado, MD. Dr. Netter was a surgeon and Dr. Machado is a cardiologist. Their clinical insights and perspectives have informed their approaches to these works of art. The collective expertise of the anatomists, educators, and clinicians guiding the selection, arrangement, labeling, and creation of the illustrations ensures the accuracy, relevancy, and educational power of this outstanding collection.

You have a copy of the regionally organized 8th edition with Latin terminology. This is the traditional organization and presentation that has been used since the first edition. Also available is an English language terminology option that is also regionally organized, as well as an option with English terminology organized by body system. In all cases, the same beautiful and instructive Art Plates and Table information are included.

New to this Edition

New Art

More than 20 new illustrations have been added and over 30 art modifications have been made throughout this edition. Highlights include new views of the temporal and infratemporal fossa, pelvic fascia, nasal cavity and paranasal sinuses, plus multiple new perspectives of the heart, a cross-section of the foot, enhanced surface anatomy plates, and overviews of many body systems. In these pages you will find the most robust illustrated coverage to date for modern clinical anatomy courses.

Terminology and Label Updates

This 8th edition incorporates terms of the *Terminologia Anatomica* (2nd edition), as published by the Federative International Programme on Anatomical Terminology (FIPAT) in 2019 (https://fipat.library.dal.ca/ta2) and adopted by the International Federation of Associations of Anatomy in 2020. A fully searchable database of the updated *Terminologia Anatomica* can be accessed at https://ta2viewer.openanatomy.org. Common clinical eponyms and former terminologies are selectively included, parenthetically, for clarity. In addition, a strong effort has been made to reduce label text on the page while maximizing label information through the use of abbreviations and focusing on the labels most relevant to the subject of each Plate.

Nerve Tables

The muscle tables and clinical tables of previous editions have been so positively received that brand new tables have been added to cover four major nerve groups: cranial nerves and the nerves of the cervical, brachial, and lumbosacral plexuses.

Latin Nomenclature

This is the second English-Latin Netter: *Atlas of Human Anatomy*. It contains Latin anatomical terms from the second edition of *Terminologia Anatomica* (TA) (https://FIPAT.library.dal.ca/TA2). The revision of TA includes spelling and grammar corrections and changes recommended by FIPAT's Informatics subcommittee (*Clin Anat* 30:300-2, 2017; *Clin Anat* 33:327-31, 2020) to eliminate appositions and to adopt word order rules that simplify the terms. Every effort has been made to ensure consistency in usage of English and Latin in the plates and tables, including use of complete Latin terms, English conjunctions, and punctuation between terms.

Latin Abbreviations

SINGULAR		PLURAL	
A., a.	Arteria, arteriae	Aa., aa.	Arteriae, arteriarum
Art., art.	Articulatio, articulationis	Artt., artt.	Articulationes, articulationum
dex.	dexter, -tra, -trum; dextri, -ae, -i	dex.	dextri, -ae, -a; dextrorum, -arum, -orum
Lig., lig.	Ligamentum, ligamenti	Ligg., ligg.	Ligamenta, ligamentorum
M., m.	Musculus, musculi	Mm., mm.	Musculi, musculorum
N., n.	Nervus, nervi	Nn., nn.	Nervi, nervorum
Proc., proc.	Processus, processus	Procc., procc.	Processus, processuum
R., r.	Ramus, rami	Rr., rr.	Rami, ramorum
sin.	sinister, -tra, -trum; sinistri, -ae, -i	sin.	sinistri, -ae, -a; sinistrorum, -arum, -orum
V., v.	Vena, venae	Vv., vv.	Venae, venarum

Each column contains the nominative and genitive forms.

The Future of the Netter Anatomy Atlas

As the Netter Atlas continues to evolve to meet the needs of students, educators, and clinicians, we welcome suggestions! Please use the following form to provide your feedback:

https://tinyurl.com/NetterAtlas8

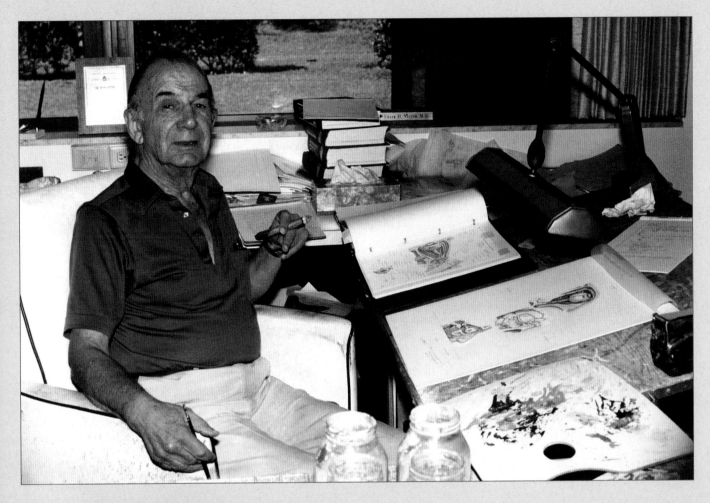

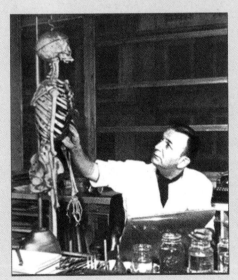

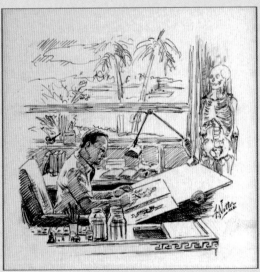

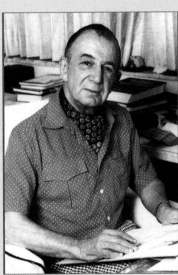

To my dear wife, Vera

PREFACE TO THE FIRST EDITION

I have often said that my career as a medical artist for almost 50 years has been a sort of "command performance" in the sense that it has grown in response to the desires and requests of the medical profession. Over these many years, I have produced almost 4,000 illustrations, mostly for *The CIBA* (now *Netter*) *Collection of Medical Illustrations* but also for *Clinical Symposia*. These pictures have been concerned with the varied subdivisions of medical knowledge such as gross anatomy, histology, embryology, physiology, pathology, diagnostic modalities, surgical and therapeutic techniques, and clinical manifestations of a multitude of diseases. As the years went by, however, there were more and more requests from physicians and students for me to produce an atlas purely of gross anatomy. Thus, this atlas has come about, not through any inspiration on my part but rather, like most of my previous works, as a fulfillment of the desires of the medical profession.

It involved going back over all the illustrations I had made over so many years, selecting those pertinent to gross anatomy, classifying them and organizing them by system and region, adapting them to page size and space, and arranging them in logical sequence. Anatomy of course does not change, but our understanding of anatomy and its clinical significance does change, as do anatomical terminology and nomenclature. This therefore required much updating of many of the older pictures and even revision of a number of them in order to make them more pertinent to today's ever-expanding scope of medical and surgical practice. In addition, I found that there were gaps in the portrayal of medical knowledge as pictorialized in the illustrations I had previously done, and this necessitated my making a number of new pictures that are included in this volume.

In creating an atlas such as this, it is important to achieve a happy medium between complexity and simplification. If the pictures are too complex, they may be difficult and confusing to read; if oversimplified, they may not be adequately definitive or may even be misleading. I have therefore striven for a middle course of realism without the clutter of confusing minutiae. I hope that the students and members of the medical and allied professions will find the illustrations readily understandable, yet instructive and useful.

At one point, the publisher and I thought it might be nice to include a foreword by a truly outstanding and renowned anatomist, but there are so many in that category that we could not make a choice. We did think of men like Vesalius, Leonardo da Vinci, William Hunter, and Henry Gray, who of course are unfortunately unavailable, but I do wonder what their comments might have been about this atlas.

Frank H. Netter, MD
(1906–1991)

FRANK H. NETTER, MD

Frank H. Netter was born in New York City in 1906. He studied art at the Art Students League and the National Academy of Design before entering medical school at New York University, where he received his Doctor of Medicine degree in 1931. During his student years, Dr. Netter's notebook sketches attracted the attention of the medical faculty and other physicians, allowing him to augment his income by illustrating articles and textbooks. He continued illustrating as a sideline after establishing a surgical practice in 1933, but he ultimately opted to give up his practice in favor of a full-time commitment to art. After service in the United States Army during World War II, Dr. Netter began his long collaboration with the CIBA Pharmaceutical Company (now Novartis Pharmaceuticals). This 45-year partnership resulted in the production of the extraordinary collection of medical art so familiar to physicians and other medical professionals worldwide.

Icon Learning Systems acquired the Netter Collection in July 2000 and continued to update Dr. Netter's original paintings and to add newly commissioned paintings by artists trained in the style of Dr. Netter. In 2005, Elsevier Inc. purchased the Netter Collection and all publications from Icon Learning Systems. There are now over 50 publications featuring the art of Dr. Netter available through Elsevier Inc.

Dr. Netter's works are among the finest examples of the use of illustration in the teaching of medical concepts. The 13-book *Netter Collection of Medical Illustrations,* which includes the greater part of the more than 20,000 paintings created by Dr. Netter, became and remains one of the most famous medical works ever published. *The Netter Atlas of Human Anatomy,* first published in 1989, presents the anatomic paintings from the Netter Collection. Now translated into 16 languages, it is the anatomy atlas of choice among medical and health professions students the world over.

The Netter illustrations are appreciated not only for their aesthetic qualities, but, more importantly, for their intellectual content. As Dr. Netter wrote in 1949 "clarification of a subject is the aim and goal of illustration. No matter how beautifully painted, how delicately and subtly rendered a subject may be, it is of little value as a *medical illustration* if it does not serve to make clear some medical point." Dr. Netter's planning, conception, point of view, and approach are what inform his paintings and what make them so intellectually valuable.

Frank H. Netter, MD, physician and artist, died in 1991.

Carlos A.G. Machado, MD was chosen by Novartis to be Dr. Netter's successor. He continues to be the main artist who contributes to the Netter collection of medical illustrations.

Self-taught in medical illustration, cardiologist Carlos Machado has contributed meticulous updates to some of Dr. Netter's original plates and has created many paintings of his own in the style of Netter as an extension of the Netter collection. Dr. Machado's photorealistic expertise and his keen insight into the physician/patient relationship inform his vivid and unforgettable visual style. His dedication to researching each topic and subject he paints places him among the premier medical illustrators at work today.

Learn more about his background and see more of his art at: https://netterimages.com/artist-carlos-a-g-machado.html

Paul E. Neumann, MD was clinically trained in anatomical pathology and neuropathology. Most of his research publications have been in mouse neurogenetics and molecular human genetics. In the past several years, he has concentrated on the anatomical sciences, and has frequently written about anatomical terminology and anatomical ontology in the journal Clinical Anatomy. As an officer of the Federative International Programme for Anatomical Terminology (FIPAT), he participated in the production of *Terminologia Anatomica* (2nd edition), *Terminologia Embryologica* (2nd edition), and *Terminologia Neuroanatomica*. In addition to serving as the lead Latin editor of the 8th edition of Netter's Atlas, he was a contributor to the 33rd edition of Dorland's Illustrated Medical Dictionary.

R. Shane Tubbs, MS, PA-C, PhD is a native of Birmingham, Alabama and a clinical anatomist. His research interests are centered around clinical/surgical problems that are identified and solved with anatomical studies. This investigative paradigm in anatomy as resulted in over 1,700 peer reviewed publications. Dr. Tubbs' laboratory has made novel discoveries in human anatomy including a new nerve to the skin of the lower eyelid, a new space of the face, a new venous sinus over the spinal cord, new connections between the parts of the sciatic nerve, new ligaments of the neck, a previously undescribed cutaneous branch of the inferior gluteal nerve, and an etiology for postoperative C5 nerve palsies. Moreover, many anatomical feasibility studies from Dr. Tubbs' laboratory have gone on to be used by surgeons from around the world and have thus resulted in new surgical/clinical procedures such as treating hydrocephalus by shunting cerebrospinal fluid into various bones, restoration of upper limb function in paralyzed patients with neurotization procedures using the contralateral spinal accessory nerve, and harvesting of clavicle for anterior cervical discectomy and fusion procedures in patients with cervical instability or degenerative spine disease.

Dr. Tubbs sits on the editorial board of over 15 anatomical journals and has reviewed for over 150 scientific journals. He has been a visiting professor to major institutions in the United States and worldwide. Dr. Tubbs has authored over 40 books and over 75 book chapters. His published books by Elsevier include *Gray's Anatomy Review*, *Gray's Clinical Photographic Dissector of the Human Body*, *Netter's Introduction to Clinical Procedures*, and *Nerves and Nerve Injuries* volumes I and II. He is an editor for the 41st and 42nd editions of the over 150-year-old *Gray's Anatomy*, the 5th through 8th editions of *Netter's Atlas of Anatomy*, and is the editor-in-chief of the journal *Clinical Anatomy*. He is the Chair of the Federative International Programme on Anatomical Terminologies (FIPAT).

Jennifer K. Brueckner-Collins, PhD is a proud Kentucky native. She pursued her undergraduate and graduate training at the University of Kentucky. During her second year of graduate school there, she realized that her professional calling was not basic science research in skeletal muscle biology, but was instead was helping medical students master the anatomical sciences. She discovered this during a required teaching assistantship in medical histology, where working with students at the 10-headed microscope changed her career path.

The next semester of graduate school, she assisted in teaching dissection-based gross anatomy, although she had taken anatomy when the lab component was prosection based. After teaching in the first lab, she knew that she needed to learn anatomy more thoroughly through dissection on her own, so she dissected one to two labs ahead of the students that semester; that was when she really learned anatomy and was inspired to teach this discipline as a profession. All of this occurred in the early 1990s when pursuing a teaching career was frowned upon by many; it was thought that you only pursued this track if you were unsuccessful in research. She taught anatomy part-time during the rest of her graduate training, on her own time, to gain requisite experience to ultimately secure a faculty position.

Dr. Brueckner-Collins spent 10 years at the University of Kentucky as a full-time faculty member teaching dissection-based gross anatomy to medical, dental and allied health students. Then, after meeting the love of her life, she moved to the University of Louisville and has taught medical and dental students there for more than a decade. Over 20 years of teaching full time at two medical schools in the state, her teaching efforts have been recognized through receipt of the highest teaching honor at each medical school in the state, the Provost's Teaching Award at University of Kentucky, and the Distinguished Teaching Professorship at University of Louisville.

Martha Johnson Gdowski, PhD earned her BS in Biology cum laude from Gannon University in 1990, followed by a PhD in Anatomy from the Pennsylvania State University College of Medicine in 1995. She completed postdoctoral fellowships at the Cleveland Clinic and Northwestern University School of Medicine prior to accepting a faculty position in the Department of Neuroscience at the University of Rochester School of Medicine and Dentistry in

2001. Previous research interests include the development of an adult model of hydrocephalus, sensorimotor integration in the basal ganglia, and sensorimotor integration in normal and pathological aging.

Her passion throughout her career has been in her service as an educator. Her teaching has encompassed a variety of learning formats including didactic lecture, laboratory, journal club, and problem-based learning. She has taught for four academic institutions in different capacities (The Pennsylvania State University School of Medicine, Northwestern University School of Medicine, Ithaca College, and The University of Rochester School of Medicine and Dentistry). She has taught in the following curricula: Undergraduate and Graduate Neuroscience, Graduate Neuroanatomy, Graduate Human Anatomy and Physiology for Physical Therapists, Undergraduate Medical Human Anatomy and Histology, and Undergraduate and Graduate Human Anatomy. These experiences have provided an opportunity to instruct students that vary in age, life experience, race, ethnicity and economic background, revealing how diversity in student populations enriches learning environments in ways that benefit everyone. She has been honored to be the recipient of numerous awards for her teaching and mentoring of students during their undergraduate medical education. Martha enjoys gardening, hiking, and swimming with her husband, Greg Gdowski, PhD and their dogs, Sophie and Ivy.

Virginia T. Lyons, PhD, is an Associate Professor of Medical Education and the Associate Dean for Preclinical Education at the Geisel School of Medicine at Dartmouth. She received her BS in Biology from Rochester Institute of Technology and her PhD in Cell Biology and Anatomy from the University of North Carolina at Chapel Hill. Dr. Lyons has devoted her career to education in the anatomical sciences, teaching gross anatomy, histology, embryology, and neuroanatomy to medical students and other health professions students. She has led courses and curricula in human gross anatomy and embryology for more than 20 years and is a strong advocate for incorporating engaged pedagogies into preclinical medical education. Dr. Lyons has been recognized with numerous awards for teaching and mentoring students, and was elected to the Dartmouth chapter of the Alpha Omega Alpha Honor Medical Society. She is the author of Netter's Essential Systems-Based Anatomy and co-author of the Human Anatomy Learning Modules website accessed by students worldwide. Dr. Lyons also serves as the Discipline Editor for Anatomy on the Aquifer Sciences Curriculum Editorial Board, working to integrate anatomical concepts into virtual patient cases that are used in multiple settings including clerkships and residency training.

Peter J. Ward, PhD grew up in Casper, Wyoming, graduating from Kelly Walsh High School and then attending Carnegie Mellon University in Pittsburgh, Pennsylvania. He began graduate school at Purdue University, where he first encountered gross anatomy, histology, embryology, and neuroanatomy. Having found a course of study that engrossed him, he helped teach those courses in the veterinary and medical programs at Purdue. Dr. Ward completed a PhD program in anatomy education and, in 2005, he joined the faculty at the West Virginia School of Osteopathic Medicine (WVSOM) in Lewisburg, West Virginia. There he has taught gross anatomy, embryology, neuroscience, histology, and the history of medicine. Dr. Ward has received numerous teaching awards, including the WVSOM Golden Key Award, the Basmajian Award from the American Association of Anatomists, and has been a two-time finalist in the West Virginia Merit Foundation's Professor of the Year selection. Dr. Ward has also been director of the WVSOM plastination facility, coordinator of the anatomy graduate teaching assistants, chair of the curriculum committee, chair of the faculty council, creator and director of a clinical anatomy elective course, and host of many anatomy-centered events between WVSOM and two Japanese Colleges of Osteopathy. Dr. Ward has also served as council member and association secretary for the American Association of Clinical Anatomists. In conjunction with Bone Clones, Inc., Dr. Ward has produced tactile models that mimic the feel of anatomical structures when intact and when ruptured during the physical examination. He created the YouTube channel, Clinical Anatomy Explained! and continues to pursue interesting ways to present the anatomical sciences to the public. Dr. Ward was the Senior Associate Editor for the three volumes of *The Netter Collection: The Digestive System,* 2nd Edition, a contributor to *Gray's Anatomy,* 42nd Edition, and is author of *Netter's Integrated Musculoskeletal System: Clinical Anatomy Explained.*

Brion Benninger, MD, MBChB, MSc currently teaches surgical, imaging, and dynamic anatomy to medical students and residents in several countries (United States, New Zealand, China, Japan, Korea, The Caribbean, Mexico). He develops, invents, and assesses ultrasound probes, medical equipment, simulations, and software while identifying dynamic anatomy. He enjoys mixing educational techniques integrating macro imaging and surgical anatomy. Dr. Benninger developed the teaching theory of anatomy deconstruction/reconstruction and was the first to combine ultrasound with Google Glass during physical examination, coining the term "triple feedback examination." An early user of ultrasound, he continues to develop eFAST teaching and training techniques, has developed and shares a patent on a novel ultrasound finger probe, and is currently developing a new revolutionary ultrasound probe for breast screening. He is a reviewer for several ultrasound, clinical anatomy, surgical, and radiology journals and edits and writes medical textbooks. His research interests integrate clinical anatomy with conventional and emerging technologies to improve training techniques in situ and simulation. Dr. Benninger pioneered and coined the term "dynamic anatomy," developed a technique to deliver novel contrast medium to humans and was the first to reveal vessels and nerves not previously seen using CT and MRI imaging. He has mentored more than 200 students on over 350 research projects presented at national and international conferences and has received numerous awards for projects related to emergency procedures, ultrasound, sports medicine, clinical anatomy, medical simulation, reverse translational research, medical education, and technology. He is proud to have received medical teaching awards from several countries and institutions, including being the first recipient in more than 25 years to receive the Commendation Medal Award from the Commission of Osteopathic Accreditation for innovative clinical anatomy teaching that he designed and facilitated in Lebanon, Oregon. Dr. Benninger has received sports medicine accolades from Sir Roger Bannister regarding his medical invention on shoulder proprioception. He is also Executive Director of the Medical Anatomy Center and collaborates with colleagues globally from surgical and nonsurgical specialties. He is also an invited course speaker for surgical anatomy in New Zealand. Dr. Benninger collects medical history books, loves mountains and sports, and is an anonymous restaurant critic. British mentors directly responsible for his training include Prof. Peter Bell (surgery), Prof. Sir Alec Jeffreys (genetic fingerprinting), Profs. David deBono and Tony Gershlick (cardiology), Prof. Roger Greenhalgh (vascular surgery), Profs. Chris Colton, John Webb, and Angus Wallace (orthopaedics), Prof. Harold Ellis CBE (surgery and clinical anatomy), and Prof. Susan Standring (Guys Hospital/Kings College).

Todd M. Hoagland, PhD, is Clinical Professor of Biomedical Sciences and Occupational Therapy at Marquette University in the College of Health Sciences. Previously he was Professor of Anatomy at the Medical College of Wisconsin (MCW). Prior to MCW, Dr. Hoagland was at Boston University School of Medicine (BUSM) and he still holds an adjunct faculty position at Boston University Goldman School of Dental Medicine. Dr. Hoagland is a passionate teacher and is dedicated to helping students achieve their goals. He believes in being a strong steward of the anatomical sciences, which involves teaching it to students while contemporaneously developing resources to improve the transfer of knowledge and preparing the next generation to be even better teachers. While at BUSM, Dr. Hoagland was a leader for the Carnegie Initiative on the Doctorate in Neuroscience and helped develop the Vesalius Program (teacher training) for graduate students. The program ensures that graduate students learn about effective teaching, receive experiences in the classroom, and understand how to share what they learn via scholarship.

Dr. Hoagland's dedication to health professions education has been richly rewarded by numerous teaching awards from the University of Notre Dame, BUSM, and MCW. Dr. Hoagland received the Award for Outstanding Ethical Leadership in 2009, was inducted into the Alpha Omega Alpha Honor Medical Society in 2010, received the American Association of Anatomists Basmajian Award in 2012, and was inducted into the Society of Teaching Scholars in 2012 and was their director from 2016–2020.

Dr. Hoagland's scholarly activity centers on (1) evaluating content and instructional/learning methodology in Clinical Human Anatomy and Neuroanatomy courses, especially as relevant to clinical practice, (2) translating basic anatomical science research findings into clinically meaningful information, and (3) evaluating professionalism in students to enhance their self-awareness and improve patient care outcomes. Dr. Hoagland is also consulting editor for Netter's *Atlas of Human Anatomy,* co-author for the digital anatomy textbook *AnatomyOne,* and lead author for *Clinical Human Anatomy Dissection Guide.*

ACKNOWLEDGMENTS

Carlos A. G. Machado, MD

With the completion of this 8th edition, I celebrate 27 years contributing to the Netter brand of educational products, 25 years of which have been dedicated to the update—seven editions—of this highly prestigious, from birth, Atlas of Human Anatomy. For these 25 years I have had the privilege and honor of working with some of the most knowledgeable anatomists, educators, and consulting editors—my treasured friends—from whom I have learned considerably.

For the last 16 years it has also been a great privilege to be part of the Elsevier team and be under the skillful coordination and orientation of Marybeth Thiel, Elsevier's Senior Content Development Specialist, and Elyse O'Grady, Executive Content Strategist. I thank both for their friendship, support, sensibility, and very dedicated work.

Once more I thank my wife Adriana and my daughter Beatriz for all their love and encouragement, and for patiently steering me back on track when I get lost in philosophical divagations about turning scientific research into artistic inspiration—and vice-versa!

It is impossible to put in words how thankful I am to my much-loved parents, Carlos and Neide, for their importance in my education and in the formation of my moral and ethical values.

I am eternally grateful to the body donors for their inestimable contribution to the correct understanding of human anatomy; to the students, teachers, health professionals, colleagues, educational institutions, and friends who have, anonymously or not, directly or indirectly, been an enormous source of motivation and invaluable scientific references, constructive comments, and relevant suggestions.

My last thanks, but far from being the least, go to my teachers Eugênio Cavalcante, Mário Fortes, and Paulo Carneiro, for their inspiring teachings on the practical application of the knowledge of anatomy.

Paul E. Neumann, MD

It has been a privilege to work on the English and Latin editions of Netter's Atlas of Human Anatomy. I thank the staff at Elsevier (especially Elyse O'Grady, Marybeth Thiel and Carrie Stetz), Dr. Carlos Machado, and the other editors for their efforts to produce a new, improved edition. I am also grateful to my wife, Sandra Powell, and my daughter, Eve, for their support of my academic work.

R. Shane Tubbs, MS, PA-C, PhD

I thank Elyse O'Grady and Marybeth Thiel for their dedication and hard work on this edition. As always, I thank my wife, Susan, and son, Isaiah, for their patience with me on such projects. Additionally, I thank Drs. George and Frank Salter who inspired and encouraged me along my path to anatomy.

Jennifer K. Brueckner-Collins, PhD

Reba McEntire once said "To succeed in life, you need three things: a wishbone, a backbone and a funny bone."

My work with the Netter Atlas and the people associated with it over the past 15 years has played an instrumental role in helping me develop and sustain these three metaphorical bones in my professional and personal life.

I am forever grateful to John Hansen who believed in my ability to serve as an editor starting with the 4th edition.

I extend my sincere thanks to Marybeth Thiel and Elyse O'Grady for not only being the finest of colleagues but part of my professional family as well. Thanks to you both for your professionalism, support, patience and collegiality.

To Carlos Machado, you continue to amaze me and inspire me with your special gift of bringing anatomy to life through your art.

For this edition, I also count in my blessings, the ability to work closely with the talented team of educational leaders, including Martha Gdowski, Virginia Lyons and Peter Ward. It is humbling to work with such brilliant and dedicated teachers as we collectively assembled the systems-based Netter Atlas concept.

Finally, I dedicate my work on this edition with unconditional and infinite love to Kurt, Lincoln, my Dad in Heaven, as well as my dog boys, Bingo and Biscuit.

Martha Johnson Gdowski, PhD

I am grateful for the honor to work with the team of editors that Elsevier has selected for the preparation of this 8th edition; they are exceptional in their knowledge, passion as educators, and collegiality. I especially would like to thank Elyse O'Grady and Marybeth Thiel, who have been outstanding in their expertise, patience, and guidance. I am grateful to John T. Hansen, PhD, for his guidance, mentorship, and friendship as a colleague at the University of Rochester and for giving me the opportunity to participate in this work. He continues to be an outstanding role model who has shaped my career as an anatomical sciences educator. Special thanks to Carlos Machado for his gift for making challenging anatomical dissections and difficult concepts accessible to students of anatomy through his artistry, research of the details, and thoughtful discussions. I am indebted to the selfless individuals who have gifted their bodies for anatomical study, the students of anatomy, and my colleagues at the University of Rochester, all of whom motivate me to work to be the best educator I can be. I am most grateful for my loving husband and best friend, Greg, who is my greatest source of support and inspiration.

Virginia T. Lyons, PhD

It has been a joy to work with members of the editorial team on the iconic Atlas of Human Anatomy by Frank Netter. I would like to thank Elyse O'Grady and Marybeth Thiel for their expert guidance and ability to nourish the creative process while also keeping us focused (otherwise we would have reveled in debating anatomy minutiae for hours!). I am amazed by the talent of Carlos Machado, who is able to transform our ideas into beautiful, detailed illustrations that simplify concepts for students. I appreciate the patience and support of my husband, Patrick, and my children, Sean and Nora, who keep me sane when things get busy. Finally, I am grateful for the opportunity to teach and learn from the outstanding medical students at the Geisel School of Medicine at Dartmouth. I am fulfilled by their energy, curiosity, and love of learning.

Peter J. Ward, PhD

It is a thrill and honor to contribute to the 8th edition of *Netter's Atlas of Human Anatomy*. It still amazes me that I am helping to showcase the incomparable illustrations of Frank Netter and Carlos Machado. I hope that this atlas continues to bring these works of medical art to a new generation of students as they begin investigating the awesome enigma of the human body. Thanks to all the amazing contributors and to the hardworking team at Elsevier, especially Marybeth Thiel and Elyse O'Grady, for keeping all of us moving forward. Thank you especially to Todd Hoagland for recommending me to the team. I have immense gratitude to James Walker and Kevin Hannon, who introduced me to the world of anatomy. They both seamlessly combined high expectations for their students along with enthusiastic teaching that made the topic fascinating and rewarding. Great thanks to my parents, Robert and Lucinda Ward, for their lifelong support of my education and for the many formative museum trips to stare at dinosaur bones. Sarah, Archer, and Dashiell, you are all the reason I work hard and try to make the world a slightly better place. Your love and enthusiasm mean everything to me.

Brion Benninger, MD, MBChB, MSc

I thank all the healthcare institutions worldwide and the allopathic and osteopathic associations who have provided me the privilege to wake up each day and focus on how to improve our knowledge of teaching and healing the anatomy of the mind, body, and soul while nurturing humanism. I am grateful and fortunate to have my lovely wife, Alison, and thoughtful son, Jack, support my efforts during late nights and long weekends. Their laughs and experiences complete my life. I thank Elsevier, especially Marybeth Thiel, Elyse O'Grady, and Madelene Hyde for expecting the highest standards and providing guidance, enabling my fellow coeditors to work in a fluid diverse environment. Many thanks to Carlos Machado and Frank Netter; the world is proud. I thank clinicians who trained me, especially my early gifted surgeon/anatomist/teacher mentors, Drs. Gerald Tressidor and Harold Ellis CBE (Cambridge & Guy's Hospital); Dr. S. Standring and Dr. M. Englund, who embody professionalism; Drs. P. Crone, E. Szeto, and J. Heatherington, for supporting innovative medical education; my past, current and future students and patients; and clinical colleagues from all corners of the world who keep medicine and anatomy dynamic, fresh, and wanting. Special thanks to Drs. J.L. Horn, S. Echols, J. Anderson, and J. Underwood, friends, mentors and fellow visionaries who also see "outside the box," challenging the status quo. Heartfelt tribute to my late mentors, friends, and sister, Jim McDaniel, Bill Bryan, and Gail Hendricks, who represent what is good in teaching, caring, and healing. They made this world a wee bit better. Lastly, I thank my mother for her love of education and equality and my father for his inquisitive and creative mind.

Todd M. Hoagland, PhD

It is a privilege to teach clinical human anatomy, and I am eternally grateful to all the body donors and their families for enabling healthcare professionals to train in the dissection laboratory. It is my honor to work with occupational therapy and health professions students and colleagues at Marquette University. I am grateful to John Hansen and the professionals of the Elsevier team for the opportunity to be a steward of the incomparable *Netter Atlas*. Marybeth Thiel and Elyse O'Grady were especially helpful and a pleasure to work with. It was an honor to collaborate with the brilliant Carlos Machado and all the consulting editors. I thank Dave Bolender, Brian Bear, and Rebecca Lufler for being outstanding colleagues, and I thank all the graduate students I've worked with for helping me grow as a person; it is such a pleasure to see them flourish. I am deeply appreciative of Stan Hillman and Jack O'Malley for inspiring me with masterful teaching and rigorous expectations. I am indebted to Gary Kolesari and Richard Hoyt Jr for helping me become a competent clinical anatomist, and to Rob Bouchie for the intangibles and is camaraderie. I am most grateful to my brother, Bill, for his unwavering optimism and for always being there. I thank my mother, Liz, for her dedication and love, and for instilling a strong work ethic. I am humbled by my three awesome children, Ella, Caleb, and Gregory, for helping me redefine love, wonder, and joy. Ola, ty moye solntse!

CONTENTS

7th Edition to 8th Edition Plate Number Conversion Chart Available Online at **https://tinyurl.com/Netter7to8conversion**

SECTION 1 INTRODUCTION · Plates 1–21

General Anatomy · Plates 1–3

1	Plana Referentiae and Termini Generales
2	Partes Corporis Human: Anterior View of Female
3	Partes Corporis Human: Posterior View of Male

Systematic Anatomy · Plates 4–21

4	Systema Nervosum: Overview
5	Dermatomata: Membra Superius and Inferius
6	Pars Sympathica Systematis Nervosi: Schema
7	Pars Parasympathica Systematis Nervosi: Schema
8	Systema Skeletale: Overview
9	Juncturae Synoviales: Types
10	Systema Musculare: Overview
11	Systema Nervosum: Segmental Motor Function
12	Cutis: Cross Section
13	Systema Cardiovasculare: Overview
14	Arteriae Majores: Pulse Points
15	Systema Cardiovasculare: Venae Systematicae Majores
16	Vasa Lymphatica and Organa Lymphoidea: Overview
17	Systema Respiratorium: Overview
18	Systema Digestorium: Overview
19	Systema Urinarium: Overview
20	Systemata Genitalia: Overview
21	Systema Endocrinum: Overview

Electronic Bonus Plates · Plates BP 1– BP 13

BP 1	Apparatus Pilosebaceus
BP 2	Cavitates Majores Corporis Humani
BP 3	Neuron and Synapsis
BP 4	Nervus Periphericus: Typical Features
BP 5	Sites of Visceral Referred Pain
BP 6	Pars Sympathica Systematis Nervosi: General Topography
BP 7	Pars Parasympathica Systematis Nervosi: General Topography
BP 8	Synapses Cholinergicae and Adrenergicae: Schema
BP 9	Os: Architecture
BP 10	Musculus: Structure
BP 11	Juncturae: Textus Connectivi and Cartilago Articularis
BP 12	Systema Cardiovasculare: Composition of Blood
BP 13	Arteria: Structure of Wall

SECTION 2   CAPUT AND COLLUM · Plates 22–177

Surface Anatomy · Plates 22–24

22	Caput and Collum: Surface Anatomy
23	Caput and Collum: Nervi Cutanei
24	Facies and Epicranium: Arteriae and Venae Superficiales

Ossa and Juncturae · Plates 25–47

25	Cranium and Mandibula: Anterior View
26	Cranium and Mandibula: Radiographs
27	Cranium and Mandibula: Lateral View
28	Cranium and Mandibula: Lateral Radiograph
29	Cranium: Median Section
30	Calvaria
31	Basis Cranii: Inferior View
32	Basis Cranii: Superior View
33	Basis Cranii: Foramina and Canales (Inferior View)
34	Basis Cranii: Foramina and Canales (Superior View)
35	Cranium: Newborn
36	Caput and Collum: Skeleton
37	Skeleton Nasi and Sinus Paranasales
38	Cranium: Posterior and Lateral Views
39	Mandibula
40	Dentes
41	Dens
42	Articulatio Temporomandibularis
43	Vertebrae Cervicales: Atlas and Axis
44	Vertebrae Cervicales
45	Pars Cervicalis Columnae Vertebralis
46	Ligamenta Craniocervicalia Externa
47	Ligamenta Craniocervicalia Interna

Collum · Plates 48–58

48	Musculi Superficiales Capitis: Lateral View
49	Musculi Colli: Anterior View
50	Venae Superficiales Colli
51	Fasciae Cervicales: Schema
52	Fasciae Cervicales
53	Musculi Infrahyoidei and Suprahyoidei
54	Musculi Colli: Lateral View
55	Musculi Colli Anteriores and Laterales
56	Nervi Colli
57	Nervi Cervicales and Plexus Cervicalis
58	Carotides

Nasus • Plates 59–82

59	Skeleton Nasi
60	Facies: Musculi, Nervi, and Arteriae
61	Paries Lateralis Cavitatis Nasi
62	Paries Lateralis Cavitatis Nasalis Cranii
63	Paries Medialis Cavitatis Nasi: Septum Nasi
64	Cavitas Nasi: Nervi
65	Cavitas Nasi: Vasa Saguinea
66	Cavitas Nasalis Cranii: Nervi (Septum Nasalis Turned Up)
67	Sinus Paranasales: Paramedian Views
68	Sinus Paranasales: Changes with Age
69	Sinus Paranasales: Coronal and Transverse Sections
70	Glandulae Salivariae
71	Rami Nervi Facialis and Glandula Parotidea
72	Musculi Masticatorii: Masseter and Musculus Temporalis
73	Musculi Masticatorii: Musculi Pterygoidei
74	Arteria Maxillaris
75	Fossa Temporalis and Fossa Infratemporalis
76	Arteria Temporalis Superficialis and Arteria Maxillaris
77	Nervus Mandibularis (CN V$_3$)
78	Fossa Infratemporalis
79	Nervus Ophthalmicus and Nervus Maxillaris
80	Cavitas Nasi: Autonomic Innervation
81	Pars Media Faciei: Nervi and Arteriae
82	Basis Cranii: Nervi and Vasa Sanguinea

Stoma • Plates 83–90

83	Cavitas Oris: Inspection
84	Cavitas Oris and Lingua: Afferent Innervation
85	Palatum: Paries Superior Cavitatis Oris
86	Lingua and Glandulae Salivariae: Sections
87	Musculi Suprahyoidei
88	Lingua
89	Dorsum Linguae
90	Fauces

Pharynx • Plates 91–102

91	Pharynx: Nervi and Vasa Sanguinea (Posterior View)
92	Musculi Pharyngis: Partially Opened Posterior View
93	Pharynx: Opened Posterior View
94	Junctio Pharyngooesophagea
95	Pharynx: Medial View
96	Musculi Pharyngis: Medial View
97	Musculi Pharyngis: Lateral View
98	Stoma and Pharynx: Nervi
99	Caput and Collum: Arteriae

100 Caput and Collum: Venae
101 Caput and Collum: Nodi Lymphoidei
102 Pharynx and Lingua: Nodi Lymphoidei

Larynx and Glandulae Endocrinae • Plates 103–109

103 Glandula Thyreoidea: Anterior View
104 Glandula Thyreoidea: Posterior View
105 Glandula Thyreoidea and Glandulae Parathyreoideae
106 Cartilagines Laryngis
107 Musculi Interni Laryngis
108 Larynx: Nervi and Coronal Section
109 Larynx: Action of Intrinsic Muscles

Oculus • Plates 110–120

110 Palpebrae
111 Apparatus Lacrimalis
112 Musculi Externae Bulbi Oculi
113 Orbita: Nervi
114 Orbita: Superior and Anterior Views
115 Orbita and Palpebrae: Arteriae and Venae
116 Bulbus Oculi: Transverse Section
117 Bulbus Oculi: Camera Anterior and Camera Posterior
118 Lens, Fibrae Zonulares, and Corpus Ciliare
119 Bulbus Oculi: Vasa Sanguinea Interna
120 Bulbus Oculi: Vasa Sanguinea Externa

Auris • Plates 121–126

121 Auris: Course of Sound in Cochlea
122 Auris Externa and Cavitas Tympani
123 Cavitas Tympani
124 Auris Interna: Labyrinthus Osseus and Labyrinthus Membranaceus
125 Labyrinthus Osseus and Labyrinthus Membranaceus: Schema and Section
126 Auris Interna: Orientation of Labyrinths in Cranium

Encephalon and Meninges • Plates 127–142

127 Meninges and Venae Diploicae
128 Arteriae Meningeae
129 Meninges and Venae Superficiales Cerebri
130 Sinus Venosi Durales: Sagittal Section
131 Sinus Venosi Durales: Basis Cranii
132 Encephalon: Lateral Views
133 Encephalon: Medial Views
134 Encephalon: Inferior View
135 Ventriculi Encephali
136 Liquor Cerebrospinalis: Circulation

137 Nuclei Basales: Corpus Striatum
138 Thalamus
139 Hippocampus and Fornix
140 Truncus Encephali
141 Ventriculi and Cerebellum
142 Cerebellum

Nervi Craniales and Nervi Cervicales · Plates 143–162

143 Truncus Encephali: Nuclei Nervorum Cranialium (Posterior View)
144 Truncus Encephali: Nuclei Nervorum Cranialium (Medial View)
145 Nervi Craniales: Schema of Motor and Sensory Distribution
146 Nervus Olfactorius (CN I) and Olfactory Pathways: Schema
147 Nervus Opticus (CN II) and Visual Pathway: Schema
148 Nervi Oculomotorius (CN III), Trochlearis (CN IV), and Abducens (CN VI): Schema
149 Nervus Trigeminus (CN V): Schema
150 Nervus Facialis (CN VII): Schema
151 Nervus Vestibulocochlearis (CN VIII): Schema
152 Nervus Glossopharyngeus (CN IX): Schema
153 Nervus Vagus (CN X): Schema
154 Nervus Accessorius (CN XI): Schema
155 Nervus Hypoglossus (CN XII): Schema
156 Plexus Cervicalis: Schema
157 Collum: Nervi Autonomici
158 Caput: Nervi Autonomici
159 Ganglion Ciliare: Schema
160 Ganglion Pterygopalatinum and Ganglion Submandibulare: Schema
161 Ganglion Oticum: Schema
162 Taste Pathways: Schema

Vasa Sanguinea Encephali · Plates 163–175

163 Arteriae: Blood Supply to Encephalon and Meninges
164 Pars Petrosa Carotidis Internae
165 Arteriae: Schema of Blood Supply to Encephalon
166 Arteriae Encephali: Inferior Views
167 Circulus Arteriosus Cerebri (Willisii)
168 Arteriae Encephali: Frontal View and Section
169 Arteriae Encephali: Lateral and Medial Views
170 Arteriae Encephali: Rami of Arteria Vertebralis and Arteria Basilaris
171 Fossa Posterior Cranii: Venae
172 Venae Profundae Encephali
173 Venae Subependymales Encephali
174 Hypothalamus and Hypophysis
175 Hypothalamus and Hypophysis: Vasculature

Regional Imaging • Plates 176–177

    176   Cranial Imaging (MRA and MRV)
    177   Cranial Imaging (MRI)

Structures with High Clinical Significance • Tables 2.1–2.5

Nervi Craniales • Tables 2.6–2.8

Nervi Plexus Cervicalis • Table 2.9

Musculi • Tables 2.10–2.14

Electronic Bonus Plates • Plates BP 14–BP 32

    BP 14   Somatosensory System: Trunk and Limbs
    BP 15   Pyramidal System
    BP 16   3D Skull Reconstruction CTs
    BP 17   Vertebrae Cervicales: Degenerative Changes
    BP 18   Articulatio Atlantooccipitalis
    BP 19   Musculi Faciales: Anterior View
    BP 20   Musculi Faciales
    BP 21   Cavitas Nasalis Cranii: Arteriae (Septum Nasi Turned Up)
    BP 22   Nasus and Sinus Maxillaris: Transverse Section
    BP 23   Sinus Paranasales
    BP 24   Arteria Subclavia
    BP 25   Opening the Mouth: Musculus Pterygoideus Lateralis
    BP 26   Cavitas Oris and Pharynx: Afferent Innervation
    BP 27   Orbita and Bulbus Oculi: Fasciae
    BP 28   Cavitas Tympani: Medial and Lateral Views
    BP 29   Auris: Anatomy of the Pediatric Ear
    BP 30   Tuba Auditiva (Eustachii)
    BP 31   Cranial Imaging (MRV and MRA)
    BP 32   Encephalon: Axial and Coronal MRIs

SECTION 3   DORSUM • Plates 178–201

Surface Anatomy • Plate 178

    178   Dorsum: Surface Anatomy

Columna Vertebralis • Plates 179–185

    179   Columna Vertebralis
    180   Vertebrae Thoracicae
    181   Vertebrae Lumbales
    182   Vertebrae: Radiograph and MRI
    183   Os Sacrum and Os Coccygis

184   Ligamenta Columnae Vertebralis: Lumbosacral Region
185   Juncturae Columnae Vertebralis: Lumbar Region

Medulla Spinalis • Plates 186–194

186   Medulla Spinalis and Nervi Spinales
187   Radices Nervorum Spinalium and Vertebrae
188   Dermatomata
189   Meninges Spinales and Radices Nervorum Spinales
190   Nervi Spinales, Radices and Rami
191   Arteriae Medullae Spinalis: Schema
192   Arteriae Medullae Spinalis: Intrinsic Distribution
193   Venae Columnae Vertebralis and Venae Medullae Spinalis
194   Venae Columnae Vertebralis: Venae Vertebrales

Musculi and Nervi • Plates 195–199

195   Musculi Superficiales Dorsi
196   Musculi Dorsi: Intermediate Layer
197   Musculi Profundi Dorsi
198   Nervi Dorsi
199   Nervi Dorsales Colli

Cross-Sectional Anatomy • Plates 200–201

200   Dorsum: Cross Section of Regio Lumbalis
201   Nervus Spinalis Thoracicus

Structures with High Clinical Significance • Table 3.1

Musculi • Tables 3.2–3.4

Electronic Bonus Plates • Plates BP 33–BP 40

BP 33   Ligamenta Columnae Vertebralis
BP 34   Pars Cervicalis Columnae Vertebralis: Radiographs
BP 35   Pars Cervicalis Columnae Vertebralis: MRI and Radiograph
BP 36   Pars Thoracolumbalis Columnae Vertebralis: Lateral Radiograph
BP 37   Pars Lumbalis Columnae Vertebralis: Radiographs
BP 38   Pars Lumbalis Columnae Vertebralis: MRIs
BP 39   Venae Columnae Vertebralis: Detail Showing Venous Communications
BP 40   Medulla Spinalis: Fiber Tracts in Cross Sections

SECTION 4   THORAX • Plates 202–266

Surface Anatomy • Plate 202

202   Thorax: Surface Anatomy

Skeleton Thoracis • Plates 203–204

203 Thorax: Bony Framework
204 Costae and Juncturae Thoracicae

Glandulae Mammariae • Plates 205–208

205 Glandula Mammaria
206 Mamma: Arteriae
207 Mamma: Vasa Lymphatica and Nodi Lymphoidei
208 Mamma: Lymphatic Drainage

Paries Thoracis and Diaphragma • Plates 209–216

209 Paries Anterior Thoracis: Superficial Dissection
210 Paries Anterior Thoracis: Deeper Dissection
211 Paries Anterior Thoracis: Internal View
212 Nervi Intercostales and Arteriae Intercostales
213 Paries Thoracis: Venae
214 Nervus Phrenicus and Pericardium
215 Diaphragma: Facies Superior
216 Diaphragma: Facies Inferior

Pulmones, Trachea, and Bronchi • Plates 217–230

217 Pulmones in Thorax: Anterior View
218 Pulmones in Thorax: Posterior View
219 Pulmones in Situ: Anterior View
220 Mediastinum
221 Pulmones: Medial Views
222 Arteriae Bronchiales and Venae Bronchiales
223 Segmenta Bronchopulmonalia: Anterior and Posterior Views
224 Segmenta Bronchopulmonalia: Medial and Lateral Views
225 Trachea and Bronchi Majores
226 Arbor Tracheobronchialis and Lobulus Pulmonis
227 Lobulus Pulmonis: Schema of Blood Circulation
228 Thorax: Vasa Lymphatica and Nodi Lymphoidei
229 Nervi Autonomici of Thorax
230 Arbor Tracheobronchialis: Schema of Innervation

Cor • Plates 231–250

231 Cor in Situ
232 Cor: Anterior Exposure
233 Cor: Regiones Precordiales Auscultationis
234 Cor: Radiographs and CT Angiogram
235 Cor: Basis Cordis and Facies Diaphragmatica
236 Saccus Pericardiacus and Cavitas Pericardiaca
237 Mediastinum: Cross Section
238 Thorax: Coronal Section of Cor and Aorta Ascendens
239 Arteriae Coronariae and Venae Cardiacae

240 Arteriae Coronariae: Imaging
241 Atrium Dextrum and Ventriculus Dexter
242 Atrium Sinistrum and Ventriculus Sinister
243 Complexus Valvularis Cordis
244 Complexus Valvularis Cordis (Continued)
245 Atria, Ventriculi, and Septum Interventriculare
246 Valvae Cordis
247 Prenatal and Postnatal Circulation
248 Complexus Stimulans Cordis
249 Thorax: Nervi
250 Cor: Schema of Innervation

Mediastinum • Plates 251–261

251 Mediastinum: Right Lateral View
252 Mediastinum: Left Lateral View
253 Nervus Phrenicus
254 Oesophagus in Situ
255 Oesophagus: Constrictions and Relations
256 Oesophagus: Musculi
257 Junctio Oesophagogastrica
258 Oesophagus: Arteriae
259 Oesophagus: Venae
260 Oesophagus: Vasa Lymphatica and Nodi Lymphoidei
261 Oesophagus: Nervi

Cross-Sectional Anatomy • Plates 262–266

262 Thorax: Axial CT Images
263 Thorax: Cross Section at T3 Vertebral Level
264 Thorax: Cross Section at T3/T4 Disc Level
265 Thorax: Cross Section at T4/T5 Disc Level
266 Thorax: Cross Section at T7 Vertebral Level

Structures with High Clinical Significance • Tables 4.1–4.3

Musculi • Table 4.4

Electronic Bonus Plates • Plates BP 41–BP 52

BP 41 Costae Cervicales and Related Variations
BP 42 Costae: Muscle Attachments
BP 43 Musculi Respiratorii
BP 44 Bronchiolus Terminalis and Acinus Pulmonis: Schema
BP 45 Anatomy of Ventilation and Respiration
BP 46 Arteriae Coronariae: Right Anterolateral Views with Arteriograms
BP 47 Arteriae Coronariae and Venae Cardiacae: Variations
BP 48 Oesophagus: Intrinsic Nerves and Variations
BP 49 Oesophagus: Arterial Variations

BP 50   Thorax: Coronal Sections
BP 51   Thorax: Coronal CTs
BP 52   Vasa Sanguinea: Schema of Innervation

SECTION 5   ABDOMEN · Plates 267–351

Surface Anatomy · Plate 267

267   Abdomen: Surface Anatomy

Paries Abdominis · Plates 268–287

268   Abdomen: Bony Framework
269   Abdomen: Regiones, Plana, and Lineae
270   Paries Anterior Abdominis: Superficial Dissection
271   Paries Anterior Abdominis: Intermediate Dissection
272   Paries Anterior Abdominis: Deep Dissection
273   Vagina Musculi Recti Abdominis: Cross Section
274   Paries Anterior Abdominis: Internal View
275   Paries Posterolateralis Abdominis
276   Paries Anterior Abdominis: Arteriae
277   Paries Anterior Abdominis: Venae
278   Paries Anterior Abdominis: Nervi
279   Nervi Intercostales
280   Regio Inguinalis: Dissections
281   Canalis Inguinalis and Funiculus Spermaticus
282   Vagina Femoralis and Canalis Inguinalis
283   Paries Posterior Abdominis: Internal View
284   Paries Posterior Abdominis: Arteriae
285   Paries Posterior Abdominis: Venae
286   Paries Posterior Abdominis: Vasa Lymphatica and Nodi
        Lymphoidei
287   Paries Posterior Abdominis: Nervi

Cavitas Peritonealis · Plates 288–293

288   Omentum Majus and Viscera Abdominis
289   Mesenteria and Musculus Suspensorius Duodeni
290   Mesocola and Radix Mesenterii
291   Bursa Omentalis: Gaster Reflected
292   Bursa Omentalis: Cross Section
293   Paries Posterior Abdominis: Peritoneum

Gaster and Intestina · Plates 294–301

294   Gaster in Situ
295   Tunica Muscosa Gastris
296   Duodenum in Situ
297   Intestinum Tenue: Tunica Mucosa and Tunica Muscularis

298	Junctio Ileocaecalis
299	Caecum and Ostium Ileale
300	Vermiform Appendix
301	Intestinum Crassum: Tunica Mucosa and Tunica Muscularis

Hepar, Vesica Biliaris, Pancreas, and Splen · Plates 302–307

302	Hepar: Surfaces and Bed
303	Hepar in Situ: Trias Portae Hepatis and Tractus Portales
304	Hepar: Schema of Structure
305	Vesica Biliaris, Ductus Biliares Extrahepatici, Ductus Pancreaticus
306	Pancreas in Situ
307	Splen

Vasa Sanguinea Visceralia · Plates 308–318

308	Gaster, Hepar, and Splen: Arteriae
309	Truncus Coeliacus and Rami
310	Hepar, Pancreas, Duodenum, and Splen: Arteriae
311	Celiac Arteriogram and CT Angiogram
312	Duodenum and Caput Pancreatis: Arteriae
313	Intestinum Tenue: Arteriae
314	Intestinum Crassum: Arteriae
315	Gaster, Duodenum, Pancreas, and Splen: Venae
316	Intestinum Tenue: Venae
317	Intestinum Crassum: Venae
318	Vena Portae Hepatis, Affluentes, and Anastomoses Portocavales

Nervi Viscerales and Plexus Viscerales · Plates 319–329

319	Abdomen: Nervi Autonomici and Ganglia Autonomica
320	Gaster and Duodenum: Autonomic Innervation
321	Gaster and Duodenum: Autonomic Innervation (Continued)
322	Intestinum Tenue: Autonomic Innervation
323	Intestinum Crassum: Autonomic Innervation
324	Intestina: Schema of Autonomic Innervation
325	Oesophagus, Gaster, and Duodenum: Schema of Autonomic Innervation
326	Autonomic Reflex Pathways: Schema
327	Intestinum: Plexus Enterici
328	Hepar: Schema of Autonomic Innervation
329	Pancreas: Schema of Autonomic Innervation

Renes and Glandulae Suprarenales · Plates 330–343

330	Renes in Situ: Anterior Views
331	Renes in Situ: Posterior Views
332	Glandulae Suprarenales
333	Ren: Gross Structure

334   Arteriae Intrarenales and Segmenta Renis
335   Ureteres in Abdomen and Pelvis
336   Ureteres and Vesica Urinaria: Arteriae
337   Fascia Renalis
338   Renes and Vesica Urinaria: Vasa Lymphatica and Nodi Lymphoidei
339   Renes, Ureteres, and Vesica Urinaria: Nervi Autonomici
340   Ren and Pars Abdominalis Ureteris: Schema of Autonomic Innervation
341   Glandulae Suprarenales: Dissection and Schema of Autonomic Innervation
342   Glandulae Suprarenales in Situ: Arteriae and Venae
343   Abdomen: Paramedian Section

Vasa Lymphatica and Nodi Lymphoidei · Plate 344

344   Abdomen and Pelvis: Schema of Lymphatic Drainage

Regional Imaging · Plates 345–346

345   Abdominal Scans: Axial CT Images
346   Abdominal Scans: Axial CT Images (Continued)

Cross-Sectional Anatomy · Plates 347–351

347   Cross Section at T10 Vertebral Level, Through Junctio Oesophagogastrica
348   Cross Section at T12 Vertebral Level, Inferior to Processus Xiphoideus
349   Cross Section at T12/L1 Disc Level
350   Cross Section at L1/L2 Disc Level
351   Cross Section at L3/L4 Disc Level

Structures with High Clinical Significance · Tables 5.1–5.3

Musculi · Table 5.4

Electronic Bonus Plates · Plates BP 53–BP 83

BP 53   Regio Inguinalis and Trigonum Femorale
BP 54   Indirect Inguinal Hernia
BP 55   Gaster: Variations in Position and Contour in Relation to Body Habitus
BP 56   Duodenum: Laminae
BP 57   Appendix Vermiformis in Coronal CT image and Vesica Biliaris in MRCP
BP 58   Hepar: Topography
BP 59   Hepar: Variations in Form
BP 60   Colon Sigmoideum: Variations in Position
BP 61   Caecum: Variations in Arterial Supply and Posterior Peritoneal Attachment
BP 62   Ductus Pancreaticus: Variations

BP 63	Ductus Cysticus, Ductus Hepatici, and Ductus Pancreaticus: Variations
BP 64	Arteria Cystica: Variations
BP 65	Arteriae Hepaticae: Variations
BP 66	Vena Portae Hepatis: Variations and Anomalies
BP 67	Truncus Coeliacus: Variations
BP 68	Arteriae Colicae: Variations
BP 69	Arteriae Colicae: Variations (Continued)
BP 70	Arteria Renalis and Vena Renalis: Variations
BP 71	Corpusculum Renale: Histology
BP 72	Nephron and Tubulus Colligens: Schema
BP 73	Ren: Schema of Vasa Sanguinea Intrarenalia
BP 74	Gaster: Vasa Lymphatica and Nodi Lymphoidei
BP 75	Pancreas: Vasa Lymphatica and Nodi Lymphoidei
BP 76	Intestinum Tenue: Vasa Lymphatica and Nodi Lymphoidei
BP 77	Intestinum Crassum: Vasa Lymphatica and Nodi Lymphoidei
BP 78	Hepar: Vasa Lymphatica and Nodi Lymphoidei
BP 79	Abdomen: Cross Section at T12 Vertebral Level
BP 80	Abdomen: Cross Section at L5 Vertebral Level, Near Planum Intertuberculare
BP 81	Abdomen: Cross Section at S1 Vertebral Level, Near Spina Iliaca Anterior Superior
BP 82	Axial CT Image of Upper Abdomen
BP 83	Hepar and Vesica Biliaris: Variations in Arterial Blood Supply

SECTION 6 PELVIS · Plates 352–421

Surface Anatomy · Plate 352

352	Pelvis: Surface Anatomy

Pelvis Ossea · Plates 353–357

353	Pelvis: Bony Framework
354	Radiographs of Pelvis: Male and Female
355	Sex Differences of Pelvis Ossea: Measurements
356	Ligamenta of Pelvis Ossea
357	Ligamenta of Os Coxae

Diaphragma Pelvis and Organa Visceralia Pelvis · Plates 358–368

358	Diaphragma Pelvis: Female
359	Diaphragma Pelvis: Female (Medial and Superior Views)
360	Diaphragma Pelvis: Female (Inferior Views)
361	Diaphragma Pelvis: Male (Superior View)
362	Diaphragma Pelvis: Male (Inferior View)
363	Cavitas Pelvis: Female
364	Viscera Pelvis and Perineum: Female
365	Organa Genitalia Interna Feminina

366   Fasciae Endopelvicae
367   Cavitas Pelvis: Male
368   Viscera Pelvis and Perineum: Male

Vesica Urinaria • Plates 369–371

369   Vesica Urinaria: Orientation and Supports
370   Sphincteres Urethrae: Female
371   Vesica Urinaria: Female and Male

Organa Genitalia Feminina Interna • Plates 372–376

372   Uterus, Vagina, and Supporting Structures
373   Uterus: Ligamenta
374   Uterus and Adnexa
375   Viscera Pelvis: Female
376   Ligamenta Pelvis

Perineum Femininum and Organa Genitalia Feminina Externa • Plates 377–380

377   Perineum and Organa Genitalia Externa: Female
378   Perineum: Female (Superficial Dissection)
379   Perineum: Female (Deeper Dissection)
380   Spatia Perinei: Female

Perineum Masculinum and Organa Genitalia Masculina Externa • Plates 381–388

381   Perineum and Organa Genitalia Externa: Male (Superficial Dissection)
382   Perineum and Organa Genitalia Externa: Male (Deeper Dissection)
383   Penis
384   Spatia Perinei: Male
385   Prostata and Glandula Seminalis
386   Urethra
387   Descent of Testis
388   Scrotum and Contents

Homologies of Organa Genitalia Masculina and Organa Genitalis Feminina • Plates 389–390

389   Homologues of Organa Genitalia Externa
390   Homologues of Organa Genitalia Interna

Organa Genitalia Masculina Interna • Plates 391–392

391   Testes
392   Testis, Epididymis, and Ductus Deferens

Rectum and Canalis Analis • Plates 393–399

393   Rectum in Situ: Female and Male

394 Fossae Ischioanales
395 Rectum and Canalis Analis
396 Musculi Anorectales
397 Sphincter Externus Ani: Perineal Views
398 Spatia Perinei and Spatia Extraperitonealia Pelvis: Actual and Potential
399 Pelvic Scans: Sagittal T2-Weighted MRIs

Vasa Sanguinea, Vasa Lymphatica, and Nodi Lymphoidei · Plates 400–410

400 Arteriae of Rectum and Canalis Analis: Male (Posterior View)
401 Venae of Rectum and Canalis Analis: Female (Anterior View)
402 Arteriae and Venae of Viscera Pelvis: Female (Anterior View)
403 Arteriae and Venae of Testis: Anterior View
404 Arteriae of Pelvis: Female
405 Arteriae and Venae of Pelvis: Male
406 Arteriae and Venae of Perineum and Uterus
407 Arteriae and Venae of Perineum: Male
408 Vasa Lymphatica and Nodi Lymphoidei of Pelvis and Organa Genitalia: Female
409 Nodi Inguinales and Vasa Lymphatica of Perineum: Female
410 Vasa Lymphatica and Nodi Lymphoidei of Pelvis and Organa Genitalia: Male

Nervi Perinei and Nervi Viscerales Pelvis · Plates 411–419

411 Nervi of Organa Genitalia Externa: Male
412 Nervi of Viscera Pelvis: Male
413 Nervi of Perineum: Male
414 Nervi of Viscera Pelvis: Female
415 Nervi of Perineum and Organa Genitalia Externa: Female
416 Neuropathways in Parturition
417 Innervation of Organa Genitalia Feminina: Schema
418 Innervation of Organa Genitalia Masculina: Schema
419 Innervation of Vesica Urinaria and Pars Pelvica Ureteris: Schema

Cross-Sectional Anatomy · Plates 420–421

420 Pelvis Masculina: Cross Section of Junctio Vesicoprostatica
421 Pelvis Feminina: Cross Section of Vagina and Urethra

Structures with High Clinical Significance · Tables 6.1–6.2

Musculi · Table 6.3

Electronic Bonus Plates · Plates BP 84–BP 95

BP 84 Fasciae of Pelvis and Perineum: Male and Female
BP 85 Cystourethrograms: Male and Female
BP 86 Urethra Feminina

BP 87   Genetics of Reproduction
BP 88   Menstrual Cycle
BP 89   Development of Uterus
BP 90   Ovarium, Oocytia, and Folliculi
BP 91   Variations in Hymen
BP 92   Cross Section of Pelvis Through Prostata
BP 93   Arteriae and Venae of Pelvis: Male (Featuring Prostata)
BP 94   Cross Section of Lower Pelvis
BP 95   Endocrine Glands, Hormones, and Puberty

SECTION 7   MEMBRUM SUPERIUS · Plates 422–490

Surface Anatomy · Plates 422–426

422   Membrum Superius: Surface Anatomy
423   Membrum Superius: Cutaneous Innervation
424   Omos and Brachium: Venae Superficiales
425   Antebrachium and Manus: Venae Superficiales
426   Membrum Superius: Vasa Lymphatica and Nodi Lymphoidei

Omos and Axilla · Plates 427–439

427   Humerus and Scapula
428   Humerus, Scapula, and Clavicula: Muscle Attachment Sites
429   Clavicula and Articulatio Sternoclavicularis
430   Omos: Anteroposterior Radiograph
431   Omos: Juncturae
432   Omos: Musculi
433   Axilla: Posterior Wall
434   Musculi Cuffiae Musculotendineae (Rotator Cuff Muscles)
435   Fasciae Pectoralis, Clavipectoralis, and Axillaris
436   Omos: Musculi and Tendines
437   Arteria Axillaris and Arteriae Anastomoticae Scapulae
438   Axilla: Anterior View
439   Plexus Brachialis: Schema

Brachium · Plates 440–445

440   Musculi Brachii: Compartimentum Anterius
441   Musculi Brachii: Compartimentum Posterius
442   Arteria Brachialis in Situ
443   Membrum Superius: Arteriae
444   Membrum Superius: Venae
445   Brachium: Serial Cross Sections

Cubitus and Antebrachium · Plates 446–461

446   Cubitus: Ossa
447   Cubitus: Radiographs

448   Cubitus: Ligamenta
449   Ossa Antebrachii
450   Musculi Antebrachii: Pronatores and Supinator
451   Musculi Antebrachii: Extensores Carpi and Digitorum
452   Musculi Antebrachii: Flexores Carpi
453   Musculi Antebrachii: Flexores Digitorum
454   Musculi Antebrachii: Pars Superficialis Compartimenti Posterioris
455   Musculi Antebrachii: Pars Profunda Compartimenti Posterioris
456   Musculi Antebrachii: Pars Superficialis Compartimenti Anterioris
457   Musculi Antebrachii: Compartimentum Anterius
458   Musculi Antebrachii: Pars Profunda Compartimenti Anterioris
459   Musculi Antebrachii: Attachments (Anterior View)
460   Musculi Antebrachii: Attachments (Posterior View)
461   Antebrachium: Serial Cross Sections

Carpus and Manus • Plates 462–481

462   Ossa Carpi
463   Ossa Carpi: Movements
464   Ligamenta Carpi: Anterior View
465   Ligamenta Carpi: Posterior View
466   Ossa Manus
467   Carpus and Manus: Radiographs
468   Ligamenta Metacarpophalangea and Interphalangea
469   Carpus and Manus: Superficial Palmar Dissections
470   Carpus and Manus: Deeper Palmar Dissections
471   Manus: Musculi Lumbricales, Spatia Palmare Medium and Thenaris, Vaginae Tendinum
472   Carpus: Tendines Flexoris, Arteriae, and Nervi
473   Manus: Spatia and Vaginae Tendinum
474   Digiti: Tendines Flexoris and Extensoris
475   Musculi Manus
476   Arteriae Manus: Palmar Views
477   Carpus and Manus: Superficial Lateral Dissection
478   Carpus and Manus: Superficial Dorsal Dissection
479   Dorsum Manus and Carpus: Nervi and Arteriae
480   Carpus: Tendines Extensorum
481   Digiti

Nervi • Plates 482–489

482   Carpus and Manus: Cutaneous Innervation
483   Membrum Superius: Arteriae and Nervi (Anterior View)
484   Membrum Superius: Nervi
485   Nervus Musculocutaneus
486   Nervus Medianus

487   Nervus Ulnaris
488   Nervus Radialis (in Brachium) and Nervus Axillaris
489   Nervus Radialis in Antebrachium and Manus

Regional Imaging • Plate 490

490   Omos: MRI and CT

Structures with High Clinical Significance • Tables 7.1–7.2

Nervi Plexus Brachialis • Tables 7.3–7.5

Musculi • Tables 7.6–7.8

Electronic Bonus Plates • Plates BP 96–BP 102

BP 96   Brachium: Arteriae
BP 97   Antebrachium and Manus: Arteriae
BP 98   Ligamenta Carpi: Posterior and Anterior Views
BP 99   Flexor and Extensor Zones of Hand
BP 100   Cross Sections Through Ossa Metacarpi and Carpi
BP 101   Cross Section of Manus: Axial View
BP 102   Cross Section of Manus: Axial View (Continued)

SECTION 8   MEMBRUM INFERIUS • Plates 491–556

Surface Anatomy • Plates 491–494

491   Membrum Inferius: Surface Anatomy
492   Vena Superficiales Membri Inferioris: Anterior View
493   Vena Superficiales Membri Inferioris: Posterior View
494   Membrum Inferius: Vasa Lymphatica and Nodi Lymphoidei

Coxa, Natis, and Femur • Plates 495–515

495   Os Coxae
496   Articulatio Coxae
497   Articulatio Coxae: Anteroposterior Radiograph
498   Musculi Glutei and Musculi Femoris: Attachments (Anterior View)
499   Musculi Glutei and Musculi Femoris: Attachments (Posterior View)
500   Os Femoris
501   Musculi Glutei and Musculi Femoris: Lateral View
502   Musculi Femoris: Compartimentum Anterius
503   Musculi Femoris: Compartimentum Mediale
504   Musculi Glutei and Musculi Femoris: Posterior Views
505   Psoas and Musculus Iliacus
506   Plexus Lumbosacralis

507 Plexus Lumbalis
508 Plexus Sacralis and Plexus Coccygeus
509 Arteriae Femoris: Anterior Views
510 Arteriae Femoris: Anterior View of Deeper Dissection
511 Arteriae Femoris: Posterior View
512 Nervi Glutei
513 Bursae Coxae: Posterior and Anterolateral Views
514 Caput and Collum Ossis Femoris: Arteriae
515 Femur: Serial Cross Sections

Genu • Plates 516–523

516 Genu: Medial and Lateral Views
517 Genu: Anterior Views
518 Genu: Interior Views
519 Genu: Ligamenta Cruciata and Collateralia
520 Genu: Anteroposterior Radiograph and Posterior View
521 Genu: Posterior and Sagittal Views
522 Arteriae Membri Inferioris
523 Venae Membri Inferioris

Crus • Plates 524–534

524 Tibia and Fibula: Anterior and Posterior Views
525 Tibia and Fibula: Additional Views and Cross Section
526 Musculi Cruris: Attachments
527 Musculi Cruris: Pars Superficialis Compartimenti Posterioris
528 Musculi Cruris: Pars Superficialis Compartimenti Posterioris (Partial Dissection)
529 Musculi Cruris: Pars Profunda Compartimenti Posterioris
530 Musculi Cruris: Compartimentum Laterale
531 Musculi Cruris: Compartimentum Anterius
532 Musculi Cruris: Compartimentum Anterius (Partial Dissection)
533 Venae Cruris
534 Crus: Cross Sections and Compartimenta

Talus and Pes • Plates 535–549

535 Ossa Pedis: Superior and Inferior Views
536 Ossa Pedis: Lateral and Medial Views
537 Calcaneus
538 Ligamenta Tali and Pedis
539 Ligamenta Pedis: Plantar View
540 Vaginae Tendinum Tali
541 Musculi Dorsales Pedis: Superficial Dissection
542 Musculi Dorsales Pedis: Deep Dissection
543 Planta: Superficial Dissection
544 Musculi Plantares Pedis: First Layer
545 Musculi Plantares Pedis: Second Layer
546 Musculi Plantares Pedis: Third Layer

547   Musculi Interossei and Arteriae Profundae Pedis
548   Musculi Interossei Pedis
549   Pes: Cross Section

Nervi • Plates 550–554

550   Nervus Femoralis and Nervus Cutaneus Lateralis Femoris
551   Nervus Obturatorius
552   Nervus Ischiadicus and Nervus Cutaneus Posterior Femoris
553   Nervus Tibialis
554   Nervus Fibularis Communis

Regional Imaging • Plates 555–556

555   Coxa: MRI and 3D CT
556   Talus: Radiographs

Structures with High Clinical Significance • Tables 8.1–8.2

Nervi Plexus Lumbosacralis • Tables 8.3–8.5

Musculi • Tables 8.6–8.9

Electronic Bonus Plates • Plates BP 103–BP 112

BP 103 Genu and Pes: Arteriae
BP 104 Coxa: Cross-Sectional Anatomy
BP 105 Femur and Genu: Arteriae
BP 106 Crus: Serial Cross Sections
BP 107 Genu: Osteology
BP 108 Genu: Lateral View Radiograph
BP 109 Pes: Nervi and Arteriae
BP 110 Talus and Pes: Cross-Sectional Anatomy
BP 111 Pes: Cross-Sectional Anatomy
BP 112 Unguis Digiti Pedis: Anatomy

References

Index

INTRODUCTION

General Anatomy 1–3   **Electronic Bonus Plates**   BP 1– BP 13

Systematic Anatomy 4–21

ELECTRONIC BONUS PLATES

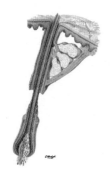

BP 1 Apparatus Pilosebaceus

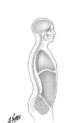

BP 2 Cavitates Majores Corporis Humani

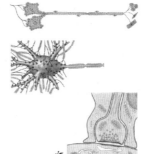

BP 3 Neuron and Synapsis

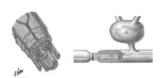

BP 4 Nervus Periphericus: Typical Features

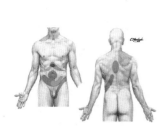

BP 5 Sites of Visceral Referred Pain

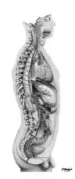

BP 6 Divisio Sympathica: General Topography

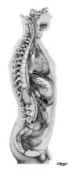

BP 7 Divisio Parasympathica: General Topography

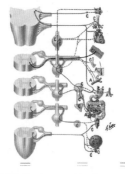

BP 8 Synapses Cholinergicae and Adrenergicae: Schema

ELECTRONIC BONUS PLATES—*cont'd*

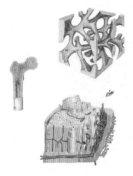

BP 9 Os: Architecture

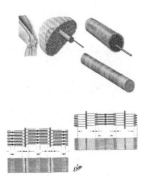

BP 10 Musculus: Structure

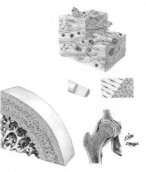

BP 11 Juncturae: Textus Connectivi and Cartilago Articularis

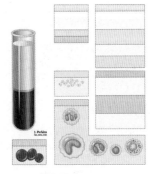

BP 12 Systema Cardiovasculare: Composition of Blood

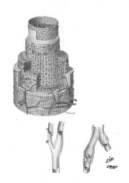

BP 13 Arteria: Structure of Wall

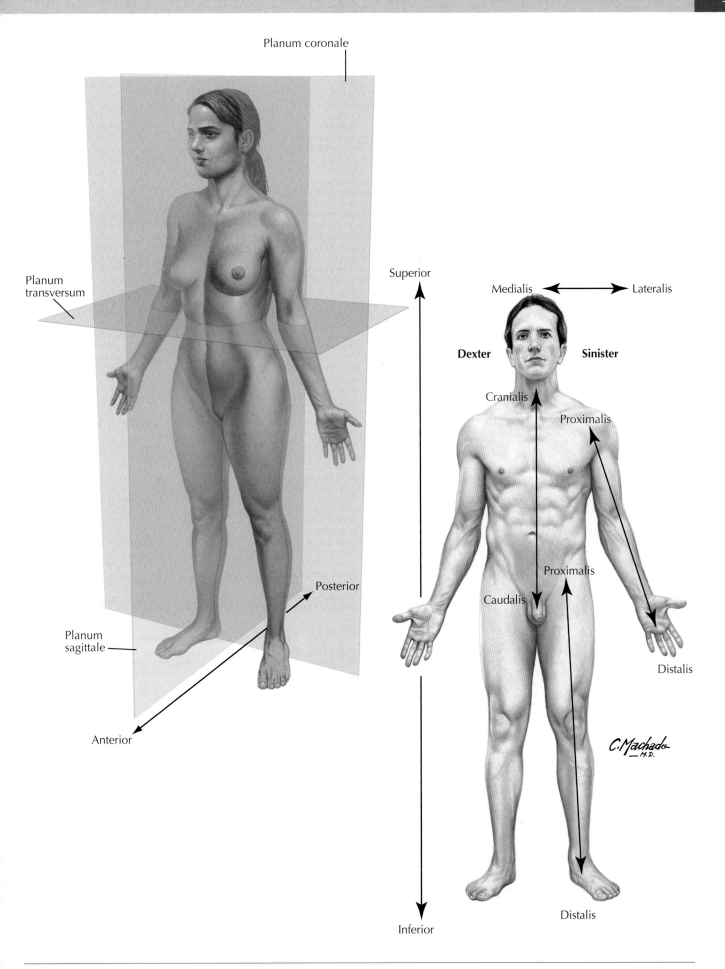

Planum coronale

Planum transversum

Planum sagittale

Anterior

Posterior

Superior

Inferior

Medialis ⟷ Lateralis

Dexter   **Sinister**

Cranialis

Proximalis

Proximalis

Caudalis

Distalis

Distalis

C. Machado
— M.D.

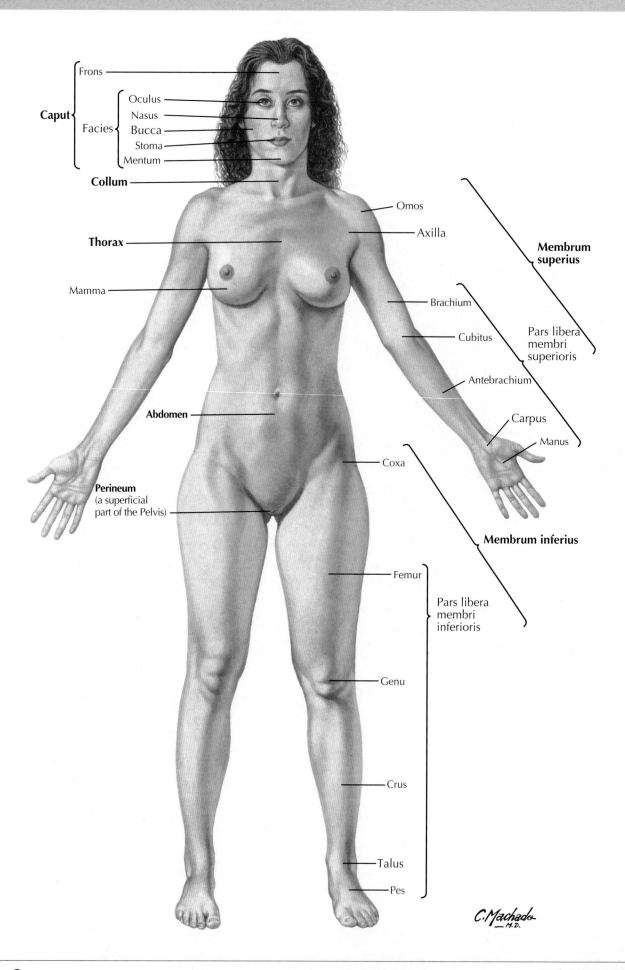

Frons

Caput

Facies
Oculus
Nasus
Bucca
Stoma
Mentum

Collum

Thorax

Mamma

Abdomen

Perineum
(a superficial
part of the Pelvis)

Omos

Axilla

**Membrum
superius**

Brachium

Cubitus

Pars libera
membri
superioris

Antebrachium

Carpus

Manus

Coxa

Membrum inferius

Femur

Pars libera
membri
inferioris

Genu

Crus

Talus

Pes

C.Machado
M.D.

Plate 2

General Anatomy

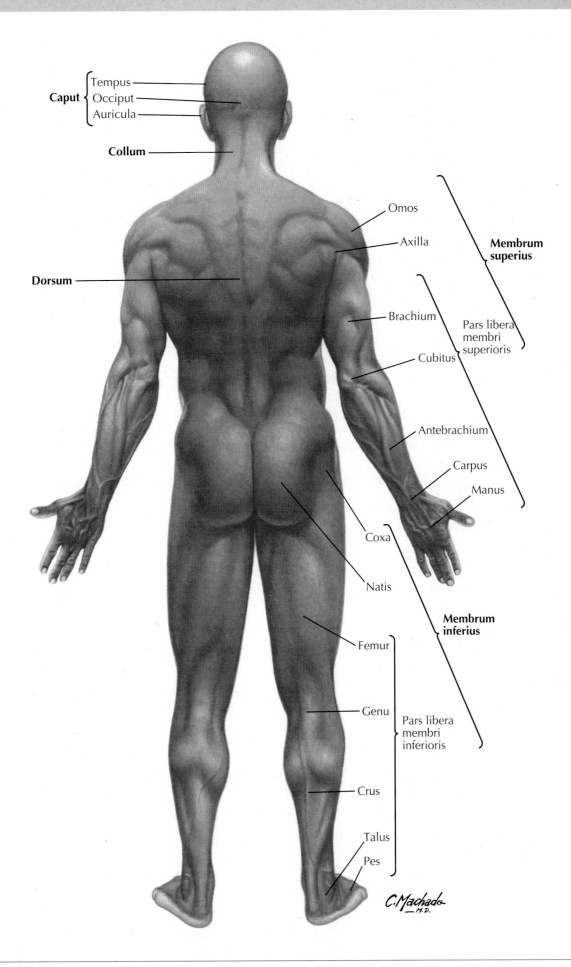

Caput { Tempus
Occiput
Auricula

Collum

Omos

Axilla

Membrum superius

Dorsum

Brachium

Pars libera membri superioris

Cubitus

Antebrachium

Carpus

Manus

Coxa

Natis

Membrum inferius

Femur

Genu

Pars libera membri inferioris

Crus

Talus

Pes

C. Machado
_M.D.

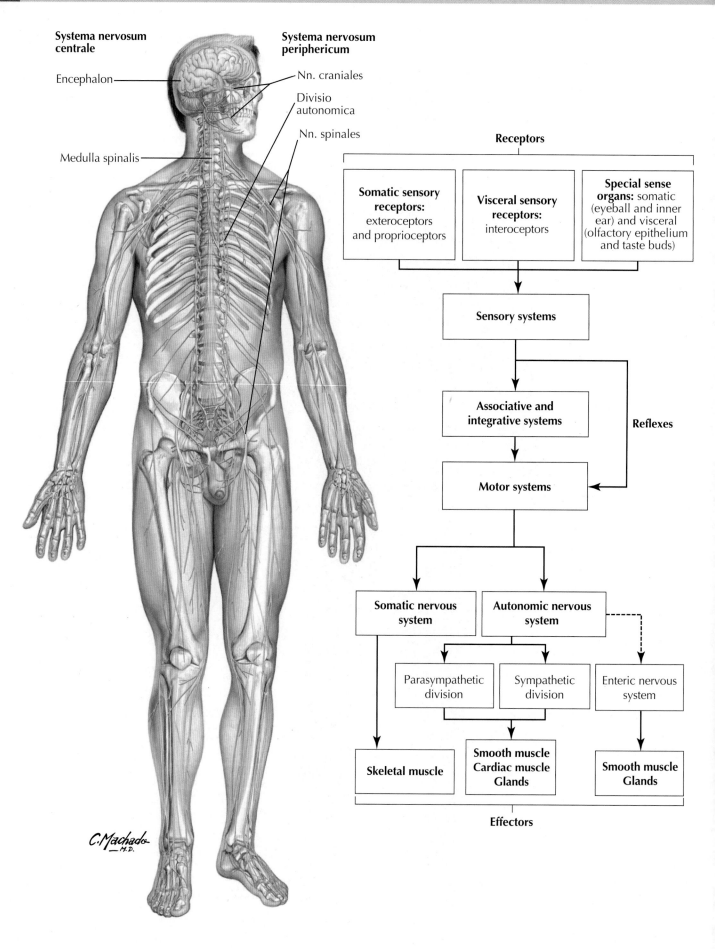

Systema nervosum centrale

Encephalon

Medulla spinalis

Systema nervosum periphericum

Nn. craniales

Divisio autonomica

Nn. spinales

C. Machado, M.D.

Receptors

| **Somatic sensory receptors:** exteroceptors and proprioceptors | **Visceral sensory receptors:** interoceptors | **Special sense organs:** somatic (eyeball and inner ear) and visceral (olfactory epithelium and taste buds) |

Sensory systems

Associative and integrative systems

Reflexes

Motor systems

Somatic nervous system

Autonomic nervous system

Parasympathetic division

Sympathetic division

Enteric nervous system

Skeletal muscle

Smooth muscle Cardiac muscle Glands

Smooth muscle Glands

Effectors

Plate 4

Systematic Anatomy

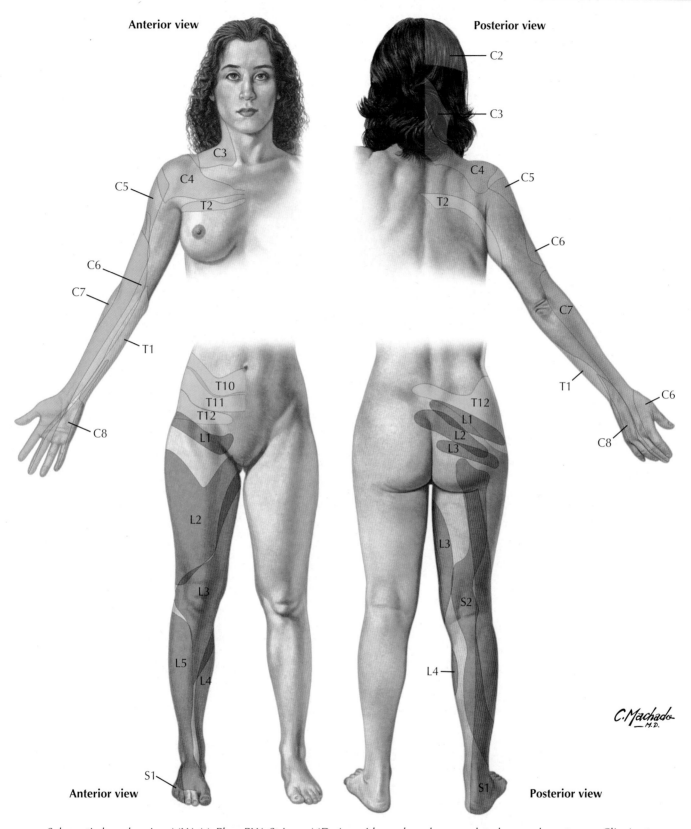

Anterior view

Posterior view

C2

C3

C3

C4

C5

C4

C5

C5

T2

T2

C6

C6

C7

C7

T1

T1

T10

T12

T11

T1

T12

L1

L1

L2

C8

L3

C6

L2

C8

L3

L3

S2

L5

L4

L4

S1

S1

Anterior view

Posterior view

C.Machado
M.D.

Schematic based on Lee MW, McPhee RW, Stringer MD. An evidence-based approach to human dermatomes. Clin Anat. 2008 Jul;21(5):363-73. doi: 10.1002/ca.20636. PMID: 18470936. Please note that these areas are not absolute and vary from person to person. S3, S4, S5, Co supply the perineum but are not shown for reasons of clarity. Of note, the dermatomes are larger than illustrated as the figure is based on best evidence; gaps represent areas in which the data are inconclusive.

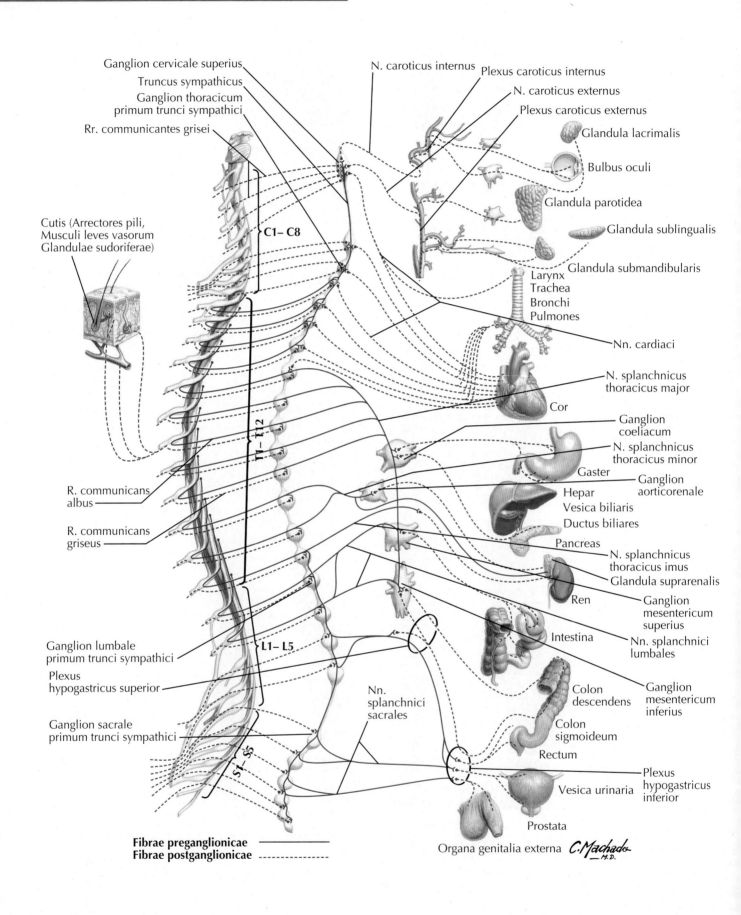

Ganglion cervicale superius

Truncus sympathicus

Ganglion thoracicum primum trunci sympathici

Rr. communicantes grisei

Cutis (Arrectores pili, Musculi leves vasorum Glandulae sudoriferae)

C1– C8

R. communicans albus

R. communicans griseus

T1– T12

Ganglion lumbale primum trunci sympathici

Plexus hypogastricus superior

Ganglion sacrale primum trunci sympathici

L1– L5

S1– S5

Nn. splanchnici sacrales

N. caroticus internus

Plexus caroticus internus

N. caroticus externus

Plexus caroticus externus

Glandula lacrimalis

Bulbus oculi

Glandula parotidea

Glandula sublingualis

Glandula submandibularis

Larynx
Trachea
Bronchi
Pulmones

Nn. cardiaci

N. splanchnicus thoracicus major

Cor

Ganglion coeliacum

N. splanchnicus thoracicus minor

Gaster

Ganglion aorticorenale

Hepar

Vesica biliaris

Ductus biliares

Pancreas

N. splanchnicus thoracicus imus

Glandula suprarenalis

Ren

Ganglion mesentericum superius

Intestina

Nn. splanchnici lumbales

Colon descendens

Ganglion mesentericum inferius

Colon sigmoideum

Rectum

Plexus hypogastricus inferior

Vesica urinaria

Prostata

Organa genitalia externa

C.Machado
_M.D.

Fibrae preganglionicae ——————

Fibrae postganglionicae - - - - - - - -

Plate 6

Systematic Anatomy

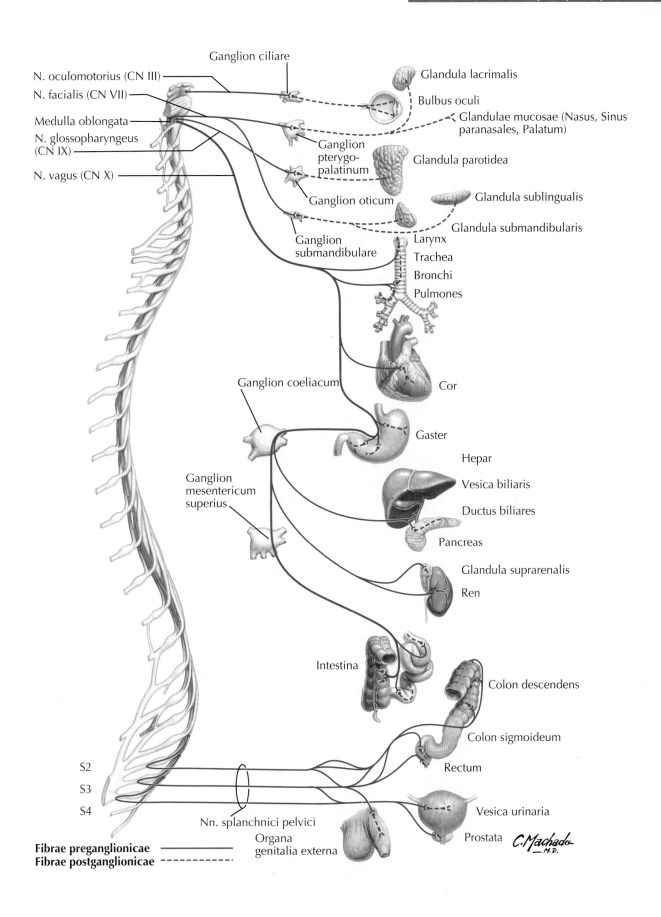

Ganglion ciliare

N. oculomotorius (CN III)

N. facialis (CN VII)

Medulla oblongata

N. glossopharyngeus (CN IX)

N. vagus (CN X)

Ganglion pterygo-palatinum

Ganglion oticum

Ganglion submandibulare

Glandula lacrimalis

Bulbus oculi

Glandulae mucosae (Nasus, Sinus paranasales, Palatum)

Glandula parotidea

Glandula sublingualis

Glandula submandibularis

Larynx

Trachea

Bronchi

Pulmones

Cor

Ganglion coeliacum

Gaster

Hepar

Vesica biliaris

Ductus biliares

Ganglion mesentericum superius

Pancreas

Glandula suprarenalis

Ren

Intestina

Colon descendens

Colon sigmoideum

Rectum

Vesica urinaria

S2

S3

S4

Nn. splanchnici pelvici

Organa genitalia externa

Prostata

C.Machado
_M.D.

Fibrae preganglionicae ——————

Fibrae postganglionicae - - - - - - - -

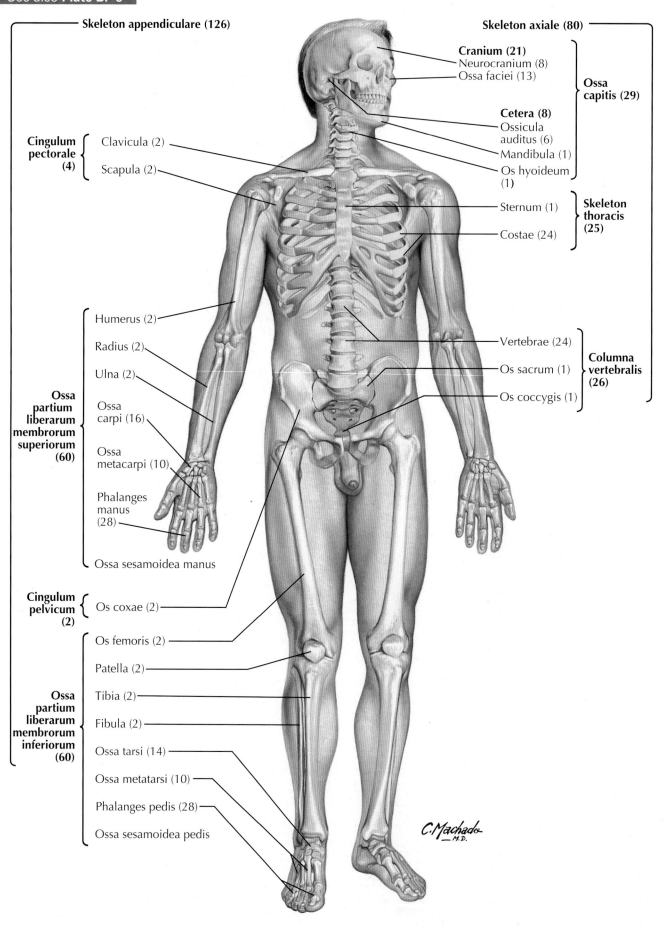

Skeleton appendiculare (126)

Skeleton axiale (80)

Cranium (21)
Neurocranium (8)
Ossa faciei (13)

Ossa capitis (29)

Cetera (8)
Ossicula auditus (6)
Mandibula (1)
Os hyoideum (1)

Cingulum pectorale (4)
Clavicula (2)
Scapula (2)

Sternum (1)
Costae (24)

Skeleton thoracis (25)

Ossa partium liberarum membrorum superiorum (60)
Humerus (2)
Radius (2)
Ulna (2)
Ossa carpi (16)
Ossa metacarpi (10)
Phalanges manus (28)
Ossa sesamoidea manus

Vertebrae (24)
Os sacrum (1)
Os coccygis (1)

Columna vertebralis (26)

Cingulum pelvicum (2)
Os coxae (2)

Ossa partium liberarum membrorum inferiorum (60)
Os femoris (2)
Patella (2)
Tibia (2)
Fibula (2)
Ossa tarsi (14)
Ossa metatarsi (10)
Phalanges pedis (28)
Ossa sesamoidea pedis

C.Machado
M.D.

Plate 8

Systematic Anatomy

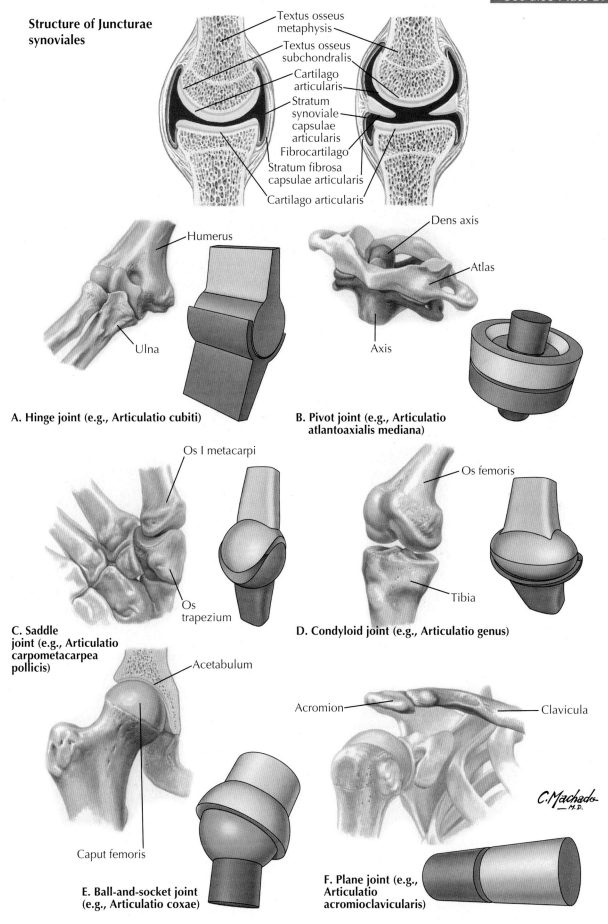

Structure of Juncturae synoviales

Textus osseus metaphysis
Textus osseus subchondralis
Cartilago articularis
Stratum synoviale capsulae articularis
Fibrocartilago
Stratum fibrosa capsulae articularis
Cartilago articularis

Humerus
Ulna

A. Hinge joint (e.g., Articulatio cubiti)

Dens axis
Atlas
Axis

B. Pivot joint (e.g., Articulatio atlantoaxialis mediana)

Os I metacarpi
Os trapezium

C. Saddle joint (e.g., Articulatio carpometacarpea pollicis)

Os femoris
Tibia

D. Condyloid joint (e.g., Articulatio genus)

Acetabulum
Caput femoris

E. Ball-and-socket joint (e.g., Articulatio coxae)

Acromion
Clavicula

F. Plane joint (e.g., Articulatio acromioclavicularis)

C. Machado M.D.

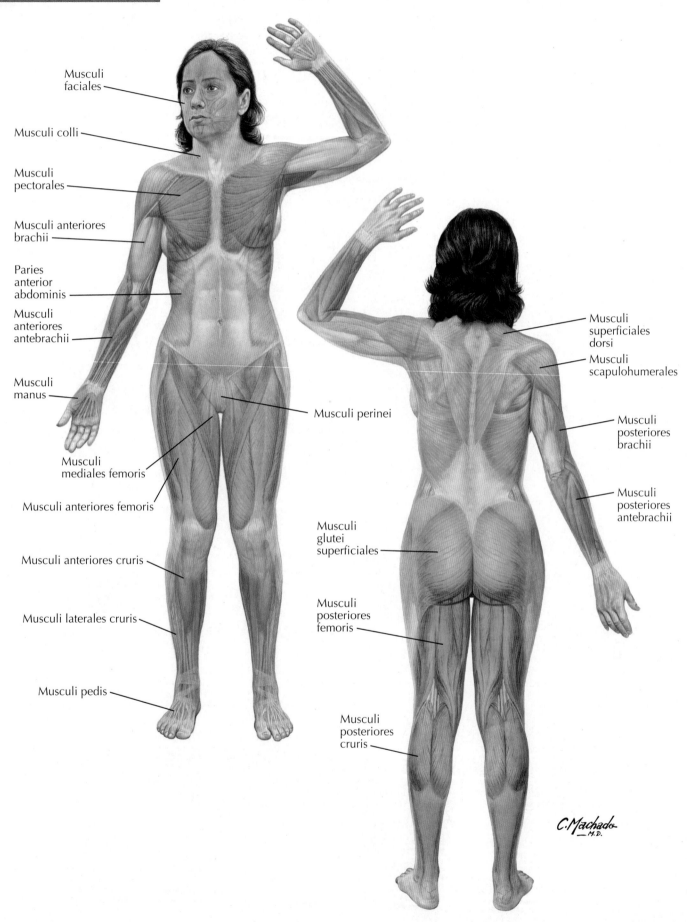

Musculi
faciales

Musculi colli

Musculi
pectorales

Musculi anteriores
brachii

Paries
anterior
abdominis

Musculi
anteriores
antebrachii

Musculi
manus

Musculi
mediales femoris

Musculi anteriores femoris

Musculi anteriores cruris

Musculi laterales cruris

Musculi pedis

Musculi perinei

Musculi
superficiales
dorsi

Musculi
scapulohumerales

Musculi
posteriores
brachii

Musculi
posteriores
antebrachii

Musculi
glutei
superficiales

Musculi
posteriores
femoris

Musculi
posteriores
cruris

C. Machado
_M.D.

Plate 10

Systematic Anatomy

Segmental innervation of upper limb movements

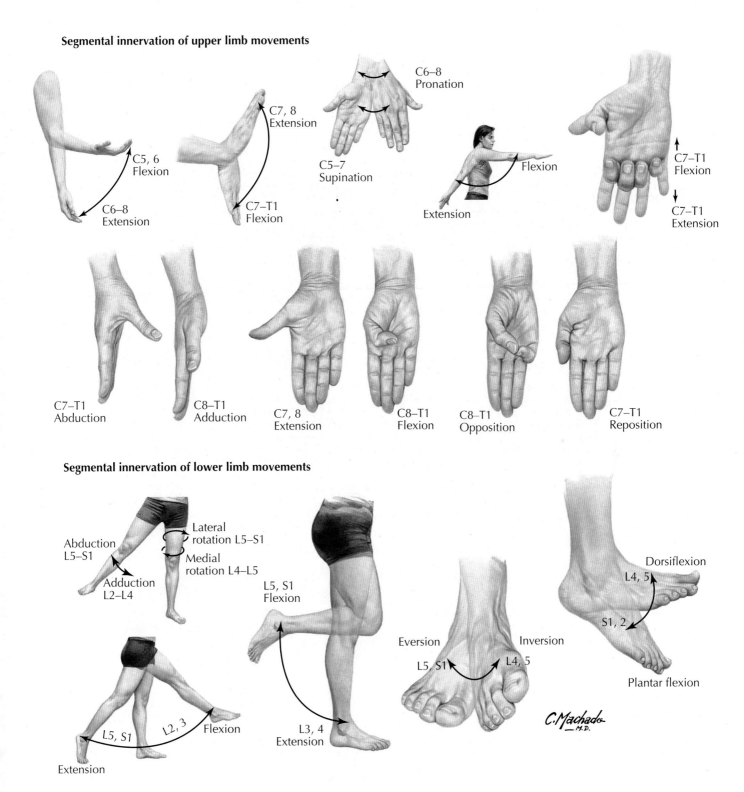

C5, 6 Flexion
C6–8 Extension

C7, 8 Extension
C7–T1 Flexion

C6–8 Pronation

C5–7 Supination

Flexion
Extension

C7–T1 Flexion
C7–T1 Extension

C7–T1 Abduction

C8–T1 Adduction

C7, 8 Extension

C8–T1 Flexion

C8–T1 Opposition

C7–T1 Reposition

Segmental innervation of lower limb movements

Abduction L5–S1
Adduction L2–L4

Lateral rotation L5–S1
Medial rotation L4–L5

L5, S1 Flexion

Eversion
L5, S1

Inversion
L4, 5

Dorsiflexion
L4, 5

S1, 2
Plantar flexion

L5, S1
L2, 3 Flexion
Extension

L3, 4 Extension

C. Machado M.D.

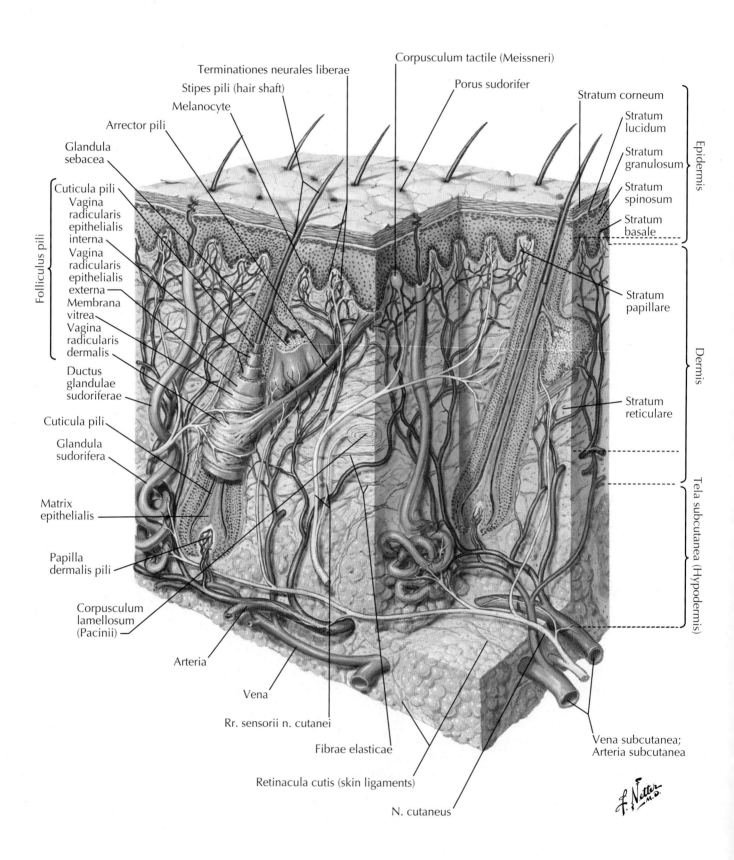

Terminationes neurales liberae

Corpusculum tactile (Meissneri)

Stipes pili (hair shaft)

Porus sudorifer

Melanocyte

Stratum corneum

Arrector pili

Stratum lucidum

Glandula sebacea

Stratum granulosum

Cuticula pili

Stratum spinosum

Vagina radicularis epithelialis interna

Stratum basale

Epidermis

Vagina radicularis epithelialis externa

Stratum papillare

Membrana vitrea

Vagina radicularis dermalis

Dermis

Ductus glandulae sudoriferae

Stratum reticulare

Cuticula pili

Glandula sudorifera

Matrix epithelialis

Papilla dermalis pili

Tela subcutanea (Hypodermis)

Corpusculum lamellosum (Pacinii)

Arteria

Vena

Rr. sensorii n. cutanei

Vena subcutanea;
Arteria subcutanea

Fibrae elasticae

Retinacula cutis (skin ligaments)

N. cutaneus

Folliculus pili

Plate 12

Systematic Anatomy

Volume distribution

Lungs (9%)

Small arteries and arterioles (8%)

Heart in diastole (7%)

Large arteries (7%)

Capillaries (5%)

Veins (64%)

Distribution of vascular resistance

Small arteries and arterioles (47%)

Veins (7%)

Large arteries (19%)

Capillaries (27%)

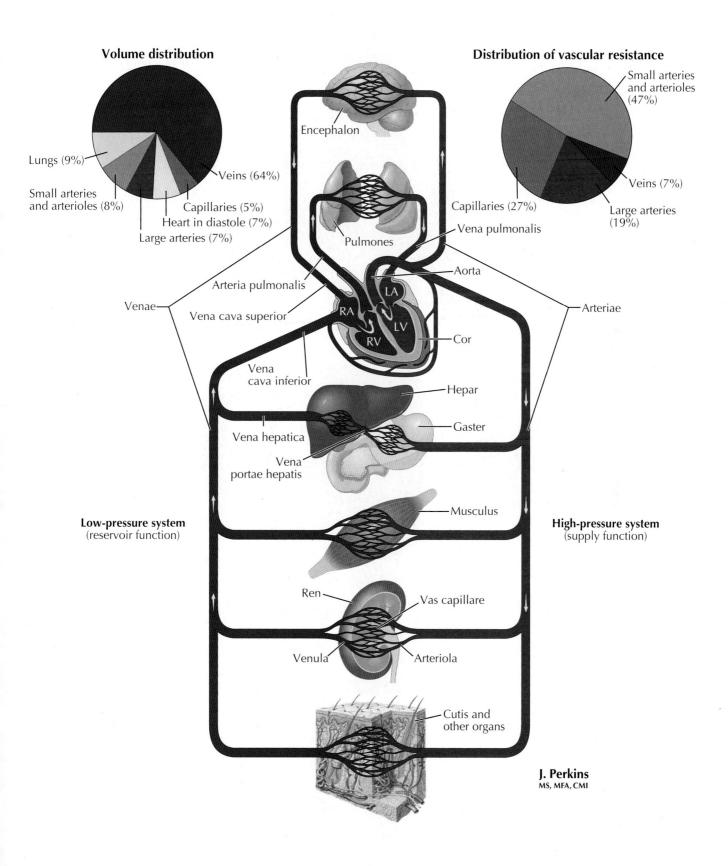

Encephalon

Pulmones

Vena pulmonalis

Arteria pulmonalis

Aorta

Vena cava superior

LA

RA

LV

RV

Cor

Venae

Arteriae

Vena cava inferior

Hepar

Gaster

Vena hepatica

Vena portae hepatis

Musculus

Low-pressure system
(reservoir function)

High-pressure system
(supply function)

Ren

Vas capillare

Venula

Arteriola

Cutis and other organs

J. Perkins
MS, MFA, CMI

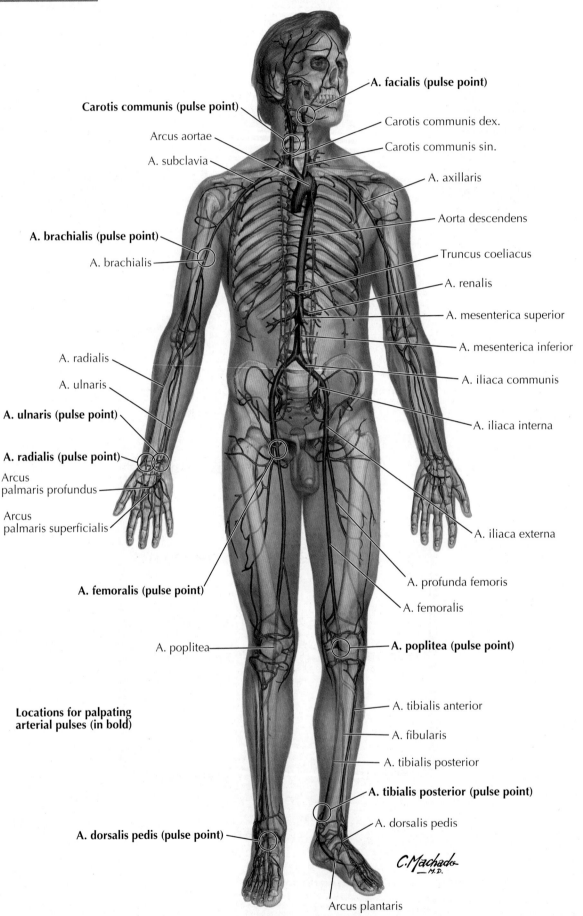

A. facialis (pulse point)

Carotis communis (pulse point)

Carotis communis dex.

Arcus aortae

Carotis communis sin.

A. subclavia

A. axillaris

Aorta descendens

A. brachialis (pulse point)

Truncus coeliacus

A. brachialis

A. renalis

A. mesenterica superior

A. mesenterica inferior

A. radialis

A. iliaca communis

A. ulnaris

A. ulnaris (pulse point)

A. iliaca interna

A. radialis (pulse point)

Arcus
palmaris profundus

Arcus
palmaris superficialis

A. iliaca externa

A. profunda femoris

A. femoralis (pulse point)

A. femoralis

A. poplitea

A. poplitea (pulse point)

**Locations for palpating
arterial pulses (in bold)**

A. tibialis anterior

A. fibularis

A. tibialis posterior

A. tibialis posterior (pulse point)

A. dorsalis pedis

A. dorsalis pedis (pulse point)

C. Machado
_M.D._

Arcus plantaris

Plate 14

Systematic Anatomy

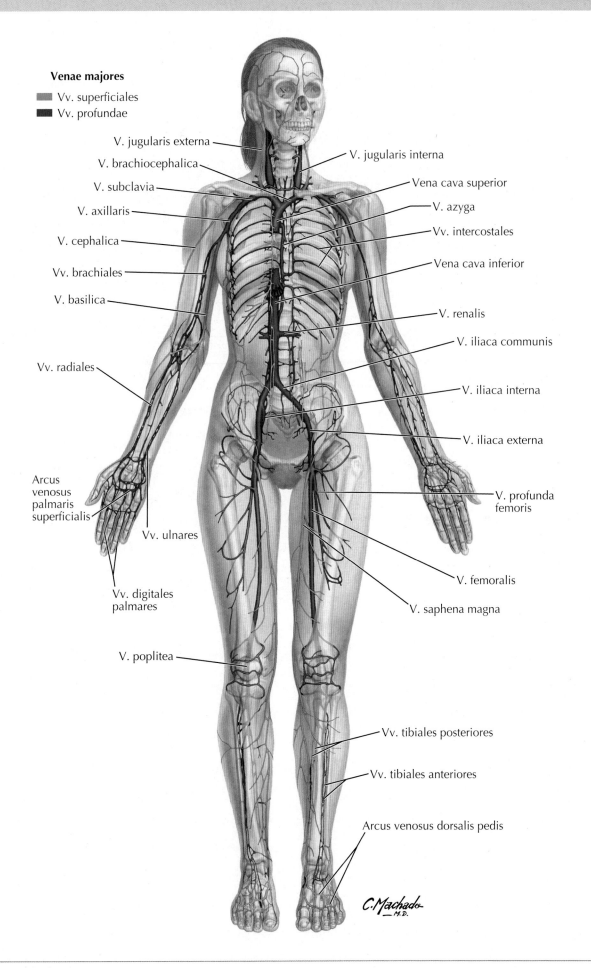

Venae majores

Vv. superficiales

Vv. profundae

V. jugularis externa

V. brachiocephalica

V. subclavia

V. axillaris

V. cephalica

Vv. brachiales

V. basilica

Vv. radiales

Arcus venosus palmaris superficialis

Vv. ulnares

Vv. digitales palmares

V. poplitea

V. jugularis interna

Vena cava superior

V. azyga

Vv. intercostales

Vena cava inferior

V. renalis

V. iliaca communis

V. iliaca interna

V. iliaca externa

V. profunda femoris

V. femoralis

V. saphena magna

Vv. tibiales posteriores

Vv. tibiales anteriores

Arcus venosus dorsalis pedis

C.Machado
M.D.

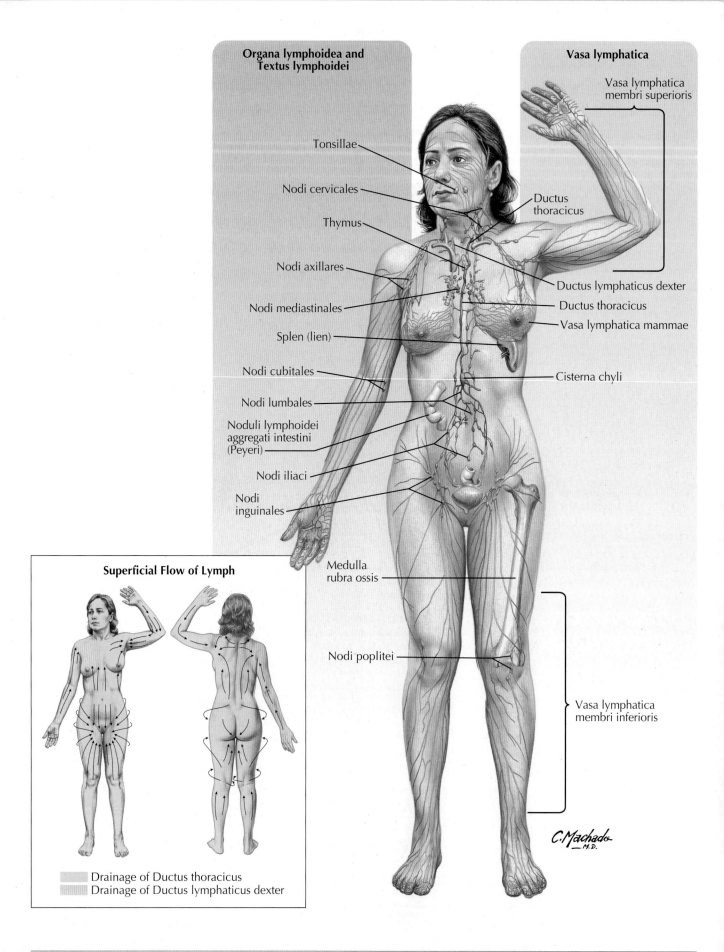

Organa lymphoidea and Textus lymphoidei

Vasa lymphatica

Vasa lymphatica membri superioris

Tonsillae

Nodi cervicales

Thymus

Nodi axillares

Nodi mediastinales

Splen (lien)

Nodi cubitales

Nodi lumbales

Noduli lymphoidei aggregati intestini (Peyeri)

Nodi iliaci

Nodi inguinales

Ductus thoracicus

Ductus lymphaticus dexter

Ductus thoracicus

Vasa lymphatica mammae

Cisterna chyli

Medulla rubra ossis

Nodi poplitei

Vasa lymphatica membri inferioris

Superficial Flow of Lymph

Drainage of Ductus thoracicus
Drainage of Ductus lymphaticus dexter

C. Machado M.D.

Plate 16   **Systematic Anatomy**

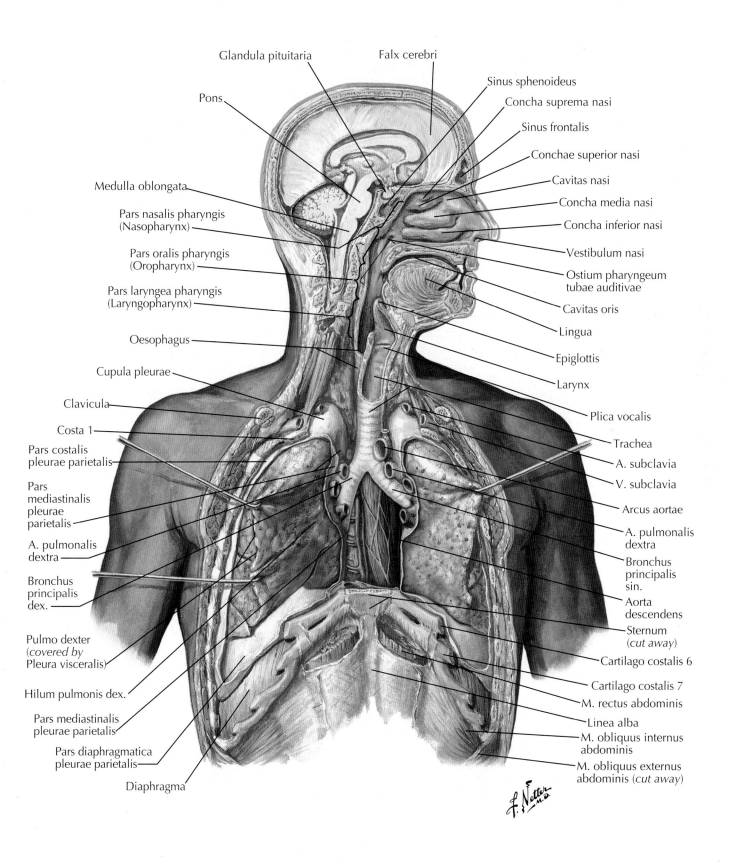

Glandula pituitaria

Falx cerebri

Pons

Sinus sphenoideus

Concha suprema nasi

Sinus frontalis

Medulla oblongata

Conchae superior nasi

Cavitas nasi

Pars nasalis pharyngis (Nasopharynx)

Concha media nasi

Concha inferior nasi

Pars oralis pharyngis (Oropharynx)

Vestibulum nasi

Ostium pharyngeum tubae auditivae

Pars laryngea pharyngis (Laryngopharynx)

Cavitas oris

Oesophagus

Lingua

Cupula pleurae

Epiglottis

Larynx

Clavicula

Plica vocalis

Costa 1

Trachea

Pars costalis pleurae parietalis

A. subclavia

V. subclavia

Pars mediastinalis pleurae parietalis

Arcus aortae

A. pulmonalis dextra

A. pulmonalis dextra

Bronchus principalis sin.

Bronchus principalis dex.

Aorta descendens

Pulmo dexter (*covered by* Pleura visceralis)

Sternum (*cut away*)

Cartilago costalis 6

Hilum pulmonis dex.

Cartilago costalis 7

Pars mediastinalis pleurae parietalis

M. rectus abdominis

Linea alba

Pars diaphragmatica pleurae parietalis

M. obliquus internus abdominis

M. obliquus externus abdominis (*cut away*)

Diaphragma

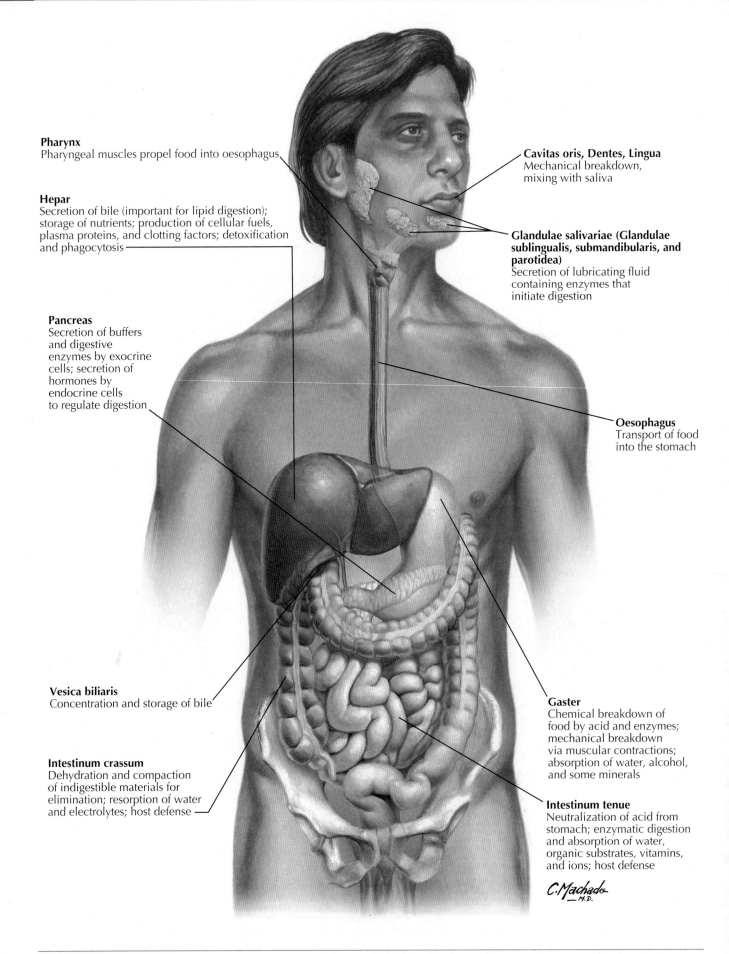

Pharynx
Pharyngeal muscles propel food into oesophagus

Hepar
Secretion of bile (important for lipid digestion); storage of nutrients; production of cellular fuels, plasma proteins, and clotting factors; detoxification and phagocytosis

Pancreas
Secretion of buffers and digestive enzymes by exocrine cells; secretion of hormones by endocrine cells to regulate digestion

Vesica biliaris
Concentration and storage of bile

Intestinum crassum
Dehydration and compaction of indigestible materials for elimination; resorption of water and electrolytes; host defense

Cavitas oris, Dentes, Lingua
Mechanical breakdown, mixing with saliva

Glandulae salivariae (Glandulae sublingualis, submandibularis, and parotidea)
Secretion of lubricating fluid containing enzymes that initiate digestion

Oesophagus
Transport of food into the stomach

Gaster
Chemical breakdown of food by acid and enzymes; mechanical breakdown via muscular contractions; absorption of water, alcohol, and some minerals

Intestinum tenue
Neutralization of acid from stomach; enzymatic digestion and absorption of water, organic substrates, vitamins, and ions; host defense

Plate 18 **Systematic Anatomy**

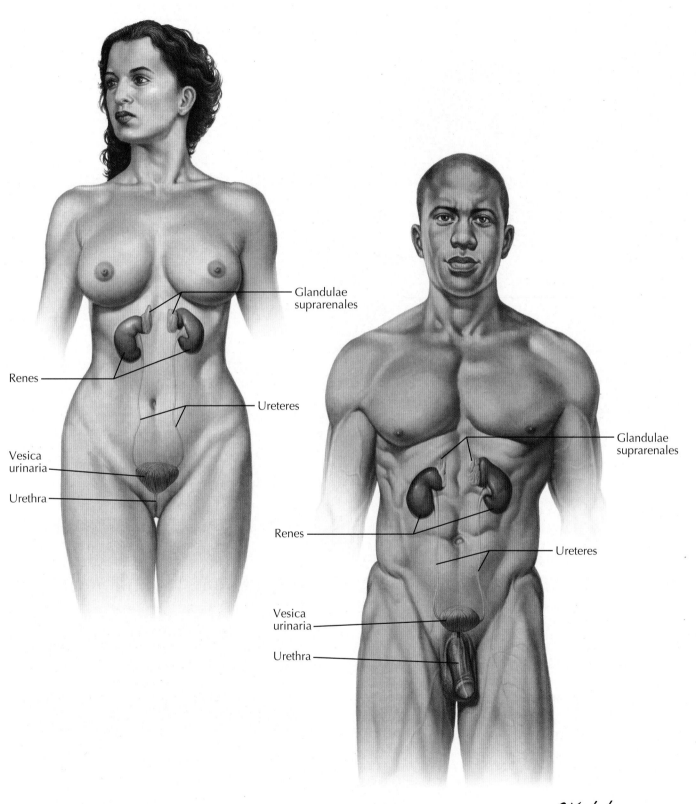

Glandulae
suprarenales

Renes

Ureteres

Vesica
urinaria

Urethra

Glandulae
suprarenales

Renes

Ureteres

Vesica
urinaria

Urethra

C. Machado
_M.D._

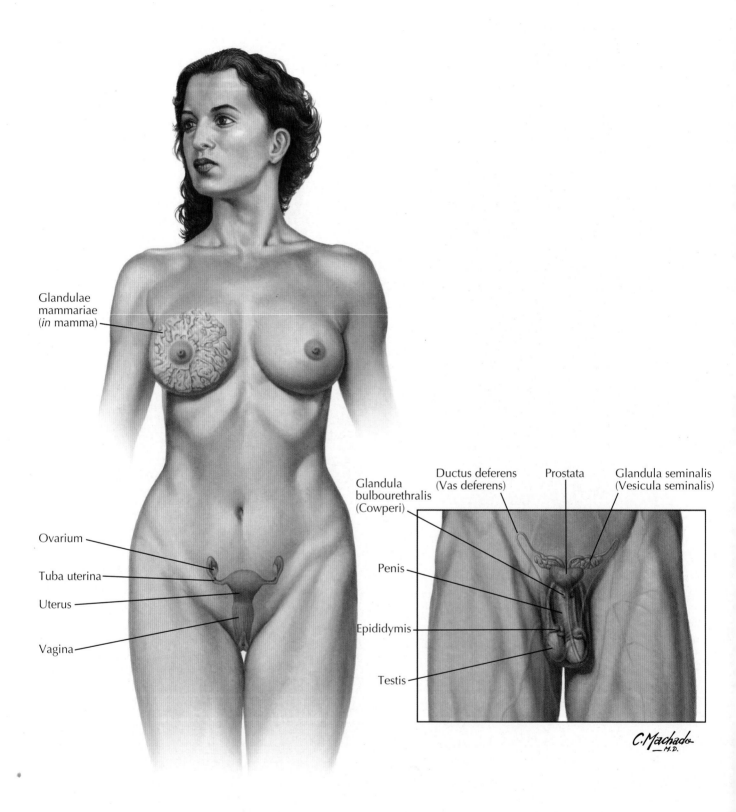

Glandulae
mammariae
(*in* mamma)

Ovarium

Tuba uterina

Uterus

Vagina

Glandula
bulbourethralis
(Cowperi)

Ductus deferens
(Vas deferens)

Prostata

Glandula seminalis
(Vesicula seminalis)

Penis

Epididymis

Testis

C.Machado
_M.D._

Plate 20   **Systematic Anatomy**

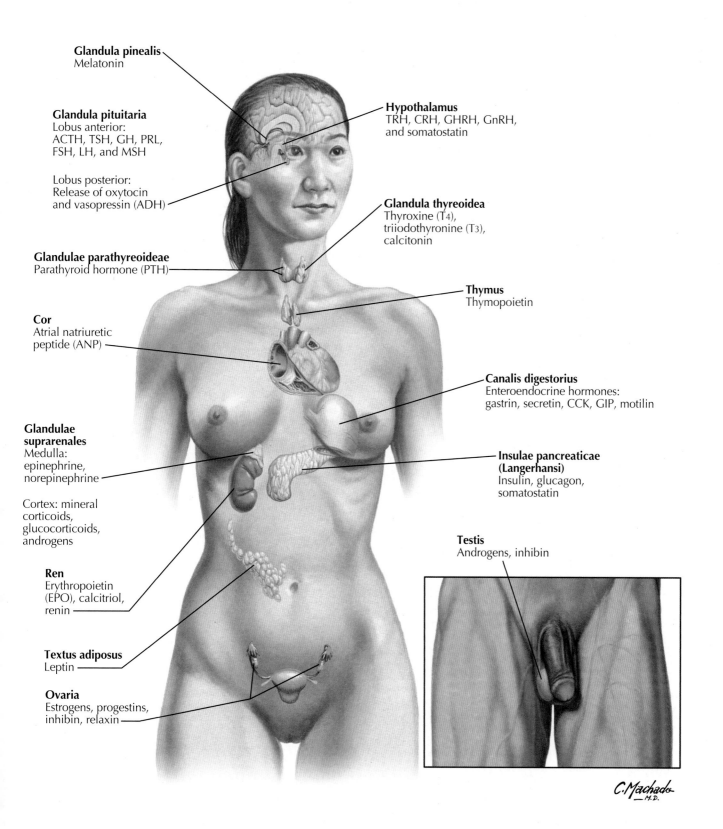

Glandula pinealis
Melatonin

Glandula pituitaria
Lobus anterior:
ACTH, TSH, GH, PRL,
FSH, LH, and MSH

Lobus posterior:
Release of oxytocin
and vasopressin (ADH)

Glandulae parathyreoideae
Parathyroid hormone (PTH)

Cor
Atrial natriuretic
peptide (ANP)

**Glandulae
suprarenales**
Medulla:
epinephrine,
norepinephrine

Cortex: mineral
corticoids,
glucocorticoids,
androgens

Ren
Erythropoietin
(EPO), calcitriol,
renin

Textus adiposus
Leptin

Ovaria
Estrogens, progestins,
inhibin, relaxin

Hypothalamus
TRH, CRH, GHRH, GnRH,
and somatostatin

Glandula thyreoidea
Thyroxine (T4),
triiodothyronine (T3),
calcitonin

Thymus
Thymopoietin

Canalis digestorius
Enteroendocrine hormones:
gastrin, secretin, CCK, GIP, motilin

**Insulae pancreaticae
(Langerhansi)**
Insulin, glucagon,
somatostatin

Testis
Androgens, inhibin

C.Machado
—M.D.

CAPUT AND COLLUM 2

Surface Anatomy   22–24
Ossa and Juncturae   25–47
Collum   48–58
Nasus   59–82
Stoma   83–90
Pharynx   91–102
Larynx and Glandulae
  Endocrinae   103–109
Oculus   110–120
Auris   121–126
Encephalon and Meninges   127–142

Nervi Craniales and
  Nervi Cervicales   143–162
Vasa Sanguinea Encephali   163–175
Regional Imaging   176–177
Structures with High
  Clinical Significance   Tables 2.1–2.5
Nervi Craniales   Tables 2.6–2.8
Nervi Plexus Cervicalis   Table 2.9
Musculi   Tables 2.10–2.14
Electronic Bonus Plates   Plates BP 14–BP 32

ELECTRONIC BONUS PLATES

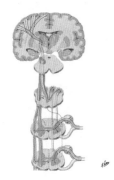

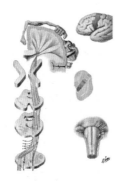

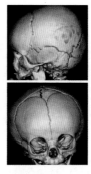

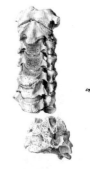

BP 14 Somatosensory System: Trunk and Limbs

BP 15 Pyramidal System

BP 16 3D Skull Reconstruction CTs

BP 17 Vertebrae Cervicales: Degenerative Changes

ELECTRONIC BONUS PLATES—*cont'd*

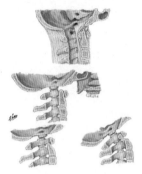

BP 18 Articulatio Atlantooccipitalis

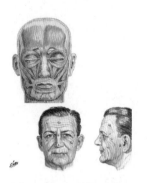

BP 19 Musculi Faciales: Anterior View

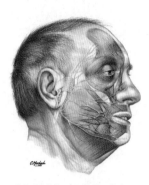

BP 20 Musculi Faciales

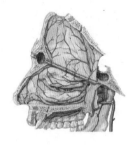

BP 21 Cavitas Nasalis Cranii: Arteriae (Septum Nasalis Turned Up)

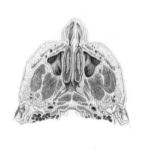

BP 22 Nasus and Sinus Maxillaris: Transverse Section

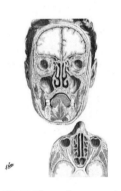

BP 23 Sinus Paranasales

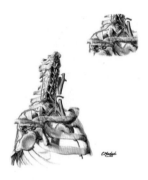

BP 24 Arteria Subclavia

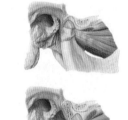
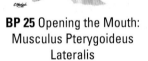

BP 25 Opening the Mouth: Musculus Pterygoideus Lateralis

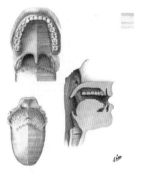

BP 26 Cavitas Oris and Pharynx: Afferent Innervation

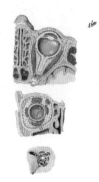

BP 27 Orbita and Bulbus Oculi: Fasciae

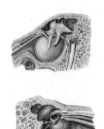

BP 28 Cavitas Tympani: Medial and Lateral Views

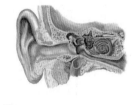

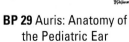

BP 29 Auris: Anatomy of the Pediatric Ear

ELECTRONIC BONUS PLATES—*cont'd*

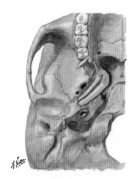

BP 30 Tuba Auditiva
(Eustachii)

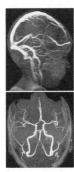

BP 31 Cranial Imaging (MRV
and MRA)

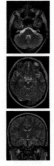

BP 32 Axial and Coronal MRIs
of Brain

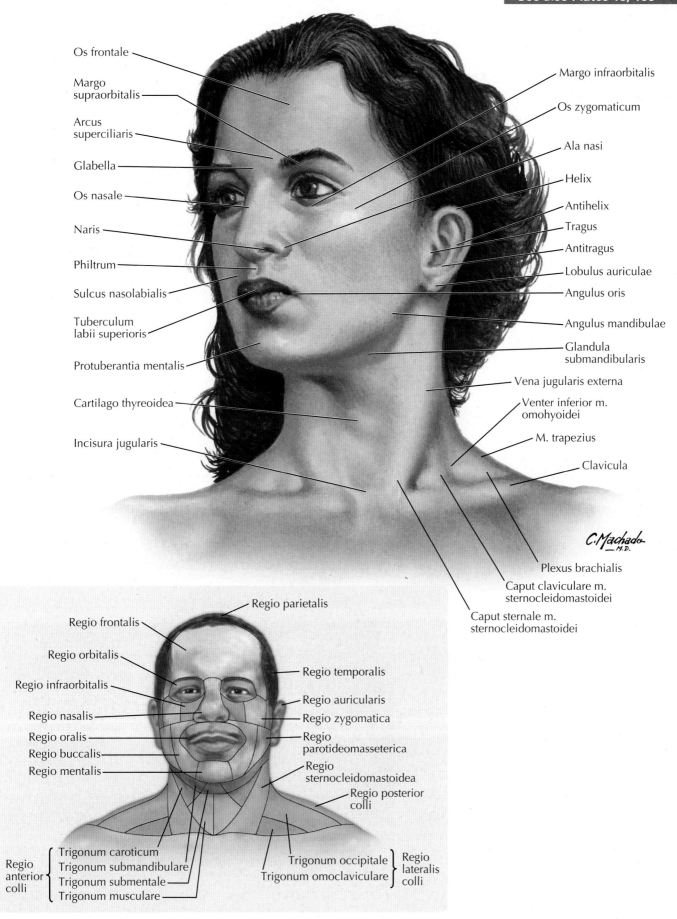

Os frontale

Margo
supraorbitalis

Arcus
superciliaris

Glabella

Os nasale

Naris

Philtrum

Sulcus nasolabialis

Tuberculum
labii superioris

Protuberantia mentalis

Cartilago thyreoidea

Incisura jugularis

Margo infraorbitalis

Os zygomaticum

Ala nasi

Helix

Antihelix

Tragus

Antitragus

Lobulus auriculae

Angulus oris

Angulus mandibulae

Glandula
submandibularis

Vena jugularis externa

Venter inferior m.
omohyoidei

M. trapezius

Clavicula

Plexus brachialis

Caput claviculare m.
sternocleidomastoidei

Caput sternale m.
sternocleidomastoidei

C. Machado
M.D.

Regio parietalis

Regio frontalis

Regio orbitalis

Regio infraorbitalis

Regio nasalis

Regio oralis

Regio buccalis

Regio mentalis

Regio temporalis

Regio auricularis

Regio zygomatica

Regio
parotideomasseterica

Regio
sternocleidomastoidea

Regio posterior
colli

Regio
anterior
colli

{ Trigonum caroticum
Trigonum submandibulare
Trigonum submentale
Trigonum musculare

Trigonum occipitale
Trigonum omoclaviculare

} Regio
lateralis
colli

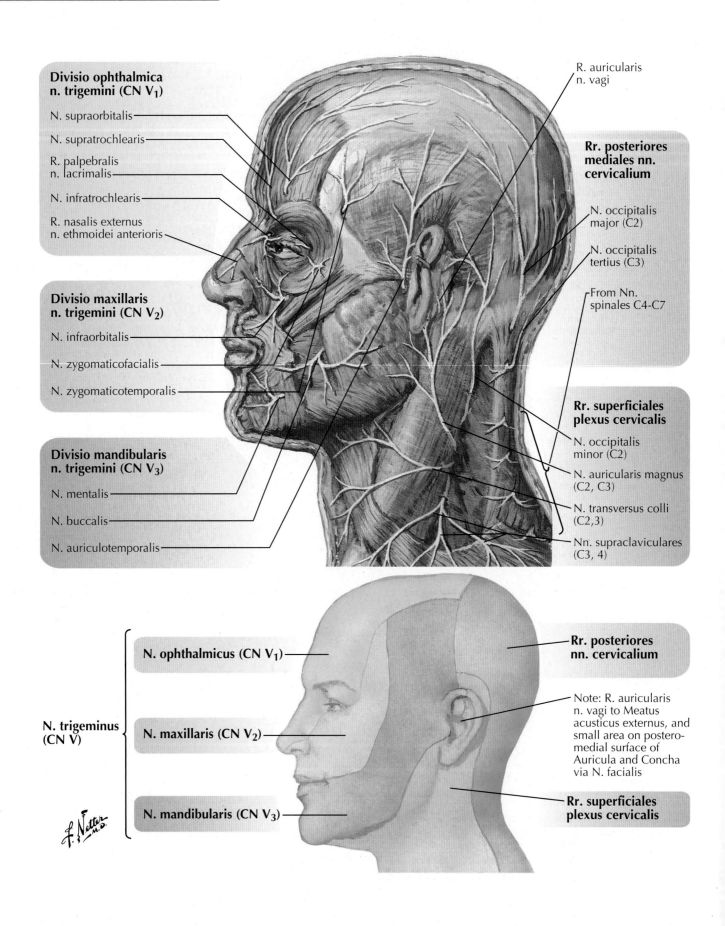

Divisio ophthalmica n. trigemini (CN V₁)

N. supraorbitalis

N. supratrochlearis

R. palpebralis n. lacrimalis

N. infratrochlearis

R. nasalis externus n. ethmoidei anterioris

Divisio maxillaris n. trigemini (CN V₂)

N. infraorbitalis

N. zygomaticofacialis

N. zygomaticotemporalis

Divisio mandibularis n. trigemini (CN V₃)

N. mentalis

N. buccalis

N. auriculotemporalis

R. auricularis n. vagi

Rr. posteriores mediales nn. cervicalium

N. occipitalis major (C2)

N. occipitalis tertius (C3)

From Nn. spinales C4-C7

Rr. superficiales plexus cervicalis

N. occipitalis minor (C2)

N. auricularis magnus (C2, C3)

N. transversus colli (C2,3)

Nn. supraclaviculares (C3, 4)

N. ophthalmicus (CN V₁)

N. maxillaris (CN V₂)

N. trigeminus (CN V)

N. mandibularis (CN V₃)

Rr. posteriores nn. cervicalium

Note: R. auricularis n. vagi to Meatus acusticus externus, and small area on postero-medial surface of Auricula and Concha via N. facialis

Rr. superficiales plexus cervicalis

Plate 23

Surface Anatomy

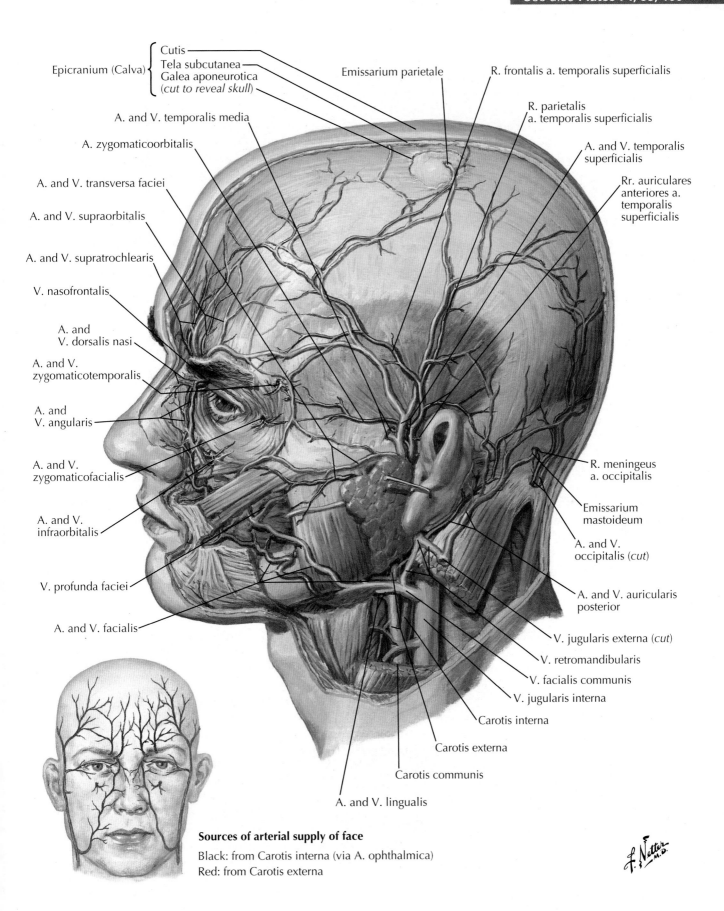

Epicranium (Calva) { Cutis
Tela subcutanea
Galea aponeurotica
(cut to reveal skull)

Emissarium parietale

R. frontalis a. temporalis superficialis

R. parietalis a. temporalis superficialis

A. and V. temporalis media

A. zygomaticoorbitalis

A. and V. temporalis superficialis

A. and V. transversa faciei

Rr. auriculares anteriores a. temporalis superficialis

A. and V. supraorbitalis

A. and V. supratrochlearis

V. nasofrontalis

A. and V. dorsalis nasi

A. and V. zygomaticotemporalis

A. and V. angularis

R. meningeus a. occipitalis

A. and V. zygomaticofacialis

Emissarium mastoideum

A. and V. occipitalis *(cut)*

A. and V. infraorbitalis

A. and V. auricularis posterior

V. profunda faciei

A. and V. facialis

V. jugularis externa *(cut)*

V. retromandibularis

V. facialis communis

V. jugularis interna

Carotis interna

Carotis externa

Carotis communis

A. and V. lingualis

Sources of arterial supply of face

Black: from Carotis interna (via A. ophthalmica)

Red: from Carotis externa

f. Netter M.D.

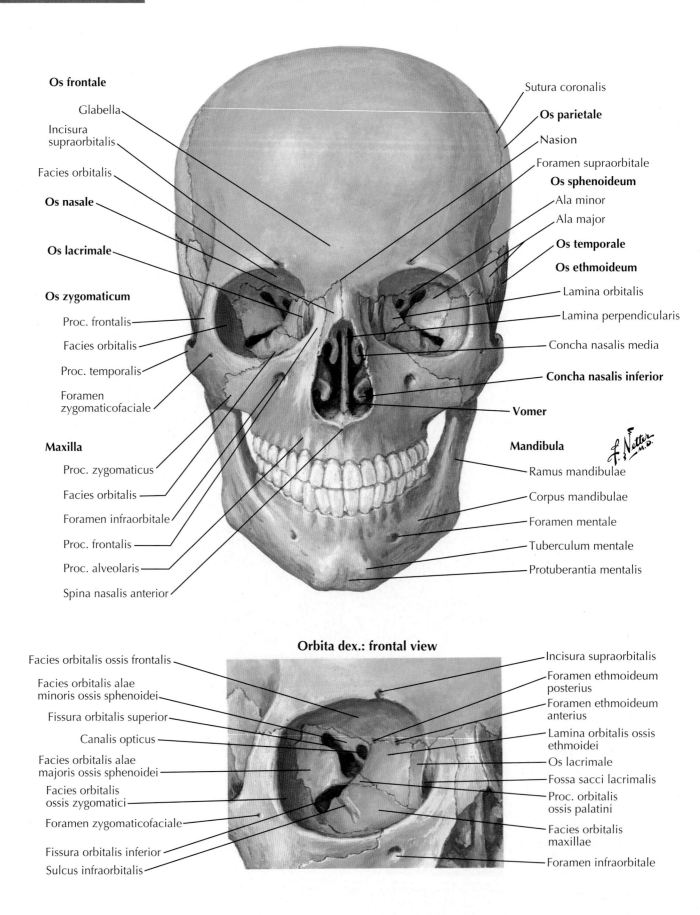

Os frontale

Glabella

Incisura supraorbitalis

Facies orbitalis

Os nasale

Os lacrimale

Os zygomaticum

Proc. frontalis

Facies orbitalis

Proc. temporalis

Foramen zygomaticofaciale

Maxilla

Proc. zygomaticus

Facies orbitalis

Foramen infraorbitale

Proc. frontalis

Proc. alveolaris

Spina nasalis anterior

Sutura coronalis

Os parietale

Nasion

Foramen supraorbitale

Os sphenoideum

Ala minor

Ala major

Os temporale

Os ethmoideum

Lamina orbitalis

Lamina perpendicularis

Concha nasalis media

Concha nasalis inferior

Vomer

Mandibula

Ramus mandibulae

Corpus mandibulae

Foramen mentale

Tuberculum mentale

Protuberantia mentalis

Orbita dex.: frontal view

Facies orbitalis ossis frontalis

Facies orbitalis alae minoris ossis sphenoidei

Fissura orbitalis superior

Canalis opticus

Facies orbitalis alae majoris ossis sphenoidei

Facies orbitalis ossis zygomatici

Foramen zygomaticofaciale

Fissura orbitalis inferior

Sulcus infraorbitalis

Incisura supraorbitalis

Foramen ethmoideum posterius

Foramen ethmoideum anterius

Lamina orbitalis ossis ethmoidei

Os lacrimale

Fossa sacci lacrimalis

Proc. orbitalis ossis palatini

Facies orbitalis maxillae

Foramen infraorbitale

Plate 25

Ossa and Juncturae

Posterior anterior view

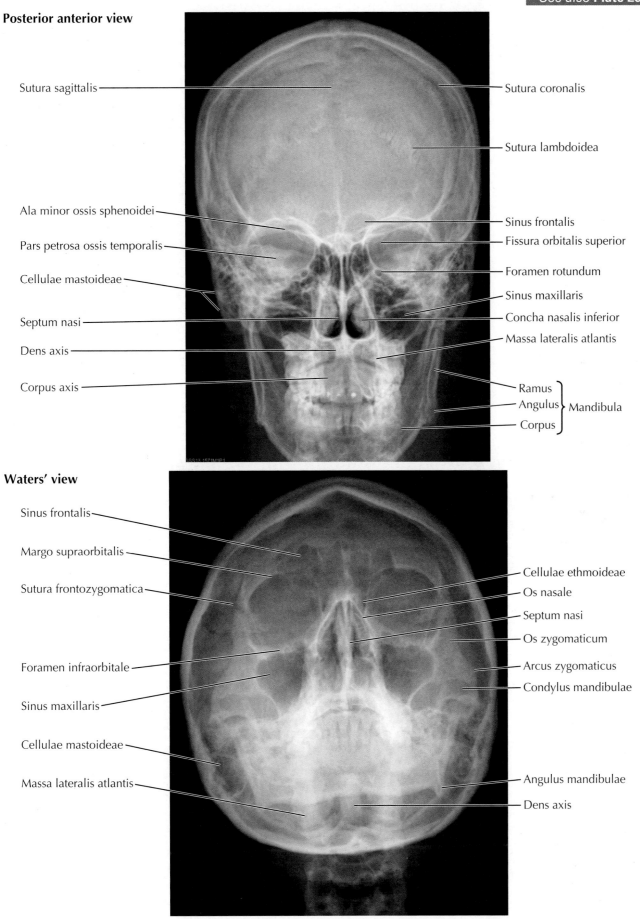

Sutura sagittalis

Sutura coronalis

Sutura lambdoidea

Ala minor ossis sphenoidei

Pars petrosa ossis temporalis

Cellulae mastoideae

Septum nasi

Dens axis

Corpus axis

Sinus frontalis

Fissura orbitalis superior

Foramen rotundum

Sinus maxillaris

Concha nasalis inferior

Massa lateralis atlantis

Ramus
Angulus } Mandibula
Corpus

Waters' view

Sinus frontalis

Margo supraorbitalis

Sutura frontozygomatica

Foramen infraorbitale

Sinus maxillaris

Cellulae mastoideae

Massa lateralis atlantis

Cellulae ethmoideae

Os nasale

Septum nasi

Os zygomaticum

Arcus zygomaticus

Condylus mandibulae

Angulus mandibulae

Dens axis

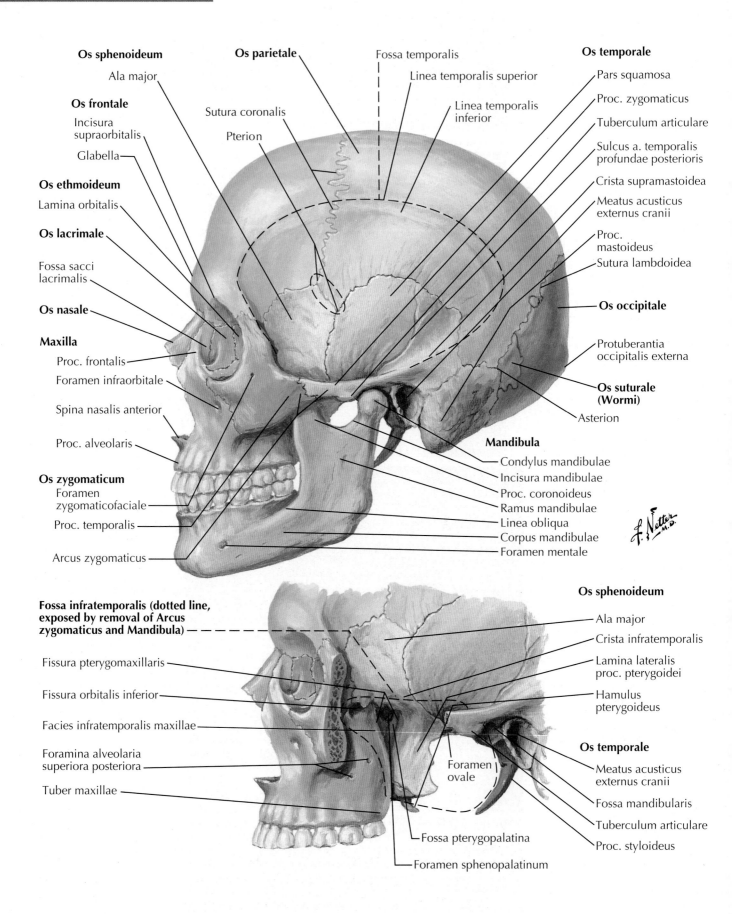

Os sphenoideum
Ala major

Os frontale
Incisura supraorbitalis
Glabella

Os ethmoideum
Lamina orbitalis

Os lacrimale
Fossa sacci lacrimalis

Os nasale

Maxilla
Proc. frontalis
Foramen infraorbitale
Spina nasalis anterior
Proc. alveolaris

Os zygomaticum
Foramen zygomaticofaciale
Proc. temporalis
Arcus zygomaticus

Os parietale
Sutura coronalis
Pterion

Fossa temporalis
Linea temporalis superior
Linea temporalis inferior

Os temporale
Pars squamosa
Proc. zygomaticus
Tuberculum articulare
Sulcus a. temporalis profundae posterioris
Crista supramastoidea
Meatus acusticus externus cranii
Proc. mastoideus
Sutura lambdoidea

Os occipitale
Protuberantia occipitalis externa

Os suturale (Wormi)
Asterion

Mandibula
Condylus mandibulae
Incisura mandibulae
Proc. coronoideus
Ramus mandibulae
Linea obliqua
Corpus mandibulae
Foramen mentale

Fossa infratemporalis (dotted line, exposed by removal of Arcus zygomaticus and Mandibula)

Fissura pterygomaxillaris
Fissura orbitalis inferior
Facies infratemporalis maxillae
Foramina alveolaria superiora posteriora
Tuber maxillae

Os sphenoideum
Ala major
Crista infratemporalis
Lamina lateralis proc. pterygoidei
Hamulus pterygoideus

Os temporale
Meatus acusticus externus cranii
Fossa mandibularis
Tuberculum articulare
Proc. styloideus

Foramen ovale
Fossa pterygopalatina
Foramen sphenopalatinum

Plate 27

Ossa and Juncturae

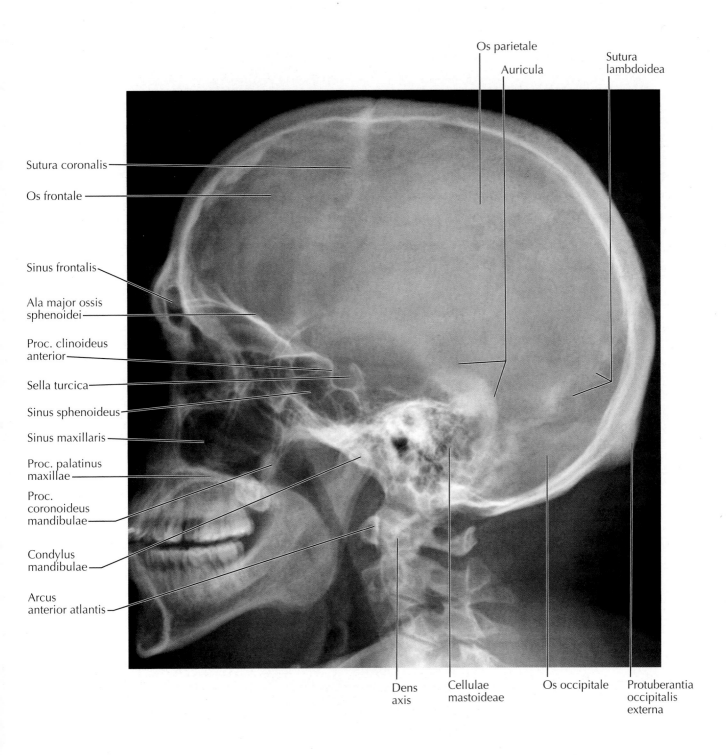

Os parietale

Auricula

Sutura lambdoidea

Sutura coronalis

Os frontale

Sinus frontalis

Ala major ossis sphenoidei

Proc. clinoideus anterior

Sella turcica

Sinus sphenoideus

Sinus maxillaris

Proc. palatinus maxillae

Proc. coronoideus mandibulae

Condylus mandibulae

Arcus anterior atlantis

Dens axis

Cellulae mastoideae

Os occipitale

Protuberantia occipitalis externa

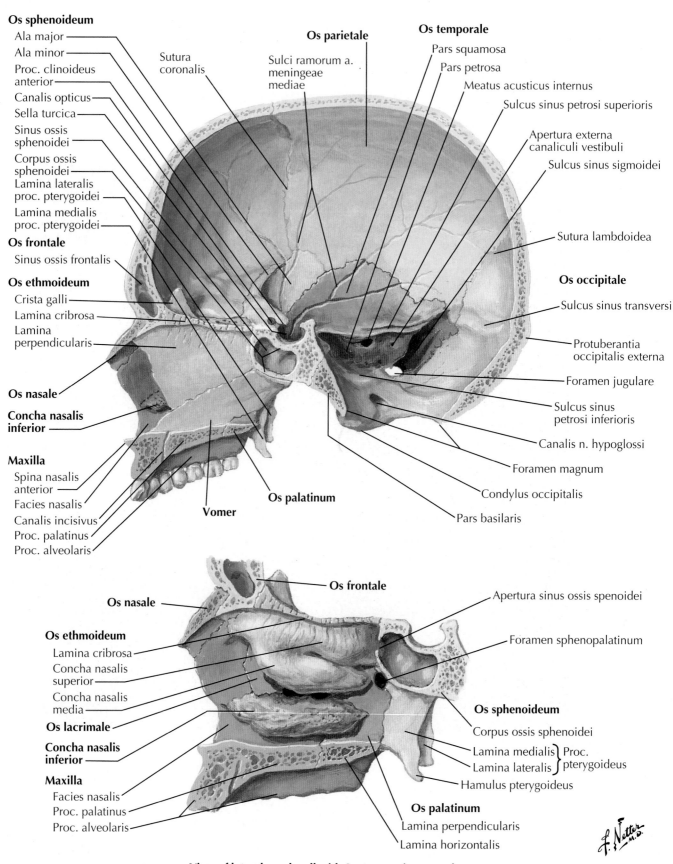

Os sphenoideum
Ala major
Ala minor
Proc. clinoideus anterior
Canalis opticus
Sella turcica
Sinus ossis sphenoidei
Corpus ossis sphenoidei
Lamina lateralis proc. pterygoidei
Lamina medialis proc. pterygoidei
Os frontale
Sinus ossis frontalis
Os ethmoideum
Crista galli
Lamina cribrosa
Lamina perpendicularis
Os nasale
Concha nasalis inferior
Maxilla
Spina nasalis anterior
Facies nasalis
Canalis incisivus
Proc. palatinus
Proc. alveolaris

Sutura coronalis

Os parietale
Sulci ramorum a. meningeae mediae

Os temporale
Pars squamosa
Pars petrosa
Meatus acusticus internus
Sulcus sinus petrosi superioris
Apertura externa canaliculi vestibuli
Sulcus sinus sigmoidei
Sutura lambdoidea

Os occipitale
Sulcus sinus transversi
Protuberantia occipitalis externa
Foramen jugulare
Sulcus sinus petrosi inferioris
Canalis n. hypoglossi
Foramen magnum
Condylus occipitalis
Pars basilaris

Os palatinum
Vomer

Os nasale

Os ethmoideum
Lamina cribrosa
Concha nasalis superior
Concha nasalis media
Os lacrimale
Concha nasalis inferior
Maxilla
Facies nasalis
Proc. palatinus
Proc. alveolaris

Os frontale
Apertura sinus ossis spenoidei
Foramen sphenopalatinum

Os sphenoideum
Corpus ossis sphenoidei
Lamina medialis ⎫ Proc.
Lamina lateralis ⎭ pterygoideus
Hamulus pterygoideus

Os palatinum
Lamina perpendicularis
Lamina horizontalis

View of lateral nasal wall with Septum nasi removed

Plate 29

Ossa and Juncturae

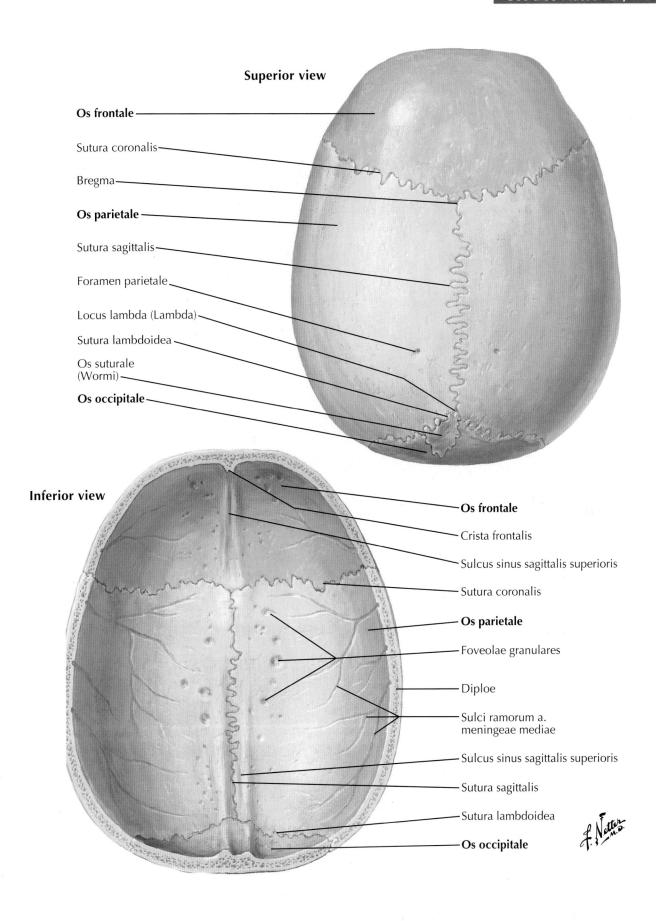

Superior view

Os frontale

Sutura coronalis

Bregma

Os parietale

Sutura sagittalis

Foramen parietale

Locus lambda (Lambda)

Sutura lambdoidea

Os suturale
(Wormi)

Os occipitale

Inferior view

Os frontale

Crista frontalis

Sulcus sinus sagittalis superioris

Sutura coronalis

Os parietale

Foveolae granulares

Diploe

Sulci ramorum a.
meningeae mediae

Sulcus sinus sagittalis superioris

Sutura sagittalis

Sutura lambdoidea

Os occipitale

Maxilla
Fossa incisiva
Proc. palatinus
Sutura intermaxillaris
Proc. zygomaticus

Os zygomaticum

Os frontale

Os sphenoideum
Proc. pterygoideus
Hamulus pterygiodeus
Lamina medialis
Fossa pterygoidea
Lamina lateralis
Fossa scaphoidea
Ala major
Foramen ovale
Foramen spinosum
Spina ossis sphenoidei

Os temporale
Proc. zygomaticus
Tuberculum articulare
Fossa mandibularis
Proc. styloideus
Fissura petrotympanica
Apertura externa canalis carotidis
Pars petrosa
Meatus acusticus externus cranii
Canaliculus tympanicus inferior
Canaliculus mastoideus
Proc. mastoideus
Foramen stylomastoideum
Fossa jugularis
Foramen jugulare
Incisura mastoidea
Sulcus a. occipitalis
Foramen mastoideum

Os parietale

Os occipitale
Canalis n. hypoglossi
Pars basilaris
Condylus occipitalis
Tuberculum pharyngeum
Canalis condylaris
Fossa condylaris
Foramen magnum
Linea nuchalis inferior
Crista occipitalis externa
Linea nuchalis superior
Protuberantia occipitalis vexterna

Sutura palatomaxillaris

Os palatinum
Lamina horizontalis
Foramen palatinum majus
Proc. pyramidalis
Foramina palatina minora
Spina nasalis posterior

Choanae

Vomer
Ala vomeris

Sulcus tubae auditivae

Foramen lacerum

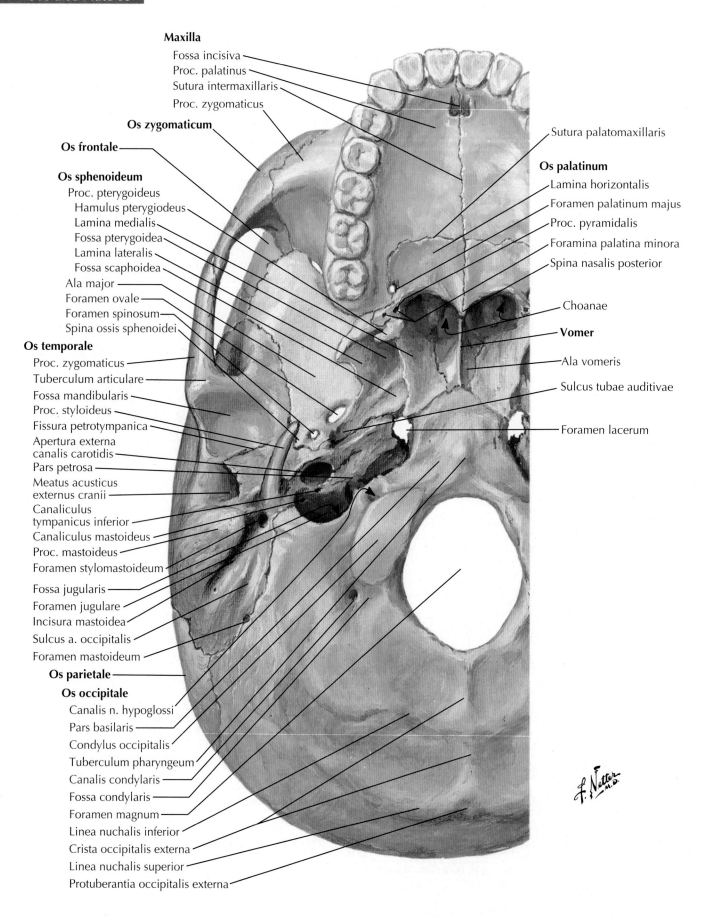

Plate 31

Ossa and Juncturae

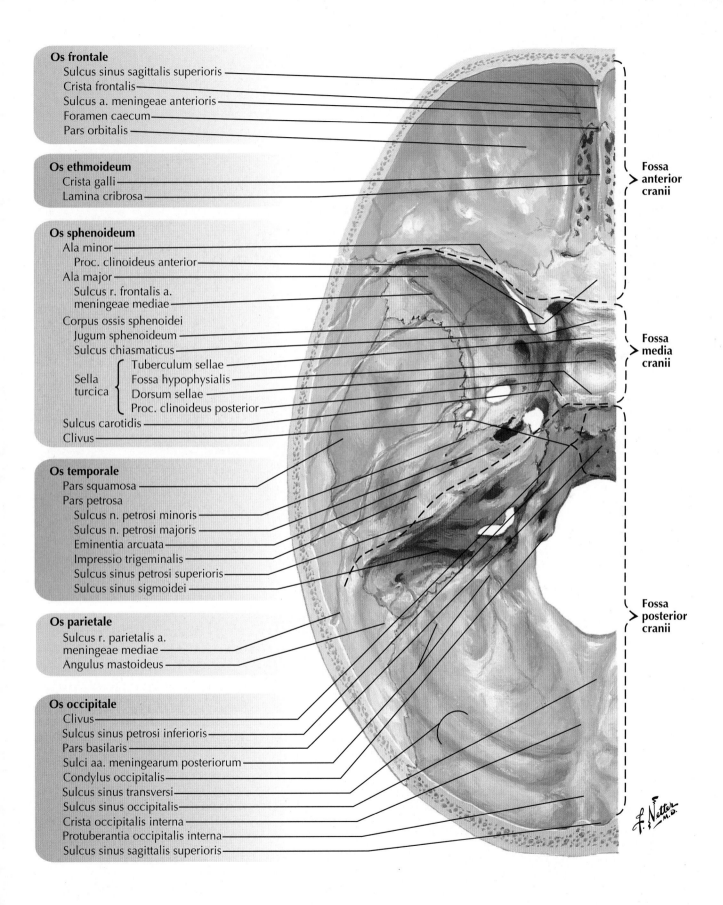

Os frontale
- Sulcus sinus sagittalis superioris
- Crista frontalis
- Sulcus a. meningeae anterioris
- Foramen caecum
- Pars orbitalis

Os ethmoideum
- Crista galli
- Lamina cribrosa

Os sphenoideum
- Ala minor
- Proc. clinoideus anterior
- Ala major
- Sulcus r. frontalis a. meningeae mediae
- Corpus ossis sphenoidei
- Jugum sphenoideum
- Sulcus chiasmaticus
- Sella turcica
  - Tuberculum sellae
  - Fossa hypophysialis
  - Dorsum sellae
  - Proc. clinoideus posterior
- Sulcus carotidis
- Clivus

Os temporale
- Pars squamosa
- Pars petrosa
  - Sulcus n. petrosi minoris
  - Sulcus n. petrosi majoris
  - Eminentia arcuata
  - Impressio trigeminalis
  - Sulcus sinus petrosi superioris
  - Sulcus sinus sigmoidei

Os parietale
- Sulcus r. parietalis a. meningeae mediae
- Angulus mastoideus

Os occipitale
- Clivus
- Sulcus sinus petrosi inferioris
- Pars basilaris
- Sulci aa. meningearum posteriorum
- Condylus occipitalis
- Sulcus sinus transversi
- Sulcus sinus occipitalis
- Crista occipitalis interna
- Protuberantia occipitalis interna
- Sulcus sinus sagittalis superioris

Fossa anterior cranii

Fossa media cranii

Fossa posterior cranii

F. Netter M.D.

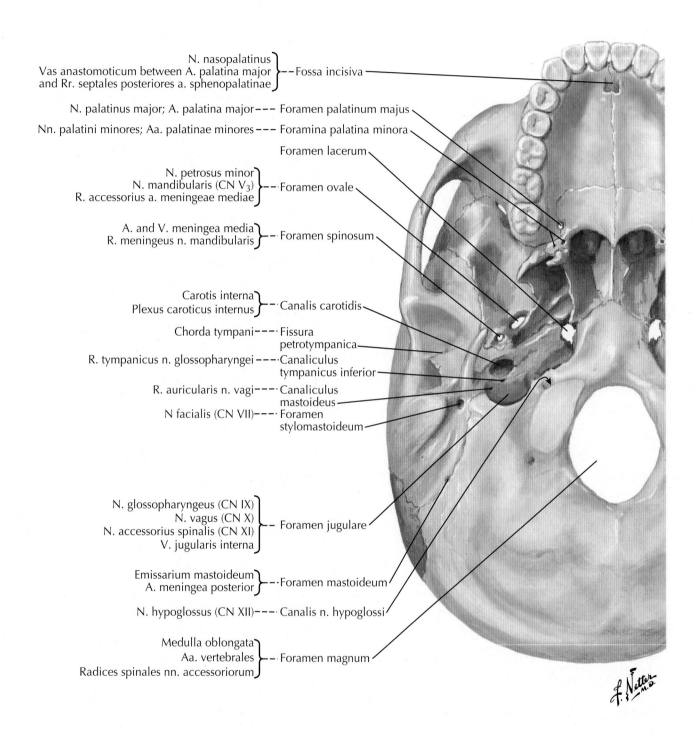

N. nasopalatinus
Vas anastomoticum between A. palatina major
and Rr. septales posteriores a. sphenopalatinae } --- Fossa incisiva

N. palatinus major; A. palatina major --- Foramen palatinum majus

Nn. palatini minores; Aa. palatinae minores --- Foramina palatina minora

Foramen lacerum

N. petrosus minor
N. mandibularis (CN V₃) } --- Foramen ovale
R. accessorius a. meningeae mediae

A. and V. meningea media } --- Foramen spinosum
R. meningeus n. mandibularis

Carotis interna } --- Canalis carotidis
Plexus caroticus internus

Chorda tympani --- Fissura petrotympanica

R. tympanicus n. glossopharyngei --- Canaliculus tympanicus inferior

R. auricularis n. vagi --- Canaliculus mastoideus

N facialis (CN VII) --- Foramen stylomastoideum

N. glossopharyngeus (CN IX)
N. vagus (CN X)
N. accessorius spinalis (CN XI) } --- Foramen jugulare
V. jugularis interna

Emissarium mastoideum } --- Foramen mastoideum
A. meningea posterior

N. hypoglossus (CN XII) --- Canalis n. hypoglossi

Medulla oblongata
Aa. vertebrales } --- Foramen magnum
Radices spinales nn. accessoriorum

Plate 33   **Ossa and Juncturae**

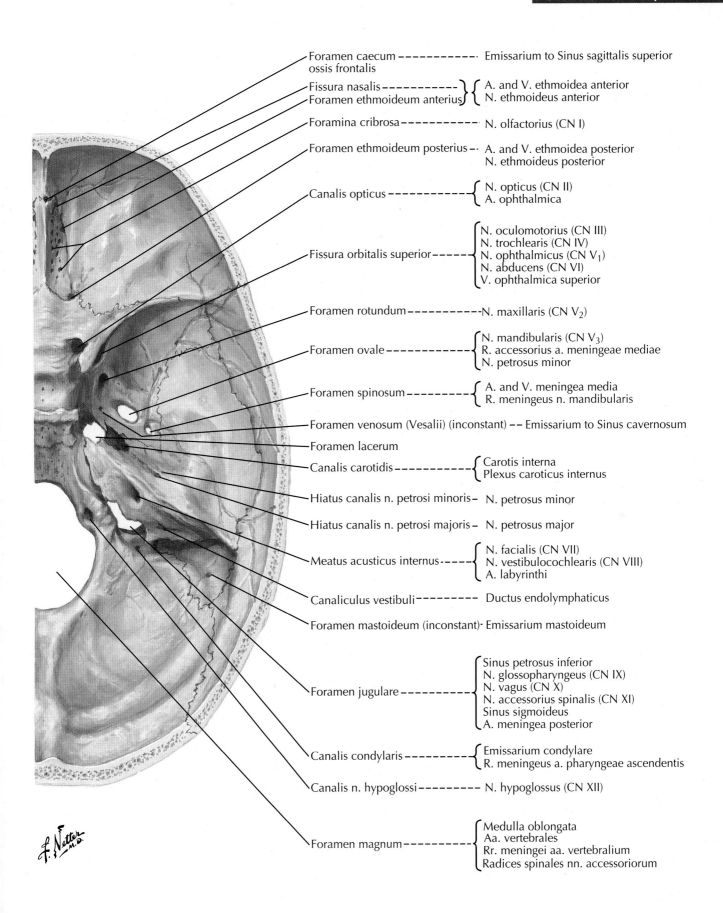

Foramen caecum ossis frontalis ----------- Emissarium to Sinus sagittalis superior

Fissura nasalis ----------- } { A. and V. ethmoidea anterior
Foramen ethmoideum anterius } { N. ethmoideus anterior

Foramina cribrosa ----------- N. olfactorius (CN I)

Foramen ethmoideum posterius -- A. and V. ethmoidea posterior
N. ethmoideus posterior

Canalis opticus ----------- { N. opticus (CN II)
{ A. ophthalmica

Fissura orbitalis superior ----- { N. oculomotorius (CN III)
{ N. trochlearis (CN IV)
{ N. ophthalmicus (CN V₁)
{ N. abducens (CN VI)
{ V. ophthalmica superior

Foramen rotundum ----------- N. maxillaris (CN V₂)

Foramen ovale ----------- { N. mandibularis (CN V₃)
{ R. accessorius a. meningeae mediae
{ N. petrosus minor

Foramen spinosum --------- { A. and V. meningea media
{ R. meningeus n. mandibularis

Foramen venosum (Vesalii) (inconstant) -- Emissarium to Sinus cavernosum

Foramen lacerum

Canalis carotidis ----------- { Carotis interna
{ Plexus caroticus internus

Hiatus canalis n. petrosi minoris - N. petrosus minor

Hiatus canalis n. petrosi majoris - N. petrosus major

Meatus acusticus internus ----- { N. facialis (CN VII)
{ N. vestibulocochlearis (CN VIII)
{ A. labyrinthi

Canaliculus vestibuli -------- Ductus endolymphaticus

Foramen mastoideum (inconstant)· Emissarium mastoideum

Foramen jugulare --------- { Sinus petrosus inferior
{ N. glossopharyngeus (CN IX)
{ N. vagus (CN X)
{ N. accessorius spinalis (CN XI)
{ Sinus sigmoideus
{ A. meningea posterior

Canalis condylaris --------- { Emissarium condylare
{ R. meningeus a. pharyngeae ascendentis

Canalis n. hypoglossi --------- N. hypoglossus (CN XII)

Foramen magnum --------- { Medulla oblongata
{ Aa. vertebrales
{ Rr. meningei aa. vertebralium
{ Radices spinales nn. accessoriorum

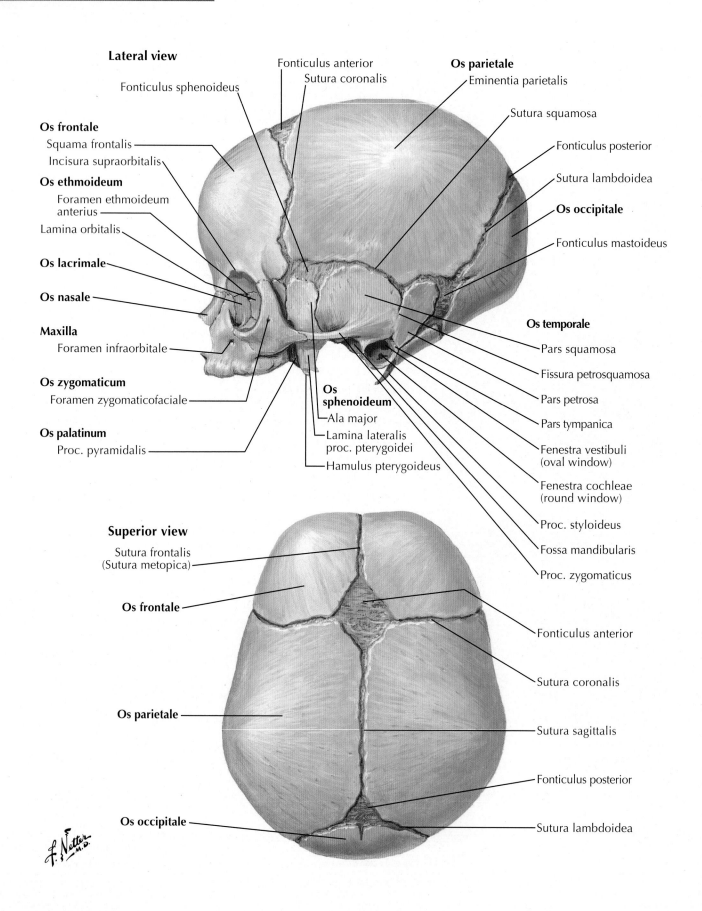

Lateral view

Fonticulus sphenoideus

Fonticulus anterior
Sutura coronalis

Os parietale
Eminentia parietalis

Os frontale
Squama frontalis
Incisura supraorbitalis

Os ethmoideum
Foramen ethmoideum anterius
Lamina orbitalis

Os lacrimale

Os nasale

Maxilla
Foramen infraorbitale

Os zygomaticum
Foramen zygomaticofaciale

Os palatinum
Proc. pyramidalis

Os sphenoideum
Ala major
Lamina lateralis proc. pterygoidei
Hamulus pterygoideus

Sutura squamosa
Fonticulus posterior
Sutura lambdoidea

Os occipitale
Fonticulus mastoideus

Os temporale
Pars squamosa
Fissura petrosquamosa
Pars petrosa
Pars tympanica
Fenestra vestibuli (oval window)
Fenestra cochleae (round window)
Proc. styloideus
Fossa mandibularis
Proc. zygomaticus

Superior view
Sutura frontalis (Sutura metopica)

Os frontale

Os parietale

Os occipitale

Fonticulus anterior

Sutura coronalis

Sutura sagittalis

Fonticulus posterior

Sutura lambdoidea

Plate 35

Ossa and Juncturae

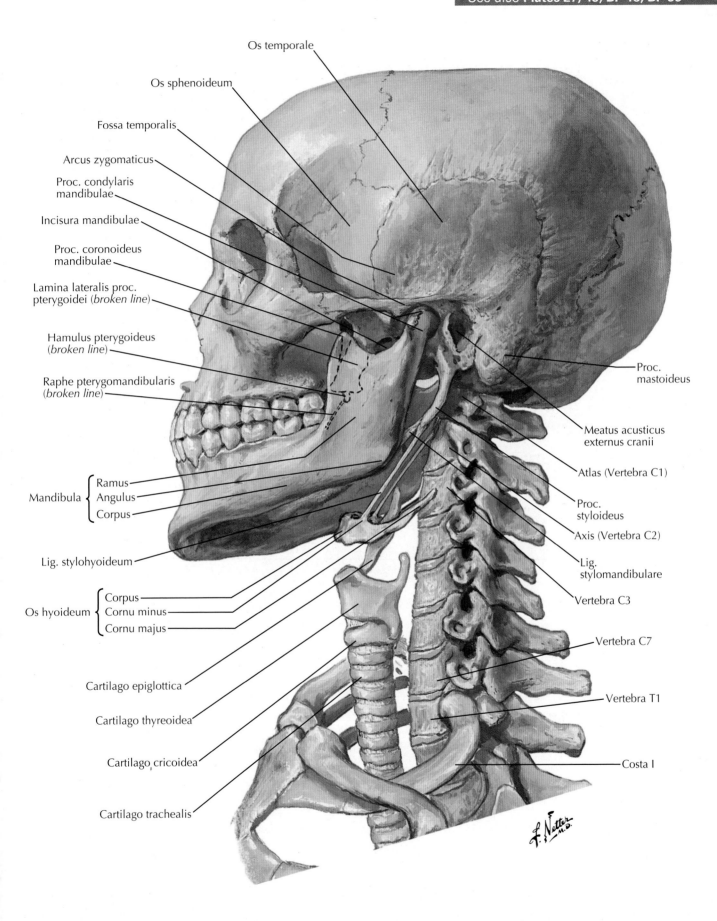

Os temporale

Os sphenoideum

Fossa temporalis

Arcus zygomaticus

Proc. condylaris
mandibulae

Incisura mandibulae

Proc. coronoideus
mandibulae

Lamina lateralis proc.
pterygoidei (*broken line*)

Hamulus pterygoideus
(*broken line*)

Raphe pterygomandibularis
(*broken line*)

Mandibula { Ramus
Angulus
Corpus

Lig. stylohyoideum

Os hyoideum { Corpus
Cornu minus
Cornu majus

Cartilago epiglottica

Cartilago thyreoidea

Cartilago cricoidea

Cartilago trachealis

Proc.
mastoideus

Meatus acusticus
externus cranii

Atlas (Vertebra C1)

Proc.
styloideus

Axis (Vertebra C2)

Lig.
stylomandibulare

Vertebra C3

Vertebra C7

Vertebra T1

Costa I

Plane of section   1 Os ethmoideum
                    2 Concha nasalis
                      inferior

Crista galli

Lamina cribrosa

Fossa anterior
cranii

Cellulae
ethmoideae

Fissura
orbitalis
superior

Orbita

Concha
nasalis
superior

Fissura
orbitalis
inferior

SM

Os
zygomaticum

MM

MM

Concha
nasalis
media
(cut)

Sinus maxillae

IM

IM

Maxilla

Concha nasalis inferior (cut)

Cavitas nasalis

Pars ossea septi nasi

Dens molaris 1

C. Machado
_M.D.

Palatum osseum

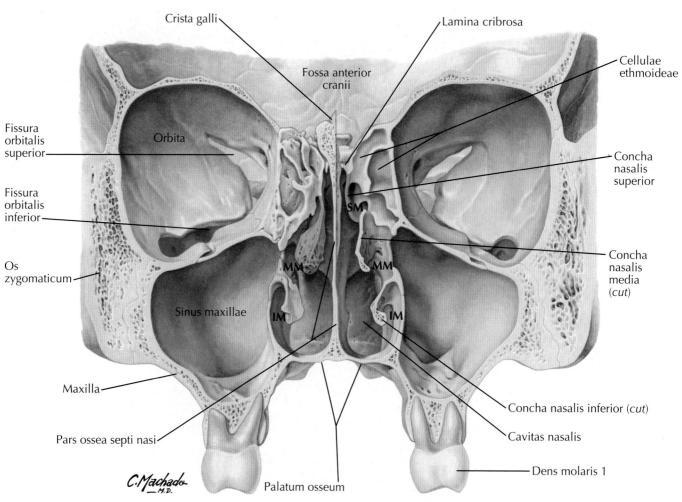

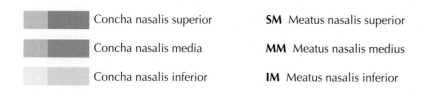

	Concha nasalis superior	**SM**	Meatus nasalis superior
	Concha nasalis media	**MM**	Meatus nasalis medius
	Concha nasalis inferior	**IM**	Meatus nasalis inferior

Plate 37

Ossa and Juncturae

Posterior view

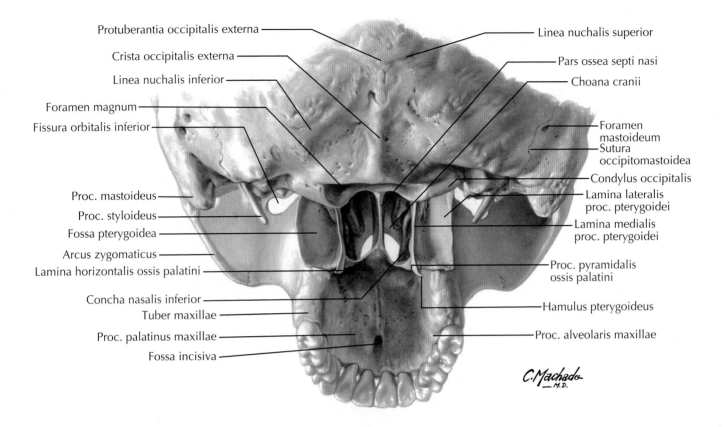

Protuberantia occipitalis externa

Crista occipitalis externa

Linea nuchalis inferior

Foramen magnum

Fissura orbitalis inferior

Proc. mastoideus

Proc. styloideus

Fossa pterygoidea

Arcus zygomaticus

Lamina horizontalis ossis palatini

Concha nasalis inferior

Tuber maxillae

Proc. palatinus maxillae

Fossa incisiva

Linea nuchalis superior

Pars ossea septi nasi

Choana cranii

Foramen mastoideum

Sutura occipitomastoidea

Condylus occipitalis

Lamina lateralis proc. pterygoidei

Lamina medialis proc. pterygoidei

Proc. pyramidalis ossis palatini

Hamulus pterygoideus

Proc. alveolaris maxillae

C. Machado —M.D.

Lateral view

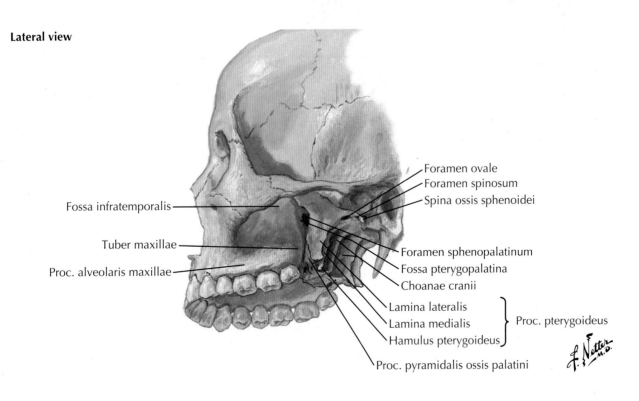

Fossa infratemporalis

Tuber maxillae

Proc. alveolaris maxillae

Foramen ovale

Foramen spinosum

Spina ossis sphenoidei

Foramen sphenopalatinum

Fossa pterygopalatina

Choanae cranii

Lamina lateralis ⎫
Lamina medialis ⎬ Proc. pterygoideus
Hamulus pterygoideus ⎭

Proc. pyramidalis ossis palatini

f. Netter M.D.

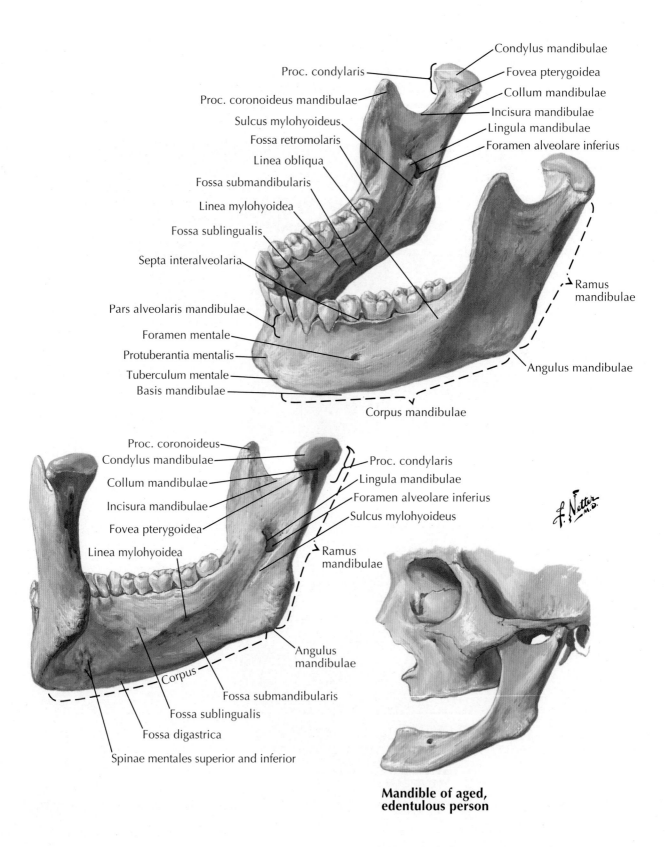

Condylus mandibulae
Fovea pterygoidea
Collum mandibulae
Incisura mandibulae
Lingula mandibulae
Foramen alveolare inferius

Proc. condylaris
Proc. coronoideus mandibulae
Sulcus mylohyoideus
Fossa retromolaris
Linea obliqua
Fossa submandibularis
Linea mylohyoidea
Fossa sublingualis
Septa interalveolaria
Pars alveolaris mandibulae
Foramen mentale
Protuberantia mentalis
Tuberculum mentale
Basis mandibulae

Ramus mandibulae
Angulus mandibulae
Corpus mandibulae

Proc. coronoideus
Condylus mandibulae
Collum mandibulae
Incisura mandibulae
Fovea pterygoidea
Linea mylohyoidea

Proc. condylaris
Lingula mandibulae
Foramen alveolare inferius
Sulcus mylohyoideus
Ramus mandibulae
Angulus mandibulae
Corpus
Fossa submandibularis
Fossa sublingualis
Fossa digastrica
Spinae mentales superior and inferior

Mandible of aged, edentulous person

Plate 39

Ossa and Juncturae

**Dentes decidui
(usual age of eruption)**

**Dentes permanentes
(usual age of eruption)**

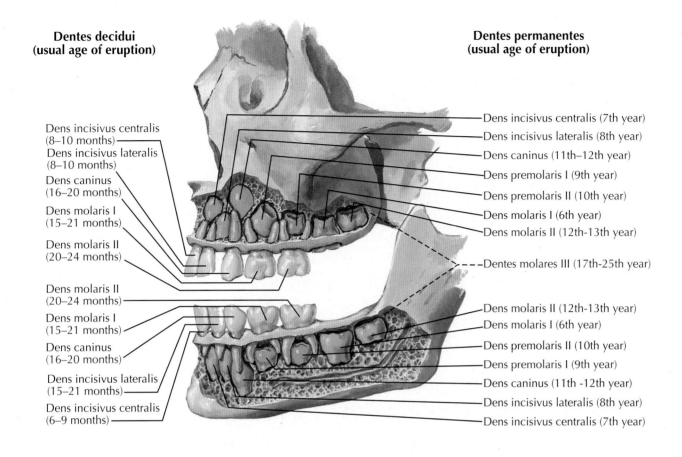

Dens incisivus centralis
(8–10 months)

Dens incisivus lateralis
(8–10 months)

Dens caninus
(16–20 months)

Dens molaris I
(15–21 months)

Dens molaris II
(20–24 months)

Dens molaris II
(20–24 months)

Dens molaris I
(15–21 months)

Dens caninus
(16–20 months)

Dens incisivus lateralis
(15–21 months)

Dens incisivus centralis
(6–9 months)

Dens incisivus centralis (7th year)

Dens incisivus lateralis (8th year)

Dens caninus (11th–12th year)

Dens premolaris I (9th year)

Dens premolaris II (10th year)

Dens molaris I (6th year)

Dens molaris II (12th-13th year)

Dentes molares III (17th-25th year)

Dens molaris II (12th-13th year)

Dens molaris I (6th year)

Dens premolaris II (10th year)

Dens premolaris I (9th year)

Dens caninus (11th -12th year)

Dens incisivus lateralis (8th year)

Dens incisivus centralis (7th year)

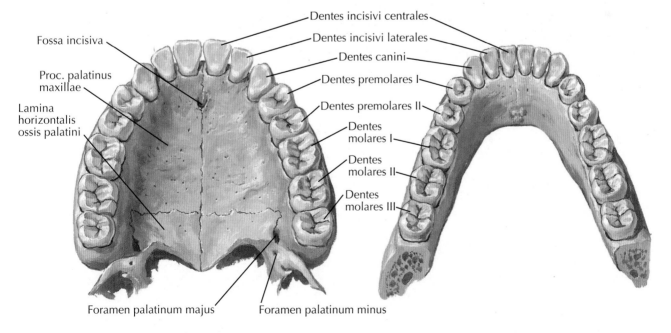

Fossa incisiva

Proc. palatinus
maxillae

Lamina
horizontalis
ossis palatini

Dentes incisivi centrales

Dentes incisivi laterales

Dentes canini

Dentes premolares I

Dentes premolares II

Dentes
molares I

Dentes
molares II

Dentes
molares III

Foramen palatinum majus

Foramen palatinum minus

Dentes permanentes superiores

Dentes permanentes inferiores

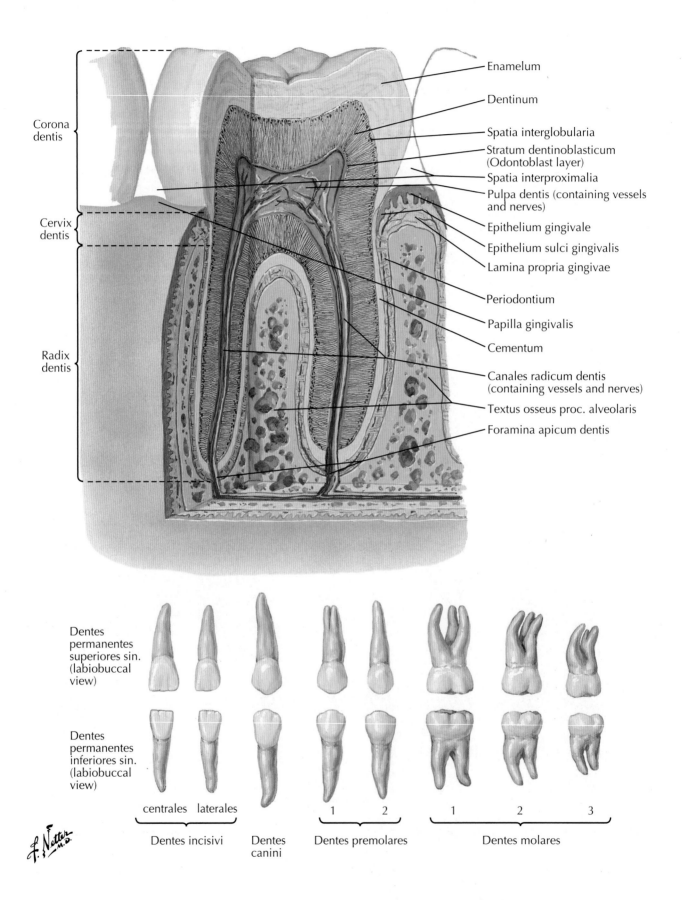

Enamelum

Dentinum

Spatia interglobularia

Stratum dentinoblasticum
(Odontoblast layer)

Spatia interproximalia

Pulpa dentis (containing vessels
and nerves)

Epithelium gingivale

Epithelium sulci gingivalis

Lamina propria gingivae

Periodontium

Papilla gingivalis

Cementum

Canales radicum dentis
(containing vessels and nerves)

Textus osseus proc. alveolaris

Foramina apicum dentis

Corona
dentis

Cervix
dentis

Radix
dentis

Dentes
permanentes
superiores sin.
(labiobuccal
view)

Dentes
permanentes
inferiores sin.
(labiobuccal
view)

centrales   laterales

1   2

1   2   3

Dentes incisivi

Dentes
canini

Dentes premolares

Dentes molares

Plate 41   **Ossa and Juncturae**

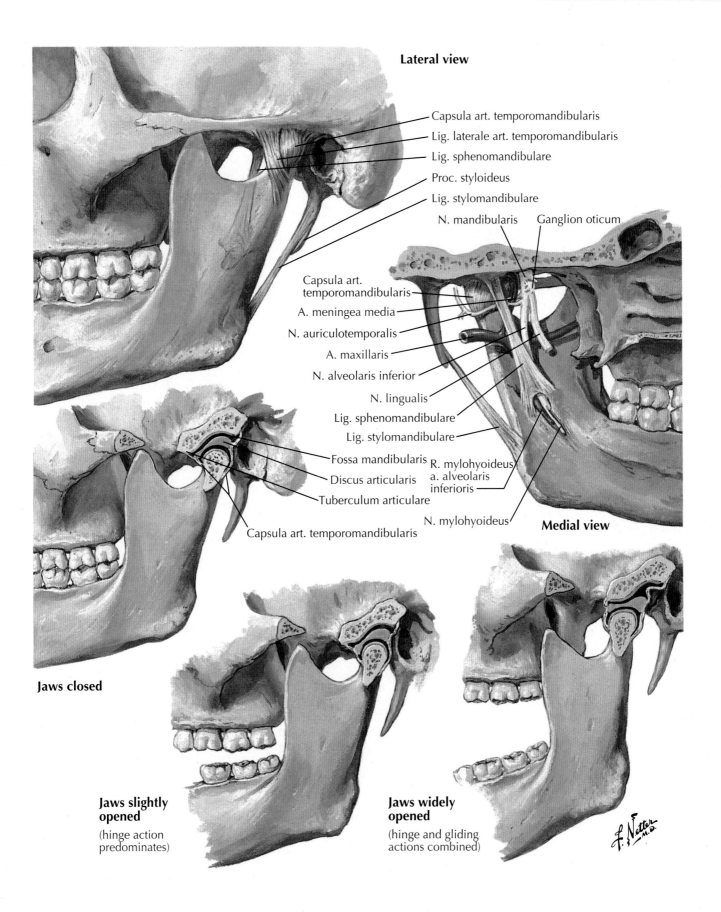

Lateral view

Capsula art. temporomandibularis
Lig. laterale art. temporomandibularis
Lig. sphenomandibulare
Proc. styloideus
Lig. stylomandibulare
N. mandibularis   Ganglion oticum

Capsula art. temporomandibularis
A. meningea media
N. auriculotemporalis
A. maxillaris
N. alveolaris inferior
N. lingualis
Lig. sphenomandibulare
Lig. stylomandibulare
Fossa mandibularis
Discus articularis
Tuberculum articulare
Capsula art. temporomandibularis

R. mylohyoideus
a. alveolaris
inferioris
N. mylohyoideus   **Medial view**

Jaws closed

Jaws slightly opened
(hinge action predominates)

Jaws widely opened
(hinge and gliding actions combined)

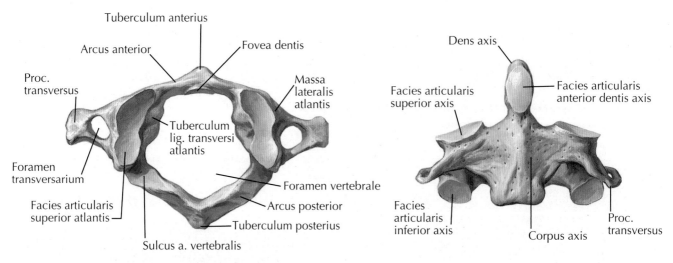

Tuberculum anterius

Arcus anterior

Fovea dentis

Proc. transversus

Massa lateralis atlantis

Tuberculum lig. transversi atlantis

Foramen transversarium

Facies articularis superior atlantis

Foramen vertebrale

Arcus posterior

Tuberculum posterius

Sulcus a. vertebralis

Atlas: superior view

Dens axis

Facies articularis superior axis

Facies articularis anterior dentis axis

Facies articularis inferior axis

Corpus axis

Proc. transversus

Axis: anterior view

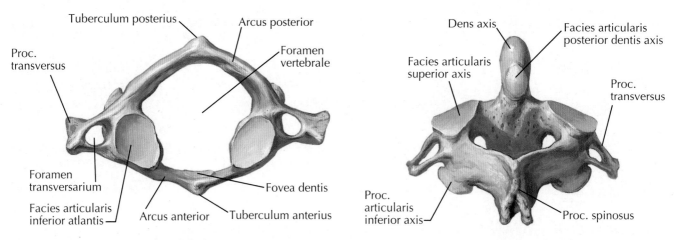

Tuberculum posterius

Arcus posterior

Proc. transversus

Foramen vertebrale

Foramen transversarium

Fovea dentis

Facies articularis inferior atlantis

Arcus anterior

Tuberculum anterius

Atlas: inferior view

Dens axis

Facies articularis posterior dentis axis

Facies articularis superior axis

Proc. transversus

Proc. articularis inferior axis

Proc. spinosus

Axis: posterosuperior view

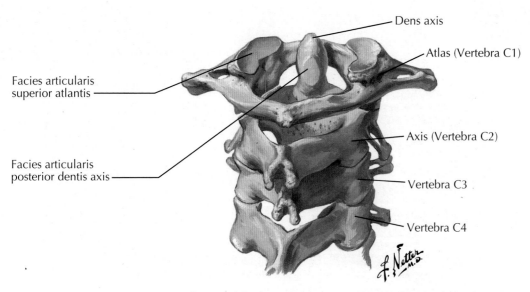

Dens axis

Atlas (Vertebra C1)

Facies articularis superior atlantis

Facies articularis posterior dentis axis

Axis (Vertebra C2)

Vertebra C3

Vertebra C4

Vertebrae cervicales superiores: posterosuperior view

Plate 43

Ossa and Juncturae

Inferior aspect of vertebra C3 and superior aspect of vertebra C4 showing the sites of the articular surfaces of the articulationes uncovertebrales

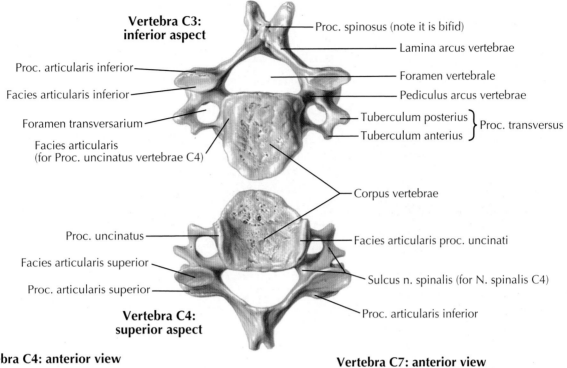

Vertebra C3: inferior aspect

Proc. articularis inferior

Facies articularis inferior

Foramen transversarium

Facies articularis (for Proc. uncinatus vertebrae C4)

Proc. spinosus (note it is bifid)

Lamina arcus vertebrae

Foramen vertebrale

Pediculus arcus vertebrae

Tuberculum posterius } Proc. transversus
Tuberculum anterius

Corpus vertebrae

Proc. uncinatus

Facies articularis superior

Proc. articularis superior

Facies articularis proc. uncinati

Sulcus n. spinalis (for N. spinalis C4)

Proc. articularis inferior

Vertebra C4: superior aspect

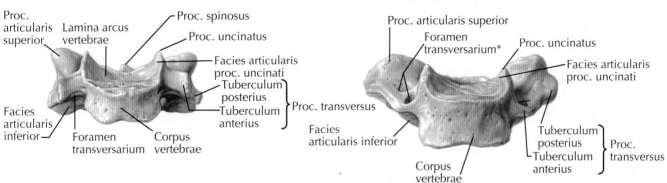

Vertebra C4: anterior view

Proc. articularis superior

Lamina arcus vertebrae

Proc. spinosus

Proc. uncinatus

Facies articularis proc. uncinati

Tuberculum posterius
Tuberculum anterius } Proc. transversus

Facies articularis inferior

Foramen transversarium

Corpus vertebrae

Vertebra C7: anterior view

Proc. articularis superior

Foramen transversarium*

Proc. uncinatus

Facies articularis proc. uncinati

Facies articularis inferior

Tuberculum posterius
Tuberculum anterius } Proc. transversus

Corpus vertebrae

Vertebra C7 (Vertebra prominens): superior view

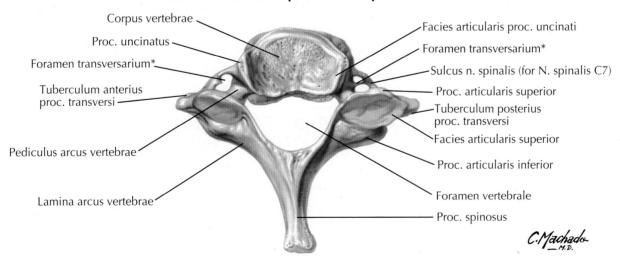

Corpus vertebrae

Proc. uncinatus

Foramen transversarium*

Tuberculum anterius proc. transversi

Pediculus arcus vertebrae

Lamina arcus vertebrae

Facies articularis proc. uncinati

Foramen transversarium*

Sulcus n. spinalis (for N. spinalis C7)

Proc. articularis superior

Tuberculum posterius proc. transversi

Facies articularis superior

Proc. articularis inferior

Foramen vertebrale

Proc. spinosus

C.Machado
M.D.

The foramina transversaria vertebrae C7 transmit vv. vertebrales, but usually not the a. vertebralis, and are asymmetrical in these drawings. Note the foramen transversarium dexter is septated.

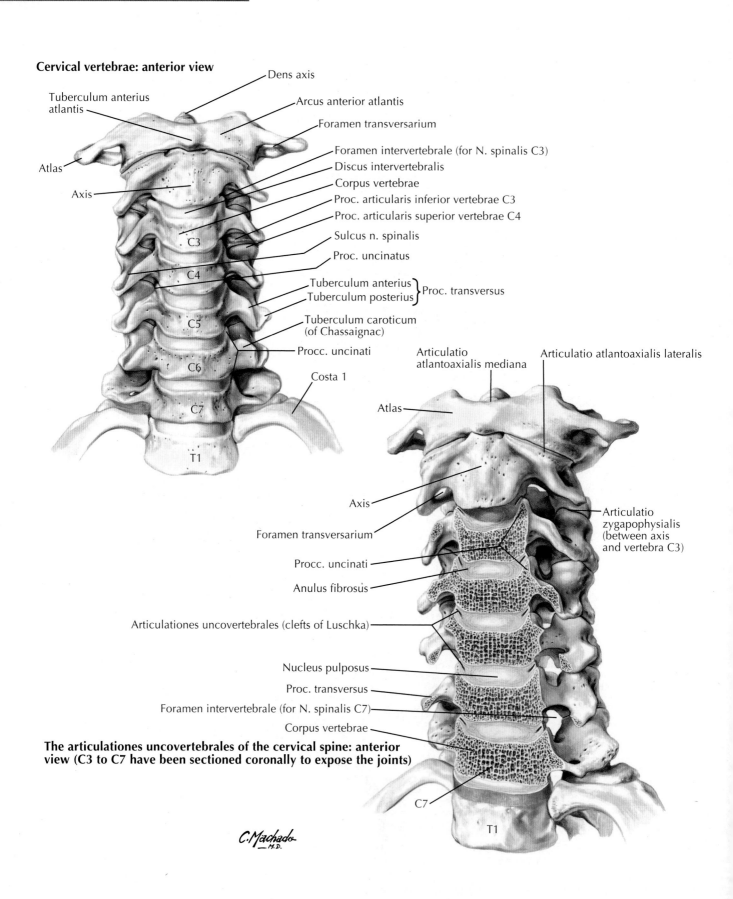

Cervical vertebrae: anterior view

Dens axis

Tuberculum anterius atlantis

Arcus anterior atlantis

Foramen transversarium

Atlas

Foramen intervertebrale (for N. spinalis C3)

Discus intervertebralis

Axis

Corpus vertebrae

Proc. articularis inferior vertebrae C3

Proc. articularis superior vertebrae C4

Sulcus n. spinalis

Proc. uncinatus

C3

C4

Tuberculum anterius }
Tuberculum posterius } Proc. transversus

Tuberculum caroticum (of Chassaignac)

C5

Procc. uncinati

C6

Costa 1

C7

Articulatio atlantoaxialis mediana

Articulatio atlantoaxialis lateralis

Atlas

T1

Axis

Articulatio zygapophysialis (between axis and vertebra C3)

Foramen transversarium

Procc. uncinati

Anulus fibrosus

Articulationes uncovertebrales (clefts of Luschka)

Nucleus pulposus

Proc. transversus

Foramen intervertebrale (for N. spinalis C7)

Corpus vertebrae

The articulationes uncovertebrales of the cervical spine: anterior view (C3 to C7 have been sectioned coronally to expose the joints)

C7

T1

C. Machado
M.D.

Plate 45

Ossa and Juncturae

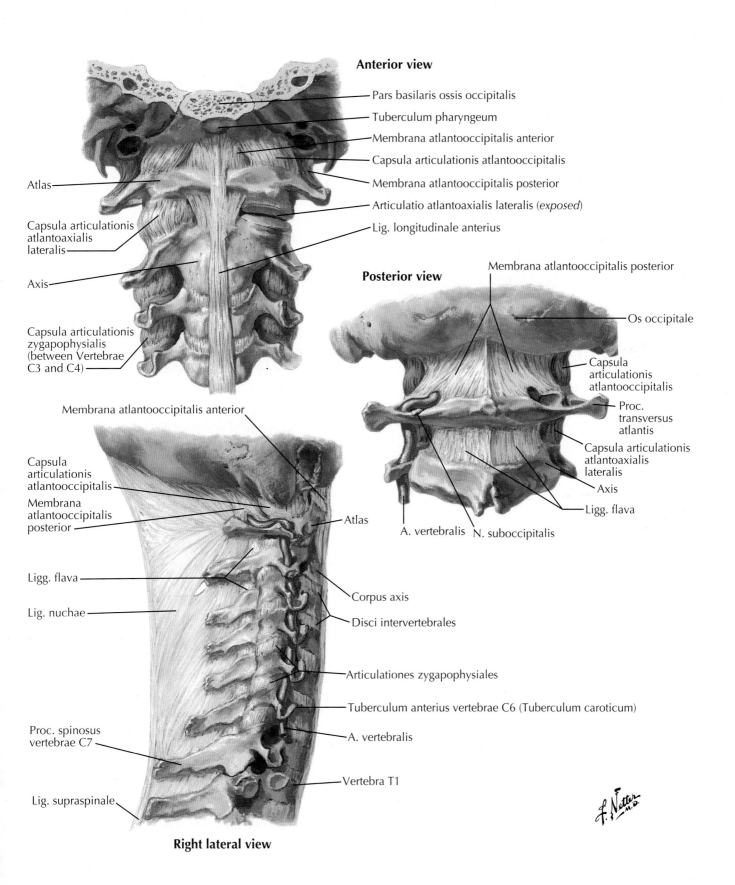

Anterior view

Pars basilaris ossis occipitalis

Tuberculum pharyngeum

Membrana atlantooccipitalis anterior

Capsula articulationis atlantooccipitalis

Membrana atlantooccipitalis posterior

Articulatio atlantoaxialis lateralis (*exposed*)

Lig. longitudinale anterius

Atlas

Capsula articulationis atlantoaxialis lateralis

Axis

Capsula articulationis zygapophysialis (between Vertebrae C3 and C4)

Posterior view

Membrana atlantooccipitalis posterior

Os occipitale

Capsula articulationis atlantooccipitalis

Proc. transversus atlantis

Capsula articulationis atlantoaxialis lateralis

Axis

Ligg. flava

A. vertebralis   N. suboccipitalis

Membrana atlantooccipitalis anterior

Capsula articulationis atlantooccipitalis

Membrana atlantooccipitalis posterior

Atlas

Ligg. flava

Lig. nuchae

Corpus axis

Disci intervertebrales

Articulationes zygapophysiales

Tuberculum anterius vertebrae C6 (Tuberculum caroticum)

A. vertebralis

Proc. spinosus vertebrae C7

Vertebra T1

Lig. supraspinale

Right lateral view

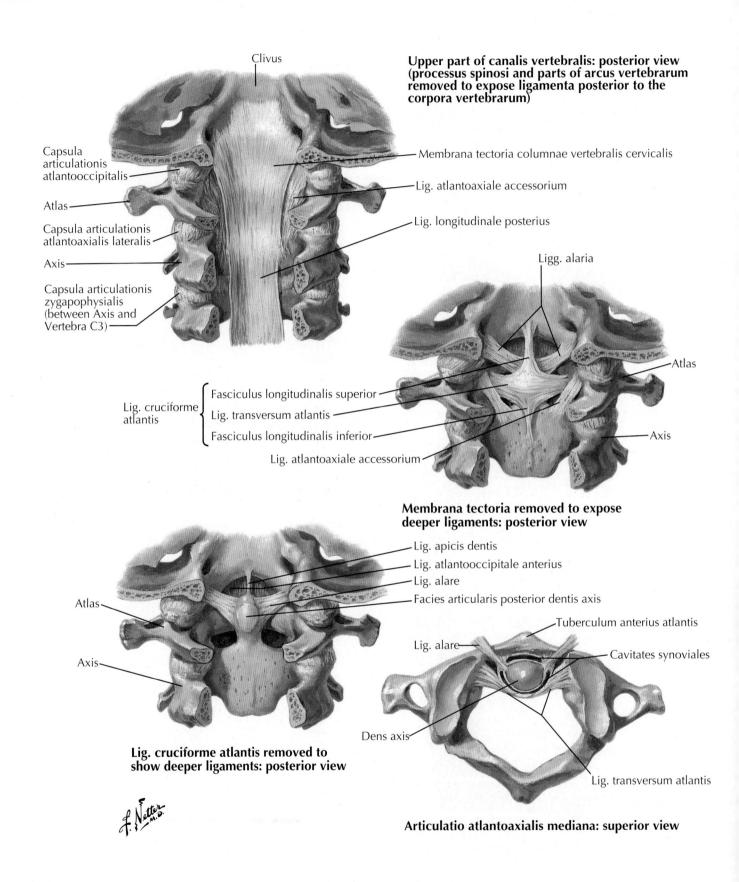

Clivus

Upper part of canalis vertebralis: posterior view
(processus spinosi and parts of arcus vertebrarum
removed to expose ligamenta posterior to the
corpora vertebrarum)

Capsula articulationis atlantooccipitalis

Atlas

Capsula articulationis atlantoaxialis lateralis

Axis

Capsula articulationis zygapophysialis (between Axis and Vertebra C3)

Membrana tectoria columnae vertebralis cervicalis

Lig. atlantoaxiale accessorium

Lig. longitudinale posterius

Ligg. alaria

Lig. cruciforme atlantis
- Fasciculus longitudinalis superior
- Lig. transversum atlantis
- Fasciculus longitudinalis inferior

Lig. atlantoaxiale accessorium

Atlas

Axis

Membrana tectoria removed to expose deeper ligaments: posterior view

Lig. apicis dentis
Lig. atlantooccipitale anterius
Lig. alare
Facies articularis posterior dentis axis

Atlas

Axis

Tuberculum anterius atlantis

Lig. alare

Cavitates synoviales

Dens axis

Lig. transversum atlantis

Lig. cruciforme atlantis removed to show deeper ligaments: posterior view

Articulatio atlantoaxialis mediana: superior view

Plate 47

Ossa and Juncturae

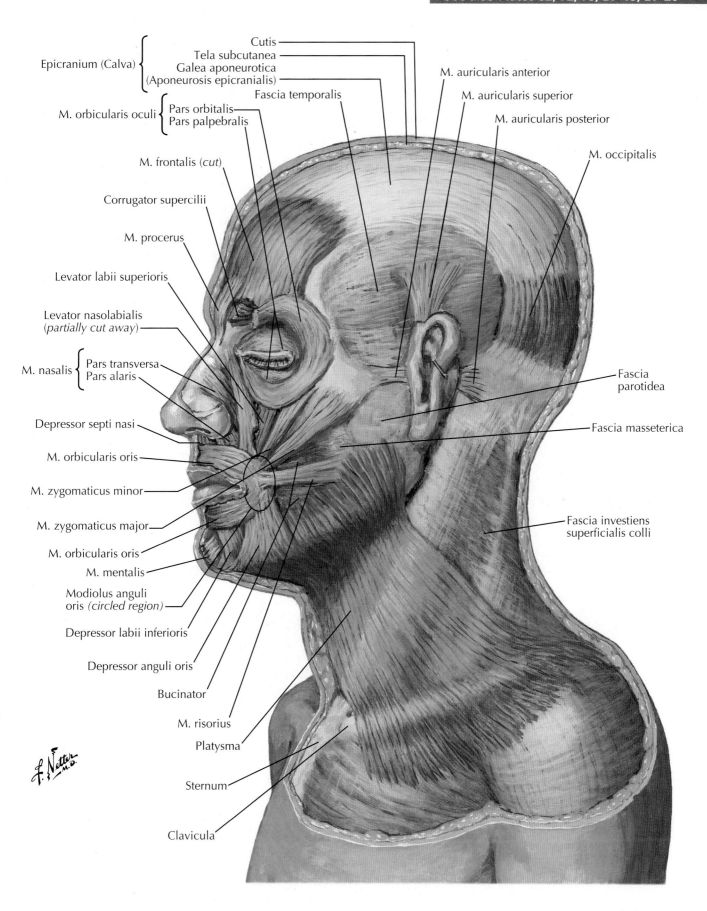

Cutis

Tela subcutanea

Epicranium (Calva)

Galea aponeurotica
(Aponeurosis epicranialis)

Fascia temporalis

M. orbicularis oculi — Pars orbitalis
Pars palpebralis

M. frontalis (*cut*)

Corrugator supercilii

M. procerus

Levator labii superioris

Levator nasolabialis
(*partially cut away*)

M. nasalis — Pars transversa
Pars alaris

Depressor septi nasi

M. orbicularis oris

M. zygomaticus minor

M. zygomaticus major

M. orbicularis oris

M. mentalis

Modiolus anguli
oris (*circled region*)

Depressor labii inferioris

Depressor anguli oris

Bucinator

M. risorius

Platysma

Sternum

Clavicula

M. auricularis anterior

M. auricularis superior

M. auricularis posterior

M. occipitalis

Fascia
parotidea

Fascia masseterica

Fascia investiens
superficialis colli

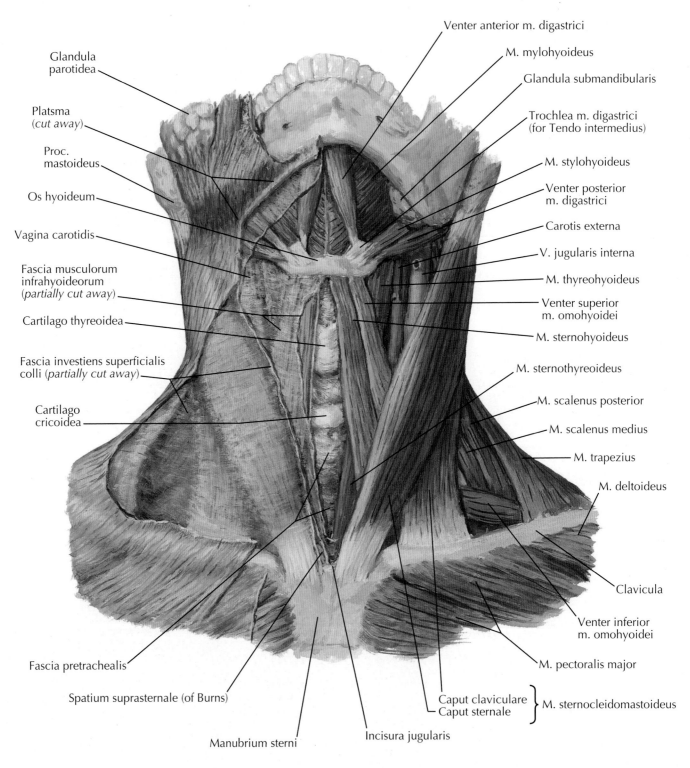

Glandula parotidea

Platsma (*cut away*)

Proc. mastoideus

Os hyoideum

Vagina carotidis

Fascia musculorum infrahyoideorum (*partially cut away*)

Cartilago thyreoidea

Fascia investiens superficialis colli (*partially cut away*)

Cartilago cricoidea

Fascia pretrachealis

Spatium suprasternale (of Burns)

Manubrium sterni

Venter anterior m. digastrici

M. mylohyoideus

Glandula submandibularis

Trochlea m. digastrici (for Tendo intermedius)

M. stylohyoideus

Venter posterior m. digastrici

Carotis externa

V. jugularis interna

M. thyreohyoideus

Venter superior m. omohyoidei

M. sternohyoideus

M. sternothyreoideus

M. scalenus posterior

M. scalenus medius

M. trapezius

M. deltoideus

Clavicula

Venter inferior m. omohyoidei

M. pectoralis major

Caput claviculare
Caput sternale } M. sternocleidomastoideus

Incisura jugularis

Plate 49

Collum

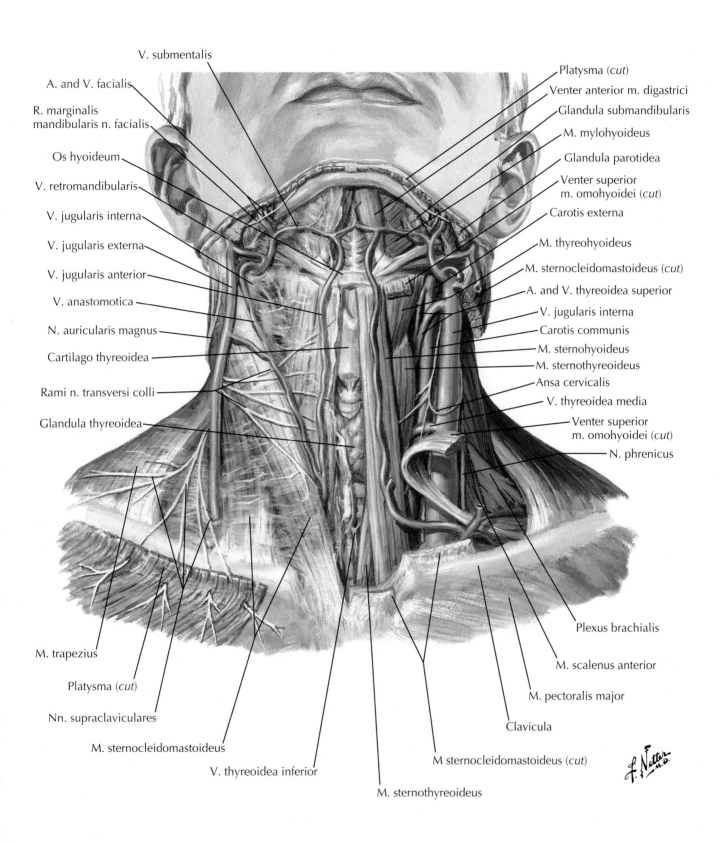

V. submentalis

A. and V. facialis

R. marginalis
mandibularis n. facialis

Os hyoideum

V. retromandibularis

V. jugularis interna

V. jugularis externa

V. jugularis anterior

V. anastomotica

N. auricularis magnus

Cartilago thyreoidea

Rami n. transversi colli

Glandula thyreoidea

M. trapezius

Platysma (*cut*)

Nn. supraclaviculares

M. sternocleidomastoideus

V. thyreoidea inferior

M. sternothyreoideus

Platysma (*cut*)

Venter anterior m. digastrici

Glandula submandibularis

M. mylohyoideus

Glandula parotidea

Venter superior
m. omohyoidei (*cut*)

Carotis externa

M. thyreohyoideus

M. sternocleidomastoideus (*cut*)

A. and V. thyreoidea superior

V. jugularis interna

Carotis communis

M. sternohyoideus

M. sternothyreoideus

Ansa cervicalis

V. thyreoidea media

Venter superior
m. omohyoidei (*cut*)

N. phrenicus

Plexus brachialis

M. scalenus anterior

M. pectoralis major

Clavicula

M sternocleidomastoideus (*cut*)

Cross section

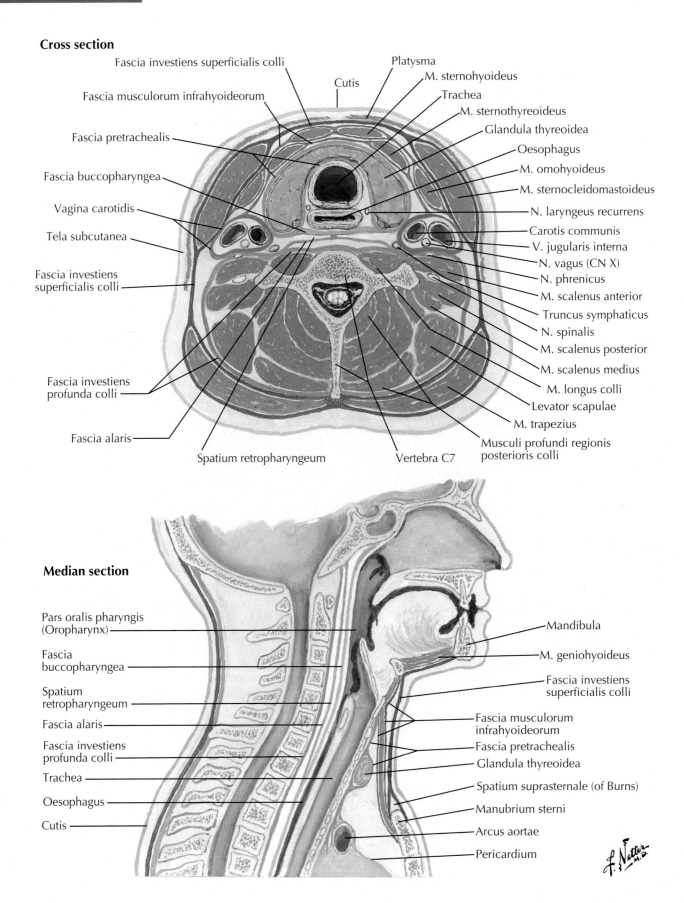

Fascia investiens superficialis colli

Platysma

Cutis

M. sternohyoideus

Fascia musculorum infrahyoideorum

Trachea

M. sternothyreoideus

Fascia pretrachealis

Glandula thyreoidea

Oesophagus

Fascia buccopharyngea

M. omohyoideus

M. sternocleidomastoideus

Vagina carotidis

N. laryngeus recurrens

Tela subcutanea

Carotis communis

V. jugularis interna

N. vagus (CN X)

Fascia investiens superficialis colli

N. phrenicus

M. scalenus anterior

Truncus symphaticus

N. spinalis

M. scalenus posterior

Fascia investiens profunda colli

M. scalenus medius

M. longus colli

Levator scapulae

Fascia alaris

M. trapezius

Spatium retropharyngeum

Vertebra C7

Musculi profundi regionis posterioris colli

Median section

Pars oralis pharyngis (Oropharynx)

Mandibula

Fascia buccopharyngea

M. geniohyoideus

Spatium retropharyngeum

Fascia investiens superficialis colli

Fascia alaris

Fascia musculorum infrahyoideorum

Fascia investiens profunda colli

Fascia pretrachealis

Trachea

Glandula thyreoidea

Oesophagus

Spatium suprasternale (of Burns)

Cutis

Manubrium sterni

Arcus aortae

Pericardium

Plate 51

Collum

Fascia investiens superficialis colli
Fascia musculorum infrahyoideorum
Fascia pretrachealis
Fascia buccopharyngea
Vagina carotidis
Fascia investiens profunda colli

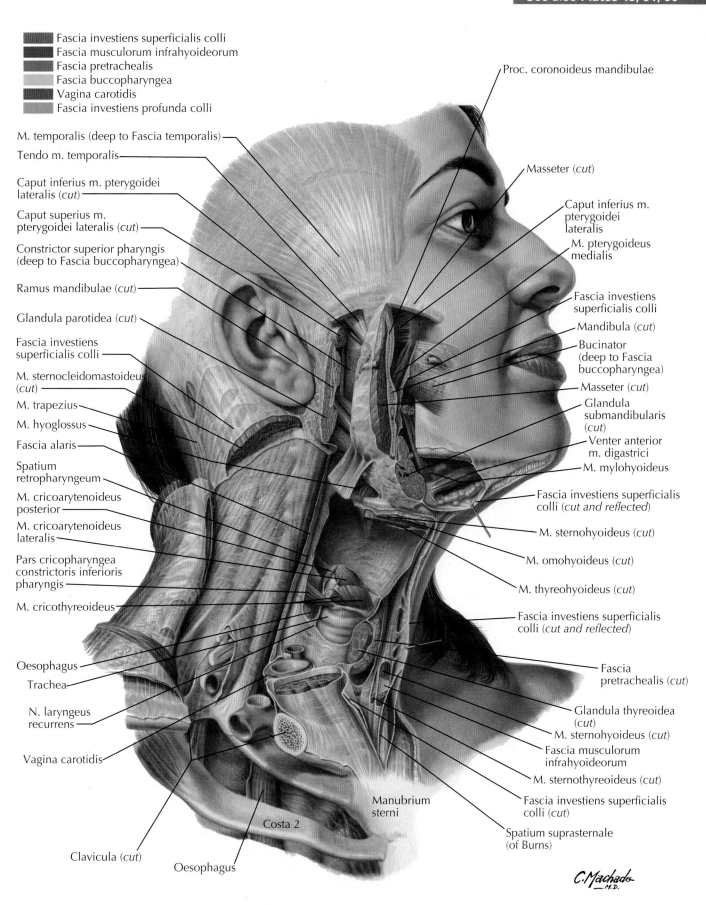

Proc. coronoideus mandibulae

M. temporalis (deep to Fascia temporalis)
Tendo m. temporalis
Caput inferius m. pterygoidei lateralis (*cut*)
Caput superius m. pterygoidei lateralis (*cut*)
Constrictor superior pharyngis (deep to Fascia buccopharyngea)
Ramus mandibulae (*cut*)
Glandula parotidea (*cut*)
Fascia investiens superficialis colli
M. sternocleidomastoideus (*cut*)
M. trapezius
M. hyoglossus
Fascia alaris
Spatium retropharyngeum
M. cricoarytenoideus posterior
M. cricoarytenoideus lateralis
Pars cricopharyngea constrictoris inferioris pharyngis
M. cricothyreoideus
Oesophagus
Trachea
N. laryngeus recurrens
Vagina carotidis
Clavicula (*cut*)
Costa 2
Oesophagus

Masseter (*cut*)
Caput inferius m. pterygoidei lateralis
M. pterygoideus medialis
Fascia investiens superficialis colli
Mandibula (*cut*)
Bucinator (deep to Fascia buccopharyngea)
Masseter (*cut*)
Glandula submandibularis (*cut*)
Venter anterior m. digastrici
M. mylohyoideus
Fascia investiens superficialis colli (*cut and reflected*)
M. sternohyoideus (*cut*)
M. omohyoideus (*cut*)
M. thyreohyoideus (*cut*)
Fascia investiens superficialis colli (*cut and reflected*)
Fascia pretrachealis (*cut*)
Glandula thyreoidea (*cut*)
M. sternohyoideus (*cut*)
Fascia musculorum infrahyoideorum
M. sternothyreoideus (*cut*)
Fascia investiens superficialis colli (*cut*)
Spatium suprasternale (of Burns)

Manubrium sterni

C. Machado
_M.D.

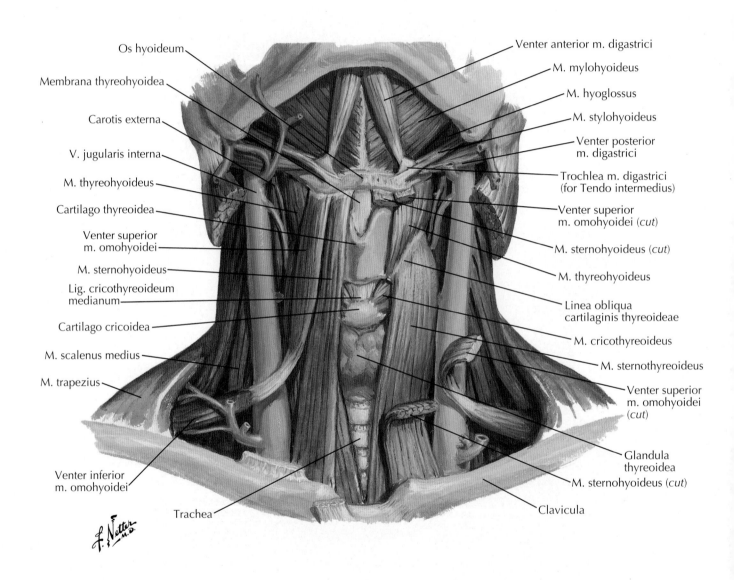

Os hyoideum

Membrana thyreohyoidea

Carotis externa

V. jugularis interna

M. thyreohyoideus

Cartilago thyreoidea

Venter superior
m. omohyoidei

M. sternohyoideus

Lig. cricothyreoideum
medianum

Cartilago cricoidea

M. scalenus medius

M. trapezius

Venter inferior
m. omohyoidei

Trachea

Venter anterior m. digastrici

M. mylohyoideus

M. hyoglossus

M. stylohyoideus

Venter posterior
m. digastrici

Trochlea m. digastrici
(for Tendo intermedius)

Venter superior
m. omohyoidei (cut)

M. sternohyoideus (cut)

M. thyreohyoideus

Linea obliqua
cartilaginis thyreoideae

M. cricothyreoideus

M. sternothyreoideus

Venter superior
m. omohyoidei
(cut)

Glandula
thyreoidea

M. sternohyoideus (cut)

Clavicula

Plate 53

Collum

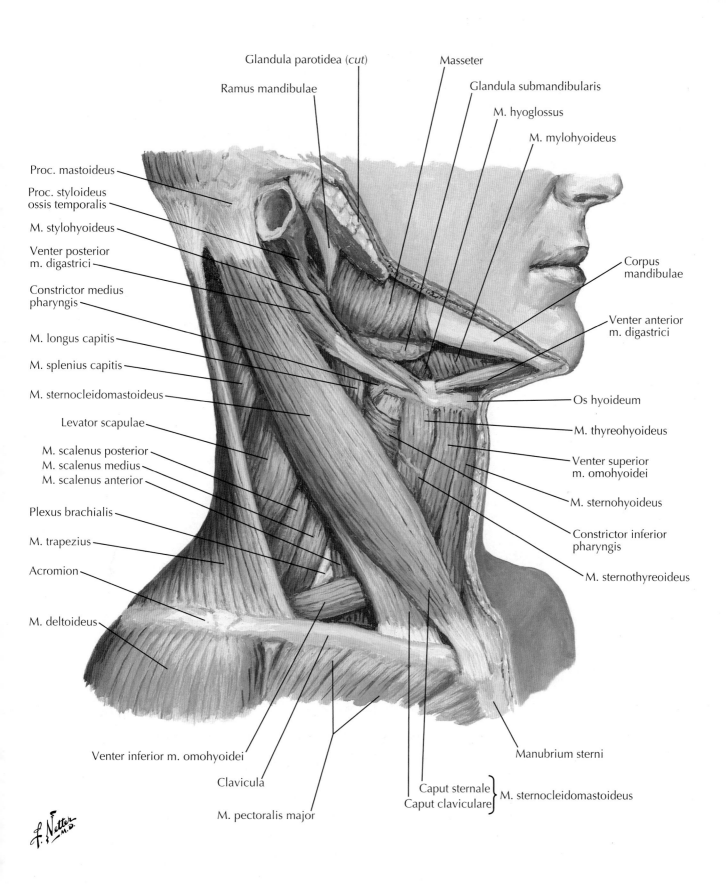

Glandula parotidea (*cut*)

Ramus mandibulae

Masseter

Glandula submandibularis

M. hyoglossus

M. mylohyoideus

Proc. mastoideus

Proc. styloideus ossis temporalis

M. stylohyoideus

Venter posterior m. digastrici

Constrictor medius pharyngis

M. longus capitis

M. splenius capitis

M. sternocleidomastoideus

Levator scapulae

M. scalenus posterior

M. scalenus medius

M. scalenus anterior

Plexus brachialis

M. trapezius

Acromion

M. deltoideus

Corpus mandibulae

Venter anterior m. digastrici

Os hyoideum

M. thyreohyoideus

Venter superior m. omohyoidei

M. sternohyoideus

Constrictor inferior pharyngis

M. sternothyreoideus

Venter inferior m. omohyoidei

Clavicula

M. pectoralis major

Manubrium sterni

Caput sternale
Caput claviculare } M. sternocleidomastoideus

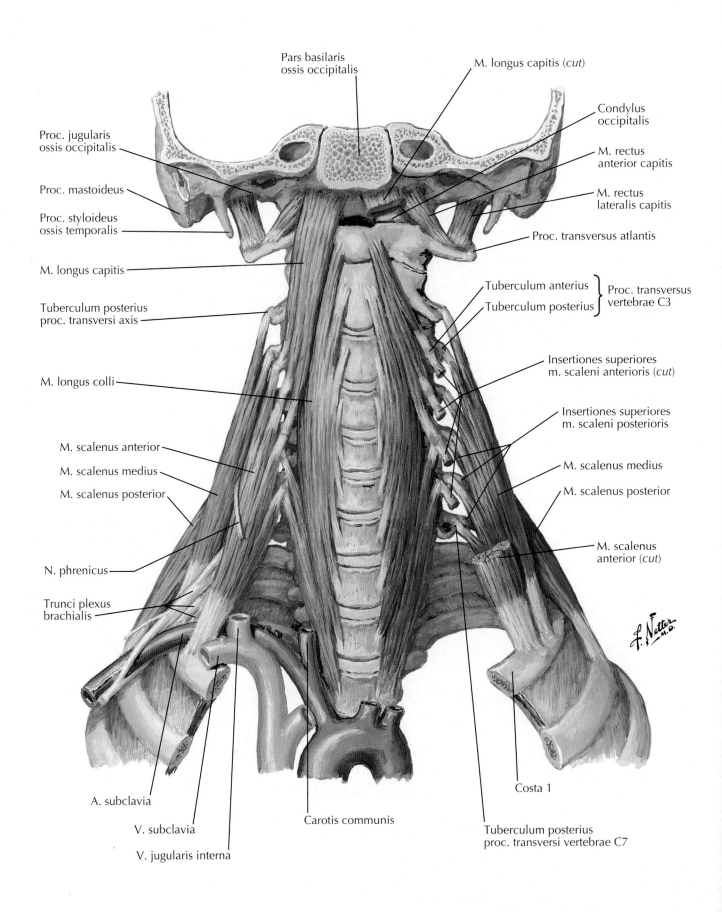

Pars basilaris
ossis occipitalis

M. longus capitis (*cut*)

Condylus
occipitalis

Proc. jugularis
ossis occipitalis

M. rectus
anterior capitis

Proc. mastoideus

M. rectus
lateralis capitis

Proc. styloideus
ossis temporalis

Proc. transversus atlantis

M. longus capitis

Tuberculum anterius
Tuberculum posterius } Proc. transversus
vertebrae C3

Tuberculum posterius
proc. transversi axis

Insertiones superiores
m. scaleni anterioris (*cut*)

M. longus colli

Insertiones superiores
m. scaleni posterioris

M. scalenus anterior

M. scalenus medius

M. scalenus medius

M. scalenus posterior

M. scalenus posterior

M. scalenus
anterior (*cut*)

N. phrenicus

Trunci plexus
brachialis

A. subclavia

Costa 1

V. subclavia

Carotis communis

Tuberculum posterius
proc. transversi vertebrae C7

V. jugularis interna

Plate 55

Collum

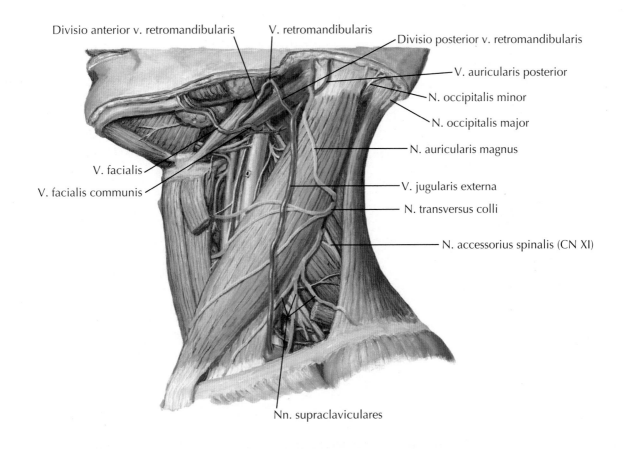

Divisio anterior v. retromandibularis
V. retromandibularis
Divisio posterior v. retromandibularis
V. auricularis posterior
N. occipitalis minor
N. occipitalis major
N. auricularis magnus
V. facialis
V. facialis communis
V. jugularis externa
N. transversus colli
N. accessorius spinalis (CN XI)
Nn. supraclaviculares

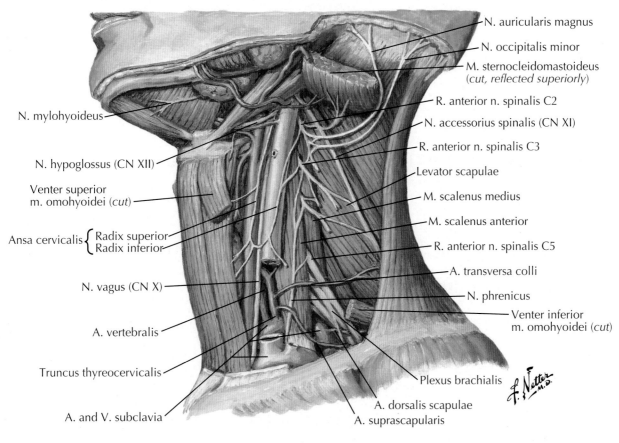

N. auricularis magnus
N. occipitalis minor
M. sternocleidomastoideus
(cut, reflected superiorly)
R. anterior n. spinalis C2
N. accessorius spinalis (CN XI)
R. anterior n. spinalis C3
Levator scapulae
M. scalenus medius
M. scalenus anterior
R. anterior n. spinalis C5
A. transversa colli
N. phrenicus
Venter inferior
m. omohyoidei (cut)
Plexus brachialis
A. dorsalis scapulae
A. suprascapularis
N. mylohyoideus
N. hypoglossus (CN XII)
Venter superior
m. omohyoidei (cut)
Ansa cervicalis { Radix superior
Radix inferior
N. vagus (CN X)
A. vertebralis
Truncus thyreocervicalis
A. and V. subclavia

Plexus cervicalis: schema

(S = Ramus communicans griseus from Ganglion cervicale superius)

R. geniohyoideus n. hypoglossi

R. thyreohyoideus n. hypoglossi

N. transversus colli

Nervus to Venter superior m. omohyoidei

Ansa cervicalis { Radix superior / Radix inferior

N. sternothyreoideus

N. sternohyoideus

Nervus to Venter inferior m. omohyoidei

Nn. supraclaviculares

N. hypoglossus (CN XII)

S
C1
S
S   C3
S   C4

N. phrenicus

N. accessorius spinalis (CN XI)

N. auricularis magnus

N. occipitalis minor

Nervi to Mm. rectus lateralis capitis, longus capitis, and rectus anterior capitis

Nervi to Mm. longus capitis and longus colli

Nervi to Mm. scaleni and Levator scapulae

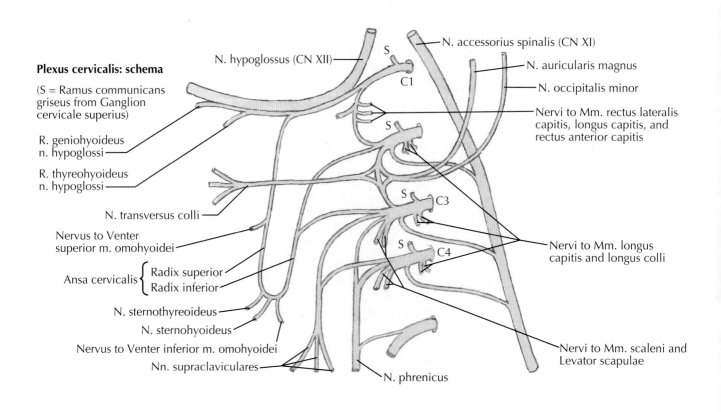

Right anterior view

V. jugularis interna

Carotis communis

A. cervicalis ascendens

N. phrenicus

M. scalenus anterior

A. thyreoidea inferior

A. transversa colli

Plexus brachialis

A. suprascapularis

A. dorsalis scapulae

Truncus costocervicalis

Truncus thyreocervicalis

A. and V. subclavia

Glandula thyreoidea (*retracted*)

Ganglion cervicale medium

N. vagus (CN X)

A. vertebralis

Carotis communis

N. laryngeus recurrens

Truncus brachiocephalicus

V. jugularis interna (*cut*)

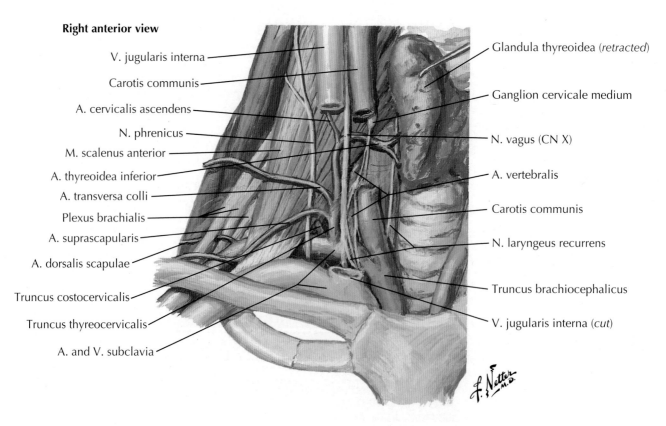

Plate 57   **Collum**

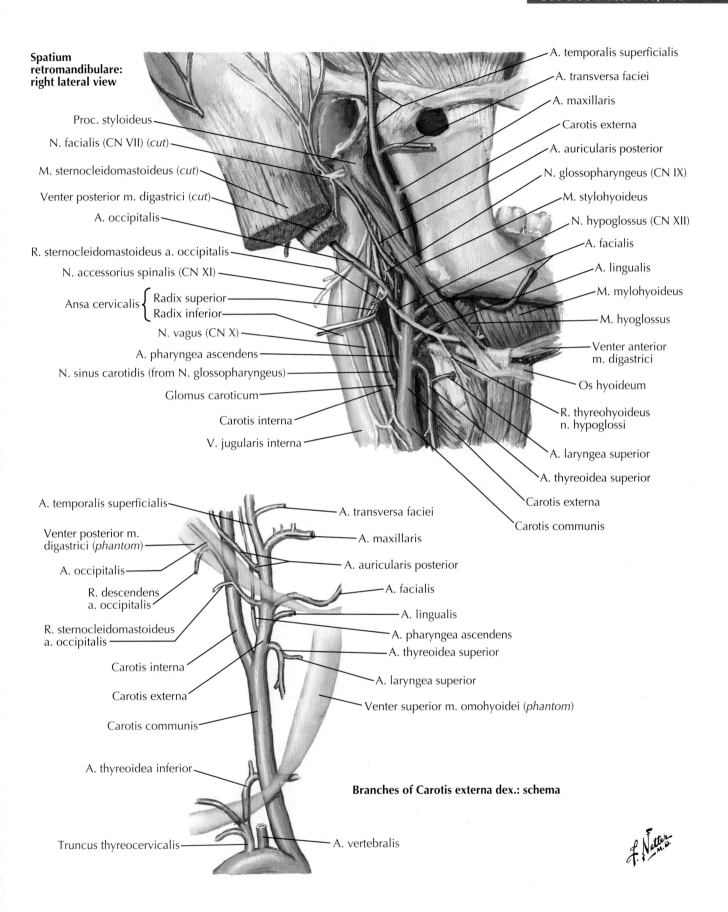

Spatium retromandibulare: right lateral view

Proc. styloideus

N. facialis (CN VII) (*cut*)

M. sternocleidomastoideus (*cut*)

Venter posterior m. digastrici (*cut*)

A. occipitalis

R. sternocleidomastoideus a. occipitalis

N. accessorius spinalis (CN XI)

Ansa cervicalis { Radix superior
Radix inferior

N. vagus (CN X)

A. pharyngea ascendens

N. sinus carotidis (from N. glossopharyngeus)

Glomus caroticum

Carotis interna

V. jugularis interna

A. temporalis superficialis

A. transversa faciei

A. maxillaris

Carotis externa

A. auricularis posterior

N. glossopharyngeus (CN IX)

M. stylohyoideus

N. hypoglossus (CN XII)

A. facialis

A. lingualis

M. mylohyoideus

M. hyoglossus

Venter anterior m. digastrici

Os hyoideum

R. thyreohyoideus n. hypoglossi

A. laryngea superior

A. thyreoidea superior

Carotis externa

Carotis communis

A. temporalis superficialis

Venter posterior m. digastrici (*phantom*)

A. occipitalis

R. descendens a. occipitalis

R. sternocleidomastoideus a. occipitalis

Carotis interna

Carotis externa

Carotis communis

A. thyreoidea inferior

Truncus thyreocervicalis

A. transversa faciei

A. maxillaris

A. auricularis posterior

A. facialis

A. lingualis

A. pharyngea ascendens

A. thyreoidea superior

A. laryngea superior

Venter superior m. omohyoidei (*phantom*)

Branches of Carotis externa dex.: schema

A. vertebralis

Collum

Plate 58

Anterolateral view

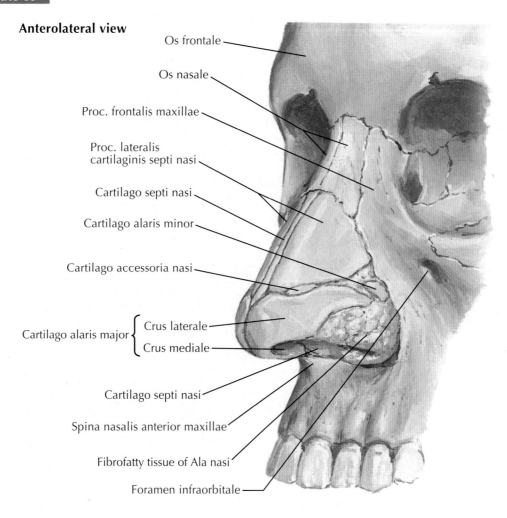

Os frontale

Os nasale

Proc. frontalis maxillae

Proc. lateralis cartilaginis septi nasi

Cartilago septi nasi

Cartilago alaris minor

Cartilago accessoria nasi

Cartilago alaris major { Crus laterale / Crus mediale

Cartilago septi nasi

Spina nasalis anterior maxillae

Fibrofatty tissue of Ala nasi

Foramen infraorbitale

Inferior view

Cartilago alaris major

Crus laterale

Crus mediale

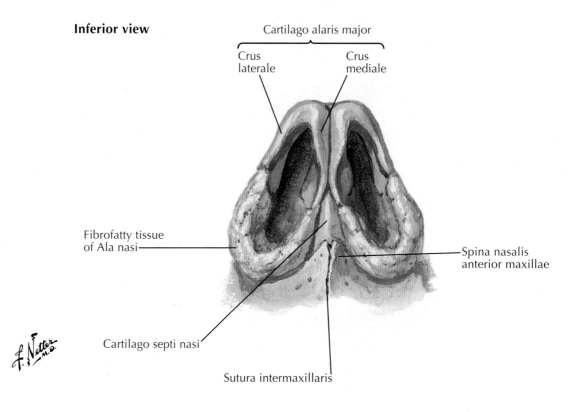

Fibrofatty tissue of Ala nasi

Spina nasalis anterior maxillae

Cartilago septi nasi

Sutura intermaxillaris

Plate 59   **Nasus**

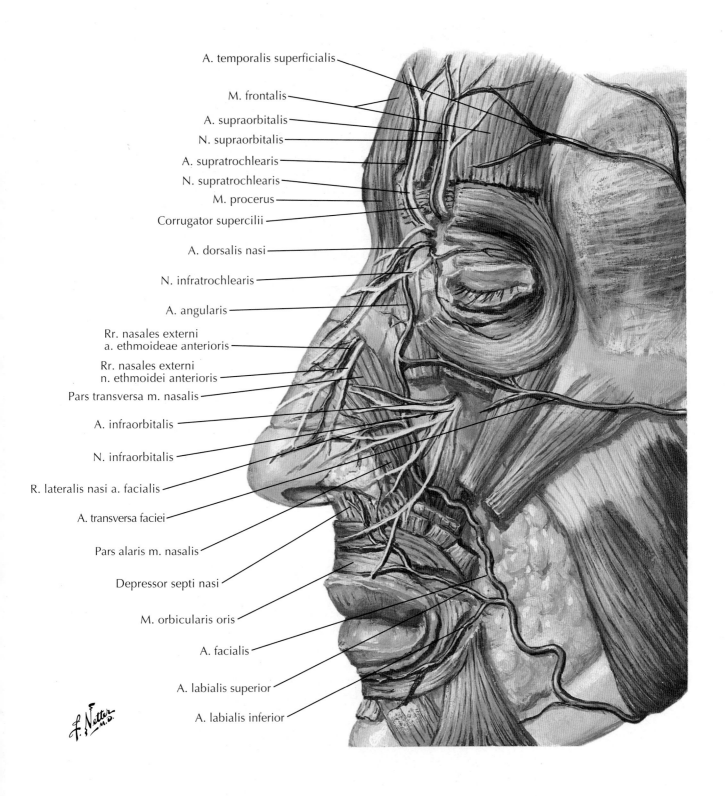

A. temporalis superficialis

M. frontalis

A. supraorbitalis

N. supraorbitalis

A. supratrochlearis

N. supratrochlearis

M. procerus

Corrugator supercilii

A. dorsalis nasi

N. infratrochlearis

A. angularis

Rr. nasales externi
a. ethmoideae anterioris

Rr. nasales externi
n. ethmoidei anterioris

Pars transversa m. nasalis

A. infraorbitalis

N. infraorbitalis

R. lateralis nasi a. facialis

A. transversa faciei

Pars alaris m. nasalis

Depressor septi nasi

M. orbicularis oris

A. facialis

A. labialis superior

A. labialis inferior

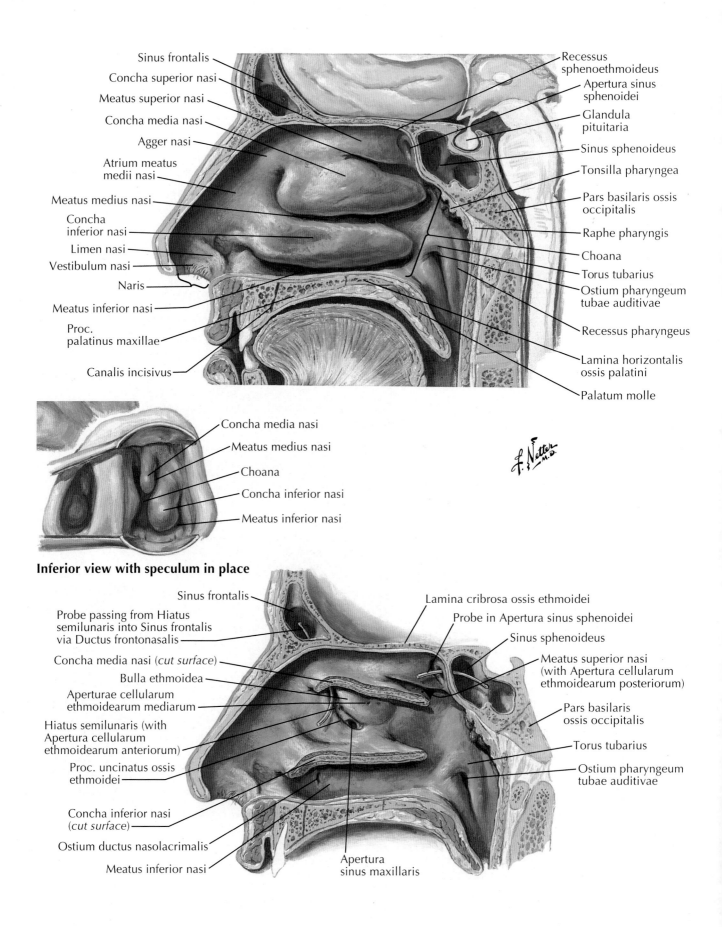

Sinus frontalis

Concha superior nasi

Meatus superior nasi

Concha media nasi

Agger nasi

Atrium meatus medii nasi

Meatus medius nasi

Concha inferior nasi

Limen nasi

Vestibulum nasi

Naris

Meatus inferior nasi

Proc. palatinus maxillae

Canalis incisivus

Recessus sphenoethmoideus

Apertura sinus sphenoidei

Glandula pituitaria

Sinus sphenoideus

Tonsilla pharyngea

Pars basilaris ossis occipitalis

Raphe pharyngis

Choana

Torus tubarius

Ostium pharyngeum tubae auditivae

Recessus pharyngeus

Lamina horizontalis ossis palatini

Palatum molle

Concha media nasi

Meatus medius nasi

Choana

Concha inferior nasi

Meatus inferior nasi

Inferior view with speculum in place

Sinus frontalis

Probe passing from Hiatus semilunaris into Sinus frontalis via Ductus frontonasalis

Concha media nasi (*cut surface*)

Bulla ethmoidea

Aperturae cellularum ethmoidearum mediarum

Hiatus semilunaris (with Apertura cellularum ethmoidearum anteriorum)

Proc. uncinatus ossis ethmoidei

Concha inferior nasi (*cut surface*)

Ostium ductus nasolacrimalis

Meatus inferior nasi

Lamina cribrosa ossis ethmoidei

Probe in Apertura sinus sphenoidei

Sinus sphenoideus

Meatus superior nasi (with Apertura cellularum ethmoidearum posteriorum)

Pars basilaris ossis occipitalis

Torus tubarius

Ostium pharyngeum tubae auditivae

Apertura sinus maxillaris

Plate 61

Nasus

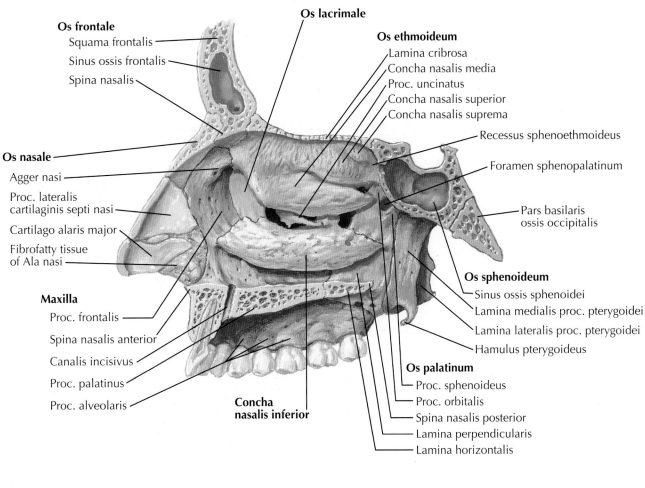

Os frontale
Squama frontalis
Sinus ossis frontalis
Spina nasalis

Os lacrimale

Os ethmoideum
Lamina cribrosa
Concha nasalis media
Proc. uncinatus
Concha nasalis superior
Concha nasalis suprema

Recessus sphenoethmoideus

Foramen sphenopalatinum

Pars basilaris
ossis occipitalis

Os nasale
Agger nasi
Proc. lateralis
cartilaginis septi nasi
Cartilago alaris major
Fibrofatty tissue
of Ala nasi

Os sphenoideum
Sinus ossis sphenoidei
Lamina medialis proc. pterygoidei
Lamina lateralis proc. pterygoidei
Hamulus pterygoideus

Maxilla
Proc. frontalis
Spina nasalis anterior
Canalis incisivus
Proc. palatinus
Proc. alveolaris

Os palatinum
Proc. sphenoideus
Proc. orbitalis
Spina nasalis posterior
Lamina perpendicularis
Lamina horizontalis

**Concha
nasalis inferior**

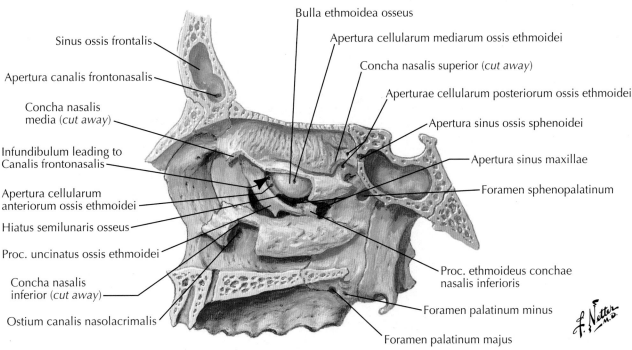

Sinus ossis frontalis

Apertura canalis frontonasalis

Concha nasalis
media (*cut away*)

Infundibulum leading to
Canalis frontonasalis

Apertura cellularum
anteriorum ossis ethmoidei

Hiatus semilunaris osseus

Proc. uncinatus ossis ethmoidei

Concha nasalis
inferior (*cut away*)

Ostium canalis nasolacrimalis

Bulla ethmoidea osseus

Apertura cellularum mediarum ossis ethmoidei

Concha nasalis superior (*cut away*)

Aperturae cellularum posteriorum ossis ethmoidei

Apertura sinus ossis sphenoidei

Apertura sinus maxillae

Foramen sphenopalatinum

Proc. ethmoideus conchae
nasalis inferioris

Foramen palatinum minus

Foramen palatinum majus

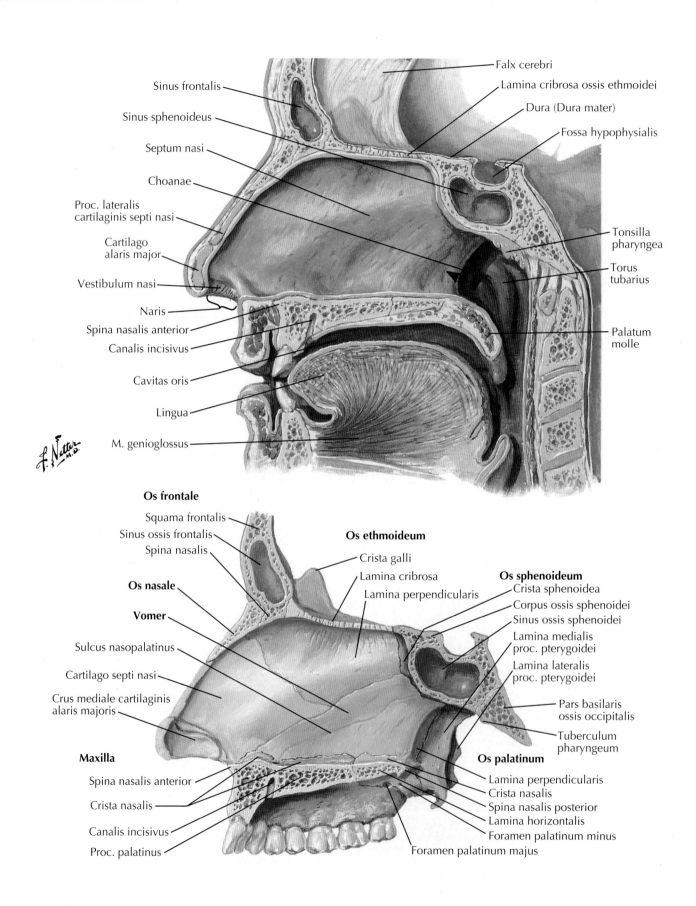

Sinus frontalis

Sinus sphenoideus

Septum nasi

Choanae

Proc. lateralis
cartilaginis septi nasi

Cartilago
alaris major

Vestibulum nasi

Naris

Spina nasalis anterior

Canalis incisivus

Cavitas oris

Lingua

M. genioglossus

Falx cerebri

Lamina cribrosa ossis ethmoidei

Dura (Dura mater)

Fossa hypophysialis

Tonsilla
pharyngea

Torus
tubarius

Palatum
molle

Os frontale

Squama frontalis

Sinus ossis frontalis

Spina nasalis

Os nasale

Vomer

Sulcus nasopalatinus

Cartilago septi nasi

Crus mediale cartilaginis
alaris majoris

Maxilla

Spina nasalis anterior

Crista nasalis

Canalis incisivus

Proc. palatinus

Os ethmoideum

Crista galli

Lamina cribrosa

Lamina perpendicularis

Os sphenoideum

Crista sphenoidea

Corpus ossis sphenoidei

Sinus ossis sphenoidei

Lamina medialis
proc. pterygoidei

Lamina lateralis
proc. pterygoidei

Pars basilaris
ossis occipitalis

Tuberculum
pharyngeum

Os palatinum

Lamina perpendicularis

Crista nasalis

Spina nasalis posterior

Lamina horizontalis

Foramen palatinum minus

Foramen palatinum majus

Plate 63

Nasus

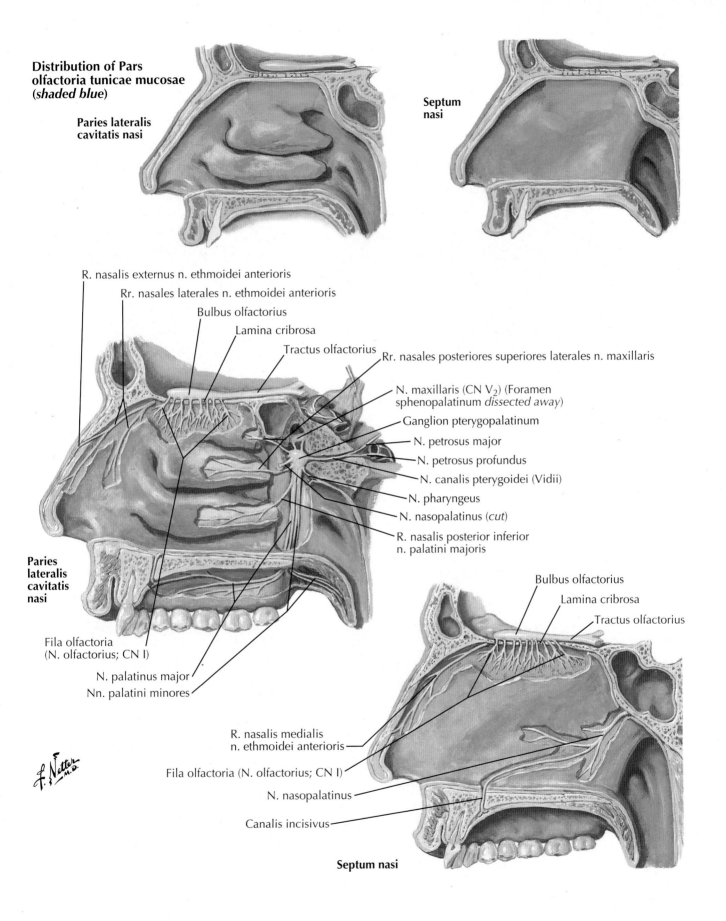

Distribution of Pars olfactoria tunicae mucosae (*shaded blue*)

Paries lateralis cavitatis nasi

Septum nasi

R. nasalis externus n. ethmoidei anterioris

Rr. nasales laterales n. ethmoidei anterioris

Bulbus olfactorius

Lamina cribrosa

Tractus olfactorius

Rr. nasales posteriores superiores laterales n. maxillaris

N. maxillaris (CN V₂) (Foramen sphenopalatinum *dissected away*)

Ganglion pterygopalatinum

N. petrosus major

N. petrosus profundus

N. canalis pterygoidei (Vidii)

N. pharyngeus

N. nasopalatinus (*cut*)

R. nasalis posterior inferior n. palatini majoris

Paries lateralis cavitatis nasi

Fila olfactoria (N. olfactorius; CN I)

N. palatinus major

Nn. palatini minores

Bulbus olfactorius

Lamina cribrosa

Tractus olfactorius

R. nasalis medialis n. ethmoidei anterioris

Fila olfactoria (N. olfactorius; CN I)

N. nasopalatinus

Canalis incisivus

Septum nasi

Paries lateralis cavitatis nasi

Septum nasi

R. nasalis lateralis anterior a. ethmoideae anterioris

A. ethmoidea anterior

A. ethmoidea posterior

A. ophthalmica

Carotis interna

A. sphenopalatina

A. palatina descendens

A. maxillaris

Rr. nasales laterales posteriores a. sphenopalatinae

Rr. nasales laterales a. facialis

A. palatina major

A. palatina minor

Carotis externa

Carotis interna

Rr. septales anteriores a. ethmoideae anterioris

Plexus arteriosus septi nasi (Kisselbachi)

R. septalis posterior a. sphenopalatinae

A. palatina major

Vas anastomoticum between R. septalis posterior a. sphenopalatinae and A. palatina major in Canalis incisivus

Rr. septales a. labialis superioris

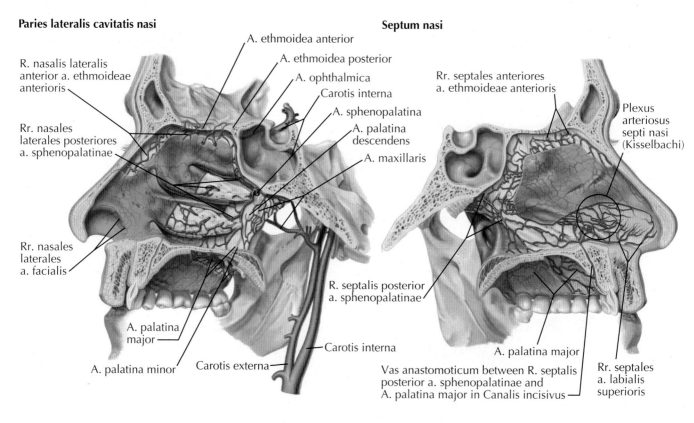

Paries lateralis cavitatis nasi

Septum nasi

V. ethmoidea anterior

V. ethmoidea posterior

V. ophthalmica superior

V. ophthalmica inferior

Sinus cavernosus

V. sphenopalatina

Plexus venosus pterygoideus

V. nasofrontalis

Affluens nasalis lateralis anterior v. ethmoideae anterioris

V. nasalis externa

Affluentes nasales laterales posteriores v. sphenopalatinae

V. palatina descendens

Affluens septalis posterior v. sphenopalatinae

V. facialis

V. retromandibularis

Vv. anastomoticae between Cavitas oris and Cavitas nasi in Canalis incisivus

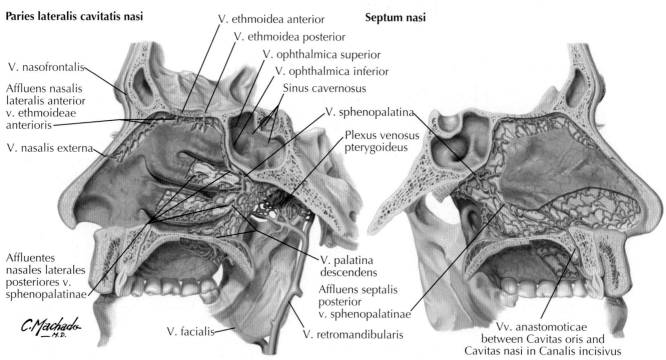

Plate 65

Nasus

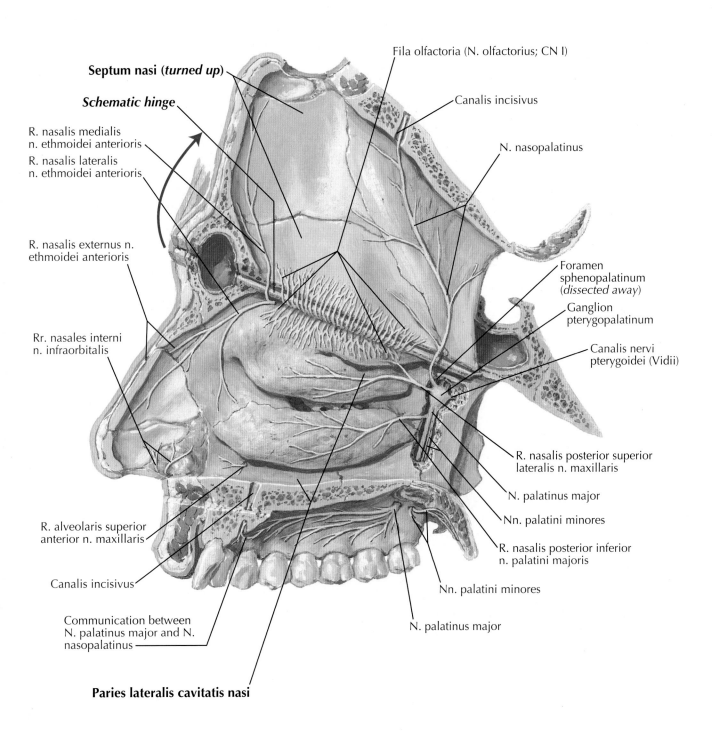

Septum nasi (*turned up*)

Schematic hinge

R. nasalis medialis
n. ethmoidei anterioris

R. nasalis lateralis
n. ethmoidei anterioris

R. nasalis externus n.
ethmoidei anterioris

Rr. nasales interni
n. infraorbitalis

R. alveolaris superior
anterior n. maxillaris

Canalis incisivus

Communication between
N. palatinus major and N.
nasopalatinus

Paries lateralis cavitatis nasi

Fila olfactoria (N. olfactorius; CN I)

Canalis incisivus

N. nasopalatinus

Foramen
sphenopalatinum
(*dissected away*)

Ganglion
pterygopalatinum

Canalis nervi
pterygoidei (Vidii)

R. nasalis posterior superior
lateralis n. maxillaris

N. palatinus major

Nn. palatini minores

R. nasalis posterior inferior
n. palatini majoris

Nn. palatini minores

N. palatinus major

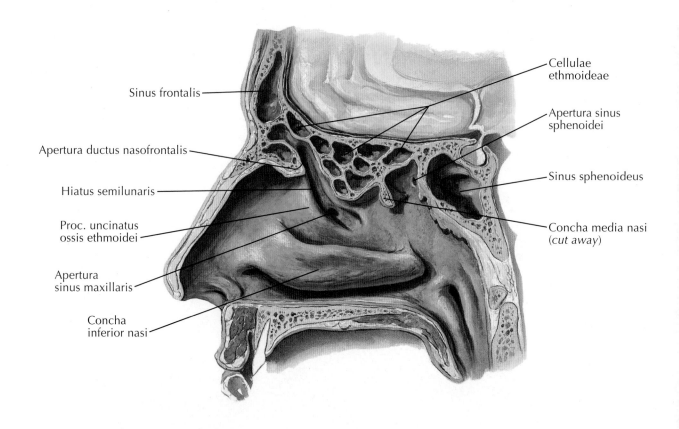

Sinus frontalis

Cellulae
ethmoideae

Apertura ductus nasofrontalis

Apertura sinus
sphenoidei

Hiatus semilunaris

Sinus sphenoideus

Proc. uncinatus
ossis ethmoidei

Concha media nasi
(*cut away*)

Apertura
sinus maxillaris

Concha
inferior nasi

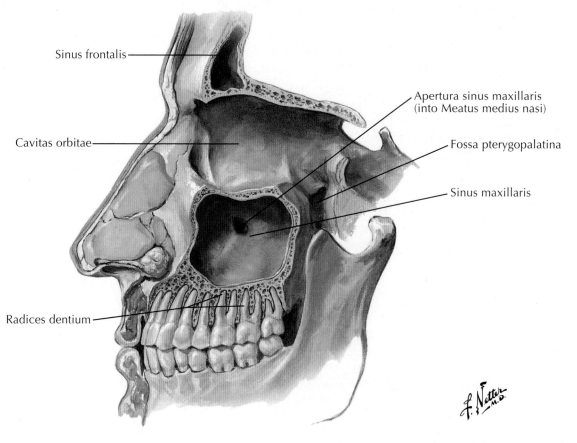

Sinus frontalis

Apertura sinus maxillaris
(into Meatus medius nasi)

Cavitas orbitae

Fossa pterygopalatina

Sinus maxillaris

Radices dentium

Plate 67

Nasus

Bones of Cavitas nasi and Sinus paranasales at birth

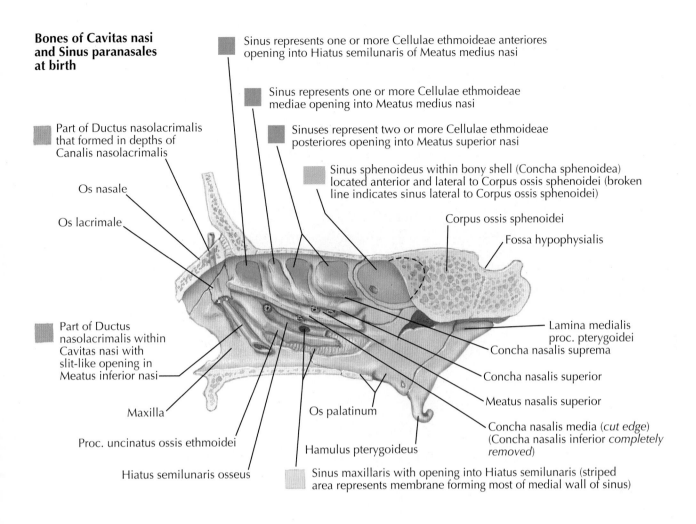

Sinus represents one or more Cellulae ethmoideae anteriores opening into Hiatus semilunaris of Meatus medius nasi

Sinus represents one or more Cellulae ethmoideae mediae opening into Meatus medius nasi

Sinuses represent two or more Cellulae ethmoideae posteriores opening into Meatus superior nasi

Sinus sphenoideus within bony shell (Concha sphenoidea) located anterior and lateral to Corpus ossis sphenoidei (broken line indicates sinus lateral to Corpus ossis sphenoidei)

Part of Ductus nasolacrimalis that formed in depths of Canalis nasolacrimalis

Os nasale

Os lacrimale

Part of Ductus nasolacrimalis within Cavitas nasi with slit-like opening in Meatus inferior nasi

Maxilla

Proc. uncinatus ossis ethmoidei

Hiatus semilunaris osseus

Os palatinum

Hamulus pterygoideus

Corpus ossis sphenoidei

Fossa hypophysialis

Lamina medialis proc. pterygoidei

Concha nasalis suprema

Concha nasalis superior

Meatus nasalis superior

Concha nasalis media (*cut edge*) (Concha nasalis inferior *completely removed*)

Sinus maxillaris with opening into Hiatus semilunaris (striped area represents membrane forming most of medial wall of sinus)

Growth of sinuses in Os frontale and Maxilla throughout life

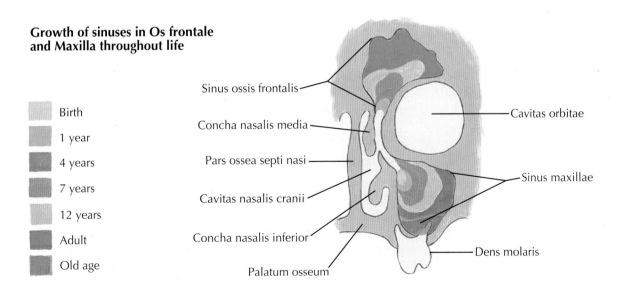

Birth

1 year

4 years

7 years

12 years

Adult

Old age

Sinus ossis frontalis

Concha nasalis media

Pars ossea septi nasi

Cavitas nasalis cranii

Concha nasalis inferior

Palatum osseum

Cavitas orbitae

Sinus maxillae

Dens molaris

Coronal section

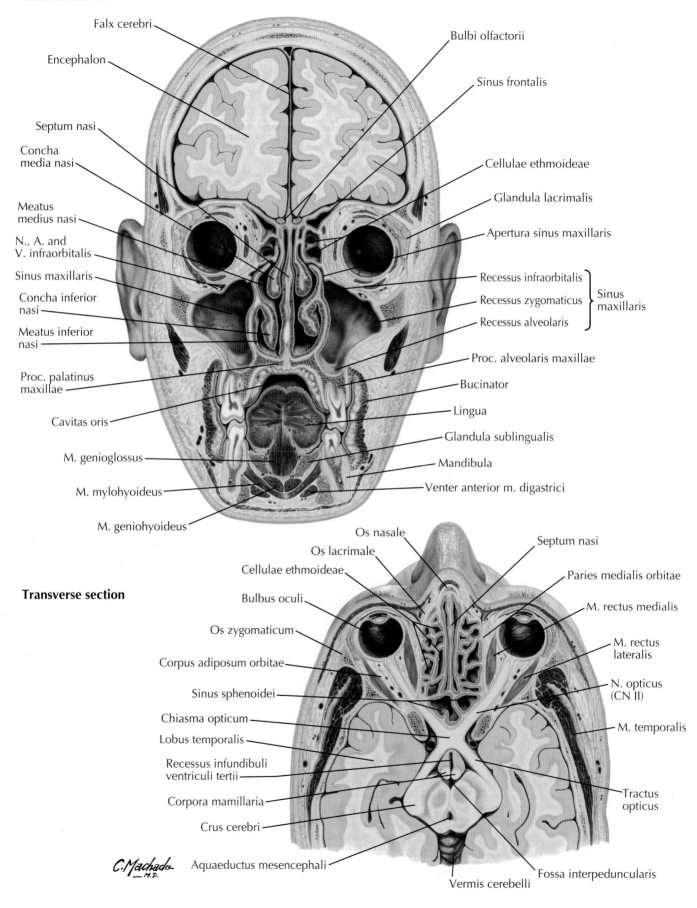

Falx cerebri

Encephalon

Septum nasi

Concha
media nasi

Meatus
medius nasi

N., A. and
V. infraorbitalis

Sinus maxillaris

Concha inferior
nasi

Meatus inferior
nasi

Proc. palatinus
maxillae

Cavitas oris

M. genioglossus

M. mylohyoideus

M. geniohyoideus

Bulbi olfactorii

Sinus frontalis

Cellulae ethmoideae

Glandula lacrimalis

Apertura sinus maxillaris

Recessus infraorbitalis ⎱
Recessus zygomaticus ⎰ Sinus
 maxillaris
Recessus alveolaris ⎰

Proc. alveolaris maxillae

Bucinator

Lingua

Glandula sublingualis

Mandibula

Venter anterior m. digastrici

Transverse section

Os nasale

Os lacrimale

Cellulae ethmoideae

Bulbus oculi

Os zygomaticum

Corpus adiposum orbitae

Sinus sphenoidei

Chiasma opticum

Lobus temporalis

Recessus infundibuli
ventriculi tertii

Corpora mamillaria

Crus cerebri

Septum nasi

Paries medialis orbitae

M. rectus medialis

M. rectus
lateralis

N. opticus
(CN II)

M. temporalis

Tractus
opticus

C. Machado
_M.D._

Aquaeductus mesencephali

Vermis cerebelli

Fossa interpeduncularis

Plate 69

Nasus

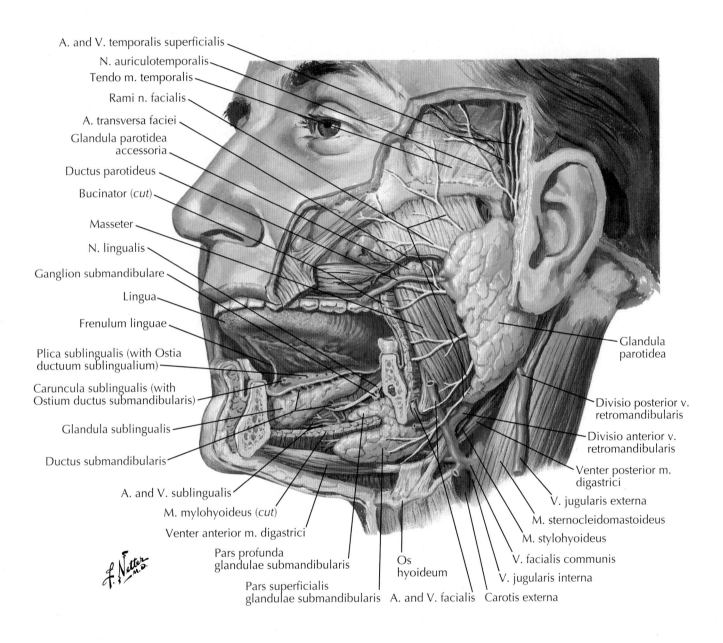

A. and V. temporalis superficialis

N. auriculotemporalis

Tendo m. temporalis

Rami n. facialis

A. transversa faciei

Glandula parotidea accessoria

Ductus parotideus

Bucinator (*cut*)

Masseter

N. lingualis

Ganglion submandibulare

Lingua

Frenulum linguae

Plica sublingualis (with Ostia ductuum sublingualium)

Caruncula sublingualis (with Ostium ductus submandibularis)

Glandula sublingualis

Ductus submandibularis

A. and V. sublingualis

M. mylohyoideus (*cut*)

Venter anterior m. digastrici

Pars profunda glandulae submandibularis

Pars superficialis glandulae submandibularis

Os hyoideum

A. and V. facialis

Carotis externa

Glandula parotidea

Divisio posterior v. retromandibularis

Divisio anterior v. retromandibularis

Venter posterior m. digastrici

V. jugularis externa

M. sternocleidomastoideus

M. stylohyoideus

V. facialis communis

V. jugularis interna

F. Netter M.D.

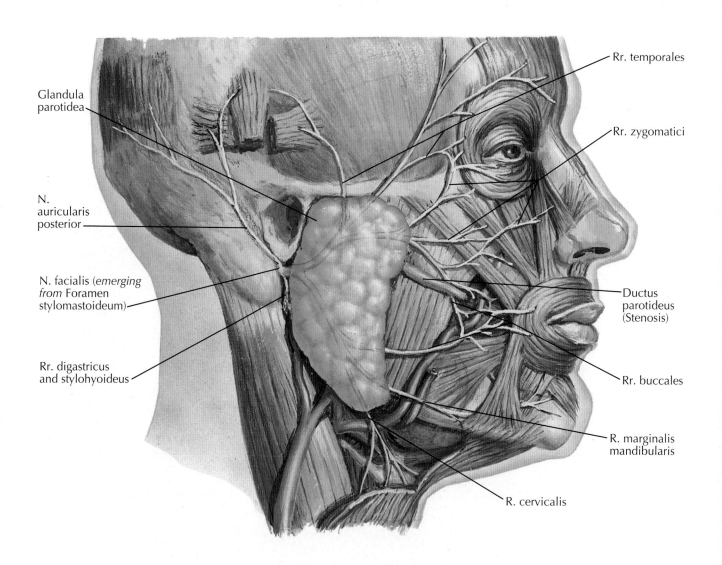

Glandula parotidea

N. auricularis posterior

N. facialis (*emerging from* Foramen stylomastoideum)

Rr. digastricus and stylohyoideus

Rr. temporales

Rr. zygomatici

Ductus parotideus (Stenosis)

Rr. buccales

R. marginalis mandibularis

R. cervicalis

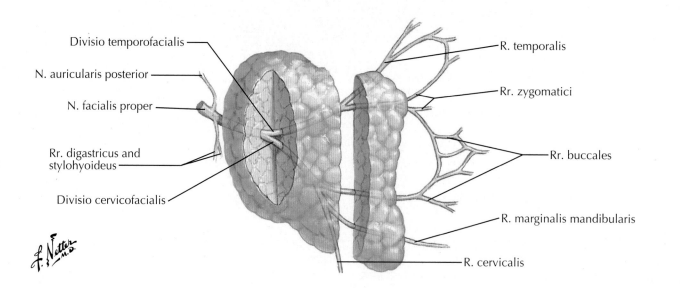

Divisio temporofacialis

N. auricularis posterior

N. facialis proper

Rr. digastricus and stylohyoideus

Divisio cervicofacialis

R. temporalis

Rr. zygomatici

Rr. buccales

R. marginalis mandibularis

R. cervicalis

Plate 71

Nasus

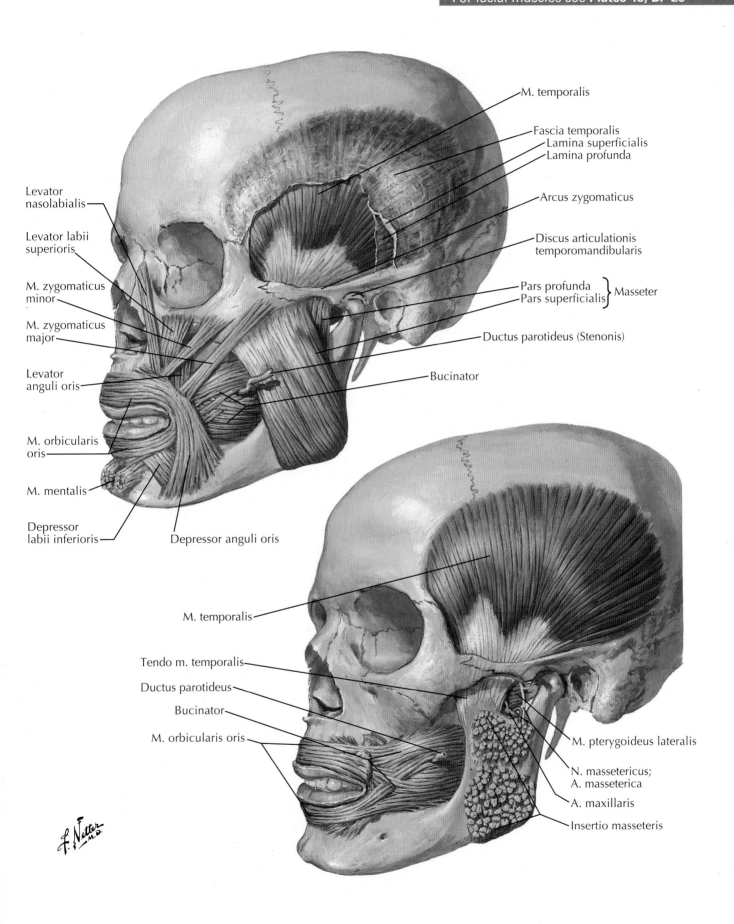

M. temporalis

Fascia temporalis
Lamina superficialis
Lamina profunda

Arcus zygomaticus

Discus articulationis
temporomandibularis

Pars profunda
Pars superficialis } Masseter

Ductus parotideus (Stenonis)

Bucinator

Levator
nasolabialis

Levator labii
superioris

M. zygomaticus
minor

M. zygomaticus
major

Levator
anguli oris

M. orbicularis
oris

M. mentalis

Depressor
labii inferioris

Depressor anguli oris

M. temporalis

Tendo m. temporalis

Ductus parotideus

Bucinator

M. orbicularis oris

M. pterygoideus lateralis

N. massetericus;
A. masseterica

A. maxillaris

Insertio masseteris

Lateral view

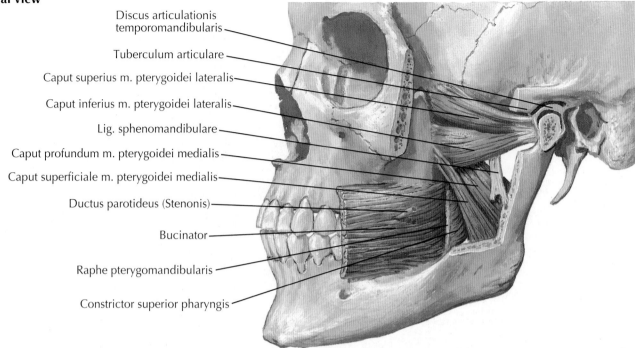

Discus articulationis temporomandibularis

Tuberculum articulare

Caput superius m. pterygoidei lateralis

Caput inferius m. pterygoidei lateralis

Lig. sphenomandibulare

Caput profundum m. pterygoidei medialis

Caput superficiale m. pterygoidei medialis

Ductus parotideus (Stenonis)

Bucinator

Raphe pterygomandibularis

Constrictor superior pharyngis

Posterior view

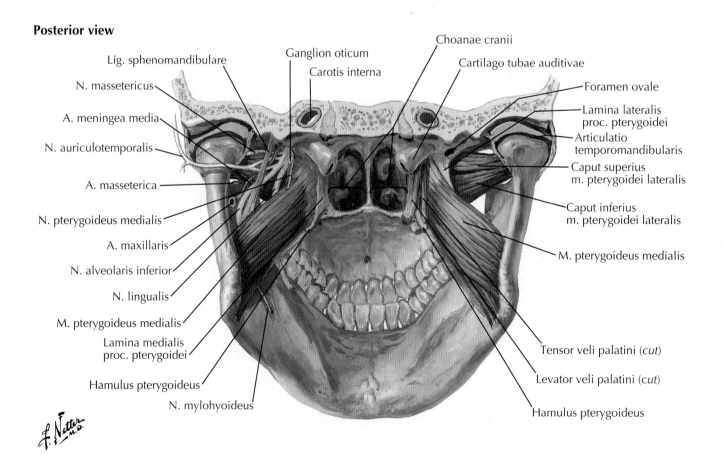

Lig. sphenomandibulare

N. massetericus

A. meningea media

N. auriculotemporalis

A. masseterica

N. pterygoideus medialis

A. maxillaris

N. alveolaris inferior

N. lingualis

M. pterygoideus medialis

Lamina medialis proc. pterygoidei

Hamulus pterygoideus

N. mylohyoideus

Ganglion oticum

Carotis interna

Choanae cranii

Cartilago tubae auditivae

Foramen ovale

Lamina lateralis proc. pterygoidei

Articulatio temporomandibularis

Caput superius m. pterygoidei lateralis

Caput inferius m. pterygoidei lateralis

M. pterygoideus medialis

Tensor veli palatini (*cut*)

Levator veli palatini (*cut*)

Hamulus pterygoideus

Plate 73

Nasus

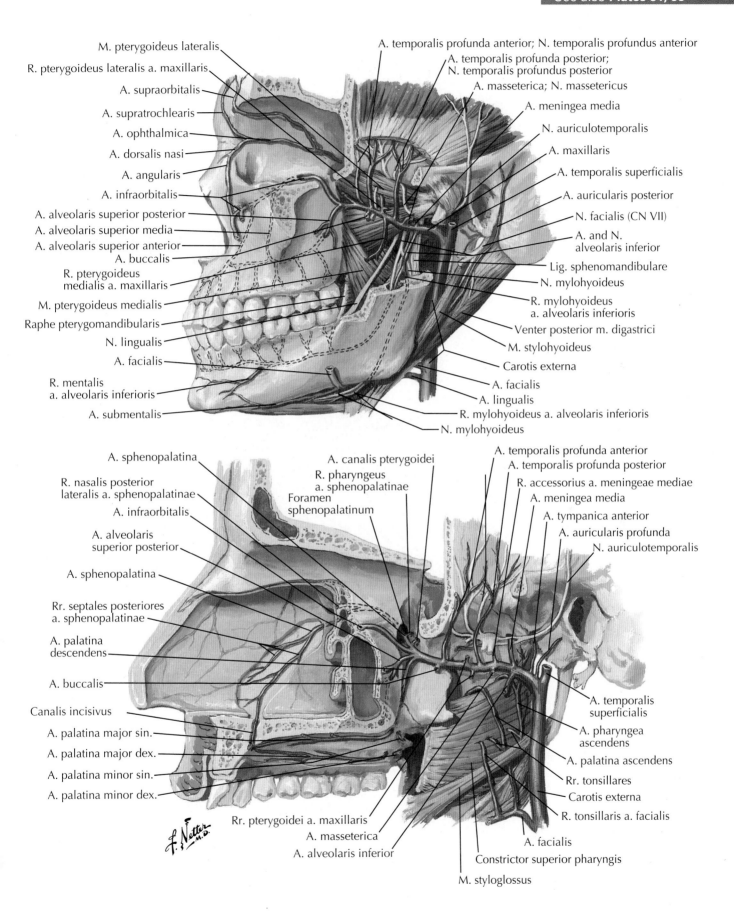

M. pterygoideus lateralis

R. pterygoideus lateralis a. maxillaris

A. supraorbitalis

A. supratrochlearis

A. ophthalmica

A. dorsalis nasi

A. angularis

A. infraorbitalis

A. alveolaris superior posterior

A. alveolaris superior media

A. alveolaris superior anterior

A. buccalis

R. pterygoideus medialis a. maxillaris

M. pterygoideus medialis

Raphe pterygomandibularis

N. lingualis

A. facialis

R. mentalis a. alveolaris inferioris

A. submentalis

A. temporalis profunda anterior; N. temporalis profundus anterior

A. temporalis profunda posterior; N. temporalis profundus posterior

A. masseterica; N. massetericus

A. meningea media

N. auriculotemporalis

A. maxillaris

A. temporalis superficialis

A. auricularis posterior

N. facialis (CN VII)

A. and N. alveolaris inferior

Lig. sphenomandibulare

N. mylohyoideus

R. mylohyoideus a. alveolaris inferioris

Venter posterior m. digastrici

M. stylohyoideus

Carotis externa

A. facialis

A. lingualis

R. mylohyoideus a. alveolaris inferioris

N. mylohyoideus

A. sphenopalatina

R. nasalis posterior lateralis a. sphenopalatinae

A. infraorbitalis

A. alveolaris superior posterior

A. sphenopalatina

Rr. septales posteriores a. sphenopalatinae

A. palatina descendens

A. buccalis

Canalis incisivus

A. palatina major sin.

A. palatina major dex.

A. palatina minor sin.

A. palatina minor dex.

A. canalis pterygoidei

R. pharyngeus a. sphenopalatinae

Foramen sphenopalatinum

A. temporalis profunda anterior

A. temporalis profunda posterior

R. accessorius a. meningeae mediae

A. meningea media

A. tympanica anterior

A. auricularis profunda

N. auriculotemporalis

A. temporalis superficialis

A. pharyngea ascendens

A. palatina ascendens

Rr. tonsillares

Carotis externa

R. tonsillaris a. facialis

A. facialis

Constrictor superior pharyngis

M. styloglossus

A. alveolaris inferior

A. masseterica

Rr. pterygoidei a. maxillaris

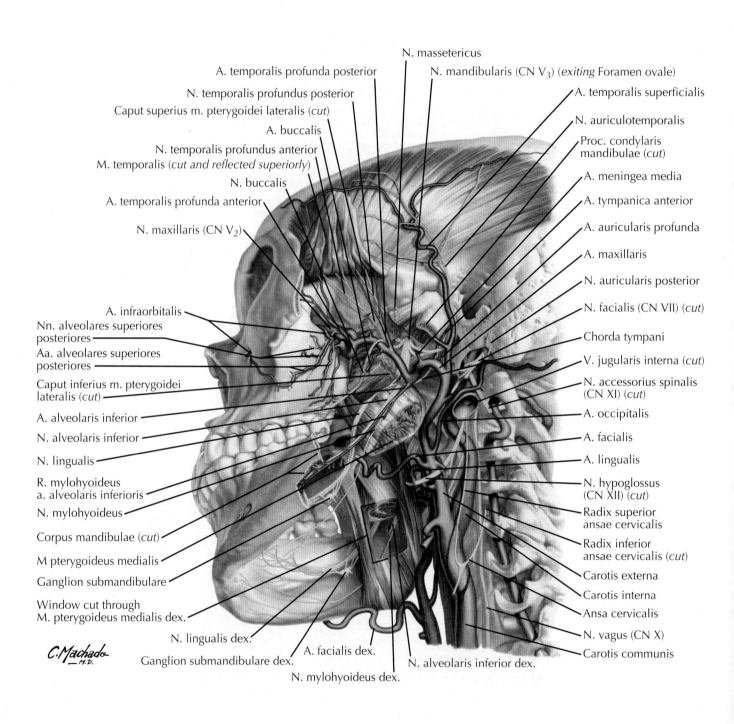

N. massetericus

A. temporalis profunda posterior

N. mandibularis (CN V₃) (*exiting* Foramen ovale)

N. temporalis profundus posterior

A. temporalis superficialis

Caput superius m. pterygoidei lateralis (*cut*)

N. auriculotemporalis

A. buccalis

Proc. condylaris mandibulae (*cut*)

N. temporalis profundus anterior

A. meningea media

M. temporalis (*cut and reflected superiorly*)

A. tympanica anterior

N. buccalis

A. auricularis profunda

A. temporalis profunda anterior

A. maxillaris

N. maxillaris (CN V₂)

N. auricularis posterior

N. facialis (CN VII) (*cut*)

A. infraorbitalis

Chorda tympani

Nn. alveolares superiores posteriores

V. jugularis interna (*cut*)

Aa. alveolares superiores posteriores

N. accessorius spinalis (CN XI) (*cut*)

Caput inferius m. pterygoidei lateralis (*cut*)

A. occipitalis

A. alveolaris inferior

A. facialis

N. alveolaris inferior

A. lingualis

N. lingualis

N. hypoglossus (CN XII) (*cut*)

R. mylohyoideus a. alveolaris inferioris

Radix superior ansae cervicalis

N. mylohyoideus

Radix inferior ansae cervicalis (*cut*)

Corpus mandibulae (*cut*)

Carotis externa

M pterygoideus medialis

Carotis interna

Ganglion submandibulare

Ansa cervicalis

Window cut through M. pterygoideus medialis dex.

N. vagus (CN X)

N. lingualis dex.

Carotis communis

A. facialis dex.

Ganglion submandibulare dex.

N. alveolaris inferior dex.

N. mylohyoideus dex.

C. Machado M.D.

Plate 75

Nasus

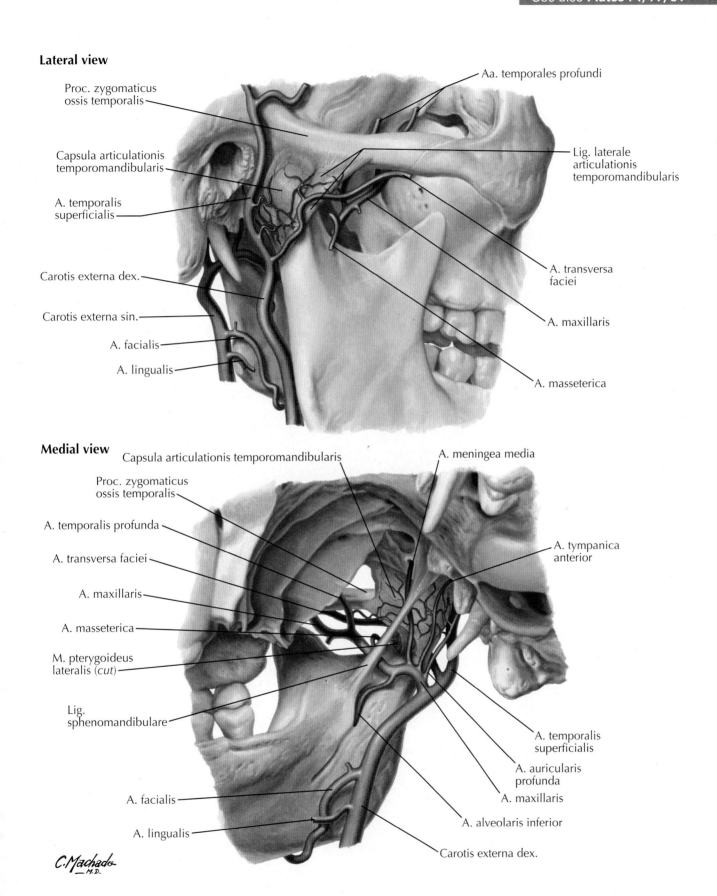

Lateral view

Proc. zygomaticus ossis temporalis

Capsula articulationis temporomandibularis

A. temporalis superficialis

Carotis externa dex.

Carotis externa sin.

A. facialis

A. lingualis

Aa. temporales profundi

Lig. laterale articulationis temporomandibularis

A. transversa faciei

A. maxillaris

A. masseterica

Medial view

Capsula articulationis temporomandibularis

Proc. zygomaticus ossis temporalis

A. temporalis profunda

A. transversa faciei

A. maxillaris

A. masseterica

M. pterygoideus lateralis (cut)

Lig. sphenomandibulare

A. facialis

A. lingualis

A. meningea media

A. tympanica anterior

A. temporalis superficialis

A. auricularis profunda

A. maxillaris

A. alveolaris inferior

Carotis externa dex.

C. Machado
—M.D.

Nasus

Plate 76

Lateral view

Divisio anterior n. mandibularis

Divisio posterior n. mandibularis

Foramen ovale

R. meningeus n. mandibularis

Foramen spinosum

A. meningea media

N. auriculo-temporalis

N. auricularis posterior

N. facialis (CN VII)

Chorda tympani

N. lingualis

N. alveolaris inferior (*cut*)

N. mylohyoideus

M. pterygoideus medialis (*cut*)

Venter posterior m. digastrici

M. stylohyoideus

N. hypoglossus (CN XII)

Glandula submandibularis

Fascia temporalis

M. temporalis

N. temporalis profundus posterior

N. temporalis profundus anterior

N. massetericus

N. pterygoideus lateralis

M. pterygoideus lateralis

N. buccalis

Bucinator (*cut*)

Ganglion submandibulare

Glandula sublingualis

N. mylohyoideus (*cut*)

N. mentalis

N. alveolaris inferior (*cut*)

Venter anterior m. digastrici

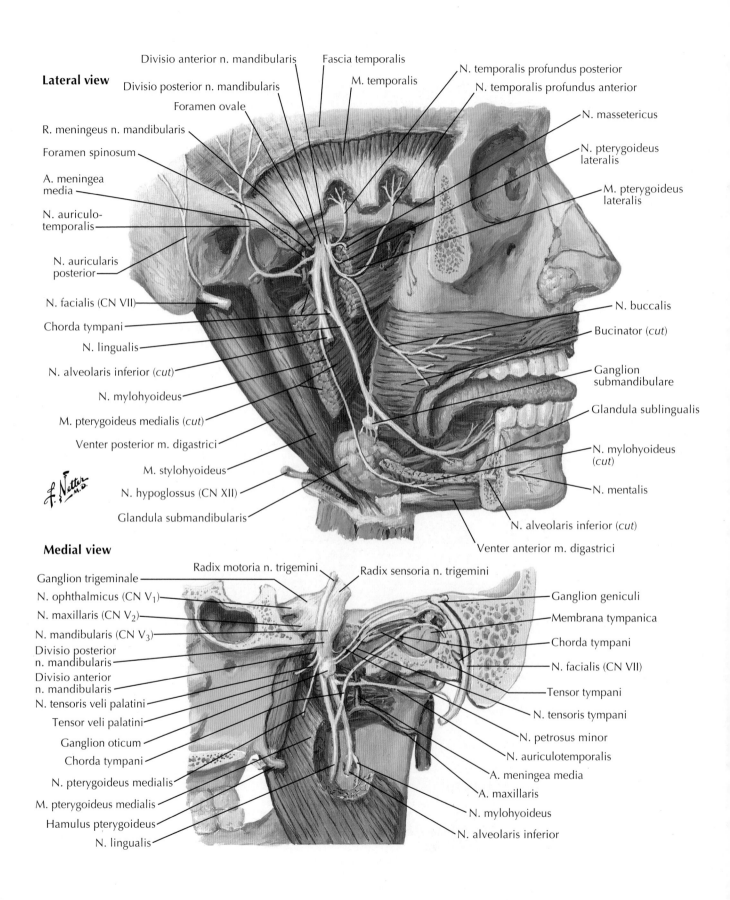

Medial view

Ganglion trigeminale

N. ophthalmicus (CN V₁)

N. maxillaris (CN V₂)

N. mandibularis (CN V₃)

Divisio posterior n. mandibularis

Divisio anterior n. mandibularis

N. tensoris veli palatini

Tensor veli palatini

Ganglion oticum

Chorda tympani

N. pterygoideus medialis

M. pterygoideus medialis

Hamulus pterygoideus

N. lingualis

Radix motoria n. trigemini

Radix sensoria n. trigemini

Ganglion geniculi

Membrana tympanica

Chorda tympani

N. facialis (CN VII)

Tensor tympani

N. tensoris tympani

N. petrosus minor

N. auriculotemporalis

A. meningea media

A. maxillaris

N. mylohyoideus

N. alveolaris inferior

Plate 77

Nasus

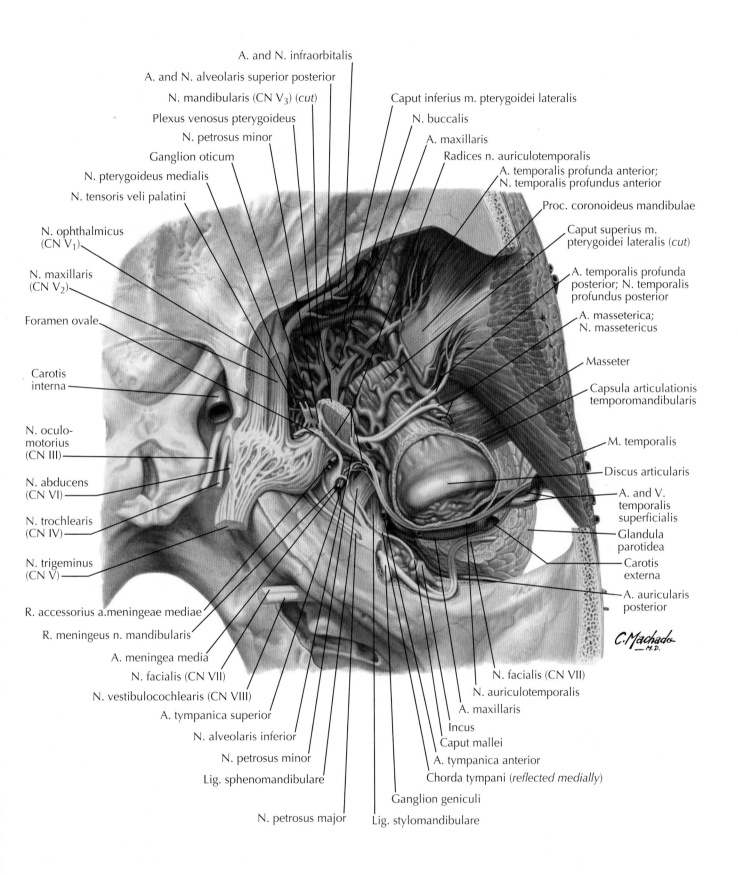

A. and N. infraorbitalis

A. and N. alveolaris superior posterior

N. mandibularis (CN V₃) (cut)

Plexus venosus pterygoideus

N. petrosus minor

Ganglion oticum

N. pterygoideus medialis

N. tensoris veli palatini

N. ophthalmicus (CN V₁)

N. maxillaris (CN V₂)

Foramen ovale

Carotis interna

N. oculo-motorius (CN III)

N. abducens (CN VI)

N. trochlearis (CN IV)

N. trigeminus (CN V)

R. accessorius a.meningeae mediae

R. meningeus n. mandibularis

A. meningea media

N. facialis (CN VII)

N. vestibulocochlearis (CN VIII)

A. tympanica superior

N. alveolaris inferior

N. petrosus minor

Lig. sphenomandibulare

N. petrosus major

Lig. stylomandibulare

Ganglion geniculi

Chorda tympani (reflected medially)

A. tympanica anterior

Caput mallei

Incus

A. maxillaris

N. auriculotemporalis

N. facialis (CN VII)

Caput inferius m. pterygoidei lateralis

N. buccalis

A. maxillaris

Radices n. auriculotemporalis

A. temporalis profunda anterior;
N. temporalis profundus anterior

Proc. coronoideus mandibulae

Caput superius m. pterygoidei lateralis (cut)

A. temporalis profunda posterior; N. temporalis profundus posterior

A. masseterica;
N. massetericus

Masseter

Capsula articulationis temporomandibularis

M. temporalis

Discus articularis

A. and V. temporalis superficialis

Glandula parotidea

Carotis externa

A. auricularis posterior

C.Machado
_M.D._

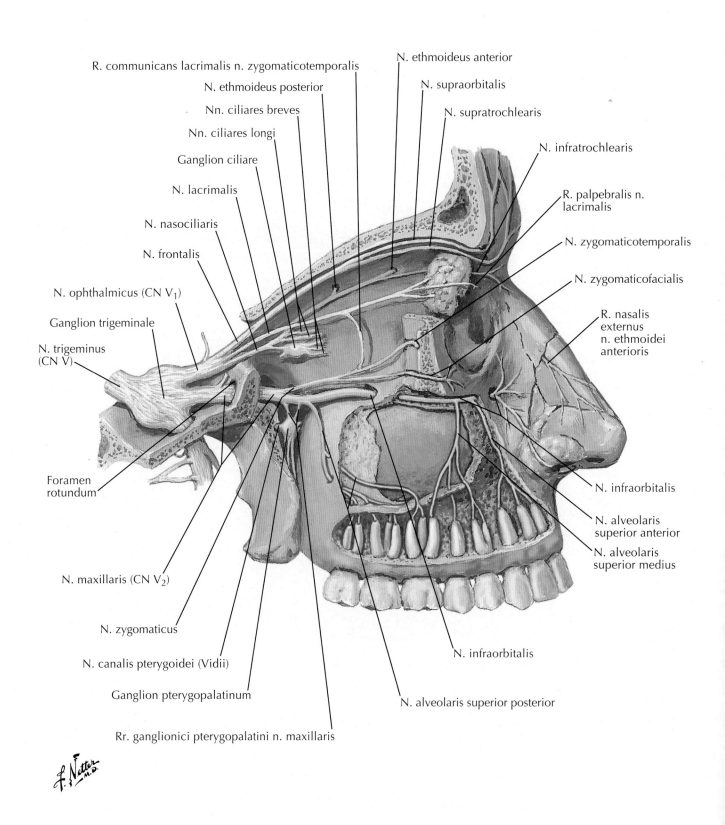

R. communicans lacrimalis n. zygomaticotemporalis

N. ethmoideus posterior

Nn. ciliares breves

Nn. ciliares longi

Ganglion ciliare

N. lacrimalis

N. nasociliaris

N. frontalis

N. ophthalmicus (CN V₁)

Ganglion trigeminale

N. trigeminus (CN V)

Foramen rotundum

N. maxillaris (CN V₂)

N. zygomaticus

N. canalis pterygoidei (Vidii)

Ganglion pterygopalatinum

Rr. ganglionici pterygopalatini n. maxillaris

N. ethmoideus anterior

N. supraorbitalis

N. supratrochlearis

N. infratrochlearis

R. palpebralis n. lacrimalis

N. zygomaticotemporalis

N. zygomaticofacialis

R. nasalis externus n. ethmoidei anterioris

N. infraorbitalis

N. alveolaris superior anterior

N. alveolaris superior medius

N. infraorbitalis

N. alveolaris superior posterior

Plate 79

Nasus

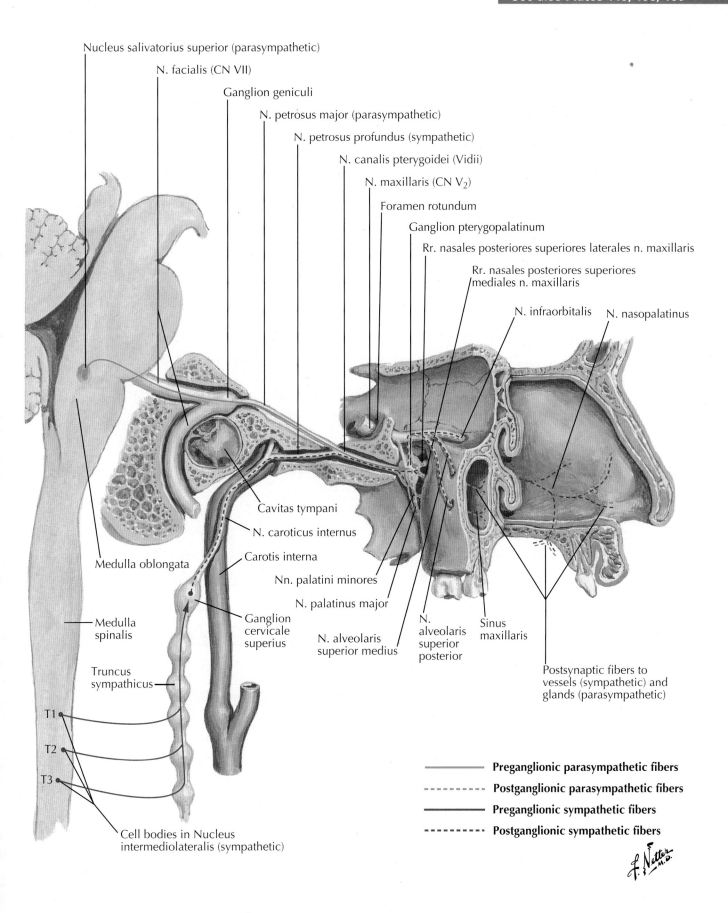

Nucleus salivatorius superior (parasympathetic)

N. facialis (CN VII)

Ganglion geniculi

N. petrosus major (parasympathetic)

N. petrosus profundus (sympathetic)

N. canalis pterygoidei (Vidii)

N. maxillaris (CN V₂)

Foramen rotundum

Ganglion pterygopalatinum

Rr. nasales posteriores superiores laterales n. maxillaris

Rr. nasales posteriores superiores mediales n. maxillaris

N. infraorbitalis

N. nasopalatinus

Cavitas tympani

N. caroticus internus

Carotis interna

Medulla oblongata

Nn. palatini minores

N. palatinus major

N. alveolaris superior posterior

Sinus maxillaris

Medulla spinalis

Ganglion cervicale superius

N. alveolaris superior medius

Truncus sympathicus

Postsynaptic fibers to vessels (sympathetic) and glands (parasympathetic)

T1

T2

T3

Cell bodies in Nucleus intermediolateralis (sympathetic)

———— Preganglionic parasympathetic fibers

- - - - - - - Postganglionic parasympathetic fibers

———— Preganglionic sympathetic fibers

- - - - - - Postganglionic sympathetic fibers

f. Netter m.d.

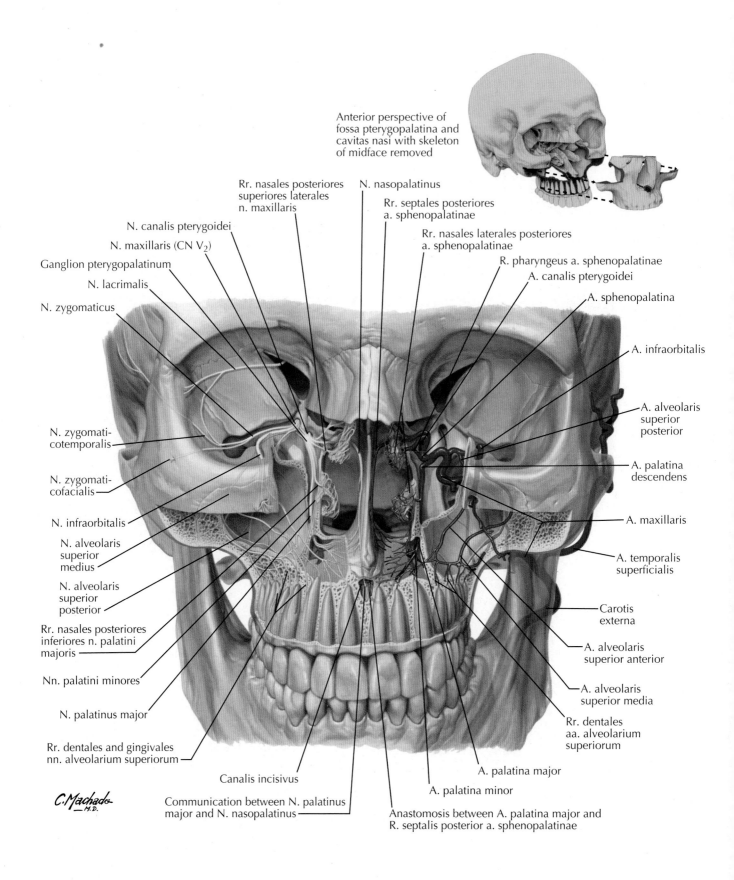

Anterior perspective of
fossa pterygopalatina and
cavitas nasi with skeleton
of midface removed

Rr. nasales posteriores
superiores laterales
n. maxillaris

N. nasopalatinus

Rr. septales posteriores
a. sphenopalatinae

N. canalis pterygoidei

Rr. nasales laterales posteriores
a. sphenopalatinae

N. maxillaris (CN V₂)

R. pharyngeus a. sphenopalatinae

Ganglion pterygopalatinum

A. canalis pterygoidei

N. lacrimalis

A. sphenopalatina

N. zygomaticus

A. infraorbitalis

A. alveolaris
superior
posterior

N. zygomati-
cotemporalis

A. palatina
descendens

N. zygomati-
cofacialis

A. maxillaris

N. infraorbitalis

A. temporalis
superficialis

N. alveolaris
superior
medius

Carotis
externa

N. alveolaris
superior
posterior

A. alveolaris
superior anterior

Rr. nasales posteriores
inferiores n. palatini
majoris

A. alveolaris
superior media

Nn. palatini minores

Rr. dentales
aa. alveolarium
superiorum

N. palatinus major

Rr. dentales and gingivales
nn. alveolarium superiorum

A. palatina major

Canalis incisivus

A. palatina minor

Communication between N. palatinus
major and N. nasopalatinus

Anastomosis between A. palatina major and
R. septalis posterior a. sphenopalatinae

C. Machado
—M.D.—

Plate 81

Nasus

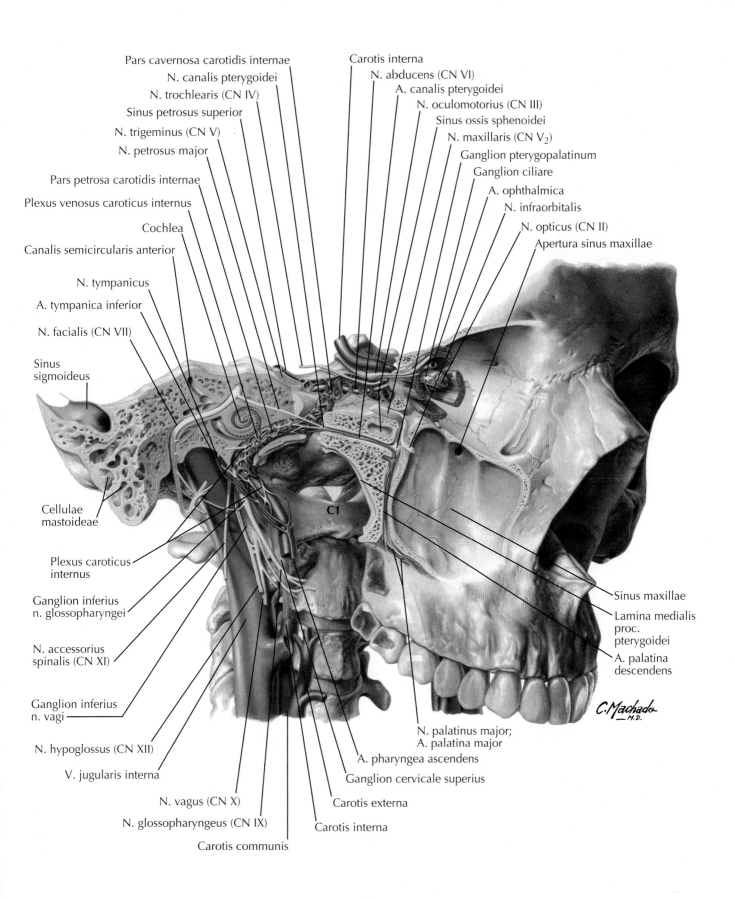

Pars cavernosa carotidis internae

N. canalis pterygoidei

N. trochlearis (CN IV)

Sinus petrosus superior

N. trigeminus (CN V)

N. petrosus major

Pars petrosa carotidis internae

Plexus venosus caroticus internus

Cochlea

Canalis semicircularis anterior

N. tympanicus

A. tympanica inferior

N. facialis (CN VII)

Sinus sigmoideus

Cellulae mastoideae

Plexus caroticus internus

Ganglion inferius n. glossopharyngei

N. accessorius spinalis (CN XI)

Ganglion inferius n. vagi

N. hypoglossus (CN XII)

V. jugularis interna

N. vagus (CN X)

N. glossopharyngeus (CN IX)

Carotis communis

Carotis interna

N. abducens (CN VI)

A. canalis pterygoidei

N. oculomotorius (CN III)

Sinus ossis sphenoidei

N. maxillaris (CN V$_2$)

Ganglion pterygopalatinum

Ganglion ciliare

A. ophthalmica

N. infraorbitalis

N. opticus (CN II)

Apertura sinus maxillae

C1

Sinus maxillae

Lamina medialis proc. pterygoidei

A. palatina descendens

N. palatinus major; A. palatina major

A. pharyngea ascendens

Ganglion cervicale superius

Carotis externa

Carotis interna

C.Machado M.D.

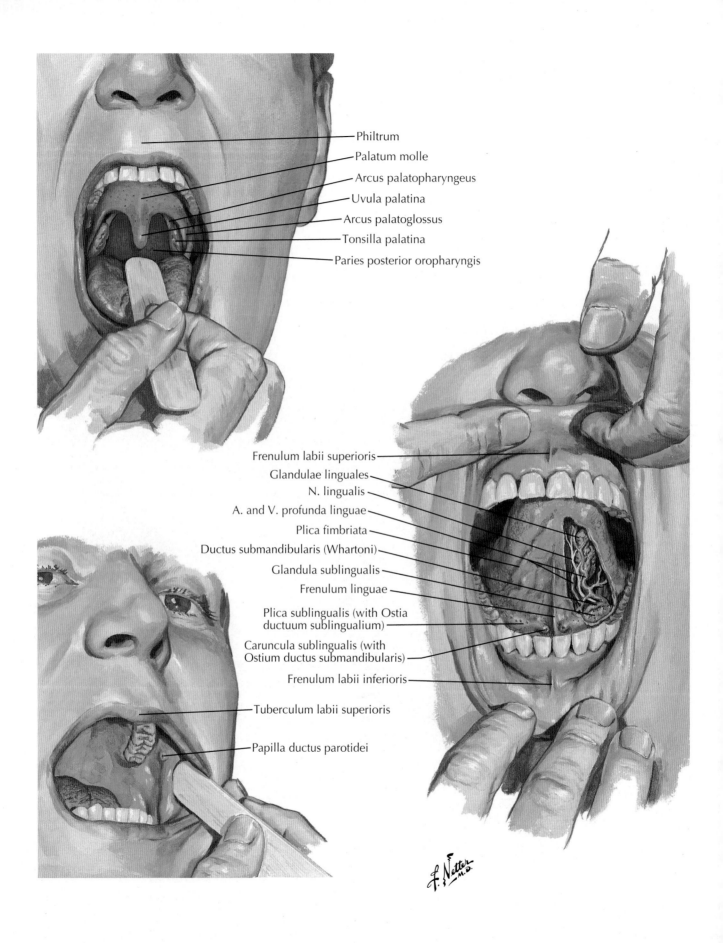

Philtrum

Palatum molle

Arcus palatopharyngeus

Uvula palatina

Arcus palatoglossus

Tonsilla palatina

Paries posterior oropharyngis

Frenulum labii superioris

Glandulae linguales

N. lingualis

A. and V. profunda linguae

Plica fimbriata

Ductus submandibularis (Whartoni)

Glandula sublingualis

Frenulum linguae

Plica sublingualis (with Ostia ductuum sublingualium)

Caruncula sublingualis (with Ostium ductus submandibularis)

Frenulum labii inferioris

Tuberculum labii superioris

Papilla ductus parotidei

Plate 83   **Stoma**

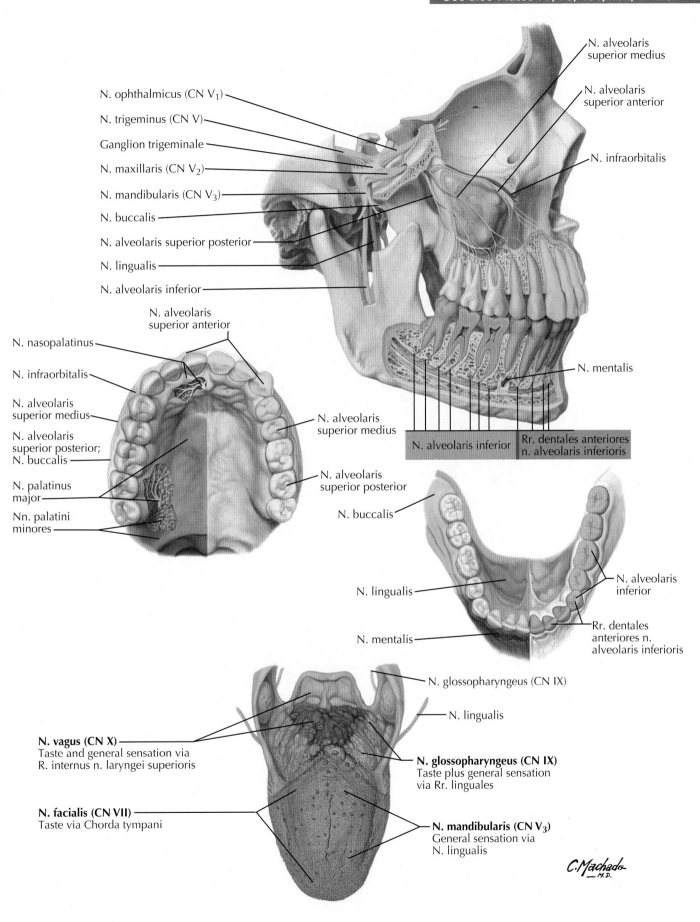

N. alveolaris superior medius

N. alveolaris superior anterior

N. ophthalmicus (CN V₁)

N. trigeminus (CN V)

Ganglion trigeminale

N. maxillaris (CN V₂)

N. mandibularis (CN V₃)

N. buccalis

N. alveolaris superior posterior

N. lingualis

N. alveolaris inferior

N. infraorbitalis

N. mentalis

N. alveolaris inferior

Rr. dentales anteriores n. alveolaris inferioris

N. alveolaris superior anterior

N. nasopalatinus

N. infraorbitalis

N. alveolaris superior medius

N. alveolaris superior posterior; N. buccalis

N. palatinus major

Nn. palatini minores

N. alveolaris superior medius

N. alveolaris superior posterior

N. buccalis

N. lingualis

N. mentalis

N. alveolaris inferior

Rr. dentales anteriores n. alveolaris inferioris

N. glossopharyngeus (CN IX)

N. lingualis

N. vagus (CN X)
Taste and general sensation via R. internus n. laryngei superioris

N. glossopharyngeus (CN IX)
Taste plus general sensation via Rr. linguales

N. facialis (CN VII)
Taste via Chorda tympani

N. mandibularis (CN V₃)
General sensation via N. lingualis

C. Machado
_M.D.

Stoma

Plate 84

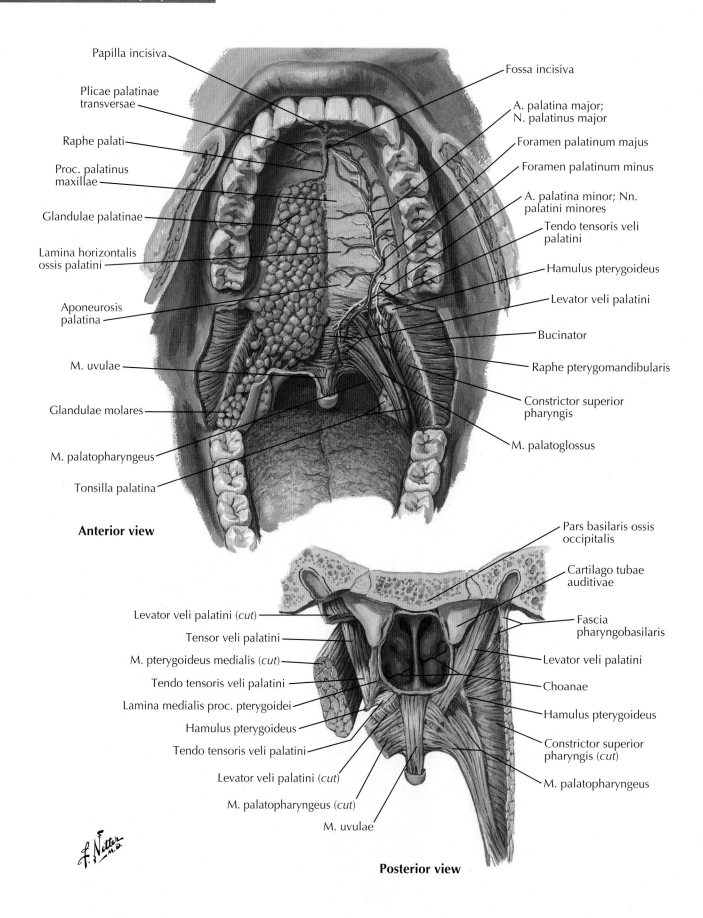

Papilla incisiva

Plicae palatinae transversae

Raphe palati

Proc. palatinus maxillae

Glandulae palatinae

Lamina horizontalis ossis palatini

Aponeurosis palatina

M. uvulae

Glandulae molares

M. palatopharyngeus

Tonsilla palatina

Anterior view

Fossa incisiva

A. palatina major; N. palatinus major

Foramen palatinum majus

Foramen palatinum minus

A. palatina minor; Nn. palatini minores

Tendo tensoris veli palatini

Hamulus pterygoideus

Levator veli palatini

Bucinator

Raphe pterygomandibularis

Constrictor superior pharyngis

M. palatoglossus

Levator veli palatini (*cut*)

Tensor veli palatini

M. pterygoideus medialis (*cut*)

Tendo tensoris veli palatini

Lamina medialis proc. pterygoidei

Hamulus pterygoideus

Tendo tensoris veli palatini

Levator veli palatini (*cut*)

M. palatopharyngeus (*cut*)

M. uvulae

Pars basilaris ossis occipitalis

Cartilago tubae auditivae

Fascia pharyngobasilaris

Levator veli palatini

Choanae

Hamulus pterygoideus

Constrictor superior pharyngis (*cut*)

M. palatopharyngeus

Posterior view

Plate 85

Stoma

Horizontal section below Lingula mandibulae (superior view)

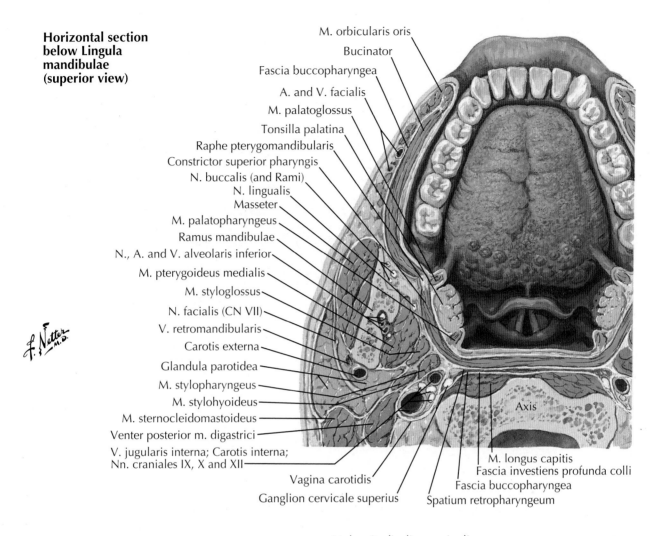

M. orbicularis oris

Bucinator

Fascia buccopharyngea

A. and V. facialis

M. palatoglossus

Tonsilla palatina

Raphe pterygomandibularis

Constrictor superior pharyngis

N. buccalis (and Rami)

N. lingualis

Masseter

M. palatopharyngeus

Ramus mandibulae

N., A. and V. alveolaris inferior

M. pterygoideus medialis

M. styloglossus

N. facialis (CN VII)

V. retromandibularis

Carotis externa

Glandula parotidea

M. stylopharyngeus

M. stylohyoideus

M. sternocleidomastoideus

Venter posterior m. digastrici

V. jugularis interna; Carotis interna; Nn. craniales IX, X and XII

Vagina carotidis

Ganglion cervicale superius

Axis

M. longus capitis

Fascia investiens profunda colli

Fascia buccopharyngea

Spatium retropharyngeum

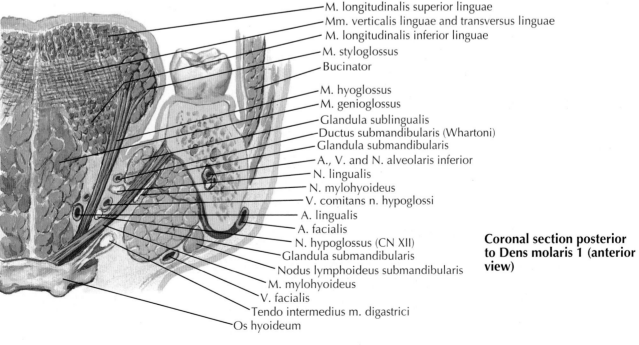

M. longitudinalis superior linguae

Mm. verticalis linguae and transversus linguae

M. longitudinalis inferior linguae

M. styloglossus

Bucinator

M. hyoglossus

M. genioglossus

Glandula sublingualis

Ductus submandibularis (Whartoni)

Glandula submandibularis

A., V. and N. alveolaris inferior

N. lingualis

N. mylohyoideus

V. comitans n. hypoglossi

A. lingualis

A. facialis

N. hypoglossus (CN XII)

Glandula submandibularis

Nodus lymphoideus submandibularis

M. mylohyoideus

V. facialis

Tendo intermedius m. digastrici

Os hyoideum

Coronal section posterior to Dens molaris 1 (anterior view)

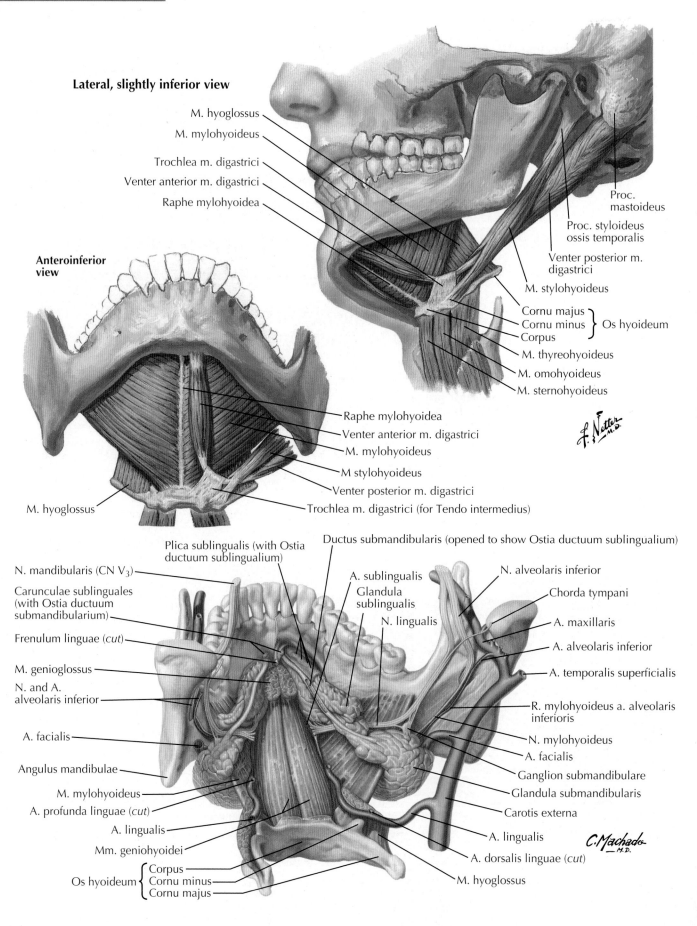

Lateral, slightly inferior view

M. hyoglossus
M. mylohyoideus
Trochlea m. digastrici
Venter anterior m. digastrici
Raphe mylohyoidea

Proc. mastoideus
Proc. styloideus ossis temporalis
Venter posterior m. digastrici
M. stylohyoideus
Cornu majus
Cornu minus } Os hyoideum
Corpus
M. thyreohyoideus
M. omohyoideus
M. sternohyoideus

Anteroinferior view

Raphe mylohyoidea
Venter anterior m. digastrici
M. mylohyoideus
M stylohyoideus
Venter posterior m. digastrici
Trochlea m. digastrici (for Tendo intermedius)

M. hyoglossus

Plica sublingualis (with Ostia ductuum sublingualium)
Ductus submandibularis (opened to show Ostia ductuum sublingualium)

N. mandibularis (CN V₃)
Carunculae sublinguales (with Ostia ductuum submandibularium)
Frenulum linguae (cut)
M. genioglossus
N. and A. alveolaris inferior
A. facialis
Angulus mandibulae
M. mylohyoideus
A. profunda linguae (cut)
A. lingualis
Mm. geniohyoidei
Os hyoideum { Corpus / Cornu minus / Cornu majus

A. sublingualis
Glandula sublingualis
N. lingualis

N. alveolaris inferior
Chorda tympani
A. maxillaris
A. alveolaris inferior
A. temporalis superficialis
R. mylohyoideus a. alveolaris inferioris
N. mylohyoideus
A. facialis
Ganglion submandibulare
Glandula submandibularis
Carotis externa
A. lingualis
A. dorsalis linguae (cut)
M. hyoglossus

Plate 87

Stoma

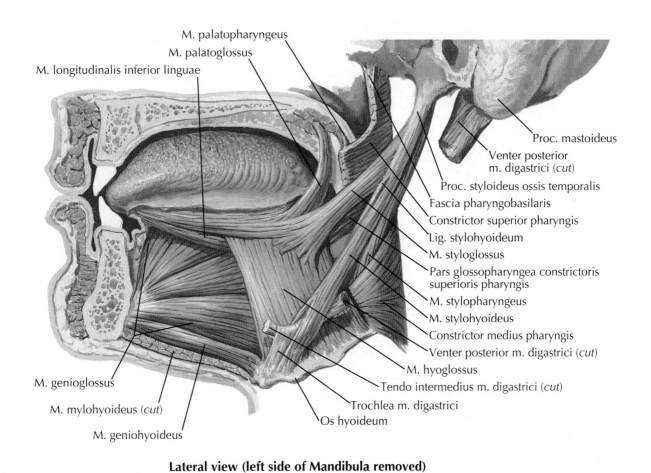

M. palatopharyngeus

M. palatoglossus

M. longitudinalis inferior linguae

Proc. mastoideus

Venter posterior m. digastrici (*cut*)

Proc. styloideus ossis temporalis

Fascia pharyngobasilaris

Constrictor superior pharyngis

Lig. stylohyoideum

M. styloglossus

Pars glossopharyngea constrictoris superioris pharyngis

M. stylopharyngeus

M. stylohyoideus

Constrictor medius pharyngis

Venter posterior m. digastrici (*cut*)

M. hyoglossus

Tendo intermedius m. digastrici (*cut*)

Trochlea m. digastrici

Os hyoideum

M. genioglossus

M. mylohyoideus (*cut*)

M. geniohyoideus

Lateral view (left side of Mandibula removed)

N. lingualis

Ganglion submandibulare

A. and V. profunda linguae

Constrictor superior pharyngis

M. styloglossus

M. palatoglossus (*cut*)

Lig. stylohyoideum

M. stylopharyngeus

M. hyoglossus (*cut*)

A. lingualis

Carotis externa

V. jugularis interna

V. retromandibularis

V. facialis

V. facialis communis

Ductus submandibularis (Whartoni)

V. lingualis

M. genioglossus

A. and V. sublingualis

M. geniohyoideus

Os hyoideum

R. suprahyoideus a. lingualis

A. and V. dorsalis linguae

N. hypoglossus (CN XII)

Vena comitans n. hypoglossi

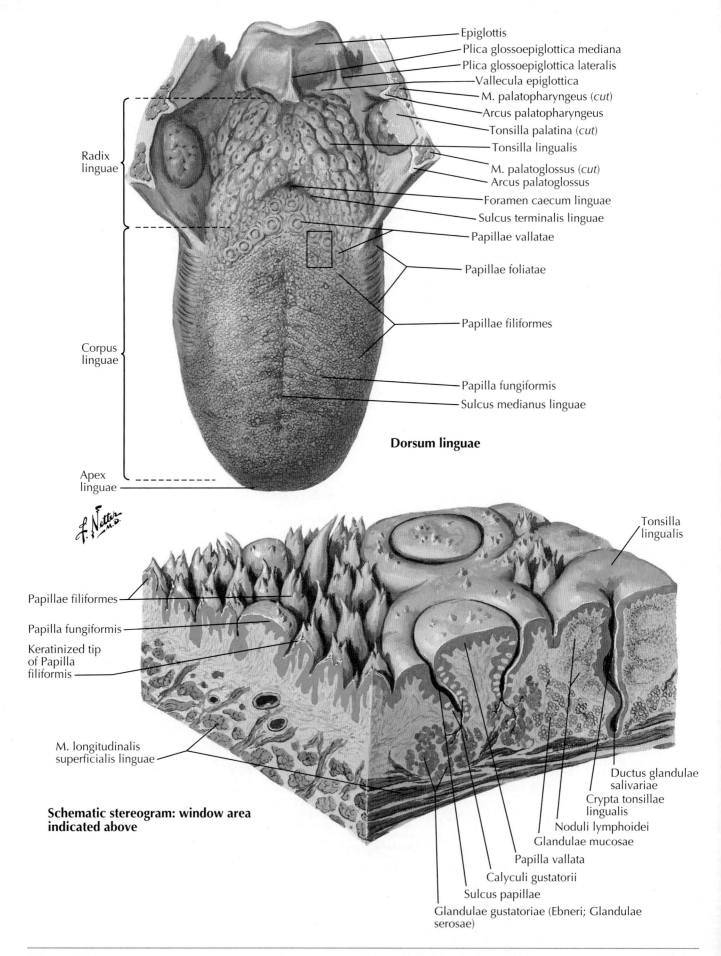

Epiglottis

Plica glossoepiglottica mediana

Plica glossoepiglottica lateralis

Vallecula epiglottica

M. palatopharyngeus (*cut*)

Arcus palatopharyngeus

Tonsilla palatina (*cut*)

Tonsilla lingualis

M. palatoglossus (*cut*)

Arcus palatoglossus

Foramen caecum linguae

Sulcus terminalis linguae

Papillae vallatae

Papillae foliatae

Papillae filiformes

Papilla fungiformis

Sulcus medianus linguae

Radix linguae

Corpus linguae

Apex linguae

Dorsum linguae

Papillae filiformes

Papilla fungiformis

Keratinized tip of Papilla filiformis

Tonsilla lingualis

M. longitudinalis superficialis linguae

Schematic stereogram: window area indicated above

Ductus glandulae salivariae

Crypta tonsillae lingualis

Noduli lymphoidei

Glandulae mucosae

Papilla vallata

Calyculi gustatorii

Sulcus papillae

Glandulae gustatoriae (Ebneri; Glandulae serosae)

Plate 89   **Stoma**

**Medial view
sagittal section**

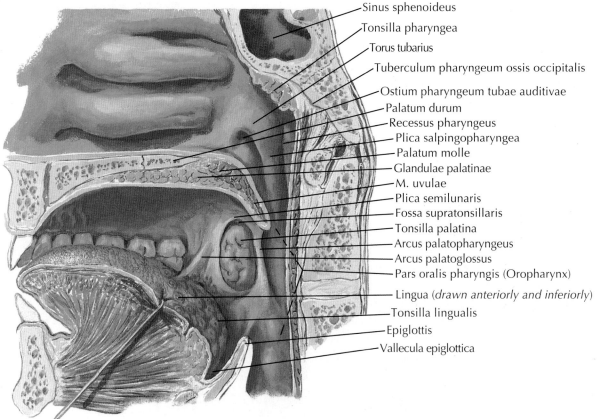

Sinus sphenoideus
Tonsilla pharyngea
Torus tubarius
Tuberculum pharyngeum ossis occipitalis
Ostium pharyngeum tubae auditivae
Palatum durum
Recessus pharyngeus
Plica salpingopharyngea
Palatum molle
Glandulae palatinae
M. uvulae
Plica semilunaris
Fossa supratonsillaris
Tonsilla palatina
Arcus palatopharyngeus
Arcus palatoglossus
Pars oralis pharyngis (Oropharynx)
Lingua (*drawn anteriorly and inferiorly*)
Tonsilla lingualis
Epiglottis
Vallecula epiglottica

Tunica muscosa pharyngis removed

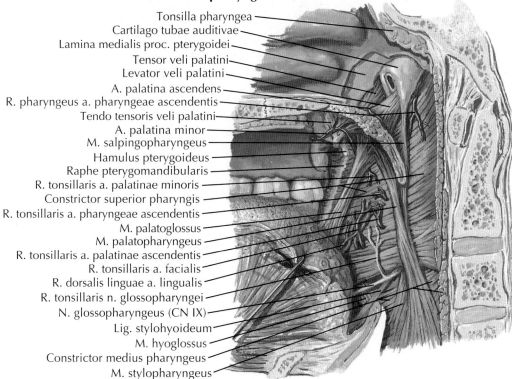

Tonsilla pharyngea
Cartilago tubae auditivae
Lamina medialis proc. pterygoidei
Tensor veli palatini
Levator veli palatini
A. palatina ascendens
R. pharyngeus a. pharyngeae ascendentis
Tendo tensoris veli palatini
A. palatina minor
M. salpingopharyngeus
Hamulus pterygoideus
Raphe pterygomandibularis
R. tonsillaris a. palatinae minoris
Constrictor superior pharyngis
R. tonsillaris a. pharyngeae ascendentis
M. palatoglossus
M. palatopharyngeus
R. tonsillaris a. palatinae ascendentis
R. tonsillaris a. facialis
R. dorsalis linguae a. lingualis
R. tonsillaris n. glossopharyngei
N. glossopharyngeus (CN IX)
Lig. stylohyoideum
M. hyoglossus
Constrictor medius pharyngeus
M. stylopharyngeus

Stoma

Plate 90

Superior view of the basis cranii showing line of cut and the removed part

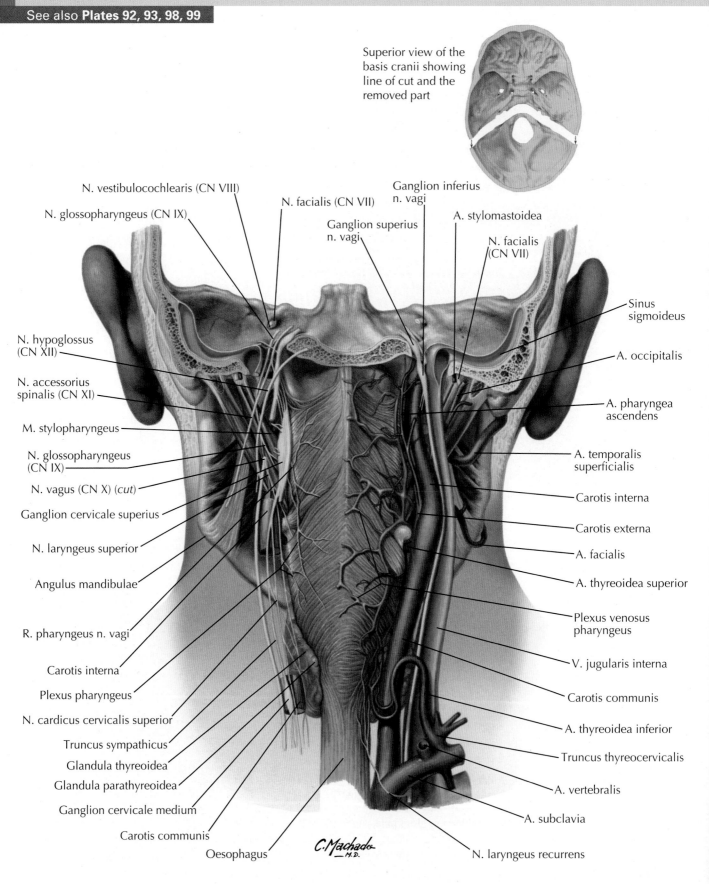

N. vestibulocochlearis (CN VIII)

N. glossopharyngeus (CN IX)

N. facialis (CN VII)

Ganglion inferius n. vagi

Ganglion superius n. vagi

A. stylomastoidea

N. facialis (CN VII)

Sinus sigmoideus

N. hypoglossus (CN XII)

A. occipitalis

N. accessorius spinalis (CN XI)

A. pharyngea ascendens

M. stylopharyngeus

N. glossopharyngeus (CN IX)

A. temporalis superficialis

N. vagus (CN X) (cut)

Carotis interna

Ganglion cervicale superius

Carotis externa

N. laryngeus superior

A. facialis

Angulus mandibulae

A. thyreoidea superior

R. pharyngeus n. vagi

Plexus venosus pharyngeus

Carotis interna

V. jugularis interna

Plexus pharyngeus

Carotis communis

N. cardicus cervicalis superior

A. thyreoidea inferior

Truncus sympathicus

Truncus thyreocervicalis

Glandula thyreoidea

A. vertebralis

Glandula parathyreoidea

Ganglion cervicale medium

A. subclavia

Carotis communis

N. laryngeus recurrens

Oesophagus

C. Machado
M.D.

Plate 91

Pharynx

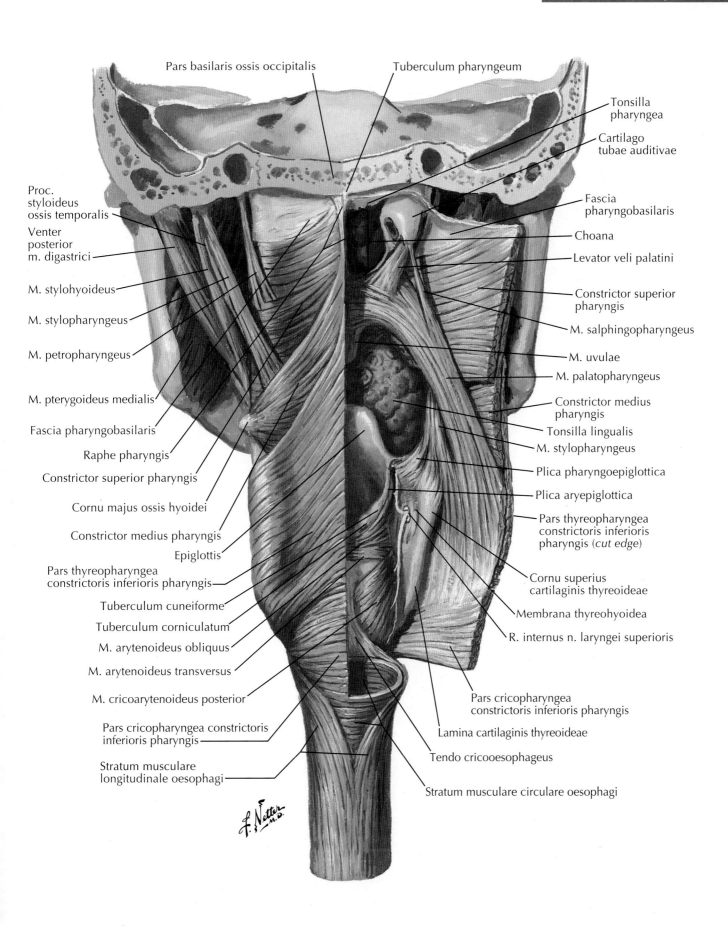

Pars basilaris ossis occipitalis

Tuberculum pharyngeum

Tonsilla pharyngea

Cartilago tubae auditivae

Proc. styloideus ossis temporalis

Venter posterior m. digastrici

M. stylohyoideus

M. stylopharyngeus

M. petropharyngeus

M. pterygoideus medialis

Fascia pharyngobasilaris

Raphe pharyngis

Constrictor superior pharyngis

Cornu majus ossis hyoidei

Constrictor medius pharyngis

Epiglottis

Pars thyreopharyngea constrictoris inferioris pharyngis

Tuberculum cuneiforme

Tuberculum corniculatum

M. arytenoideus obliquus

M. arytenoideus transversus

M. cricoarytenoideus posterior

Pars cricopharyngea constrictoris inferioris pharyngis

Stratum musculare longitudinale oesophagi

Fascia pharyngobasilaris

Choana

Levator veli palatini

Constrictor superior pharyngis

M. salphingopharyngeus

M. uvulae

M. palatopharyngeus

Constrictor medius pharyngis

Tonsilla lingualis

M. stylopharyngeus

Plica pharyngoepiglottica

Plica aryepiglottica

Pars thyreopharyngea constrictoris inferioris pharyngis (cut edge)

Cornu superius cartilaginis thyreoideae

Membrana thyreohyoidea

R. internus n. laryngei superioris

Pars cricopharyngea constrictoris inferioris pharyngis

Lamina cartilaginis thyreoideae

Tendo cricooesophageus

Stratum musculare circulare oesophagi

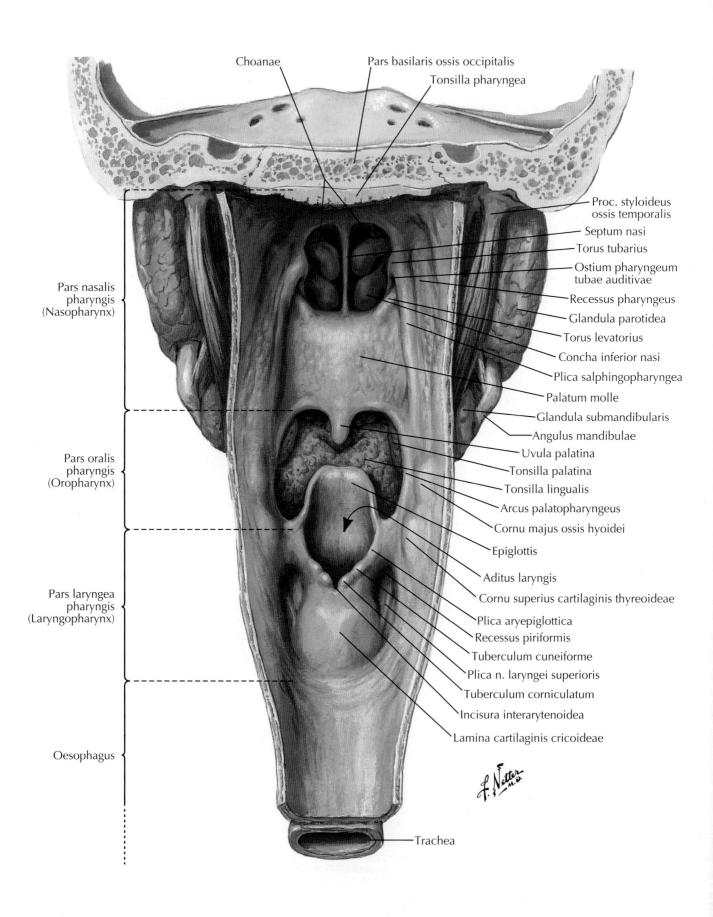

Choanae

Pars basilaris ossis occipitalis

Tonsilla pharyngea

Proc. styloideus ossis temporalis

Septum nasi

Torus tubarius

Ostium pharyngeum tubae auditivae

Recessus pharyngeus

Glandula parotidea

Torus levatorius

Concha inferior nasi

Plica salphingopharyngea

Palatum molle

Glandula submandibularis

Angulus mandibulae

Uvula palatina

Tonsilla palatina

Tonsilla lingualis

Arcus palatopharyngeus

Cornu majus ossis hyoidei

Epiglottis

Aditus laryngis

Cornu superius cartilaginis thyreoideae

Plica aryepiglottica

Recessus piriformis

Tuberculum cuneiforme

Plica n. laryngei superioris

Tuberculum corniculatum

Incisura interarytenoidea

Lamina cartilaginis cricoideae

Pars nasalis pharyngis (Nasopharynx)

Pars oralis pharyngis (Oropharynx)

Pars laryngea pharyngis (Laryngopharynx)

Oesophagus

Trachea

Plate 93   **Pharynx**

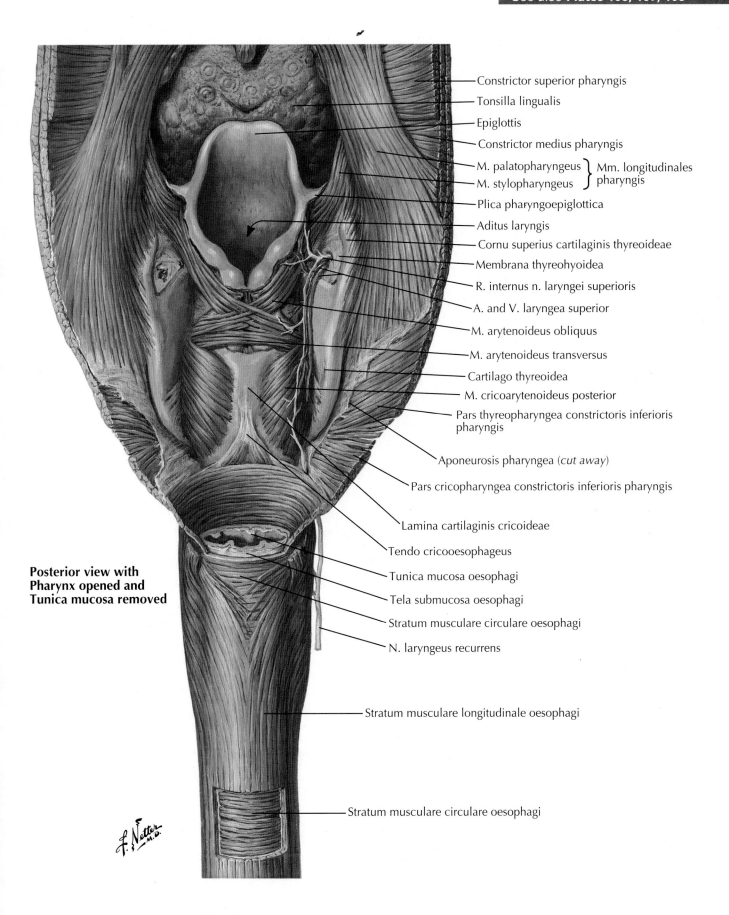

Constrictor superior pharyngis

Tonsilla lingualis

Epiglottis

Constrictor medius pharyngis

M. palatopharyngeus ⎫ Mm. longitudinales
M. stylopharyngeus ⎭ pharyngis

Plica pharyngoepiglottica

Aditus laryngis

Cornu superius cartilaginis thyreoideae

Membrana thyreohyoidea

R. internus n. laryngei superioris

A. and V. laryngea superior

M. arytenoideus obliquus

M. arytenoideus transversus

Cartilago thyreoidea

M. cricoarytenoideus posterior

Pars thyreopharyngea constrictoris inferioris pharyngis

Aponeurosis pharyngea (*cut away*)

Pars cricopharyngea constrictoris inferioris pharyngis

Lamina cartilaginis cricoideae

Tendo cricooesophageus

Tunica mucosa oesophagi

Tela submucosa oesophagi

Stratum musculare circulare oesophagi

N. laryngeus recurrens

Stratum musculare longitudinale oesophagi

Stratum musculare circulare oesophagi

Posterior view with Pharynx opened and Tunica mucosa removed

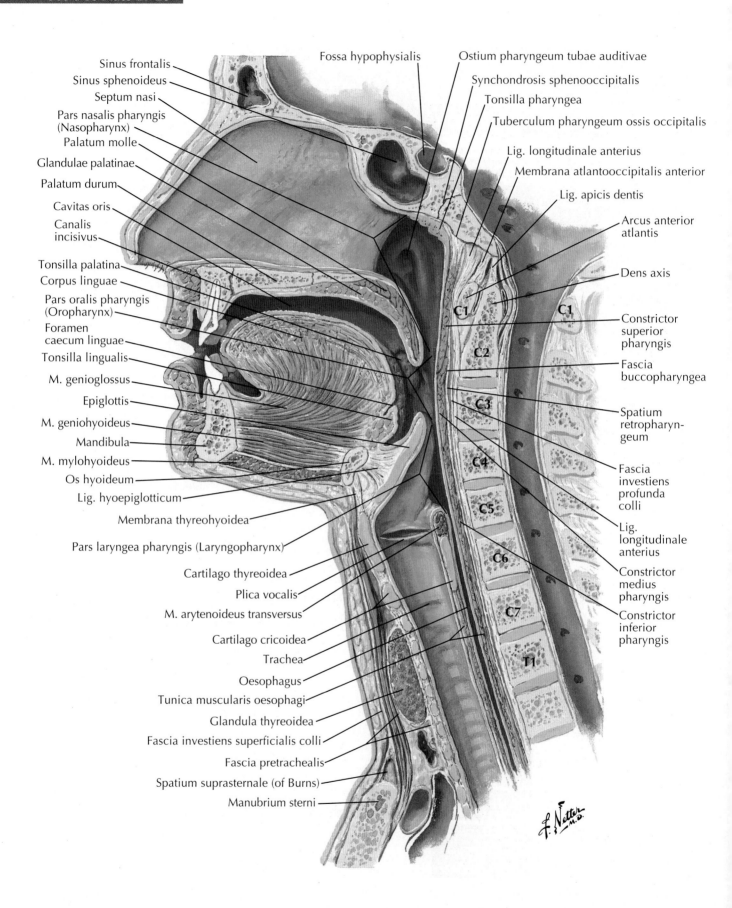

Sinus frontalis

Sinus sphenoideus

Septum nasi

Pars nasalis pharyngis
(Nasopharynx)

Palatum molle

Glandulae palatinae

Palatum durum

Cavitas oris

Canalis
incisivus

Tonsilla palatina

Corpus linguae

Pars oralis pharyngis
(Oropharynx)

Foramen
caecum linguae

Tonsilla lingualis

M. genioglossus

Epiglottis

M. geniohyoideus

Mandibula

M. mylohyoideus

Os hyoideum

Lig. hyoepiglotticum

Membrana thyreohyoidea

Pars laryngea pharyngis (Laryngopharynx)

Cartilago thyreoidea

Plica vocalis

M. arytenoideus transversus

Cartilago cricoidea

Trachea

Oesophagus

Tunica muscularis oesophagi

Glandula thyreoidea

Fascia investiens superficialis colli

Fascia pretrachealis

Spatium suprasternale (of Burns)

Manubrium sterni

Fossa hypophysialis

Ostium pharyngeum tubae auditivae

Synchondrosis sphenooccipitalis

Tonsilla pharyngea

Tuberculum pharyngeum ossis occipitalis

Lig. longitudinale anterius

Membrana atlantooccipitalis anterior

Lig. apicis dentis

Arcus anterior
atlantis

Dens axis

Constrictor
superior
pharyngis

Fascia
buccopharyngea

Spatium
retropharyn-
geum

Fascia
investiens
profunda
colli

Lig.
longitudinale
anterius

Constrictor
medius
pharyngis

Constrictor
inferior
pharyngis

C1

C1

C2

C3

C4

C5

C6

C7

T1

Plate 95

Pharynx

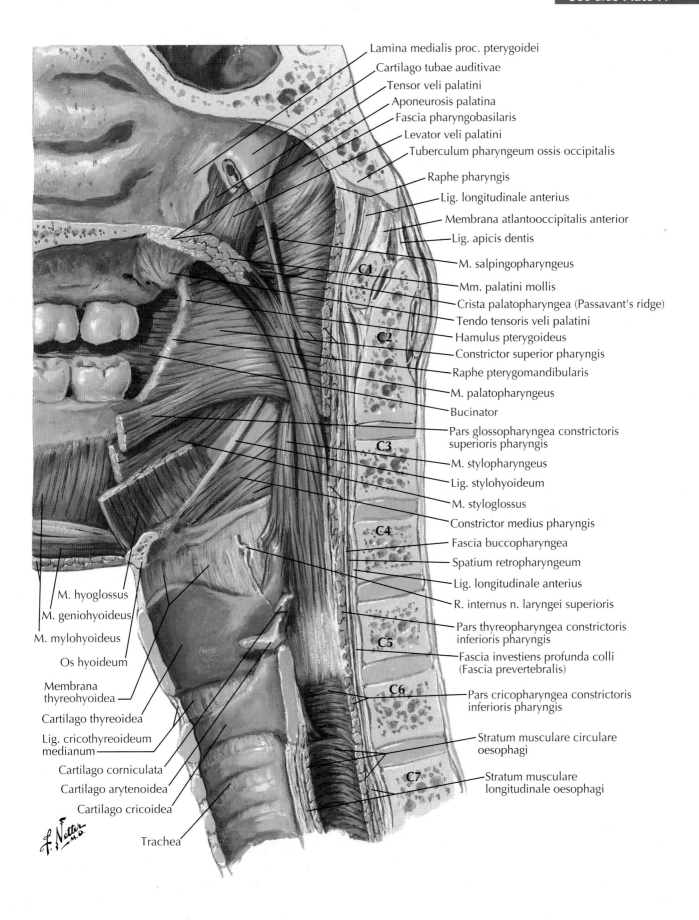

Lamina medialis proc. pterygoidei
Cartilago tubae auditivae
Tensor veli palatini
Aponeurosis palatina
Fascia pharyngobasilaris
Levator veli palatini
Tuberculum pharyngeum ossis occipitalis
Raphe pharyngis
Lig. longitudinale anterius
Membrana atlantooccipitalis anterior
Lig. apicis dentis
M. salpingopharyngeus
Mm. palatini mollis
Crista palatopharyngea (Passavant's ridge)
Tendo tensoris veli palatini
Hamulus pterygoideus
Constrictor superior pharyngis
Raphe pterygomandibularis
M. palatopharyngeus
Bucinator
Pars glossopharyngea constrictoris superioris pharyngis
M. stylopharyngeus
Lig. stylohyoideum
M. styloglossus
Constrictor medius pharyngis
Fascia buccopharyngea
Spatium retropharyngeum
Lig. longitudinale anterius
R. internus n. laryngei superioris
Pars thyreopharyngea constrictoris inferioris pharyngis
Fascia investiens profunda colli (Fascia prevertebralis)
Pars cricopharyngea constrictoris inferioris pharyngis
Stratum musculare circulare oesophagi
Stratum musculare longitudinale oesophagi

C1
C2
C3
C4
C5
C6
C7

M. hyoglossus
M. geniohyoideus
M. mylohyoideus
Os hyoideum
Membrana thyreohyoidea
Cartilago thyreoidea
Lig. cricothyreoideum medianum
Cartilago corniculata
Cartilago arytenoidea
Cartilago cricoidea
Trachea

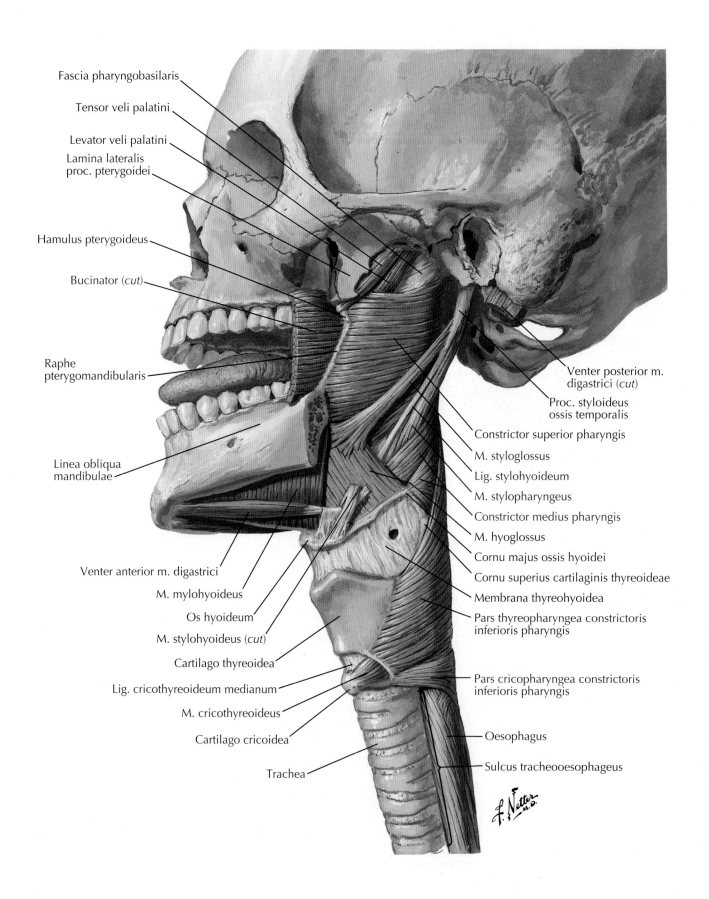

Fascia pharyngobasilaris

Tensor veli palatini

Levator veli palatini

Lamina lateralis
proc. pterygoidei

Hamulus pterygoideus

Bucinator (*cut*)

Raphe
pterygomandibularis

Linea obliqua
mandibulae

Venter anterior m. digastrici

M. mylohyoideus

Os hyoideum

M. stylohyoideus (*cut*)

Cartilago thyreoidea

Lig. cricothyreoideum medianum

M. cricothyreoideus

Cartilago cricoidea

Trachea

Venter posterior m.
digastrici (*cut*)

Proc. styloideus
ossis temporalis

Constrictor superior pharyngis

M. styloglossus

Lig. stylohyoideum

M. stylopharyngeus

Constrictor medius pharyngis

M. hyoglossus

Cornu majus ossis hyoidei

Cornu superius cartilaginis thyreoideae

Membrana thyreohyoidea

Pars thyreopharyngea constrictoris
inferioris pharyngis

Pars cricopharyngea constrictoris
inferioris pharyngis

Oesophagus

Sulcus tracheooesophageus

Plate 97

Pharynx

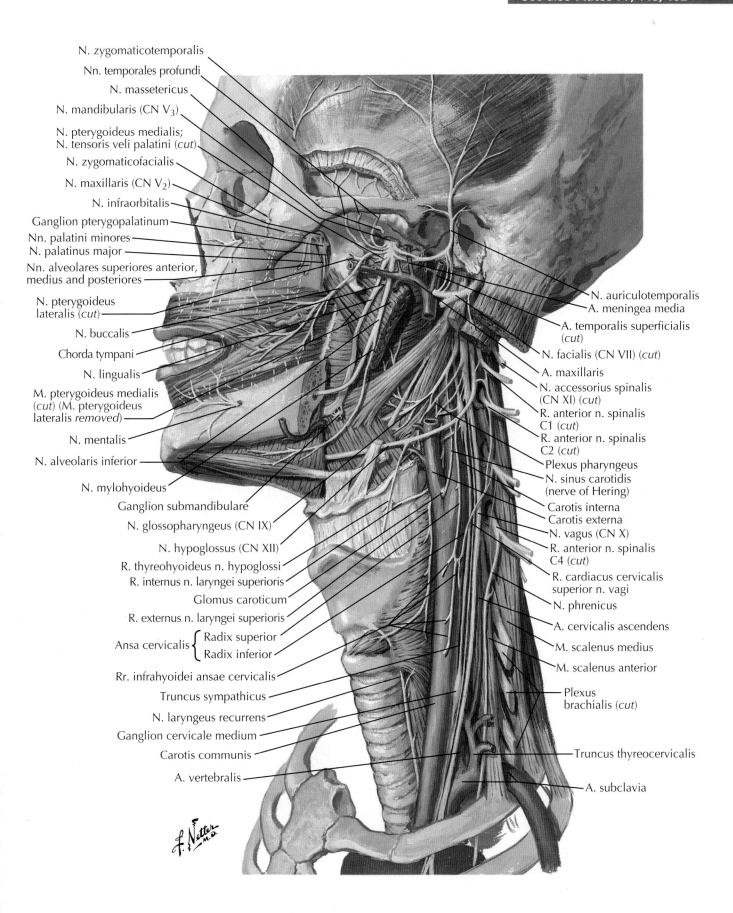

N. zygomaticotemporalis

Nn. temporales profundi

N. massetericus

N. mandibularis (CN V₃)

N. pterygoideus medialis;
N. tensoris veli palatini (cut)

N. zygomaticofacialis

N. maxillaris (CN V₂)

N. infraorbitalis

Ganglion pterygopalatinum

Nn. palatini minores

N. palatinus major

Nn. alveolares superiores anterior,
medius and posteriores

N. pterygoideus
lateralis (cut)

N. buccalis

Chorda tympani

N. lingualis

M. pterygoideus medialis
(cut) (M. pterygoideus
lateralis removed)

N. mentalis

N. alveolaris inferior

N. mylohyoideus

Ganglion submandibulare

N. glossopharyngeus (CN IX)

N. hypoglossus (CN XII)

R. thyreohyoideus n. hypoglossi

R. internus n. laryngei superioris

Glomus caroticum

R. externus n. laryngei superioris

Ansa cervicalis { Radix superior
Radix inferior

Rr. infrahyoidei ansae cervicalis

Truncus sympathicus

N. laryngeus recurrens

Ganglion cervicale medium

Carotis communis

A. vertebralis

N. auriculotemporalis

A. meningea media

A. temporalis superficialis
(cut)

N. facialis (CN VII) (cut)

A. maxillaris

N. accessorius spinalis
(CN XI) (cut)

R. anterior n. spinalis
C1 (cut)

R. anterior n. spinalis
C2 (cut)

Plexus pharyngeus

N. sinus carotidis
(nerve of Hering)

Carotis interna

Carotis externa

N. vagus (CN X)

R. anterior n. spinalis
C4 (cut)

R. cardiacus cervicalis
superior n. vagi

N. phrenicus

A. cervicalis ascendens

M. scalenus medius

M. scalenus anterior

Plexus
brachialis (cut)

Truncus thyreocervicalis

A. subclavia

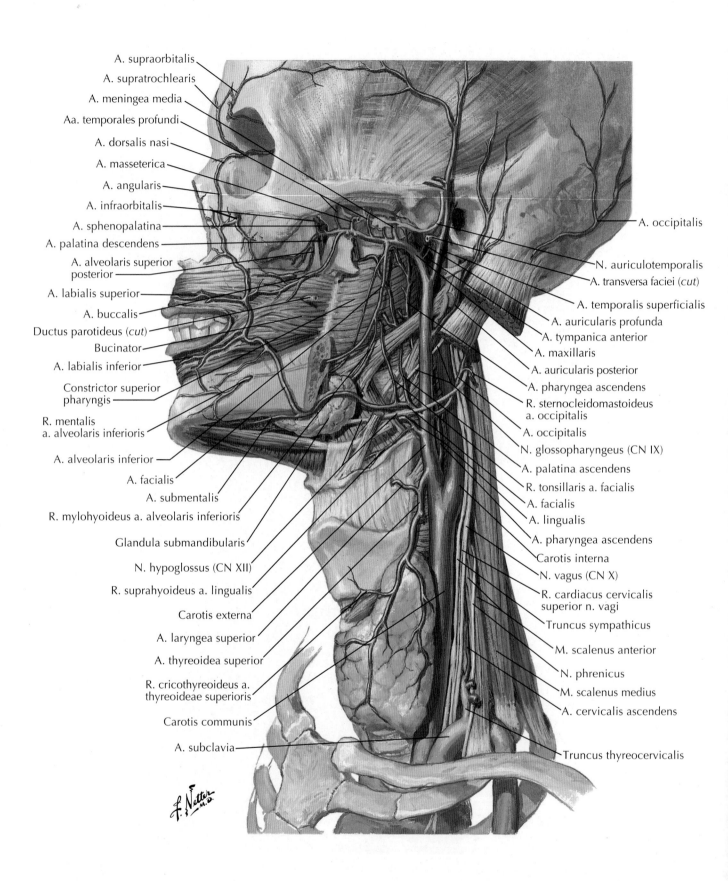

A. supraorbitalis

A. supratrochlearis

A. meningea media

Aa. temporales profundi

A. dorsalis nasi

A. masseterica

A. angularis

A. infraorbitalis

A. sphenopalatina

A. palatina descendens

A. alveolaris superior posterior

A. labialis superior

A. buccalis

Ductus parotideus (*cut*)

Bucinator

A. labialis inferior

Constrictor superior pharyngis

R. mentalis a. alveolaris inferioris

A. alveolaris inferior

A. facialis

A. submentalis

R. mylohyoideus a. alveolaris inferioris

Glandula submandibularis

N. hypoglossus (CN XII)

R. suprahyoideus a. lingualis

Carotis externa

A. laryngea superior

A. thyreoidea superior

R. cricothyreoideus a. thyreoideae superioris

Carotis communis

A. subclavia

A. occipitalis

N. auriculotemporalis

A. transversa faciei (*cut*)

A. temporalis superficialis

A. auricularis profunda

A. tympanica anterior

A. maxillaris

A. auricularis posterior

A. pharyngea ascendens

R. sternocleidomastoideus a. occipitalis

A. occipitalis

N. glossopharyngeus (CN IX)

A. palatina ascendens

R. tonsillaris a. facialis

A. facialis

A. lingualis

A. pharyngea ascendens

Carotis interna

N. vagus (CN X)

R. cardiacus cervicalis superior n. vagi

Truncus sympathicus

M. scalenus anterior

N. phrenicus

M. scalenus medius

A. cervicalis ascendens

Truncus thyreocervicalis

Plate 99

Pharynx

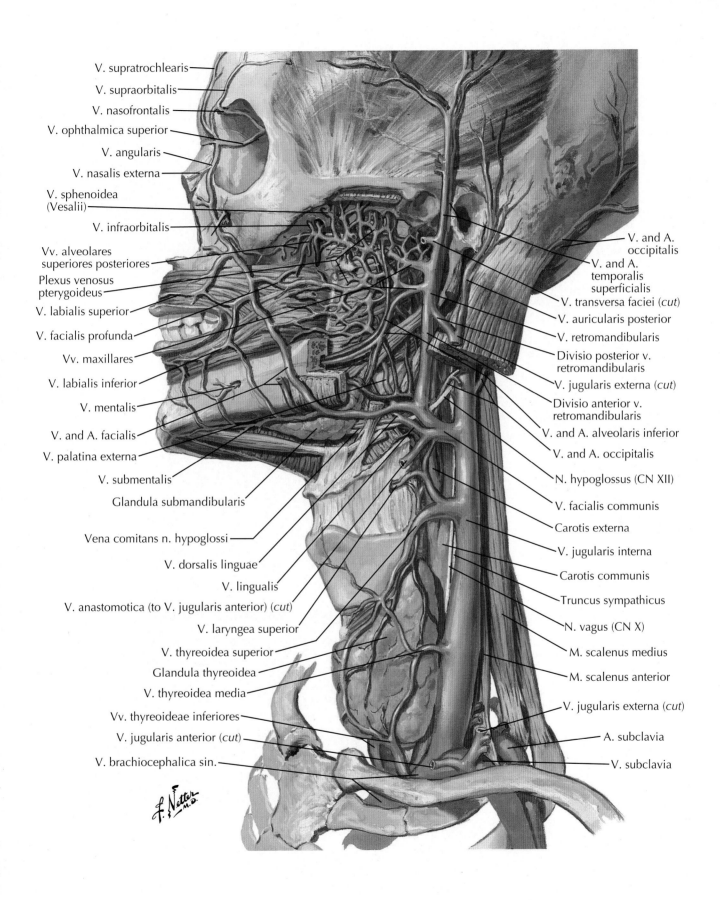

V. supratrochlearis

V. supraorbitalis

V. nasofrontalis

V. ophthalmica superior

V. angularis

V. nasalis externa

V. sphenoidea (Vesalii)

V. infraorbitalis

Vv. alveolares superiores posteriores

Plexus venosus pterygoideus

V. labialis superior

V. facialis profunda

Vv. maxillares

V. labialis inferior

V. mentalis

V. and A. facialis

V. palatina externa

V. submentalis

Glandula submandibularis

Vena comitans n. hypoglossi

V. dorsalis linguae

V. lingualis

V. anastomotica (to V. jugularis anterior) (cut)

V. laryngea superior

V. thyreoidea superior

Glandula thyreoidea

V. thyreoidea media

Vv. thyreoideae inferiores

V. jugularis anterior (cut)

V. brachiocephalica sin.

V. and A. occipitalis

V. and A. temporalis superficialis

V. transversa faciei (cut)

V. auricularis posterior

V. retromandibularis

Divisio posterior v. retromandibularis

V. jugularis externa (cut)

Divisio anterior v. retromandibularis

V. and A. alveolaris inferior

V. and A. occipitalis

N. hypoglossus (CN XII)

V. facialis communis

Carotis externa

V. jugularis interna

Carotis communis

Truncus sympathicus

N. vagus (CN X)

M. scalenus medius

M. scalenus anterior

V. jugularis externa (cut)

A. subclavia

V. subclavia

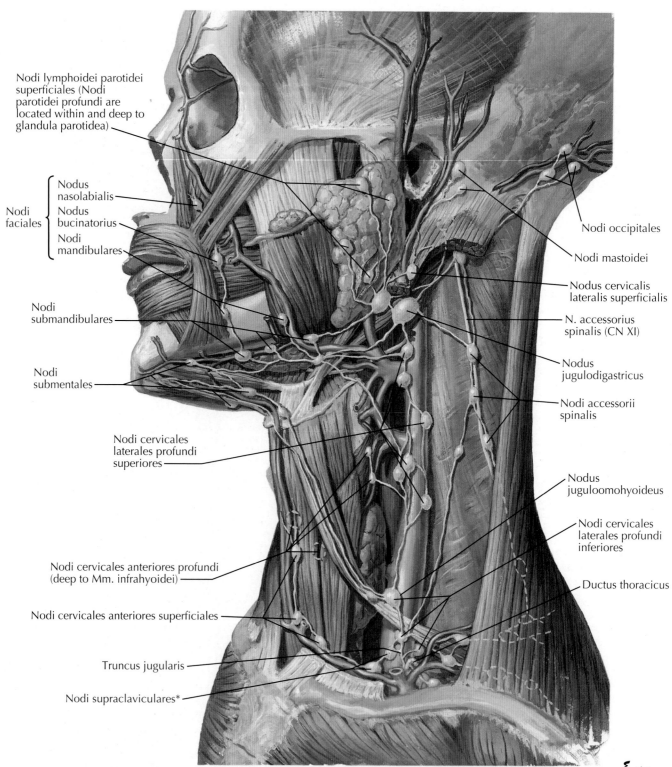

Nodi lymphoidei parotidei superficiales (Nodi parotidei profundi are located within and deep to glandula parotidea)

Nodi faciales
- Nodus nasolabialis
- Nodus bucinatorius
- Nodi mandibulares

Nodi submandibulares

Nodi submentales

Nodi cervicales laterales profundi superiores

Nodi cervicales anteriores profundi (deep to Mm. infrahyoidei)

Nodi cervicales anteriores superficiales

Truncus jugularis

Nodi supraclaviculares*

Nodi occipitales

Nodi mastoidei

Nodus cervicalis lateralis superficialis

N. accessorius spinalis (CN XI)

Nodus jugulodigastricus

Nodi accessorii spinalis

Nodus juguloomohyoideus

Nodi cervicales laterales profundi inferiores

Ductus thoracicus

*Nodi supraclaviculares, especially on the left, are also sometimes referred to as the signal or sentinel lymph nodes of Virchow or Troisier, especially when sufficiently enlarged and palpable. These nodes (or a single node) are so termed because they may be the first recognized presumptive evidence of malignant disease in the viscera.

Plate 101

Pharynx

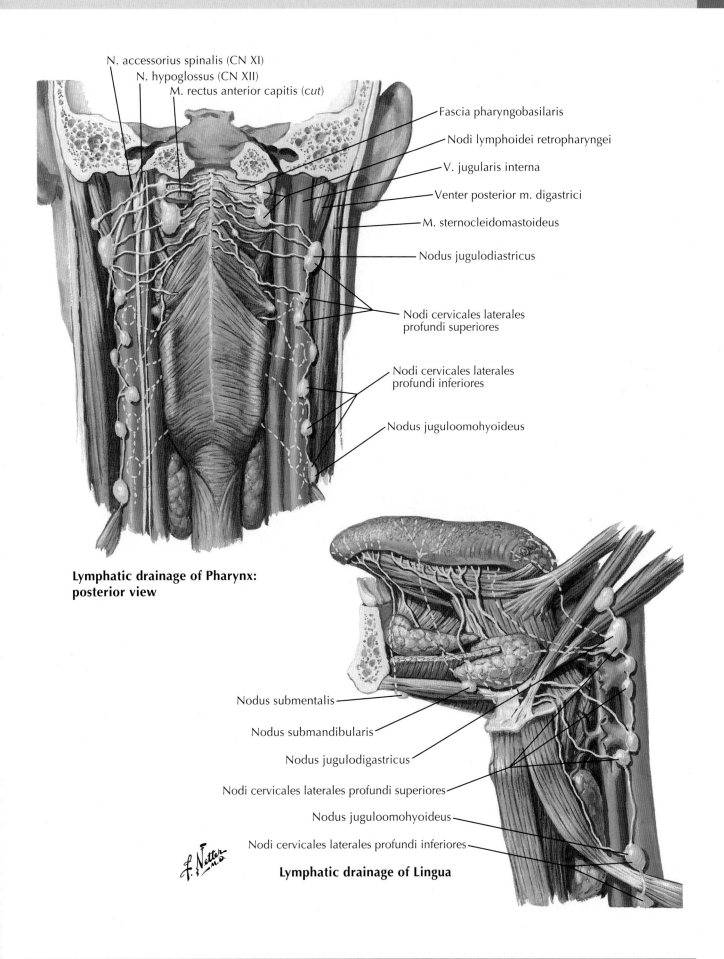

N. accessorius spinalis (CN XI)
N. hypoglossus (CN XII)
M. rectus anterior capitis (*cut*)

Fascia pharyngobasilaris

Nodi lymphoidei retropharyngei

V. jugularis interna

Venter posterior m. digastrici

M. sternocleidomastoideus

Nodus jugulodiastricus

Nodi cervicales laterales profundi superiores

Nodi cervicales laterales profundi inferiores

Nodus juguloomohyoideus

Lymphatic drainage of Pharynx: posterior view

Nodus submentalis

Nodus submandibularis

Nodus jugulodigastricus

Nodi cervicales laterales profundi superiores

Nodus juguloomohyoideus

Nodi cervicales laterales profundi inferiores

Lymphatic drainage of Lingua

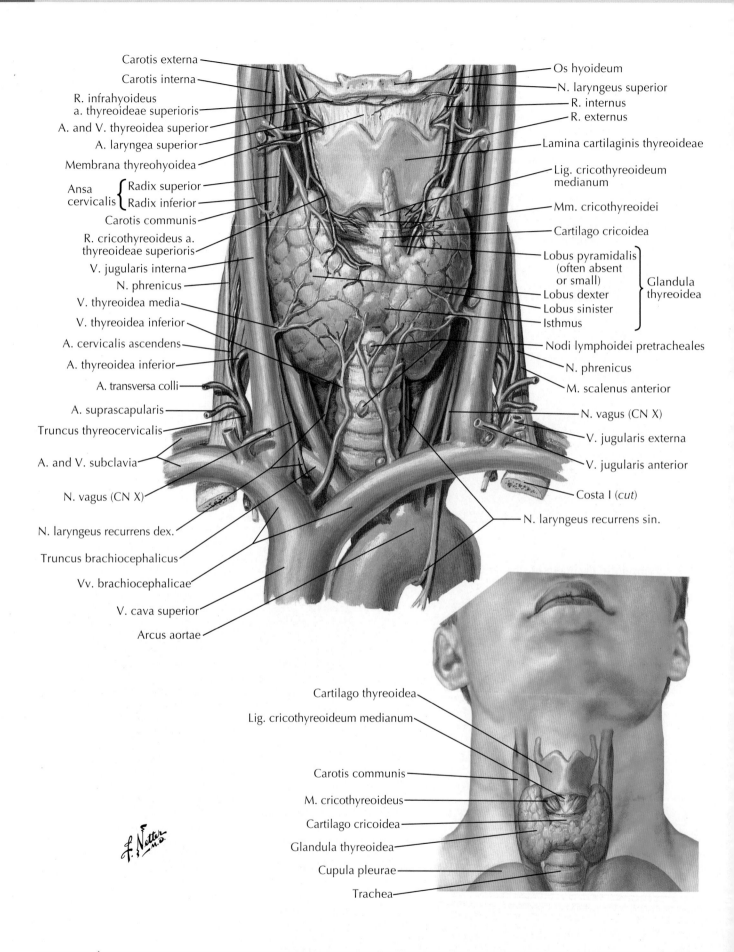

Carotis externa

Carotis interna

R. infrahyoideus
a. thyreoideae superioris

A. and V. thyreoidea superior

A. laryngea superior

Membrana thyreohyoidea

Ansa { Radix superior
cervicalis { Radix inferior

Carotis communis

R. cricothyreoideus a.
thyreoideae superioris

V. jugularis interna

N. phrenicus

V. thyreoidea media

V. thyreoidea inferior

A. cervicalis ascendens

A. thyreoidea inferior

A. transversa colli

A. suprascapularis

Truncus thyreocervicalis

A. and V. subclavia

N. vagus (CN X)

N. laryngeus recurrens dex.

Truncus brachiocephalicus

Vv. brachiocephalicae

V. cava superior

Arcus aortae

Os hyoideum

N. laryngeus superior

R. internus

R. externus

Lamina cartilaginis thyreoideae

Lig. cricothyreoideum
medianum

Mm. cricothyreoidei

Cartilago cricoidea

Lobus pyramidalis
(often absent
or small)

Lobus dexter

Lobus sinister

Isthmus

} Glandula
thyreoidea

Nodi lymphoidei pretracheales

N. phrenicus

M. scalenus anterior

N. vagus (CN X)

V. jugularis externa

V. jugularis anterior

Costa I (cut)

N. laryngeus recurrens sin.

Cartilago thyreoidea

Lig. cricothyreoideum medianum

Carotis communis

M. cricothyreoideus

Cartilago cricoidea

Glandula thyreoidea

Cupula pleurae

Trachea

Plate 103

Larynx and Glandulae Endocrinae

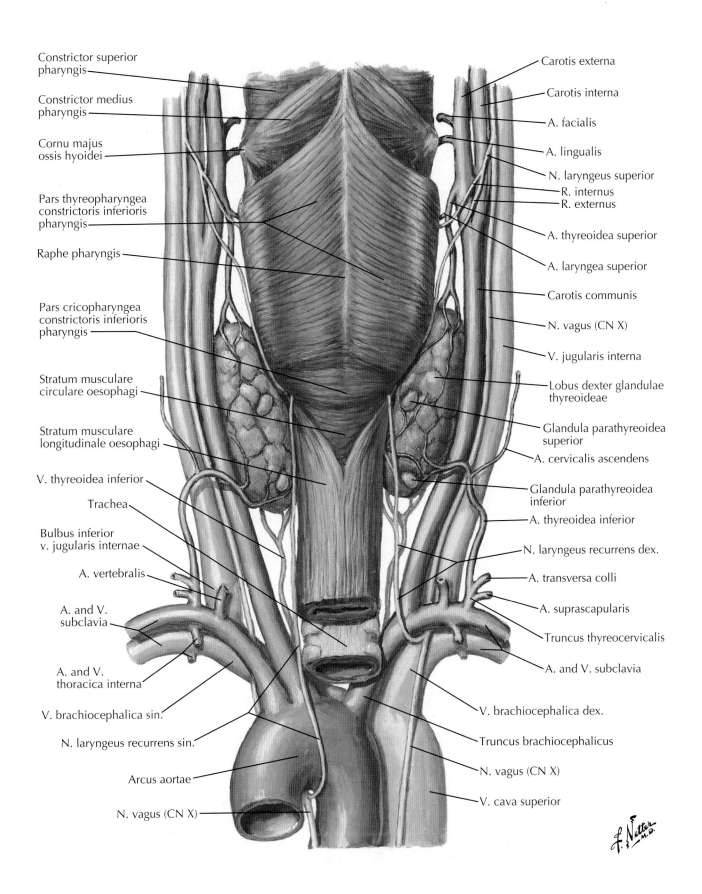

Constrictor superior pharyngis

Constrictor medius pharyngis

Cornu majus ossis hyoidei

Pars thyreopharyngea constrictoris inferioris pharyngis

Raphe pharyngis

Pars cricopharyngea constrictoris inferioris pharyngis

Stratum musculare circulare oesophagi

Stratum musculare longitudinale oesophagi

V. thyreoidea inferior

Trachea

Bulbus inferior v. jugularis internae

A. vertebralis

A. and V. subclavia

A. and V. thoracica interna

V. brachiocephalica sin.

N. laryngeus recurrens sin.

Arcus aortae

N. vagus (CN X)

Carotis externa

Carotis interna

A. facialis

A. lingualis

N. laryngeus superior

R. internus
R. externus

A. thyreoidea superior

A. laryngea superior

Carotis communis

N. vagus (CN X)

V. jugularis interna

Lobus dexter glandulae thyreoideae

Glandula parathyreoidea superior

A. cervicalis ascendens

Glandula parathyreoidea inferior

A. thyreoidea inferior

N. laryngeus recurrens dex.

A. transversa colli

A. suprascapularis

Truncus thyreocervicalis

A. and V. subclavia

V. brachiocephalica dex.

Truncus brachiocephalicus

N. vagus (CN X)

V. cava superior

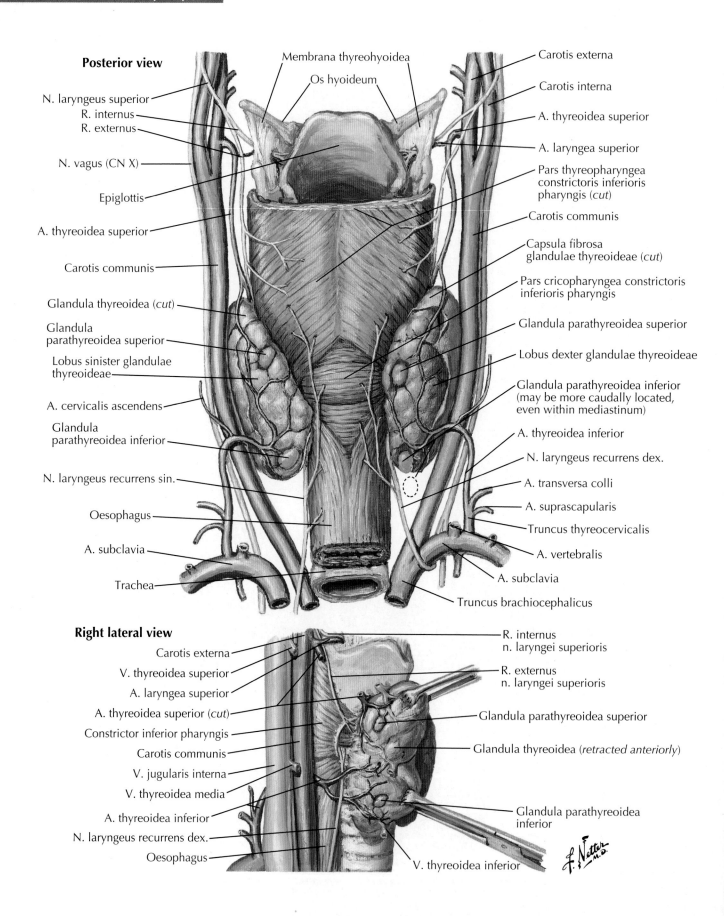

Posterior view

N. laryngeus superior
R. internus
R. externus

N. vagus (CN X)

Epiglottis

A. thyreoidea superior

Carotis communis

Glandula thyreoidea (*cut*)

Glandula parathyreoidea superior

Lobus sinister glandulae thyreoideae

A. cervicalis ascendens

Glandula parathyreoidea inferior

N. laryngeus recurrens sin.

Oesophagus

A. subclavia

Trachea

Membrana thyreohyoidea
Os hyoideum

Carotis externa

Carotis interna

A. thyreoidea superior

A. laryngea superior

Pars thyreopharyngea constrictoris inferioris pharyngis (*cut*)

Carotis communis

Capsula fibrosa glandulae thyreoideae (*cut*)

Pars cricopharyngea constrictoris inferioris pharyngis

Glandula parathyreoidea superior

Lobus dexter glandulae thyreoideae

Glandula parathyreoidea inferior (may be more caudally located, even within mediastinum)

A. thyreoidea inferior

N. laryngeus recurrens dex.

A. transversa colli

A. suprascapularis

Truncus thyreocervicalis

A. vertebralis

A. subclavia

Truncus brachiocephalicus

Right lateral view

Carotis externa
V. thyreoidea superior
A. laryngea superior
A. thyreoidea superior (*cut*)
Constrictor inferior pharyngis
Carotis communis
V. jugularis interna
V. thyreoidea media
A. thyreoidea inferior
N. laryngeus recurrens dex.
Oesophagus

R. internus n. laryngei superioris

R. externus n. laryngei superioris

Glandula parathyreoidea superior

Glandula thyreoidea (*retracted anteriorly*)

Glandula parathyreoidea inferior

V. thyreoidea inferior

Plate 105

Larynx and Glandulae Endocrinae

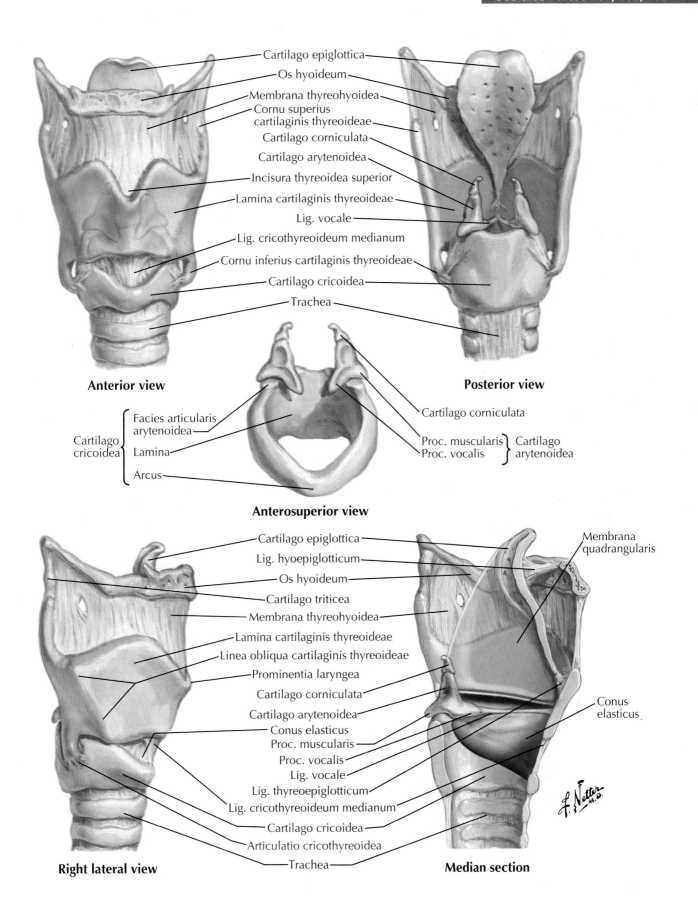

Cartilago epiglottica
Os hyoideum
Membrana thyreohyoidea
Cornu superius cartilaginis thyreoideae
Cartilago corniculata
Cartilago arytenoidea
Incisura thyreoidea superior
Lamina cartilaginis thyreoideae
Lig. vocale
Lig. cricothyreoideum medianum
Cornu inferius cartilaginis thyreoideae
Cartilago cricoidea
Trachea

Anterior view

Posterior view

Cartilago cricoidea { Facies articularis arytenoidea · Lamina · Arcus

Cartilago corniculata

Proc. muscularis · Proc. vocalis } Cartilago arytenoidea

Anterosuperior view

Cartilago epiglottica
Lig. hyoepiglotticum
Os hyoideum
Cartilago triticea
Membrana thyreohyoidea
Lamina cartilaginis thyreoideae
Linea obliqua cartilaginis thyreoideae
Prominentia laryngea
Cartilago corniculata
Cartilago arytenoidea
Conus elasticus
Proc. muscularis
Proc. vocalis
Lig. vocale
Lig. thyreoepiglotticum
Lig. cricothyreoideum medianum
Cartilago cricoidea
Articulatio cricothyreoidea
Trachea

Membrana quadrangularis

Conus elasticus

Right lateral view

Median section

Larynx and Glandulae Endocrinae

Plate 106

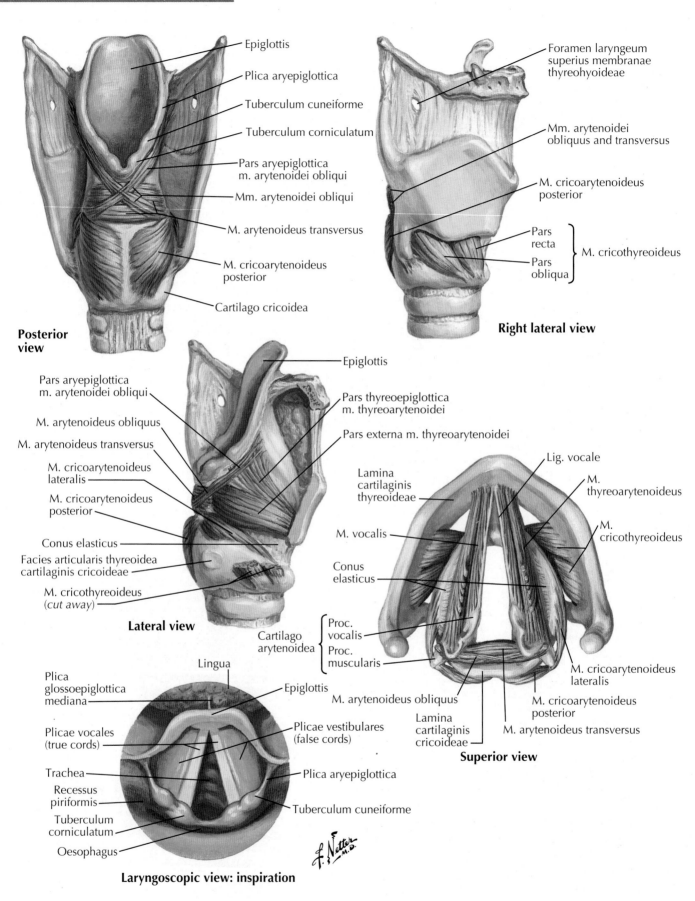

Epiglottis

Plica aryepiglottica

Tuberculum cuneiforme

Tuberculum corniculatum

**Pars aryepiglottica
m. arytenoidei obliqui**

Mm. arytenoidei obliqui

M. arytenoideus transversus

**M. cricoarytenoideus
posterior**

Cartilago cricoidea

**Posterior
view**

**Foramen laryngeum
superius membranae
thyreohyoideae**

**Mm. arytenoidei
obliquus and transversus**

**M. cricoarytenoideus
posterior**

**Pars
recta**

**Pars
obliqua**

} M. cricothyreoideus

Right lateral view

Epiglottis

**Pars aryepiglottica
m. arytenoidei obliqui**

M. arytenoideus obliquus

M. arytenoideus transversus

**M. cricoarytenoideus
lateralis**

**M. cricoarytenoideus
posterior**

Conus elasticus

**Facies articularis thyreoidea
cartilaginis cricoideae**

**M. cricothyreoideus
(cut away)**

**Pars thyreoepiglottica
m. thyreoarytenoidei**

Pars externa m. thyreoarytenoidei

Lateral view

Lig. vocale

**M.
thyreoarytenoideus**

**Lamina
cartilaginis
thyreoideae**

M. vocalis

**Conus
elasticus**

**M.
cricothyreoideus**

**Cartilago
arytenoidea**

**Proc.
vocalis**

**Proc.
muscularis**

M. arytenoideus obliquus

**Lamina
cartilaginis
cricoideae**

**M. cricoarytenoideus
lateralis**

**M. cricoarytenoideus
posterior**

M. arytenoideus transversus

Superior view

Lingua

**Plica
glossoepiglottica
mediana**

Epiglottis

**Plicae vocales
(true cords)**

**Plicae vestibulares
(false cords)**

Trachea

**Recessus
piriformis**

Plica aryepiglottica

**Tuberculum
corniculatum**

Tuberculum cuneiforme

Oesophagus

Laryngoscopic view: inspiration

Plate 107

Larynx and Glandulae Endocrinae

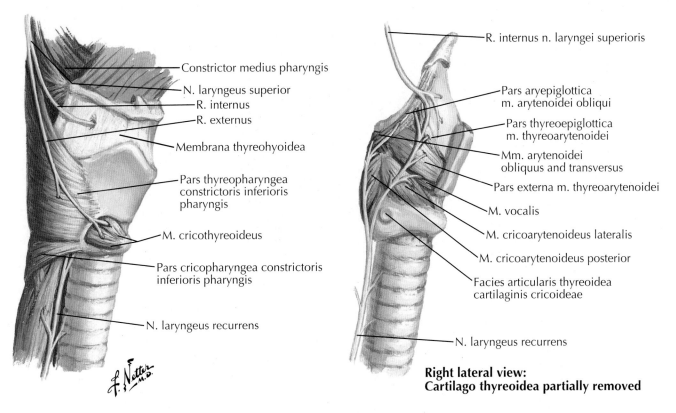

Constrictor medius pharyngis
N. laryngeus superior
R. internus
R. externus
Membrana thyreohyoidea

Pars thyreopharyngea
constrictoris inferioris
pharyngis

M. cricothyreoideus

Pars cricopharyngea constrictoris
inferioris pharyngis

N. laryngeus recurrens

R. internus n. laryngei superioris

Pars aryepiglottica
m. arytenoidei obliqui

Pars thyreoepiglottica
m. thyreoarytenoidei

Mm. arytenoidei
obliquus and transversus

Pars externa m. thyreoarytenoidei

M. vocalis

M. cricoarytenoideus lateralis

M. cricoarytenoideus posterior

Facies articularis thyreoidea
cartilaginis cricoideae

N. laryngeus recurrens

Right lateral view:
Cartilago thyreoidea partially removed

Coronal section through Larynx

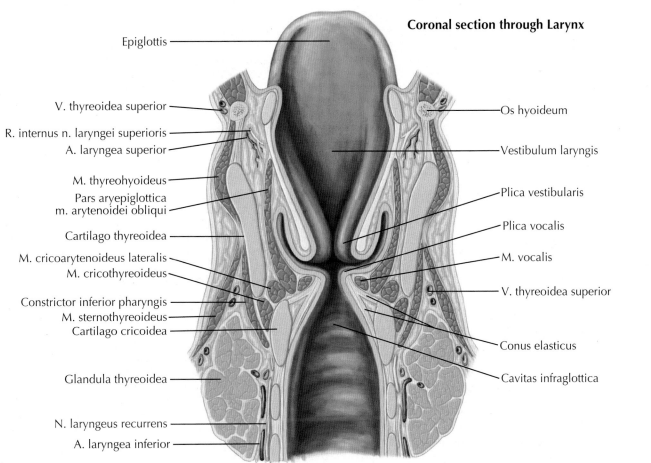

Epiglottis

V. thyreoidea superior
R. internus n. laryngei superioris
A. laryngea superior
M. thyreohyoideus
Pars aryepiglottica
m. arytenoidei obliqui
Cartilago thyreoidea
M. cricoarytenoideus lateralis
M. cricothyreoideus
Constrictor inferior pharyngis
M. sternothyreoideus
Cartilago cricoidea
Glandula thyreoidea
N. laryngeus recurrens
A. laryngea inferior

Os hyoideum
Vestibulum laryngis
Plica vestibularis
Plica vocalis
M. vocalis
V. thyreoidea superior
Conus elasticus
Cavitas infraglottica

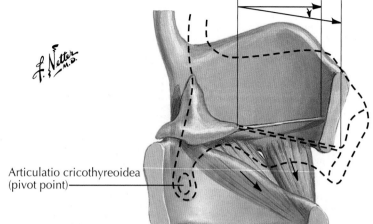

Articulatio cricothyreoidea
(pivot point)

Action of M. cricothyreoideus
Stretching of Ligg. vocalia

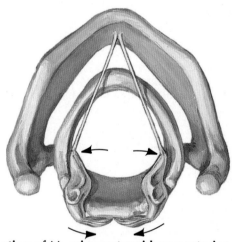

Action of M. cricoarytenoideus posterior
Abduction of Ligg. vocalia

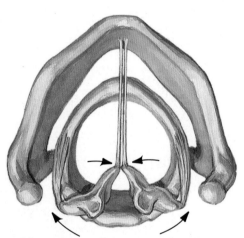

Action of M. cricoarytenoideus lateralis
Adduction of Ligg. vocalia

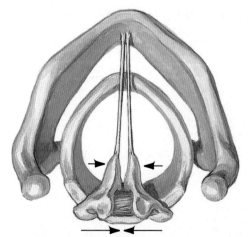

Action of Mm. arytenoidei transversus and obliquus
Adduction of Ligg. vocalia

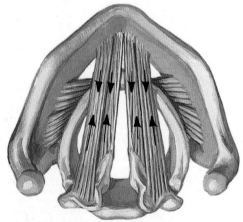

Action of Mm. vocalis and thyreoarytenoideus
Shortening (relaxation) of Ligg. vocalia

Plate 109

Larynx and Glandulae Endocrinae

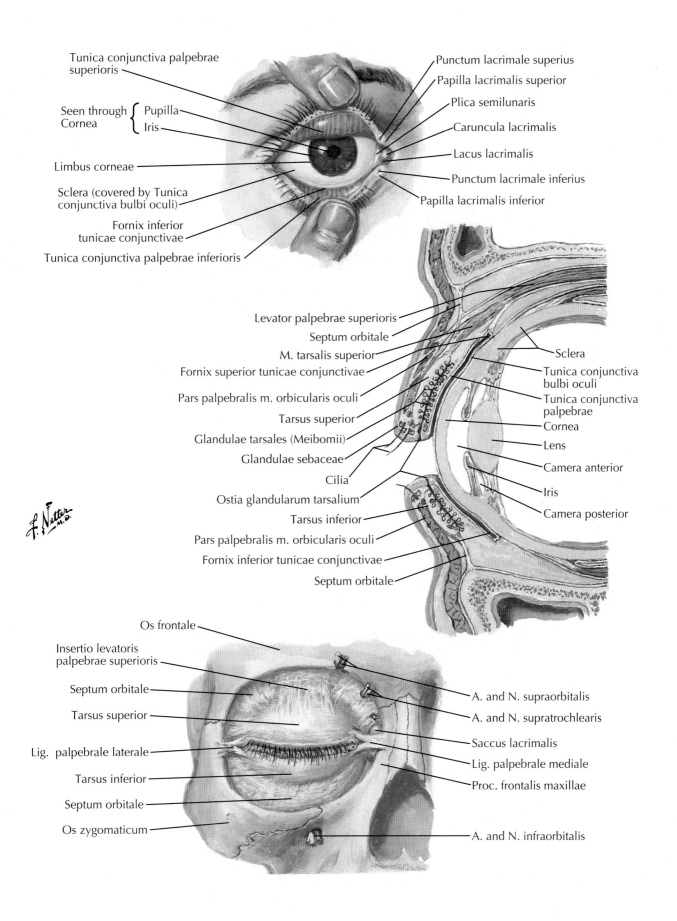

Tunica conjunctiva palpebrae superioris

Seen through Cornea { Pupilla / Iris

Limbus corneae

Sclera (covered by Tunica conjunctiva bulbi oculi)

Fornix inferior tunicae conjunctivae

Tunica conjunctiva palpebrae inferioris

Punctum lacrimale superius

Papilla lacrimalis superior

Plica semilunaris

Caruncula lacrimalis

Lacus lacrimalis

Punctum lacrimale inferius

Papilla lacrimalis inferior

Levator palpebrae superioris

Septum orbitale

M. tarsalis superior

Fornix superior tunicae conjunctivae

Pars palpebralis m. orbicularis oculi

Tarsus superior

Glandulae tarsales (Meibomii)

Glandulae sebaceae

Cilia

Ostia glandularum tarsalium

Tarsus inferior

Pars palpebralis m. orbicularis oculi

Fornix inferior tunicae conjunctivae

Septum orbitale

Sclera

Tunica conjunctiva bulbi oculi

Tunica conjunctiva palpebrae

Cornea

Lens

Camera anterior

Iris

Camera posterior

Os frontale

Insertio levatoris palpebrae superioris

Septum orbitale

Tarsus superior

Lig. palpebrale laterale

Tarsus inferior

Septum orbitale

Os zygomaticum

A. and N. supraorbitalis

A. and N. supratrochlearis

Saccus lacrimalis

Lig. palpebrale mediale

Proc. frontalis maxillae

A. and N. infraorbitalis

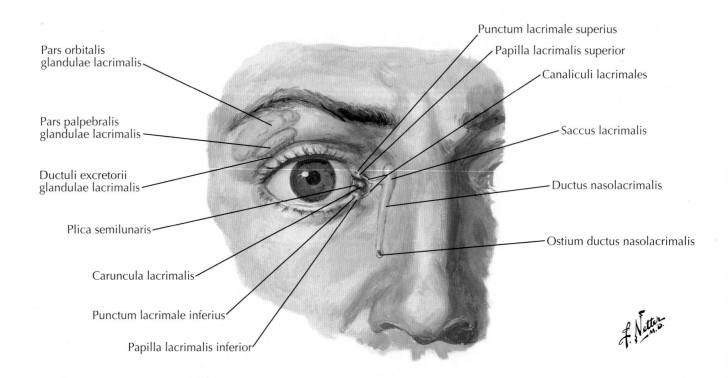

Pars orbitalis
glandulae lacrimalis

Pars palpebralis
glandulae lacrimalis

Ductuli excretorii
glandulae lacrimalis

Plica semilunaris

Caruncula lacrimalis

Punctum lacrimale inferius

Papilla lacrimalis inferior

Punctum lacrimale superius

Papilla lacrimalis superior

Canaliculi lacrimales

Saccus lacrimalis

Ductus nasolacrimalis

Ostium ductus nasolacrimalis

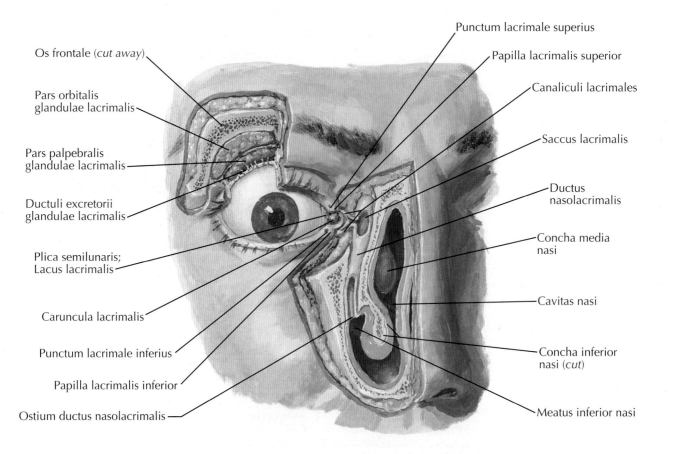

Os frontale (*cut away*)

Pars orbitalis
glandulae lacrimalis

Pars palpebralis
glandulae lacrimalis

Ductuli excretorii
glandulae lacrimalis

Plica semilunaris;
Lacus lacrimalis

Caruncula lacrimalis

Punctum lacrimale inferius

Papilla lacrimalis inferior

Ostium ductus nasolacrimalis

Punctum lacrimale superius

Papilla lacrimalis superior

Canaliculi lacrimales

Saccus lacrimalis

Ductus
nasolacrimalis

Concha media
nasi

Cavitas nasi

Concha inferior
nasi (*cut*)

Meatus inferior nasi

Plate 111

Oculus

Right lateral view

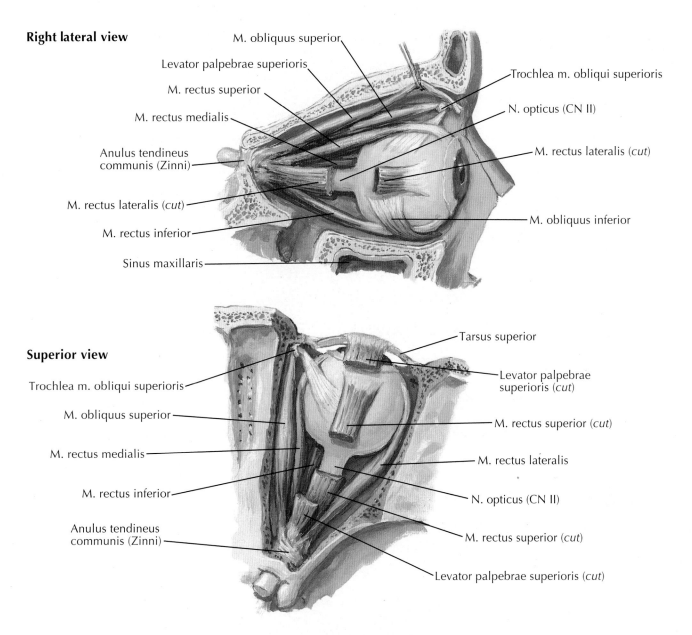

M. obliquus superior

Levator palpebrae superioris

M. rectus superior

M. rectus medialis

Anulus tendineus communis (Zinni)

M. rectus lateralis (*cut*)

M. rectus inferior

Sinus maxillaris

Trochlea m. obliqui superioris

N. opticus (CN II)

M. rectus lateralis (*cut*)

M. obliquus inferior

Superior view

Trochlea m. obliqui superioris

M. obliquus superior

M. rectus medialis

M. rectus inferior

Anulus tendineus communis (Zinni)

Tarsus superior

Levator palpebrae superioris (*cut*)

M. rectus superior (*cut*)

M. rectus lateralis

N. opticus (CN II)

M. rectus superior (*cut*)

Levator palpebrae superioris (*cut*)

Innervation of extrinsic eye muscles: anterior view

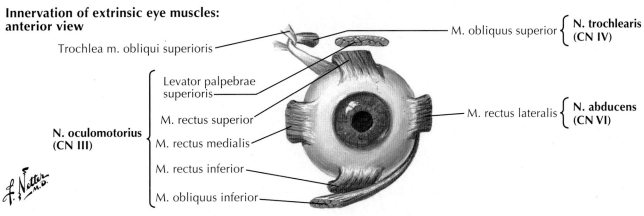

Trochlea m. obliqui superioris

M. obliquus superior $\left\{\begin{array}{c}\end{array}\right.$ **N. trochlearis (CN IV)**

N. oculomotorius (CN III) $\left\{\begin{array}{c}\end{array}\right.$

Levator palpebrae superioris

M. rectus superior

M. rectus medialis

M. rectus inferior

M. obliquus inferior

M. rectus lateralis $\left\{\begin{array}{c}\end{array}\right.$ **N. abducens (CN VI)**

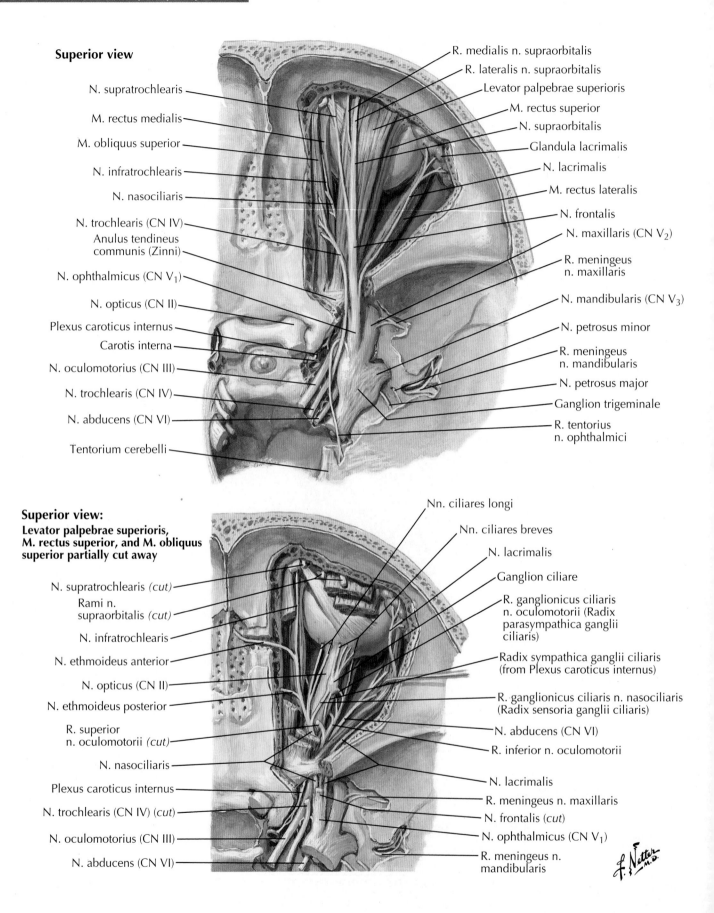

Superior view

N. supratrochlearis

M. rectus medialis

M. obliquus superior

N. infratrochlearis

N. nasociliaris

N. trochlearis (CN IV)

Anulus tendineus communis (Zinni)

N. ophthalmicus (CN V₁)

N. opticus (CN II)

Plexus caroticus internus

Carotis interna

N. oculomotorius (CN III)

N. trochlearis (CN IV)

N. abducens (CN VI)

Tentorium cerebelli

R. medialis n. supraorbitalis

R. lateralis n. supraorbitalis

Levator palpebrae superioris

M. rectus superior

N. supraorbitalis

Glandula lacrimalis

N. lacrimalis

M. rectus lateralis

N. frontalis

N. maxillaris (CN V₂)

R. meningeus n. maxillaris

N. mandibularis (CN V₃)

N. petrosus minor

R. meningeus n. mandibularis

N. petrosus major

Ganglion trigeminale

R. tentorius n. ophthalmici

Superior view:
Levator palpebrae superioris,
M. rectus superior, and M. obliquus
superior partially cut away

N. supratrochlearis *(cut)*

Rami n. supraorbitalis *(cut)*

N. infratrochlearis

N. ethmoideus anterior

N. opticus (CN II)

N. ethmoideus posterior

R. superior n. oculomotorii *(cut)*

N. nasociliaris

Plexus caroticus internus

N. trochlearis (CN IV) *(cut)*

N. oculomotorius (CN III)

N. abducens (CN VI)

Nn. ciliares longi

Nn. ciliares breves

N. lacrimalis

Ganglion ciliare

R. ganglionicus ciliaris n. oculomotorii (Radix parasympathica ganglii ciliaris)

Radix sympathica ganglii ciliaris (from Plexus caroticus internus)

R. ganglionicus ciliaris n. nasociliaris (Radix sensoria ganglii ciliaris)

N. abducens (CN VI)

R. inferior n. oculomotorii

N. lacrimalis

R. meningeus n. maxillaris

N. frontalis *(cut)*

N. ophthalmicus (CN V₁)

R. meningeus n. mandibularis

Plate 113

Oculus

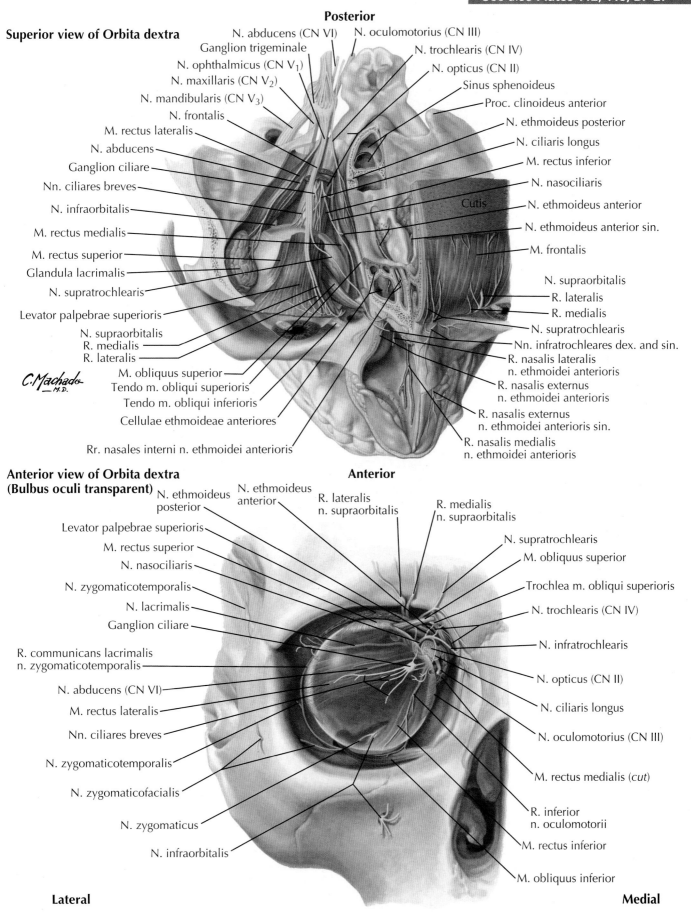

Superior view of Orbita dextra

Posterior

N. abducens (CN VI)
N. oculomotorius (CN III)
Ganglion trigeminale
N. trochlearis (CN IV)
N. ophthalmicus (CN V₁)
N. opticus (CN II)
N. maxillaris (CN V₂)
Sinus sphenoideus
N. mandibularis (CN V₃)
Proc. clinoideus anterior
N. frontalis
N. ethmoideus posterior
M. rectus lateralis
N. ciliaris longus
N. abducens
M. rectus inferior
Ganglion ciliare
N. nasociliaris
Nn. ciliares breves
Cutis
N. ethmoideus anterior
N. infraorbitalis
N. ethmoideus anterior sin.
M. rectus medialis
M. frontalis
M. rectus superior
N. supraorbitalis
Glandula lacrimalis
R. lateralis
N. supratrochlearis
R. medialis
Levator palpebrae superioris
N. supratrochlearis
N. supraorbitalis
Nn. infratrochleares dex. and sin.
R. medialis
R. nasalis lateralis
R. lateralis
n. ethmoidei anterioris
M. obliquus superior
R. nasalis externus
Tendo m. obliqui superioris
n. ethmoidei anterioris
Tendo m. obliqui inferioris
R. nasalis externus
Cellulae ethmoideae anteriores
n. ethmoidei anterioris sin.
R. nasalis medialis
Rr. nasales interni n. ethmoidei anterioris
n. ethmoidei anterioris

Anterior view of Orbita dextra
(Bulbus oculi transparent)

Anterior

N. ethmoideus posterior
N. ethmoideus anterior
R. lateralis n. supraorbitalis
R. medialis n. supraorbitalis
Levator palpebrae superioris
N. supratrochlearis
M. rectus superior
M. obliquus superior
N. nasociliaris
Trochlea m. obliqui superioris
N. zygomaticotemporalis
N. trochlearis (CN IV)
N. lacrimalis
N. infratrochlearis
Ganglion ciliare
N. opticus (CN II)
R. communicans lacrimalis
n. zygomaticotemporalis
N. ciliaris longus
N. abducens (CN VI)
N. oculomotorius (CN III)
M. rectus lateralis
Nn. ciliares breves
M. rectus medialis (cut)
N. zygomaticotemporalis
R. inferior
N. zygomaticofacialis
n. oculomotorii
N. zygomaticus
M. rectus inferior
N. infraorbitalis
M. obliquus inferior

Lateral

Medial

C. Machado
M.D.

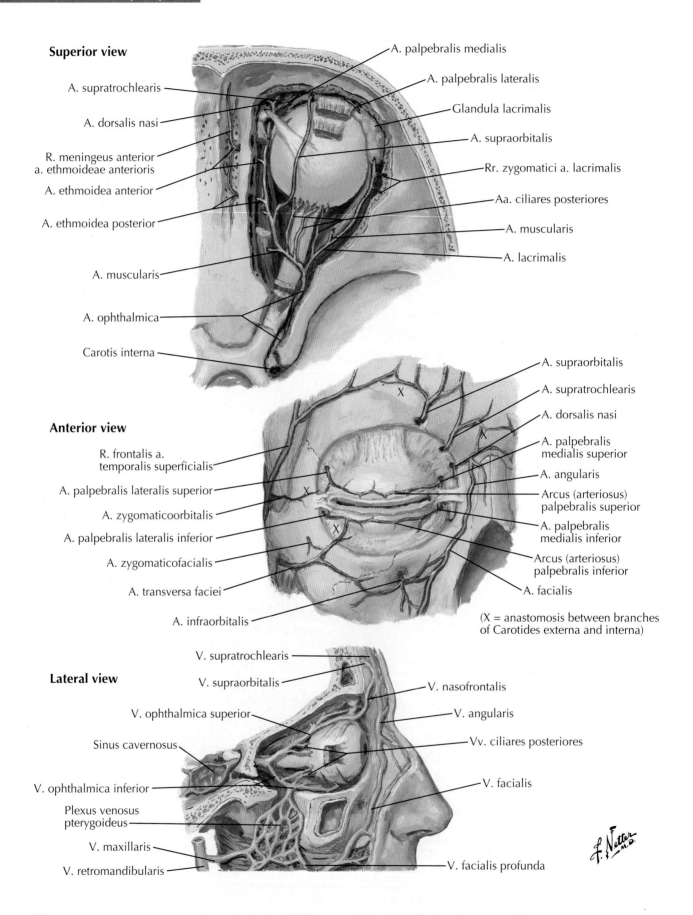

Superior view

A. palpebralis medialis

A. supratrochlearis

A. palpebralis lateralis

A. dorsalis nasi

Glandula lacrimalis

R. meningeus anterior
a. ethmoideae anterioris

A. supraorbitalis

A. ethmoidea anterior

Rr. zygomatici a. lacrimalis

A. ethmoidea posterior

Aa. ciliares posteriores

A. muscularis

A. lacrimalis

A. muscularis

A. ophthalmica

Carotis interna

A. supraorbitalis

A. supratrochlearis

Anterior view

A. dorsalis nasi

A. palpebralis
medialis superior

R. frontalis a.
temporalis superficialis

A. angularis

A. palpebralis lateralis superior

Arcus (arteriosus)
palpebralis superior

A. zygomaticoorbitalis

A. palpebralis
medialis inferior

A. palpebralis lateralis inferior

Arcus (arteriosus)
palpebralis inferior

A. zygomaticofacialis

A. transversa faciei

A. facialis

A. infraorbitalis

(X = anastomosis between branches
of Carotides externa and interna)

V. supratrochlearis

Lateral view

V. supraorbitalis

V. nasofrontalis

V. ophthalmica superior

V. angularis

Sinus cavernosus

Vv. ciliares posteriores

V. ophthalmica inferior

V. facialis

Plexus venosus
pterygoideus

V. maxillaris

V. retromandibularis

V. facialis profunda

Plate 115

Oculus

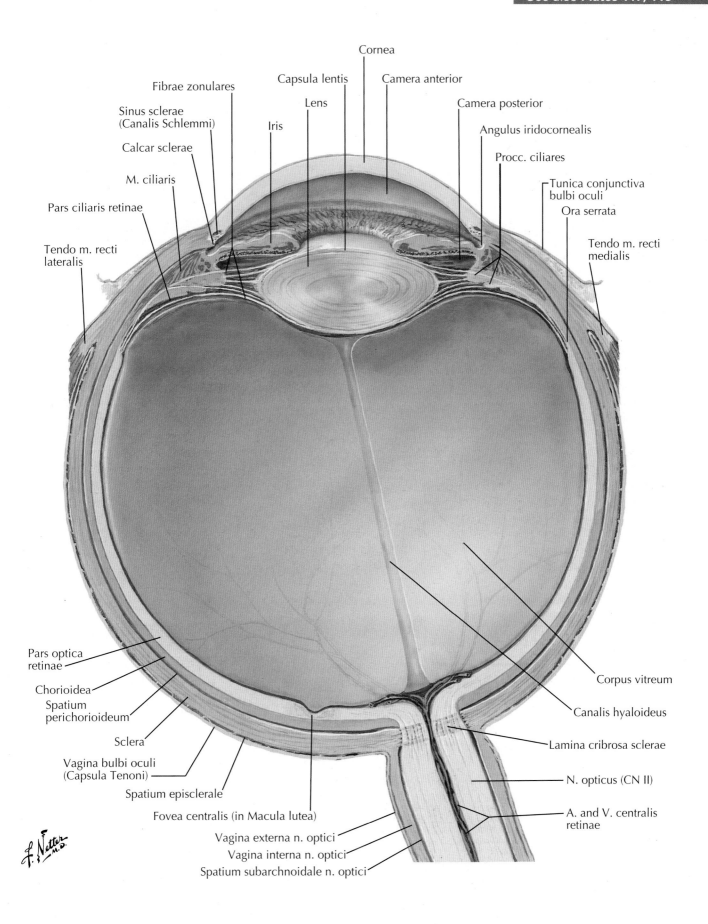

Cornea

Capsula lentis

Camera anterior

Fibrae zonulares

Lens

Camera posterior

Sinus sclerae
(Canalis Schlemmi)

Iris

Angulus iridocornealis

Calcar sclerae

Procc. ciliares

M. ciliaris

Tunica conjunctiva
bulbi oculi

Pars ciliaris retinae

Ora serrata

Tendo m. recti
lateralis

Tendo m. recti
medialis

Pars optica
retinae

Corpus vitreum

Chorioidea

Canalis hyaloideus

Spatium
perichorioideum

Sclera

Lamina cribrosa sclerae

Vagina bulbi oculi
(Capsula Tenoni)

N. opticus (CN II)

Spatium episclerale

Fovea centralis (in Macula lutea)

A. and V. centralis
retinae

Vagina externa n. optici

Vagina interna n. optici

Spatium subarchnoidale n. optici

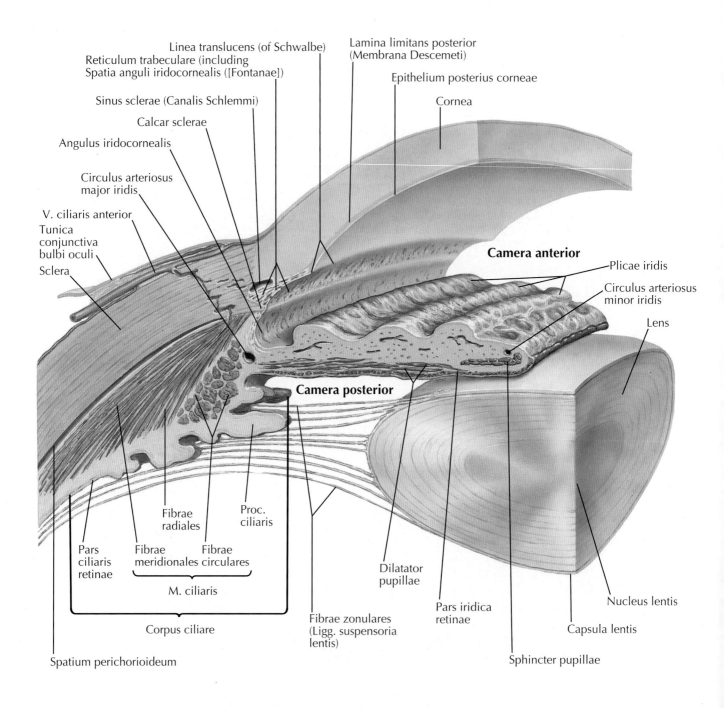

Linea translucens (of Schwalbe)

Reticulum trabeculare (including
Spatia anguli iridocornealis ([Fontanae])

Lamina limitans posterior
(Membrana Descemeti)

Sinus sclerae (Canalis Schlemmi)

Epithelium posterius corneae

Calcar sclerae

Cornea

Angulus iridocornealis

Circulus arteriosus
major iridis

Camera anterior

V. ciliaris anterior

Plicae iridis

Tunica
conjunctiva
bulbi oculi

Circulus arteriosus
minor iridis

Sclera

Lens

Camera posterior

Fibrae
radiales

Proc.
ciliaris

Pars
ciliaris
retinae

Fibrae
meridionales

Fibrae
circulares

M. ciliaris

Dilatator
pupillae

Nucleus lentis

Corpus ciliare

Fibrae zonulares
(Ligg. suspensoria
lentis)

Pars iridica
retinae

Capsula lentis

Spatium perichorioideum

Sphincter pupillae

*Note: For clarity, only single plane of fibrae zonulares shown;
actually, fibers surround entire circumference of lens.*

Plate 117

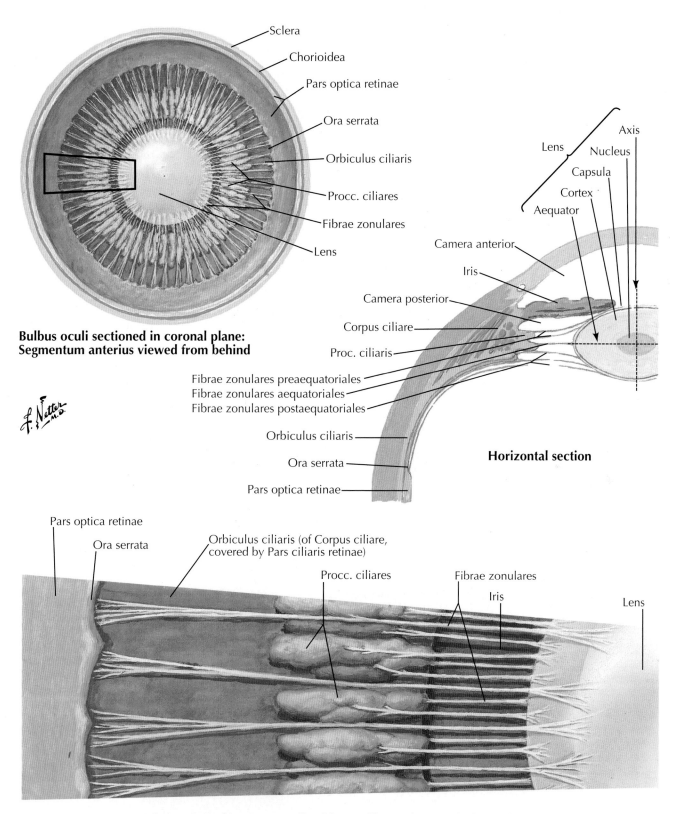

Sclera

Chorioidea

Pars optica retinae

Ora serrata

Orbiculus ciliaris

Procc. ciliares

Fibrae zonulares

Lens

**Bulbus oculi sectioned in coronal plane:
Segmentum anterius viewed from behind**

Axis

Lens

Nucleus

Capsula

Cortex

Aequator

Camera anterior

Iris

Camera posterior

Corpus ciliare

Proc. ciliaris

Fibrae zonulares preaequatoriales

Fibrae zonulares aequatoriales

Fibrae zonulares postaequatoriales

Orbiculus ciliaris

Ora serrata

Pars optica retinae

Horizontal section

Pars optica retinae

Ora serrata

Orbiculus ciliaris (of Corpus ciliare,
covered by Pars ciliaris retinae)

Procc. ciliares

Fibrae zonulares

Iris

Lens

Enlargement of segment outlined in top illustration (semischematic)

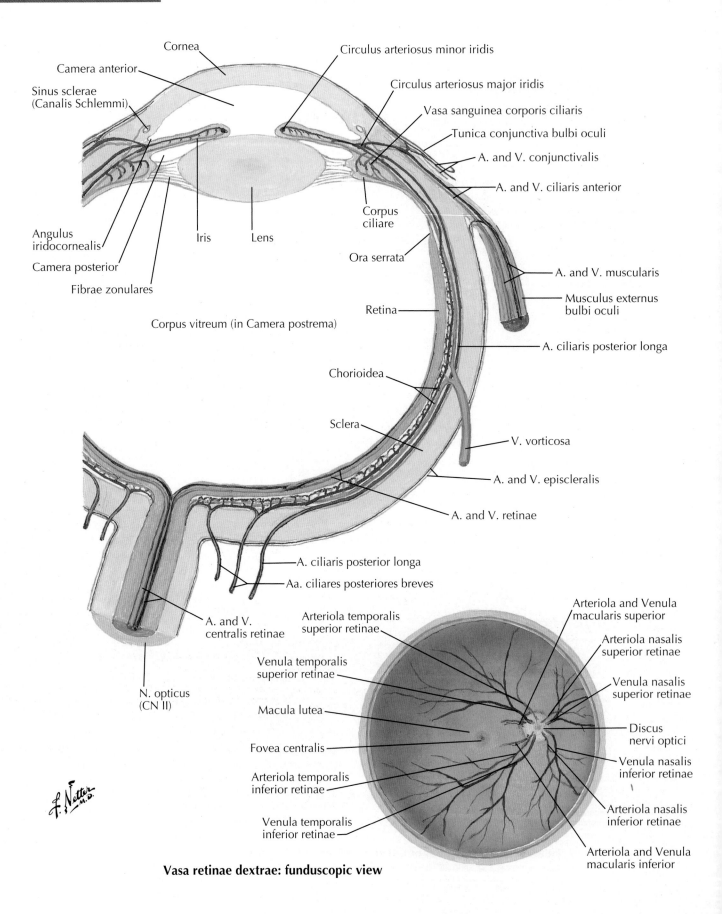

Cornea

Circulus arteriosus minor iridis

Camera anterior

Sinus sclerae
(Canalis Schlemmi)

Circulus arteriosus major iridis

Vasa sanguinea corporis ciliaris

Tunica conjunctiva bulbi oculi

A. and V. conjunctivalis

A. and V. ciliaris anterior

Angulus
iridocornealis

Iris   Lens

Camera posterior

Corpus
ciliare

Fibrae zonulares

Ora serrata

A. and V. muscularis

Musculus externus
bulbi oculi

Retina

Corpus vitreum (in Camera postrema)

A. ciliaris posterior longa

Chorioidea

Sclera

V. vorticosa

A. and V. episcleralis

A. and V. retinae

A. ciliaris posterior longa

Aa. ciliares posteriores breves

A. and V.
centralis retinae

Arteriola temporalis
superior retinae

Arteriola and Venula
macularis superior

Arteriola nasalis
superior retinae

Venula temporalis
superior retinae

Venula nasalis
superior retinae

Macula lutea

Discus
nervi optici

N. opticus
(CN II)

Fovea centralis

Venula nasalis
inferior retinae

Arteriola temporalis
inferior retinae

Arteriola nasalis
inferior retinae

Venula temporalis
inferior retinae

Arteriola and Venula
macularis inferior

Vasa retinae dextrae: funduscopic view

Plate 119

Oculus

Vascular arrangements within the tunica vasculosa bulbi oculi

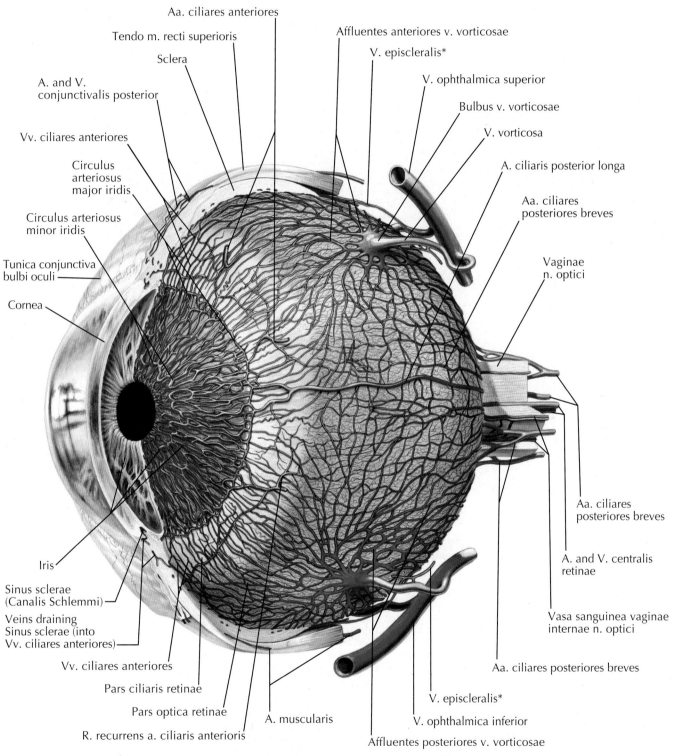

Aa. ciliares anteriores

Tendo m. recti superioris

Sclera

A. and V. conjunctivalis posterior

Vv. ciliares anteriores

Circulus arteriosus major iridis

Circulus arteriosus minor iridis

Tunica conjunctiva bulbi oculi

Cornea

Iris

Sinus sclerae (Canalis Schlemmi)

Veins draining Sinus sclerae (into Vv. ciliares anteriores)

Vv. ciliares anteriores

Pars ciliaris retinae

Pars optica retinae

R. recurrens a. ciliaris anterioris

A. muscularis

Affluentes anteriores v. vorticosae

V. episcleralis*

V. ophthalmica superior

Bulbus v. vorticosae

V. vorticosa

A. ciliaris posterior longa

Aa. ciliares posteriores breves

Vaginae n. optici

Aa. ciliares posteriores breves

A. and V. centralis retinae

Vasa sanguinea vaginae internae n. optici

Aa. ciliares posteriores breves

V. episcleralis*

V. ophthalmica inferior

Affluentes posteriores v. vorticosae

Vv. episclerales are shown here anastomosing with the Vv. vorticosae, which they do; however, they also drain into the Vv. ciliares anteriores.

C. Machado M.D.

Frontal section

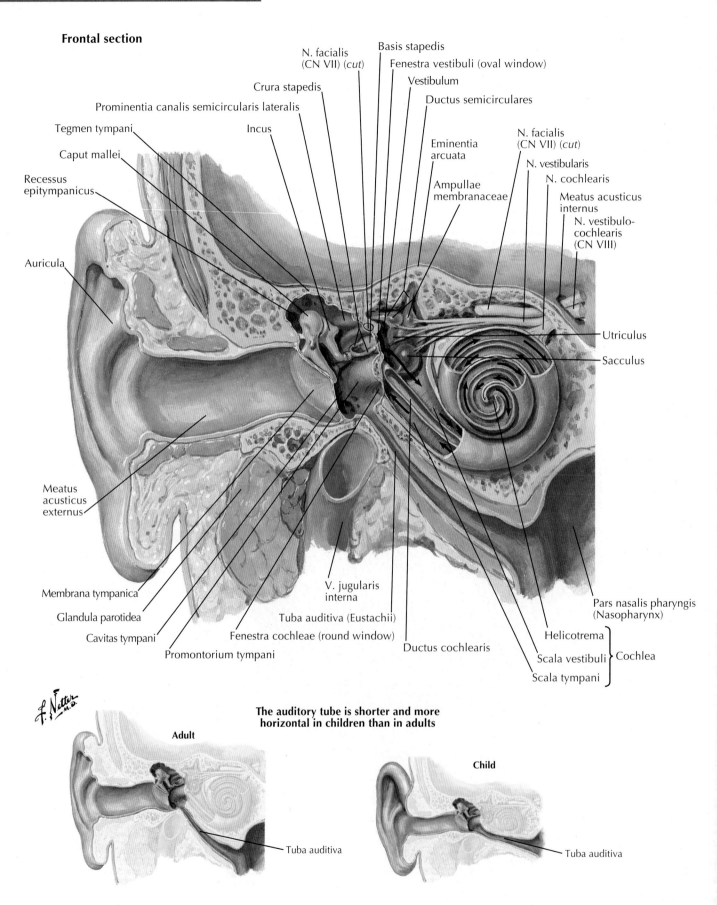

N. facialis (CN VII) (cut)

Basis stapedis

Fenestra vestibuli (oval window)

Crura stapedis

Vestibulum

Prominentia canalis semicircularis lateralis

Incus

Ductus semicirculares

Tegmen tympani

Eminentia arcuata

N. facialis (CN VII) (cut)

Caput mallei

N. vestibularis

Ampullae membranaceae

N. cochlearis

Recessus epitympanicus

Meatus acusticus internus

N. vestibulo-cochlearis (CN VIII)

Auricula

Utriculus

Sacculus

Meatus acusticus externus

Membrana tympanica

V. jugularis interna

Pars nasalis pharyngis (Nasopharynx)

Glandula parotidea

Tuba auditiva (Eustachii)

Cavitas tympani

Helicotrema

Fenestra cochleae (round window)

Ductus cochlearis

Scala vestibuli

Cochlea

Promontorium tympani

Scala tympani

The auditory tube is shorter and more horizontal in children than in adults

Adult

Child

Tuba auditiva

Tuba auditiva

Plate 121

Auris

Auricula dextra

Fossa triangularis

Helix

Scapha

Crura antihelicis

Tuberculum auriculare (tubercule of Darwin)

Antihelix

Concha auriculae

Lobulus auriculae

Crus helicis

Meatus acusticus externus

Tragus

Incisura intertragica

Antitragus

Otoscopic view of membrana tympanica dextra

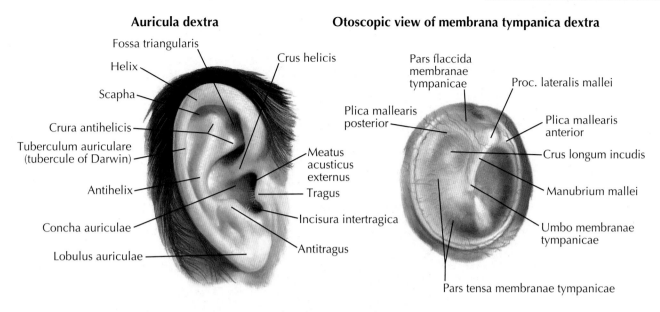

Pars flaccida membranae tympanicae

Plica mallearis posterior

Proc. lateralis mallei

Plica mallearis anterior

Crus longum incudis

Manubrium mallei

Umbo membranae tympanicae

Pars tensa membranae tympanicae

Coronal oblique section of meatus acusticus externus and auris media

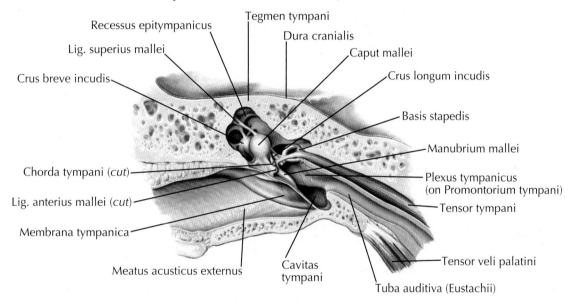

Recessus epitympanicus

Lig. superius mallei

Crus breve incudis

Chorda tympani (*cut*)

Lig. anterius mallei (*cut*)

Membrana tympanica

Meatus acusticus externus

Tegmen tympani

Dura cranialis

Caput mallei

Crus longum incudis

Basis stapedis

Manubrium mallei

Plexus tympanicus (on Promontorium tympani)

Tensor tympani

Tensor veli palatini

Cavitas tympani

Tuba auditiva (Eustachii)

Cavitas tympani dex. after removal of membrana tympanica (lateral view)

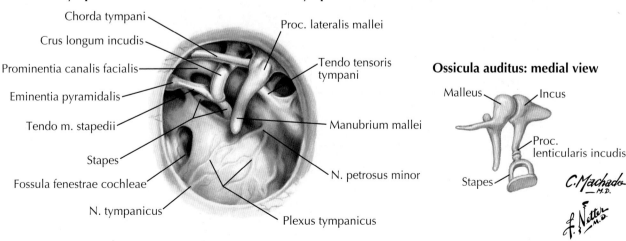

Chorda tympani

Crus longum incudis

Prominentia canalis facialis

Eminentia pyramidalis

Tendo m. stapedii

Stapes

Fossula fenestrae cochleae

N. tympanicus

Proc. lateralis mallei

Tendo tensoris tympani

Manubrium mallei

N. petrosus minor

Plexus tympanicus

Ossicula auditus: medial view

Malleus

Incus

Proc. lenticularis incudis

Stapes

C. Machado
_M.D._

F. Netter
_M.D._

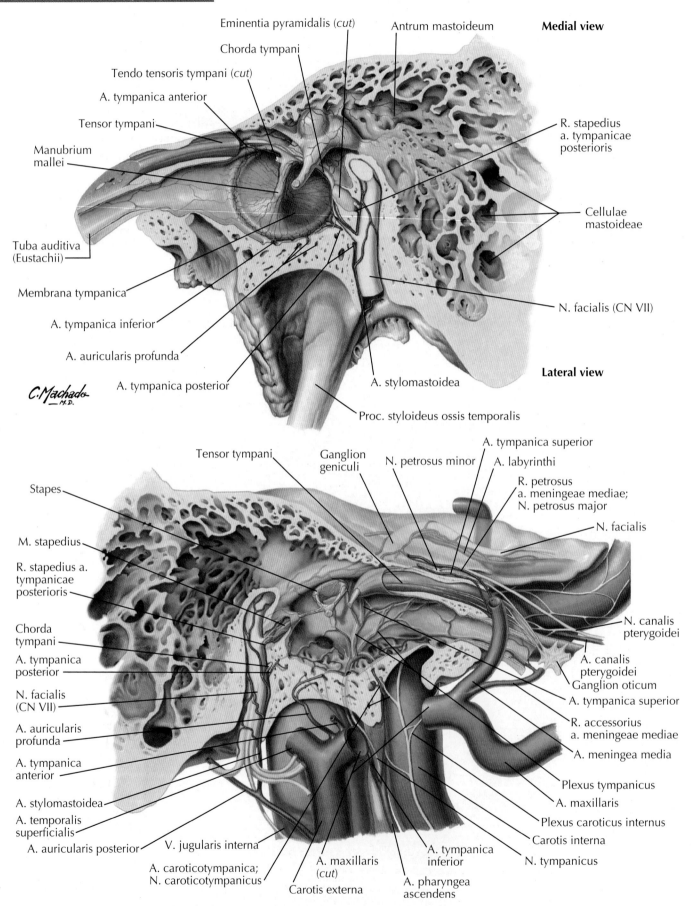

Eminentia pyramidalis (*cut*)

Chorda tympani

Tendo tensoris tympani (*cut*)

A. tympanica anterior

Tensor tympani

Manubrium mallei

Tuba auditiva (Eustachii)

Membrana tympanica

A. tympanica inferior

A. auricularis profunda

A. tympanica posterior

Antrum mastoideum

Medial view

R. stapedius a. tympanicae posterioris

Cellulae mastoideae

N. facialis (CN VII)

Lateral view

A. stylomastoidea

Proc. styloideus ossis temporalis

Stapes

M. stapedius

R. stapedius a. tympanicae posterioris

Chorda tympani

A. tympanica posterior

N. facialis (CN VII)

A. auricularis profunda

A. tympanica anterior

A. stylomastoidea

A. temporalis superficialis

A. auricularis posterior

V. jugularis interna

A. caroticotympanica; N. caroticotympanicus

Carotis externa

A. maxillaris (*cut*)

Tensor tympani

Ganglion geniculi

N. petrosus minor

A. tympanica superior

A. labyrinthi

R. petrosus a. meningeae mediae; N. petrosus major

N. facialis

N. canalis pterygoidei

A. canalis pterygoidei

Ganglion oticum

A. tympanica superior

R. accessorius a. meningeae mediae

A. meningea media

Plexus tympanicus

A. maxillaris

Plexus caroticus internus

Carotis interna

N. tympanicus

A. tympanica inferior

A. pharyngea ascendens

Plate 123

Auris

Labyrinthus osseus dexter (capsula otica), anterolateral view: surrounding cancellous bone removed

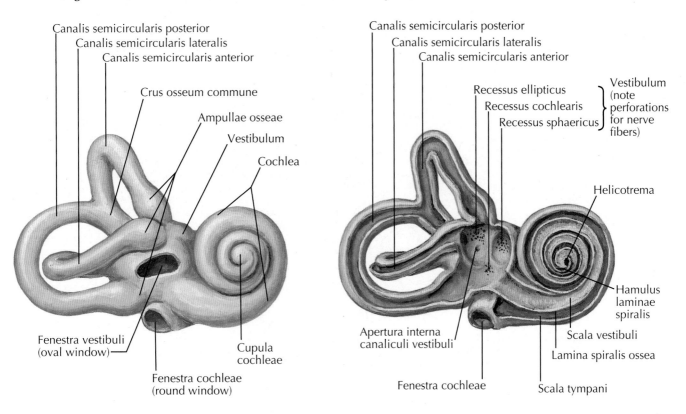

Canalis semicircularis posterior
Canalis semicircularis lateralis
Canalis semicircularis anterior
Crus osseum commune
Ampullae osseae
Vestibulum
Cochlea
Fenestra vestibuli (oval window)
Fenestra cochleae (round window)
Cupula cochleae

Dissected Labyrinthus osseus dexter (capsula otica): labyrinthus membranaceus removed

Canalis semicircularis posterior
Canalis semicircularis lateralis
Canalis semicircularis anterior
Recessus ellipticus
Recessus cochlearis
Recessus sphaericus
Vestibulum (note perforations for nerve fibers)
Helicotrema
Apertura interna canaliculi vestibuli
Fenestra cochleae
Hamulus laminae spiralis
Scala vestibuli
Lamina spiralis ossea
Scala tympani

Labyrinthus membranaceus dexter with nerves: medial view

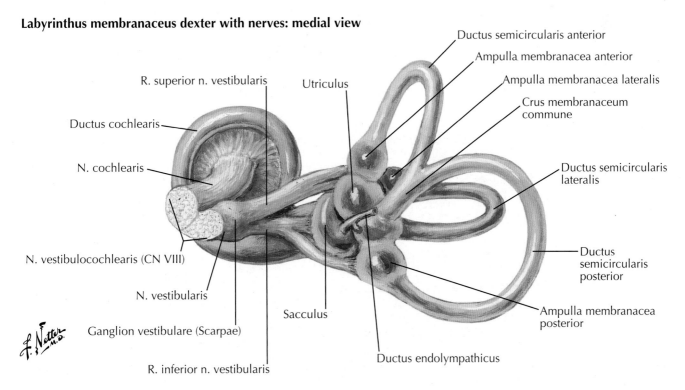

R. superior n. vestibularis
Utriculus
Ductus semicircularis anterior
Ampulla membranacea anterior
Ampulla membranacea lateralis
Crus membranaceum commune
Ductus cochlearis
N. cochlearis
Ductus semicircularis lateralis
N. vestibulocochlearis (CN VIII)
N. vestibularis
Ganglion vestibulare (Scarpae)
Sacculus
Ductus semicircularis posterior
Ampulla membranacea posterior
R. inferior n. vestibularis
Ductus endolympathicus

Labyrinthus osseus and labyrinthus membranaceus: schema

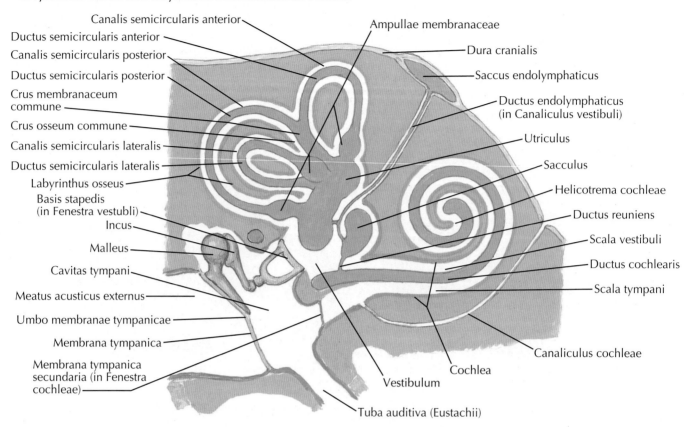

Canalis semicircularis anterior
Ductus semicircularis anterior
Canalis semicircularis posterior
Ductus semicircularis posterior
Crus membranaceum commune
Crus osseum commune
Canalis semicircularis lateralis
Ductus semicircularis lateralis
Labyrinthus osseus
Basis stapedis (in Fenestra vestubli)
Incus
Malleus
Cavitas tympani
Meatus acusticus externus
Umbo membranae tympanicae
Membrana tympanica
Membrana tympanica secundaria (in Fenestra cochleae)

Ampullae membranaceae
Dura cranialis
Saccus endolymphaticus
Ductus endolymphaticus (in Canaliculus vestibuli)
Utriculus
Sacculus
Helicotrema cochleae
Ductus reuniens
Scala vestibuli
Ductus cochlearis
Scala tympani
Canaliculus cochleae
Cochlea
Vestibulum
Tuba auditiva (Eustachii)

Section through turn of cochlea

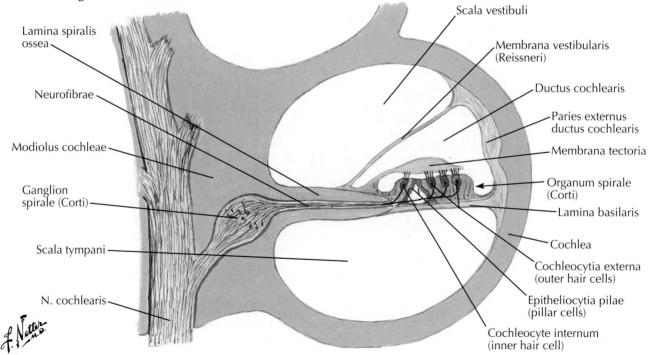

Lamina spiralis ossea
Neurofibrae
Modiolus cochleae
Ganglion spirale (Corti)
Scala tympani
N. cochlearis

Scala vestibuli
Membrana vestibularis (Reissneri)
Ductus cochlearis
Paries externus ductus cochlearis
Membrana tectoria
Organum spirale (Corti)
Lamina basilaris
Cochlea
Cochleocytia externa (outer hair cells)
Epitheliocytia pilae (pillar cells)
Cochleocyte internum (inner hair cell)

Plate 125   **Auris**

Superior projection of labyrinthus osseus dexter on floor of cranium

Cochlea

N. cochlearis

N. facialis (CN VII)

Porus acusticus internus

N. vestibulocochlearis (CN VIII)

N. vestibularis

Pars petrosa ossis temporalis

Apertura externa canaliculi vestibuli

Sulcus n. petrosi majoris

Ganglion geniculi

Canalis semicircularis anterior

Canalis semicircularis lateralis

Canalis semicircularis posterior

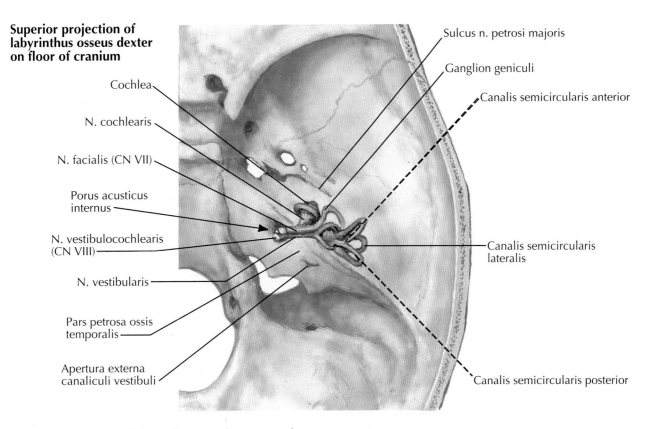

Lateral projection of labyrinthus membranaceus dexter

Ganglion geniculi

N. trigeminus (CN V)

N. facialis (CN VII)

N. vestibulocochlearis (CN VIII)

Ductus semicircularis anterior

Cerebellum

Sinus petrosus superior

Sinus rectus

Confluens sinuum

Auricula (*retracted anteriorly*)

Ductus cochlearis

N. cochlearis

R. superior n. vestibularis

V. jugularis interna

R. inferior n. vestibularis

Ductus semicircularis lateralis

Ductus semicircularis posterior

Sinus sigmoideus

Sinus transversus

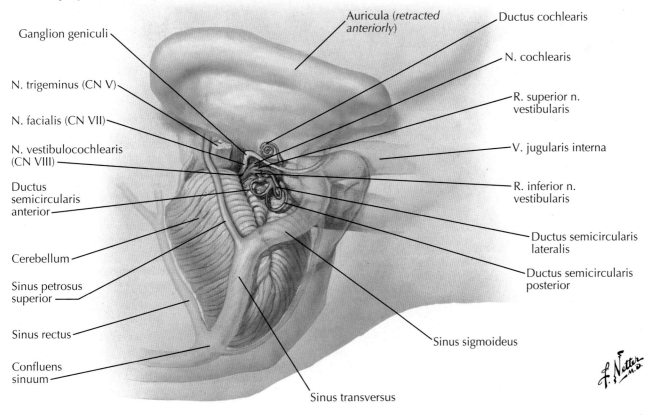

Auris

Plate 126

Coronal view

Vv. diploicae

Sinus sagittalis superior

Emissarium

Vv. temporales superficiales

Rami a. temporalis superficialis

Foveola granularis

Lacuna lateralis (Trolardi)

V. superior cerebri

Sinus sagittalis inferior

Cavum septi pellucidi

Granulatio arachnoideae

Bridging vein

Partes periostea durae cranialis

Partes meningea durae cranialis

Arachnoidea cranialis

Spatium subarachnoidale

Pia cranialis

A. and V. meningea media

M. temporalis

A. and V. temporalis profunda

A. and V. temporalis superficialis

A. and V. temporalis media

V. media superficialis cerebri

V. media profunda cerebri

V. thalamostriata superior

V. chorioidea superior

V. interna cerebri

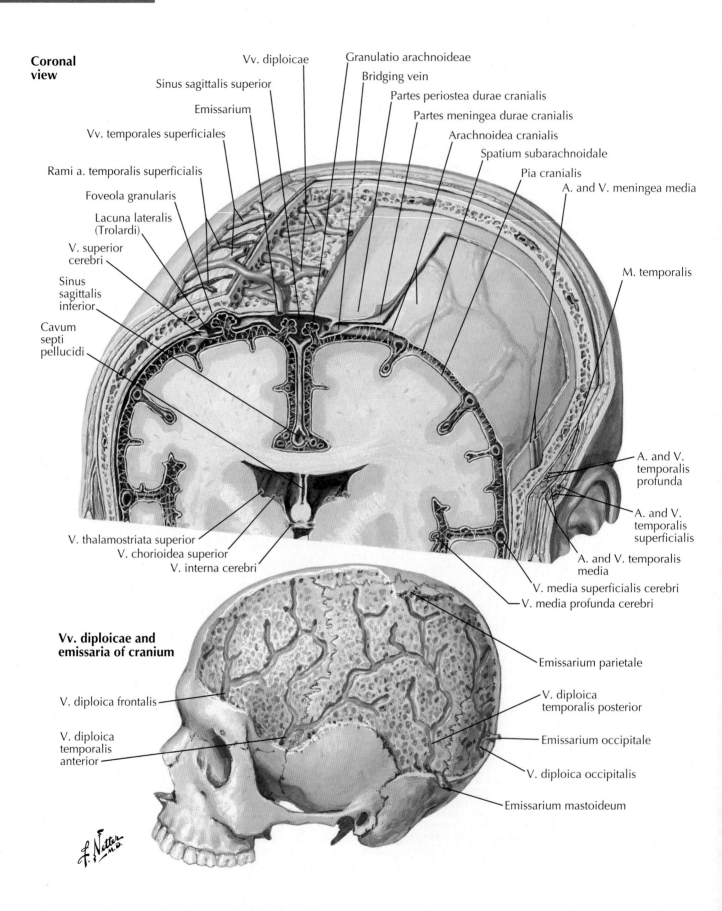

Vv. diploicae and emissaria of cranium

V. diploica frontalis

V. diploica temporalis anterior

Emissarium parietale

V. diploica temporalis posterior

Emissarium occipitale

V. diploica occipitalis

Emissarium mastoideum

Plate 127

Encephalon and Meninges

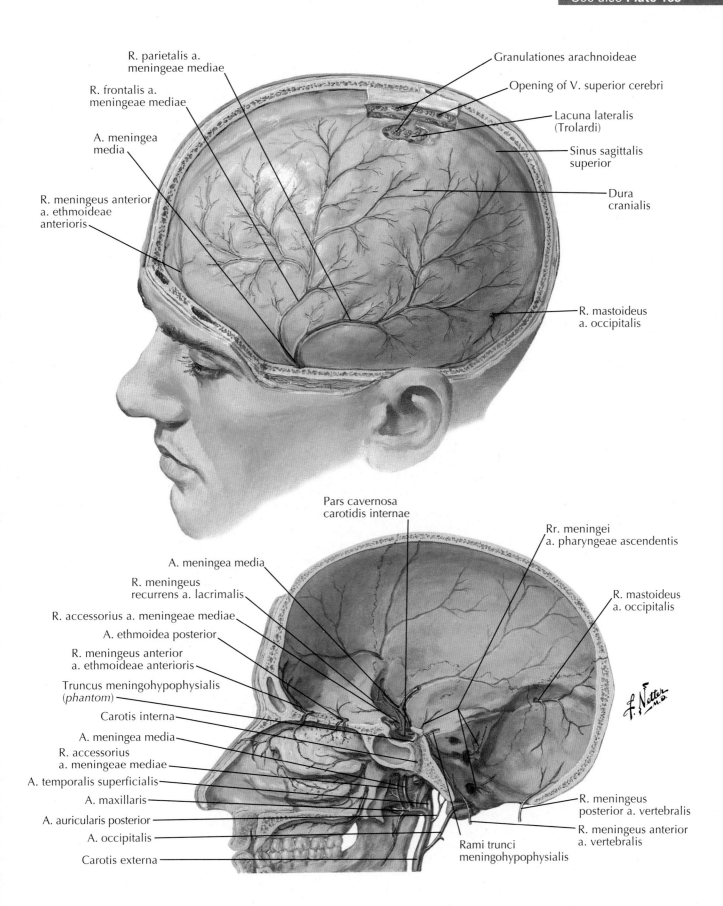

R. parietalis a. meningeae mediae

R. frontalis a. meningeae mediae

A. meningea media

R. meningeus anterior a. ethmoideae anterioris

Granulationes arachnoideae

Opening of V. superior cerebri

Lacuna lateralis (Trolardi)

Sinus sagittalis superior

Dura cranialis

R. mastoideus a. occipitalis

Pars cavernosa carotidis internae

A. meningea media

R. meningeus recurrens a. lacrimalis

R. accessorius a. meningeae mediae

A. ethmoidea posterior

R. meningeus anterior a. ethmoideae anterioris

Truncus meningohypophysialis (*phantom*)

Carotis interna

A. meningea media

R. accessorius a. meningeae mediae

A. temporalis superficialis

A. maxillaris

A. auricularis posterior

A. occipitalis

Carotis externa

Rr. meningei a. pharyngeae ascendentis

R. mastoideus a. occipitalis

R. meningeus posterior a. vertebralis

R. meningeus anterior a. vertebralis

Rami trunci meningohypophysialis

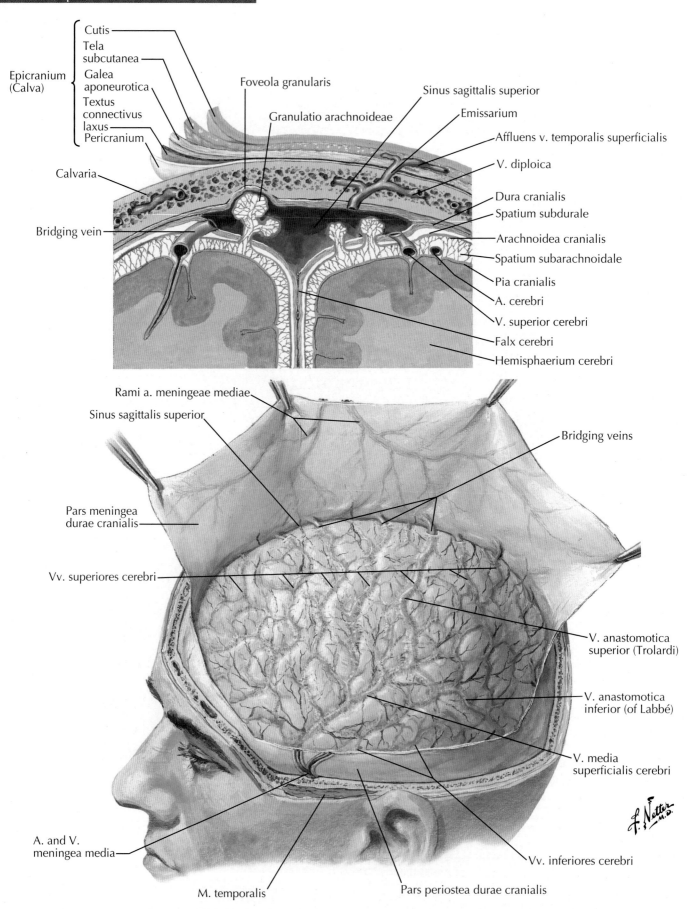

Epicranium (Calva)
- Cutis
- Tela subcutanea
- Galea aponeurotica
- Textus connectivus laxus
- Pericranium

Foveola granularis

Granulatio arachnoideae

Sinus sagittalis superior

Emissarium

Affluens v. temporalis superficialis

V. diploica

Calvaria

Bridging vein

Dura cranialis

Spatium subdurale

Arachnoidea cranialis

Spatium subarachnoidale

Pia cranialis

A. cerebri

V. superior cerebri

Falx cerebri

Hemisphaerium cerebri

Rami a. meningeae mediae

Sinus sagittalis superior

Bridging veins

Pars meningea durae cranialis

Vv. superiores cerebri

V. anastomotica superior (Trolardi)

V. anastomotica inferior (of Labbé)

V. media superficialis cerebri

A. and V. meningea media

Vv. inferiores cerebri

M. temporalis

Pars periostea durae cranialis

Plate 129

Encephalon and Meninges

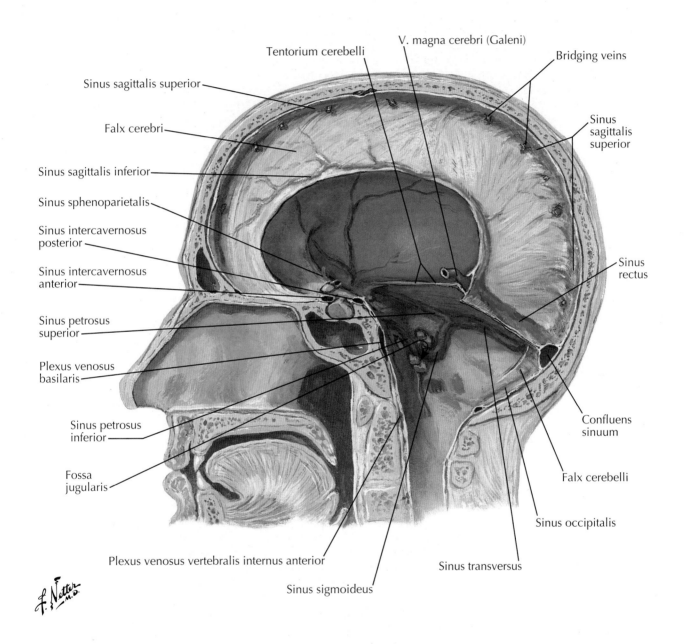

Tentorium cerebelli

V. magna cerebri (Galeni)

Bridging veins

Sinus sagittalis superior

Sinus sagittalis superior

Falx cerebri

Sinus sagittalis inferior

Sinus sphenoparietalis

Sinus intercavernosus posterior

Sinus intercavernosus anterior

Sinus petrosus superior

Plexus venosus basilaris

Sinus petrosus inferior

Fossa jugularis

Sinus rectus

Confluens sinuum

Falx cerebelli

Sinus occipitalis

Plexus venosus vertebralis internus anterior

Sinus sigmoideus

Sinus transversus

Cranium sectioned horizontally: superior view

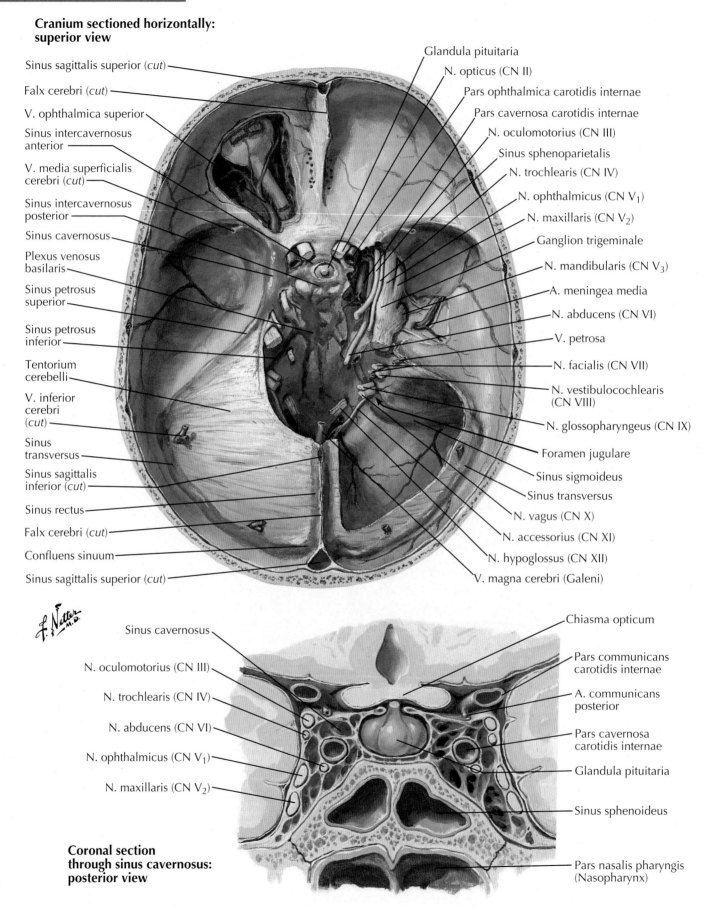

Sinus sagittalis superior (*cut*)

Falx cerebri (*cut*)

V. ophthalmica superior

Sinus intercavernosus anterior

V. media superficialis cerebri (*cut*)

Sinus intercavernosus posterior

Sinus cavernosus

Plexus venosus basilaris

Sinus petrosus superior

Sinus petrosus inferior

Tentorium cerebelli

V. inferior cerebri (*cut*)

Sinus transversus

Sinus sagittalis inferior (*cut*)

Sinus rectus

Falx cerebri (*cut*)

Confluens sinuum

Sinus sagittalis superior (*cut*)

Glandula pituitaria

N. opticus (CN II)

Pars ophthalmica carotidis internae

Pars cavernosa carotidis internae

N. oculomotorius (CN III)

Sinus sphenoparietalis

N. trochlearis (CN IV)

N. ophthalmicus (CN V_1)

N. maxillaris (CN V_2)

Ganglion trigeminale

N. mandibularis (CN V_3)

A. meningea media

N. abducens (CN VI)

V. petrosa

N. facialis (CN VII)

N. vestibulocochlearis (CN VIII)

N. glossopharyngeus (CN IX)

Foramen jugulare

Sinus sigmoideus

Sinus transversus

N. vagus (CN X)

N. accessorius (CN XI)

N. hypoglossus (CN XII)

V. magna cerebri (Galeni)

Sinus cavernosus

N. oculomotorius (CN III)

N. trochlearis (CN IV)

N. abducens (CN VI)

N. ophthalmicus (CN V_1)

N. maxillaris (CN V_2)

Chiasma opticum

Pars communicans carotidis internae

A. communicans posterior

Pars cavernosa carotidis internae

Glandula pituitaria

Sinus sphenoideus

Pars nasalis pharyngis (Nasopharynx)

Coronal section through sinus cavernosus: posterior view

Plate 131

Encephalon and Meninges

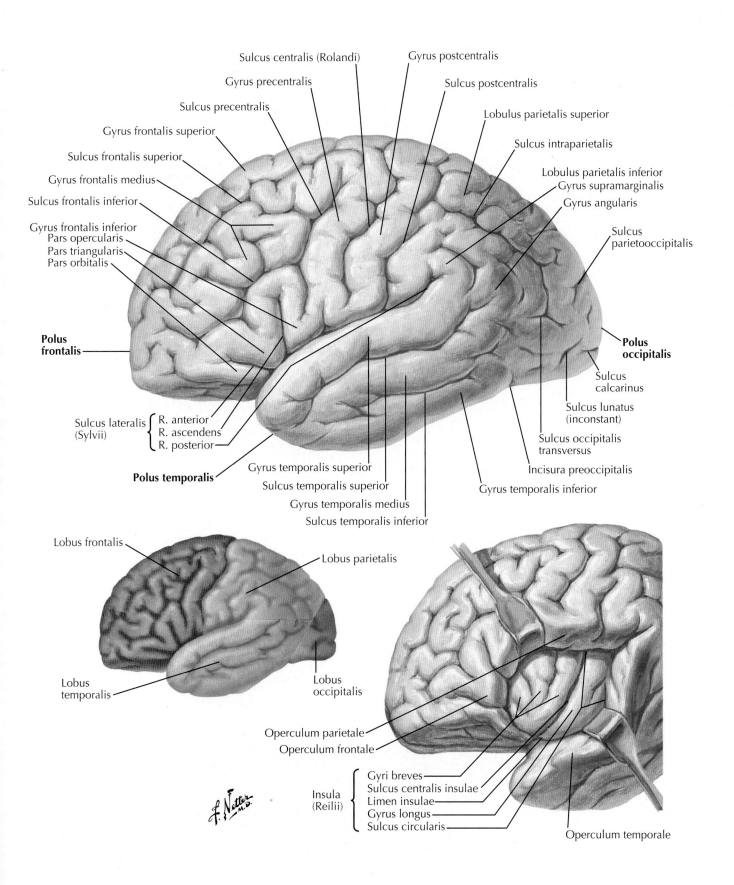

Sulcus centralis (Rolandi)

Gyrus postcentralis

Gyrus precentralis

Sulcus postcentralis

Sulcus precentralis

Lobulus parietalis superior

Gyrus frontalis superior

Sulcus intraparietalis

Sulcus frontalis superior

Lobulus parietalis inferior

Gyrus frontalis medius

Gyrus supramarginalis

Sulcus frontalis inferior

Gyrus angularis

Gyrus frontalis inferior
Pars opercularis
Pars triangularis
Pars orbitalis

Sulcus
parietooccipitalis

**Polus
frontalis**

**Polus
occipitalis**

Sulcus
calcarinus

Sulcus lunatus
(inconstant)

Sulcus lateralis
(Sylvii) {
R. anterior
R. ascendens
R. posterior

Sulcus occipitalis
transversus

Polus temporalis

Incisura preoccipitalis

Gyrus temporalis superior

Gyrus temporalis inferior

Sulcus temporalis superior

Gyrus temporalis medius

Sulcus temporalis inferior

Lobus frontalis

Lobus parietalis

Lobus
temporalis

Lobus
occipitalis

Operculum parietale

Operculum frontale

Insula
(Reilii) {
Gyri breves
Sulcus centralis insulae
Limen insulae
Gyrus longus
Sulcus circularis

Operculum temporale

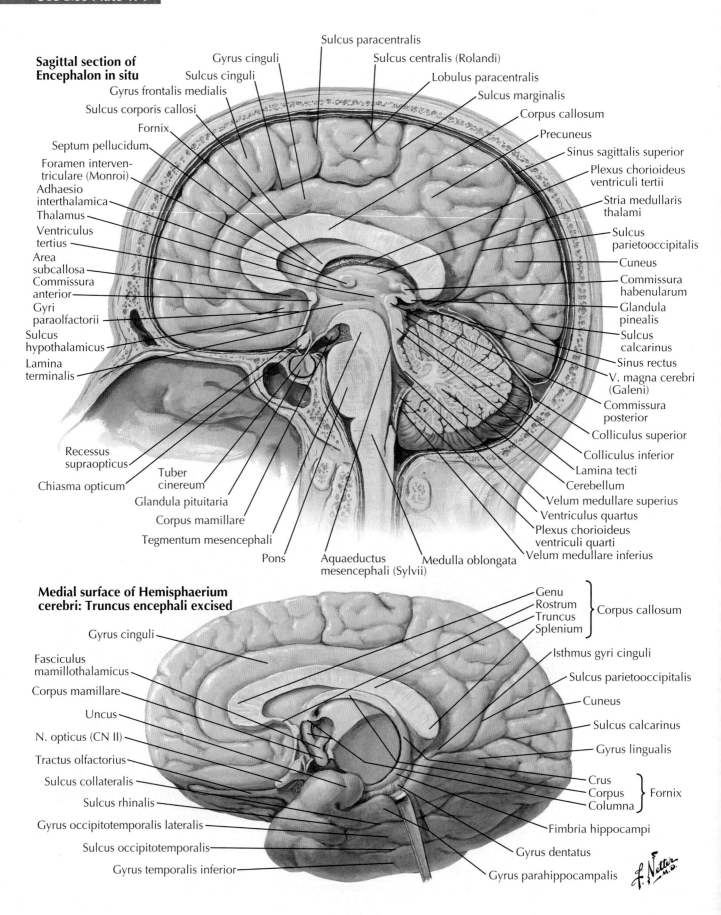

Sagittal section of Encephalon in situ

Sulcus paracentralis

Gyrus cinguli

Sulcus centralis (Rolandi)

Sulcus cinguli

Lobulus paracentralis

Gyrus frontalis medialis

Sulcus marginalis

Sulcus corporis callosi

Corpus callosum

Fornix

Precuneus

Septum pellucidum

Sinus sagittalis superior

Foramen interventriculare (Monroi)

Plexus chorioideus ventriculi tertii

Adhaesio interthalamica

Stria medullaris thalami

Thalamus

Ventriculus tertius

Sulcus parietooccipitalis

Area subcallosa

Cuneus

Commissura anterior

Commissura habenularum

Gyri paraolfactorii

Glandula pinealis

Sulcus hypothalamicus

Sulcus calcarinus

Lamina terminalis

Sinus rectus

V. magna cerebri (Galeni)

Recessus supraopticus

Commissura posterior

Chiasma opticum

Tuber cinereum

Colliculus superior

Colliculus inferior

Lamina tecti

Glandula pituitaria

Cerebellum

Corpus mamillare

Velum medullare superius

Tegmentum mesencephali

Ventriculus quartus

Pons

Plexus chorioideus ventriculi quarti

Aquaeductus mesencephali (Sylvii)

Medulla oblongata

Velum medullare inferius

Medial surface of Hemisphaerium cerebri: Truncus encephali excised

Gyrus cinguli

Genu
Rostrum
Truncus
Splenium } Corpus callosum

Fasciculus mamillothalamicus

Isthmus gyri cinguli

Corpus mamillare

Sulcus parietooccipitalis

Uncus

Cuneus

N. opticus (CN II)

Sulcus calcarinus

Tractus olfactorius

Gyrus lingualis

Sulcus collateralis

Crus
Corpus
Columna } Fornix

Sulcus rhinalis

Gyrus occipitotemporalis lateralis

Fimbria hippocampi

Sulcus occipitotemporalis

Gyrus dentatus

Gyrus temporalis inferior

Gyrus parahippocampalis

Plate 133

Encephalon and Meninges

Sectioned Truncus encephali

Polus frontalis hemisphaerii cerebri

Gyrus rectus

Sulcus olfactorius

Sulci orbitales

Gyri orbitales

Polus temporalis hemisphaerii cerebri

Sulcus lateralis (Sylvii)

Sulcus temporalis inferior

Gyrus temporalis inferior

Margo inferolateralis hemisphaerii cerebri

Sulcus rhinalis

Uncus

Gyrus temporalis inferior

Sulcus occipitotemporalis

Gyrus occipitotemporalis lateralis

Sulcus collateralis

Gyrus parahippocampalis

Gyrus occipitotemporalis medialis

Sulcus calcarinus

Isthmus gyri cinguli

Fissura longitudinalis cerebri

Genu corporis callosi

Lamina terminalis

Bulbus olfactorius

Tractus olfactorius

Chiasma opticum

N. opticus (CN II) (cut)

Glandula pituitaria

Substantia perforata anterior

Tractus opticus

Tuber cinereum

Corpus mamillare

Substantia perforata posterior

Crus cerebri

Corpus geniculatum laterale

Substantia nigra

Corpus geniculatum mediale

Nucleus ruber

Pulvinar

Colliculus superior

Aquaeductus mesencephali

Splenium corporis callosi

Gyrus lingualis

Polus occipitalis hemisphaerii cerebri

Fissura longitudinalis cerebri

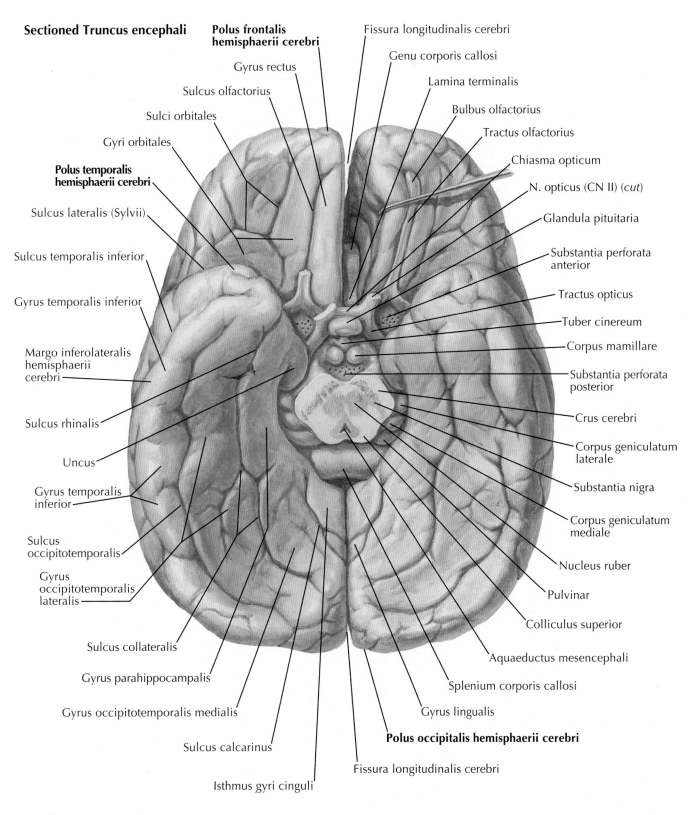

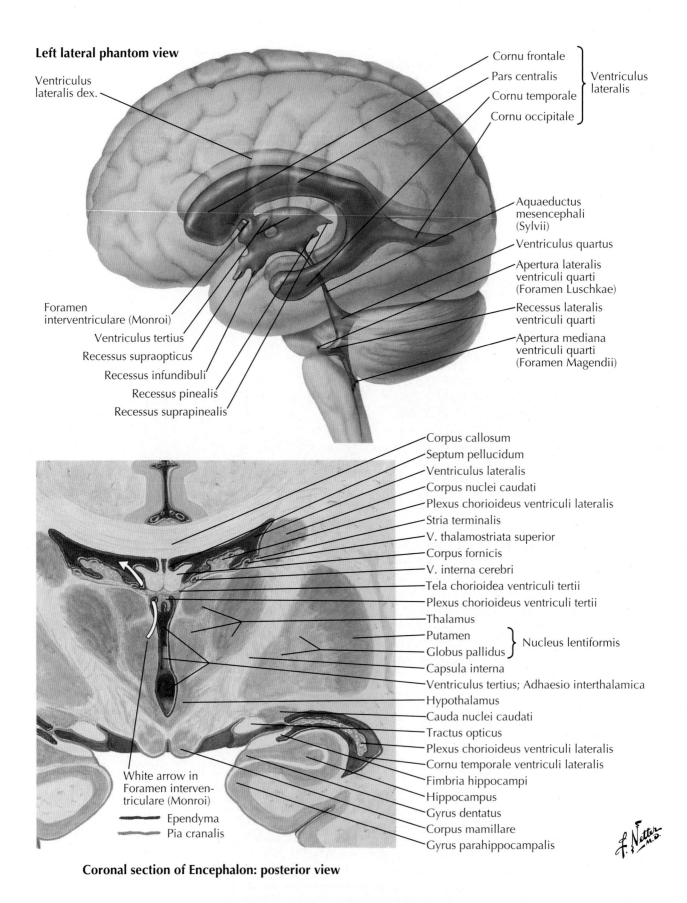

Left lateral phantom view

Ventriculus lateralis dex.

Cornu frontale
Pars centralis
Cornu temporale
Cornu occipitale
} Ventriculus lateralis

Aquaeductus mesencephali (Sylvii)
Ventriculus quartus
Apertura lateralis ventriculi quarti (Foramen Luschkae)
Recessus lateralis ventriculi quarti
Apertura mediana ventriculi quarti (Foramen Magendii)

Foramen interventriculare (Monroi)
Ventriculus tertius
Recessus supraopticus
Recessus infundibuli
Recessus pinealis
Recessus suprapinealis

Corpus callosum
Septum pellucidum
Ventriculus lateralis
Corpus nuclei caudati
Plexus chorioideus ventriculi lateralis
Stria terminalis
V. thalamostriata superior
Corpus fornicis
V. interna cerebri
Tela chorioidea ventriculi tertii
Plexus chorioideus ventriculi tertii
Thalamus
Putamen
Globus pallidus
} Nucleus lentiformis
Capsula interna
Ventriculus tertius; Adhaesio interthalamica
Hypothalamus
Cauda nuclei caudati
Tractus opticus
Plexus chorioideus ventriculi lateralis
Cornu temporale ventriculi lateralis
Fimbria hippocampi
Hippocampus
Gyrus dentatus
Corpus mamillare
Gyrus parahippocampalis

White arrow in Foramen interventriculare (Monroi)

Ependyma
Pia cranalis

Coronal section of Encephalon: posterior view

Plate 135   **Encephalon and Meninges**

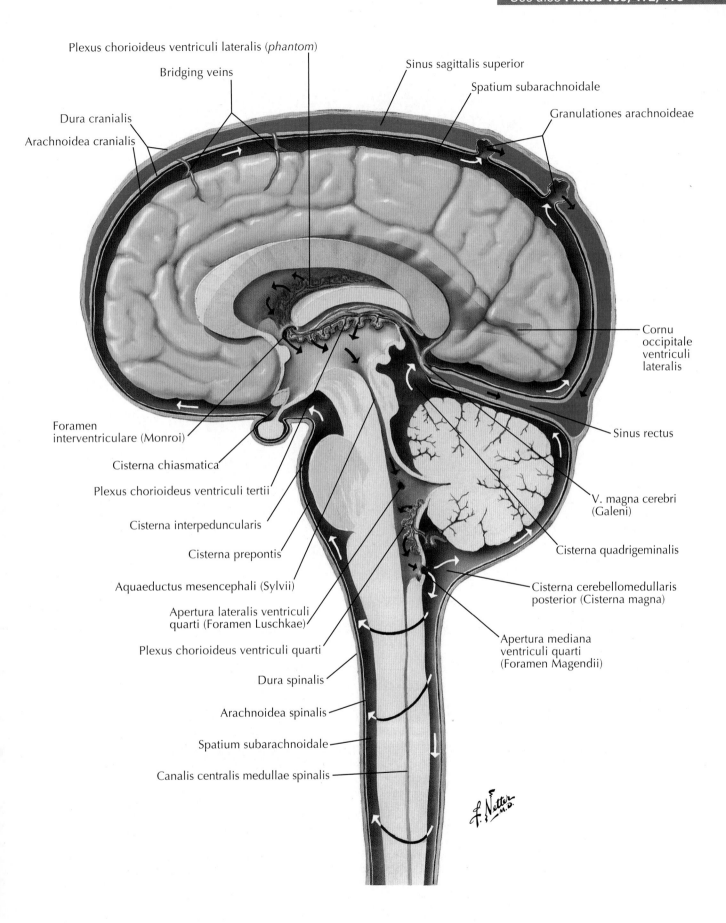

Plexus chorioideus ventriculi lateralis (*phantom*)

Bridging veins

Dura cranialis

Arachnoidea cranialis

Sinus sagittalis superior

Spatium subarachnoidale

Granulationes arachnoideae

Cornu occipitale ventriculi lateralis

Sinus rectus

Foramen interventriculare (Monroi)

Cisterna chiasmatica

Plexus chorioideus ventriculi tertii

Cisterna interpeduncularis

Cisterna prepontis

Aquaeductus mesencephali (Sylvii)

Apertura lateralis ventriculi quarti (Foramen Luschkae)

Plexus chorioideus ventriculi quarti

Dura spinalis

Arachnoidea spinalis

Spatium subarachnoidale

Canalis centralis medullae spinalis

V. magna cerebri (Galeni)

Cisterna quadrigeminalis

Cisterna cerebellomedullaris posterior (Cisterna magna)

Apertura mediana ventriculi quarti (Foramen Magendii)

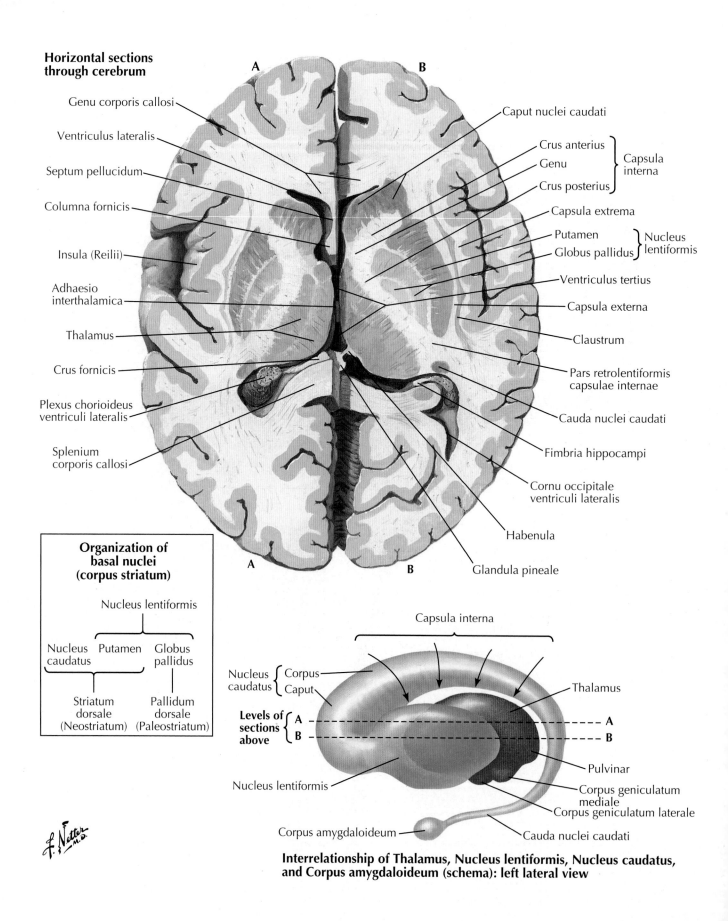

Horizontal sections through cerebrum

A B

- Genu corporis callosi
- Ventriculus lateralis
- Septum pellucidum
- Columna fornicis
- Insula (Reilii)
- Adhaesio interthalamica
- Thalamus
- Crus fornicis
- Plexus chorioideus ventriculi lateralis
- Splenium corporis callosi

- Caput nuclei caudati
- Crus anterius ⎫
- Genu   ⎬ Capsula interna
- Crus posterius ⎭
- Capsula extrema
- Putamen ⎫ Nucleus lentiformis
- Globus pallidus ⎭
- Ventriculus tertius
- Capsula externa
- Claustrum
- Pars retrolentiformis capsulae internae
- Cauda nuclei caudati
- Fimbria hippocampi
- Cornu occipitale ventriculi lateralis
- Habenula
- Glandula pineale

A B

Organization of basal nuclei (corpus striatum)

Nucleus lentiformis

| Nucleus caudatus | Putamen | Globus pallidus |

Striatum dorsale (Neostriatum)   Pallidum dorsale (Paleostriatum)

Capsula interna

Nucleus caudatus { Corpus / Caput }
Thalamus

Levels of sections above { A / B }

A
B

Pulvinar
Corpus geniculatum mediale
Corpus geniculatum laterale
Cauda nuclei caudati

Nucleus lentiformis

Corpus amygdaloideum

Interrelationship of Thalamus, Nucleus lentiformis, Nucleus caudatus, and Corpus amygdaloideum (schema): left lateral view

Plate 137   **Encephalon and Meninges**

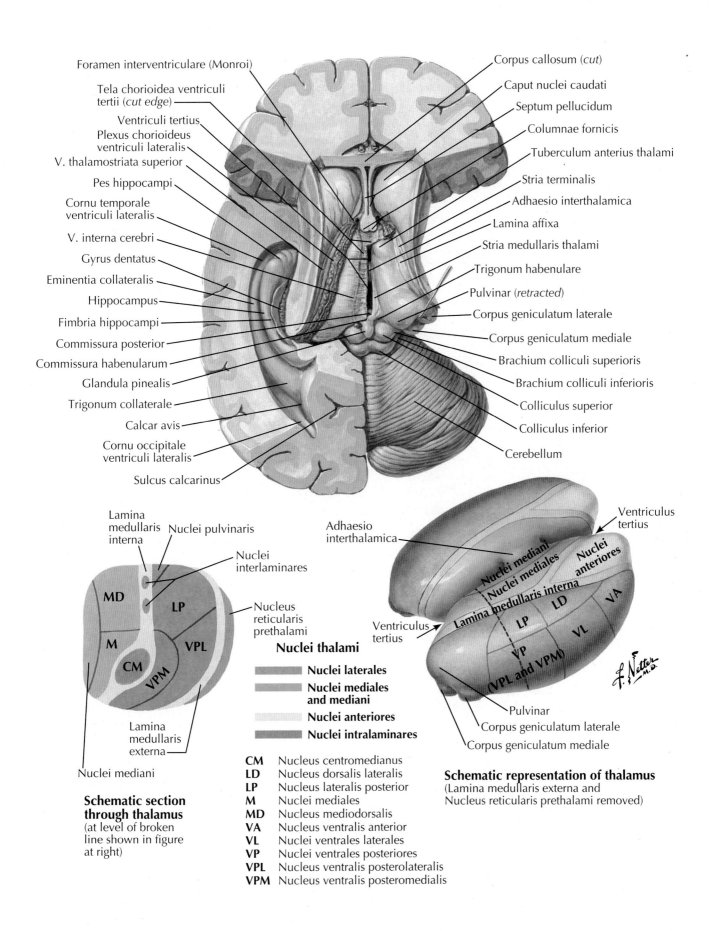

Foramen interventriculare (Monroi)

Tela chorioidea ventriculi tertii (*cut edge*)

Ventriculi tertius

Plexus chorioideus ventriculi lateralis

V. thalamostriata superior

Pes hippocampi

Cornu temporale ventriculi lateralis

V. interna cerebri

Gyrus dentatus

Eminentia collateralis

Hippocampus

Fimbria hippocampi

Commissura posterior

Commissura habenularum

Glandula pinealis

Trigonum collaterale

Calcar avis

Cornu occipitale ventriculi lateralis

Sulcus calcarinus

Corpus callosum (*cut*)

Caput nuclei caudati

Septum pellucidum

Columnae fornicis

Tuberculum anterius thalami

Stria terminalis

Adhaesio interthalamica

Lamina affixa

Stria medullaris thalami

Trigonum habenulare

Pulvinar (*retracted*)

Corpus geniculatum laterale

Corpus geniculatum mediale

Brachium colliculi superioris

Brachium colliculi inferioris

Colliculus superior

Colliculus inferior

Cerebellum

Lamina medullaris interna

Nuclei pulvinaris

Nuclei interlaminares

Nucleus reticularis prethalami

MD

LP

M

VPL

CM

VPM

Lamina medullaris externa

Nuclei mediani

Schematic section through thalamus
(at level of broken line shown in figure at right)

Adhaesio interthalamica

Nuclei mediani

Nuclei mediales

Nuclei anteriores

Lamina medullaris interna

Ventriculus tertius

Ventriculus tertius

LD

VA

LP

VL

VP
(VPL and VPM)

Pulvinar

Corpus geniculatum laterale

Corpus geniculatum mediale

Nuclei thalami

Nuclei laterales

Nuclei mediales and mediani

Nuclei anteriores

Nuclei intralaminares

CM	Nucleus centromedianus
LD	Nucleus dorsalis lateralis
LP	Nucleus lateralis posterior
M	Nuclei mediales
MD	Nucleus mediodorsalis
VA	Nucleus ventralis anterior
VL	Nuclei ventrales laterales
VP	Nuclei ventrales posteriores
VPL	Nucleus ventralis posterolateralis
VPM	Nucleus ventralis posteromedialis

Schematic representation of thalamus
(Lamina medullaris externa and Nucleus reticularis prethalami removed)

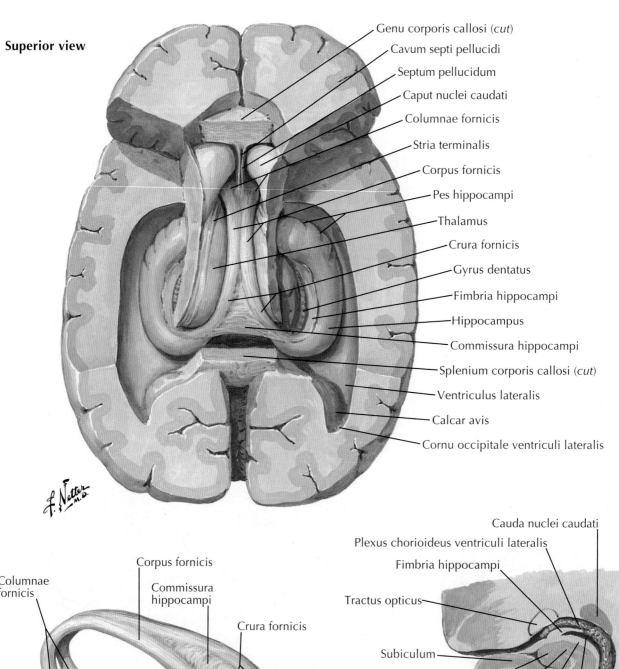

Superior view

Genu corporis callosi (*cut*)

Cavum septi pellucidi

Septum pellucidum

Caput nuclei caudati

Columnae fornicis

Stria terminalis

Corpus fornicis

Pes hippocampi

Thalamus

Crura fornicis

Gyrus dentatus

Fimbria hippocampi

Hippocampus

Commissura hippocampi

Splenium corporis callosi (*cut*)

Ventriculus lateralis

Calcar avis

Cornu occipitale ventriculi lateralis

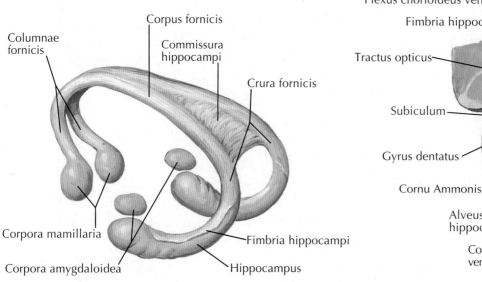

Columnae fornicis

Corpus fornicis

Commissura hippocampi

Crura fornicis

Corpora mamillaria

Corpora amygdaloidea

Fimbria hippocampi

Hippocampus

Fornix: schema

Cauda nuclei caudati

Plexus chorioideus ventriculi lateralis

Fimbria hippocampi

Tractus opticus

Subiculum

Gyrus dentatus

Cornu Ammonis

Alveus hippocampi

Cornu temporale ventriculi lateralis

Coronal section: posterior view

Plate 139

Encephalon and Meninges

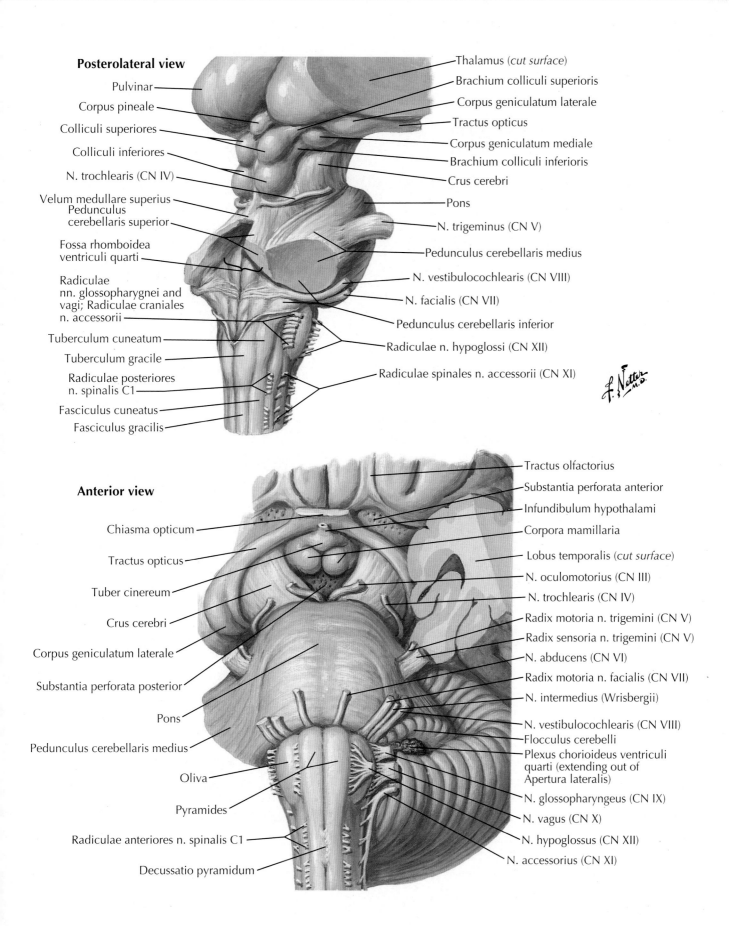

Posterolateral view

Pulvinar

Corpus pineale

Colliculi superiores

Colliculi inferiores

N. trochlearis (CN IV)

Velum medullare superius
Pedunculus
cerebellaris superior

Fossa rhomboidea
ventriculi quarti

Radiculae
nn. glossopharygnei and
vagi; Radiculae craniales
n. accessorii

Tuberculum cuneatum

Tuberculum gracile

Radiculae posteriores
n. spinalis C1

Fasciculus cuneatus

Fasciculus gracilis

Thalamus (cut surface)

Brachium colliculi superioris

Corpus geniculatum laterale

Tractus opticus

Corpus geniculatum mediale

Brachium colliculi inferioris

Crus cerebri

Pons

N. trigeminus (CN V)

Pedunculus cerebellaris medius

N. vestibulocochlearis (CN VIII)

N. facialis (CN VII)

Pedunculus cerebellaris inferior

Radiculae n. hypoglossi (CN XII)

Radiculae spinales n. accessorii (CN XI)

Anterior view

Chiasma opticum

Tractus opticus

Tuber cinereum

Crus cerebri

Corpus geniculatum laterale

Substantia perforata posterior

Pons

Pedunculus cerebellaris medius

Oliva

Pyramides

Radiculae anteriores n. spinalis C1

Decussatio pyramidum

Tractus olfactorius

Substantia perforata anterior

Infundibulum hypothalami

Corpora mamillaria

Lobus temporalis (cut surface)

N. oculomotorius (CN III)

N. trochlearis (CN IV)

Radix motoria n. trigemini (CN V)

Radix sensoria n. trigemini (CN V)

N. abducens (CN VI)

Radix motoria n. facialis (CN VII)

N. intermedius (Wrisbergii)

N. vestibulocochlearis (CN VIII)

Flocculus cerebelli

Plexus chorioideus ventriculi
quarti (extending out of
Apertura lateralis)

N. glossopharyngeus (CN IX)

N. vagus (CN X)

N. hypoglossus (CN XII)

N. accessorius (CN XI)

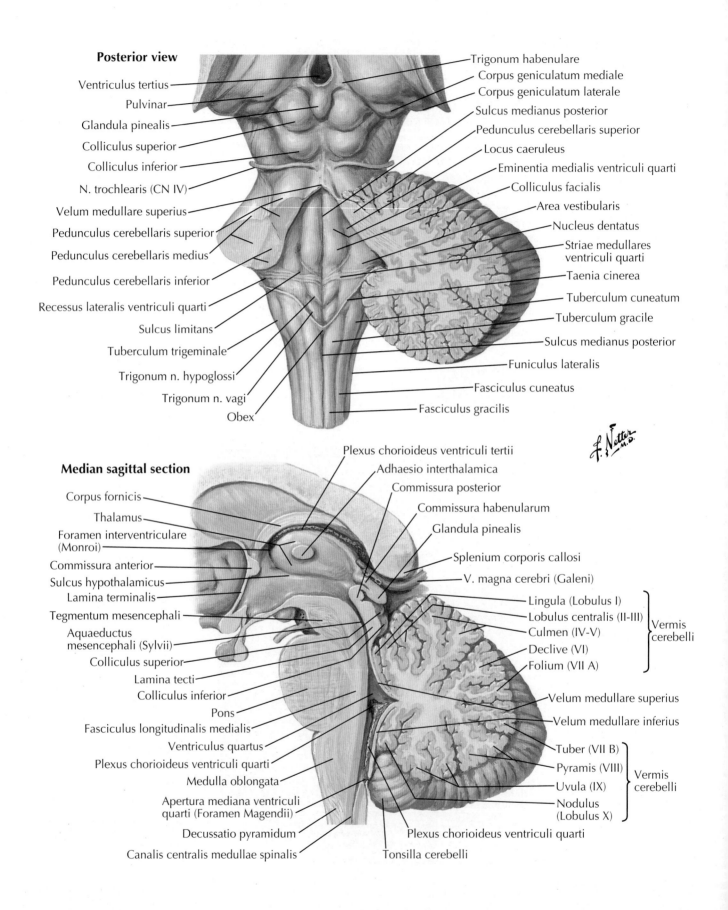

Posterior view

Ventriculus tertius

Pulvinar

Glandula pinealis

Colliculus superior

Colliculus inferior

N. trochlearis (CN IV)

Velum medullare superius

Pedunculus cerebellaris superior

Pedunculus cerebellaris medius

Pedunculus cerebellaris inferior

Recessus lateralis ventriculi quarti

Sulcus limitans

Tuberculum trigeminale

Trigonum n. hypoglossi

Trigonum n. vagi

Obex

Trigonum habenulare

Corpus geniculatum mediale

Corpus geniculatum laterale

Sulcus medianus posterior

Pedunculus cerebellaris superior

Locus caeruleus

Eminentia medialis ventriculi quarti

Colliculus facialis

Area vestibularis

Nucleus dentatus

Striae medullares ventriculi quarti

Taenia cinerea

Tuberculum cuneatum

Tuberculum gracile

Sulcus medianus posterior

Funiculus lateralis

Fasciculus cuneatus

Fasciculus gracilis

Median sagittal section

Corpus fornicis

Thalamus

Foramen interventriculare (Monroi)

Commissura anterior

Sulcus hypothalamicus

Lamina terminalis

Tegmentum mesencephali

Aquaeductus mesencephali (Sylvii)

Colliculus superior

Lamina tecti

Colliculus inferior

Pons

Fasciculus longitudinalis medialis

Ventriculus quartus

Plexus chorioideus ventriculi quarti

Medulla oblongata

Apertura mediana ventriculi quarti (Foramen Magendii)

Decussatio pyramidum

Canalis centralis medullae spinalis

Plexus chorioideus ventriculi tertii

Adhaesio interthalamica

Commissura posterior

Commissura habenularum

Glandula pinealis

Splenium corporis callosi

V. magna cerebri (Galeni)

Lingula (Lobulus I)

Lobulus centralis (II-III)

Culmen (IV-V)

Declive (VI)

Folium (VII A)

Vermis cerebelli

Velum medullare superius

Velum medullare inferius

Tuber (VII B)

Pyramis (VIII)

Uvula (IX)

Nodulus (Lobulus X)

Vermis cerebelli

Plexus chorioideus ventriculi quarti

Tonsilla cerebelli

Plate 141　　　　　　　　　　　　　　　　　　　**Encephalon and Meninges**

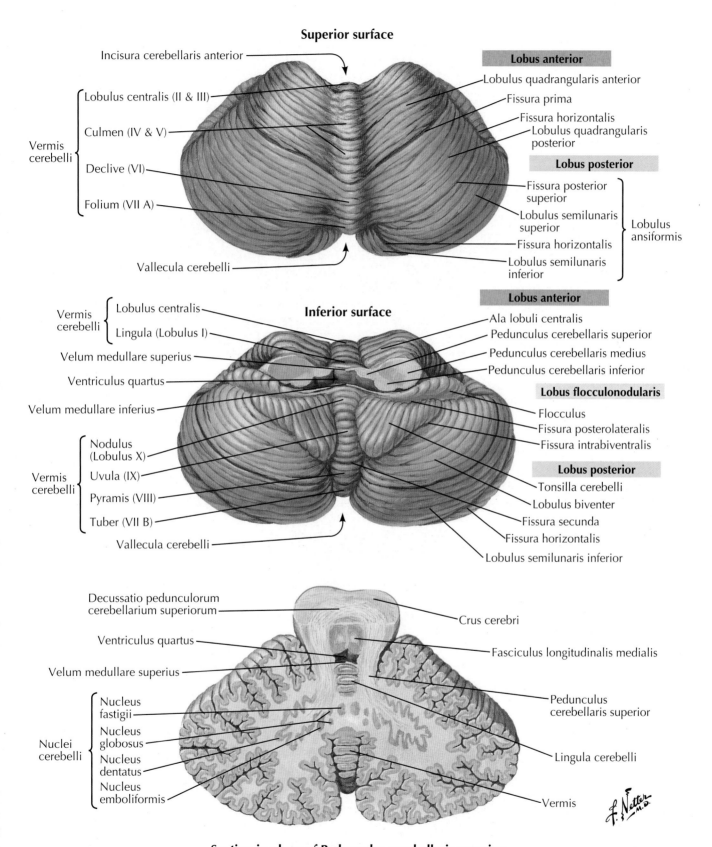

Superior surface

Incisura cerebellaris anterior

Lobus anterior

Lobulus quadrangularis anterior

Fissura prima

Fissura horizontalis

Lobulus quadrangularis posterior

Vermis cerebelli
- Lobulus centralis (II & III)
- Culmen (IV & V)
- Declive (VI)
- Folium (VII A)

Lobus posterior

Fissura posterior superior

Lobulus semilunaris superior

Fissura horizontalis

Lobulus semilunaris inferior

Lobulus ansiformis

Vallecula cerebelli

Inferior surface

Vermis cerebelli
- Lobulus centralis
- Lingula (Lobulus I)

Velum medullare superius

Ventriculus quartus

Velum medullare inferius

Vermis cerebelli
- Nodulus (Lobulus X)
- Uvula (IX)
- Pyramis (VIII)
- Tuber (VII B)

Vallecula cerebelli

Lobus anterior

Ala lobuli centralis

Pedunculus cerebellaris superior

Pedunculus cerebellaris medius

Pedunculus cerebellaris inferior

Lobus flocculonodularis

Flocculus

Fissura posterolateralis

Fissura intrabiventralis

Lobus posterior

Tonsilla cerebelli

Lobulus biventer

Fissura secunda

Fissura horizontalis

Lobulus semilunaris inferior

Decussatio pedunculorum cerebellarium superiorum

Ventriculus quartus

Velum medullare superius

Nuclei cerebelli
- Nucleus fastigii
- Nucleus globosus
- Nucleus dentatus
- Nucleus emboliformis

Crus cerebri

Fasciculus longitudinalis medialis

Pedunculus cerebellaris superior

Lingula cerebelli

Vermis

Section in plane of Pedunculus cerebellaris superior

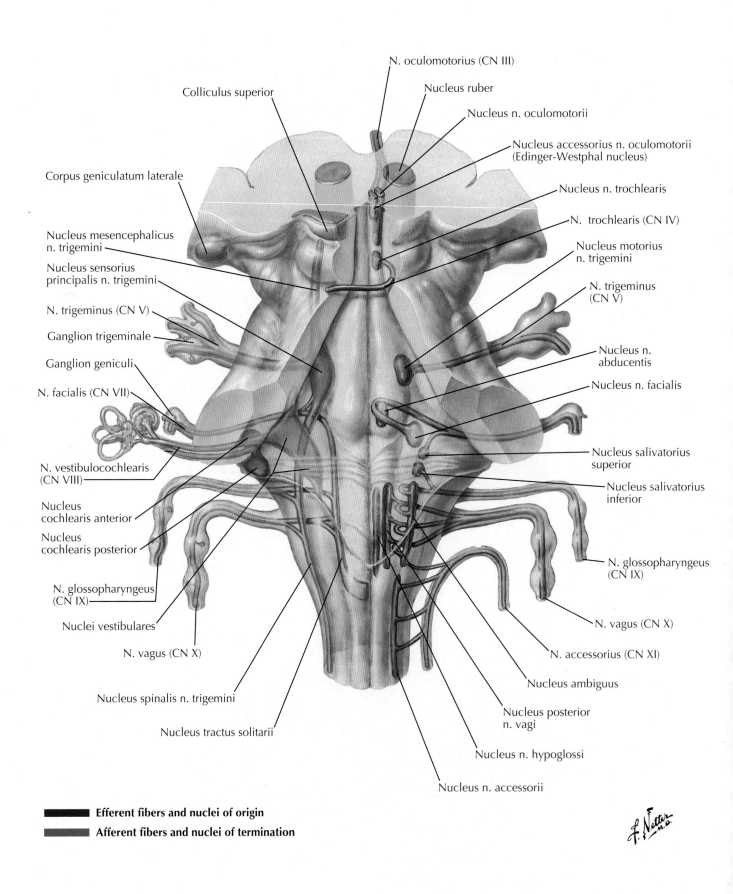

N. oculomotorius (CN III)

Colliculus superior

Nucleus ruber

Nucleus n. oculomotorii

Nucleus accessorius n. oculomotorii
(Edinger-Westphal nucleus)

Corpus geniculatum laterale

Nucleus n. trochlearis

N. trochlearis (CN IV)

Nucleus mesencephalicus
n. trigemini

Nucleus motorius
n. trigemini

Nucleus sensorius
principalis n. trigemini

N. trigeminus
(CN V)

N. trigeminus (CN V)

Ganglion trigeminale

Nucleus n.
abducentis

Ganglion geniculi

Nucleus n. facialis

N. facialis (CN VII)

N. vestibulocochlearis
(CN VIII)

Nucleus salivatorius
superior

Nucleus salivatorius
inferior

Nucleus
cochlearis anterior

Nucleus
cochlearis posterior

N. glossopharyngeus
(CN IX)

N. glossopharyngeus
(CN IX)

Nuclei vestibulares

N. vagus (CN X)

N. accessorius (CN XI)

Nucleus spinalis n. trigemini

Nucleus ambiguus

Nucleus posterior
n. vagi

Nucleus tractus solitarii

Nucleus n. hypoglossi

Nucleus n. accessorii

▬▬▬▬ **Efferent fibers and nuclei of origin**

▬▬▬▬ **Afferent fibers and nuclei of termination**

Plate 143   **Nervi Craniales and Nervi Cervicales**

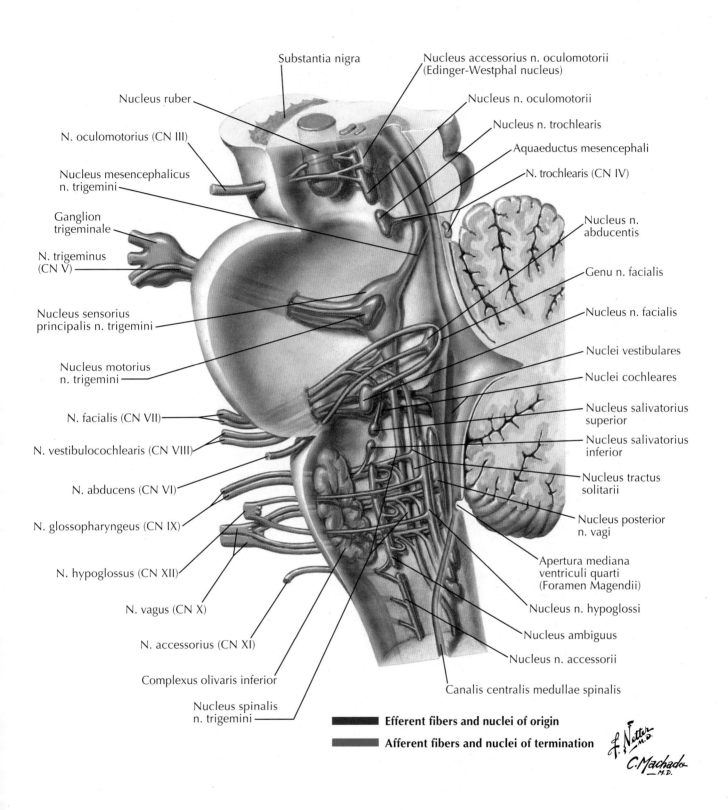

Substantia nigra

Nucleus accessorius n. oculomotorii
(Edinger-Westphal nucleus)

Nucleus ruber

Nucleus n. oculomotorii

N. oculomotorius (CN III)

Nucleus n. trochlearis

Nucleus mesencephalicus
n. trigemini

Aquaeductus mesencephali

N. trochlearis (CN IV)

Ganglion
trigeminale

Nucleus n.
abducentis

N. trigeminus
(CN V)

Genu n. facialis

Nucleus sensorius
principalis n. trigemini

Nucleus n. facialis

Nuclei vestibulares

Nucleus motorius
n. trigemini

Nuclei cochleares

Nucleus salivatorius
superior

N. facialis (CN VII)

Nucleus salivatorius
inferior

N. vestibulocochlearis (CN VIII)

Nucleus tractus
solitarii

N. abducens (CN VI)

Nucleus posterior
n. vagi

N. glossopharyngeus (CN IX)

N. hypoglossus (CN XII)

Apertura mediana
ventriculi quarti
(Foramen Magendii)

N. vagus (CN X)

Nucleus n. hypoglossi

N. accessorius (CN XI)

Nucleus ambiguus

Complexus olivaris inferior

Nucleus n. accessorii

Nucleus spinalis
n. trigemini

Canalis centralis medullae spinalis

◼◼◼ Efferent fibers and nuclei of origin

◼◼◼ Afferent fibers and nuclei of termination

F. Netter
M.D.

C. Machado
M.D.

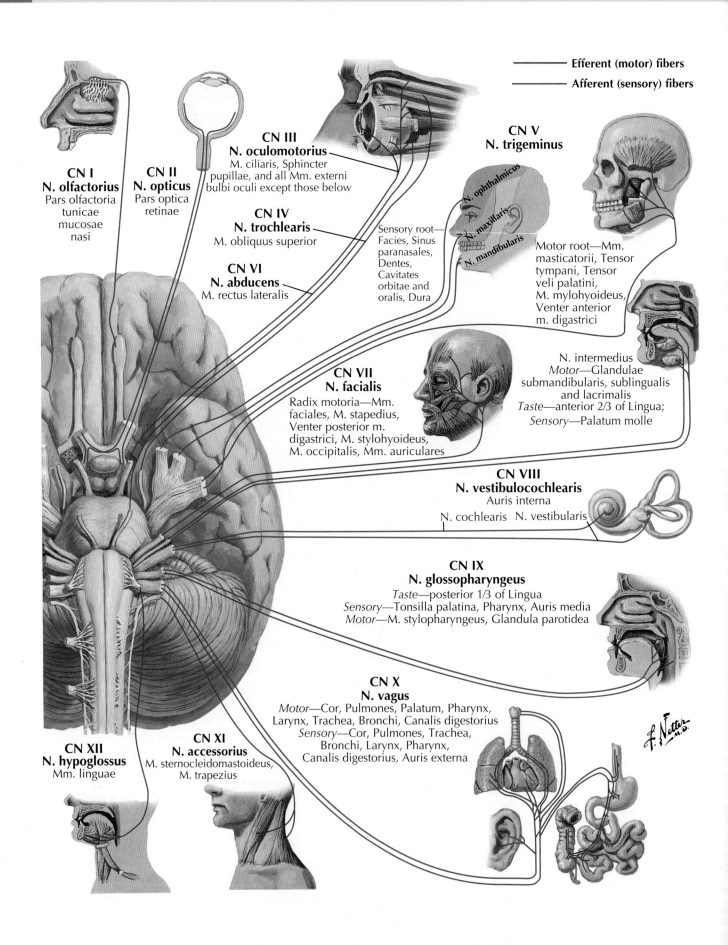

Efferent (motor) fibers
Afferent (sensory) fibers

CN III
N. oculomotorius
M. ciliaris, Sphincter pupillae, and all Mm. externi bulbi oculi except those below

CN I
N. olfactorius
Pars olfactoria tunicae mucosae nasi

CN II
N. opticus
Pars optica retinae

CN IV
N. trochlearis
M. obliquus superior

CN VI
N. abducens
M. rectus lateralis

Sensory root—Facies, Sinus paranasales, Dentes, Cavitates orbitae and oralis, Dura

CN V
N. trigeminus

N. ophthalmicus
N. maxillaris
N. mandibularis

Motor root—Mm. masticatorii, Tensor tympani, Tensor veli palatini, M. mylohyoideus, Venter anterior m. digastrici

N. intermedius
Motor—Glandulae submandibularis, sublingualis and lacrimalis
Taste—anterior 2/3 of Lingua;
Sensory—Palatum molle

CN VII
N. facialis
Radix motoria—Mm. faciales, M. stapedius, Venter posterior m. digastrici, M. stylohyoideus, M. occipitalis, Mm. auriculares

CN VIII
N. vestibulocochlearis
Auris interna
N. cochlearis   N. vestibularis

CN IX
N. glossopharyngeus
Taste—posterior 1/3 of Lingua
Sensory—Tonsilla palatina, Pharynx, Auris media
Motor—M. stylopharyngeus, Glandula parotidea

CN X
N. vagus
Motor—Cor, Pulmones, Palatum, Pharynx, Larynx, Trachea, Bronchi, Canalis digestorius
Sensory—Cor, Pulmones, Trachea, Bronchi, Larynx, Pharynx, Canalis digestorius, Auris externa

CN XII
N. hypoglossus
Mm. linguae

CN XI
N. accessorius
M. sternocleidomastoideus, M. trapezius

Plate 145

Nervi Craniales and Nervi Cervicales

Olfactory bulb cells: schema

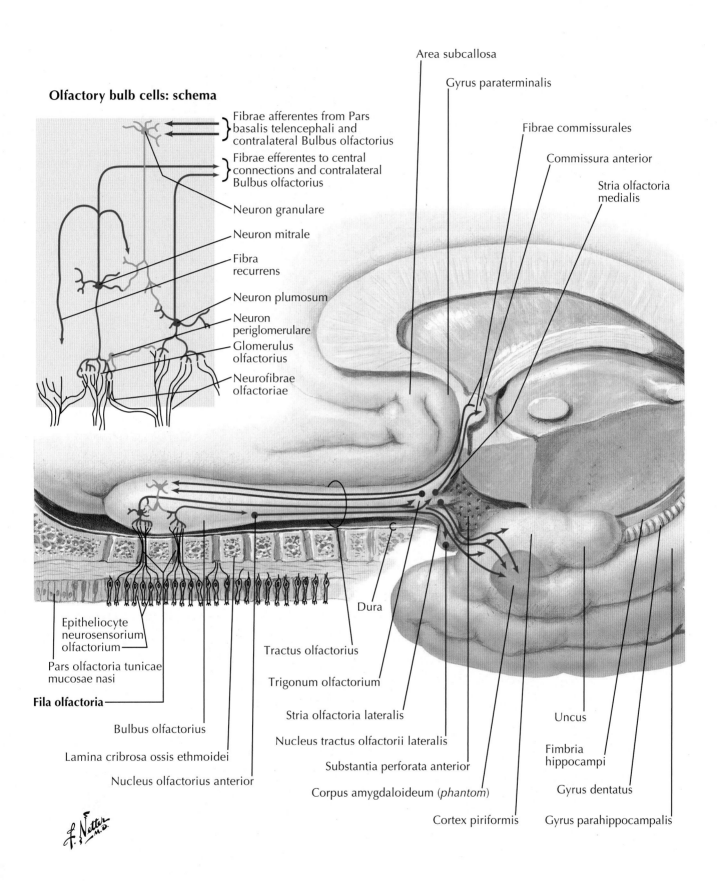

Area subcallosa

Gyrus paraterminalis

Fibrae commissurales

Commissura anterior

Stria olfactoria medialis

Fibrae afferentes from Pars basalis telencephali and contralateral Bulbus olfactorius

Fibrae efferentes to central connections and contralateral Bulbus olfactorius

Neuron granulare

Neuron mitrale

Fibra recurrens

Neuron plumosum

Neuron periglomerulare

Glomerulus olfactorius

Neurofibrae olfactoriae

Epitheliocyte neurosensorium olfactorium

Pars olfactoria tunicae mucosae nasi

Fila olfactoria

Bulbus olfactorius

Lamina cribrosa ossis ethmoidei

Nucleus olfactorius anterior

Dura

Tractus olfactorius

Trigonum olfactorium

Stria olfactoria lateralis

Nucleus tractus olfactorii lateralis

Substantia perforata anterior

Corpus amygdaloideum (*phantom*)

Cortex piriformis

Uncus

Fimbria hippocampi

Gyrus dentatus

Gyrus parahippocampalis

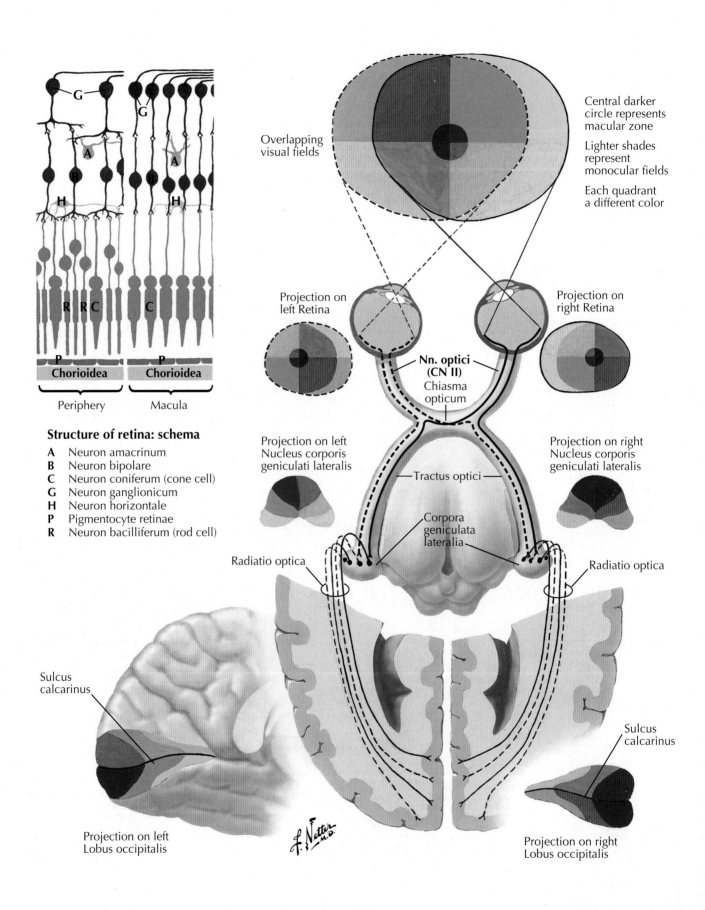

Overlapping visual fields

Central darker circle represents macular zone

Lighter shades represent monocular fields

Each quadrant a different color

Projection on left Retina

Projection on right Retina

Nn. optici (CN II)

Chiasma opticum

Projection on left Nucleus corporis geniculati lateralis

Projection on right Nucleus corporis geniculati lateralis

Tractus optici

Radiatio optica

Corpora geniculata lateralia

Radiatio optica

Sulcus calcarinus

Sulcus calcarinus

Projection on left Lobus occipitalis

Projection on right Lobus occipitalis

Structure of retina: schema

A   Neuron amacrinum
B   Neuron bipolare
C   Neuron coniferum (cone cell)
G   Neuron ganglionicum
H   Neuron horizontale
P   Pigmentocyte retinae
R   Neuron bacilliferum (rod cell)

Chorioidea

Chorioidea

Periphery

Macula

Plate 147

Nervi Craniales and Nervi Cervicales

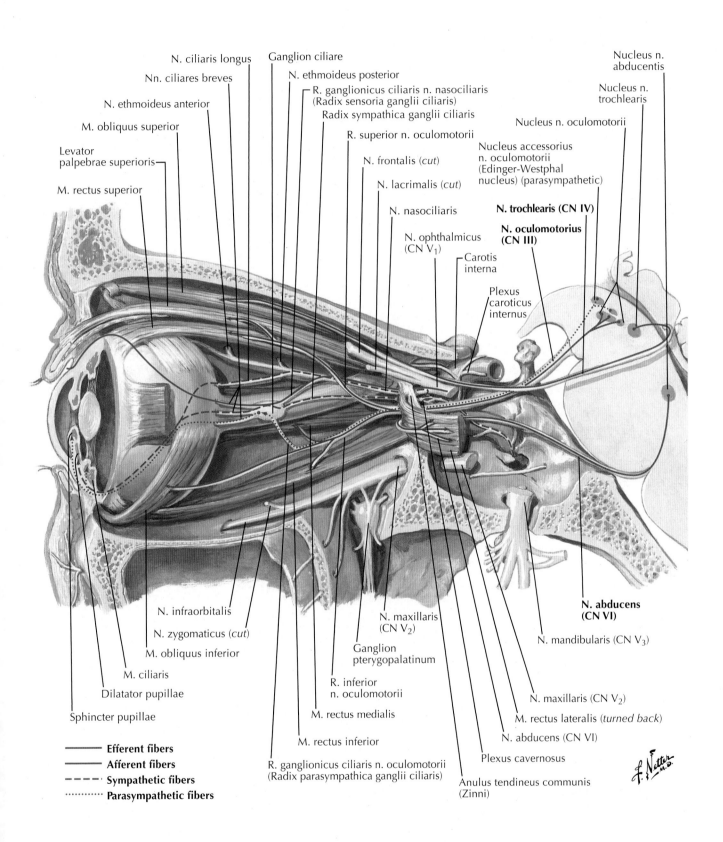

N. ciliaris longus

Nn. ciliares breves

N. ethmoideus anterior

M. obliquus superior

Levator palpebrae superioris

M. rectus superior

Ganglion ciliare

N. ethmoideus posterior

R. ganglionicus ciliaris n. nasociliaris (Radix sensoria ganglii ciliaris)

Radix sympathica ganglii ciliaris

R. superior n. oculomotorii

N. frontalis (cut)

N. lacrimalis (cut)

N. nasociliaris

N. ophthalmicus (CN V$_1$)

Carotis interna

Plexus caroticus internus

Nucleus n. abducentis

Nucleus n. trochlearis

Nucleus n. oculomotorii

Nucleus accessorius n. oculomotorii (Edinger-Westphal nucleus) (parasympathetic)

N. trochlearis (CN IV)

N. oculomotorius (CN III)

N. infraorbitalis

N. zygomaticus (cut)

M. obliquus inferior

M. ciliaris

Dilatator pupillae

Sphincter pupillae

N. maxillaris (CN V$_2$)

Ganglion pterygopalatinum

R. inferior n. oculomotorii

M. rectus medialis

M. rectus inferior

R. ganglionicus ciliaris n. oculomotorii (Radix parasympathica ganglii ciliaris)

N. abducens (CN VI)

N. mandibularis (CN V$_3$)

N. maxillaris (CN V$_2$)

M. rectus lateralis (turned back)

N. abducens (CN VI)

Plexus cavernosus

Anulus tendineus communis (Zinni)

Efferent fibers

Afferent fibers

Sympathetic fibers

Parasympathetic fibers

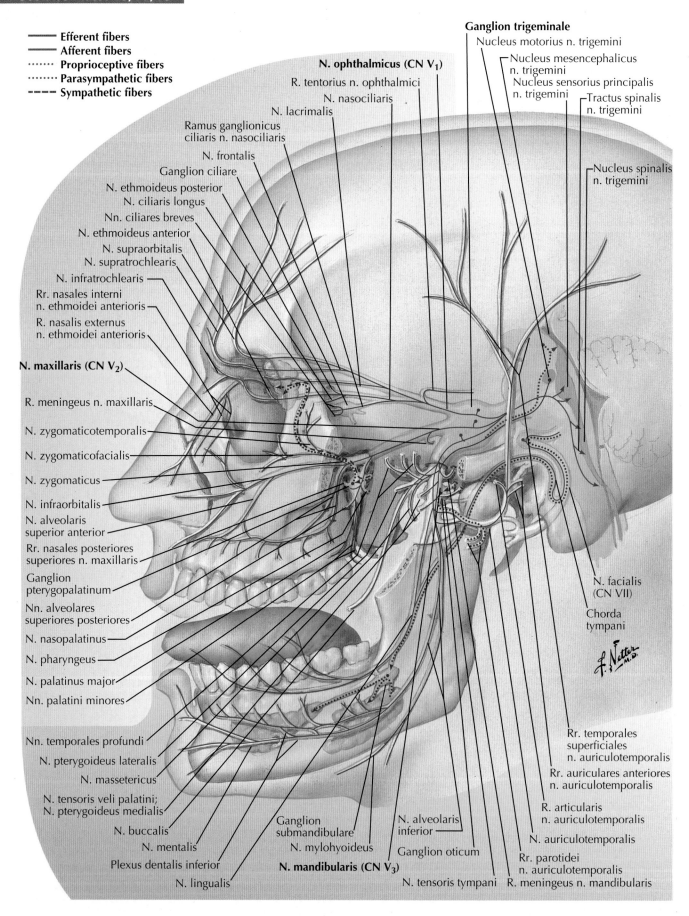

Efferent fibers
Afferent fibers
Proprioceptive fibers
Parasympathetic fibers
Sympathetic fibers

Ganglion trigeminale

Nucleus motorius n. trigemini

Nucleus mesencephalicus n. trigemini

Nucleus sensorius principalis n. trigemini

Tractus spinalis n. trigemini

Nucleus spinalis n. trigemini

N. ophthalmicus (CN V₁)

R. tentorius n. ophthalmici

N. nasociliaris

N. lacrimalis

Ramus ganglionicus ciliaris n. nasociliaris

N. frontalis

Ganglion ciliare

N. ethmoideus posterior

N. ciliaris longus

Nn. ciliares breves

N. ethmoideus anterior

N. supraorbitalis

N. supratrochlearis

N. infratrochlearis

Rr. nasales interni n. ethmoidei anterioris

R. nasalis externus n. ethmoidei anterioris

N. maxillaris (CN V₂)

R. meningeus n. maxillaris

N. zygomaticotemporalis

N. zygomaticofacialis

N. zygomaticus

N. infraorbitalis

N. alveolaris superior anterior

Rr. nasales posteriores superiores n. maxillaris

Ganglion pterygopalatinum

Nn. alveolares superiores posteriores

N. nasopalatinus

N. pharyngeus

N. palatinus major

Nn. palatini minores

Nn. temporales profundi

N. pterygoideus lateralis

N. massetericus

N. tensoris veli palatini; N. pterygoideus medialis

N. buccalis

N. mentalis

Plexus dentalis inferior

N. lingualis

Ganglion submandibulare

N. mylohyoideus

N. mandibularis (CN V₃)

N. alveolaris inferior

Ganglion oticum

N. tensoris tympani

N. facialis (CN VII)

Chorda tympani

Rr. temporales superficiales n. auriculotemporalis

Rr. auriculares anteriores n. auriculotemporalis

R. articularis n. auriculotemporalis

N. auriculotemporalis

Rr. parotidei n. auriculotemporalis

R. meningeus n. mandibularis

Plate 149

Nervi Craniales and Nervi Cervicales

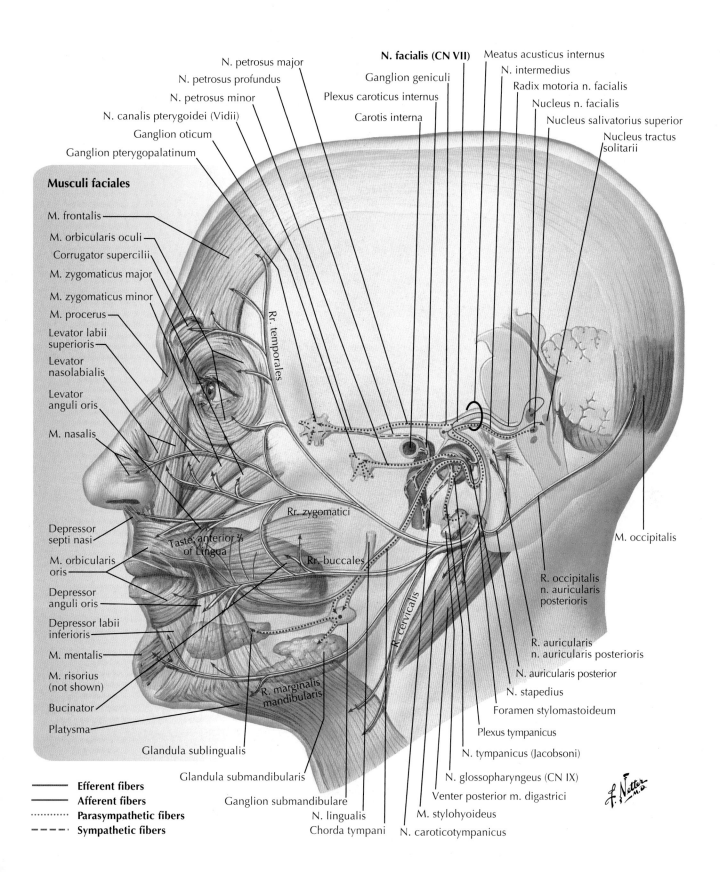

N. petrosus major

N. petrosus profundus

N. petrosus minor

N. canalis pterygoidei (Vidii)

Ganglion oticum

Ganglion pterygopalatinum

N. facialis (CN VII)

Ganglion geniculi

Plexus caroticus internus

Carotis interna

Meatus acusticus internus

N. intermedius

Radix motoria n. facialis

Nucleus n. facialis

Nucleus salivatorius superior

Nucleus tractus solitarii

Musculi faciales

M. frontalis

M. orbicularis oculi

Corrugator supercilii

M. zygomaticus major

M. zygomaticus minor

M. procerus

Levator labii superioris

Levator nasolabialis

Levator anguli oris

M. nasalis

Depressor septi nasi

M. orbicularis oris

Depressor anguli oris

Depressor labii inferioris

M. mentalis

M. risorius (not shown)

Bucinator

Platysma

Rr. temporales

Rr. zygomatici

Taste; anterior ⅔ of Lingua

Rr. buccales

R. cervicalis

R. marginalis mandibularis

Glandula sublingualis

Glandula submandibularis

Ganglion submandibulare

N. lingualis

Chorda tympani

M. occipitalis

R. occipitalis n. auricularis posterioris

R. auricularis n. auricularis posterioris

N. auricularis posterior

N. stapedius

Foramen stylomastoideum

Plexus tympanicus

N. tympanicus (Jacobsoni)

N. glossopharyngeus (CN IX)

Venter posterior m. digastrici

M. stylohyoideus

N. caroticotympanicus

—— Efferent fibers

—— Afferent fibers

········· Parasympathetic fibers

- - - - Sympathetic fibers

Afferent fibers

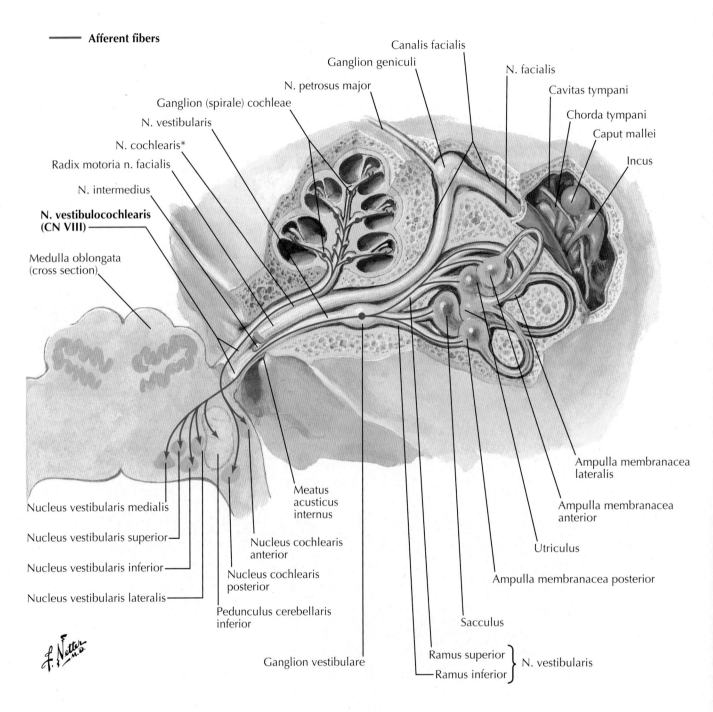

Canalis facialis

Ganglion geniculi

N. petrosus major

N. facialis

Cavitas tympani

Chorda tympani

Caput mallei

Ganglion (spirale) cochleae

Incus

N. vestibularis

N. cochlearis*

Radix motoria n. facialis

N. intermedius

N. vestibulocochlearis (CN VIII)

Medulla oblongata (cross section)

Ampulla membranacea lateralis

Ampulla membranacea anterior

Nucleus vestibularis medialis

Utriculus

Nucleus vestibularis superior

Meatus acusticus internus

Ampulla membranacea posterior

Nucleus vestibularis inferior

Nucleus cochlearis anterior

Nucleus vestibularis lateralis

Nucleus cochlearis posterior

Pedunculus cerebellaris inferior

Sacculus

Ganglion vestibulare

Ramus superior

Ramus inferior

} N. vestibularis

*Note: N. cochlearis also contains efferent fibers to the sensory epithelium.
These fibers are derived from the n. vestibularis while in the meatus acusticus internus.*

Plate 151

Nervi Craniales and Nervi Cervicales

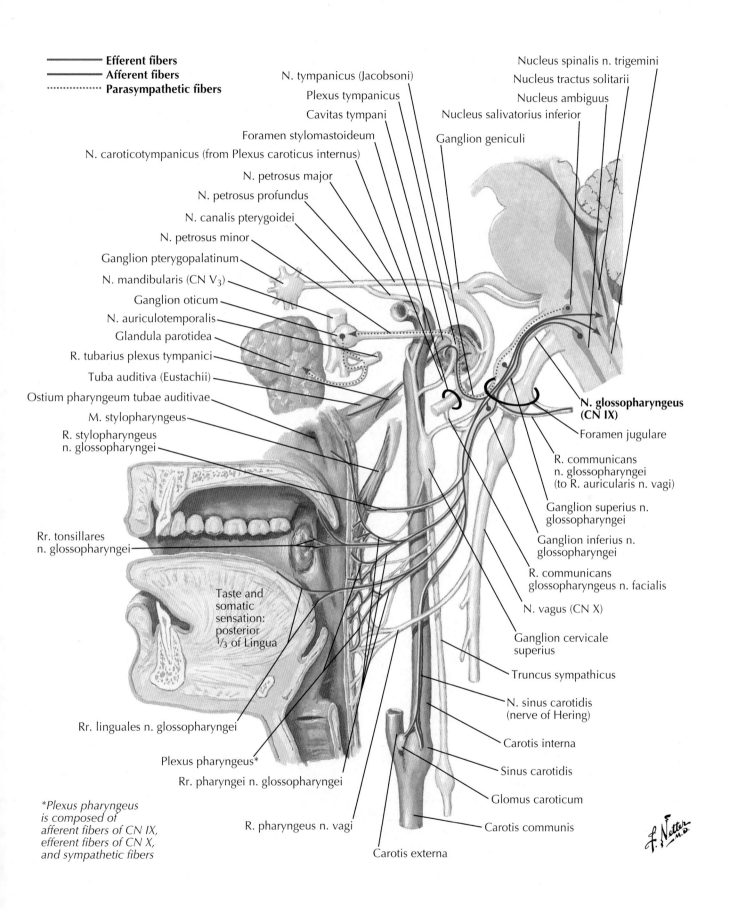

Efferent fibers
Afferent fibers
Parasympathetic fibers

N. tympanicus (Jacobsoni)
Plexus tympanicus
Cavitas tympani
Foramen stylomastoideum
N. caroticotympanicus (from Plexus caroticus internus)
N. petrosus major
N. petrosus profundus
N. canalis pterygoidei
N. petrosus minor
Ganglion pterygopalatinum
N. mandibularis (CN V₃)
Ganglion oticum
N. auriculotemporalis
Glandula parotidea
R. tubarius plexus tympanici
Tuba auditiva (Eustachii)
Ostium pharyngeum tubae auditivae
M. stylopharyngeus
R. stylopharyngeus
n. glossopharyngei

Nucleus spinalis n. trigemini
Nucleus tractus solitarii
Nucleus ambiguus
Nucleus salivatorius inferior
Ganglion geniculi

N. glossopharyngeus
(CN IX)
Foramen jugulare
R. communicans
n. glossopharyngei
(to R. auricularis n. vagi)
Ganglion superius n.
glossopharyngei
Ganglion inferius n.
glossopharyngei
R. communicans
glossopharyngeus n. facialis
N. vagus (CN X)
Ganglion cervicale
superius
Truncus sympathicus
N. sinus carotidis
(nerve of Hering)
Carotis interna
Sinus carotidis
Glomus caroticum
Carotis communis

Rr. tonsillares
n. glossopharyngei

Taste and
somatic
sensation:
posterior
¹/₃ of Lingua

Rr. linguales n. glossopharyngei

Plexus pharyngeus*

Rr. pharyngei n. glossopharyngei

*Plexus pharyngeus
is composed of
afferent fibers of CN IX,
efferent fibers of CN X,
and sympathetic fibers

R. pharyngeus n. vagi

Carotis externa

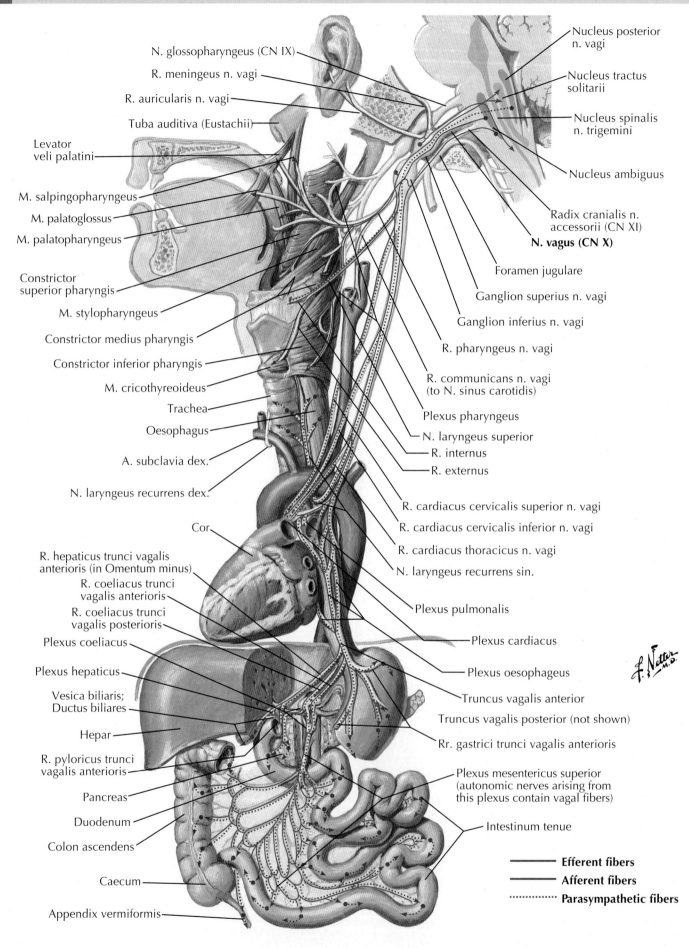

N. glossopharyngeus (CN IX)

R. meningeus n. vagi

R. auricularis n. vagi

Tuba auditiva (Eustachii)

Levator veli palatini

M. salpingopharyngeus

M. palatoglossus

M. palatopharyngeus

Constrictor superior pharyngis

M. stylopharyngeus

Constrictor medius pharyngis

Constrictor inferior pharyngis

M. cricothyreoideus

Trachea

Oesophagus

A. subclavia dex.

N. laryngeus recurrens dex.

Cor

R. hepaticus trunci vagalis anterioris (in Omentum minus)

R. coeliacus trunci vagalis anterioris

R. coeliacus trunci vagalis posterioris

Plexus coeliacus

Plexus hepaticus

Vesica biliaris; Ductus biliares

Hepar

R. pyloricus trunci vagalis anterioris

Pancreas

Duodenum

Colon ascendens

Caecum

Appendix vermiformis

Nucleus posterior n. vagi

Nucleus tractus solitarii

Nucleus spinalis n. trigemini

Nucleus ambiguus

Radix cranialis n. accessorii (CN XI)

N. vagus (CN X)

Foramen jugulare

Ganglion superius n. vagi

Ganglion inferius n. vagi

R. pharyngeus n. vagi

R. communicans n. vagi (to N. sinus carotidis)

Plexus pharyngeus

N. laryngeus superior

R. internus

R. externus

R. cardiacus cervicalis superior n. vagi

R. cardiacus cervicalis inferior n. vagi

R. cardiacus thoracicus n. vagi

N. laryngeus recurrens sin.

Plexus pulmonalis

Plexus cardiacus

Plexus oesophageus

Truncus vagalis anterior

Truncus vagalis posterior (not shown)

Rr. gastrici trunci vagalis anterioris

Plexus mesentericus superior (autonomic nerves arising from this plexus contain vagal fibers)

Intestinum tenue

————	**Efferent fibers**
————	**Afferent fibers**
··········	**Parasympathetic fibers**

Plate 153

Nervi Craniales and Nervi Cervicales

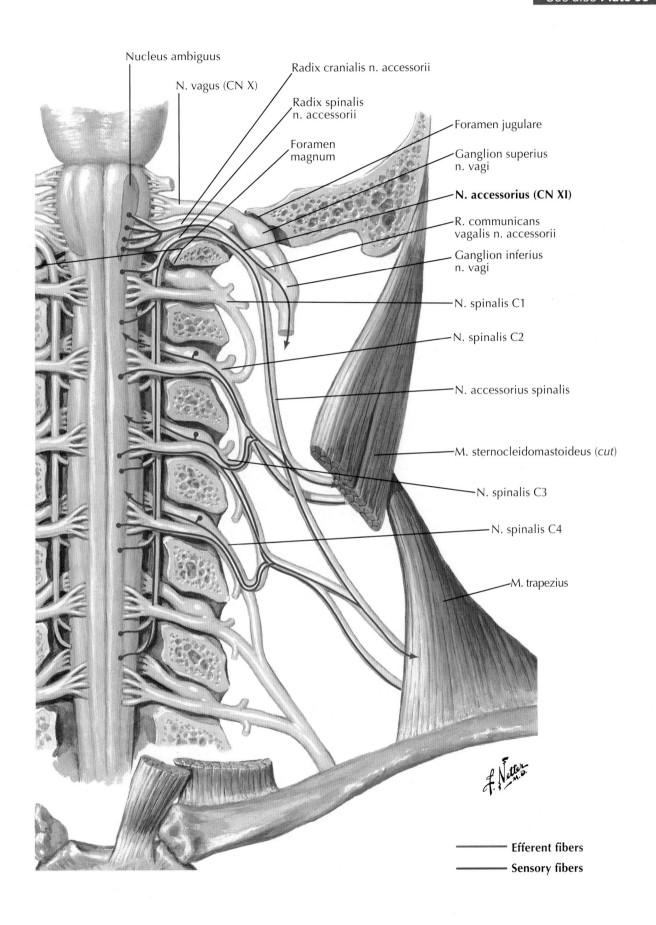

Nucleus ambiguus

N. vagus (CN X)

Radix cranialis n. accessorii

Radix spinalis
n. accessorii

Foramen
magnum

Foramen jugulare

Ganglion superius
n. vagi

N. accessorius (CN XI)

R. communicans
vagalis n. accessorii

Ganglion inferius
n. vagi

N. spinalis C1

N. spinalis C2

N. accessorius spinalis

M. sternocleidomastoideus (*cut*)

N. spinalis C3

N. spinalis C4

M. trapezius

—— Efferent fibers
—— Sensory fibers

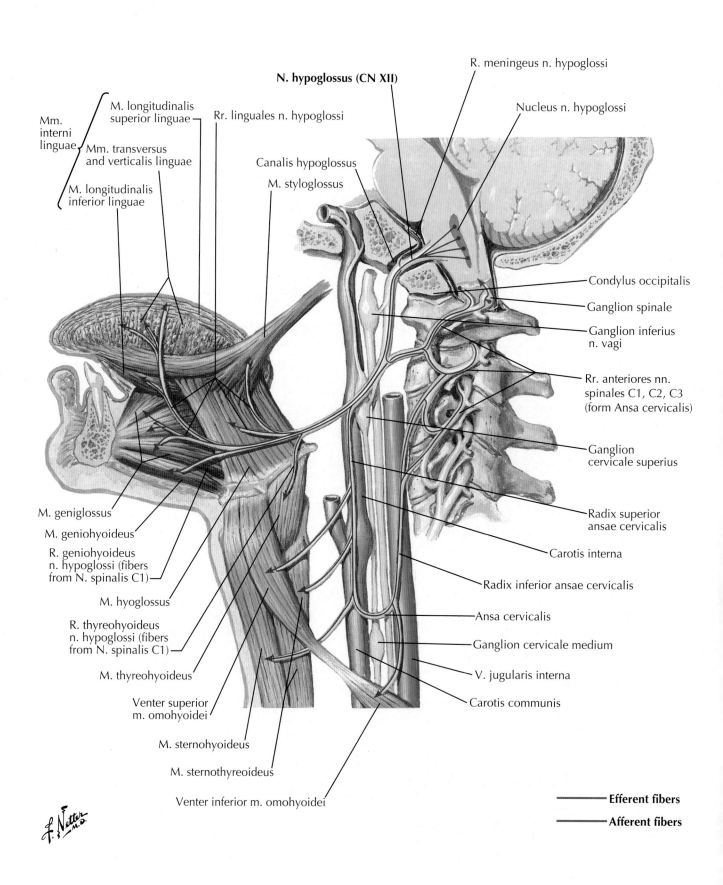

N. hypoglossus (CN XII)

R. meningeus n. hypoglossi

Nucleus n. hypoglossi

M. longitudinalis superior linguae

Rr. linguales n. hypoglossi

Mm. interni linguae

Mm. transversus and verticalis linguae

Canalis hypoglossus

M. styloglossus

M. longitudinalis inferior linguae

Condylus occipitalis

Ganglion spinale

Ganglion inferius n. vagi

Rr. anteriores nn. spinales C1, C2, C3 (form Ansa cervicalis)

Ganglion cervicale superius

M. geniglossus

M. geniohyoideus

R. geniohyoideus n. hypoglossi (fibers from N. spinalis C1)

M. hyoglossus

R. thyreohyoideus n. hypoglossi (fibers from N. spinalis C1)

M. thyreohyoideus

Venter superior m. omohyoidei

M. sternohyoideus

M. sternothyreoideus

Venter inferior m. omohyoidei

Radix superior ansae cervicalis

Carotis interna

Radix inferior ansae cervicalis

Ansa cervicalis

Ganglion cervicale medium

V. jugularis interna

Carotis communis

Efferent fibers

Afferent fibers

Plate 155

Nervi Craniales and Nervi Cervicales

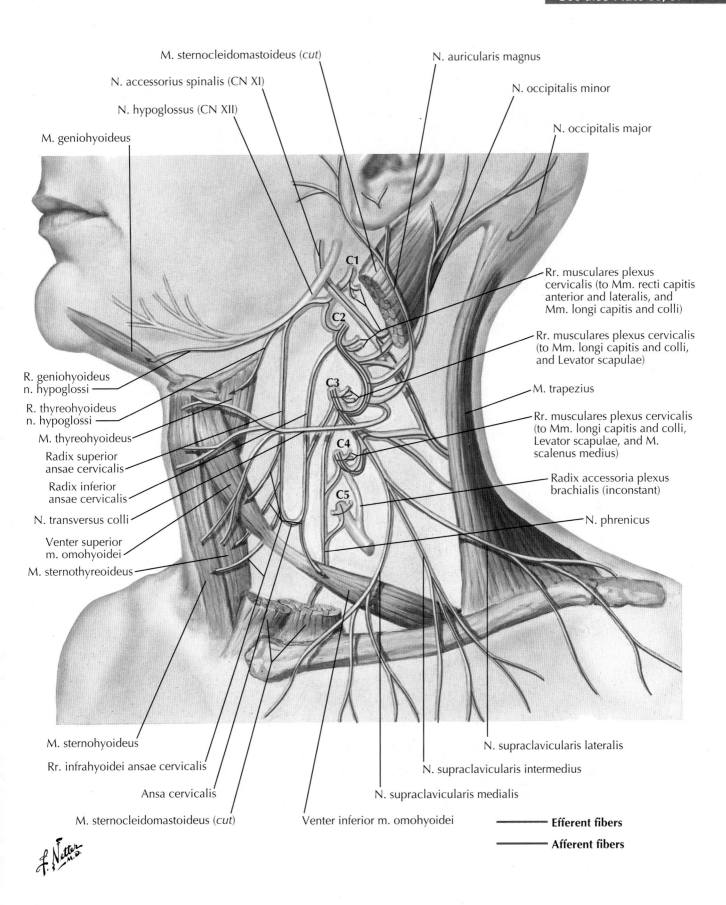

M. sternocleidomastoideus (*cut*)

N. accessorius spinalis (CN XI)

N. hypoglossus (CN XII)

M. geniohyoideus

N. auricularis magnus

N. occipitalis minor

N. occipitalis major

C1

C2

C3

C4

C5

R. geniohyoideus n. hypoglossi

R. thyreohyoideus n. hypoglossi

M. thyreohyoideus

Radix superior ansae cervicalis

Radix inferior ansae cervicalis

N. transversus colli

Venter superior m. omohyoidei

M. sternothyreoideus

Rr. musculares plexus cervicalis (to Mm. recti capitis anterior and lateralis, and Mm. longi capitis and colli)

Rr. musculares plexus cervicalis (to Mm. longi capitis and colli, and Levator scapulae)

M. trapezius

Rr. musculares plexus cervicalis (to Mm. longi capitis and colli, Levator scapulae, and M. scalenus medius)

Radix accessoria plexus brachialis (inconstant)

N. phrenicus

M. sternohyoideus

Rr. infrahyoidei ansae cervicalis

Ansa cervicalis

M. sternocleidomastoideus (*cut*)

Venter inferior m. omohyoidei

N. supraclavicularis medialis

N. supraclavicularis intermedius

N. supraclavicularis lateralis

——— **Efferent fibers**

——— **Afferent fibers**

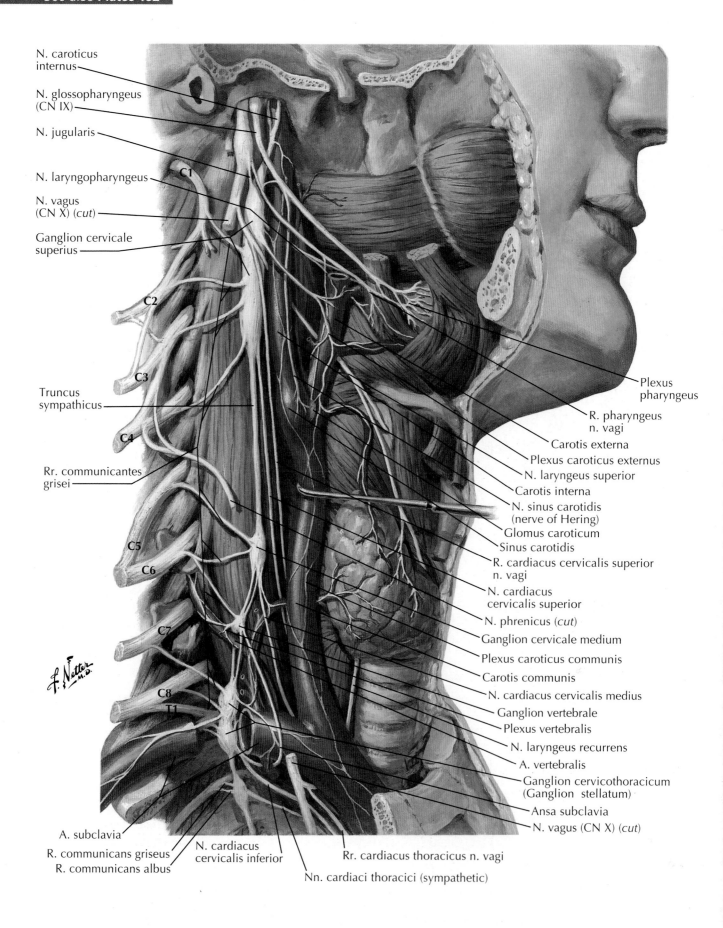

N. caroticus internus

N. glossopharyngeus (CN IX)

N. jugularis

N. laryngopharyngeus

N. vagus (CN X) *(cut)*

Ganglion cervicale superius

C1

C2

C3

Truncus sympathicus

C4

Rr. communicantes grisei

C5

C6

C7

C8
T1

A. subclavia

R. communicans griseus

R. communicans albus

N. cardiacus cervicalis inferior

Plexus pharyngeus

R. pharyngeus n. vagi

Carotis externa

Plexus caroticus externus

N. laryngeus superior

Carotis interna

N. sinus carotidis (nerve of Hering)

Glomus caroticum

Sinus carotidis

R. cardiacus cervicalis superior n. vagi

N. cardiacus cervicalis superior

N. phrenicus *(cut)*

Ganglion cervicale medium

Plexus caroticus communis

Carotis communis

N. cardiacus cervicalis medius

Ganglion vertebrale

Plexus vertebralis

N. laryngeus recurrens

A. vertebralis

Ganglion cervicothoracicum (Ganglion stellatum)

Ansa subclavia

N. vagus (CN X) *(cut)*

Rr. cardiacus thoracicus n. vagi

Nn. cardiaci thoracici (sympathetic)

Plate 157

Nervi Craniales and Nervi Cervicales

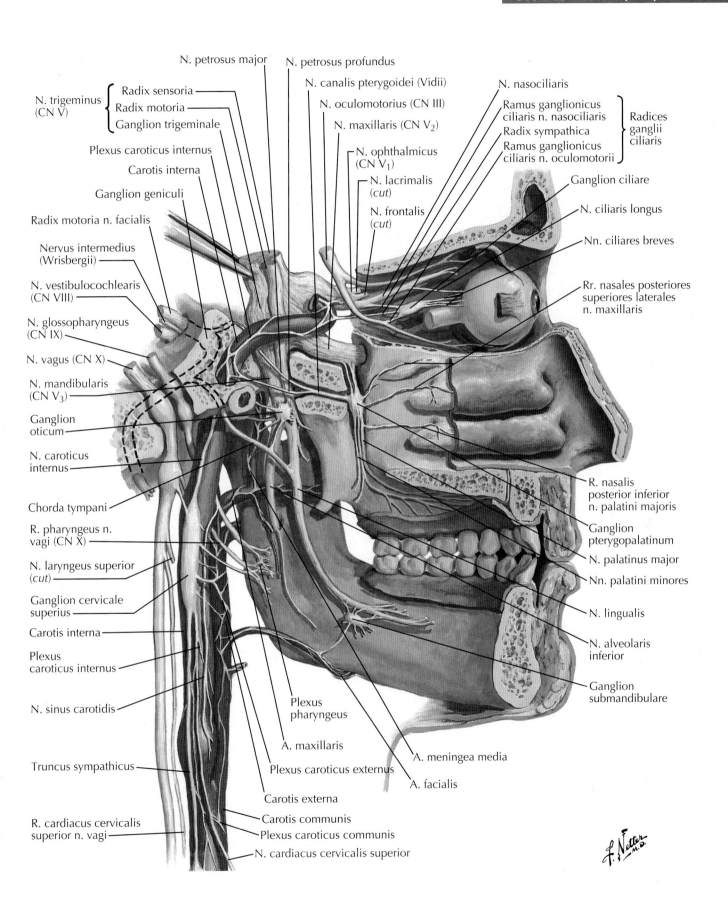

N. petrosus major

N. petrosus profundus

N. canalis pterygoidei (Vidii)

N. nasociliaris

N. trigeminus (CN V)
- Radix sensoria
- Radix motoria
- Ganglion trigeminale

N. oculomotorius (CN III)

Ramus ganglionicus ciliaris n. nasociliaris

N. maxillaris (CN V₂)

Radix sympathica

Radices ganglii ciliaris

Plexus caroticus internus

N. ophthalmicus (CN V₁)

Ramus ganglionicus ciliaris n. oculomotorii

Carotis interna

N. lacrimalis (*cut*)

Ganglion ciliare

Ganglion geniculi

N. frontalis (*cut*)

N. ciliaris longus

Radix motoria n. facialis

Nn. ciliares breves

Nervus intermedius (Wrisbergii)

N. vestibulocochlearis (CN VIII)

Rr. nasales posteriores superiores laterales n. maxillaris

N. glossopharyngeus (CN IX)

N. vagus (CN X)

N. mandibularis (CN V₃)

Ganglion oticum

N. caroticus internus

R. nasalis posterior inferior n. palatini majoris

Chorda tympani

Ganglion pterygopalatinum

R. pharyngeus n. vagi (CN X)

N. palatinus major

Nn. palatini minores

N. laryngeus superior (*cut*)

N. lingualis

Ganglion cervicale superius

Carotis interna

N. alveolaris inferior

Plexus caroticus internus

Ganglion submandibulare

N. sinus carotidis

Plexus pharyngeus

Truncus sympathicus

A. maxillaris

A. meningea media

Plexus caroticus externus

A. facialis

Carotis externa

R. cardiacus cervicalis superior n. vagi

Carotis communis

Plexus caroticus communis

N. cardiacus cervicalis superior

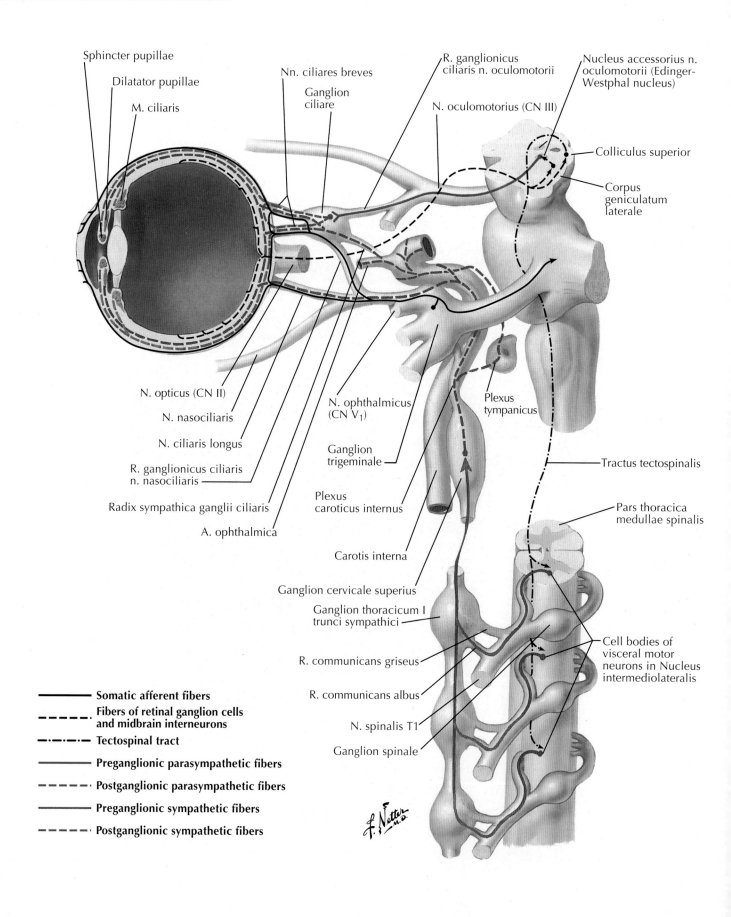

Sphincter pupillae

Dilatator pupillae

M. ciliaris

Nn. ciliares breves

Ganglion ciliare

R. ganglionicus ciliaris n. oculomotorii

N. oculomotorius (CN III)

Nucleus accessorius n. oculomotorii (Edinger-Westphal nucleus)

Colliculus superior

Corpus geniculatum laterale

N. opticus (CN II)

N. nasociliaris

N. ciliaris longus

R. ganglionicus ciliaris n. nasociliaris

Radix sympathica ganglii ciliaris

A. ophthalmica

N. ophthalmicus (CN V_1)

Ganglion trigeminale

Plexus caroticus internus

Carotis interna

Ganglion cervicale superius

Ganglion thoracicum I trunci sympathici

R. communicans griseus

R. communicans albus

N. spinalis T1

Ganglion spinale

Plexus tympanicus

Tractus tectospinalis

Pars thoracica medullae spinalis

Cell bodies of visceral motor neurons in Nucleus intermediolateralis

——— Somatic afferent fibers

– – – Fibers of retinal ganglion cells and midbrain interneurons

–·–·– Tectospinal tract

——— Preganglionic parasympathetic fibers

– – – Postganglionic parasympathetic fibers

——— Preganglionic sympathetic fibers

– – – Postganglionic sympathetic fibers

Plate 159

Nervi Craniales and Nervi Cervicales

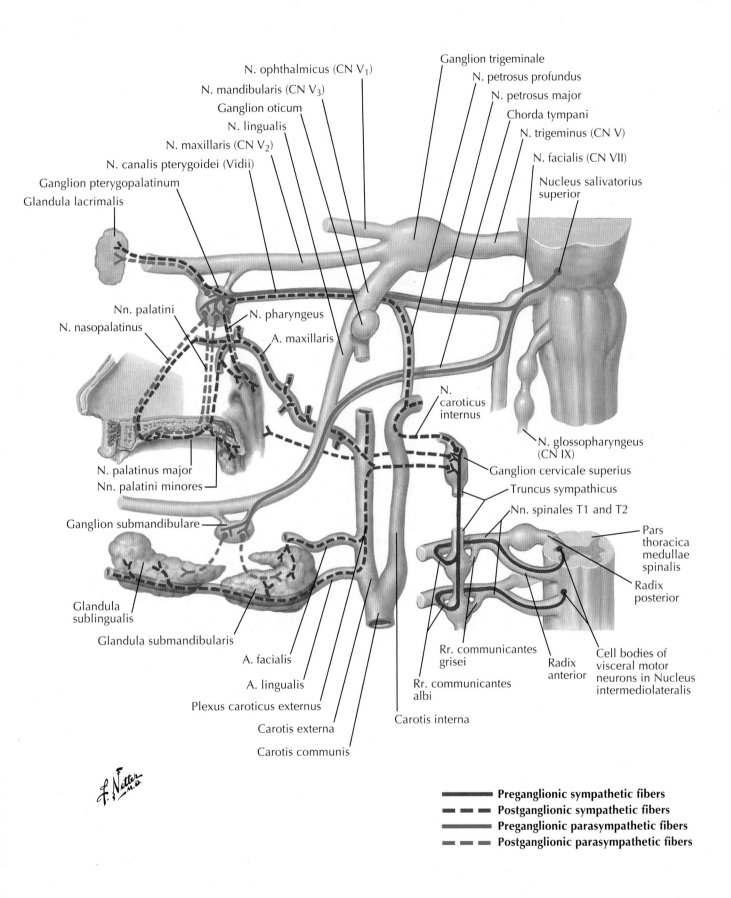

N. ophthalmicus (CN V₁)
N. mandibularis (CN V₃)
Ganglion oticum
N. lingualis
N. maxillaris (CN V₂)
N. canalis pterygoidei (Vidii)
Ganglion pterygopalatinum
Glandula lacrimalis

Ganglion trigeminale
N. petrosus profundus
N. petrosus major
Chorda tympani
N. trigeminus (CN V)
N. facialis (CN VII)
Nucleus salivatorius superior

Nn. palatini
N. nasopalatinus
N. pharyngeus
A. maxillaris

N. palatinus major
Nn. palatini minores

N. caroticus internus

N. glossopharyngeus (CN IX)
Ganglion cervicale superius
Truncus sympathicus
Nn. spinales T1 and T2

Ganglion submandibulare

Pars thoracica medullae spinalis
Radix posterior

Glandula sublingualis
Glandula submandibularis
A. facialis
A. lingualis
Plexus caroticus externus
Carotis externa
Carotis communis

Rr. communicantes grisei
Rr. communicantes albi
Carotis interna

Radix anterior

Cell bodies of visceral motor neurons in Nucleus intermediolateralis

═══ Preganglionic sympathetic fibers
━ ━ ━ Postganglionic sympathetic fibers
─── Preganglionic parasympathetic fibers
━ ━ ━ Postganglionic parasympathetic fibers

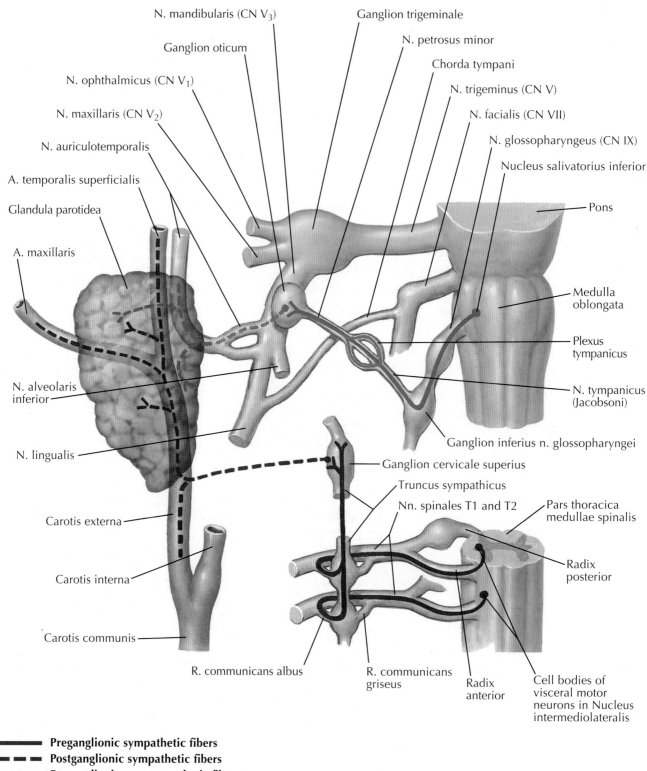

N. mandibularis (CN V₃)

Ganglion oticum

N. ophthalmicus (CN V₁)

N. maxillaris (CN V₂)

N. auriculotemporalis

A. temporalis superficialis

Glandula parotidea

A. maxillaris

N. alveolaris inferior

N. lingualis

Carotis externa

Carotis interna

Carotis communis

R. communicans albus

Ganglion trigeminale

N. petrosus minor

Chorda tympani

N. trigeminus (CN V)

N. facialis (CN VII)

N. glossopharyngeus (CN IX)

Nucleus salivatorius inferior

Pons

Medulla oblongata

Plexus tympanicus

N. tympanicus (Jacobsoni)

Ganglion inferius n. glossopharyngei

Ganglion cervicale superius

Truncus sympathicus

Nn. spinales T1 and T2

Pars thoracica medullae spinalis

Radix posterior

R. communicans griseus

Radix anterior

Cell bodies of visceral motor neurons in Nucleus intermediolateralis

▬▬▬▬▬ **Preganglionic sympathetic fibers**
▬ ▬ ▬ **Postganglionic sympathetic fibers**
▬▬▬▬▬ **Preganglionic parasympathetic fibers**
▬ ▬ ▬ **Postganglionic parasympathetic fibers**

Plate 161

Nervi Craniales and Nervi Cervicales

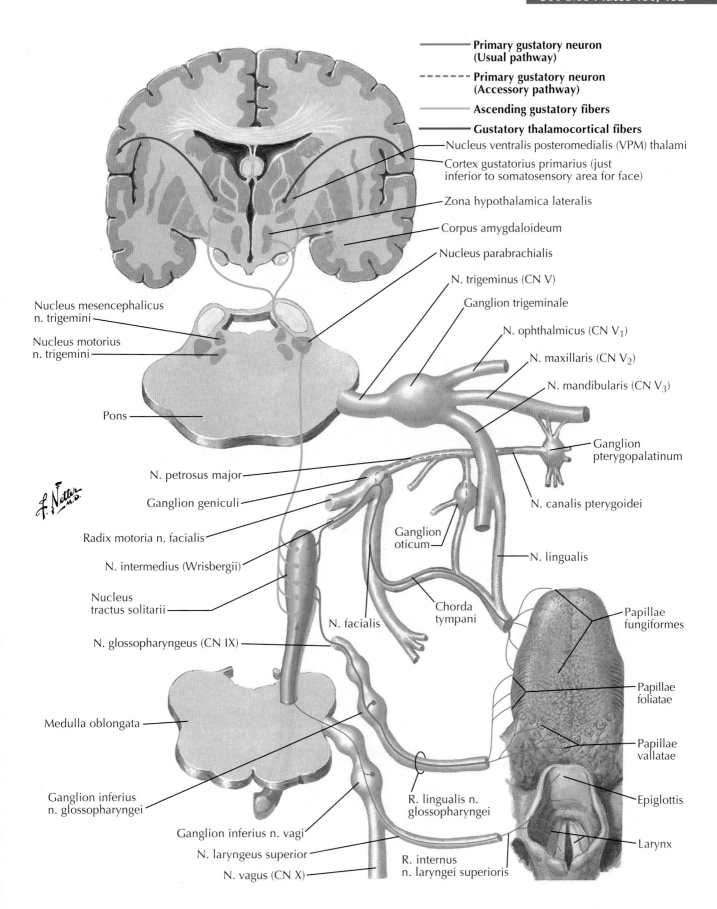

Primary gustatory neuron (Usual pathway)

Primary gustatory neuron (Accessory pathway)

Ascending gustatory fibers

Gustatory thalamocortical fibers

Nucleus ventralis posteromedialis (VPM) thalami

Cortex gustatorius primarius (just inferior to somatosensory area for face)

Zona hypothalamica lateralis

Corpus amygdaloideum

Nucleus parabrachialis

N. trigeminus (CN V)

Ganglion trigeminale

N. ophthalmicus (CN V₁)

N. maxillaris (CN V₂)

N. mandibularis (CN V₃)

Nucleus mesencephalicus n. trigemini

Nucleus motorius n. trigemini

Pons

Ganglion pterygopalatinum

N. petrosus major

Ganglion geniculi

Ganglion oticum

N. canalis pterygoidei

N. lingualis

Radix motoria n. facialis

N. intermedius (Wrisbergii)

Nucleus tractus solitarii

N. facialis

Chorda tympani

Papillae fungiformes

N. glossopharyngeus (CN IX)

Papillae foliatae

Medulla oblongata

Papillae vallatae

Ganglion inferius n. glossopharyngei

R. lingualis n. glossopharyngei

Epiglottis

Ganglion inferius n. vagi

N. laryngeus superior

N. vagus (CN X)

R. internus n. laryngei superioris

Larynx

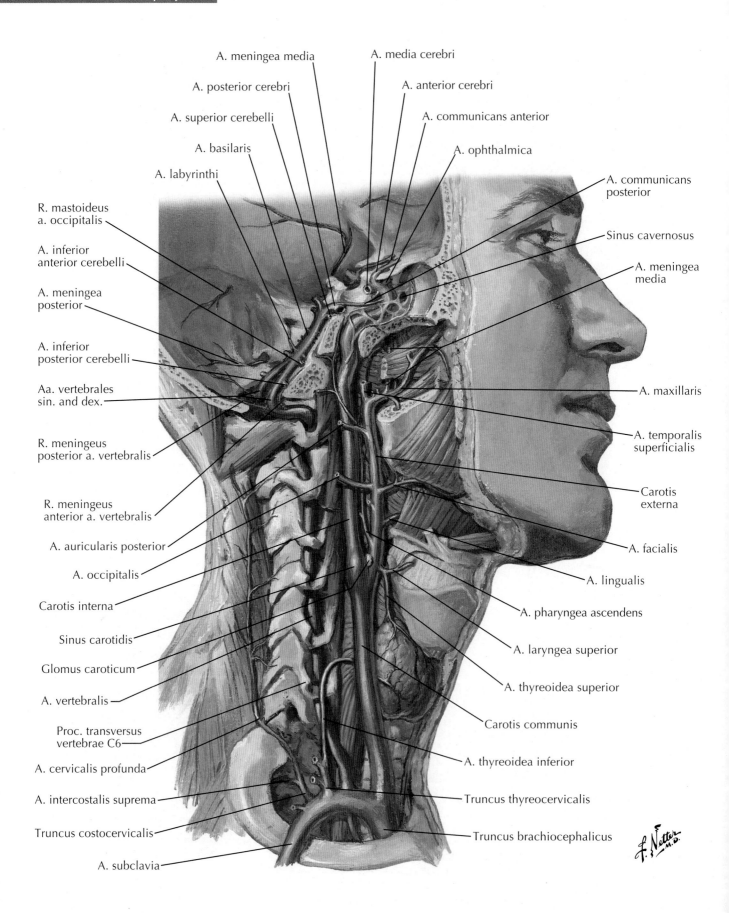

A. meningea media

A. media cerebri

A. posterior cerebri

A. anterior cerebri

A. superior cerebelli

A. communicans anterior

A. basilaris

A. ophthalmica

A. labyrinthi

A. communicans posterior

R. mastoideus a. occipitalis

Sinus cavernosus

A. inferior anterior cerebelli

A. meningea media

A. meningea posterior

A. inferior posterior cerebelli

Aa. vertebrales sin. and dex.

A. maxillaris

R. meningeus posterior a. vertebralis

A. temporalis superficialis

R. meningeus anterior a. vertebralis

Carotis externa

A. auricularis posterior

A. facialis

A. occipitalis

A. lingualis

Carotis interna

A. pharyngea ascendens

Sinus carotidis

A. laryngea superior

Glomus caroticum

A. thyreoidea superior

A. vertebralis

Carotis communis

Proc. transversus vertebrae C6

A. cervicalis profunda

A. thyreoidea inferior

A. intercostalis suprema

Truncus thyreocervicalis

Truncus costocervicalis

Truncus brachiocephalicus

A. subclavia

Plate 163

Vasa Sanguinea Encephali

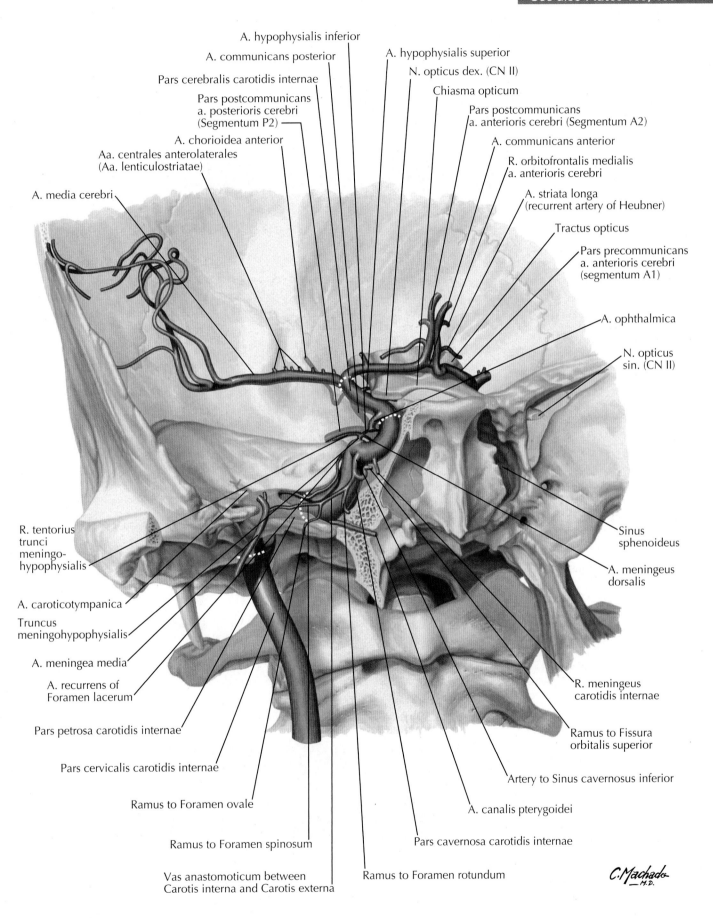

A. hypophysialis inferior

A. communicans posterior

Pars cerebralis carotidis internae

Pars postcommunicans
a. posterioris cerebri
(Segmentum P2)

A. chorioidea anterior

Aa. centrales anterolaterales
(Aa. lenticulostriatae)

A. media cerebri

A. hypophysialis superior

N. opticus dex. (CN II)

Chiasma opticum

Pars postcommunicans
a. anterioris cerebri (Segmentum A2)

A. communicans anterior

R. orbitofrontalis medialis
a. anterioris cerebri

A. striata longa
(recurrent artery of Heubner)

Tractus opticus

Pars precommunicans
a. anterioris cerebri
(segmentum A1)

A. ophthalmica

N. opticus
sin. (CN II)

Sinus
sphenoideus

A. meningeus
dorsalis

R. tentorius
trunci
meningo-
hypophysialis

A. caroticotympanica

Truncus
meningohypophysialis

A. meningea media

A. recurrens of
Foramen lacerum

Pars petrosa carotidis internae

Pars cervicalis carotidis internae

Ramus to Foramen ovale

Ramus to Foramen spinosum

Vas anastomoticum between
Carotis interna and Carotis externa

Ramus to Foramen rotundum

Pars cavernosa carotidis internae

A. canalis pterygoidei

Artery to Sinus cavernosus inferior

Ramus to Fissura
orbitalis superior

R. meningeus
carotidis internae

C. Machado
_M.D.

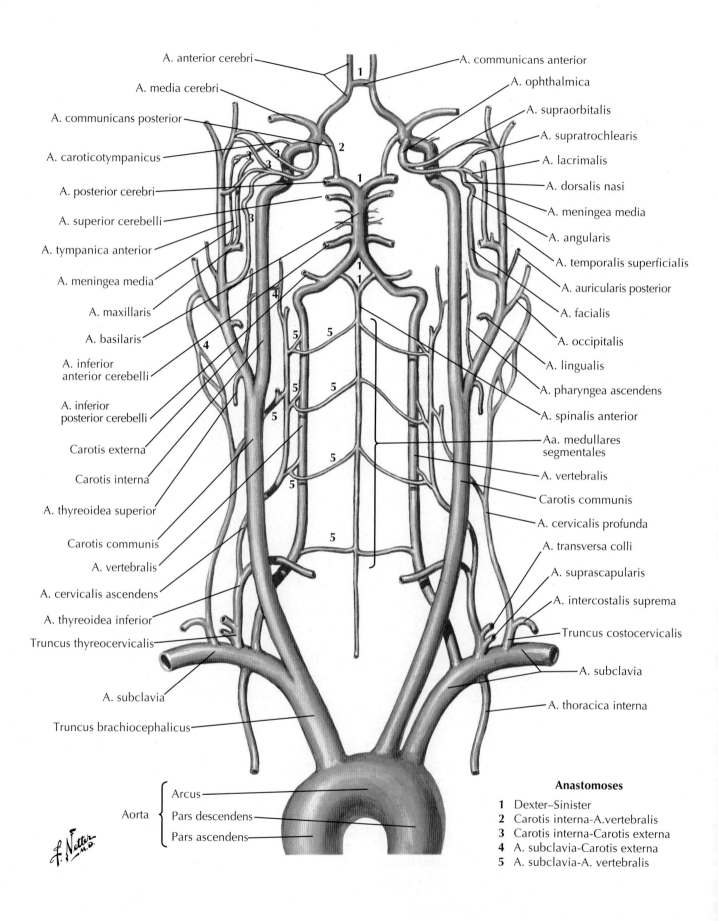

A. anterior cerebri
A. media cerebri
A. communicans posterior
A. caroticotympanicus
A. posterior cerebri
A. superior cerebelli
A. tympanica anterior
A. meningea media
A. maxillaris
A. basilaris
A. inferior anterior cerebelli
A. inferior posterior cerebelli
Carotis externa
Carotis interna
A. thyreoidea superior
Carotis communis
A. vertebralis
A. cervicalis ascendens
A. thyreoidea inferior
Truncus thyreocervicalis
A. subclavia
Truncus brachiocephalicus

A. communicans anterior
A. ophthalmica
A. supraorbitalis
A. supratrochlearis
A. lacrimalis
A. dorsalis nasi
A. meningea media
A. angularis
A. temporalis superficialis
A. auricularis posterior
A. facialis
A. occipitalis
A. lingualis
A. pharyngea ascendens
A. spinalis anterior
Aa. medullares segmentales
A. vertebralis
Carotis communis
A. cervicalis profunda
A. transversa colli
A. suprascapularis
A. intercostalis suprema
Truncus costocervicalis
A. subclavia
A. thoracica interna

Aorta {
Arcus
Pars descendens
Pars ascendens

Anastomoses

1 Dexter–Sinister
2 Carotis interna-A.vertebralis
3 Carotis interna-Carotis externa
4 A. subclavia-Carotis externa
5 A. subclavia-A. vertebralis

Plate 165

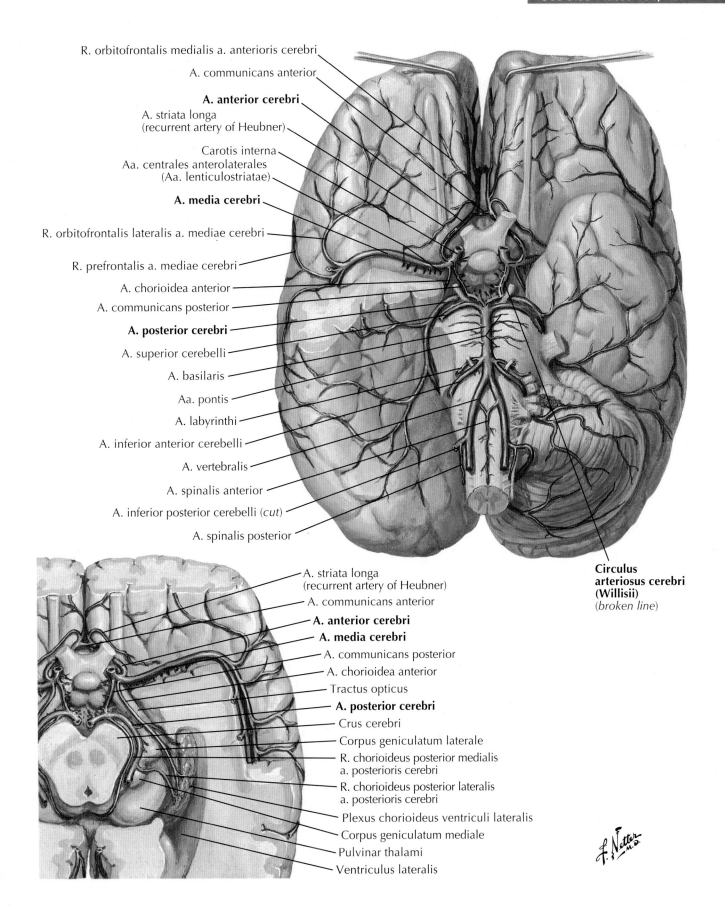

R. orbitofrontalis medialis a. anterioris cerebri

A. communicans anterior

A. anterior cerebri

A. striata longa
(recurrent artery of Heubner)

Carotis interna
Aa. centrales anterolaterales
(Aa. lenticulostriatae)

A. media cerebri

R. orbitofrontalis lateralis a. mediae cerebri

R. prefrontalis a. mediae cerebri

A. chorioidea anterior

A. communicans posterior

A. posterior cerebri

A. superior cerebelli

A. basilaris

Aa. pontis

A. labyrinthi

A. inferior anterior cerebelli

A. vertebralis

A. spinalis anterior

A. inferior posterior cerebelli (*cut*)

A. spinalis posterior

Circulus arteriosus cerebri (Willisii)
(*broken line*)

A. striata longa
(recurrent artery of Heubner)

A. communicans anterior

A. anterior cerebri

A. media cerebri

A. communicans posterior

A. chorioidea anterior

Tractus opticus

A. posterior cerebri

Crus cerebri

Corpus geniculatum laterale

R. chorioideus posterior medialis
a. posterioris cerebri

R. chorioideus posterior lateralis
a. posterioris cerebri

Plexus chorioideus ventriculi lateralis

Corpus geniculatum mediale

Pulvinar thalami

Ventriculus lateralis

Vessels dissected out: inferior view

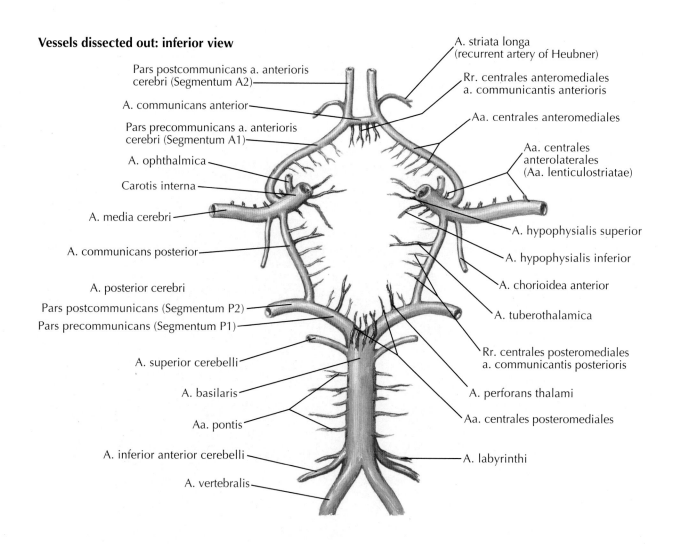

Pars postcommunicans a. anterioris cerebri (Segmentum A2)

A. communicans anterior

Pars precommunicans a. anterioris cerebri (Segmentum A1)

A. ophthalmica

Carotis interna

A. media cerebri

A. communicans posterior

A. posterior cerebri

Pars postcommunicans (Segmentum P2)

Pars precommunicans (Segmentum P1)

A. superior cerebelli

A. basilaris

Aa. pontis

A. inferior anterior cerebelli

A. vertebralis

A. striata longa (recurrent artery of Heubner)

Rr. centrales anteromediales a. communicantis anterioris

Aa. centrales anteromediales

Aa. centrales anterolaterales (Aa. lenticulostriatae)

A. hypophysialis superior

A. hypophysialis inferior

A. chorioidea anterior

A. tuberothalamica

Rr. centrales posteromediales a. communicantis posterioris

A. perforans thalami

Aa. centrales posteromediales

A. labyrinthi

Vessels in situ: inferior view

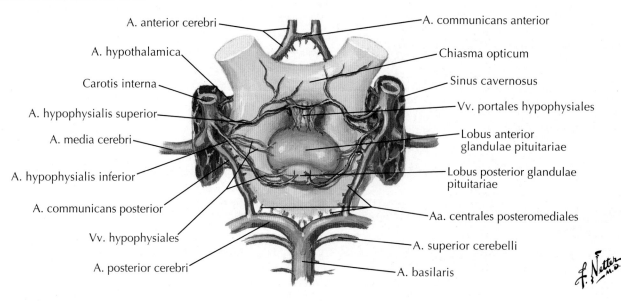

A. anterior cerebri

A. hypothalamica

Carotis interna

A. hypophysialis superior

A. media cerebri

A. hypophysialis inferior

A. communicans posterior

Vv. hypophysiales

A. posterior cerebri

A. communicans anterior

Chiasma opticum

Sinus cavernosus

Vv. portales hypophysiales

Lobus anterior glandulae pituitariae

Lobus posterior glandulae pituitariae

Aa. centrales posteromediales

A. superior cerebelli

A. basilaris

Plate 167

Vasa Sanguinea Encephali

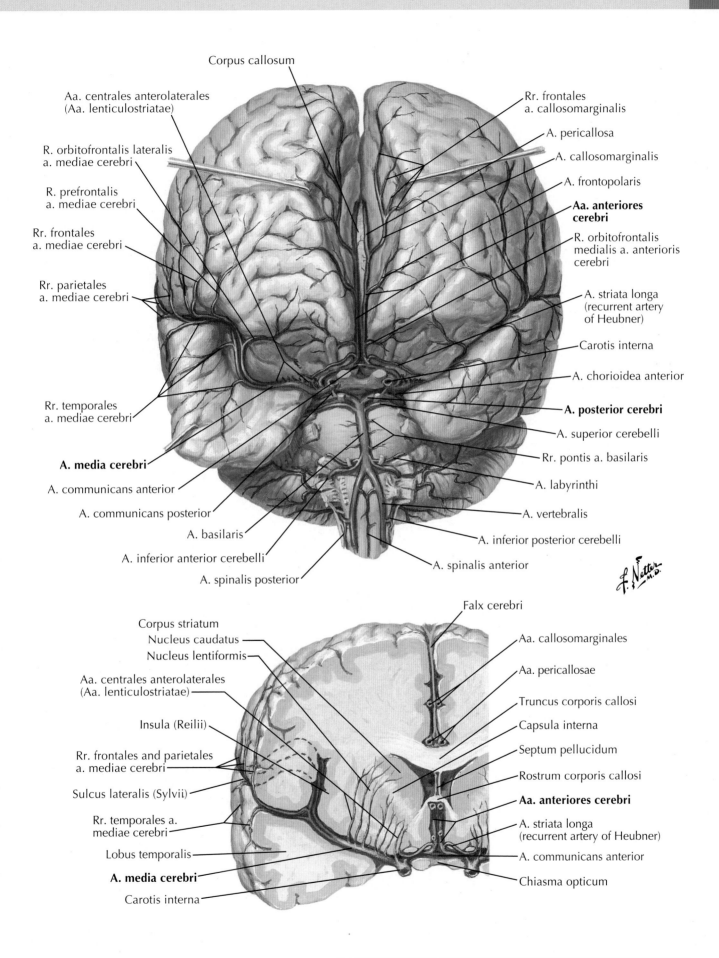

Corpus callosum

Aa. centrales anterolaterales
(Aa. lenticulostriatae)

R. orbitofrontalis lateralis
a. mediae cerebri

R. prefrontalis
a. mediae cerebri

Rr. frontales
a. mediae cerebri

Rr. parietales
a. mediae cerebri

Rr. temporales
a. mediae cerebri

A. media cerebri

A. communicans anterior

A. communicans posterior

A. basilaris

A. inferior anterior cerebelli

A. spinalis posterior

Rr. frontales
a. callosomarginalis

A. pericallosa

A. callosomarginalis

A. frontopolaris

**Aa. anteriores
cerebri**

R. orbitofrontalis
medialis a. anterioris
cerebri

A. striata longa
(recurrent artery
of Heubner)

Carotis interna

A. chorioidea anterior

A. posterior cerebri

A. superior cerebelli

Rr. pontis a. basilaris

A. labyrinthi

A. vertebralis

A. inferior posterior cerebelli

A. spinalis anterior

Corpus striatum
Nucleus caudatus
Nucleus lentiformis

Aa. centrales anterolaterales
(Aa. lenticulostriatae)

Insula (Reilii)

Rr. frontales and parietales
a. mediae cerebri

Sulcus lateralis (Sylvii)

Rr. temporales a.
mediae cerebri

Lobus temporalis

A. media cerebri

Carotis interna

Falx cerebri

Aa. callosomarginales

Aa. pericallosae

Truncus corporis callosi

Capsula interna

Septum pellucidum

Rostrum corporis callosi

Aa. anteriores cerebri

A. striata longa
(recurrent artery of Heubner)

A. communicans anterior

Chiasma opticum

Vasa Sanguinea Encephali

Plate 168

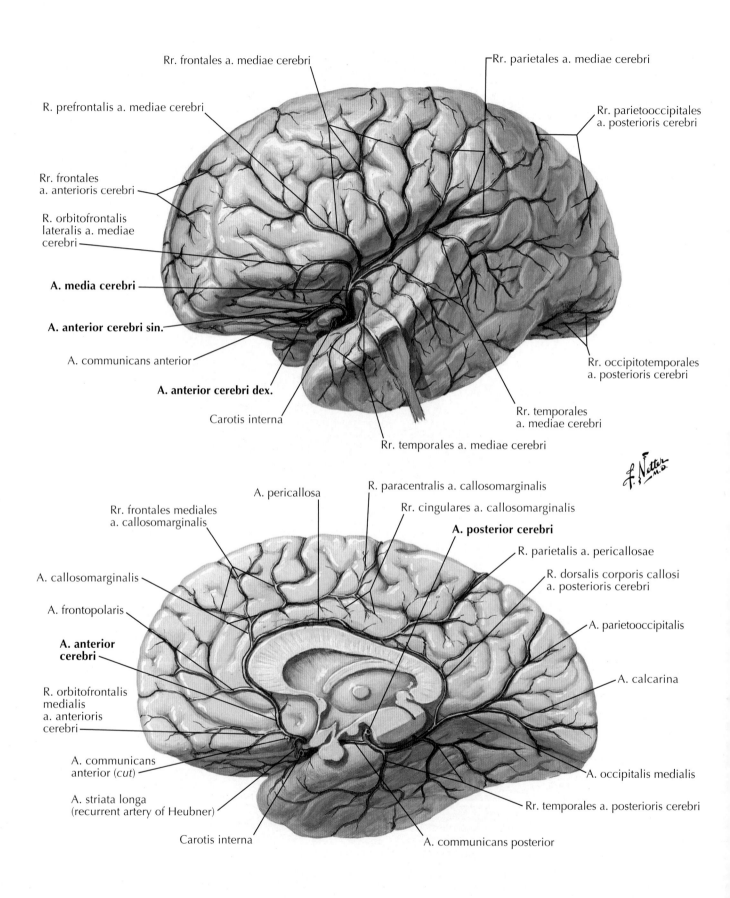

Rr. frontales a. mediae cerebri

Rr. parietales a. mediae cerebri

R. prefrontalis a. mediae cerebri

Rr. parietooccipitales
a. posterioris cerebri

Rr. frontales
a. anterioris cerebri

R. orbitofrontalis
lateralis a. mediae
cerebri

A. media cerebri

A. anterior cerebri sin.

A. communicans anterior

Rr. occipitotemporales
a. posterioris cerebri

A. anterior cerebri dex.

Carotis interna

Rr. temporales
a. mediae cerebri

Rr. temporales a. mediae cerebri

A. pericallosa

R. paracentralis a. callosomarginalis

Rr. frontales mediales
a. callosomarginalis

Rr. cingulares a. callosomarginalis

A. posterior cerebri

A. callosomarginalis

R. parietalis a. pericallosae

A. frontopolaris

R. dorsalis corporis callosi
a. posterioris cerebri

**A. anterior
cerebri**

A. parietooccipitalis

R. orbitofrontalis
medialis
a. anterioris
cerebri

A. calcarina

A. communicans
anterior (*cut*)

A. striata longa
(recurrent artery of Heubner)

A. occipitalis medialis

Rr. temporales a. posterioris cerebri

Carotis interna

A. communicans posterior

Plate 169

Vasa Sanguinea Encephali

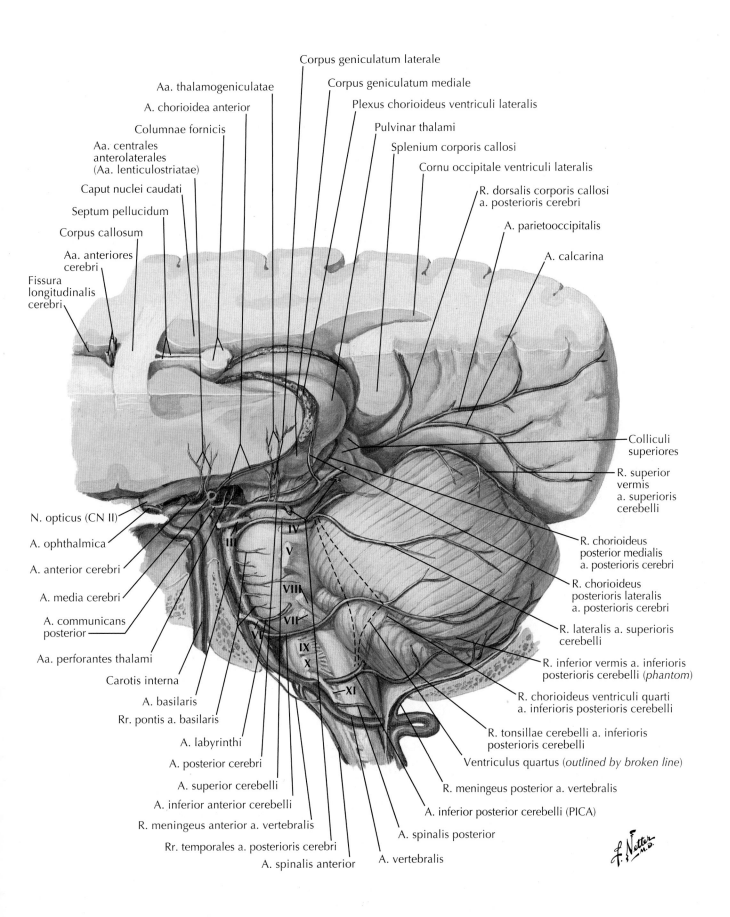

Corpus geniculatum laterale

Corpus geniculatum mediale

Aa. thalamogeniculatae

A. chorioidea anterior

Plexus chorioideus ventriculi lateralis

Columnae fornicis

Pulvinar thalami

Aa. centrales anterolaterales (Aa. lenticulostriatae)

Splenium corporis callosi

Caput nuclei caudati

Cornu occipitale ventriculi lateralis

Septum pellucidum

R. dorsalis corporis callosi a. posterioris cerebri

Corpus callosum

A. parietooccipitalis

Aa. anteriores cerebri

A. calcarina

Fissura longitudinalis cerebri

Colliculi superiores

R. superior vermis a. superioris cerebelli

N. opticus (CN II)

A. ophthalmica

R. chorioideus posterior medialis a. posterioris cerebri

A. anterior cerebri

A. media cerebri

R. chorioideus posterioris lateralis a. posterioris cerebri

A. communicans posterior

R. lateralis a. superioris cerebelli

Aa. perforantes thalami

R. inferior vermis a. inferioris posterioris cerebelli (*phantom*)

Carotis interna

R. chorioideus ventriculi quarti a. inferioris posterioris cerebelli

A. basilaris

Rr. pontis a. basilaris

R. tonsillae cerebelli a. inferioris posterioris cerebelli

A. labyrinthi

Ventriculus quartus (*outlined by broken line*)

A. posterior cerebri

A. superior cerebelli

R. meningeus posterior a. vertebralis

A. inferior anterior cerebelli

R. meningeus anterior a. vertebralis

A. inferior posterior cerebelli (PICA)

Rr. temporales a. posterioris cerebri

A. spinalis posterior

A. spinalis anterior

A. vertebralis

III IV V VIII VII VI IX X XI

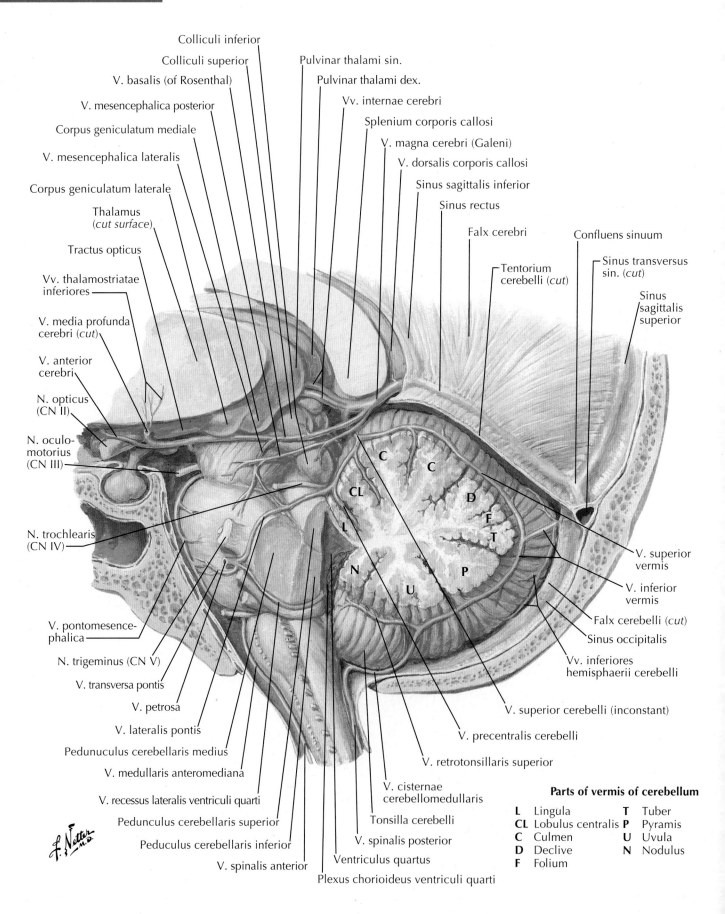

Colliculi inferior

Colliculi superior

V. basalis (of Rosenthal)

V. mesencephalica posterior

Corpus geniculatum mediale

V. mesencephalica lateralis

Corpus geniculatum laterale

Thalamus (cut surface)

Tractus opticus

Vv. thalamostriatae inferiores

V. media profunda cerebri (cut)

V. anterior cerebri

N. opticus (CN II)

N. oculo-motorius (CN III)

N. trochlearis (CN IV)

V. pontomesence-phalica

N. trigeminus (CN V)

V. transversa pontis

V. petrosa

V. lateralis pontis

Pedunuculus cerebellaris medius

V. medullaris anteromediana

V. recessus lateralis ventriculi quarti

Pedunculus cerebellaris superior

Peduculus cerebellaris inferior

V. spinalis anterior

Pulvinar thalami sin.

Pulvinar thalami dex.

Vv. internae cerebri

Splenium corporis callosi

V. magna cerebri (Galeni)

V. dorsalis corporis callosi

Sinus sagittalis inferior

Sinus rectus

Falx cerebri

Tentorium cerebelli (cut)

Confluens sinuum

Sinus transversus sin. (cut)

Sinus sagittalis superior

V. superior vermis

V. inferior vermis

Falx cerebelli (cut)

Sinus occipitalis

Vv. inferiores hemisphaerii cerebelli

V. superior cerebelli (inconstant)

V. precentralis cerebelli

V. retrotonsillaris superior

V. cisternae cerebellomedullaris

Tonsilla cerebelli

V. spinalis posterior

Ventriculus quartus

Plexus chorioideus ventriculi quarti

Parts of vermis of cerebellum

L	Lingula	**T**	Tuber
CL	Lobulus centralis	**P**	Pyramis
C	Culmen	**U**	Uvula
D	Declive	**N**	Nodulus
F	Folium		

Plate 171

Vasa Sanguinea Encephali

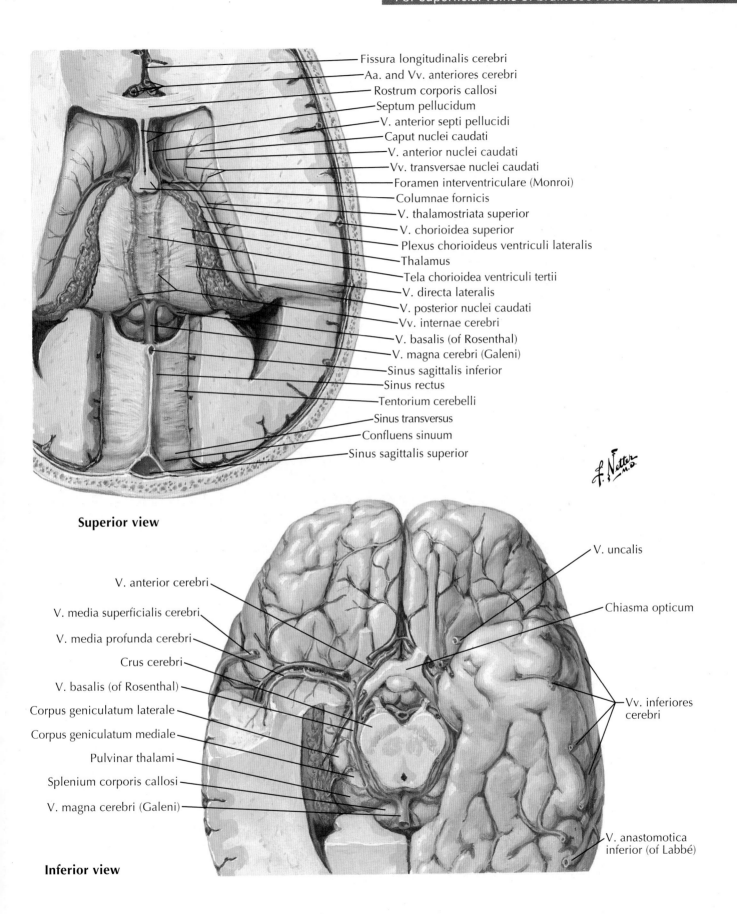

Fissura longitudinalis cerebri
Aa. and Vv. anteriores cerebri
Rostrum corporis callosi
Septum pellucidum
V. anterior septi pellucidi
Caput nuclei caudati
V. anterior nuclei caudati
Vv. transversae nuclei caudati
Foramen interventriculare (Monroi)
Columnae fornicis
V. thalamostriata superior
V. chorioidea superior
Plexus chorioideus ventriculi lateralis
Thalamus
Tela chorioidea ventriculi tertii
V. directa lateralis
V. posterior nuclei caudati
Vv. internae cerebri
V. basalis (of Rosenthal)
V. magna cerebri (Galeni)
Sinus sagittalis inferior
Sinus rectus
Tentorium cerebelli
Sinus transversus
Confluens sinuum
Sinus sagittalis superior

Superior view

V. uncalis
Chiasma opticum

V. anterior cerebri
V. media superficialis cerebri
V. media profunda cerebri
Crus cerebri
V. basalis (of Rosenthal)
Corpus geniculatum laterale
Corpus geniculatum mediale
Pulvinar thalami
Splenium corporis callosi
V. magna cerebri (Galeni)

Vv. inferiores cerebri

V. anastomotica inferior (of Labbé)

Inferior view

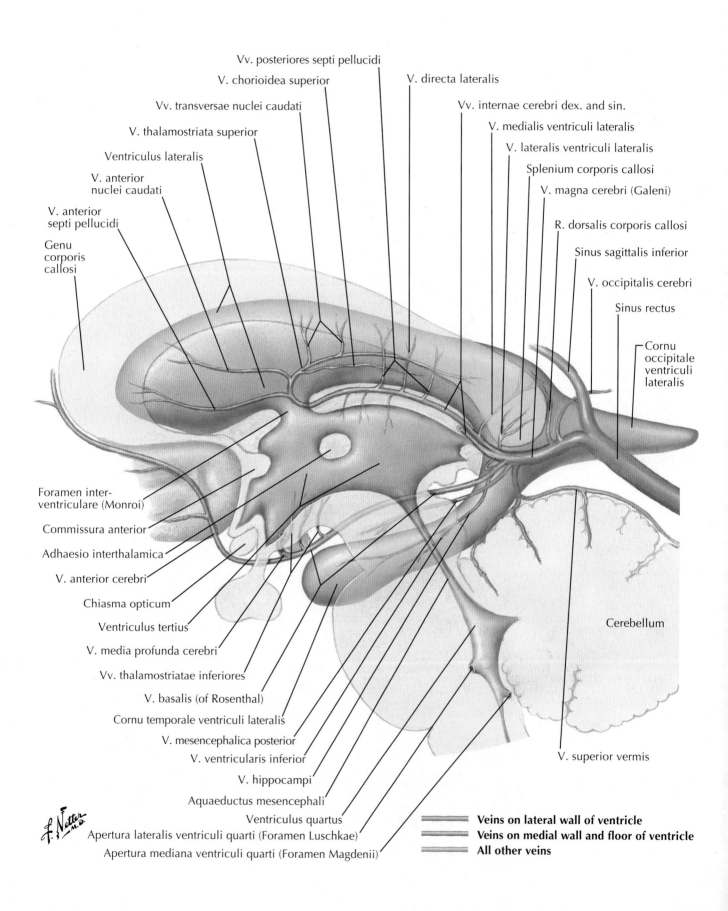

Vv. posteriores septi pellucidi

V. chorioidea superior

V. directa lateralis

Vv. transversae nuclei caudati

Vv. internae cerebri dex. and sin.

V. thalamostriata superior

V. medialis ventriculi lateralis

Ventriculus lateralis

V. lateralis ventriculi lateralis

V. anterior nuclei caudati

Splenium corporis callosi

V. anterior septi pellucidi

V. magna cerebri (Galeni)

Genu corporis callosi

R. dorsalis corporis callosi

Sinus sagittalis inferior

V. occipitalis cerebri

Sinus rectus

Cornu occipitale ventriculi lateralis

Foramen inter-ventriculare (Monroi)

Commissura anterior

Adhaesio interthalamica

V. anterior cerebri

Chiasma opticum

Ventriculus tertius

V. media profunda cerebri

Vv. thalamostriatae inferiores

V. basalis (of Rosenthal)

Cornu temporale ventriculi lateralis

V. mesencephalica posterior

V. ventricularis inferior

V. hippocampi

Aquaeductus mesencephali

Ventriculus quartus

Apertura lateralis ventriculi quarti (Foramen Luschkae)

Apertura mediana ventriculi quarti (Foramen Magdenii)

Cerebellum

V. superior vermis

≡≡≡	Veins on lateral wall of ventricle
≡≡≡	Veins on medial wall and floor of ventricle
≡≡≡	All other veins

Plate 173

Vasa Sanguinea Encephali

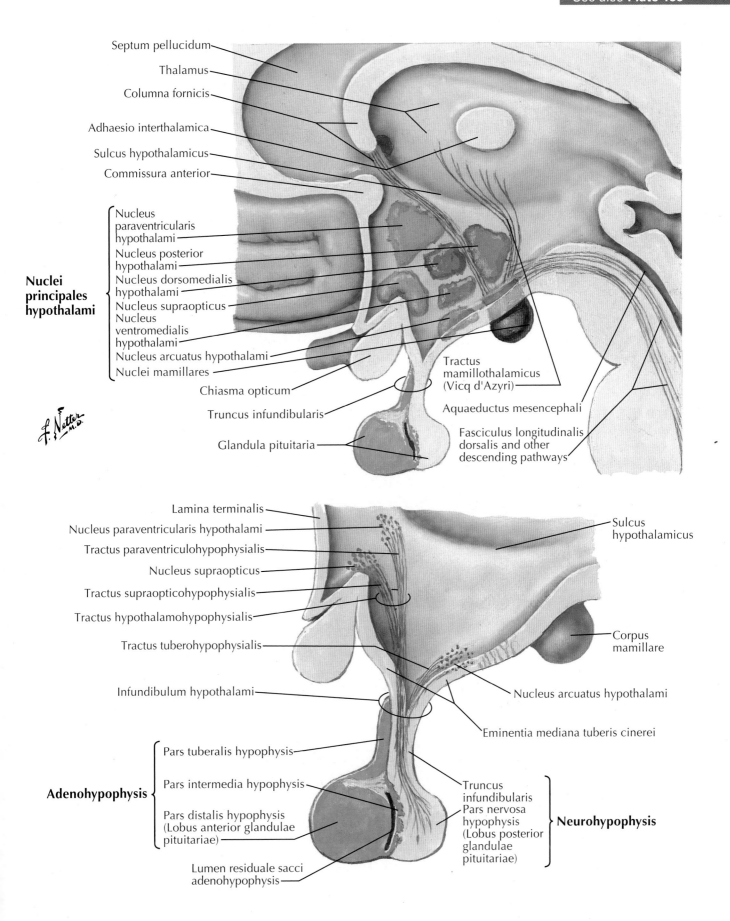

Septum pellucidum

Thalamus

Columna fornicis

Adhaesio interthalamica

Sulcus hypothalamicus

Commissura anterior

Nuclei principales hypothalami
- Nucleus paraventricularis hypothalami
- Nucleus posterior hypothalami
- Nucleus dorsomedialis hypothalami
- Nucleus supraopticus
- Nucleus ventromedialis hypothalami
- Nucleus arcuatus hypothalami
- Nuclei mamillares

Chiasma opticum

Truncus infundibularis

Glandula pituitaria

Tractus mamillothalamicus (Vicq d'Azyri)

Aquaeductus mesencephali

Fasciculus longitudinalis dorsalis and other descending pathways

Lamina terminalis

Nucleus paraventricularis hypothalami

Tractus paraventriculohypophysialis

Nucleus supraopticus

Tractus supraopticohypophysialis

Tractus hypothalamohypophysialis

Tractus tuberohypophysialis

Infundibulum hypothalami

Adenohypophysis
- Pars tuberalis hypophysis
- Pars intermedia hypophysis
- Pars distalis hypophysis (Lobus anterior glandulae pituitariae)

Lumen residuale sacci adenohypophysis

Sulcus hypothalamicus

Corpus mamillare

Nucleus arcuatus hypothalami

Eminentia mediana tuberis cinerei

Truncus infundibularis
Pars nervosa hypophysis (Lobus posterior glandulae pituitariae)

Neurohypophysis

Vasa Sanguinea Encephali

Plate 174

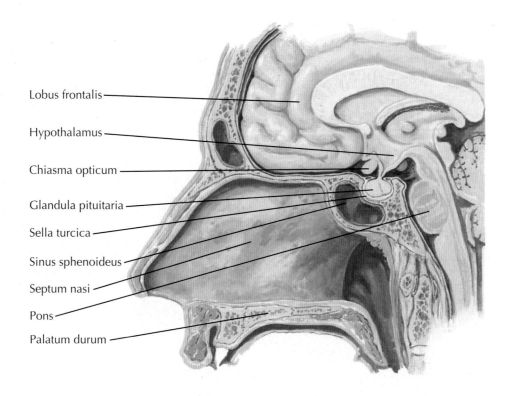

Lobus frontalis

Hypothalamus

Chiasma opticum

Glandula pituitaria

Sella turcica

Sinus sphenoideus

Septum nasi

Pons

Palatum durum

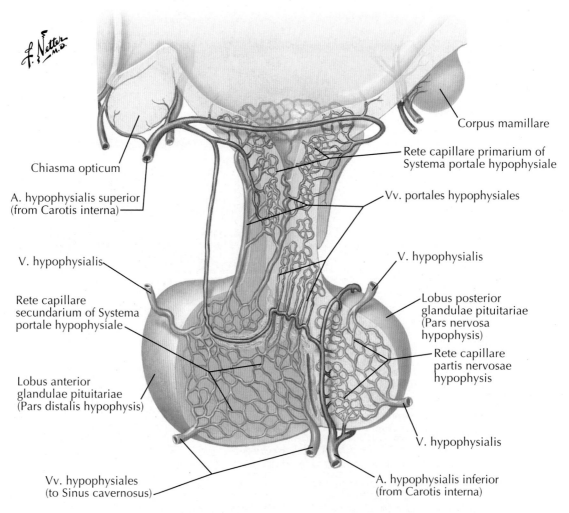

Corpus mamillare

Rete capillare primarium of
Systema portale hypophysiale

Chiasma opticum

A. hypophysialis superior
(from Carotis interna)

Vv. portales hypophysiales

V. hypophysialis

V. hypophysialis

Rete capillare
secundarium of Systema
portale hypophysiale

Lobus posterior
glandulae pituitariae
(Pars nervosa
hypophysis)

Rete capillare
partis nervosae
hypophysis

Lobus anterior
glandulae pituitariae
(Pars distalis hypophysis)

V. hypophysialis

Vv. hypophysiales
(to Sinus cavernosus)

A. hypophysialis inferior
(from Carotis interna)

Plate 175

Vasa Sanguinea Encephali

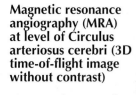

Magnetic resonance angiography (MRA) at level of Circulus arteriosus cerebri (3D time-of-flight image without contrast)

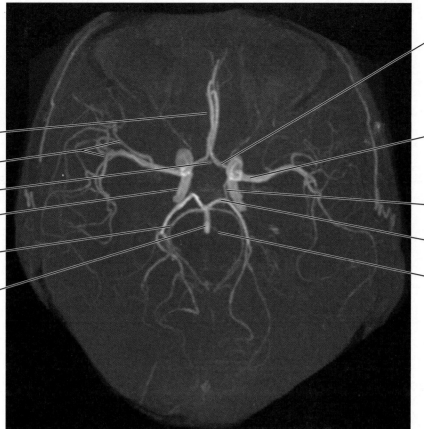

Pars precommunicans a. anterioris cerebri (Segmentum A1)

Pars postcommunicans a. anterioris cerebri (Segmentum A2)

A. media cerebri (Segmenta M2)

A. communicans anterior

Carotis interna

A. superior cerebelli

A. basilaris

A. media cerebri (Segmentum M1)

A. communicans posterior

A. posterior cerebri

A. inferior anterior cerebelli

Magnetic resonance venography (MRV) (2D time-of-flight image without contrast)

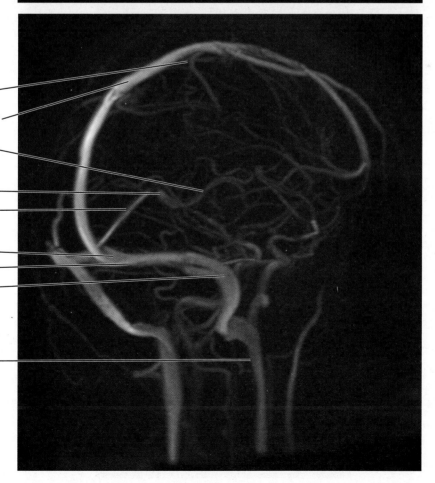

V. superior cerebri

Sinus sagittalis superior

V. interna cerebri

V. magna cerebri (Galeni)

Sinus rectus

Confluens sinuum

Sinus transversus

Sinus sigmoideus

V. jugularis interna

T1-weighted MRI, sagittal view

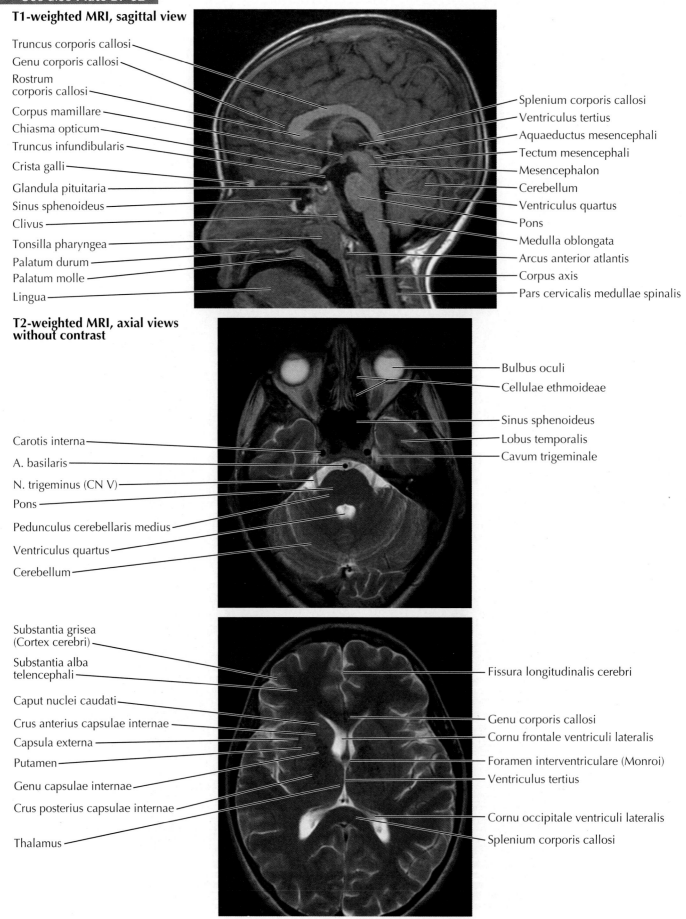

Truncus corporis callosi
Genu corporis callosi
Rostrum corporis callosi
Corpus mamillare
Chiasma opticum
Truncus infundibularis
Crista galli
Glandula pituitaria
Sinus sphenoideus
Clivus
Tonsilla pharyngea
Palatum durum
Palatum molle
Lingua

Splenium corporis callosi
Ventriculus tertius
Aquaeductus mesencephali
Tectum mesencephali
Mesencephalon
Cerebellum
Ventriculus quartus
Pons
Medulla oblongata
Arcus anterior atlantis
Corpus axis
Pars cervicalis medullae spinalis

T2-weighted MRI, axial views without contrast

Bulbus oculi
Cellulae ethmoideae
Sinus sphenoideus
Lobus temporalis
Cavum trigeminale

Carotis interna
A. basilaris
N. trigeminus (CN V)
Pons
Pedunculus cerebellaris medius
Ventriculus quartus
Cerebellum

Substantia grisea (Cortex cerebri)
Substantia alba telencephali
Caput nuclei caudati
Crus anterius capsulae internae
Capsula externa
Putamen
Genu capsulae internae
Crus posterius capsulae internae
Thalamus

Fissura longitudinalis cerebri
Genu corporis callosi
Cornu frontale ventriculi lateralis
Foramen interventriculare (Monroi)
Ventriculus tertius
Cornu occipitale ventriculi lateralis
Splenium corporis callosi

Plate 177

Regional Imaging

ANATOMICAL STRUCTURE	CLINICAL COMMENT	PLATE NUMBERS
Systema Nervosum and Organa Sensuum		
N. accessorius spinalis (CN XI)	Lymph node biopsy in posterior cervical triangle can cause iatrogenic injury of CN XI	56
Plexus cervicalis	Cervical plexus blocks are performed for neck procedures	56, 57
N. trigeminus (CN V)	Branches of CN V are anesthetized for procedures on face or anterior scalp; compression of the nerve may result in painful condition known as trigeminal neuralgia	60, 149
N. olfactorius (CN I)	One of most commonly injured cranial nerves; can be avulsed at cribriform plate following falls, resulting in anosmia	64, 146
N. facialis (CN VII)	Idiopathic unilateral facial nerve palsy (Bell's palsy) can result in inability to fully close eye and result in desiccated cornea ipsilaterally	71
N. laryngeus recurrens	May be compressed or damaged by procedures in neck (e.g., thyroidectomy), aortic arch aneurysm, or lung cancer, producing hoarseness of voice; identified by (posterior) suspensory ligament of thyroid and/or inferior thyroid artery and/or tracheoesophageal groove	104, 105
Nn. oculomotorius (CN III), trochlearis (CN IV), and abducens (CN VI)	Cavernous sinus thrombosis can result in dysfunction of extraocular muscles caused by compression of one, two, or all three nerves; abducens nerve is most commonly affected	131
Colliculus superior; aquaeductus mesencephali	Tumor of midbrain can result in compression of aqueduct of midbrain, with resultant hydrocephalus	136
N. opticus (CN II)	Pituitary gland mass may cause compression at optic chiasm and resulting bitemporal hemianopsia; optic radiations (Meyer's loop) can be affected by temporal lobe tumors; early sign of ophthalmic artery aneurysm is visual loss due to compression of overlying optic nerve.	147, 167
Fovea centralis	Location of highest density of retinal cones, making this part of macula lutea the site of greatest visual acuity and color vision	116
Utriculus; sacculus	Location of calcium carbonate crystals known as otoconia; accumulation of otoconia in semicircular canals is most common cause of vertigo, and is known as benign paroxysmal positional vertigo (BPPV)	124, 125
Lens	Degeneration and opacification, known as cataract, may lead to progressive vision loss	116
Septum orbitale	Infections anterior to this structure are known as preseptal/periorbital cellulitis and are milder than infections extending posterior to it, known as orbital cellulitis	110
Segmentum anterius bulbi oculi	Ciliary body produces aqueous humor, which flows through iris into anterior chamber and drains through scleral sinus; anterior displacement of lens may obstruct flow of aqueous humor and cause elevated intraocular pressure, a painful, vision-threatening condition known as acute angle closure glaucoma	117, 119
Membrana tympanica	Visualized with otoscope; bulging indicates middle ear infection with effusion; rupture and otorrhea may occur in severe infection; tympanostomy tubes (T-tubes) may be placed in children with recurrent effusive infections	122
Meatus acusticus externus	May become infected or inflamed in children, a condition known as otitis externa; can be diagnosed with auricle (pinna) pull technique	121

ANATOMICAL STRUCTURE	CLINICAL COMMENT	PLATE NUMBERS
Systema Skeletale		
Orbita	Most facial trauma involves orbit; traumatic fractures can occur in its rim or walls; a "blowout" fracture involves inferior wall and may injure inferior rectus muscle and/or infraorbital nerve; rim fractures affect contours of orbital rim and occur in zygomaticomaxillary fractures	25, 69
Pterion	Intersection of frontal, parietal, temporal, and sphenoid bones; thin, weak region of skull that is susceptible to fracture; frontal branch of middle meningeal artery lies immediately deep to this region and may be injured	27
Asterion	Landmark at posterior end of parietotemporal suture, used in lateral neurosurgical approaches to posterior cranial fossa	27
Articulatio temporomandibularis	Temporomandibular joint disorders are common sources of pain and joint dysfunction; poor replacement results to date; dislocations/subluxations can be reduced via retromolar fossa	42
Suturae cranii	Premature fusion may result in skull deformity known as craniosynostosis; sagittal suture is most often affected	26, 35
Vertebrae cervicales	Degenerative changes causing narrowing of intervertebral foramina may result in cervical radiculopathy; C1–C4 and C5–C7 vertebrae are common areas of pathology for children and adults, respectively; neck hyperextension from abrupt deceleration may cause bilateral pedicle fractures in axis (C2 vertebra), known as hangman's fracture; hyperflexion may cause anterior wedge vertebral fracture; axial loads may cause burst fracture; dens axis (odontoid) fractures may occur with either forceful extension or flexion; all fractures are classified as "stable" or "unstable" depending on whether structural integrity of cervical spine has been sufficiently disrupted to permit compression of spinal cord	43–45
Cartilagines laryngeae	Thyroid and cricoid cartilages are palpable landmarks of anterior neck used for cricothyrotomy, tracheostomy, and cricoid pressure during airway intubation	103, 106
Os hyoideum	Palpable anterior neck landmark at C3 vertebral level that can be fractured during sporting activities, compromising swallowing and speech; fractures may also indicate strangulation	54
Ossicula auditus	Pathologic conditions involving ossicles (e.g., otosclerosis) can cause conductive hearing loss	121, 122
Systema Musculare		
Mm. superficiales capitis (muscles of facial expression)	Used to assess function of facial nerve (CN VII) during cranial nerve examination; may become weak or paralyzed with CN VII dysfunction (e.g., Bell's palsy); often targeted with botulinum toxin injections for aesthetics (wrinkles), headache, and teeth grinding	48, 150
M. sternocleidomastoideus	Important landmark that divides neck into anterior and posterior cervical triangles; palpated to identify "nerve point of neck" for administration of anesthesia to cervical plexus and also used as landmark for insertion of central venous catheters; in children, abnormal shortening or fibrosis of sternocleidomastoid muscle results in head tilt, a condition known as torticollis	56
Mm. sternocleidomastoideus and trapezius	Used to assess function of spinal accessory nerve (CN XI) during cranial nerve examination	56, 154

Table 2.2   **Structures with High Clinical Significance**

ANATOMICAL STRUCTURE	CLINICAL COMMENT	PLATE NUMBERS
Mm. masticatorii	Used to assess function of trigeminal nerve (CN V) during cranial nerve examination; masseter is involved in teeth grinding and associated headaches, which can be treated with botulinum toxin injection	72, 73
Levator veli palatini; m. uvulae	Used to assess function of vagus nerve (CN X) during cranial nerve examination; contralateral deviation of uvula of soft palate during elevation indicates CN X dysfunction	85
M. genioglossus	Used to assess hypoglossal nerve (CN XII) function during cranial nerve examination; tongue deviates to side of lesion when protruded following CN XII injury	88, 155
M. styloglossus	Posterosuperior movement covers laryngeal inlet, protecting vocal cords and airway, which is especially crucial if epiglottis has been surgically removed because of malignancy	88, 95, 96
M. stapedius	Smallest skeletal muscle in the body, regulates movement of stapes bone to control amplitude of sound	123
Levator palpebrae superioris; m. tarsalis superior	Responsible for elevating eyelid; ptosis indicates pathological change in oculomotor nerve (CN III) or sympathetic fibers (if only superior tarsal muscle is affected)	110, 112
Mm. externi bulbi oculi	Used to assess function of oculomotor (CN III), trochlear (CN IV), and abducens (CN VI) nerves during cranial nerve examination; abnormalities in tone result in disconjugate eye movements, a condition known as strabismus	112, 114
Dilatator pupillae	Important in assessment of sympathetic function in head; lack of dilation indicates interruption in sympathetic outflow (e.g., Horner's syndrome)	117, 148
Sphincter pupillae	Involved in pupillary light reflex and accommodation reflex	117, 148
Raphe pterygomandibularis	Valuable intraoral landmark for inferior alveolar nerve blocks to anesthetize mandibular teeth	96, 97–99
Modiolus anguli oris	A fibrous intersection of facial muscles, approximately 1 cm lateral to corner of mouth; valuable landmark when considering reconstruction of injured facial muscles associated with oral region	48
Fossa retromolaris	Important clinical landmark for reducing dislocated temporomandibular joints; buccal and lingual nerves pass by the retromolar fossa and may be harmed in dental molar implant surgery	39
Systema Cardiovasculare		
Vena jugularis interna dextra; vena jugularis externa dextra	Examined to assess right atrial pressure, estimated as height of jugular pulsation above sternal angle (in centimeters) plus 5; right internal jugular vein is preferred because it is in line with superior vena cava	50
Vena jugularis interna	Thrombosis may occur secondary to local extension of inflammation from severe pharyngitis, a condition known as Lemierre's syndrome	50
Venae jugularis interna and subclavia	Used to obtain venous access via insertion of central venous catheter	50, 100
A. thyreoidea inferior	At risk during thyroidectomy; must be preserved to maintain blood supply to parathyroid glands; identified by its redundant loop shape and is landmark to identify recurrent laryngeal nerve	57, 104
Carotis communis	Palpate in neck to assess carotid pulse; bifurcation typically at C4 vertebral level	58, 165

Structures with High Clinical Significance

Table 2.3

ANATOMICAL STRUCTURE	CLINICAL COMMENT	PLATE NUMBERS
Systema Cardiovasculare—Continued		
Carotis interna	Common site for atherosclerosis, which may be treated with stent or endarterectomy for stroke prevention; carotid sinus is sensitive to changes in circulating blood volume and may be massaged to induce vagal reaction; internal carotid artery has no branches in neck; classified into seven parts: C1, cervical; C2, petrous; C3, lacerum; C4, cavernous; C5, clinoid; C6, ophthalmic; and C7, communicating	163, 164
Aa. ethmoidea anterior, sphenopalatina, and facialis	Anastomosis site of branches of these vessels in nasal vestibule, known as Kiesselbach's plexus or Little's area, is common site of anterior nosebleeds (epistaxis); sphenopalatine artery injury causes posterior nosebleeds	65
Plexus venosus pterygoideus	Common route for spread of infection due to connections between face, orbit, and venous sinuses; valveless veins allow retrograde flow	100, 115
A. ophthalmica	Primary source of blood to retina; blindness may occur if artery is occluded	115, 119
Aa. epicraniales	Scalp lacerations bleed profusely owing to rich blood supply	24, 127
Venae superiores cerebri	May be torn from their junction with superior sagittal sinus, producing subdural hematoma	129, 130, 136
A. meningea media	Trauma to pterion can tear middle meningeal artery (frontal branch), often causing epidural hematoma	128
Sinus venosi durales	Infections in head may spread to sinuses, causing dural venous sinus thrombosis; cavernous sinus is most common site	130, 131
Sinus cavernosus	Fistula (anastomosis) between internal carotid artery and cavernous sinus may form, especially following trauma	131,167
Sinus carotidis	Compressed during carotid sinus massage, which may result in bradycardia and/or hypertension; carotid sinus hypersensitivity, most common among older adults, may cause syncope	157
Circulus arteriosus cerebri (Willisi)	Common site of aneurysms and important site of collateral cerebral circulation; aneurysmal rupture produces subarachnoid hemorrhage	166
Emissaria	Valveless veins, which can convey infection extracranially to intracranially and allow alternative route for drainage when dural venous sinuses are obstructed	129
Vasa Lymphaticum and Organa Lymphoidea		
Ductus thoracicus	Thoracic duct may be injured during surgeries to neck and thorax due to multiple and frequent variants; injury in lower neck region is often at junction of left internal jugular and subclavian veins; increased risk during esophageal surgery and left central venous line placement	101, 260
Nodi lymphoidei cervicales laterales profundi superior and inferior	Palpated during neck examination to assess size and shape; if coalescent, malignancy must be excluded	101, 102
Tonsillae palatina and pharyngea	Palatine tonsils are commonly involved with viral and bacterial infections; exudative lesions combined with fever, lymphadenopathy, and lack of cough suggestive of streptococcal infection (strep throat); enlarged pharyngeal tonsils (adenoids) cause snoring and can cover auditory (Eustachian) tube opening, increasing risk of middle ear infections	90

Table 2.4   **Structures with High Clinical Significance**

ANATOMICAL STRUCTURE	CLINICAL COMMENT	PLATE NUMBERS
Systema Respiratorium		
Epiglottis	Crucial landmark during endotracheal intubation; bacterial or viral infection (e.g., with *Haemophilus influenzae*) may cause epiglottitis, which presents with respiratory distress, sore throat, and hoarse voice	93–95
Sinus paranasales (sinus maxillaris, ethmoidei, frontalis, and sphenoideus)	Cavities in skull prone to mucosal inflammation due to bacterial or viral infection	67, 69
Septum nasi	Congenital or acquired deviation may lead to nasal obstruction, treated with septoplasty; perforations may occur with cocaine use or in granulomatosis with polyangiitis	37, 69
Systema Digestorium		
Glandula parotidea	Swelling of gland due to infection (parotitis), such as from viruses or bacteria, may cause pain and compress branches of facial nerve, producing facial muscle weakness; external carotid, superficial temporal, and maxillary arteries also pass through the gland	70, 71
Organa Endocrina		
Glandula thyreoidea	Enlargement is known as goiter; may be partially or completely removed in malignancy or hyperthyroidism; during examination should move relatively equally bilaterally with hyoid bone and laryngeal cartilages; malignancy may anchor portion of gland and cause asymmetrical movement	103

*Selections were based largely on clinical data and commonly discussed clinical correlations in macroscopic ("gross") anatomy courses.

Cranial nerves are traditionally described as tree-like structures that emerge from the brain and branch peripherally. This matches the direction that action potentials travel in efferent fibers in nerves. It must be remembered that action potentials travel in the opposite direction in afferent fibers within these nerves.

NERVE	ORIGIN	COURSE	BRANCHES	MOTOR	SENSORY
N. olfactorius (CN I)	Bulbus olfactorius	Neurons of olfactory mucosa send approximately 20 axon bundles through cribriform plate to synapse on olfactory bulb neurons			SVA (smell): olfactory epithelium
N. opticus (CN II)	Chiasma opticum	Axons of retinal ganglion neurons exit orbit through optic canal to enter cranial cavity			SSA (vision): optic part of retina
N. oculomotorius (CN III)	Fossa interpeduncularis mesencephali	Exits midbrain into posterior cranial fossa and then middle cranial fossa; traverses cavernous sinus to enter orbit via superior orbital fissure	Rr. superior and inferior	GSE: Mm. recti medialis, superior, and inferior; M. obliquus inferior; Levator palpebrae superioris GVE: Ganglion ciliare	
N. trochlearis (CN IV)	Facies posterior mesencephali	Exits dorsal midbrain, coursing lateral to cerebral peduncle to anterior surface of brainstem; follows medial edge of tentorium cerebelli to enter middle cranial fossa; traverses cavernous sinus to enter orbit via superior orbital fissure		GSE: M. obliquus superior	
N. trigeminus (CN V)	Radices motoria and sensoria (arising from Pons)	Exits anterolateral pons into posterior cranial fossa; large sensory and small motor roots enter middle cranial fossa; sensory root forms trigeminal ganglion, which gives rise to ophthalmic, maxillary, and mandibular nerves; motor root passes deep to ganglion and contributes only to mandibular nerve	Nn. ophthalmicus, maxillaris, and mandibularis	SVE: see N. mandibularis	GSA: see branches
N. ophthalmicus (CN V$_1$)	N. trigeminus	Exits anterior border of trigeminal ganglion and traverses cavernous sinus to leave cranium through superior orbital fissure into orbit	Nn. lacrimalis, frontalis, and nasociliaris; R. meningeus		GSA: forehead, upper eyelid, conjunctiva
N. maxillaris (CN V$_2$)	N. trigeminus	Exits trigeminal ganglion, passes through foramen rotundum into pterygopalatine fossa, and enters orbit via inferior orbital fissure	Nn. nasopalatinus, pharyngeus, palatini major and minores, zygomaticus, alveolaris superior posterior, and infraorbitalis; Rr. nasales posteriores superiores; R. meningeus		GSA: midface, nasal cavity, paranasal sinuses, palate, maxillary teeth
N. mandibularis (CN V$_3$)	N. trigeminus	Exits trigeminal ganglion inferiorly, leaves cranium through foramen ovale and enters infratemporal fossa	Nn. temporales profundi, buccalis, auriculotemporalis, lingualis, and alveolaris inferioris; R. meningeus	SVE: Mm. masticatorii, mylohyoideus, and digastricus (venter anterior); Tensor tympani; Tensor veli palatini	GSA: mandibular teeth, anterior tongue, floor of oral cavity, temporomandibular joint
N. abducens (CN VI)	Sulcus bulbopontinus (medial to CN VII)	Exits between pons and medulla near midline, pierces dura on clivus and grooves on petrous part of temporal bone to access middle cranial fossa; traverses cavernous sinus to enter orbit through superior orbital fissure		GSE: M. rectus lateralis	

Table 2.6

Nervi Craniales

NERVE	ORIGIN	COURSE	BRANCHES	MOTOR	SENSORY
N. facialis (CN VII)	Radix motoria and N. intermedius (Radix sensoria)	Exits laterally between pons and medulla oblongata as a larger motor root and smaller intermediate nerve (carrying SVA, GVE, and GSA fibers); both roots traverse internal acoustic meatus to enter facial canal, in which a sharp turn (genu) occurs just before geniculate (facial) ganglion; facial nerve gives off several branches within facial canal, before it exits through stylomastoid foramen and forms terminal branches within parotid gland	Nn. petrosus major and auricularis posterior; Chorda tympani; Rr. temporales, zygomatici, buccales, marginalis mandibularis, and cervicalis	SVE: Mm. superficiales capitis (including Mm. faciales and epicraniales, and Platysma); Mm. digastricus (venter posterior), stylohyoideus, and stapedius GVE: Ganglia pterygopalatinum and subman-dibulare	SVA (taste): anterior tongue and palate GSA: part of external ear
N. vestibulocochlearis (CN VIII)	Sulcus bulbopontinus (lateral to CN VII)	Exits brainstem between pons and medulla oblongata, near inferior cerebellar peduncle, and divides into two branches as it traverses posterior cranial fossa	Nn. vestibularis and cochlearis		SSA: internal ear (see branches)
N. cochlearis	N. vestibulocochlearis	Contains processes of cochlear ganglion cells; passes through internal acoustic meatus into internal ear			SSA (hearing): spiral organ of cochlear duct
N. vestibularis	N. vestibulocochlearis	Contains processes of vestibular ganglion cells; passes through internal acoustic meatus into internal ear	Rr. superior and inferior		SSA (equilibrium and motion): maculae and cristae ampullares of vestibular labyrinth
N. glossopharyngeus (CN IX)	Sulcus retroolivaris medullae oblongatae	Emerges from upper medulla between olive and inferior cerebral peduncle and exits cranium by traversing jugular foramen with vagus and accessory nerves; superior and inferior ganglia for afferent components of CN IX are located just inferior to jugular foramen; nerve passes inferiorly, innervating and following stylopharyngeus muscle, ultimately sending a branch into posterior oral cavity that passes deep to hyoglossus muscle and a branch that enters pharynx by passing between superior and middle pharyngeal constrictors	N. tympanicus	SVE: M. stylo-pharyngeus GVE: Ganglion oticum	SVA (taste): posterior tongue GVA: carotid body and sinus GSA: posterior tongue, oropharynx, middle ear
N. vagus (CN X)	Sulcus retroolivaris medullae oblongatae (between CN IX and radix cranialis of CN XI)	Exits from retro-olivary groove of medulla oblongata to traverse jugular foramen with accessory and glossopharyngeal nerves; initially runs between internal carotid artery and internal jugular vein; courses of right and left vagus nerves differ, with right vagus nerve coursing inferiorly between subclavian artery and vein, at which point right recurrent laryngeal nerve ascends and vagus nerve descends along trachea and root of right lung, forming pulmonary and esophageal plexuses; left vagus nerve descends between left subclavian and common carotid arteries posteriorly to left brachiocephalic vein, and anteriorly to aortic arch, at which point left recurrent laryngeal nerve ascends posteriorly to aorta and rest of vagus nerve descends posteriorly to root of lung, forming pulmonary and esophageal plexuses; vagus nerve fibers continue into abdomen via esophageal plexuses and vagal trunks	R. pharyngeus; Nn. laryngei superior and recurrens	GVE: Ganglia visceralia thoracis and abdominis SVE: see branches	GVA: aortic arch and bodies SVA (taste): epiglottis, oropharynx GSA: external ear (also see branches)

NERVE	ORIGIN	COURSE	BRANCHES	MOTOR	SENSORY
R. pharyngeus n. vagi	N. vagus	Passes between carotid arteries superficial to middle pharyngeal constrictor		SVE: Constrictores pharyngis; Mm. palatoglossus, palatopharyngeus, and salpingopharyngeus; Levator veli palatini	
N. laryngeus superior	N. vagus	Exits inferior ganglion, passing inferiorly and medially deep to internal carotid artery, dividing into external (motor) branch and internal (sensory) branch that pierces thyrohyoid membrane	Rr. internus and externus	SVE: M. cricothyreoideus	GSA: superior larynx
N. laryngeus recurrens	N. vagus	On right side, arises anterior to subclavian artery and spirals to run superiorly and posteriorly to common carotid and inferior thyroid arteries, lateral to trachea; on left side, arises inferior to aortic arch, passing posterior to arch and lateral to ligamentum arteriosum to ascend superiorly lateral to trachea; both right and left nerves enter larynx at junction of esophagus and inferior pharyngeal constrictor		SVE: Mm. interni laryngis (except M. cricothyreoideus); Textus muscularis striatus oesophagi	GSA: inferior larynx
N. accessorius (CN XI)	Radices cranialis and spinalis	Spinal roots from C1–C5 segments of spinal cord ascend and enter cranium through foramen magnum, where they course with cranial root arising from retroolivary groove of medulla oblongata; spinal accessory nerve exits from cranium via jugular foramen; it passes inferiorly and posteriorly into upper third of sternocleidomastoid muscle and then inferiorly, crossing occipital triangle to enter trapezius muscle; vagal communicating branch joins vagus nerve at jugular foramen to innervate larynx, palate, and pharyngeal muscles	N. accessorius spinalis; R. communicans vagalis	GSE: Mm. trapezius and sternocleidomastoideus	
N. hypoglossus (CN XII)	Radiculae hypoglossae and R. communicans hypoglossus n. spinalis C1	Rootlets from anterolateral sulcus of medulla oblongata exit cranium through hypoglossal canal, then pass inferiorly and anteriorly between vagus and spinal accessory nerves to inferior border of posterior belly of digastric muscle, eventually entering oral cavity by passing between mylohyoid and hyoglossus muscles	Rr. linguales; Rami conveying fibers from N. spinalis C1 (Rr. thyreohyoideus and geniohyoideus, and Radix superior ansae cervicalis)	GSE: Mm. interni linguae, genioglossus, hyoglossus, and styloglossus C1: Mm. thyreoideus, geniohyoideus, and omohyoideus (venter superior)	

Table 2.8   **Nervi Craniales**

The roots of the cervical plexus are the anterior rami of C1–C4 spinal nerves.

NERVE	ORIGIN	COURSE	BRANCHES	MOTOR	CUTANEOUS SENSORY
R. communicans hypoglossus n. spinalis C1	R. anterior n. spinalis C1	Emerges and briefly adheres to hypoglossal nerve; superior root of ansa cervicalis exits just posterior to greater horn of hyoid bone and descends along carotid sheath, where it joins inferior root at C4/5 level	Radix superior ansae cervicalis; Rr. thyreohyoideus and geniohyoideus n. hypoglossi	Mm. omohyoideus (venter superior), thyreohyoideus, and geniohyoideus	
Radix inferior ansae cervicalis	Rr. anteriores nn. spinalium C2–C3	Descends along anterolateral carotid sheath, joining superior root at C4/5 level	Rr. infrahyoidei	Mm. omohyoideus (venter inferior), sternohyoideus, and sternothyreoideus	
Rr. musculares plexus cervicalis	Rr. anteriores nn. spinalium C1–C4	Three loops form along C1–C4 vertebrae that course laterally between levator scapulae and scalenus medius muscle, deep to sternocleidomastoid muscle		Mm. recti anterior and lateralis capitis; Mm. longi capitis and colli; Mm. scaleni anterior, medius, and posterior; Levator scapulae	
N. phrenicus	Rr. anteriores nn. spinalium C3–C5	Descends on scalenus anterior muscle deep to inferior belly of omohyoid muscle and transverses cervical and suprascapular vessels; enters thorax between subclavian vein and artery, passing anterior to root of lung and along lateral border of pericardium to pierce diaphragm		Diaphragma	
N. occipitalis minor	R. anterior n. spinalis C2	Formed in posterior cervical triangle deep to sternocleidomastoid muscle, ascending along its posterior border; perforates deep fascia at mastoid process, ascending posterior to ear			Temporal, auricular, and mastoid regions
N. auricularis magnus	Rr. anteriores nn. spinalium C2–C3	Formed in posterior cervical triangle deep to sternocleidomastoid muscle, ascending obliquely between that muscle and platysma	Rr. anterior and posterior		Parotid, auricular, and mastoid regions
N. transversus colli	Rr. anteriores nn. spinalium C2–C3	Formed in posterior cervical triangle deep to sternocleidomastoid muscle, runs superficial to that muscle, passing deep to external jugular vein	Rr. superior and inferior		Anterior and lateral regions of neck
N. supraclavicularis	Rr. anteriores nn. spinalium C3–C4	Formed in posterior cervical triangle deep to mid-third of sternocleidomastoid muscle, passes lateral to external jugular vein, and descends just inferior to clavicle	Nn. supraclaviculares medialis, intermedius, and lateralis		Clavicular and infraclavicular regions

MUSCLE	MUSCLE GROUP	ORIGIN ATTACHMENT	INSERTION ATTACHMENT	INNERVATION	BLOOD SUPPLY	MAIN ACTIONS
M. arytenoideus obliquus	Mm. laryngis	Cartilago arytenoidea	Cartilago arytenoidea (opposite)	N. laryngeus recurrens	Aa. thyreoideae superior and inferior	Closes intercartilaginous portion of rima glottidis
M. arytenoideus transversus	Mm. laryngis	Cartilago arytenoidea	Cartilago arytenoidea (opposite)	N. laryngeus recurrens	Aa. thyreoideae superior and inferior	Closes intercartilaginous portion of rima glottidis
M. auricularis anterior	Mm. superficiales capitis (mm. auriculares externi)	Fascia temporalis; aponeurosis epicranialis	Facies medialis helicis auriculae (anterior part)	Rr. temporales n. facialis	Aa. auricularis posterior and temporalis superficialis	Elevates and draws auricle forward
M. auricularis posterior	Mm. superficiales capitis (mm. auriculares externi)	Proc. mastoideus	Facies medialis auriculae (inferior part)	N. auricularis posterior (branch of n. facialis)	Aa. auricularis posterior and temporalis superficialis	Retracts and elevates auricle
M. auricularis superior	Mm. superficiales capitis (mm. auriculares externi)	Fascia temporalis; aponeurosis epicranialis	Facies medialis auriculae (superior part)	Rr. temporales n. facialis	Aa. auricularis posterior and temporalis superficialis	Retracts and elevates auricle
Bucinator	Mm. superficiales capitis (mm. faciales)	Procc. alveolares maxillae and mandibulae (posterior portions); raphe pterygomandibularis (anterior border)	Modiolus anguli oris	Rr. buccales n. facialis	Aa. facialis and maxillaris	Compresses cheeks
M. ciliaris	Mm. interni bulbi oculi (smooth muscle)	Calcar sclerae	Choroidea	Nn. ciliares breves (parasympathetic fibers from ganglion ciliaris)	A. ophthalmica	Constricts ciliary body and lens rounds up (accommodation)
Constrictor inferior pharyngis	Mm. circulares pharyngis	Linea obliqua cartilaginis thyroideae; cartilago cricoidea	Raphe pharyngis	N. vagus (via plexus pharyngeus)	Aa. pharyngea ascendens and thyreoidea superior	Constricts wall of pharynx during swallowing
Constrictor medius pharyngis	Mm. circulares pharyngis	Lig. stylohyoideum; cornua ossis hyoidei	Raphe pharyngis	N. vagus (via plexus pharyngeus)	Aa. pharyngea ascendens and palatina ascendens; Rr. tonsillares a. facialis; Rr. dorsales linguae a. lingualis	Constricts wall of pharynx during swallowing
Constrictor superior pharyngis	Mm. circulares pharyngis	Hamulus pterygoideus; raphe pterygomandibularis; linea myohyoidea mandibulae	Raphe pharyngis	N. vagus (via plexus pharyngeus)	Aa. pharyngea ascendens and palatina ascendens; Rr. tonsillares a. facialis; Rr. dorsales linguae a. lingualis	Constricts wall of pharynx during swallowing
Corrugator supercilii	Mm. superficiales capitis (mm. faciales)	Margo supraorbitalis (medial part)	Cutis supercilii (medial half)	Rr. temporales n. facialis	A. temporalis superficialis	Draws eyebrows inferiorly and medially, produces vertical wrinkles of skin between eyebrows
M. cricoarytenoideus lateralis	Mm. laryngis	Arcus cartilaginis cricoideae	Proc. muscularis cartilaginis arytenoideae	N. laryngeus recurrens	Aa. thyreoideae superior and inferior	Adducts vocal folds
M. cricoarytenoideus posterior	Mm. laryngis	Facies posterior laminae cartilaginis cricoideae	Proc. muscularis cartilaginis arytenoideae	N. laryngeus recurrens	Aa. thyreoideae superior and inferior	Abducts vocal folds
M. cricothyreoideus	Mm. laryngis	Arcus cartilaginis cricoideae	Margo inferior laminae cartilaginis thyreoideae; cornu inferius cartilaginis thyreoideae	R. externus n. laryngeus superioris	Aa. thyreoideae superior and inferior	Lengthens and tenses vocal ligaments

Table 2.10   Musculi

MUSCLE	MUSCLE GROUP	ORIGIN ATTACHMENT	INSERTION ATTACHMENT	INNERVATION	BLOOD SUPPLY	MAIN ACTIONS
Depressor anguli oris	Mm. superficiales capitis (mm. faciales)	Linea obliqua mandibulae	Modiolus anguli oris	Rr. marginalis mandibularis and buccales n. facialis	A. labialis inferior	Depresses angle of mouth
Depressor labii inferioris	Mm. superficiales capitis (mm. faciales)	Facies externa mandibulae (between symphysis mandibulae and foramen mentale)	Cutis labii inferioris	R. marginalis mandibularis n. facialis	A. labialis inferior	Depresses lower lip and draws it laterally
Depressor septi nasi	Mm. superficiales capitis (mm. faciales)	Fossa incisiva maxillae	Septum nasi; Ala nasi (posterior part)	Rr. zygomatici and buccales n. facialis	A. labialis superior	Narrows nostril, draws septum inferiorly
M. digastricus	Mm. suprahyoidei	*Venter anterior*: Fossa digastrica mandibulae *Venter posterior*: Incisura mastoidea ossis temporalis	Tendo intermedius m. digastrici (attached to corpus ossis hyoidei)	*Venter anterior*: N. alveolaris inferior (branch of n. mandibularis) *Venter posterior*: R. digastricus n. facialis	*Venter anterior*: A. submentalis *Venter posterior*: Aa. auricularis posterior and occipitalis	Elevates hyoid bone and base of tongue, steadies hyoid bone, opens mouth by depressing mandible
Dilatator pupillae	Mm. interni bulbi oculi (smooth muscle)	Pars iridica retinae	Margo pupillaris iridis	Nn. ciliares longi (sympathetic fibers from ganglion cervicale superius)	A. ophthalmica	Dilates pupil
M. frontalis	Mm. superficiales capitis (m. epicranius)	Aponeurosis epicranialis (at level of sutura coronalis)	Cutis regionis frontalis; aponeurosis epicranialis	Rr. temporales n. facialis	A. temporalis superficialis	Horizontally wrinkles skin of forehead, elevates eyebrows
M. genioglossus	Mm. externi linguae	Spina mentalis superior mandibulae	Dorsum linguae; os hyoideum	N. hypoglossus (CN XII)	Aa. sublingualis and submentalis	Depresses and protrudes tongue
M. geniohyoideus	Mm. suprahyoidei	Spina mentalis inferior mandibulae	Facies anterior corporis ossis hyoidei	R. anterior n. spinalis C1 (via n. hypoglossus)	A. sublingualis	Elevates hyoid bone and depresses mandible
M. hyoglossus	Mm. externi linguae	Corpus ossis hyoidei; cornu majus ossis hyoidei	Margo linguae; facies inferior linguae	N. hypoglossus (CN XII)	Aa. sublingualis and submentalis	Depresses and retracts tongue
Levator anguli oris	Mm. superficiales capitis (mm. faciales)	Fossa canina maxillae	Modiolus anguli oris	Rr. zygomatici and buccales n. facialis	A. labialis superior	Elevates angle of mouth
Levator labii superioris	Mm. superficiales capitis (Mm. faciales)	Maxilla (superior to foramen infraorbitale)	Cutis labii superioris oris	Rr. zygomatici and buccales n. facialis	Aa. labialis superior and angularis	Elevates upper lip, dilates nares
Levator nasolabialis (levator labii superioris alaeque nasi)	Mm. superficiales capitis (mm. faciales)	Proc. frontalis maxillae (superior part)	Cartilago alaris major; Cutis nasi; labium superius oris (lateral part)	Rr. zygomatici and buccales n. facialis	Aa. labialis superior and angularis	Elevates upper lip and dilates nostril
Levator palpebrae superioris	Mm. externi bulbi oculi	Ala minor ossis sphenoidei (anterior to canalis opticus)	Tarsus superior	N. oculomotorius (CN III)	Aa. ophthalmica	Elevates upper eyelid
Levator veli palatini	Mm. palati mollis	Pars petrosa ossis temporalis; tuba auditiva (Eustachii)	Aponeurosis palatina	N. vagus (via plexus pharyngeus)	Aa. palatinae ascendens and descendens	Elevates soft palate during swallowing
M. longitudinalis inferior linguae	Mm. interni linguae	Facies inferior linguae	Apex linguae	N. hypoglossus (CN XII)	Aa. lingualis and facialis	Shortens tongue, turns tip and sides inferiorly
M. longitudinalis superior linguae	Mm. interni linguae	Tela submucosa dorsi linguae (posterior part)	Apex linguae (unites with muscle of opposite side)	N. hypoglossus (CN XII)	Aa. profunda linguae and facialis	Shortens tongue, turns tip and sides superiorly
M. longus capitis	Mm. vertebrales anteriores	Tubercula anteriora [procc. transversorum] vertebrarum C3–C6	Pars basilaris ossis occipitalis (inferior surface)	Rr. anteriores nn. spinalium C1–C3	Aa. cervicalis ascendens, pharyngea ascendens, and vertebralis	Flexes head

MUSCLE	MUSCLE GROUP	ORIGIN ATTACHMENT	INSERTION ATTACHMENT	INNERVATION	BLOOD SUPPLY	MAIN ACTIONS
M. longus colli	Mm. vertebrales anteriores	*Pars verticalis*: Vertebrae C5–T3 *Pars obliqua inferior*: Vertebrae T1–T3 *Pars obliqua superior*: Tubercula anteriora [procc. transversorum] vertebrarum C3–C5	*Pars verticalis*: Vertebrae C2–C4 *Pars obliqua inferior*: Tubercula anteriora [procc. transversorum] vertebrarum C3–C6 *Pars obliqua superior*: Tuberculum anterius atlantis	Rr. anteriores nn. spinalium C2–C8	Aa. pharyngea ascendens, cervicalis ascendens, and vertebralis	*Bilaterally*: flex and assist in rotating cervical vertebrae and head *Unilaterally*: laterally flexes vertebral column
Masseter	Mm. masticatorii	Arcus zygomaticus	Ramus mandibulae; proc. coronoideus	N. mandibularis (CN V₃)	Aa. transversa faciei, masseterica, and facialis	Elevates and protrudes mandible; deep fibers retract it
M. mentalis	Mm. superficiales capitis (mm. faciales)	Fossa incisiva mandibulae	Cutis regionis mentalis	R. marginalis mandibularis n. facialis	A. labialis inferior	Elevates and protrudes lower lip
M. mylohyoideus	Mm. suprahyoidei	Linea mylohyoidea mandibulae	Raphe mediana mylohyoidea; corpus ossis hyoidei	N. alveolaris inferior (branch of n. mandibularis)	Aa. sublingualis and submentalis	Elevates hyoid bone, base of tongue, floor of mouth; depresses mandible
M. nasalis	Mm. superficiales capitis (mm. faciales)	Eminentia canina (superior and lateral to fossa incisiva maxillae)	Aponeurosis on cartilagines nasi	Rr. buccales n. facialis	A. labialis superior; R. septalis a. facialis; R. nasalis lateralis a. facialis	Draws ala of nose toward nasal septum, compresses nostrils; alar part opens nostrils
M. obliquus inferior	Mm. externi bulbi oculi	Paries inferior orbitae (anterior part, lateral to canalis nasolacrimalis)	Sclera (lateral to limbus corneae)	N. oculomotorius (CN III)	A. ophthalmica	Abducts, elevates, and laterally rotates eyeball
M. obliquus superior	Mm. externi bulbi oculi	Corpus ossis sphenoidei (above canalis opticus)	Sclera, superior to limbus corneae (after passing through trochlea)	N. trochlearis (CN IV)	A. ophthalmica	Abducts, depresses, and medially rotates eyeball
M. occipitalis	Mm. superficiales capitis (m. epicranius)	Linea nuchalis superior (lateral two-thirds); proc. mastoideus	Cutis regionis occipitalis; aponeurosis epicranialis	N. auricularis posterior (branch of n. facialis)	Aa. auricularis posterior and occipitalis	Moves scalp backward
M. omohyoideus	Mm. infrahyoidei	*Venter inferior*: Margo superior scapulae; lig. transversum superius scapulae *Venter superior*: Corpus ossis hyoidei	Tendo intermedius m. omohyoidei	*Venter inferior*: Ansa cervicalis (C2–C3) *Venter superior*: Ansa cervicalis (C1)	Aa. lingualis and thyreoidea superior	Steadies and depresses hyoid bone
M. orbicularis oculi	Mm. superficiales capitis (mm. faciales)	Margo orbitalis medialis; lig. palpebrale mediale; os lacrimale	Cutis regionis periorbitalis; lig. palpebrale laterale; palpebrae superior and inferior	Rr. temporales and zygomatici n. facialis	Aa. facialis and temporalis superficialis	Closes eyelids
M. orbicularis oris	Mm. superficiales capitis (mm. faciales)	Maxilla; mandibula; cutis regionis perioralis; musculi periorales	Modiolus anguli oris	Rr. buccales and marginalis mandibularis n. facialis	Aa. labiales inferior and superior	Compression, contraction, and protrusion of lips
M. palatoglossus	Mm. palati mollis	Aponeurosis palatina	Margo linguae	N. vagus (via plexus pharyngeus)	A. pharyngea ascendens; Aa. palatinae ascendens and descendens	Elevates posterior tongue, depresses palate
M. palatopharyngeus	Mm. palati mollis	Palatum durum; aponeurosis palatina	Paries lateralis pharyngis	N. vagus (via plexus pharyngeus)	Aa. palatinae ascendens and descendens	Tenses soft palate; pulls walls of pharynx superiorly, anteriorly, and medially during swallowing
Platysma	Mm. superficiales capitis (mm. colli)	Cutis regionis infraclavicularis	Mandibula; musculi labii inferioris	R. cervicalis n. facialis	Aa. submentalis and suprascapularis	Tenses skin of neck

Table 2.12   **Musculi**

MUSCLE	MUSCLE GROUP	ORIGIN ATTACHMENT	INSERTION ATTACHMENT	INNERVATION	BLOOD SUPPLY	MAIN ACTIONS
M. procerus	Mm. superficiales capitis (mm. faciales)	Fascia covering Pars inferior ossis nasalis and Pars superior cartilaginis lateralis nasi	Cutis regionis frontalis (medial and superior to supercilium)	Rr. temporales and zygomatici n. facialis	A. angularis; R. nasalis lateralis a. facialis	Draws down medial angle of eyebrows, produces transverse wrinkles over bridge of nose
M. pterygoideus lateralis	Mm. masticatorii	*Caput superior*: Facies infratemporalis alae majoris ossis sphenoidei *Caput inferior*: Lamina lateralis proc. pterygoidei	Fovea pterygoidea mandibulae; capsula art. temporomandibularis; Discus art. temporomandibularis	N. mandibularis (CN V₃)	A. maxillaris	*Bilaterally*: protrudes mandible *Unilaterally and alternately*: produces side-to-side grinding
M. pterygoideus medialis	Mm. masticatorii	Lamina lateralis proc. pterygoidei (medial surface); proc. pyramidalis ossis palatini; tuber maxillae	Ramus mandibulae and angulus mandibulae (medial surfaces, inferior to foramen alveolare inferius)	N. mandibularis (CN V₃)	Aa. facialis and maxillaris	*Bilaterally*: protrudes and elevates mandible *Unilaterally and alternately*: produces side-to-side movements
M. rectus anterior capitis	Mm. vertebrales anteriores	Massa lateralis atlantis	Pars basilaris ossis occipitalis	Rr. anteriores nn. spinalium C1–C2	Aa. vertebralis and pharyngea ascendens	Flexes head
M. rectus inferior	Mm. externi bulbi oculi	Anulus tendineus communis	Sclera (inferior to limbus corneae)	N. oculomotorius (CN III)	A. ophthalmica	Depresses, adducts, and laterally rotates eyeball
M. rectus lateralis	Mm. externi bulbi oculi	Anulus tendineus communis	Sclera (lateral to limbus corneae)	N. abducens (CN VI)	A. ophthalmica	Abducts eyeball
M. rectus lateralis capitis	Mm. vertebrales anteriores	Proc. transversus atlantis (superior surface)	Proc. jugularis ossis occipitalis (inferior surface)	Rr. anteriores nn. spinalium C1–C2	Aa. vertebralis, occipitalis, and pharyngea ascendens	Flexes head laterally to same side
M. rectus medialis	Mm. externi bulbi oculi	Anulus tendineus communis	Sclera (medial to limbus corneae)	N. oculomotorius (CN III)	A. ophthalmica	Adducts eyeball
M. rectus superior	Mm. externi bulbi oculi	Anulus tendineus communis	Sclera (superior to limbus corneae)	N. oculomotorius (CN III)	A. ophthalmica	Elevates, adducts, and medially rotates eyeball
M. risorius	Mm. superficiales capitis (mm. faciales)	Fascia masseterica	Modiolus anguli oris	Rr. buccales n. facialis	A. labialis superior	Retracts angle of mouth
M. salpingopharyngeus	Mm. longitudinales pharyngis	Tuba auditiva (Eustachii)	Paries lateralis pharyngis	N. vagus (via plexus pharyngeus)	A. pharyngea ascendens	Elevates pharynx and larynx during swallowing and speaking
M. scalenus anterior	Mm. vertebrales laterales	Tubercula anteriora [procc. transversorum] vertebrarum C3–C6	Tuberculum scalenum costae 1	Rr. anteriores nn. spinalium C5–C8	A. cervicalis ascendens	Elevates 1st rib, bends neck
M. scalenus medius	Mm. vertebrales laterales	Tubercula posteriora [procc. transversorum] vertebrarum C2–C7	Facies superior costae 1 (behind sulcus subclavius)	Rr. anteriores nn. spinalium C3–C7	A. cervicalis ascendens	Elevates 1st rib, bends neck
M. scalenus posterior	Mm. vertebrales laterales	Tubercula posteriora [procc. transversorum] vertebrarum C4–C6	Facies externa costae 2	Rr. anteriores nn. spinalium C5–C8	A. cervicalis ascendens; R. superficialis a. transversae colli	Elevates 2nd rib, bends neck
Sphincter pupillae	Mm. interni bulbi oculi (smooth muscle)	Circular smooth muscle of iris that passes around pupil	Blends with fibers of dilatator pupillae	Nn. ciliares breves (parasympathetic fibers from ganglion ciliare)	A. ophthalmica	Constricts pupil
M. stapedius	Mm. ossiculorum auditus (auris media)	Eminentia pyramidalis ossis temporalis (in cavitas tympani)	Stapes	N. stapedius (branch of n. facialis)	Aa. auricularis posterior, tympanica anterior, and meningea media	Pulls stapes posteriorly to lessen oscillation of tympanic membrane
M. sternocleidomastoideus	Mm. colli	*Caput sternale*: Facies anterior manubrii sterni *Caput claviculare*: Facies superior claviculae (medial third)	Facies lateralis proc. mastoidei; linea nuchalis superior ossis occipitalis (lateral half)	N. accessorius spinalis (CN XI)	Aa. thyreoidea superior, occipitalis, suprascapularis, and auricularis posterior	*Bilaterally*: flexes head, elevates thorax *Unilaterally*: turns face toward opposite side

MUSCLE	MUSCLE GROUP	ORIGIN ATTACHMENT	INSERTION ATTACHMENT	INNERVATION	BLOOD SUPPLY	MAIN ACTIONS
M. sternohyoideus	Mm. infrahyoidei	Facies posterior manubrii sterni; lig. sternoclaviculare posterius; extremitas sternalis claviculae	Margo inferior corporis ossis hyoidei (medial part)	Ansa cervicalis (C1–C3)	Aa. thyreoidea superior and lingualis	Depresses larynx and hyoid bone, steadies hyoid bone
M. sternothyreoideus	Mm. infrahyoidei	Facies posterior manubrii sterni; margo posterior cartilaginis costalis 1	Linea obliqua cartilaginis thyreoideae	Ansa cervicalis (C1–C3)	R. cricothyreoideus a. thyreoideae superioris	Depresses larynx and thyroid cartilage
M. styloglossus	Mm. externi linguae	Proc. styloideus ossis temporalis; lig. stylohyoideum	Margo linguae; facies inferior linguae	N. hypoglossus (CN XII)	A. sublingualis	Retracts tongue and draws it up for swallowing
M. stylohyoideus	Mm. suprahyoidei	Proc. styloideus ossis temporalis (posterior border)	Corpus ossis hyoidei (at junction with cornu majus)	R. stylohyoideus n. facialis	Aa. facialis and occipitalis	Elevates and retracts hyoid bone
M. stylopharyngeus	Mm. longitudinales pharyngis	Proc. styloideus ossis temporalis (medial surface)	Paries pharyngis; margo posterior cartilaginis thyreoideae	N. glossopharyngeus (CN IX)	Aa. pharyngea ascendens and palatina ascendens; Rr. tonsillares a. facialis; Rr. dorsales linguae a. lingualis	Elevates pharynx and larynx during swallowing and speaking
M. temporalis	Mm. masticatorii	Fossa temporalis; lamina profunda fasciae temporalis	Proc. coronoideus; ramus mandibulae	Nn. temporales profundi (branches of n. mandibularis)	Aa. temporalis superficialis and maxillaris	Elevates mandible; posterior fibers retract mandible
Tensor tympani	Mm. ossiculorum auditus (auris media)	Cartilago tubae auditivae	Manubrium mallei	N. mandibularis (CN V₃)	A. tympanica superior	Tenses tympanic membrane by drawing it medially
Tensor veli palatini	Mm. palati mollis	Fossa scaphoidea ossis sphenoidei; spina ossis sphenoidei; tuba auditiva (Eustachii)	Aponeurosis palatina	N. mandibularis (CN V₃)	Aa. palatinae ascendens and descendens	Tenses soft palate, opens auditory tube during swallowing and yawning
M. thyreoarytenoideus	Mm. laryngis	Facies interna cartilaginis thyreoideae	Proc. muscularis cartilaginis arytenoideae	N. laryngeus recurrens	Aa. thyreoideae superior and inferior	Shortens and relaxes vocal cords, sphincter of vestibule
M. thyreohyoideus	Mm. infrahyoidei	Linea obliqua cartilaginis thyreoideae	Margo inferior ossis hyoidei; cornu majus ossis hyoidei	R. anterior n. spinalis C1 (via n. hypoglossus)	A. thyreoidea superior	Depresses larynx and hyoid bone, elevates larynx when hyoid bone is fixed
M. transversus linguae	Mm. interni linguae	Septum linguae	Dorsum linguae; margo linguae	N. hypoglossus (CN XII)	Aa. profunda linguae and facialis	Narrows and elongates tongue
M. uvulae	Mm. palati mollis	Spina nasalis posterior (ossis palatini), aponeurosis palatina	Tunica mucosa uvulae palatinae	N. vagus (via plexus pharyngeus)	Aa. palatinae descendens and ascendens	Shortens, elevates, and retracts uvula of the palate
M. verticalis linguae	Mm. interni linguae	Tunica mucosa dorsi linguae (anterior part)	Facies inferior linguae	N. hypoglossus (CN XII)	Aa. profunda linguae and facialis	Flattens and broadens tongue
M. vocalis	Mm. laryngis	Proc. vocalis cartilaginis arytenoideae	Lig. vocale	N. laryngeus recurrens	Aa. thyreoideae superior and inferior	Tenses anterior part of vocal ligament, relaxes posterior part of vocal ligament
M. zygomaticus major	Mm. superficiales capitis (mm. faciales)	Arcus zygomaticus	Modiolus anguli oris	Rr. zygomatici and buccales n. facialis	A. labialis superior	Draws angle of mouth posteriorly and superiorly
M. zygomaticus minor	Mm. superficiales capitis (mm. faciales)	Arcus zygomaticus	Modiolus anguli oris; labium superius oris	Rr. zygomatici and buccales n. facialis	A. labialis superior	Elevates upper lip

Variations in spinal nerve contributions to the innervation of muscles, their arterial supply, their attachments, and their actions are common themes in human anatomy. Therefore, expect differences between texts and realize that anatomical variation is normal.

Table 2.14   **Musculi**

DORSUM 3

Surface Anatomy   178
Columna Vertebralis   179–185
Medulla Spinalis   186–194
Musculi and Nervi   195–199
Cross-Sectional Anatomy   200–201

Structures with High
  Clinical Significance   Table 3.1
Musculi   Tables 3.2–3.4
Electronic Bonus Plates   BP 33–BP 40

ELECTRONIC BONUS PLATES

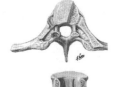

BP 33 Ligamenta Columnae Vertebralis

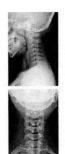
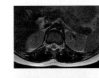

BP 34 Pars Cervicalis Columnae Vertebralis: Radiographs

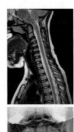
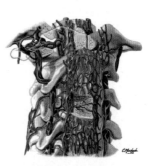

BP 35 Pars Cervicalis Columnae Vertebralis: MRI and Radiograph

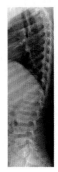
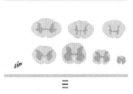

BP 36 Pars Thoracolumbalis Columnae Vertebralis: Lateral Radiograph

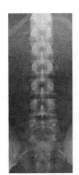

BP 37 Pars Lumbalis Columnae Vertebralis: Radiographs

BP 38 Pars Lumbalis Columnae Vertebralis: MRIs

BP 39 Venae Columnae Vertebralis: Detail Showing Venous Communications

BP 40 Medulla Spinalis: Fiber Tracts in Cross Sections

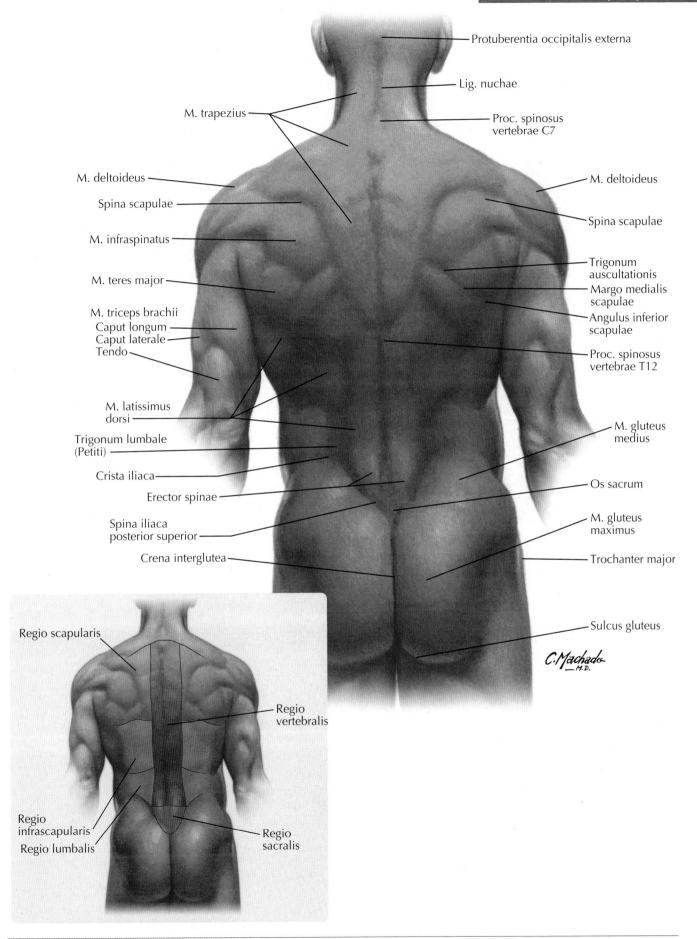

Protuberentia occipitalis externa

Lig. nuchae

M. trapezius

Proc. spinosus
vertebrae C7

M. deltoideus

M. deltoideus

Spina scapulae

Spina scapulae

M. infraspinatus

Trigonum
auscultationis

M. teres major

Margo medialis
scapulae

M. triceps brachii
Caput longum
Caput laterale
Tendo

Angulus inferior
scapulae

Proc. spinosus
vertebrae T12

M. latissimus
dorsi

Trigonum lumbale
(Petiti)

M. gluteus
medius

Crista iliaca

Os sacrum

Erector spinae

Spina iliaca
posterior superior

M. gluteus
maximus

Crena interglutea

Trochanter major

Sulcus gluteus

C. Machado
M.D.

Regio scapularis

Regio
vertebralis

Regio
infrascapularis

Regio lumbalis

Regio
sacralis

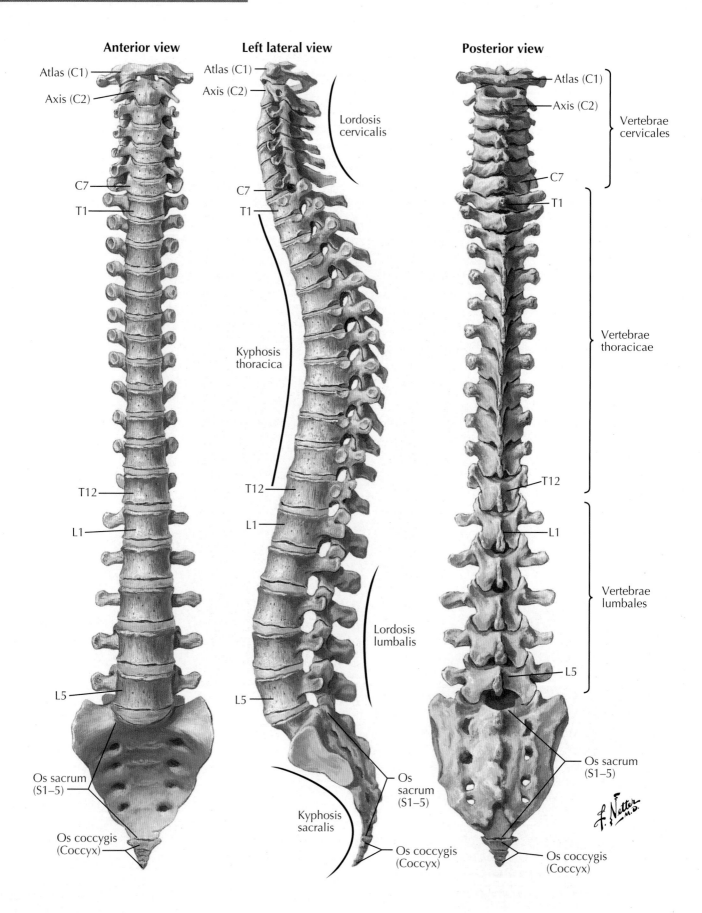

Anterior view

Atlas (C1)

Axis (C2)

C7

T1

T12

L1

L5

Os sacrum
(S1–5)

Os coccygis
(Coccyx)

Left lateral view

Atlas (C1)

Axis (C2)

Lordosis
cervicalis

C7

T1

Kyphosis
thoracica

T12

L1

L5

Lordosis
lumbalis

Os
sacrum
(S1–5)

Kyphosis
sacralis

Os coccygis
(Coccyx)

Posterior view

Atlas (C1)

Axis (C2)

Vertebrae
cervicales

C7

T1

Vertebrae
thoracicae

T12

L1

Vertebrae
lumbales

L5

Os sacrum
(S1–5)

Os coccygis
(Coccyx)

Plate 179

Columna Vertebralis

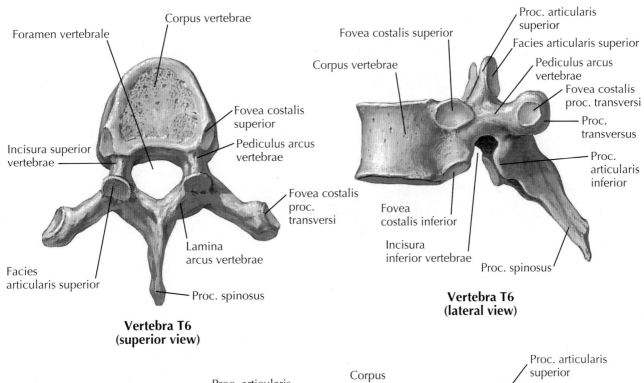

Foramen vertebrale

Corpus vertebrae

Fovea costalis superior

Pediculus arcus vertebrae

Incisura superior vertebrae

Facies articularis superior

Lamina arcus vertebrae

Fovea costalis proc. transversi

Proc. spinosus

Vertebra T6 (superior view)

Fovea costalis superior

Corpus vertebrae

Proc. articularis superior

Facies articularis superior

Pediculus arcus vertebrae

Fovea costalis proc. transversi

Proc. transversus

Proc. articularis inferior

Fovea costalis inferior

Incisura inferior vertebrae

Proc. spinosus

Vertebra T6 (lateral view)

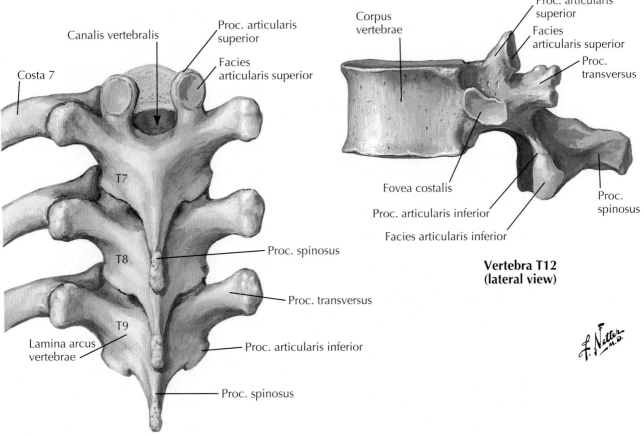

Canalis vertebralis

Proc. articularis superior

Facies articularis superior

Costa 7

T7

T8

T9

Lamina arcus vertebrae

Proc. spinosus

Proc. transversus

Proc. articularis inferior

Proc. spinosus

Vertebrae T7, T8, and T9 (posterior view)

Corpus vertebrae

Proc. articularis superior

Facies articularis superior

Proc. transversus

Fovea costalis

Proc. articularis inferior

Facies articularis inferior

Proc. spinosus

Vertebra T12 (lateral view)

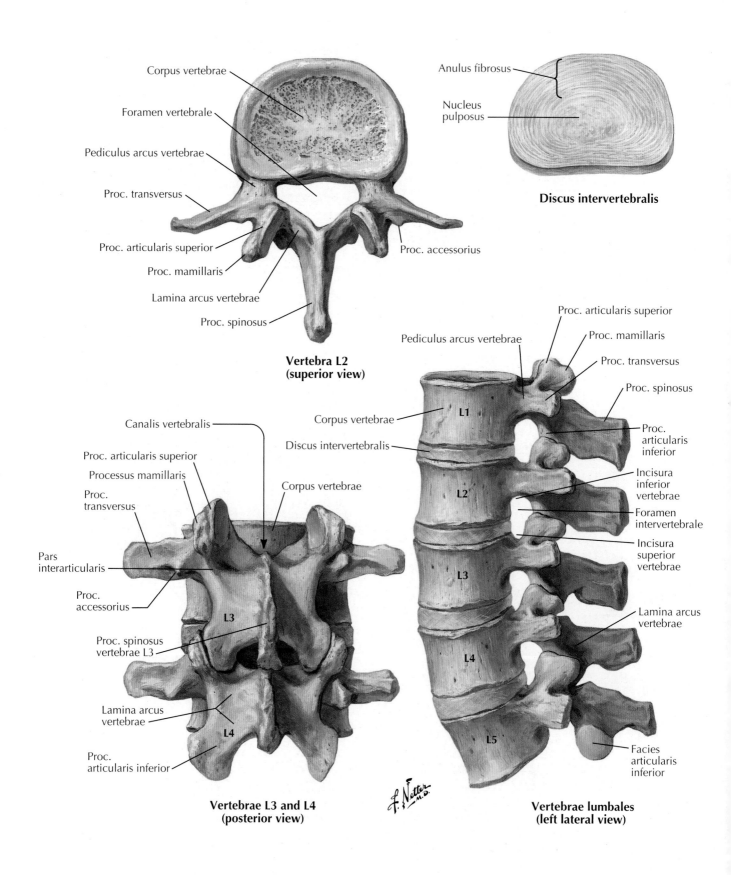

Corpus vertebrae

Foramen vertebrale

Pediculus arcus vertebrae

Proc. transversus

Proc. articularis superior

Proc. mamillaris

Lamina arcus vertebrae

Proc. spinosus

Proc. accessorius

**Vertebra L2
(superior view)**

Anulus fibrosus

Nucleus
pulposus

Discus intervertebralis

Canalis vertebralis

Proc. articularis superior

Processus mamillaris

Proc.
transversus

Pars
interarticularis

Proc.
accessorius

Corpus vertebrae

L3

Proc. spinosus
vertebrae L3

Lamina arcus
vertebrae

L4

Proc.
articularis inferior

**Vertebrae L3 and L4
(posterior view)**

Proc. articularis superior

Proc. mamillaris

Proc. transversus

Proc. spinosus

Pediculus arcus vertebrae

Corpus vertebrae

Discus intervertebralis

L1

L2

L3

L4

L5

Proc.
articularis
inferior

Incisura
inferior
vertebrae

Foramen
intervertebrale

Incisura
superior
vertebrae

Lamina arcus
vertebrae

Facies
articularis
inferior

**Vertebrae lumbales
(left lateral view)**

Plate 181

Columna Vertebralis

Anteroposterior radiograph of thoracolumbar spine

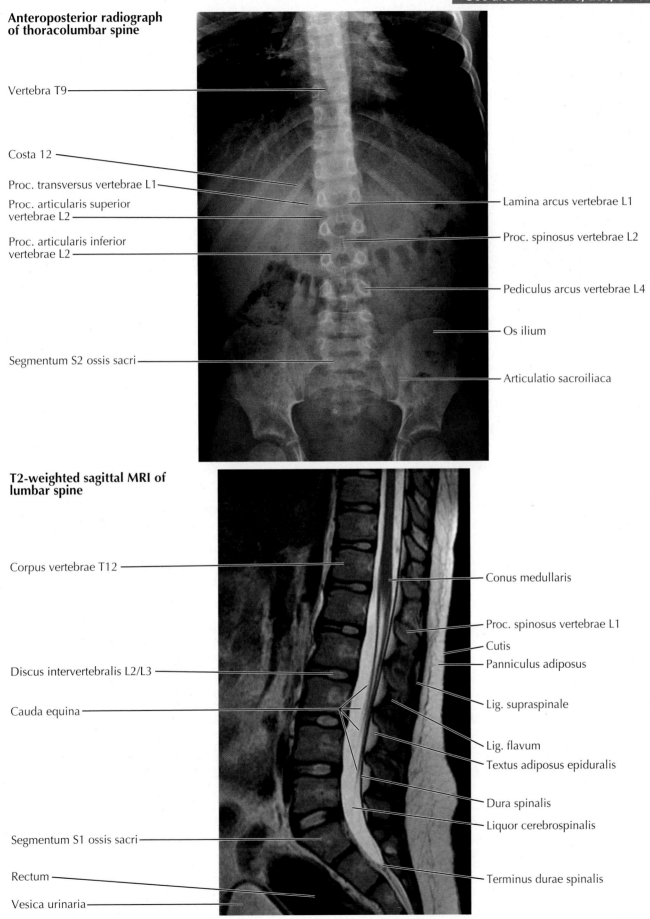

Vertebra T9

Costa 12

Proc. transversus vertebrae L1

Proc. articularis superior vertebrae L2

Proc. articularis inferior vertebrae L2

Segmentum S2 ossis sacri

Lamina arcus vertebrae L1

Proc. spinosus vertebrae L2

Pediculus arcus vertebrae L4

Os ilium

Articulatio sacroiliaca

T2-weighted sagittal MRI of lumbar spine

Corpus vertebrae T12

Discus intervertebralis L2/L3

Cauda equina

Segmentum S1 ossis sacri

Rectum

Vesica urinaria

Conus medullaris

Proc. spinosus vertebrae L1

Cutis

Panniculus adiposus

Lig. supraspinale

Lig. flavum

Textus adiposus epiduralis

Dura spinalis

Liquor cerebrospinalis

Terminus durae spinalis

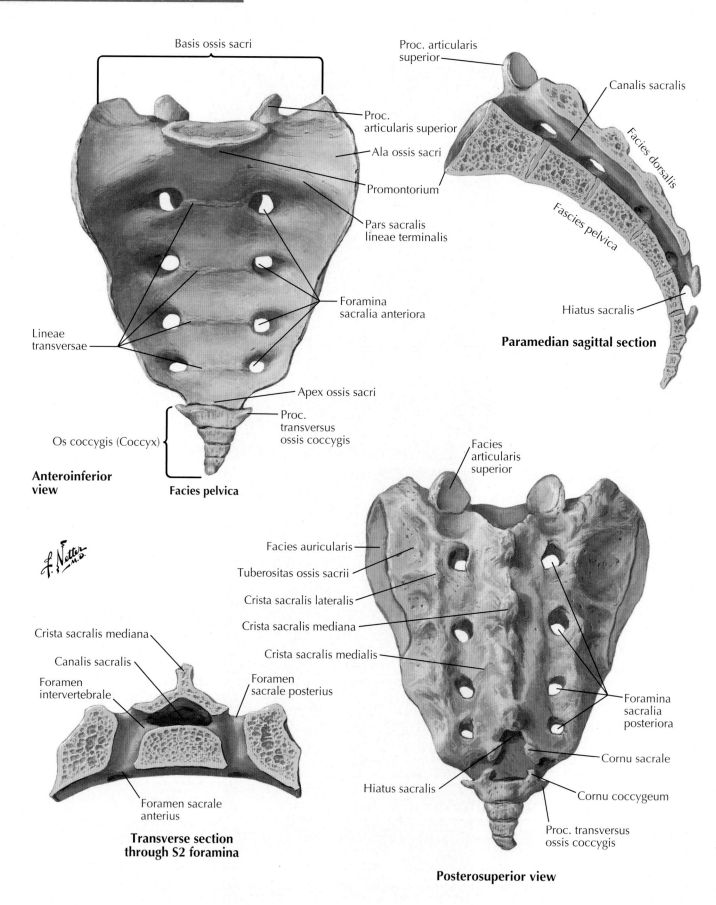

Basis ossis sacri

Proc. articularis superior

Proc. articularis superior

Canalis sacralis

Ala ossis sacri

Facies dorsalis

Promontorium

Fascies pelvica

Pars sacralis lineae terminalis

Foramina sacralia anteriora

Hiatus sacralis

Paramedian sagittal section

Lineae transversae

Apex ossis sacri

Proc. transversus ossis coccygis

Os coccygis (Coccyx)

Facies articularis superior

Anteroinferior view

Facies pelvica

Facies auricularis

Tuberositas ossis sacrii

Crista sacralis lateralis

Crista sacralis mediana

Crista sacralis medialis

Crista sacralis mediana

Canalis sacralis

Foramen intervertebrale

Foramen sacrale posterius

Foramina sacralia posteriora

Cornu sacrale

Foramen sacrale anterius

Hiatus sacralis

Cornu coccygeum

Transverse section through S2 foramina

Proc. transversus ossis coccygis

Posterosuperior view

Plate 183

Columna Vertebralis

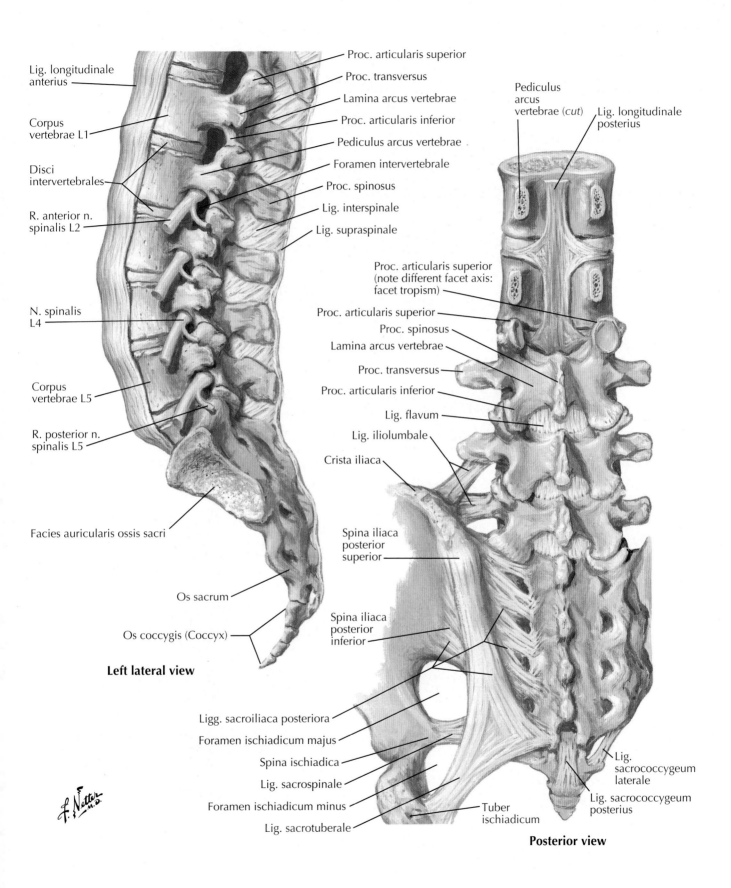

Lig. longitudinale anterius

Corpus vertebrae L1

Disci intervertebrales

R. anterior n. spinalis L2

N. spinalis L4

Corpus vertebrae L5

R. posterior n. spinalis L5

Facies auricularis ossis sacri

Os sacrum

Os coccygis (Coccyx)

Left lateral view

Proc. articularis superior

Proc. transversus

Lamina arcus vertebrae

Proc. articularis inferior

Pediculus arcus vertebrae

Foramen intervertebrale

Proc. spinosus

Lig. interspinale

Lig. supraspinale

Pediculus arcus vertebrae (cut)

Lig. longitudinale posterius

Proc. articularis superior (note different facet axis: facet tropism)

Proc. articularis superior

Proc. spinosus

Lamina arcus vertebrae

Proc. transversus

Proc. articularis inferior

Lig. flavum

Lig. iliolumbale

Crista iliaca

Spina iliaca posterior superior

Spina iliaca posterior inferior

Ligg. sacroiliaca posteriora

Foramen ischiadicum majus

Spina ischiadica

Lig. sacrospinale

Foramen ischiadicum minus

Lig. sacrotuberale

Tuber ischiadicum

Lig. sacrococcygeum laterale

Lig. sacrococcygeum posterius

Posterior view

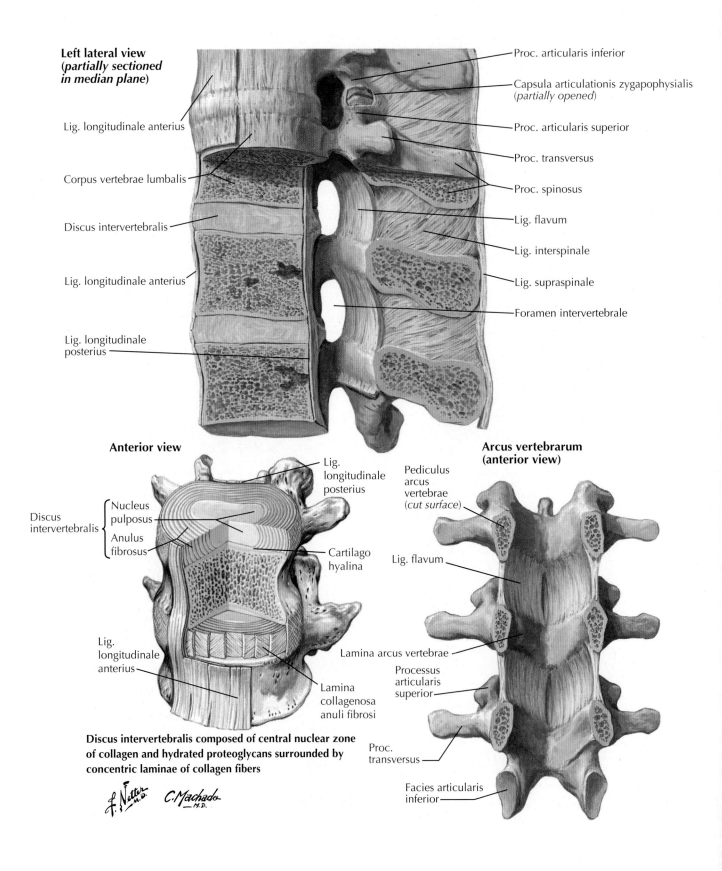

Left lateral view (*partially sectioned in median plane*)

Lig. longitudinale anterius

Corpus vertebrae lumbalis

Discus intervertebralis

Lig. longitudinale anterius

Lig. longitudinale posterius

Proc. articularis inferior

Capsula articulationis zygapophysialis (*partially opened*)

Proc. articularis superior

Proc. transversus

Proc. spinosus

Lig. flavum

Lig. interspinale

Lig. supraspinale

Foramen intervertebrale

Anterior view

Discus intervertebralis { Nucleus pulposus / Anulus fibrosus

Lig. longitudinale posterius

Cartilago hyalina

Lig. longitudinale anterius

Lamina collagenosa anuli fibrosi

Discus intervertebralis composed of central nuclear zone of collagen and hydrated proteoglycans surrounded by concentric laminae of collagen fibers

Arcus vertebrarum (anterior view)

Pediculus arcus vertebrae (*cut surface*)

Lig. flavum

Lamina arcus vertebrae

Processus articularis superior

Proc. transversus

Facies articularis inferior

Plate 185

Columna Vertebralis

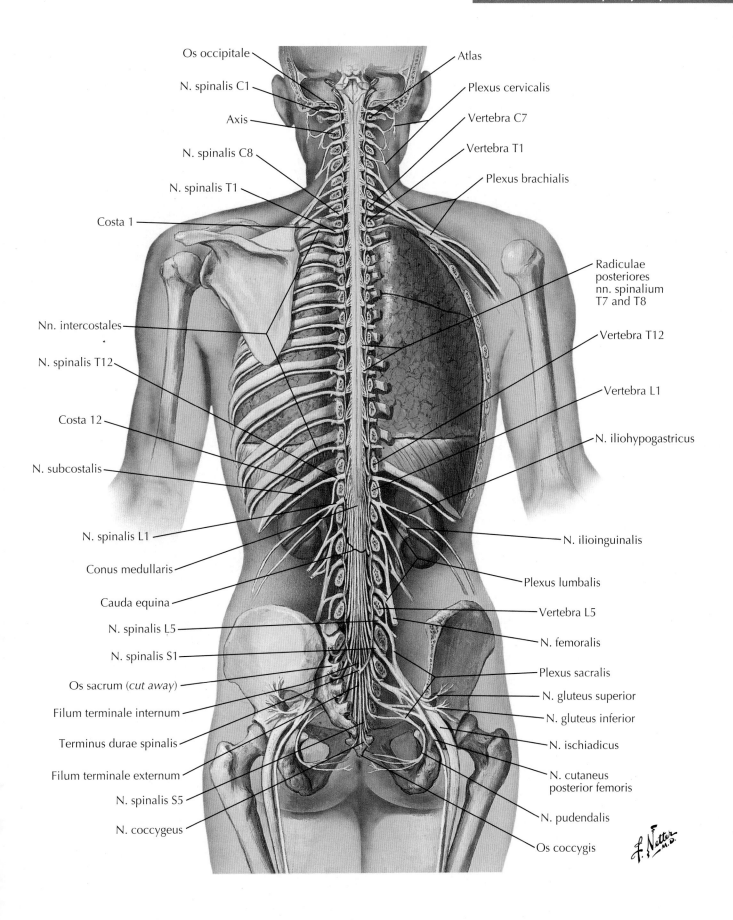

Os occipitale

N. spinalis C1

Axis

N. spinalis C8

N. spinalis T1

Costa 1

Nn. intercostales

N. spinalis T12

Costa 12

N. subcostalis

N. spinalis L1

Conus medullaris

Cauda equina

N. spinalis L5

N. spinalis S1

Os sacrum (*cut away*)

Filum terminale internum

Terminus durae spinalis

Filum terminale externum

N. spinalis S5

N. coccygeus

Atlas

Plexus cervicalis

Vertebra C7

Vertebra T1

Plexus brachialis

Radiculae posteriores nn. spinalium T7 and T8

Vertebra T12

Vertebra L1

N. iliohypogastricus

N. ilioinguinalis

Plexus lumbalis

Vertebra L5

N. femoralis

Plexus sacralis

N. gluteus superior

N. gluteus inferior

N. ischiadicus

N. cutaneus posterior femoris

N. pudendalis

Os coccygis

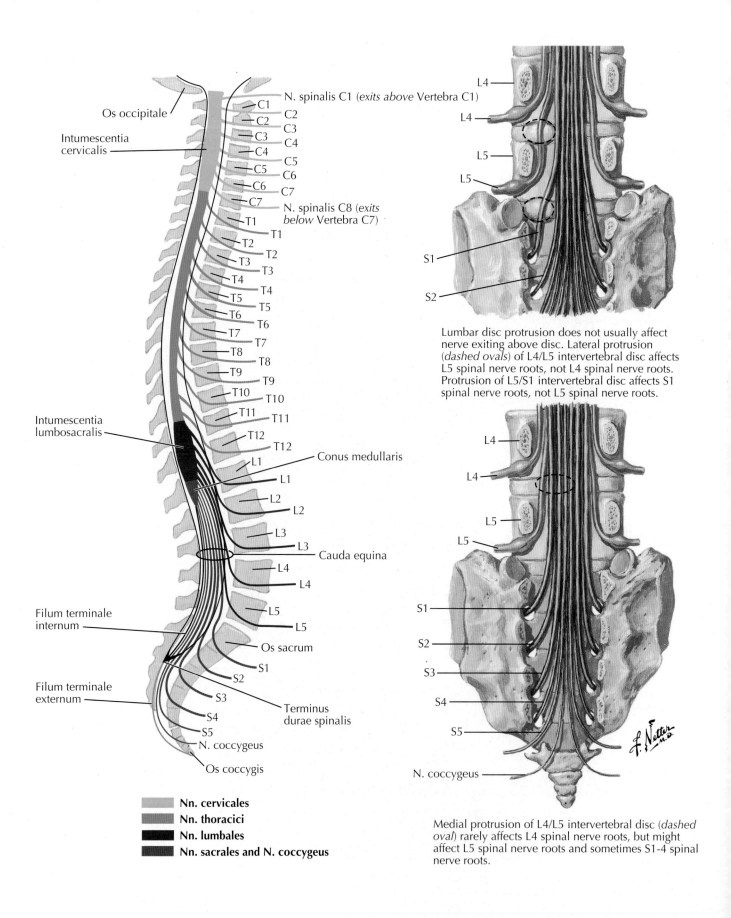

Os occipitale

Intumescentia
cervicalis

N. spinalis C1 (*exits above* Vertebra C1)

C1
C2
C3
C4
C5
C6
C7

C1
C2
C3
C4
C5
C6
C7

N. spinalis C8 (*exits below* Vertebra C7)

T1
T2
T3
T4
T5
T6
T7
T8
T9
T10
T11
T12

T1
T2
T3
T4
T5
T6
T7
T8
T9
T10
T11
T12

Intumescentia
lumbosacralis

Conus medullaris

L1
L2
L3
L4
L5

L1
L2
L3
L4
L5

Cauda equina

Filum terminale
internum

Os sacrum

S1
S2
S3
S4
S5
N. coccygeus

Terminus
durae spinalis

Filum terminale
externum

Os coccygis

Nn. cervicales
Nn. thoracici
Nn. lumbales
Nn. sacrales and N. coccygeus

L4
L4
L5
L5
S1
S2

Lumbar disc protrusion does not usually affect
nerve exiting above disc. Lateral protrusion
(*dashed ovals*) of L4/L5 intervertebral disc affects
L5 spinal nerve roots, not L4 spinal nerve roots.
Protrusion of L5/S1 intervertebral disc affects S1
spinal nerve roots, not L5 spinal nerve roots.

L4
L4
L5
L5
S1
S2
S3
S4
S5
N. coccygeus

Medial protrusion of L4/L5 intervertebral disc (*dashed
oval*) rarely affects L4 spinal nerve roots, but might
affect L5 spinal nerve roots and sometimes S1-4 spinal
nerve roots.

Plate 187

Medulla Spinalis

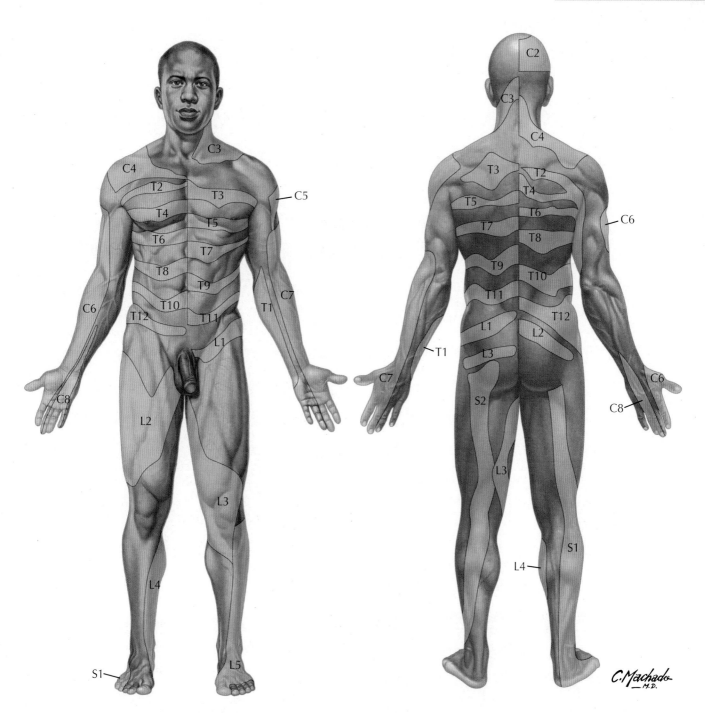

Levels of principal dermatomes

C4	Level of Clavicula	**T10**	Level of Umbilicus
C5, C6, C7	Facies laterales membri superioris	**L1**	Regio inguinalis and Pars anterior proximalis femoris
C8, T1	Facies mediales membri superioris	**L1, L2, L3, L4**	Regio glutealis and Pars anteromedialis membri inferioris
C6	Digiti laterales manus	**L4, L5, S1**	Pes
C6, C7, C8	Manus	**L4**	Pars medialis cruris
C8	Digiti mediales manus	**L5, S1**	Dorsum pedis and Pars posterolateralis membri inferioris
T4	Level of Papilla mammaria	**S1**	Pars lateralis pedis

Schematic based on Lee MW, McPhee RW, Stringer MD. An evidence-based approach to human dermatomes. Clin Anat. 2008 Jul;21(5):363-73. doi: 10.1002/ca.20636. PMID: 18470936. Please note that these areas are not absolute and vary from person to person. S3, S4, S5, Co supply the perineum but are not shown for reasons of clarity. Of note, the dermatomes are larger than illustrated as the figure is based on best evidence; gaps represent areas in which the data are inconclusive.

Medulla Spinalis

Plate 188

Posterior view

Within dural sheath {
Radix anterior n. spinalis
Radix posterior n. spinalis
Ganglion spinale

R. communicans albus
R. communicans griseus
R. anterior n. spinalis
R. posterior n. spinalis

Dura spinalis

Arachnoidea spinalis (*cut*)

Pia spinalis

Radiculae posteriores

Lig. denticulatum

Cornu posterius

Cornu anterius

Dura and arachnoidea removed: anterior view (*greatly magnified*)

Cornu laterale
Substantia grisea
Substantia alba

Radiculae posteriores

Radix posterior n. spinalis

Radiculae anteriores

Ganglion spinale

R. posterior n. spinalis

R. anterior n. spinalis

Radix anterior n. spinalis

N. spinalis

R. communicans griseus
R. communicans albus

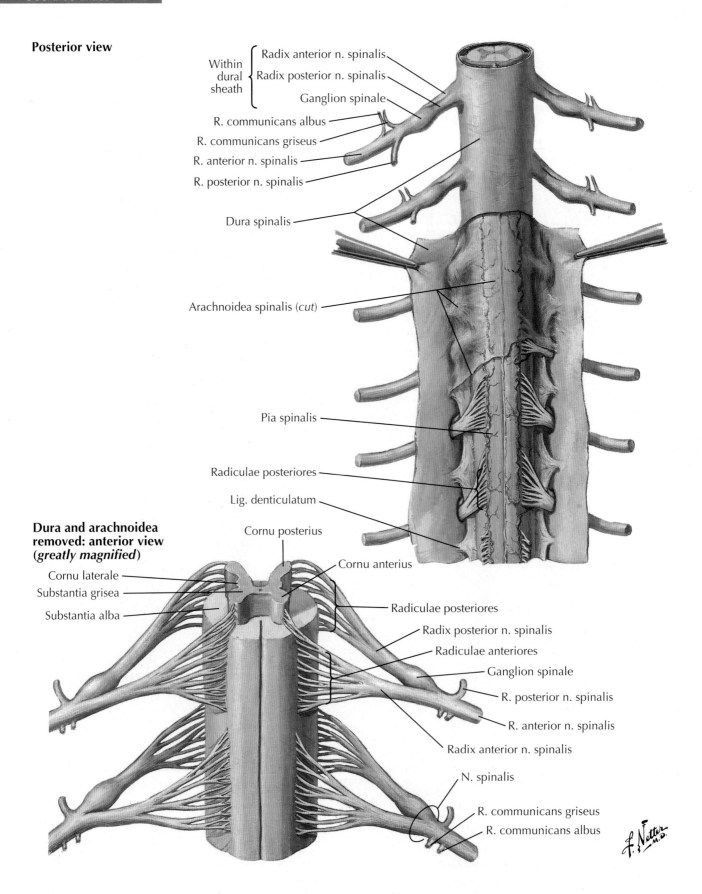

Plate 189

Medulla Spinalis

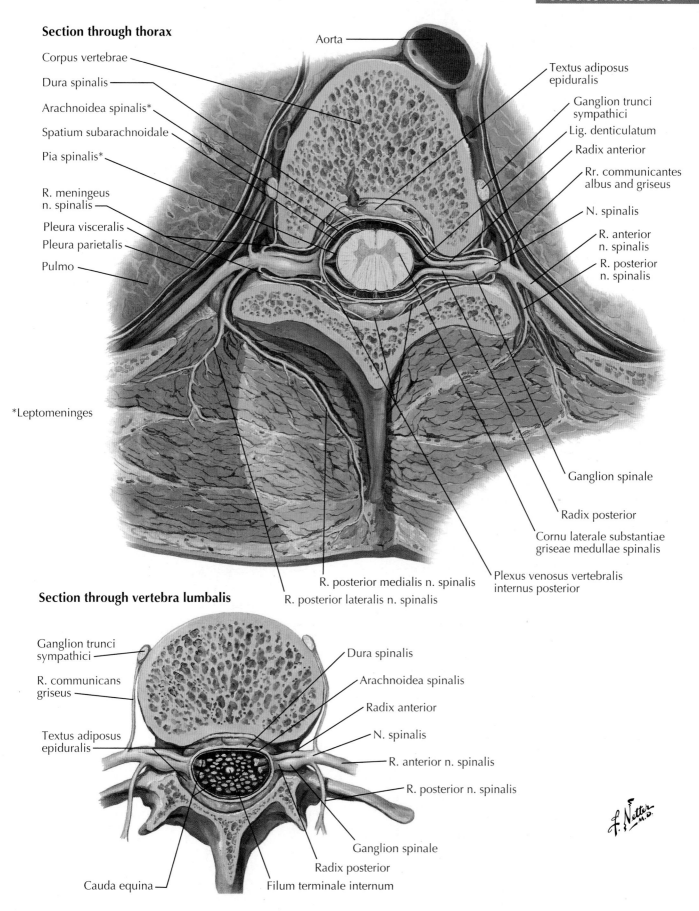

Section through thorax

Corpus vertebrae

Dura spinalis

Arachnoidea spinalis*

Spatium subarachnoidale

Pia spinalis*

R. meningeus
n. spinalis

Pleura visceralis

Pleura parietalis

Pulmo

*Leptomeninges

Aorta

Textus adiposus
epiduralis

Ganglion trunci
sympathici

Lig. denticulatum

Radix anterior

Rr. communicantes
albus and griseus

N. spinalis

R. anterior
n. spinalis

R. posterior
n. spinalis

Ganglion spinale

Radix posterior

Cornu laterale substantiae
griseae medullae spinalis

Plexus venosus vertebralis
internus posterior

R. posterior medialis n. spinalis

R. posterior lateralis n. spinalis

Section through vertebra lumbalis

Ganglion trunci
sympathici

R. communicans
griseus

Textus adiposus
epiduralis

Cauda equina

Dura spinalis

Arachnoidea spinalis

Radix anterior

N. spinalis

R. anterior n. spinalis

R. posterior n. spinalis

Ganglion spinale

Radix posterior

Filum terminale internum

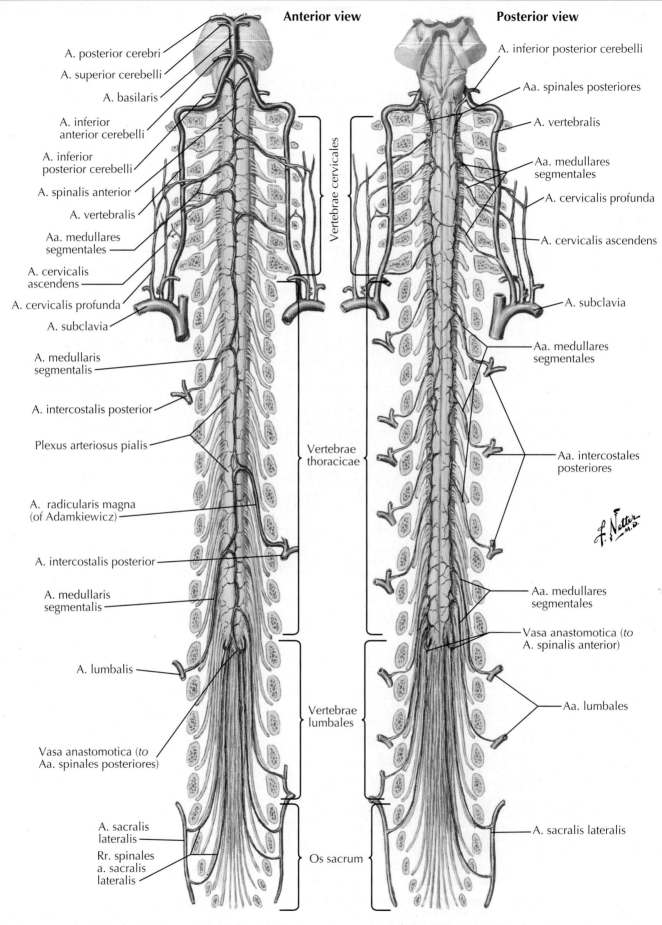

Anterior view

Posterior view

A. posterior cerebri

A. superior cerebelli

A. basilaris

A. inferior anterior cerebelli

A. inferior posterior cerebelli

A. spinalis anterior

A. vertebralis

Aa. medullares segmentales

A. cervicalis ascendens

A. cervicalis profunda

A. subclavia

A. medullaris segmentalis

A. intercostalis posterior

Plexus arteriosus pialis

A. radicularis magna (of Adamkiewicz)

A. intercostalis posterior

A. medullaris segmentalis

A. lumbalis

Vasa anastomotica (to Aa. spinales posteriores)

A. sacralis lateralis

Rr. spinales a. sacralis lateralis

Vertebrae cervicales

Vertebrae thoracicae

Vertebrae lumbales

Os sacrum

A. inferior posterior cerebelli

Aa. spinales posteriores

A. vertebralis

Aa. medullares segmentales

A. cervicalis profunda

A. cervicalis ascendens

A. subclavia

Aa. medullares segmentales

Aa. intercostales posteriores

Aa. medullares segmentales

Vasa anastomotica (to A. spinalis anterior)

Aa. lumbales

A. sacralis lateralis

Note: All spinal nerve roots have associated radicular or segmental medullary arteries. Most roots have radicular arteries (see Plate 192). Both types of arteries run along roots, but radicular arteries end before reaching anterior or posterior spinal arteries; larger segmental medullary arteries continue on to supply a segment of these arteries.

Plate 191　　　　　　　　　　　　　　　　　　　　　　　　　　**Medulla Spinalis**

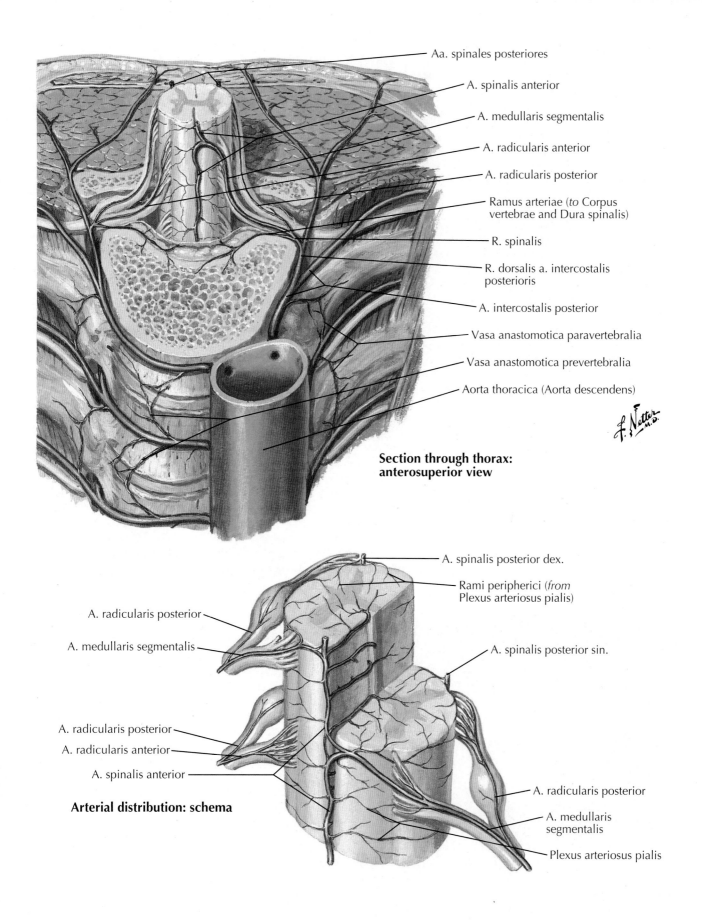

Aa. spinales posteriores

A. spinalis anterior

A. medullaris segmentalis

A. radicularis anterior

A. radicularis posterior

Ramus arteriae (*to* Corpus vertebrae and Dura spinalis)

R. spinalis

R. dorsalis a. intercostalis posterioris

A. intercostalis posterior

Vasa anastomotica paravertebralia

Vasa anastomotica prevertebralia

Aorta thoracica (Aorta descendens)

Section through thorax: anterosuperior view

A. spinalis posterior dex.

Rami peripherici (*from* Plexus arteriosus pialis)

A. radicularis posterior

A. medullaris segmentalis

A. spinalis posterior sin.

A. radicularis posterior

A. radicularis anterior

A. spinalis anterior

A. radicularis posterior

A. medullaris segmentalis

Arterial distribution: schema

Plexus arteriosus pialis

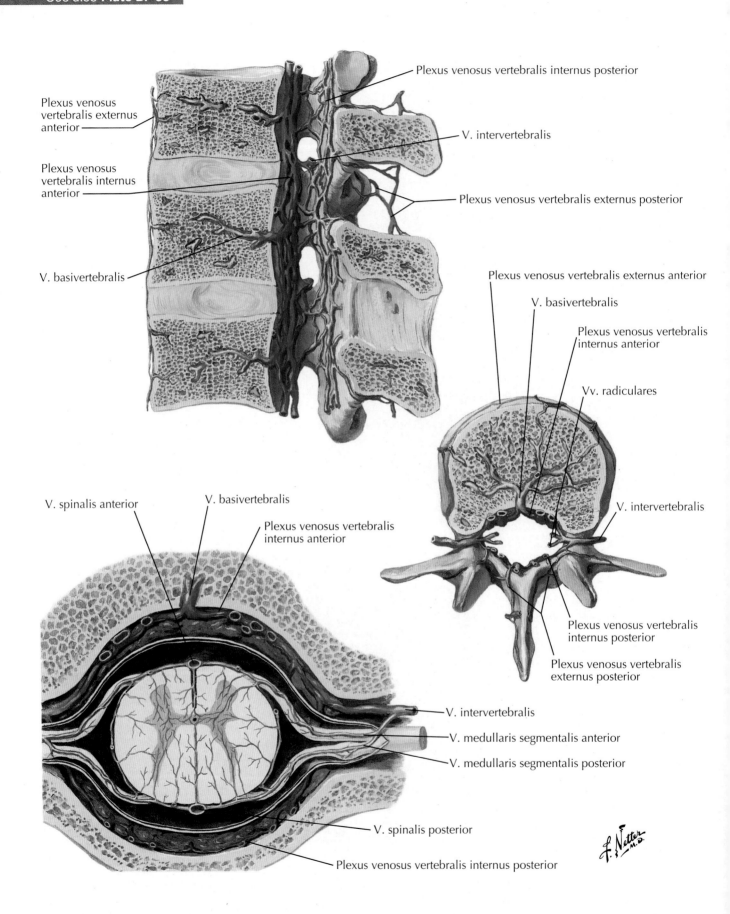

Plexus venosus vertebralis internus posterior

Plexus venosus vertebralis externus anterior

V. intervertebralis

Plexus venosus vertebralis internus anterior

Plexus venosus vertebralis externus posterior

V. basivertebralis

Plexus venosus vertebralis externus anterior

V. basivertebralis

Plexus venosus vertebralis internus anterior

Vv. radiculares

V. spinalis anterior

V. basivertebralis

Plexus venosus vertebralis internus anterior

V. intervertebralis

Plexus venosus vertebralis internus posterior

Plexus venosus vertebralis externus posterior

V. intervertebralis

V. medullaris segmentalis anterior

V. medullaris segmentalis posterior

V. spinalis posterior

Plexus venosus vertebralis internus posterior

Plate 193

Medulla Spinalis

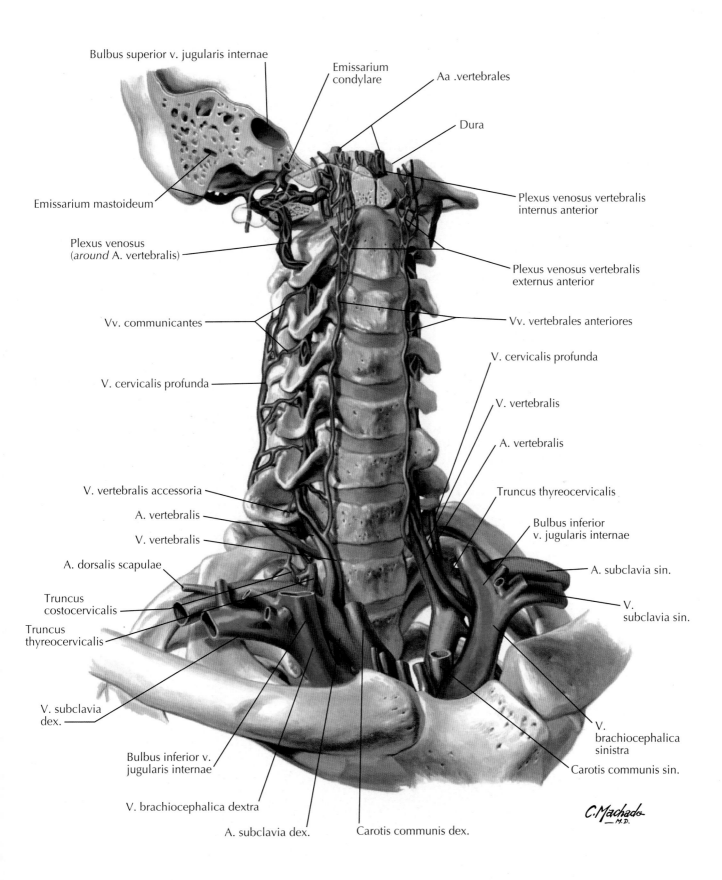

Bulbus superior v. jugularis internae

Emissarium condylare

Aa .vertebrales

Dura

Emissarium mastoideum

Plexus venosus vertebralis internus anterior

Plexus venosus (*around* A. vertebralis)

Plexus venosus vertebralis externus anterior

Vv. communicantes

Vv. vertebrales anteriores

V. cervicalis profunda

V. cervicalis profunda

V. vertebralis

A. vertebralis

V. vertebralis accessoria

Truncus thyreocervicalis

A. vertebralis

Bulbus inferior v. jugularis internae

V. vertebralis

A. dorsalis scapulae

A. subclavia sin.

Truncus costocervicalis

V. subclavia sin.

Truncus thyreocervicalis

V. subclavia dex.

V. brachiocephalica sinistra

Carotis communis sin.

Bulbus inferior v. jugularis internae

V. brachiocephalica dextra

A. subclavia dex.

Carotis communis dex.

C. Machado —M.D.

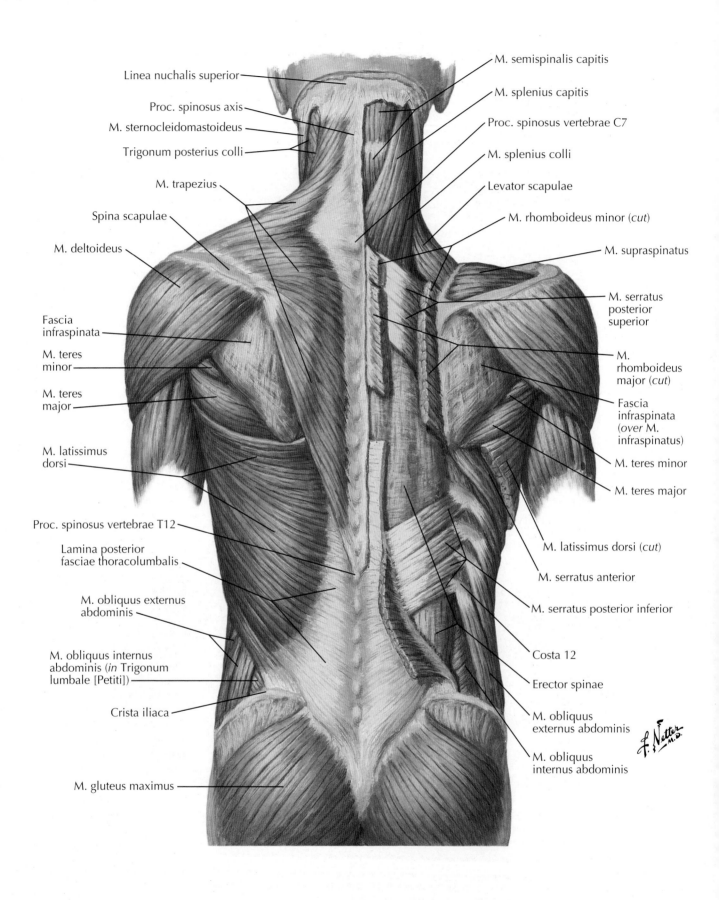

Linea nuchalis superior

Proc. spinosus axis

M. sternocleidomastoideus

Trigonum posterius colli

M. trapezius

Spina scapulae

M. deltoideus

Fascia infraspinata

M. teres minor

M. teres major

M. latissimus dorsi

Proc. spinosus vertebrae T12

Lamina posterior fasciae thoracolumbalis

M. obliquus externus abdominis

M. obliquus internus abdominis (*in* Trigonum lumbale [Petiti])

Crista iliaca

M. gluteus maximus

M. semispinalis capitis

M. splenius capitis

Proc. spinosus vertebrae C7

M. splenius colli

Levator scapulae

M. rhomboideus minor (*cut*)

M. supraspinatus

M. serratus posterior superior

M. rhomboideus major (*cut*)

Fascia infraspinata (*over* M. infraspinatus)

M. teres minor

M. teres major

M. latissimus dorsi (*cut*)

M. serratus anterior

M. serratus posterior inferior

Costa 12

Erector spinae

M. obliquus externus abdominis

M. obliquus internus abdominis

Plate 195

Musculi and Nervi

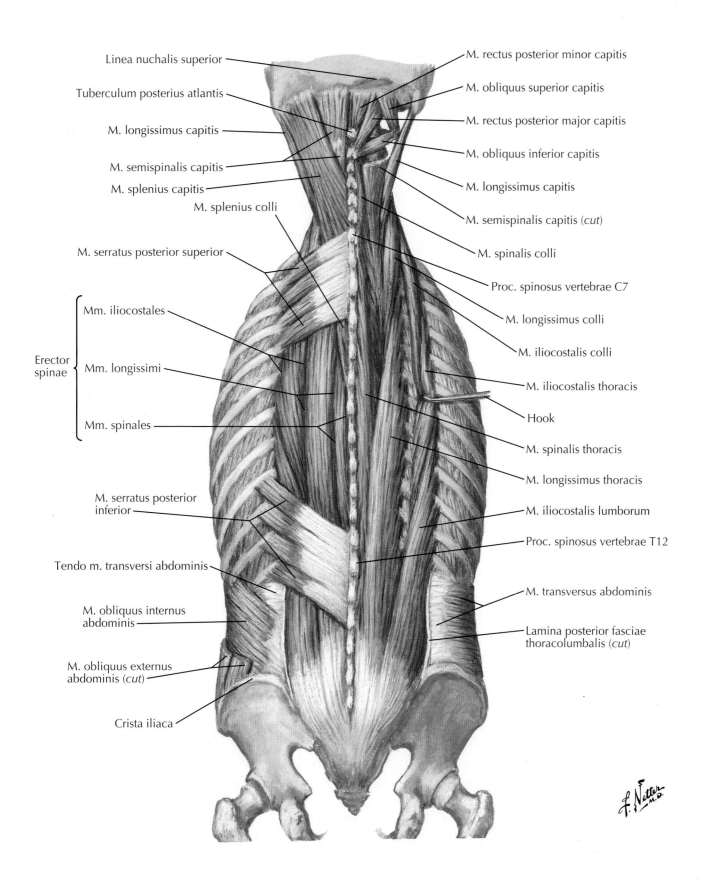

Linea nuchalis superior

Tuberculum posterius atlantis

M. longissimus capitis

M. semispinalis capitis

M. splenius capitis

M. splenius colli

M. serratus posterior superior

Mm. iliocostales

Erector spinae

Mm. longissimi

Mm. spinales

M. serratus posterior inferior

Tendo m. transversi abdominis

M. obliquus internus abdominis

M. obliquus externus abdominis (*cut*)

Crista iliaca

M. rectus posterior minor capitis

M. obliquus superior capitis

M. rectus posterior major capitis

M. obliquus inferior capitis

M. longissimus capitis

M. semispinalis capitis (*cut*)

M. spinalis colli

Proc. spinosus vertebrae C7

M. longissimus colli

M. iliocostalis colli

M. iliocostalis thoracis

Hook

M. spinalis thoracis

M. longissimus thoracis

M. iliocostalis lumborum

Proc. spinosus vertebrae T12

M. transversus abdominis

Lamina posterior fasciae thoracolumbalis (*cut*)

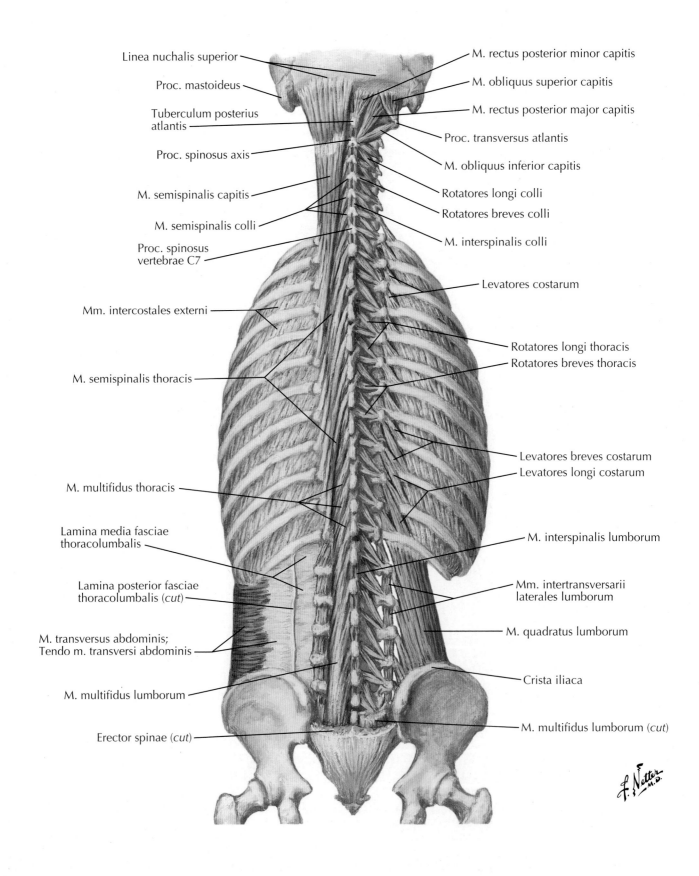

Linea nuchalis superior

Proc. mastoideus

Tuberculum posterius atlantis

Proc. spinosus axis

M. semispinalis capitis

M. semispinalis colli

Proc. spinosus vertebrae C7

Mm. intercostales externi

M. semispinalis thoracis

M. multifidus thoracis

Lamina media fasciae thoracolumbalis

Lamina posterior fasciae thoracolumbalis (cut)

M. transversus abdominis; Tendo m. transversi abdominis

M. multifidus lumborum

Erector spinae (cut)

M. rectus posterior minor capitis

M. obliquus superior capitis

M. rectus posterior major capitis

Proc. transversus atlantis

M. obliquus inferior capitis

Rotatores longi colli

Rotatores breves colli

M. interspinalis colli

Levatores costarum

Rotatores longi thoracis

Rotatores breves thoracis

Levatores breves costarum

Levatores longi costarum

M. interspinalis lumborum

Mm. intertransversarii laterales lumborum

M. quadratus lumborum

Crista iliaca

M. multifidus lumborum (cut)

Plate 197

Musculi and Nervi

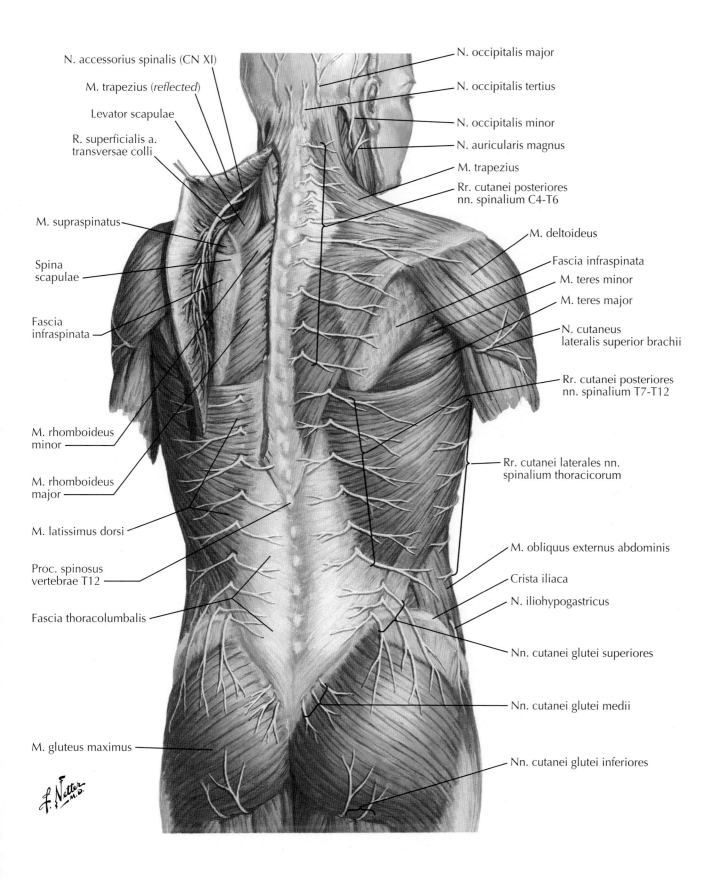

N. accessorius spinalis (CN XI)

M. trapezius (*reflected*)

Levator scapulae

R. superficialis a.
transversae colli

M. supraspinatus

Spina
scapulae

Fascia
infraspinata

M. rhomboideus
minor

M. rhomboideus
major

M. latissimus dorsi

Proc. spinosus
vertebrae T12

Fascia thoracolumbalis

M. gluteus maximus

N. occipitalis major

N. occipitalis tertius

N. occipitalis minor

N. auricularis magnus

M. trapezius

Rr. cutanei posteriores
nn. spinalium C4-T6

M. deltoideus

Fascia infraspinata

M. teres minor

M. teres major

N. cutaneus
lateralis superior brachii

Rr. cutanei posteriores
nn. spinalium T7-T12

Rr. cutanei laterales nn.
spinalium thoracicorum

M. obliquus externus abdominis

Crista iliaca

N. iliohypogastricus

Nn. cutanei glutei superiores

Nn. cutanei glutei medii

Nn. cutanei glutei inferiores

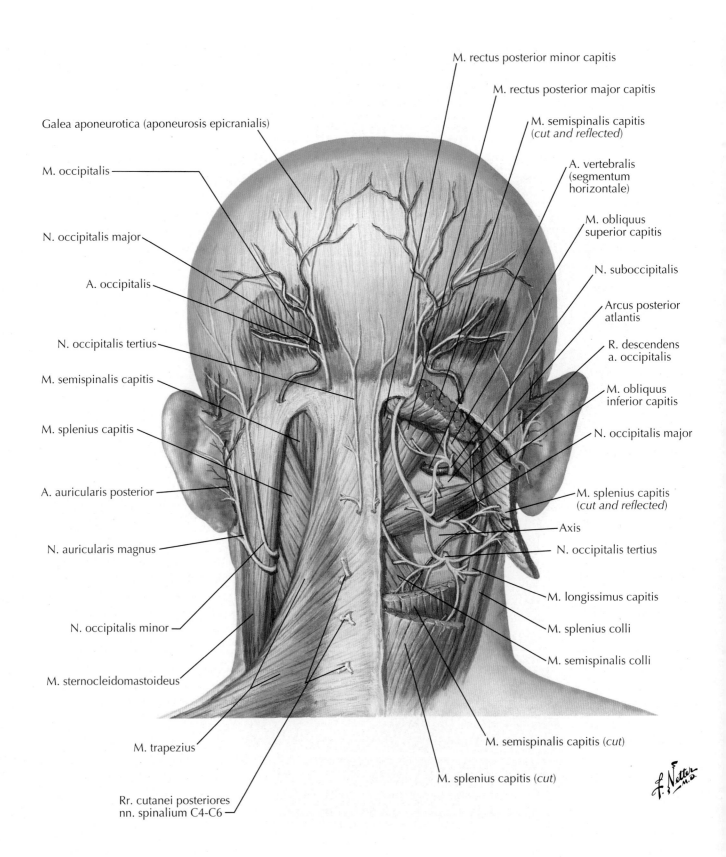

Galea aponeurotica (aponeurosis epicranialis)

M. occipitalis

N. occipitalis major

A. occipitalis

N. occipitalis tertius

M. semispinalis capitis

M. splenius capitis

A. auricularis posterior

N. auricularis magnus

N. occipitalis minor

M. sternocleidomastoideus

M. trapezius

Rr. cutanei posteriores
nn. spinalium C4-C6

M. rectus posterior minor capitis

M. rectus posterior major capitis

M. semispinalis capitis
(*cut and reflected*)

A. vertebralis
(segmentum
horizontale)

M. obliquus
superior capitis

N. suboccipitalis

Arcus posterior
atlantis

R. descendens
a. occipitalis

M. obliquus
inferior capitis

N. occipitalis major

M. splenius capitis
(*cut and reflected*)

Axis

N. occipitalis tertius

M. longissimus capitis

M. splenius colli

M. semispinalis colli

M. semispinalis capitis (*cut*)

M. splenius capitis (*cut*)

Plate 199

Musculi and Nervi

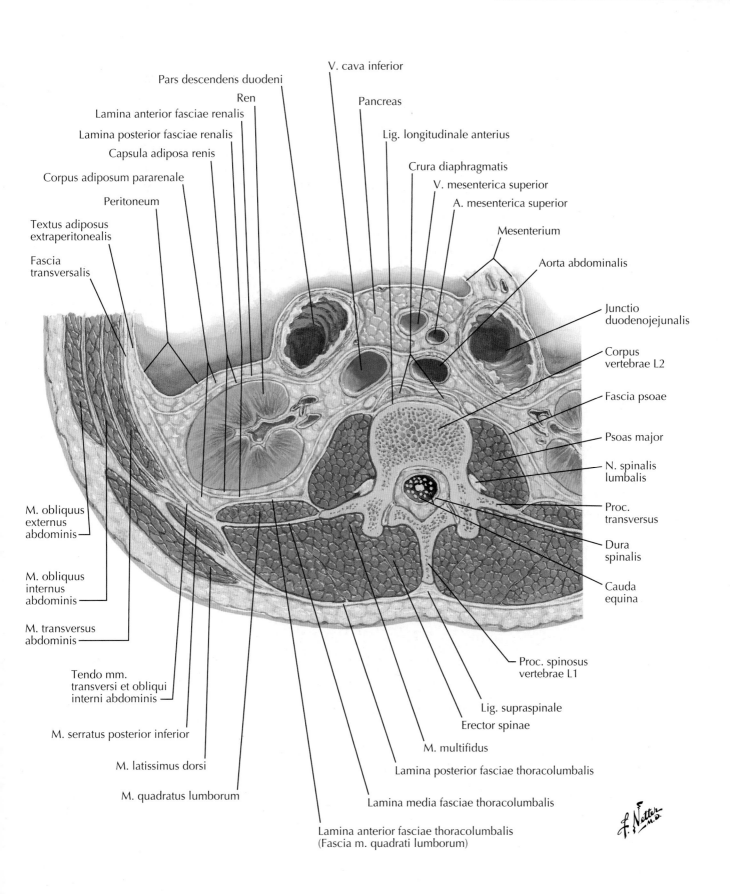

Pars descendens duodeni

V. cava inferior

Ren

Pancreas

Lamina anterior fasciae renalis

Lamina posterior fasciae renalis

Lig. longitudinale anterius

Capsula adiposa renis

Crura diaphragmatis

Corpus adiposum pararenale

V. mesenterica superior

A. mesenterica superior

Peritoneum

Mesenterium

Textus adiposus extraperitonealis

Aorta abdominalis

Fascia transversalis

Junctio duodenojejunalis

Corpus vertebrae L2

Fascia psoae

Psoas major

N. spinalis lumbalis

M. obliquus externus abdominis

Proc. transversus

Dura spinalis

M. obliquus internus abdominis

Cauda equina

M. transversus abdominis

Tendo mm. transversi et obliqui interni abdominis

Proc. spinosus vertebrae L1

M. serratus posterior inferior

Lig. supraspinale

Erector spinae

M. latissimus dorsi

M. multifidus

M. quadratus lumborum

Lamina posterior fasciae thoracolumbalis

Lamina media fasciae thoracolumbalis

Lamina anterior fasciae thoracolumbalis
(Fascia m. quadrati lumborum)

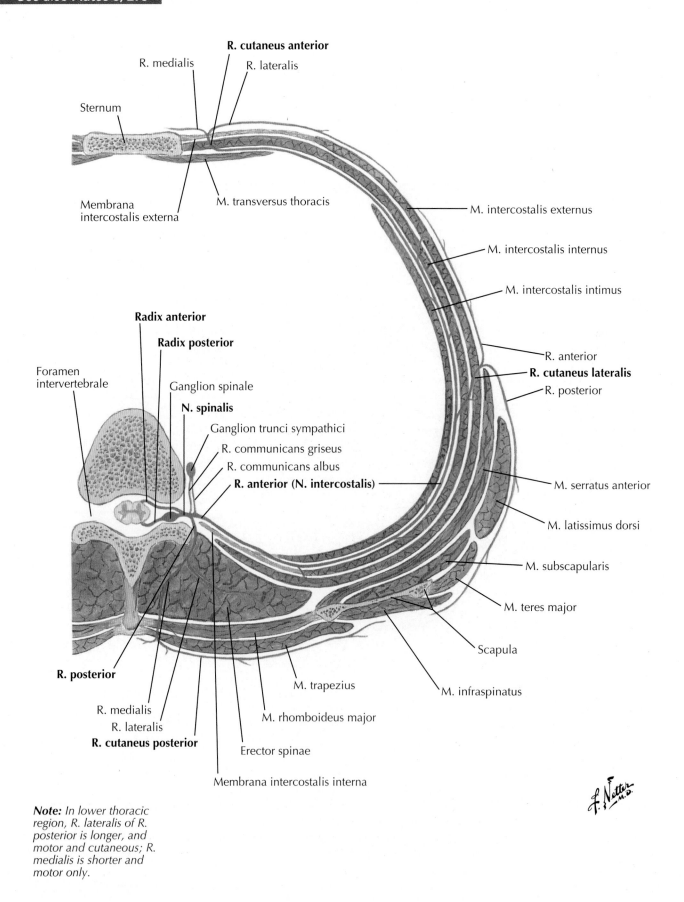

R. cutaneus anterior
R. medialis
R. lateralis
Sternum
Membrana intercostalis externa
M. transversus thoracis
M. intercostalis externus
M. intercostalis internus
M. intercostalis intimus
R. anterior
R. cutaneus lateralis
R. posterior
Radix anterior
Radix posterior
Foramen intervertebrale
Ganglion spinale
N. spinalis
Ganglion trunci sympathici
R. communicans griseus
R. communicans albus
R. anterior (N. intercostalis)
M. serratus anterior
M. latissimus dorsi
M. subscapularis
M. teres major
Scapula
M. infraspinatus
R. posterior
R. medialis
R. lateralis
R. cutaneus posterior
Erector spinae
M. trapezius
M. rhomboideus major
Membrana intercostalis interna

Note: In lower thoracic region, R. lateralis of R. posterior is longer, and motor and cutaneous; R. medialis is shorter and motor only.

Plate 201

Cross-Sectional Anatomy

ANATOMICAL STRUCTURE	CLINICAL COMMENT	PLATE NUMBERS
Systema Nervosum		
Conus medullaris	Is inferior limit of spinal cord; can lie as inferior as L4 vertebra in neonates and as superior as T12 in adults (average is L1/2); necessary to determine its location in procedures such as lumbar puncture; in adults, start at L2 or lower	186
Cauda equina	Lumbar and sacral nerve roots may be anesthetized with anesthesia injected into subarachnoid space (spinal block)	186, 187
Meninges spinales	Access to epidural and subarachnoid spaces is necessary for clinical procedures such as epidural anesthesia and lumbar puncture; meningitis is a life-threatening infection	182, 190
Systema Skeletale		
Processus spinosi	Palpable landmarks used to assess spinal curvatures and determine location of spinal cord for procedures such as lumbar puncture and injection of spinal anesthesia	178, 195
Processus spinosus vertebrae C7 (vertebra prominens)	Most prominent spinous process in cervical region; often used to begin counting vertebrae	178, 180
Discus intervertebralis	Age-related changes may produce herniation of nucleus pulposus, causing back pain; occurs most commonly in lower lumbar regions of vertebral column	181, 187
Lamina arcus vertebrae	Surgically removed in laminectomy to gain access to vertebral canal and spinal cord	181
Foramen intervertebrale	May become narrowed by age-related changes (e.g., osteophyte formation) or changes in intervertebral disc height, producing compression of its contents	181, 184, 185
Hiatus sacralis	Provides access to epidural space for administration of caudal epidural anesthesia	183
Vertebra lumbalis quinta (L5)	Spondylolysis is clinical condition in which vertebral body separates from part of its vertebral arch bearing inferior articulating process (defect is through pars interarticularis); if this occurs bilaterally, L5 vertebral body and transverse process may slide forward over sacrum, giving rise to spondylolisthesis	184
Discus intervertebralis L5/S1	Most common level of intervertebral disc herniation, which may result in nerve compression and lower back pain associated with pain and weakness in ipsilateral lower limb (sciatica)	184, 187
Foramen vertebrale	May be congenitally stenotic in cervical region, or narrowed by arthritic changes in lumbar vertebrae; can lead to back pain, sciatica, numbness or tingling, and weakness in lower limbs	180, 181
Systema Musculare		
M. trapezius	Responsible for holding scapula against thoracic wall against gravity; drooping of shoulder may indicate injury to spinal accessory nerve	195
Mm. epaxiales (mm. dorsi proprii)	Microscopic stretching or tearing of muscle fibers produces back strain, a common cause of low back pain	196, 197
Systema Cardiovasculare		
Arteriae medullae spinalis	Narrowing or damage caused by atherosclerosis, vertebral fractures, or vertebral dislocations may cause ischemia of spinal cord	191
Plexus venosi vertebrales	Mostly valveless veins along vertebral column allow retrograde flow and can act as conduits for metastasis of cancer cells to spine, lungs, and brain	194, BP 39

*Selections were based largely on clinical data and commonly discussed clinical correlations in macroscopic ("gross") anatomy courses.

Structures with High Clinical Significance **Table 3.1**

MUSCLE	MUSCLE GROUP	SUPERIOR ATTACHMENT	INFERIOR ATTACHMENT	INNERVATION	BLOOD SUPPLY	MAIN ACTIONS
Mm. iliocostales	Dorsum profundum (erector spinae)	*M. iliocostalis colli*: Tubercula posteriora vertebrarum C4–C6 *M. iliocostalis thoracis*: Anguli costarum 1–6 *M. iliocostalis lumborum*: Costae 4–12; procc. transversi vertebrarum L1–L4	*M. iliocostalis colli*: Anguli costarum 3–6 *M. iliocostalis thoracis*: Anguli costarum 7–12 *M. iliocostalis lumborum*: Os sacrum (via aponeurosis erectoris spinae); crista iliaca	Rr. posteriores nn. spinalium	*Partes cervicales*: Aa. occipitalis, cervicalis profunda, and vertebralis *Partes thoracicae*: Rr. dorsales aa. intercostales posteriores and subcostalis *Partes lumbales*: Rr. dorsales aa. lumbales and sacrales laterales	Extend and laterally bend vertebral column and head
Mm. interspinales	Dorsum profundum	*M. interspinalis colli*: procc. spinosi vertebrarum C2–C7 *M. interspinalis thoracis*: Procc. spinosi vertebrarum T1/T2 and T11/T12 *M. interspinalis lumborum*: Procc. spinosi vertebrarum L1–L4	Procc. spinosi vertebrarum subjacent to vertebrae of muscle origin	Rr. posteriores nn. spinalium	*Partes cervicales*: Aa. occipitalis, cervicalis profunda, and vertebralis *Partes thoracicae*: Rr. dorsales aa. intercostales posteriores and subcostalis *Partes lumbales*: Rr. dorsales aa. lumbales	Aid in extension of vertebral column
Mm. intertrans-versarii	Dorsum profundum	*Mm. intertransversarii mediales*: Procc. transversi vertebrarum C1–C7 and T10–T12; procc. mamillares vertebrarum L1–L4 *Mm. intertransversarii laterales and anteriores*: Procc. transversi vertebrarum C1–C7 and L1–L4	*Mm. intertransversarii mediales*: Procc. transversi vertebrarum cervicalium and thoracicarum, and procc. mamillares vertebrarum lumbalium subjacent to vertebrae of muscle origin *Mm. intertransversarii laterales and anteriores*: Procc. transversi vertebrarum subjacent to vertebrae of muscle origin	*Mm. intertransversarii mediales*: Rr. posteriores nn. spinalium *Mm. intertransversarii laterales and anteriores*: Rr. anteriores nn. spinalium	*Partes cervicales*: Aa. occipitalis, cervicalis profunda, and vertebralis *Partes thoracicae*: Rr. dorsales aa. intercostales posteriores and subcostalis *Partes lumbales*: Rr. dorsales aa. lumbales	Assist in lateral flexion of vertebral column
Mm. latissimus dorsi	Dorsum superficiale	Procc. spinosi vertebrarum T7–T12; lamina posterior fasciae thoracolumbalis (and thus to vertebrae L1–L5 and crista iliaca); costae 10–12	Sulcus intertubercularis (of humerus)	N. thoracodorsalis	A. thoracodorsalis; Rr. perforantes dorsales aa. intercostales posteriores 9-11, subcostalis, and lumbales 1-3	Extends, adducts, and medially rotates humerus
Levator scapulae	Dorsum superficiale	Procc. transversi atlantis and axis; tubercula posteriora [procc. transversorum] vertebrarum C3/C4	Margo medialis scapulae (superior to spina scapulae)	Rr. anteriores nn. spinalium C3/C4; N. dorsalis scapulae	Aa. dorsalis scapulae, transversus colli, and cervicalis ascendens	Elevates scapula medially, inferiorly rotates glenoid fossa

Table 3.2   **Musculi**

MUSCLE	MUSCLE GROUP	SUPERIOR ATTACHMENT	INFERIOR ATTACHMENT	INNERVATION	BLOOD SUPPLY	MAIN ACTIONS
Mm. longissimi	Dorsum profundum (erector spinae)	*M. longissimus capitis:* Proc. mastoideus *M. longissimus colli:* Procc. transversi vertebrarum C2–C6 *M. longissimus thoracis:* Procc. transversi vertebrarum T1–T12; costae 5–12; procc. accessorii and transversi vertebrarum L1–L5	*M. longissimus capitis:* Procc. transversi vertebrarum C4–T4 *M. longissimus colli:* Procc. transversi vertebrarum T1–T5 *M. longissimus thoracis:* Procc. spinosi vertebrarum L1–L5; facies dorsalis ossis sacri; tuberositas iliaca; lig. sacroiliacum posterius	Rr. posteriores nn. spinalium	*Partes cervicales:* Aa. occipitalis, cervicalis profunda, and vertebralis *Partes thoracicae:* Rr. dorsales aa. intercostales posteriores and subcostalis *Partes lumbales:* Rr. dorsales aa. lumbales and sacrales laterales	Extend and laterally bend vertebral column and head
Mm. multifidi	Dorsum profundum (mm. transverso-spinales)	Procc. spinosi vertebrarum C2–L5 (2–5 levels above muscle insertion)	*M. multifidus colli:* Procc. articulares superiores vertebrarum C4–C7 *M. multifidus thoracis:* Procc. transversi vertebrarum T1–T12 *M. multifidus lumborum:* Procc. mamillares vertebrarum L1–L5; os sacrum; crista iliaca	Rr. posteriores nn. spinalium	*Partes cervicales:* Aa. occipitalis, cervicalis profunda, and vertebralis *Partes thoracicae:* Rr. dorsales aa. intercostales posteriores and subcostalis *Partes lumbales:* Rr. dorsales aa. lumbales and sacrales laterales	Stabilize spine
M. obliquus inferior capitis	Mm. suboccipitales	Proc. transversus atlantis	Proc. spinosus axis	N. suboccipitalis	Aa. vertebralis and occipitalis	Rotates atlas to turn face to same side
M. obliquus superior capitis	Mm. suboccipitales	Linea nuchalis inferior (lateral part)	Proc. transversus atlantis	N. suboccipitalis	Aa. vertebralis and occipitalis	Extends and bends head laterally
M. rectus posterior major capitis	Mm. suboccipitales	Linea nuchalis inferior (middle part)	Proc. spinosus axis	N. suboccipitalis	Aa. vertebralis and occipitalis	Extends and rotates head to same side
M. rectus posterior minor capitis	Mm. suboccipitales	Linea nuchalis inferior (medial part)	Tuberculum posterius atlantis	N. suboccipitalis	Aa. vertebralis and occipitalis	Extends head
M. rhomboideus major	Dorsum superficiale	Procc. spinosi vertebrarum T2–T5	Margo medialis scapulae (inferior to spina scapulae)	N. dorsalis scapulae	Aa. dorsalis scapulae or R. profundus a. transversae colli; Rr. perforantes dorsales aa. intercostales posteriores 1–5 (or 6)	Fixes scapula to thoracic wall and retracts and rotates it to depress glenoid fossa
M. rhomboideus minor	Dorsum superficiale	Lig. nuchae; procc. spinosi vertebrarum C7 and T1	Margo medialis scapulae (at spina scapulae)	N. dorsalis scapulae	Aa. dorsalis scapulae or R. profundus a. transversae colli; Rr. perforantes dorsales aa. intercostales posteriores 1–5 (or 6)	Fixes scapula to thoracic wall and retracts and rotates it to depress glenoid fossa
Rotatores	Dorsum profundum (mm. transverso-spinales)	*Rotatores colli:* Procc. spinosi vertebrarum cervicalium *Rotatores thoracis:* Procc. spinosi and laminae vertebrarum T1–T11 *Rotatores lumborum:* Procc. spinosi vertebrarum lumbalium	*Rotatores colli:* Procc. articulares superiores vertebrarum cervicalium (1 or 2 levels below vertebra of muscle origin) *Rotatores thoracis:* Procc. transversi vertebrarum T2–T12 (*brevis* muscles insert into adjacent vertebra; *longus* muscles into vertebra 2 levels down) *Rotatores lumborum:* Procc. mamillares vertebrarum lumbalium (2 levels down)	Rr. posteriores nn. spinalium	*Partes cervicales:* Aa. occipitalis, cervicalis profunda, and vertebralis *Partes thoracicae:* Rr. dorsales aa. intercostales posteriores and subcostalis *Partes lumbales:* Rr. dorsales aa. lumbales	Stabilize, extend, and rotate spine

MUSCLE	MUSCLE GROUP	SUPERIOR ATTACHMENT	INFERIOR ATTACHMENT	INNERVATION	BLOOD SUPPLY	MAIN ACTIONS
Mm. semi-spinales	Dorsum profundum (mm. transverso-spinales)	*M. semispinalis capitis*: Os occipitale (between Lineae nuchales superior and inferior) *M. semispinalis colli*: Procc. spinosi vertebrarum C2–C5 *M. semispinalis thoracis*: Procc. spinosi vertebrarum C6–T4	*M. semispinalis capitis*: Procc. articulares superiores vertebrarum C4–C7; procc. transversi vertebrarum T1–T6 *M. semispinalis colli*: Procc. transversi vertebrarum T1–T6 *M. semispinalis thoracis*: Procc. transversi vertebrarum T6–T10	Rr. posteriores nn. spinalium	*Partes cervicales*: Aa. occipitalis, cervicalis profunda, and vertebralis *Partes thoracicae*: Rr. dorsales aa. intercostales posteriores	Extend head and neck and rotate them to opposite side
M. serratus posterior inferior	Dorsum superficiale	Margines inferiores costarum 9–12	Procc. spinosi vertebrarum T11–L2	Rr. anteriores nn. spinalium T9–T12	Aa. intercostales posteriores	Depresses ribs
M. serratus posterior superior	Dorsum superficiale	Lig. nuchae; procc. spinosi vertebrarum C7–T3	Margines superiores costarum 2–5	Rr. anteriores nn. spinalium T2–T5	Aa. intercostales posteriores	Elevates ribs
Mm. spinales	Dorsum profundum (erector spinae)	*M. spinalis capitis*: Protuberantia occipitalis externa *M. spinalis colli*: Procc. spinosi vertebrarum C2–C4 *M. spinalis thoracis*: Procc. spinosi vertebrarum T2–T8	*M. spinalis capitis*: Procc. spinosi vertebrarum C7 and T1 *M. spinalis colli*: Procc. spinosi vertebrarum C7–T2 *M. spinalis thoracis*: Procc. spinosi vertebrarum T11–L2	Rr. posteriores nn. spinalium	*Partes cervicales*: Aa. occipitalis, cervicalis profunda, and vertebralis *Partes thoracicae*: Rr. dorsales aa. intercostales posteriores and subcostalis *Partes lumbales*: Rr. dorsales aa. lumbales and sacrales laterales	Extend and laterally bend vertebral column and head
M. splenius capitis	Mm. spinotrans-versales	Processus mastoideus [ossis temporalis]; lateral one-third of linea nuchalis superior	Lig. nuchae; procc. spinosi vertebrarum C7–T4	Rr. posteriores nn. spinalium C2–C3	Aa. occipitalis and cervicalis profunda	*Bilaterally*: extends head *Unilaterally*: laterally bends (flexes) and rotates face to same side
M. splenius colli	Mm. spinotrans-versales	Procc. transversi vertebrarum C1–C3	Procc. spinosi vertebrarum T3–T6	Rr. posteriores nn. spinalium C4–C6	Aa. occipitalis and cervicalis profunda	*Bilaterally*: extends neck *Unilaterally*: laterally bends (flexes) and rotates neck toward same side
M. trapezius	Dorsum superficiale	*Pars descendens*: Linea nuchalis superior; protuberantia occipitalis externa; lig. nuchae *Pars transversa*: Procc. spinosi vertebrarum C7–T3 *Pars ascendens*: Procc. spinosi vertebrarum T4–T12	*Pars descendens*: Clavicula (lateral one-third) *Pars transversa*: Acromion *Pars ascendens*: Spina scapulae	N. accessorius spinalis (CN XI)	Aa. transversa colli and intercostales posteriores	Elevates, retracts, and rotates scapula; lower fibers depress scapula

Variations in spinal nerve contributions to the innervation of muscles, their arterial supply, their attachments, and their actions are common themes in human anatomy. Therefore, expect differences between texts and realize that anatomical variation is normal.

Table 3.4   **Musculi**

THORAX 4

Surface Anatomy	202	Mediastinum	251–261
Skeleton Thoracis	203–204	Cross-Sectional Anatomy	262–266
Glandulae Mammariae	205–208	Structures with High	
Paries Thoracis and Diaphragma	209–216	Clinical Significance	Tables 4.1–4.3
Pulmones, Trachea, and Bronchi	217–230	Musculi	Table 4.4
Cor	231–250	Electronic Bonus Plates	BP 41–BP 52

ELECTRONIC BONUS PLATES

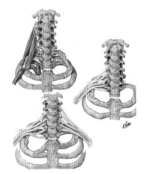

BP 41 Costae Cervicales and Related Variations

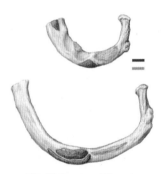

BP 42 Costae: Muscle Attachments

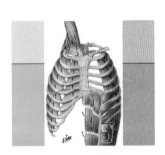

BP 43 Musculi Respiratorii

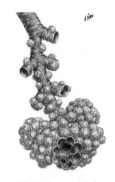

BP 44 Bronchiolus Terminalis and Acinus Pulmonis: Schema

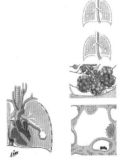

BP 45 Anatomy of Ventilation and Respiration

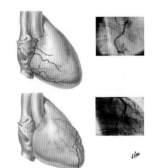

BP 46 Arteriae Coronariae: Right Anterolateral Views with Arteriograms

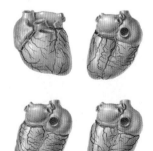

BP 47 Arteriae Coronariae and Venae Cardiacae: Variations

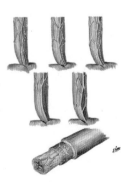

BP 48 Oesophagus: Intrinsic Nerves and Variations

ELECTRONIC BONUS PLATES—*cont'd*

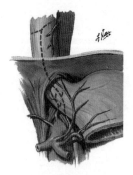

BP 49 Oesophagus: Arterial Variations

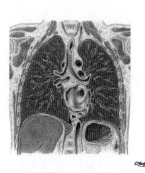

BP 50 Thorax: Coronal Sections

BP 51 Thorax: Coronal CTs

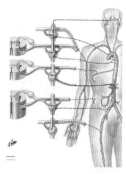

BP 52 Vasa Sanguinea: Schema of Innervation

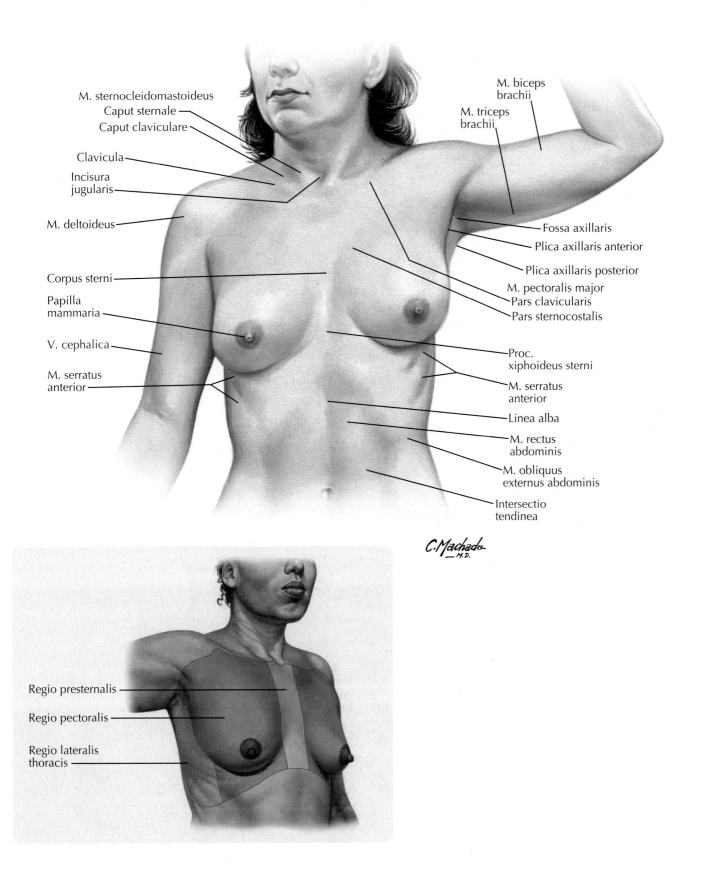

M. sternocleidomastoideus
Caput sternale
Caput claviculare

Clavicula

Incisura jugularis

M. deltoideus

Corpus sterni

Papilla mammaria

V. cephalica

M. serratus anterior

M. biceps brachii

M. triceps brachii

Fossa axillaris

Plica axillaris anterior

Plica axillaris posterior

M. pectoralis major
Pars clavicularis
Pars sternocostalis

Proc. xiphoideus sterni

M. serratus anterior

Linea alba

M. rectus abdominis

M. obliquus externus abdominis

Intersectio tendinea

C. Machado M.D.

Regio presternalis

Regio pectoralis

Regio lateralis thoracis

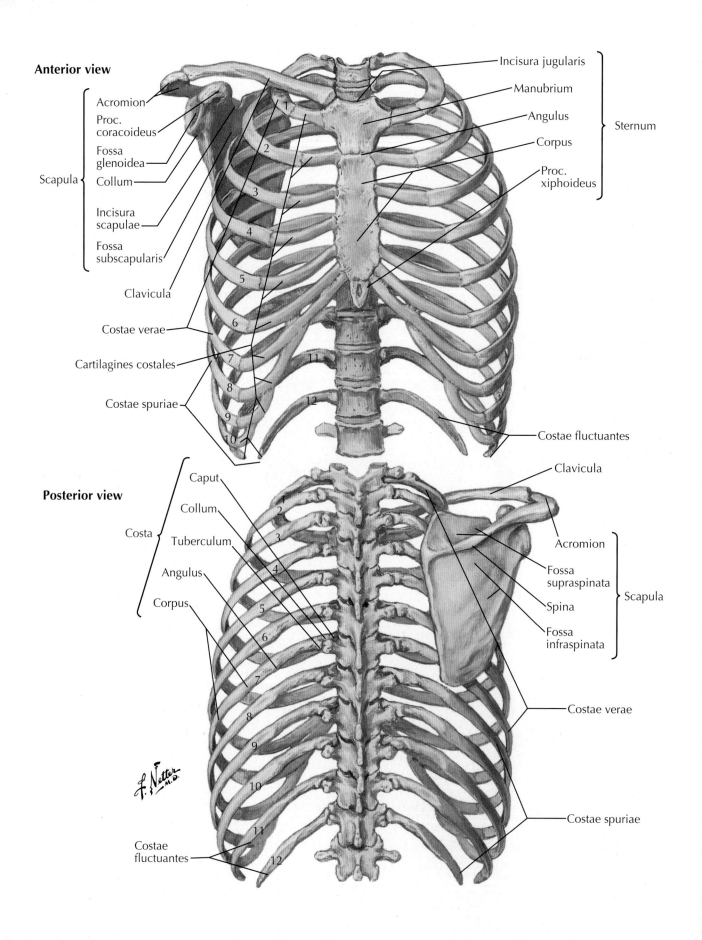

Anterior view

Acromion
Proc. coracoideus
Fossa glenoidea
Collum
Incisura scapulae
Fossa subscapularis

Scapula

Clavicula

Costae verae

Cartilagines costales

Costae spuriae

Incisura jugularis
Manubrium
Angulus
Corpus
Proc. xiphoideus

Sternum

Costae fluctuantes

Posterior view

Caput
Collum
Tuberculum
Angulus
Corpus

Costa

Clavicula

Acromion
Fossa supraspinata
Spina
Fossa infraspinata

Scapula

Costae verae

Costae spuriae

Costae fluctuantes

Plate 203   **Skeleton Thoracis**

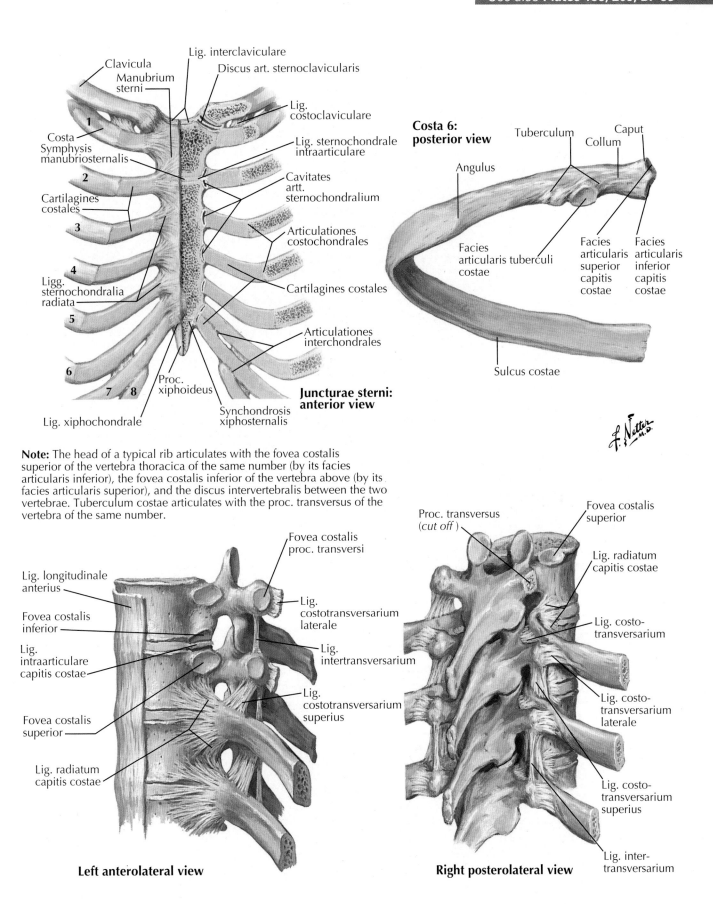

Clavicula
Manubrium sterni
Lig. interclaviculare
Discus art. sternoclavicularis
Costa
Symphysis manubriosternalis
Lig. costoclaviculare
Lig. sternochondrale intraarticulare
Cavitates artt. sternochondralium
Cartilagines costales
Articulationes costochondrales
Ligg. sternochondralia radiata
Cartilagines costales
Articulationes interchondrales
Proc. xiphoideus
Lig. xiphochondrale
Synchondrosis xiphosternalis
Juncturae sterni: anterior view

Costa 6: posterior view
Tuberculum
Caput
Collum
Angulus
Facies articularis tuberculi costae
Facies articularis superior capitis costae
Facies articularis inferior capitis costae
Sulcus costae

Note: The head of a typical rib articulates with the fovea costalis superior of the vertebra thoracica of the same number (by its facies articularis inferior), the fovea costalis inferior of the vertebra above (by its facies articularis superior), and the discus intervertebralis between the two vertebrae. Tuberculum costae articulates with the proc. transversus of the vertebra of the same number.

Lig. longitudinale anterius
Fovea costalis inferior
Lig. intraarticulare capitis costae
Fovea costalis superior
Lig. radiatum capitis costae
Fovea costalis proc. transversi
Lig. costotransversarium laterale
Lig. intertransversarium
Lig. costotransversarium superius

Left anterolateral view

Proc. transversus (*cut off*)
Fovea costalis superior
Lig. radiatum capitis costae
Lig. costo-transversarium
Lig. costo-transversarium laterale
Lig. costo-transversarium superius
Lig. inter-transversarium

Right posterolateral view

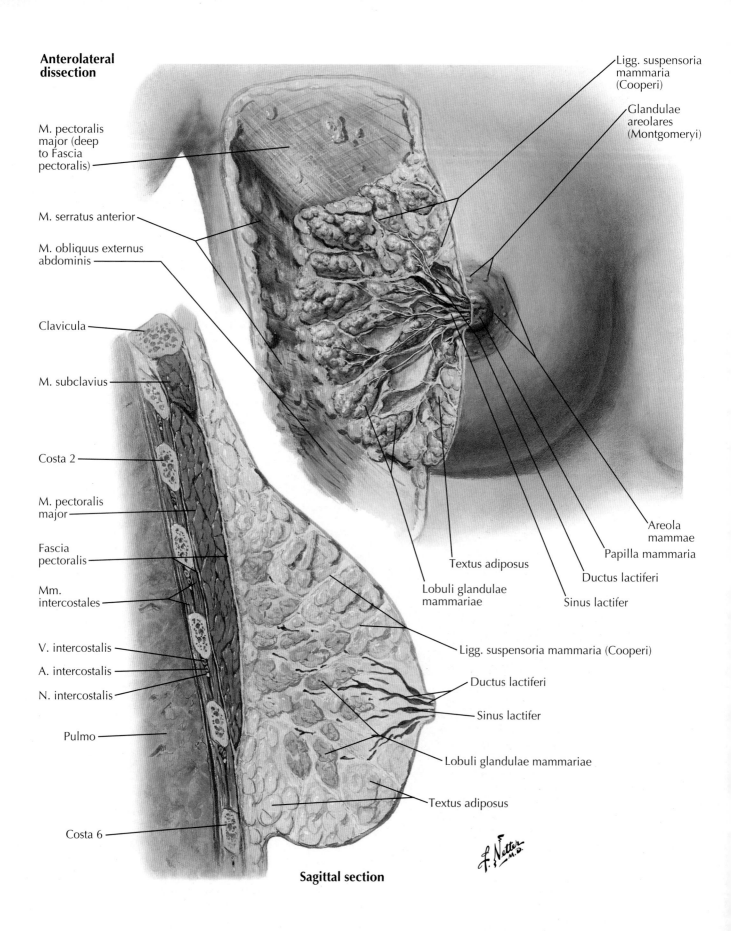

Anterolateral dissection

Ligg. suspensoria mammaria (Cooperi)

Glandulae areolares (Montgomeryi)

M. pectoralis major (deep to Fascia pectoralis)

M. serratus anterior

M. obliquus externus abdominis

Clavicula

M. subclavius

Costa 2

M. pectoralis major

Fascia pectoralis

Mm. intercostales

V. intercostalis

A. intercostalis

N. intercostalis

Pulmo

Costa 6

Areola mammae

Papilla mammaria

Ductus lactiferi

Sinus lactifer

Textus adiposus

Lobuli glandulae mammariae

Ligg. suspensoria mammaria (Cooperi)

Ductus lactiferi

Sinus lactifer

Lobuli glandulae mammariae

Textus adiposus

Sagittal section

Plate 205

Glandulae Mammariae

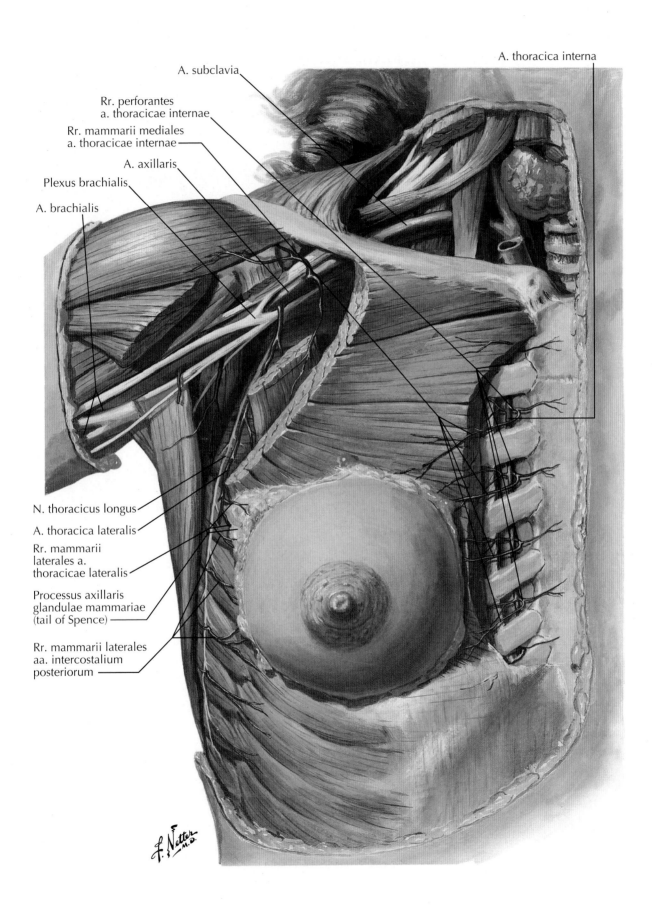

A. thoracica interna

A. subclavia

Rr. perforantes
a. thoracicae internae

Rr. mammarii mediales
a. thoracicae internae

A. axillaris

Plexus brachialis

A. brachialis

N. thoracicus longus

A. thoracica lateralis

Rr. mammarii
laterales a.
thoracicae lateralis

Processus axillaris
glandulae mammariae
(tail of Spence)

Rr. mammarii laterales
aa. intercostalium
posteriorum

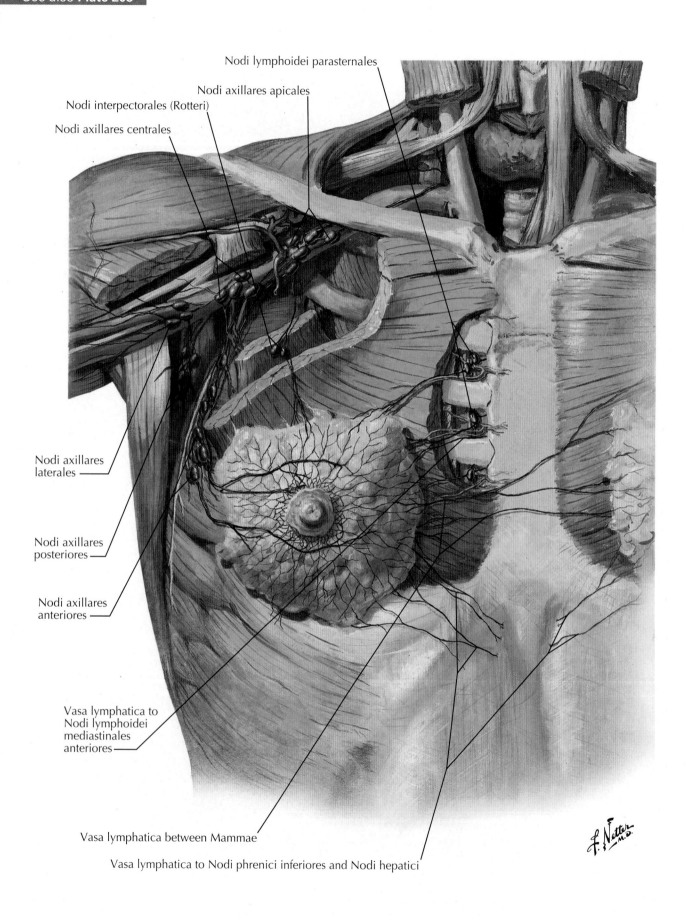

Nodi lymphoidei parasternales

Nodi axillares apicales

Nodi interpectorales (Rotteri)

Nodi axillares centrales

Nodi axillares laterales

Nodi axillares posteriores

Nodi axillares anteriores

Vasa lymphatica to Nodi lymphoidei mediastinales anteriores

Vasa lymphatica between Mammae

Vasa lymphatica to Nodi phrenici inferiores and Nodi hepatici

Plate 207

Glandulae Mammariae

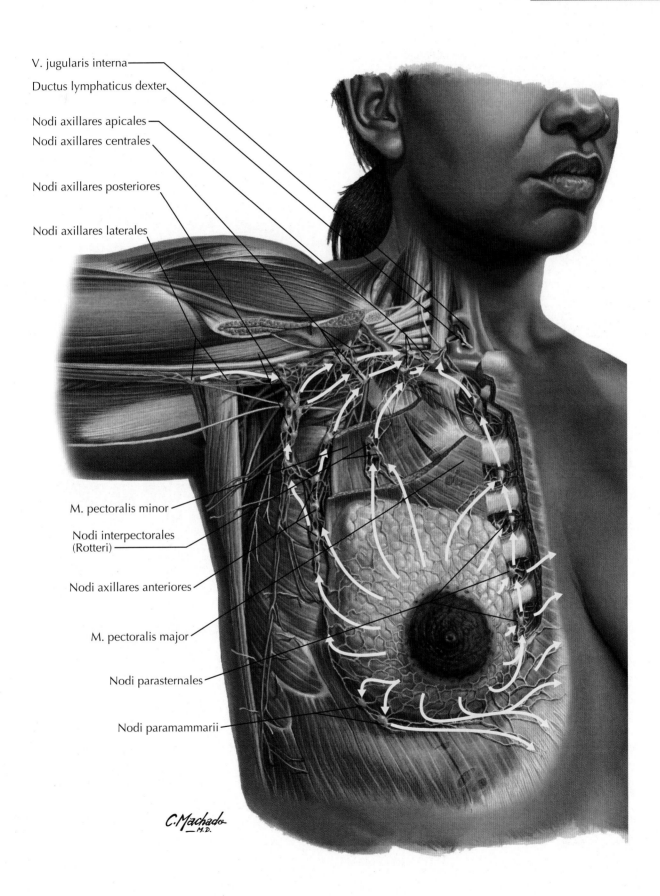

V. jugularis interna

Ductus lymphaticus dexter

Nodi axillares apicales

Nodi axillares centrales

Nodi axillares posteriores

Nodi axillares laterales

M. pectoralis minor

Nodi interpectorales
(Rotteri)

Nodi axillares anteriores

M. pectoralis major

Nodi parasternales

Nodi paramammarii

C. Machado
—M.D.

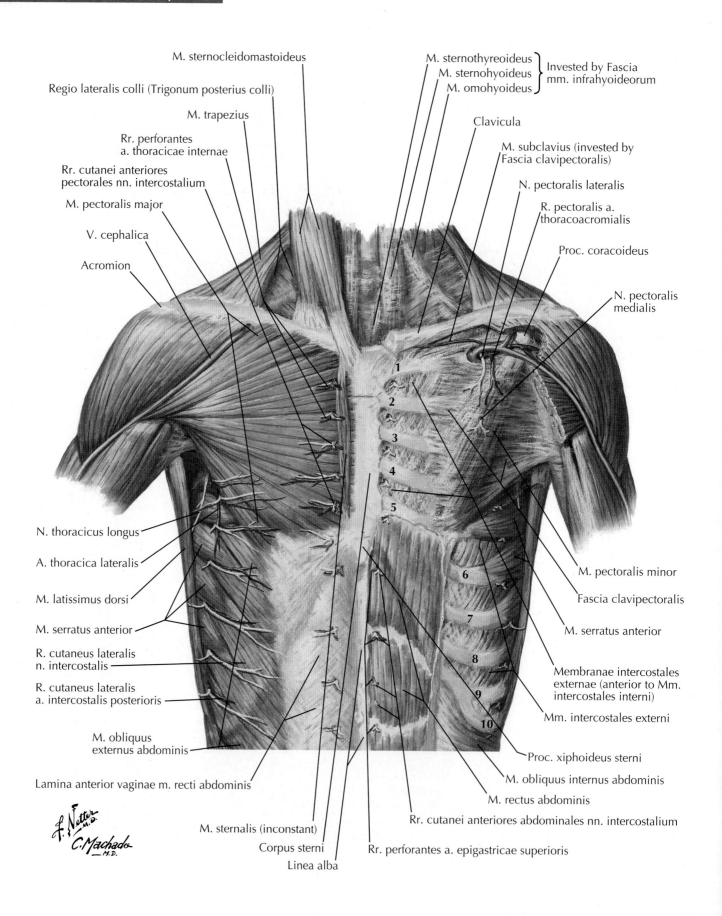

M. sternocleidomastoideus

Regio lateralis colli (Trigonum posterius colli)

M. trapezius

Rr. perforantes
a. thoracicae internae

Rr. cutanei anteriores
pectorales nn. intercostalium

M. pectoralis major

V. cephalica

Acromion

M. sternothyreoideus ⎫
M. sternohyoideus ⎬ Invested by Fascia
M. omohyoideus ⎭ mm. infrahyoideorum

Clavicula

M. subclavius (invested by
Fascia clavipectoralis)

N. pectoralis lateralis

R. pectoralis a.
thoracoacromialis

Proc. coracoideus

N. pectoralis
medialis

1
2
3
4
5

N. thoracicus longus

A. thoracica lateralis

M. latissimus dorsi

M. serratus anterior

R. cutaneus lateralis
n. intercostalis

R. cutaneus lateralis
a. intercostalis posterioris

M. obliquus
externus abdominis

Lamina anterior vaginae m. recti abdominis

6
7
8
9
10

M. pectoralis minor

Fascia clavipectoralis

M. serratus anterior

Membranae intercostales
externae (anterior to Mm.
intercostales interni)

Mm. intercostales externi

Proc. xiphoideus sterni

M. obliquus internus abdominis

M. rectus abdominis

Rr. cutanei anteriores abdominales nn. intercostalium

Rr. perforantes a. epigastricae superioris

M. sternalis (inconstant)

Corpus sterni

Linea alba

Plate 209

Paries Thoracis and Diaphragma

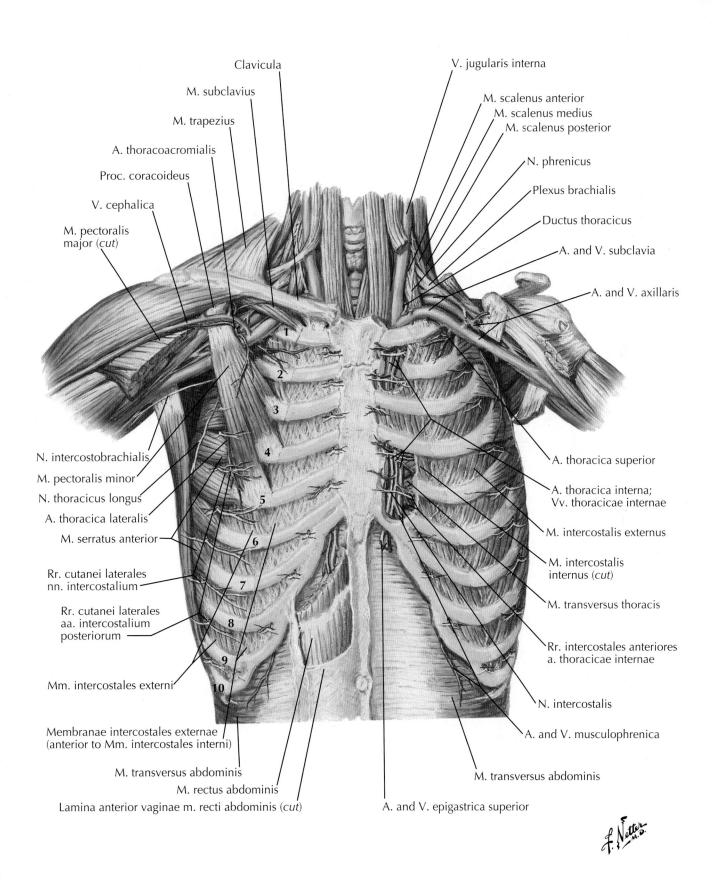

Clavicula

V. jugularis interna

M. subclavius

M. scalenus anterior
M. scalenus medius
M. scalenus posterior

M. trapezius

N. phrenicus

A. thoracoacromialis

Plexus brachialis

Proc. coracoideus

Ductus thoracicus

V. cephalica

A. and V. subclavia

M. pectoralis
major (*cut*)

A. and V. axillaris

N. intercostobrachialis

A. thoracica superior

M. pectoralis minor

N. thoracicus longus

A. thoracica interna;
Vv. thoracicae internae

A. thoracica lateralis

M. intercostalis externus

M. serratus anterior

M. intercostalis
internus (*cut*)

Rr. cutanei laterales
nn. intercostalium

M. transversus thoracis

Rr. cutanei laterales
aa. intercostalium
posteriorum

Rr. intercostales anteriores
a. thoracicae internae

Mm. intercostales externi

N. intercostalis

Membranae intercostales externae
(anterior to Mm. intercostales interni)

A. and V. musculophrenica

M. transversus abdominis

M. transversus abdominis

M. rectus abdominis

Lamina anterior vaginae m. recti abdominis (*cut*)

A. and V. epigastrica superior

1 2 3 4 5 6 7 8 9 10

M. sternothyreoideus

M. sternohyoideus

V. jugularis interna

M. scalenus anterior

A. and V. subclavia

Clavicula (*cut*)

V. brachiocephalica

N. phrenicus

A. and V.
pericardiocophrenica

A. and V. thoracica
interna

N. intercostalis

A. and V.
intercostalis anterior

R. perforans
a. thoracicae
internae

R. cutaneus
anterior pectoralis
n. intercostalis

R. collateralis
n. intercostalis

Rr. collaterales
a. and v.
intercostalis

Corpus sterni

Trigonum
sternocostale

Diaphragma

Pars costalis
diaphragmatis

M. transversus
abdominis

Manubrium sterni

Carotis communis

Truncus brachiocephalicus

A. and V. subclavia

V. brachiocephalica

A. and V. thoracica
interna

A. and V. intercostalis
anterior

N. intercostalis

Mm. intercostales
interni

Mm. intercostales
intimi

M. transversus
thoracis

A. and V.
musculophrenica

Pars sternalis diaphragmatis

Proc. xiphoideus

A. thoracica interna; Vv. thoracicae internae

A. epigastrica superior; Vv. epigastricae superiores

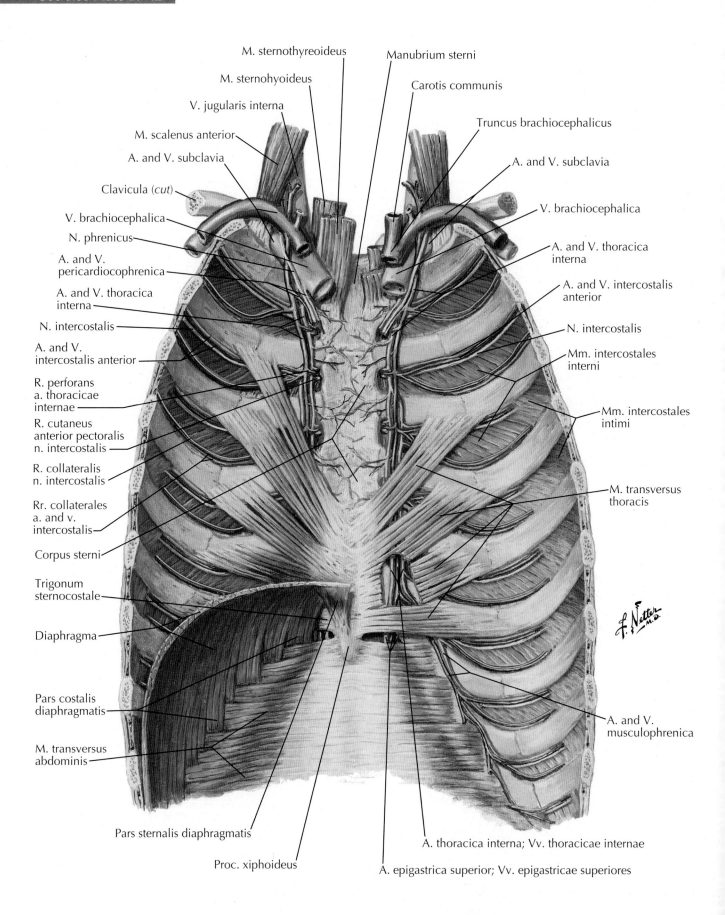

Plate 211

Paries Thoracis and Diaphragma

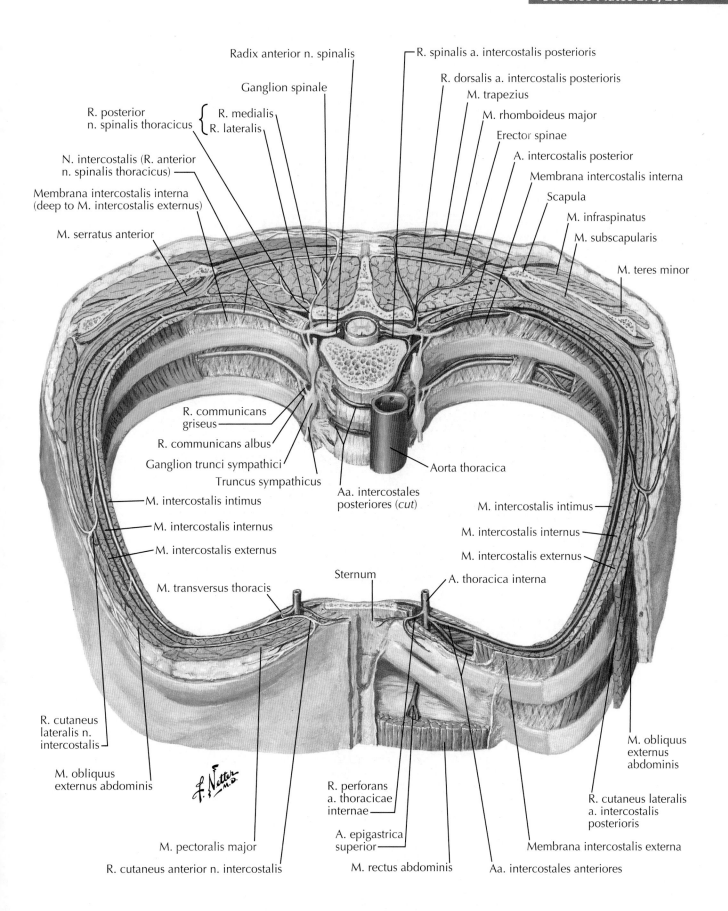

Radix anterior n. spinalis

Ganglion spinale

R. spinalis a. intercostalis posterioris

R. dorsalis a. intercostalis posterioris

M. trapezius

M. rhomboideus major

Erector spinae

A. intercostalis posterior

Membrana intercostalis interna

Scapula

M. infraspinatus

M. subscapularis

M. teres minor

R. posterior n. spinalis thoracicus
{ R. medialis
  R. lateralis

N. intercostalis (R. anterior n. spinalis thoracicus)

Membrana intercostalis interna (deep to M. intercostalis externus)

M. serratus anterior

R. communicans griseus

R. communicans albus

Ganglion trunci sympathici

Truncus sympathicus

Aa. intercostales posteriores (cut)

Aorta thoracica

M. intercostalis intimus

M. intercostalis internus

M. intercostalis externus

M. intercostalis intimus

M. intercostalis internus

M. intercostalis externus

M. transversus thoracis

Sternum

A. thoracica interna

R. cutaneus lateralis n. intercostalis

M. obliquus externus abdominis

M. pectoralis major

R. perforans a. thoracicae internae

A. epigastrica superior

M. rectus abdominis

M. obliquus externus abdominis

R. cutaneus lateralis a. intercostalis posterioris

Membrana intercostalis externa

Aa. intercostales anteriores

R. cutaneus anterior n. intercostalis

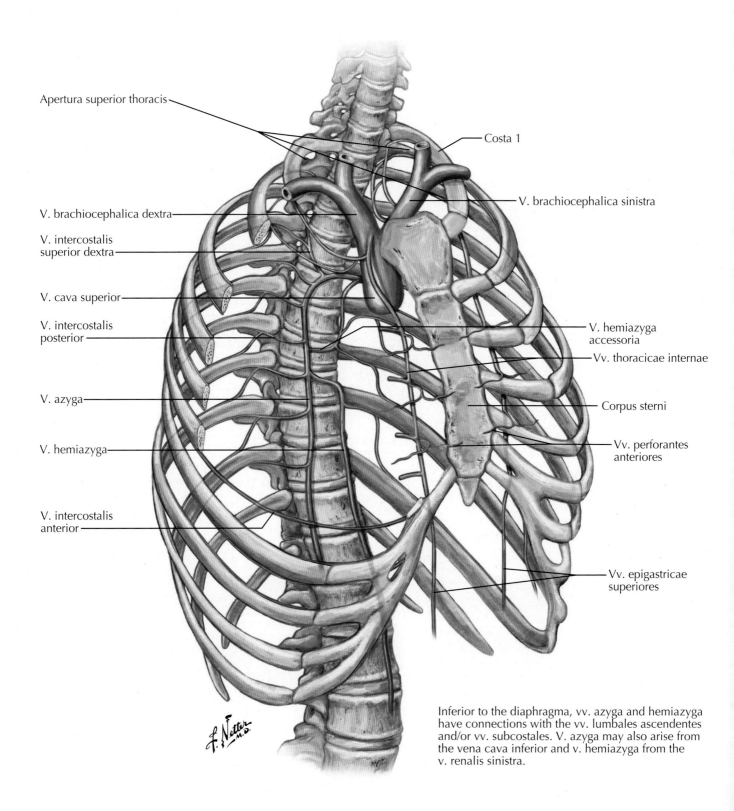

Apertura superior thoracis

Costa 1

V. brachiocephalica dextra

V. brachiocephalica sinistra

V. intercostalis superior dextra

V. cava superior

V. hemiazyga accessoria

V. intercostalis posterior

Vv. thoracicae internae

V. azyga

Corpus sterni

V. hemiazyga

Vv. perforantes anteriores

V. intercostalis anterior

Vv. epigastricae superiores

Inferior to the diaphragma, vv. azyga and hemiazyga have connections with the vv. lumbales ascendentes and/or vv. subcostales. V. azyga may also arise from the vena cava inferior and v. hemiazyga from the v. renalis sinistra.

Plate 213

Paries Thoracis and Diaphragma

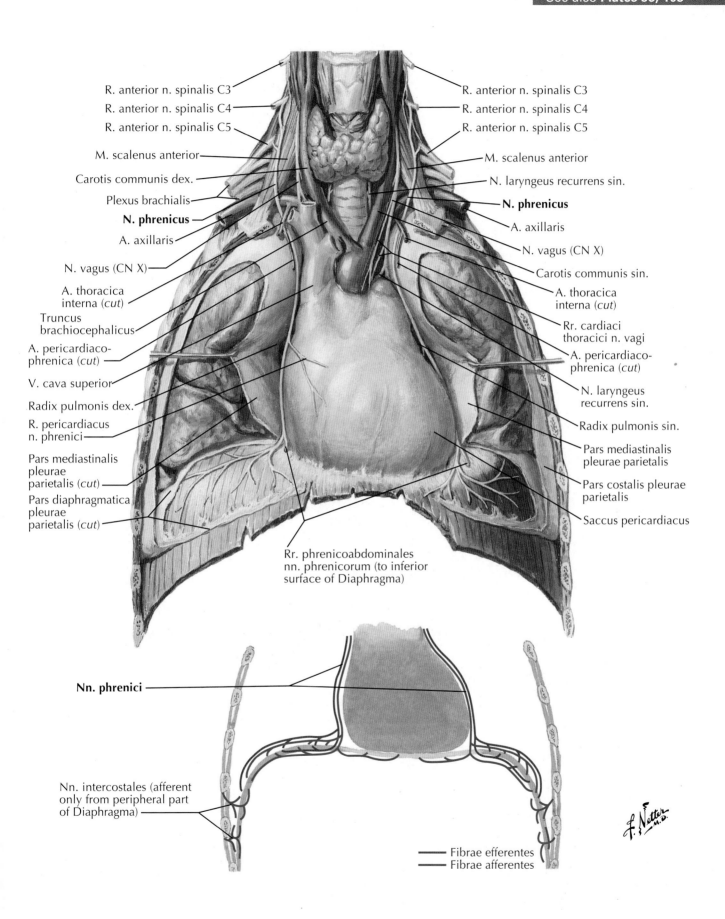

R. anterior n. spinalis C3

R. anterior n. spinalis C4

R. anterior n. spinalis C5

M. scalenus anterior

Carotis communis dex.

Plexus brachialis

N. phrenicus

A. axillaris

N. vagus (CN X)

A. thoracica interna (*cut*)

Truncus brachiocephalicus

A. pericardiaco-phrenica (*cut*)

V. cava superior

Radix pulmonis dex.

R. pericardiacus n. phrenici

Pars mediastinalis pleurae parietalis (*cut*)

Pars diaphragmatica pleurae parietalis (*cut*)

R. anterior n. spinalis C3

R. anterior n. spinalis C4

R. anterior n. spinalis C5

M. scalenus anterior

N. laryngeus recurrens sin.

N. phrenicus

A. axillaris

N. vagus (CN X)

Carotis communis sin.

A. thoracica interna (*cut*)

Rr. cardiaci thoracici n. vagi

A. pericardiaco-phrenica (*cut*)

N. laryngeus recurrens sin.

Radix pulmonis sin.

Pars mediastinalis pleurae parietalis

Pars costalis pleurae parietalis

Saccus pericardiacus

Rr. phrenicoabdominales nn. phrenicorum (to inferior surface of Diaphragma)

Nn. phrenici

Nn. intercostales (afferent only from peripheral part of Diaphragma)

Fibrae efferentes
Fibrae afferentes

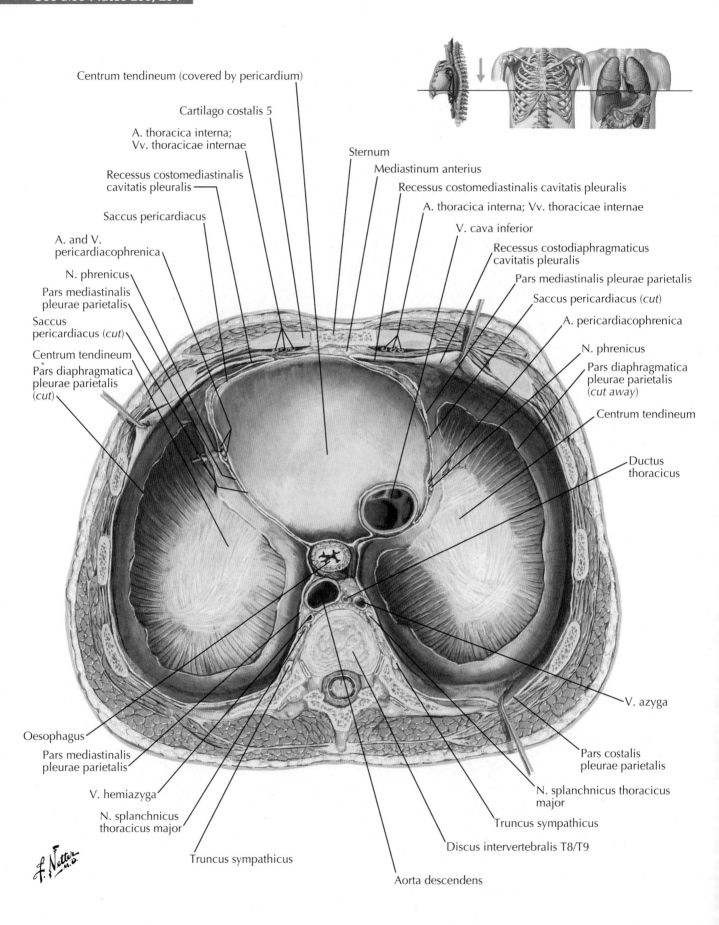

Centrum tendineum (covered by pericardium)

Cartilago costalis 5

A. thoracica interna;
Vv. thoracicae internae

Recessus costomediastinalis
cavitatis pleuralis

Saccus pericardiacus

A. and V.
pericardiacophrenica

N. phrenicus

Pars mediastinalis
pleurae parietalis

Saccus
pericardiacus (*cut*)

Centrum tendineum

Pars diaphragmatica
pleurae parietalis
(*cut*)

Sternum

Mediastinum anterius

Recessus costomediastinalis cavitatis pleuralis

A. thoracica interna; Vv. thoracicae internae

V. cava inferior

Recessus costodiaphragmaticus
cavitatis pleuralis

Pars mediastinalis pleurae parietalis

Saccus pericardiacus (*cut*)

A. pericardiacophrenica

N. phrenicus

Pars diaphragmatica
pleurae parietalis
(*cut away*)

Centrum tendineum

Ductus
thoracicus

V. azyga

Pars costalis
pleurae parietalis

Oesophagus

Pars mediastinalis
pleurae parietalis

V. hemiazyga

N. splanchnicus
thoracicus major

Truncus sympathicus

N. splanchnicus thoracicus
major

Truncus sympathicus

Discus intervertebralis T8/T9

Aorta descendens

Plate 215

Paries Thoracis and Diaphragma

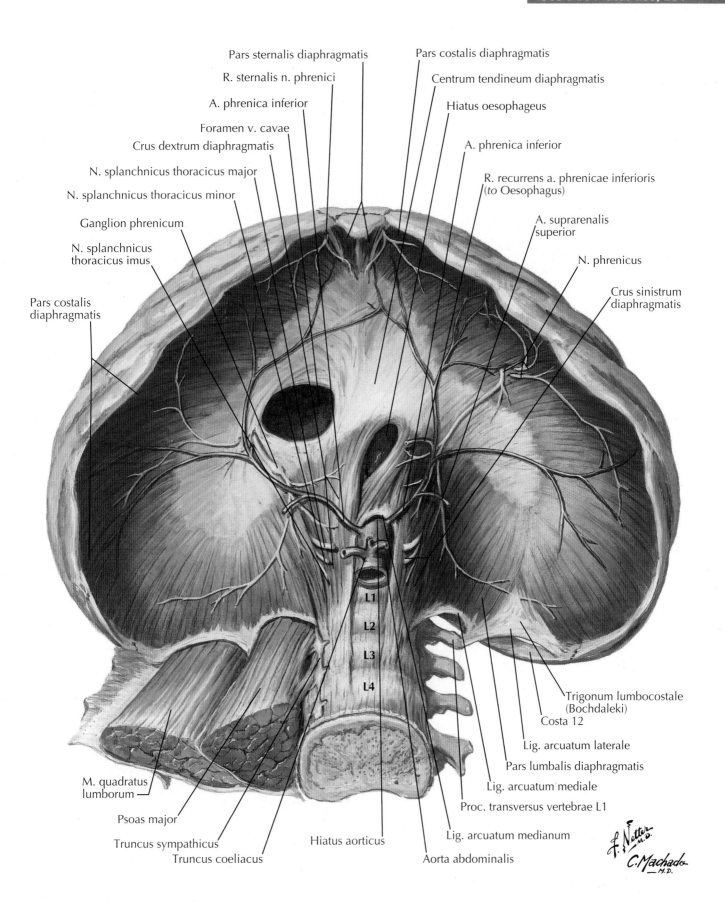

Pars sternalis diaphragmatis

R. sternalis n. phrenici

A. phrenica inferior

Foramen v. cavae

Crus dextrum diaphragmatis

N. splanchnicus thoracicus major

N. splanchnicus thoracicus minor

Ganglion phrenicum

N. splanchnicus thoracicus imus

Pars costalis diaphragmatis

Pars costalis diaphragmatis

Centrum tendineum diaphragmatis

Hiatus oesophageus

A. phrenica inferior

R. recurrens a. phrenicae inferioris (*to* Oesophagus)

A. suprarenalis superior

N. phrenicus

Crus sinistrum diaphragmatis

L1

L2

L3

L4

Trigonum lumbocostale (Bochdaleki)

Costa 12

Lig. arcuatum laterale

Pars lumbalis diaphragmatis

Lig. arcuatum mediale

Proc. transversus vertebrae L1

Lig. arcuatum medianum

Aorta abdominalis

M. quadratus lumborum

Psoas major

Truncus sympathicus

Truncus coeliacus

Hiatus aorticus

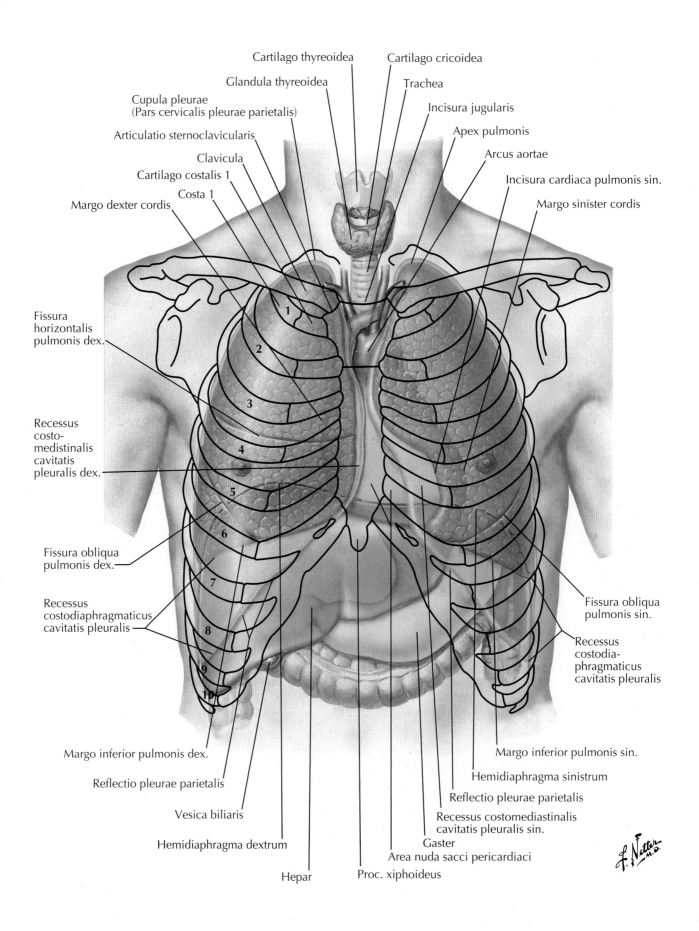

Cartilago thyreoidea

Cartilago cricoidea

Glandula thyreoidea

Trachea

Cupula pleurae
(Pars cervicalis pleurae parietalis)

Incisura jugularis

Articulatio sternoclavicularis

Apex pulmonis

Clavicula

Arcus aortae

Cartilago costalis 1

Incisura cardiaca pulmonis sin.

Costa 1

Margo sinister cordis

Margo dexter cordis

Fissura
horizontalis
pulmonis dex.

Recessus
costo-
medistinalis
cavitatis
pleuralis dex.

Fissura obliqua
pulmonis dex.

Fissura obliqua
pulmonis sin.

Recessus
costodiaphragmaticus
cavitatis pleuralis

Recessus
costodia-
phragmaticus
cavitatis pleuralis

Margo inferior pulmonis dex.

Margo inferior pulmonis sin.

Reflectio pleurae parietalis

Hemidiaphragma sinistrum

Reflectio pleurae parietalis

Vesica biliaris

Recessus costomediastinalis
cavitatis pleuralis sin.

Hemidiaphragma dextrum

Gaster

Area nuda sacci pericardiaci

Hepar

Proc. xiphoideus

Plate 217   **Pulmones, Trachea, and Bronchi**

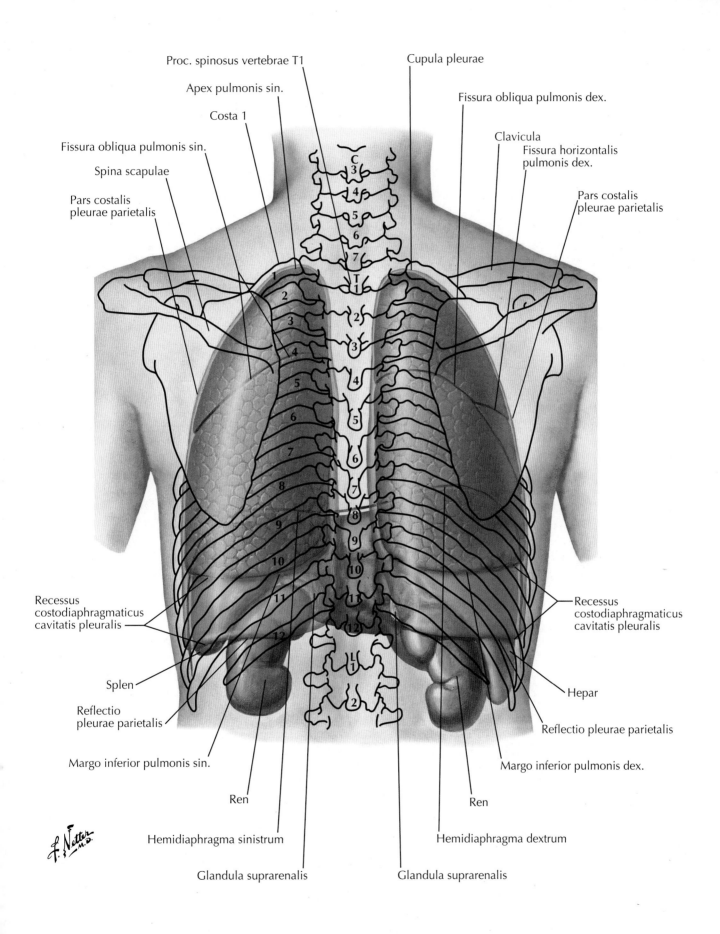

Proc. spinosus vertebrae T1

Apex pulmonis sin.

Costa 1

Cupula pleurae

Fissura obliqua pulmonis dex.

Clavicula

Fissura horizontalis pulmonis dex.

Fissura obliqua pulmonis sin.

Spina scapulae

Pars costalis pleurae parietalis

Pars costalis pleurae parietalis

Recessus costodiaphragmaticus cavitatis pleuralis

Recessus costodiaphragmaticus cavitatis pleuralis

Splen

Reflectio pleurae parietalis

Hepar

Reflectio pleurae parietalis

Margo inferior pulmonis sin.

Margo inferior pulmonis dex.

Ren

Ren

Hemidiaphragma sinistrum

Hemidiaphragma dextrum

Glandula suprarenalis

Glandula suprarenalis

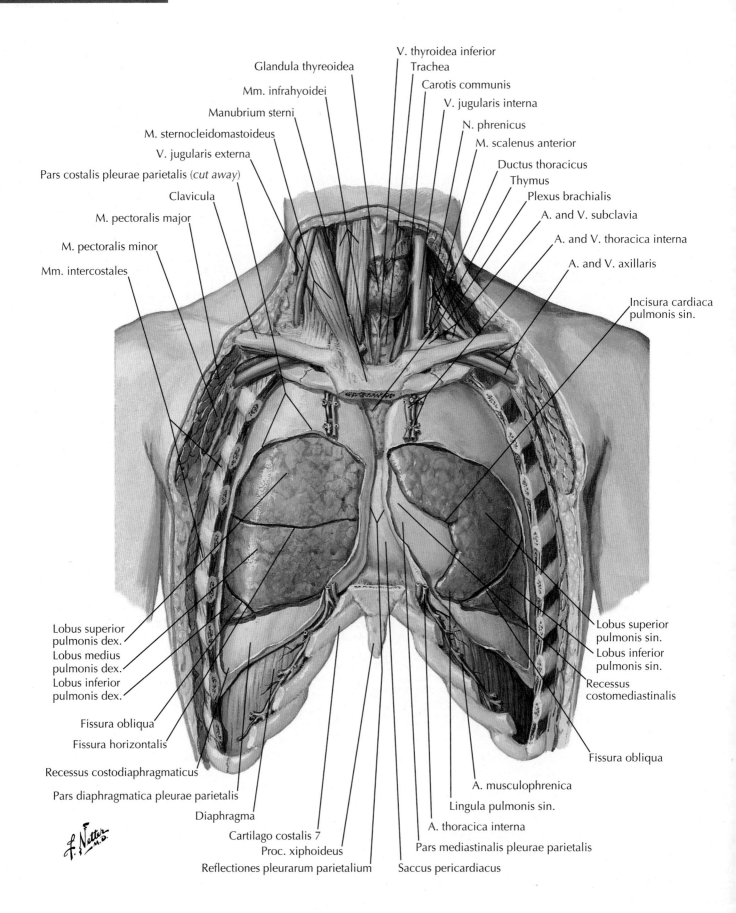

Glandula thyreoidea

Mm. infrahyoidei

Manubrium sterni

M. sternocleidomastoideus

V. jugularis externa

Pars costalis pleurae parietalis (*cut away*)

Clavicula

M. pectoralis major

M. pectoralis minor

Mm. intercostales

V. thyroidea inferior

Trachea

Carotis communis

V. jugularis interna

N. phrenicus

M. scalenus anterior

Ductus thoracicus

Thymus

Plexus brachialis

A. and V. subclavia

A. and V. thoracica interna

A. and V. axillaris

Incisura cardiaca pulmonis sin.

Lobus superior pulmonis dex.

Lobus medius pulmonis dex.

Lobus inferior pulmonis dex.

Fissura obliqua

Fissura horizontalis

Recessus costodiaphragmaticus

Pars diaphragmatica pleurae parietalis

Diaphragma

Cartilago costalis 7

Proc. xiphoideus

Reflectiones pleurarum parietalium

Lobus superior pulmonis sin.

Lobus inferior pulmonis sin.

Recessus costomediastinalis

Fissura obliqua

A. musculophrenica

Lingula pulmonis sin.

A. thoracica interna

Pars mediastinalis pleurae parietalis

Saccus pericardiacus

Plate 219

Pulmones, Trachea, and Bronchi

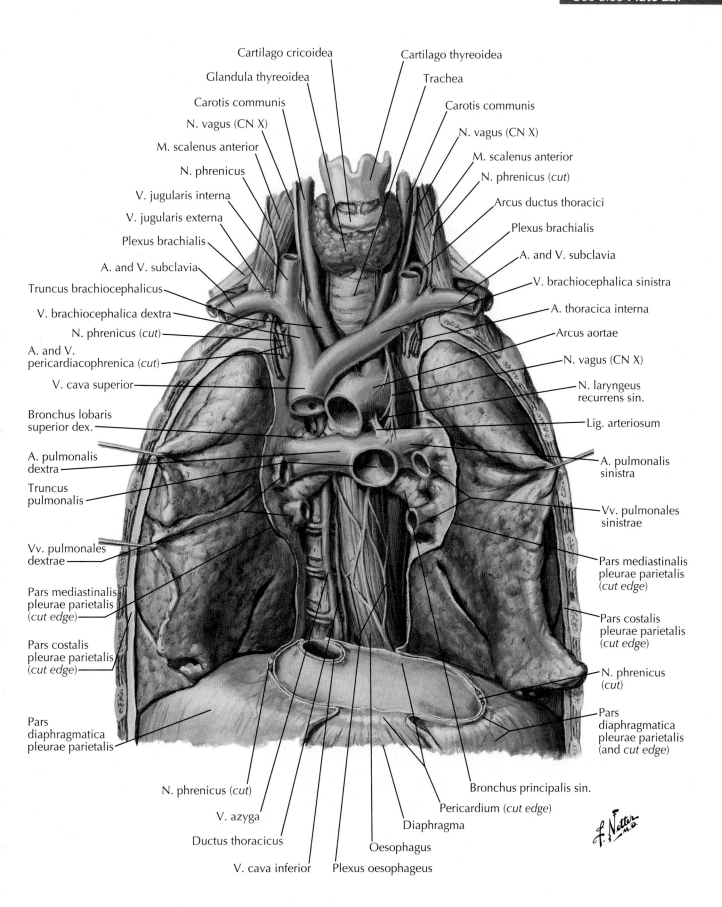

Cartilago cricoidea

Cartilago thyreoidea

Glandula thyreoidea

Trachea

Carotis communis

Carotis communis

N. vagus (CN X)

N. vagus (CN X)

M. scalenus anterior

M. scalenus anterior

N. phrenicus

N. phrenicus (*cut*)

V. jugularis interna

Arcus ductus thoracici

V. jugularis externa

Plexus brachialis

Plexus brachialis

A. and V. subclavia

A. and V. subclavia

V. brachiocephalica sinistra

Truncus brachiocephalicus

A. thoracica interna

V. brachiocephalica dextra

Arcus aortae

N. phrenicus (*cut*)

N. vagus (CN X)

A. and V.
pericardiacophrenica (*cut*)

N. laryngeus
recurrens sin.

V. cava superior

Bronchus lobaris
superior dex.

Lig. arteriosum

A. pulmonalis
dextra

A. pulmonalis
sinistra

Truncus
pulmonalis

Vv. pulmonales
sinistrae

Vv. pulmonales
dextrae

Pars mediastinalis
pleurae parietalis
(*cut edge*)

Pars mediastinalis
pleurae parietalis
(*cut edge*)

Pars costalis
pleurae parietalis
(*cut edge*)

Pars costalis
pleurae parietalis
(*cut edge*)

N. phrenicus
(*cut*)

Pars
diaphragmatica
pleurae parietalis

Pars
diaphragmatica
pleurae parietalis
(and *cut edge*)

N. phrenicus (*cut*)

Bronchus principalis sin.

V. azyga

Pericardium (*cut edge*)

Ductus thoracicus

Diaphragma

V. cava inferior

Oesophagus

Plexus oesophageus

Pulmones, Trachea, and Bronchi

Plate 220

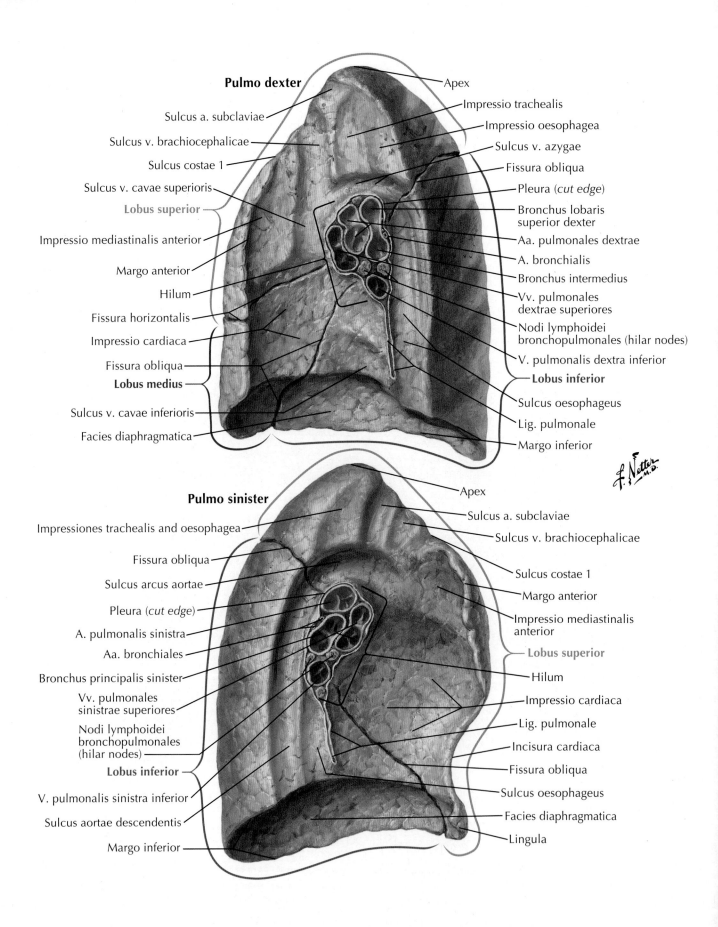

Pulmo dexter

Sulcus a. subclaviae

Sulcus v. brachiocephalicae

Sulcus costae 1

Sulcus v. cavae superioris

Lobus superior

Impressio mediastinalis anterior

Margo anterior

Hilum

Fissura horizontalis

Impressio cardiaca

Fissura obliqua

Lobus medius

Sulcus v. cavae inferioris

Facies diaphragmatica

Apex

Impressio trachealis

Impressio oesophagea

Sulcus v. azygae

Fissura obliqua

Pleura (*cut edge*)

Bronchus lobaris superior dexter

Aa. pulmonales dextrae

A. bronchialis

Bronchus intermedius

Vv. pulmonales dextrae superiores

Nodi lymphoidei bronchopulmonales (hilar nodes)

V. pulmonalis dextra inferior

Lobus inferior

Sulcus oesophageus

Lig. pulmonale

Margo inferior

Pulmo sinister

Impressiones trachealis and oesophagea

Fissura obliqua

Sulcus arcus aortae

Pleura (*cut edge*)

A. pulmonalis sinistra

Aa. bronchiales

Bronchus principalis sinister

Vv. pulmonales sinistrae superiores

Nodi lymphoidei bronchopulmonales (hilar nodes)

Lobus inferior

V. pulmonalis sinistra inferior

Sulcus aortae descendentis

Margo inferior

Apex

Sulcus a. subclaviae

Sulcus v. brachiocephalicae

Sulcus costae 1

Margo anterior

Impressio mediastinalis anterior

Lobus superior

Hilum

Impressio cardiaca

Lig. pulmonale

Incisura cardiaca

Fissura obliqua

Sulcus oesophageus

Facies diaphragmatica

Lingula

Plate 221

Pulmones, Trachea, and Bronchi

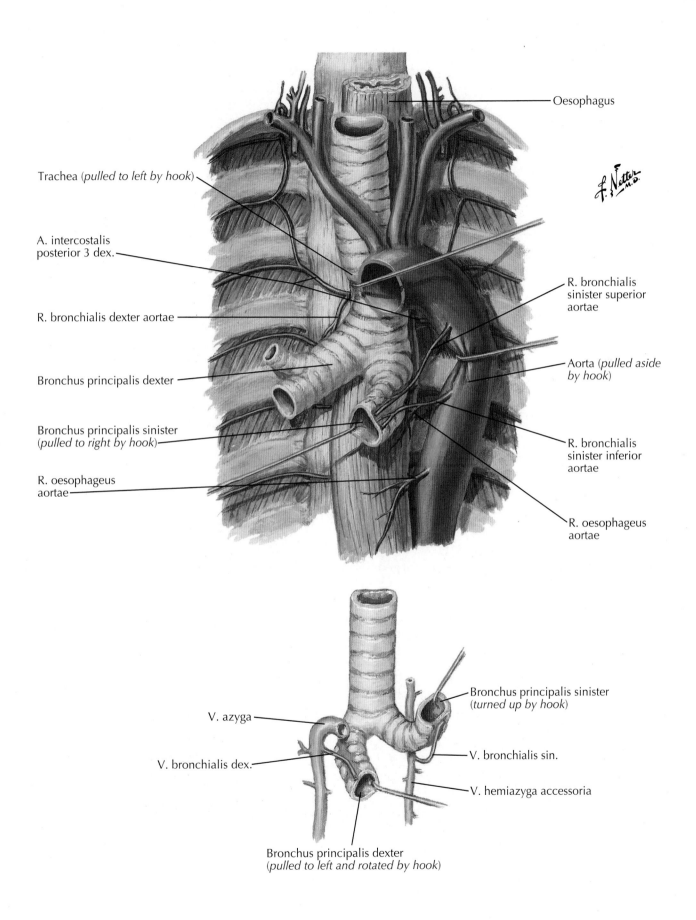

Oesophagus

Trachea (*pulled to left by hook*)

A. intercostalis posterior 3 dex.

R. bronchialis dexter aortae

Bronchus principalis dexter

Bronchus principalis sinister (*pulled to right by hook*)

R. oesophageus aortae

R. bronchialis sinister superior aortae

Aorta (*pulled aside by hook*)

R. bronchialis sinister inferior aortae

R. oesophageus aortae

V. azyga

V. bronchialis dex.

Bronchus principalis sinister (*turned up by hook*)

V. bronchialis sin.

V. hemiazyga accessoria

Bronchus principalis dexter (*pulled to left and rotated by hook*)

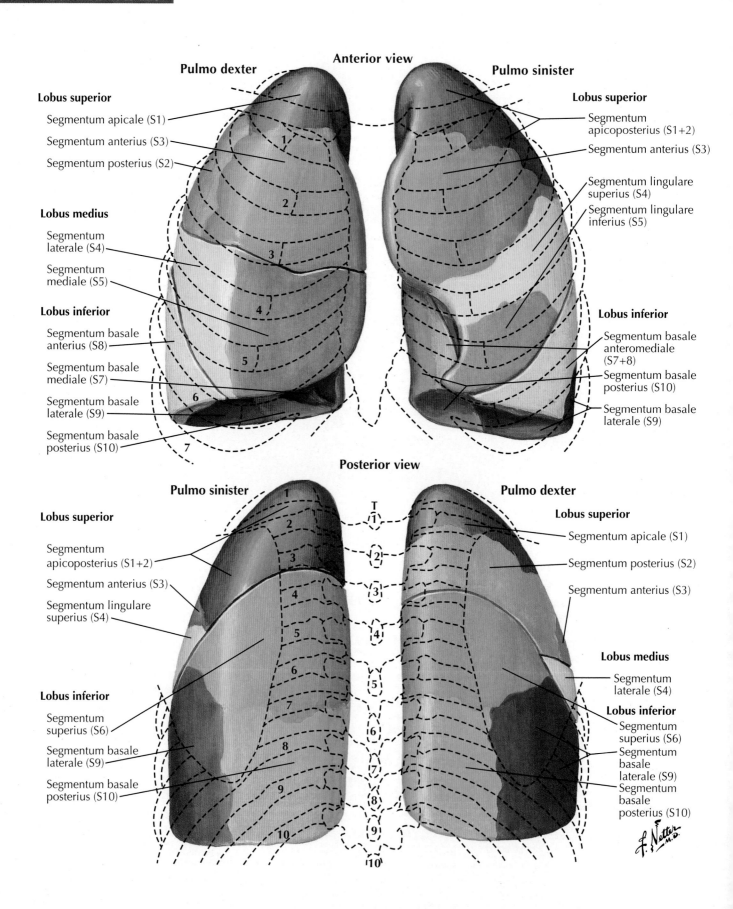

Anterior view

Pulmo dexter

Pulmo sinister

Lobus superior

Segmentum apicale (S1)

Segmentum anterius (S3)

Segmentum posterius (S2)

Lobus medius

Segmentum laterale (S4)

Segmentum mediale (S5)

Lobus inferior

Segmentum basale anterius (S8)

Segmentum basale mediale (S7)

Segmentum basale laterale (S9)

Segmentum basale posterius (S10)

Lobus superior

Segmentum apicoposterius (S1+2)

Segmentum anterius (S3)

Segmentum lingulare superius (S4)

Segmentum lingulare inferius (S5)

Lobus inferior

Segmentum basale anteromediale (S7+8)

Segmentum basale posterius (S10)

Segmentum basale laterale (S9)

Posterior view

Pulmo sinister

Pulmo dexter

Lobus superior

Segmentum apicoposterius (S1+2)

Segmentum anterius (S3)

Segmentum lingulare superius (S4)

Lobus inferior

Segmentum superius (S6)

Segmentum basale laterale (S9)

Segmentum basale posterius (S10)

Lobus superior

Segmentum apicale (S1)

Segmentum posterius (S2)

Segmentum anterius (S3)

Lobus medius

Segmentum laterale (S4)

Lobus inferior

Segmentum superius (S6)

Segmentum basale laterale (S9)

Segmentum basale posterius (S10)

Plate 223

Pulmones, Trachea, and Bronchi

Lateral views

Pulmo dexter

Lobus superior

Segmentum apicale (S1)

Segmentum posterius (S2)

Segmentum anterius (S3)

Lobus medius

Segmentum laterale (S4)

Segmentum mediale (S5)

Lobus inferior

Segmentum superius (S6)

Segmentum basale anterius (S8)

Segmentum basale laterale (S9)

Pulmo sinister

Lobus superior

Segmentum apicoposterius (S1+2)

Segmentum anterius (S3)

Segmentum lingulare superius (S4)

Segmentum lingulare inferius (S5)

Lobus inferior

Segmentum superius (S6)

Segmentum basale anteromediale (S7+8)

Segmentum basale laterale (S9)

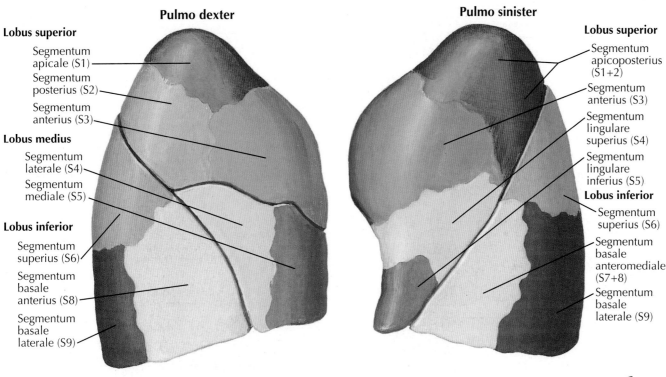

Medial views

Pulmo dexter

Lobus superior

Segmentum apicale (S1)

Segmentum posterius (S2)

Segmentum anterius (S3)

Lobus medius

Segmentum mediale (S5)

Lobus inferior

Segmentum superius (S6)

Segmentum basale mediale (S7)

Segmentum basale anterius (S8)

Segmentum basale laterale (S9)

Segmentum basale posterius (S10)

Pulmo sinister

Lobus superior

Segmentum apicoposterius (S1+2)

Segmentum anterius (S3)

Segmentum lingulare superius (S4)

Segmentum lingulare inferius (S5)

Lobus inferior

Segmentum superius (S6)

Segmentum basale anteromediale (S7+8)

Segmentum basale laterale (S9)

Segmentum basale posterius (S10)

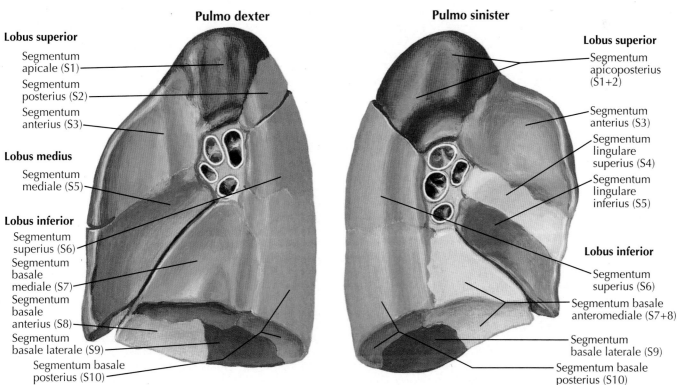

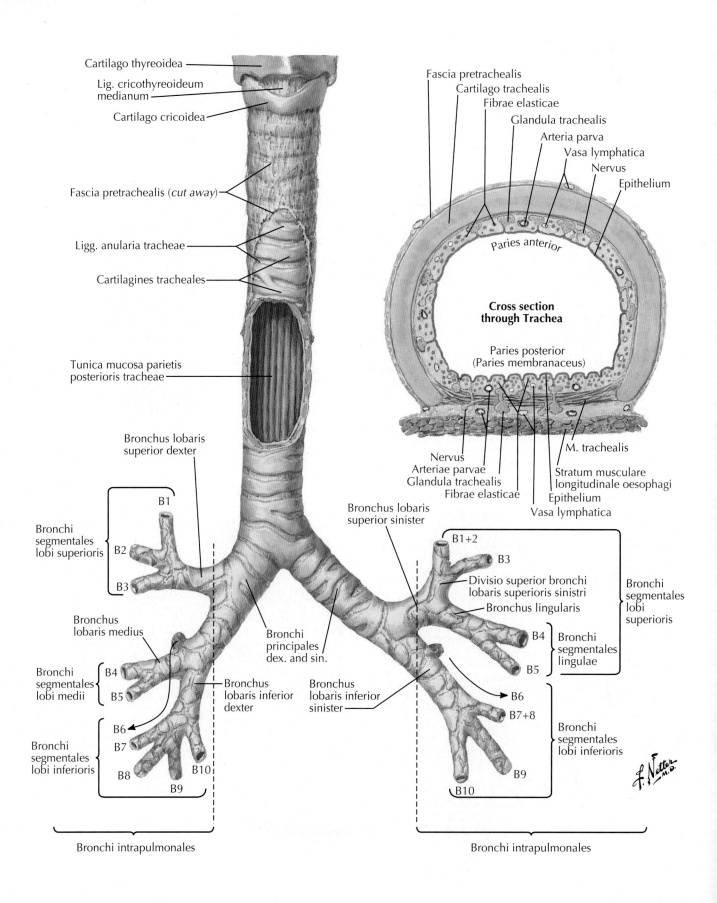

Cartilago thyreoidea

Lig. cricothyreoideum medianum

Cartilago cricoidea

Fascia pretrachealis (cut away)

Ligg. anularia tracheae

Cartilagines tracheales

Tunica mucosa parietis posterioris tracheae

Bronchus lobaris superior dexter

B1

Bronchi segmentales lobi superioris

B2

B3

Bronchus lobaris medius

Bronchi segmentales lobi medii

B4

B5

Bronchi segmentales lobi inferioris

B6

B7

B8

B9

B10

Bronchus lobaris inferior dexter

Bronchi principales dex. and sin.

Bronchus lobaris inferior sinister

Bronchi intrapulmonales

Fascia pretrachealis
Cartilago trachealis
Fibrae elasticae
Glandula trachealis
Arteria parva
Vasa lymphatica
Nervus
Epithelium

Paries anterior

Cross section through Trachea

Paries posterior (Paries membranaceus)

Nervus
Arteriae parvae
Glandula trachealis
Fibrae elasticae

M. trachealis
Stratum musculare longitudinale oesophagi
Epithelium
Vasa lymphatica

Bronchus lobaris superior sinister

B1+2
B3
Divisio superior bronchi lobaris superioris sinistri
Bronchus lingularis

B4
B5

Bronchi segmentales lobi superioris

Bronchi segmentales lingulae

B6
B7+8
B9
B10

Bronchi segmentales lobi inferioris

Bronchi intrapulmonales

Plate 225

Pulmones, Trachea, and Bronchi

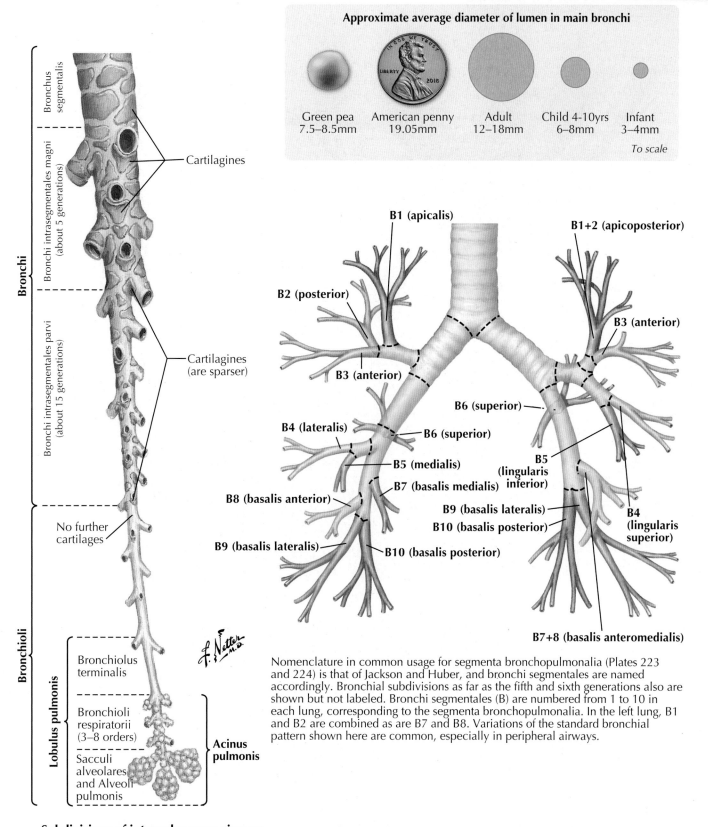

Approximate average diameter of lumen in main bronchi

Green pea
7.5–8.5mm

American penny
19.05mm

Adult
12–18mm

Child 4-10yrs
6–8mm

Infant
3–4mm

To scale

Bronchus
segmentalis

Cartilagines

Bronchi intrasegmentales magni
(about 5 generations)

Cartilagines
(are sparser)

Bronchi intrasegmentales parvi
(about 15 generations)

No further
cartilages

Bronchi

Bronchioli

Bronchiolus
terminalis

Lobulus pulmonis

Bronchioli
respiratorii
(3–8 orders)

Acinus
pulmonis

Sacculi
alveolares
and Alveoli
pulmonis

Subdivisions of intrapulmonary airways

B1 (apicalis)

B1+2 (apicoposterior)

B2 (posterior)

B3 (anterior)

B3 (anterior)

B6 (superior)

B4 (lateralis)

B6 (superior)

B5 (medialis)

B5
(lingularis
inferior)

B7 (basalis medialis)

B8 (basalis anterior)

B9 (basalis lateralis)

B10 (basalis posterior)

B4
(lingularis
superior)

B9 (basalis lateralis)

B10 (basalis posterior)

B7+8 (basalis anteromedialis)

Nomenclature in common usage for segmenta bronchopulmonalia (Plates 223 and 224) is that of Jackson and Huber, and bronchi segmentales are named accordingly. Bronchial subdivisions as far as the fifth and sixth generations also are shown but not labeled. Bronchi segmentales (B) are numbered from 1 to 10 in each lung, corresponding to the segmenta bronchopulmonalia. In the left lung, B1 and B2 are combined as are B7 and B8. Variations of the standard bronchial pattern shown here are common, especially in peripheral airways.

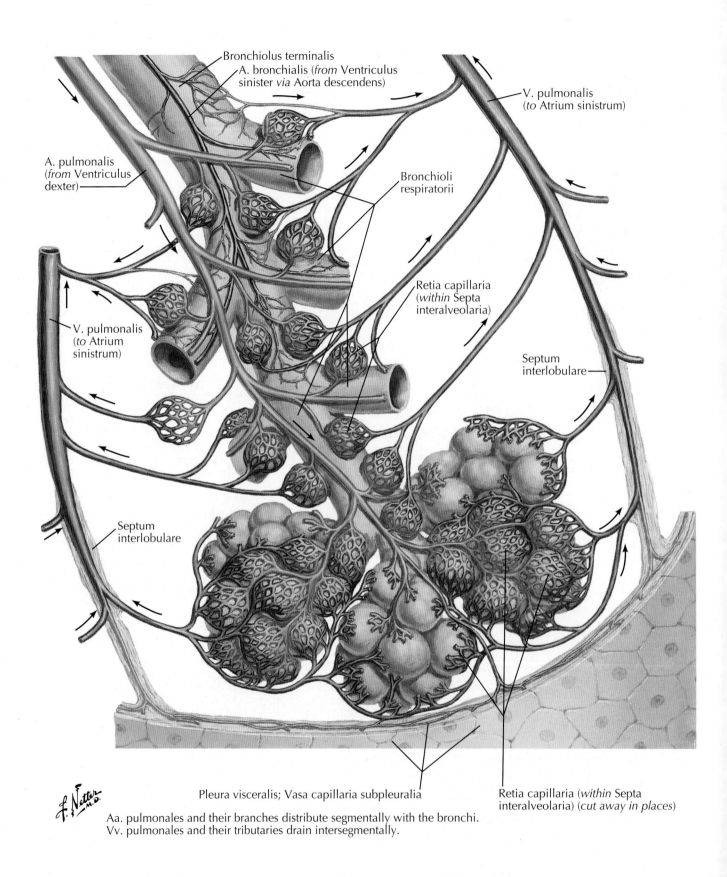

Bronchiolus terminalis
A. bronchialis (*from* Ventriculus sinister *via* Aorta descendens)

V. pulmonalis (*to* Atrium sinistrum)

A. pulmonalis (*from* Ventriculus dexter)

Bronchioli respiratorii

Retia capillaria (*within* Septa interalveolaria)

V. pulmonalis (*to* Atrium sinistrum)

Septum interlobulare

Septum interlobulare

Pleura visceralis; Vasa capillaria subpleuralia

Retia capillaria (*within* Septa interalveolaria) (*cut away in places*)

Aa. pulmonales and their branches distribute segmentally with the bronchi.
Vv. pulmonales and their tributaries drain intersegmentally.

Plate 227

Pulmones, Trachea, and Bronchi

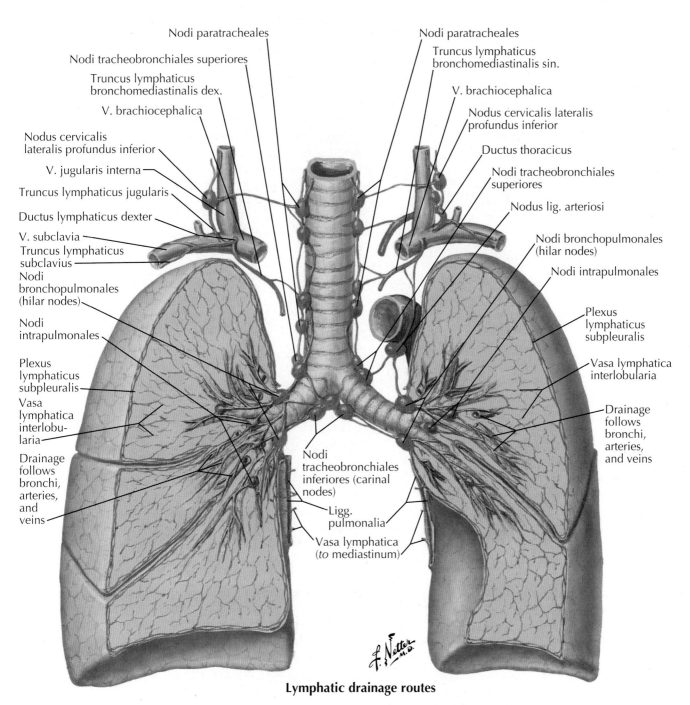

Nodi paratracheales

Nodi tracheobronchiales superiores

Truncus lymphaticus bronchomediastinalis dex.

V. brachiocephalica

Nodus cervicalis lateralis profundus inferior

V. jugularis interna

Truncus lymphaticus jugularis

Ductus lymphaticus dexter

V. subclavia

Truncus lymphaticus subclavius

Nodi bronchopulmonales (hilar nodes)

Nodi intrapulmonales

Plexus lymphaticus subpleuralis

Vasa lymphatica interlobularia

Drainage follows bronchi, arteries, and veins

Nodi paratracheales

Truncus lymphaticus bronchomediastinalis sin.

V. brachiocephalica

Nodus cervicalis lateralis profundus inferior

Ductus thoracicus

Nodi tracheobronchiales superiores

Nodus lig. arteriosi

Nodi bronchopulmonales (hilar nodes)

Nodi intrapulmonales

Plexus lymphaticus subpleuralis

Vasa lymphatica interlobularia

Drainage follows bronchi, arteries, and veins

Nodi tracheobronchiales inferiores (carinal nodes)

Ligg. pulmonalia

Vasa lymphatica (*to mediastinum*)

Lymphatic drainage routes

Right lung: All lobes drain to intrapulmonary and bronchopulmonary nodes, then to inferior tracheobronchial nodes, right superior tracheobronchial nodes, and right paratracheal nodes on the way to the brachiocephalic vein via the right bronchomediastinal and jugular lymphatic trunks.

Left lung: The superior lobe drains to intrapulmonary and bronchoplumonary nodes, then to inferior tracheobronchial nodes, left superior tracheobronchial nodes, left paratracheal nodes, and the node of the ligamentum arteriosum on the way to the brachiocephalic vein via the left bronchomediastinal lymphatic trunk and thoracic duct. The intrapulmonary and bronchopulmonary nodes of the left lung also drain to right superior tracheobronchial nodes, where the lymph follows the same route as lymph from the right lung.

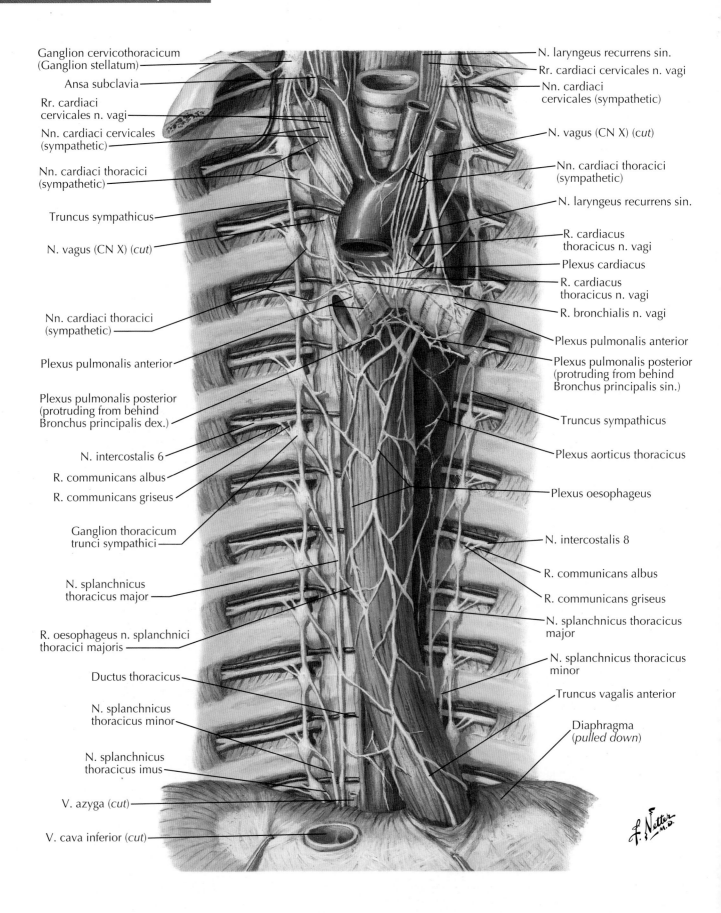

Ganglion cervicothoracicum (Ganglion stellatum)

Ansa subclavia

Rr. cardiaci cervicales n. vagi

Nn. cardiaci cervicales (sympathetic)

Nn. cardiaci thoracici (sympathetic)

Truncus sympathicus

N. vagus (CN X) (cut)

Nn. cardiaci thoracici (sympathetic)

Plexus pulmonalis anterior

Plexus pulmonalis posterior (protruding from behind Bronchus principalis dex.)

N. intercostalis 6

R. communicans albus

R. communicans griseus

Ganglion thoracicum trunci sympathici

N. splanchnicus thoracicus major

R. oesophageus n. splanchnici thoracici majoris

Ductus thoracicus

N. splanchnicus thoracicus minor

N. splanchnicus thoracicus imus

V. azyga (cut)

V. cava inferior (cut)

N. laryngeus recurrens sin.

Rr. cardiaci cervicales n. vagi

Nn. cardiaci cervicales (sympathetic)

N. vagus (CN X) (cut)

Nn. cardiaci thoracici (sympathetic)

N. laryngeus recurrens sin.

R. cardiacus thoracicus n. vagi

Plexus cardiacus

R. cardiacus thoracicus n. vagi

R. bronchialis n. vagi

Plexus pulmonalis anterior

Plexus pulmonalis posterior (protruding from behind Bronchus principalis sin.)

Truncus sympathicus

Plexus aorticus thoracicus

Plexus oesophageus

N. intercostalis 8

R. communicans albus

R. communicans griseus

N. splanchnicus thoracicus major

N. splanchnicus thoracicus minor

Truncus vagalis anterior

Diaphragma (pulled down)

Plate 229

Pulmones, Trachea, and Bronchi

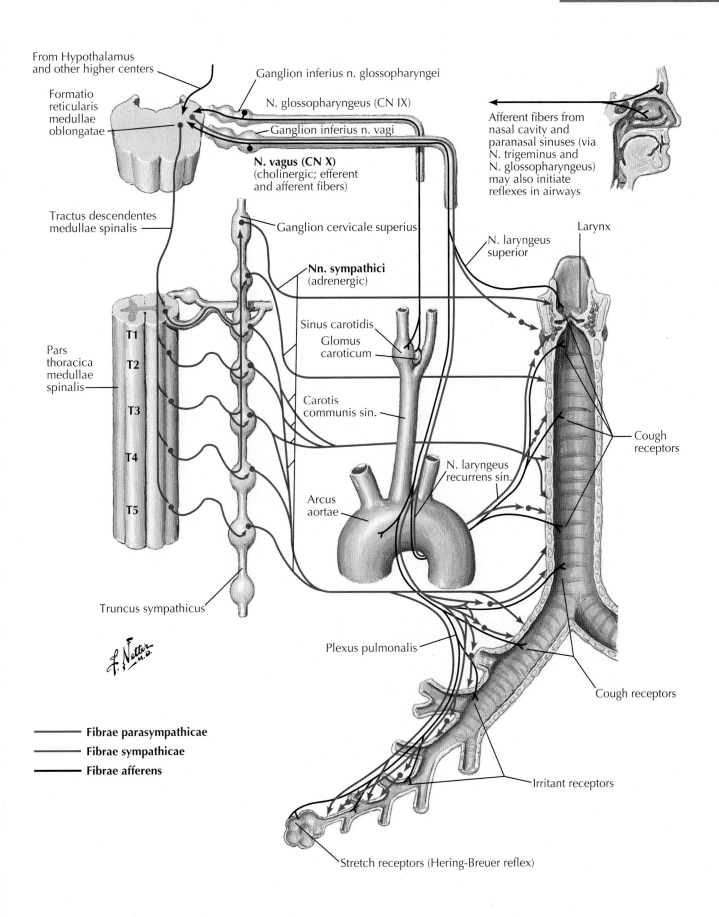

From Hypothalamus and other higher centers

Formatio reticularis medullae oblongatae

Tractus descendentes medullae spinalis

Pars thoracica medullae spinalis

Ganglion inferius n. glossopharyngei

N. glossopharyngeus (CN IX)

Ganglion inferius n. vagi

N. vagus (CN X) (cholinergic; efferent and afferent fibers)

Afferent fibers from nasal cavity and paranasal sinuses (via N. trigeminus and N. glossopharyngeus) may also initiate reflexes in airways

Ganglion cervicale superius

Nn. sympathici (adrenergic)

Sinus carotidis

Glomus caroticum

Carotis communis sin.

Arcus aortae

Larynx

N. laryngeus superior

Cough receptors

N. laryngeus recurrens sin.

T1

T2

T3

T4

T5

Truncus sympathicus

Plexus pulmonalis

Cough receptors

Irritant receptors

— Fibrae parasympathicae

— Fibrae sympathicae

— Fibrae afferens

Stretch receptors (Hering-Breuer reflex)

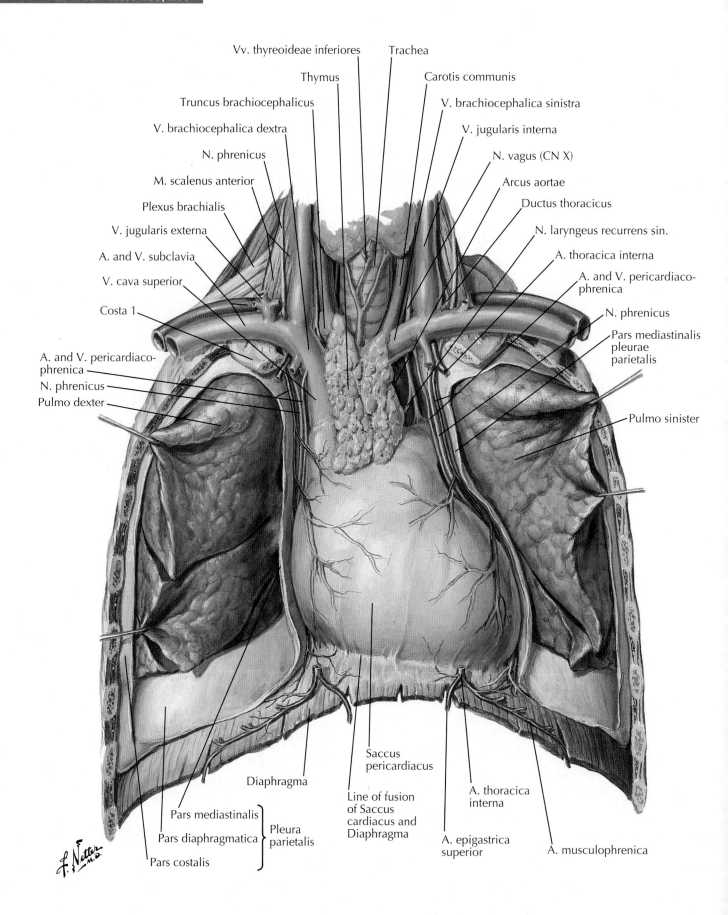

Vv. thyreoideae inferiores

Trachea

Thymus

Carotis communis

Truncus brachiocephalicus

V. brachiocephalica sinistra

V. brachiocephalica dextra

V. jugularis interna

N. phrenicus

N. vagus (CN X)

M. scalenus anterior

Arcus aortae

Plexus brachialis

Ductus thoracicus

V. jugularis externa

N. laryngeus recurrens sin.

A. and V. subclavia

A. thoracica interna

V. cava superior

A. and V. pericardiaco-
phrenica

Costa 1

N. phrenicus

A. and V. pericardiaco-
phrenica

Pars mediastinalis
pleurae
parietalis

N. phrenicus

Pulmo dexter

Pulmo sinister

Diaphragma

Saccus
pericardiacus

Pars mediastinalis

Line of fusion
of Saccus
cardiacus and
Diaphragma

A. thoracica
interna

Pars diaphragmatica

Pleura
parietalis

Pars costalis

A. epigastrica
superior

A. musculophrenica

Plate 231

Cor

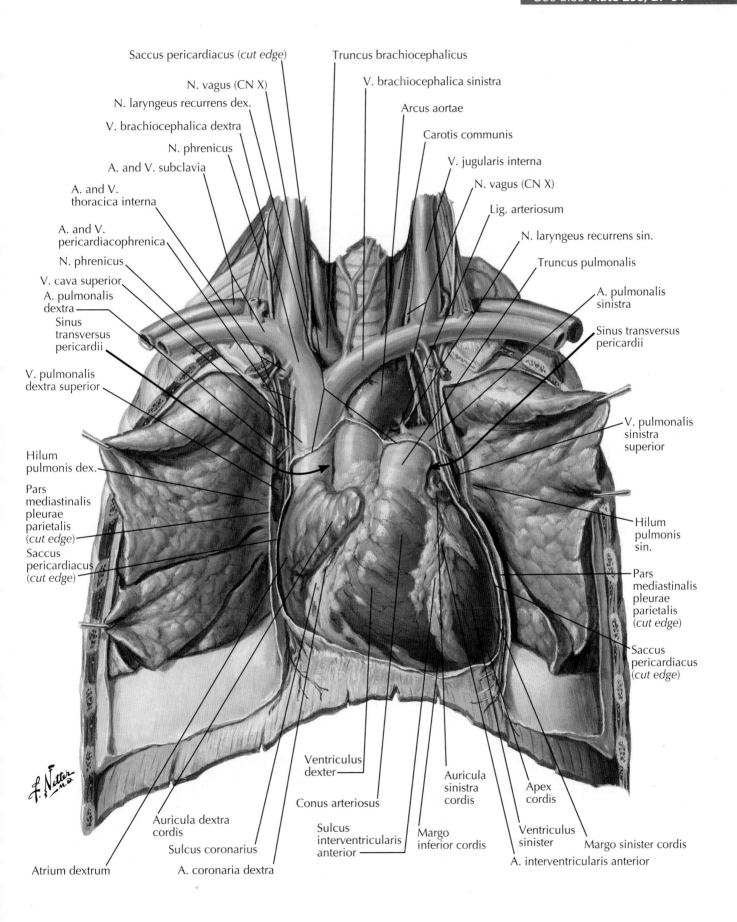

Saccus pericardiacus (*cut edge*)

N. vagus (CN X)

N. laryngeus recurrens dex.

V. brachiocephalica dextra

N. phrenicus

A. and V. subclavia

A. and V. thoracica interna

A. and V. pericardiacophrenica

N. phrenicus

V. cava superior

A. pulmonalis dextra

Sinus transversus pericardii

V. pulmonalis dextra superior

Hilum pulmonis dex.

Pars mediastinalis pleurae parietalis (*cut edge*)

Saccus pericardiacus (*cut edge*)

Truncus brachiocephalicus

V. brachiocephalica sinistra

Arcus aortae

Carotis communis

V. jugularis interna

N. vagus (CN X)

Lig. arteriosum

N. laryngeus recurrens sin.

Truncus pulmonalis

A. pulmonalis sinistra

Sinus transversus pericardii

V. pulmonalis sinistra superior

Hilum pulmonis sin.

Pars mediastinalis pleurae parietalis (*cut edge*)

Saccus pericardiacus (*cut edge*)

Ventriculus dexter

Conus arteriosus

Auricula sinistra cordis

Apex cordis

Auricula dextra cordis

Sulcus coronarius

A. coronaria dextra

Sulcus interventricularis anterior

Margo inferior cordis

Ventriculus sinister

Margo sinister cordis

A. interventricularis anterior

Atrium dextrum

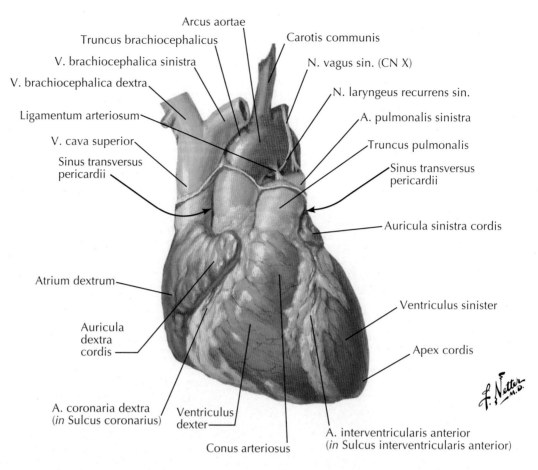

Arcus aortae

Truncus brachiocephalicus

Carotis communis

V. brachiocephalica sinistra

N. vagus sin. (CN X)

V. brachiocephalica dextra

N. laryngeus recurrens sin.

Ligamentum arteriosum

A. pulmonalis sinistra

V. cava superior

Truncus pulmonalis

Sinus transversus pericardii

Sinus transversus pericardii

Auricula sinistra cordis

Atrium dextrum

Ventriculus sinister

Auricula dextra cordis

Apex cordis

A. coronaria dextra (*in* Sulcus coronarius)

Ventriculus dexter

Conus arteriosus

A. interventricularis anterior (*in* Sulcus interventricularis anterior)

Precordial areas of auscultation:
One listens to the closing of the heart valves downstream from the heart valve, i.e, in Ventriculi dexter and sinister for the Valvae tricuspidalis and mitralis, respectively, and over the Truncus pulmonalis and Aorta ascendens for the Valvae trunci pulmonalis and aortae, respectively.

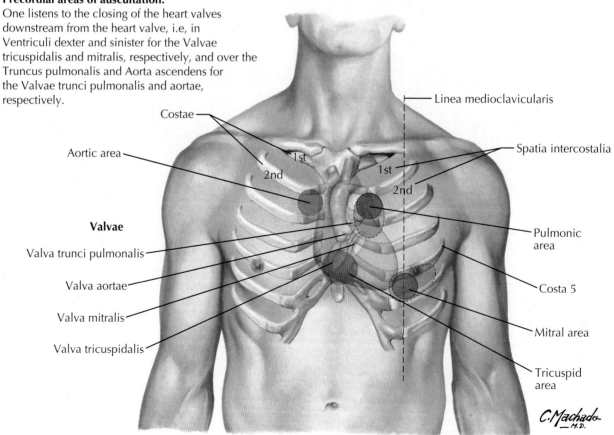

Costae

Linea medioclavicularis

Aortic area

Spatia intercostalia

1st

1st

2nd

2nd

Valvae

Pulmonic area

Valva trunci pulmonalis

Valva aortae

Costa 5

Valva mitralis

Mitral area

Valva tricuspidalis

Tricuspid area

Plate 233

Cor

See also **Plates 233, BP 51**

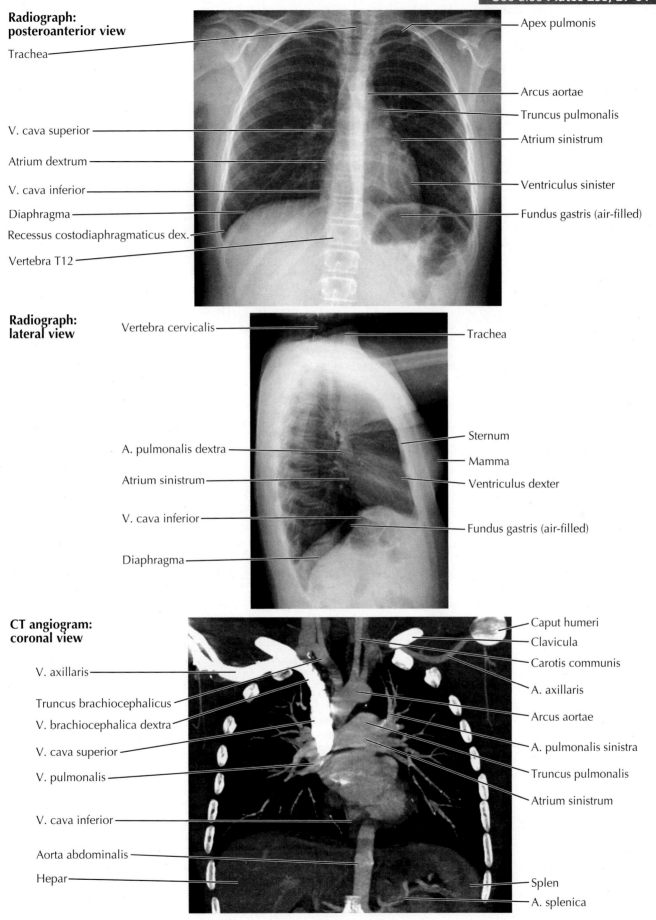

Radiograph: posteroanterior view

Trachea

V. cava superior

Atrium dextrum

V. cava inferior

Diaphragma

Recessus costodiaphragmaticus dex.

Vertebra T12

Apex pulmonis

Arcus aortae

Truncus pulmonalis

Atrium sinistrum

Ventriculus sinister

Fundus gastris (air-filled)

Radiograph: lateral view

Vertebra cervicalis

A. pulmonalis dextra

Atrium sinistrum

V. cava inferior

Diaphragma

Trachea

Sternum

Mamma

Ventriculus dexter

Fundus gastris (air-filled)

CT angiogram: coronal view

V. axillaris

Truncus brachiocephalicus

V. brachiocephalica dextra

V. cava superior

V. pulmonalis

V. cava inferior

Aorta abdominalis

Hepar

Caput humeri

Clavicula

Carotis communis

A. axillaris

Arcus aortae

A. pulmonalis sinistra

Truncus pulmonalis

Atrium sinistrum

Splen

A. splenica

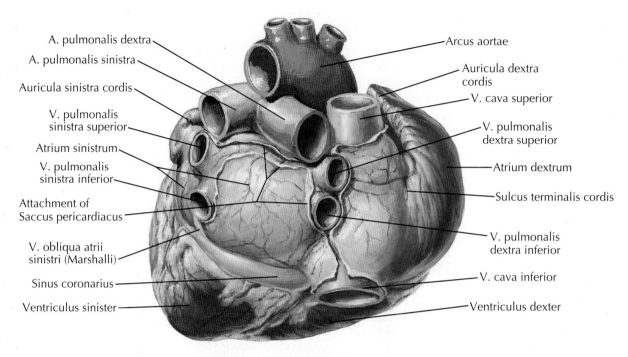

A. pulmonalis dextra

A. pulmonalis sinistra

Auricula sinistra cordis

V. pulmonalis sinistra superior

Atrium sinistrum

V. pulmonalis sinistra inferior

Attachment of Saccus pericardiacus

V. obliqua atrii sinistri (Marshalli)

Sinus coronarius

Ventriculus sinister

Arcus aortae

Auricula dextra cordis

V. cava superior

V. pulmonalis dextra superior

Atrium dextrum

Sulcus terminalis cordis

V. pulmonalis dextra inferior

V. cava inferior

Ventriculus dexter

Basis cordis: posterior view

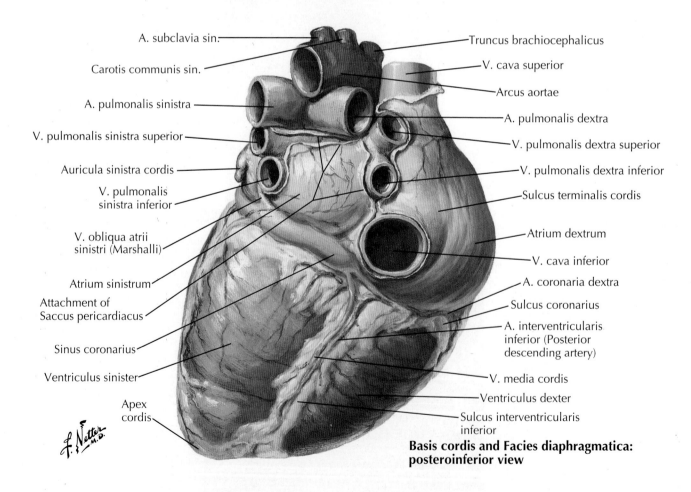

A. subclavia sin.

Carotis communis sin.

A. pulmonalis sinistra

V. pulmonalis sinistra superior

Auricula sinistra cordis

V. pulmonalis sinistra inferior

V. obliqua atrii sinistri (Marshalli)

Atrium sinistrum

Attachment of Saccus pericardiacus

Sinus coronarius

Ventriculus sinister

Apex cordis

Truncus brachiocephalicus

V. cava superior

Arcus aortae

A. pulmonalis dextra

V. pulmonalis dextra superior

V. pulmonalis dextra inferior

Sulcus terminalis cordis

Atrium dextrum

V. cava inferior

A. coronaria dextra

Sulcus coronarius

A. interventricularis inferior (Posterior descending artery)

V. media cordis

Ventriculus dexter

Sulcus interventricularis inferior

Basis cordis and Facies diaphragmatica: posteroinferior view

Plate 235

Cor

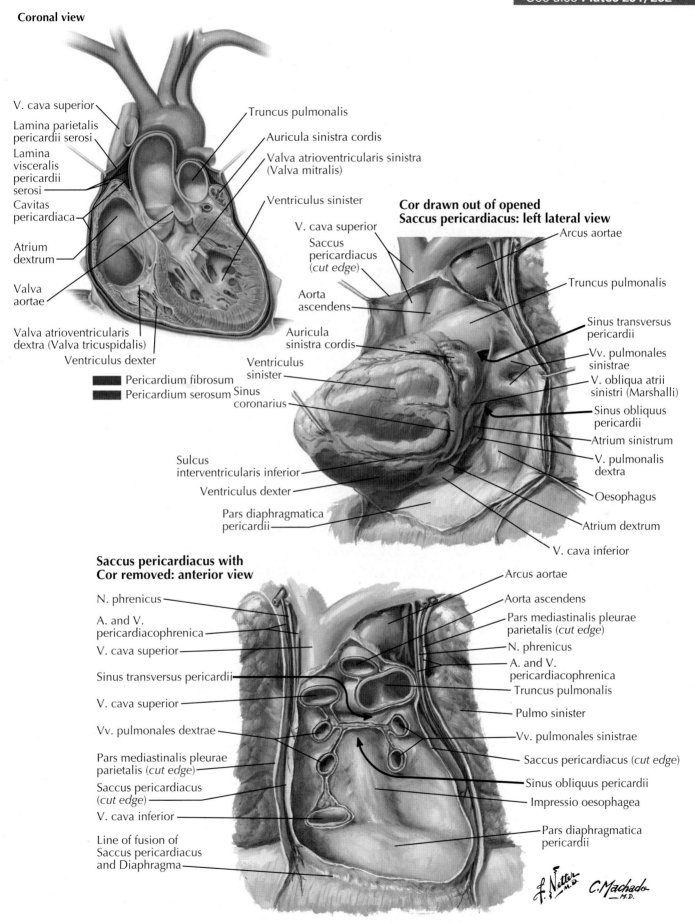

Coronal view

V. cava superior

Lamina parietalis pericardii serosi

Lamina visceralis pericardii serosi

Cavitas pericardiaca

Atrium dextrum

Valva aortae

Valva atrioventricularis dextra (Valva tricuspidalis)

Ventriculus dexter

Truncus pulmonalis

Auricula sinistra cordis

Valva atrioventricularis sinistra (Valva mitralis)

Ventriculus sinister

Pericardium fibrosum

Pericardium serosum

Cor drawn out of opened Saccus pericardiacus: left lateral view

V. cava superior

Saccus pericardiacus (*cut edge*)

Aorta ascendens

Auricula sinistra cordis

Ventriculus sinister

Sinus coronarius

Sulcus interventricularis inferior

Ventriculus dexter

Pars diaphragmatica pericardii

Arcus aortae

Truncus pulmonalis

Sinus transversus pericardii

Vv. pulmonales sinistrae

V. obliqua atrii sinistri (Marshalli)

Sinus obliquus pericardii

Atrium sinistrum

V. pulmonalis dextra

Oesophagus

Atrium dextrum

V. cava inferior

Saccus pericardiacus with Cor removed: anterior view

N. phrenicus

A. and V. pericardiacophrenica

V. cava superior

Sinus transversus pericardii

V. cava superior

Vv. pulmonales dextrae

Pars mediastinalis pleurae parietalis (*cut edge*)

Saccus pericardiacus (*cut edge*)

V. cava inferior

Line of fusion of Saccus pericardiacus and Diaphragma

Arcus aortae

Aorta ascendens

Pars mediastinalis pleurae parietalis (*cut edge*)

N. phrenicus

A. and V. pericardiacophrenica

Truncus pulmonalis

Pulmo sinister

Vv. pulmonales sinistrae

Saccus pericardiacus (*cut edge*)

Sinus obliquus pericardii

Impressio oesophagea

Pars diaphragmatica pericardii

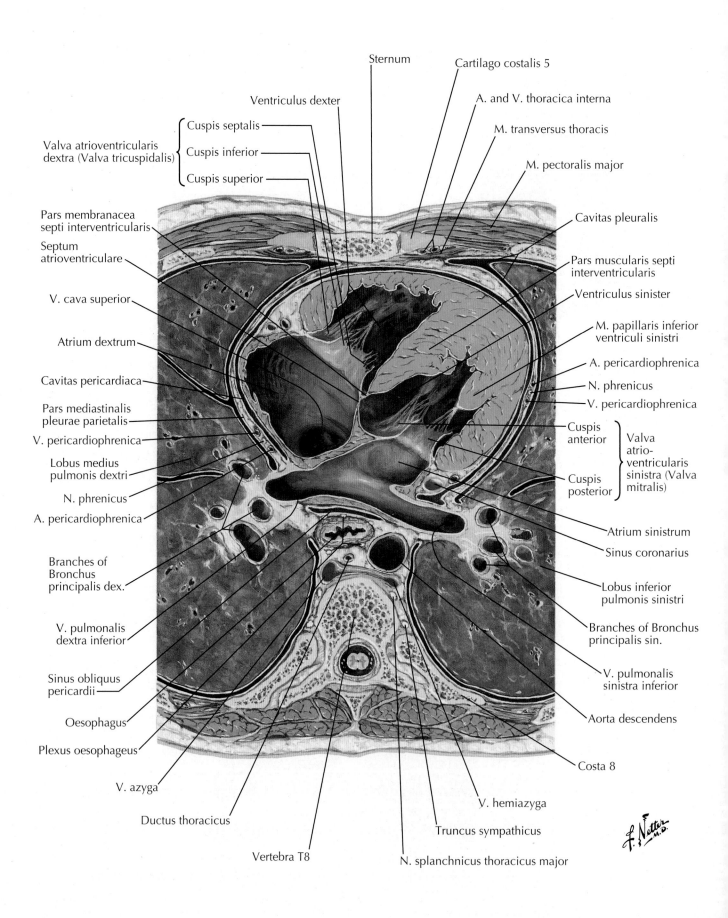

Sternum

Cartilago costalis 5

Ventriculus dexter

A. and V. thoracica interna

M. transversus thoracis

M. pectoralis major

Valva atrioventricularis dextra (Valva tricuspidalis) { Cuspis septalis

Cuspis inferior

Cuspis superior

Pars membranacea septi interventricularis

Septum atrioventriculare

V. cava superior

Atrium dextrum

Cavitas pericardiaca

Pars mediastinalis pleurae parietalis

V. pericardiophrenica

Lobus medius pulmonis dextri

N. phrenicus

A. pericardiophrenica

Branches of Bronchus principalis dex.

V. pulmonalis dextra inferior

Sinus obliquus pericardii

Oesophagus

Plexus oesophageus

V. azyga

Ductus thoracicus

Vertebra T8

Cavitas pleuralis

Pars muscularis septi interventricularis

Ventriculus sinister

M. papillaris inferior ventriculi sinistri

A. pericardiophrenica

N. phrenicus

V. pericardiophrenica

Cuspis anterior

Cuspis posterior

Valva atrio-ventricularis sinistra (Valva mitralis)

Atrium sinistrum

Sinus coronarius

Lobus inferior pulmonis sinistri

Branches of Bronchus principalis sin.

V. pulmonalis sinistra inferior

Aorta descendens

Costa 8

V. hemiazyga

Truncus sympathicus

N. splanchnicus thoracicus major

Plate 237

Cor

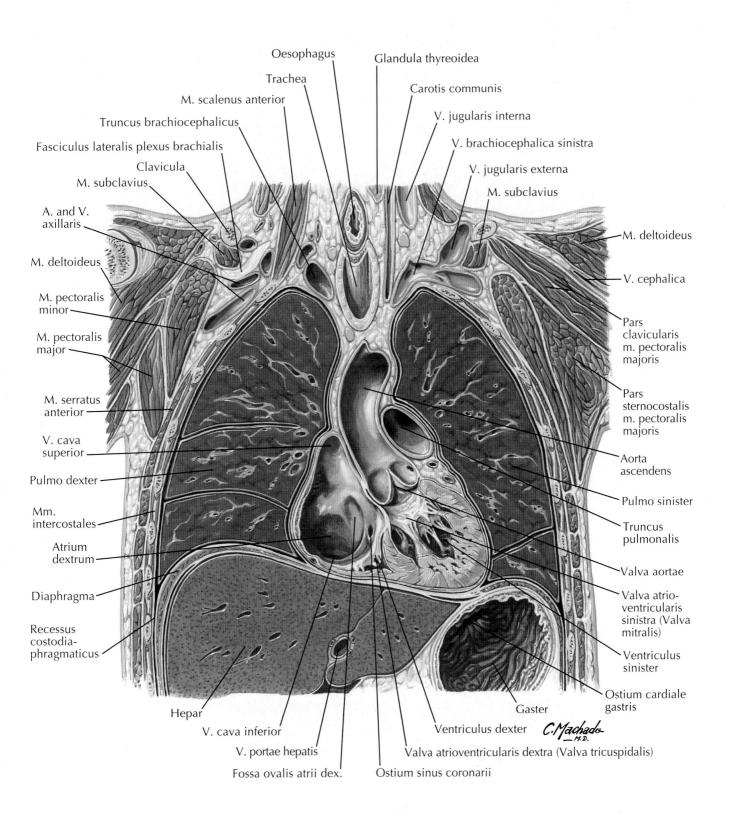

Oesophagus

Trachea

M. scalenus anterior

Truncus brachiocephalicus

Fasciculus lateralis plexus brachialis

Clavicula

M. subclavius

A. and V. axillaris

M. deltoideus

M. pectoralis minor

M. pectoralis major

M. serratus anterior

V. cava superior

Pulmo dexter

Mm. intercostales

Atrium dextrum

Diaphragma

Recessus costodia- phragmaticus

Glandula thyreoidea

Carotis communis

V. jugularis interna

V. brachiocephalica sinistra

V. jugularis externa

M. subclavius

M. deltoideus

V. cephalica

Pars clavicularis m. pectoralis majoris

Pars sternocostalis m. pectoralis majoris

Aorta ascendens

Pulmo sinister

Truncus pulmonalis

Valva aortae

Valva atrio- ventricularis sinistra (Valva mitralis)

Ventriculus sinister

Ostium cardiale gastris

Hepar

V. cava inferior

V. portae hepatis

Fossa ovalis atrii dex.

Ostium sinus coronarii

Ventriculus dexter

Gaster

Valva atrioventricularis dextra (Valva tricuspidalis)

C. Machado — M.D.

Facies sternocostalis

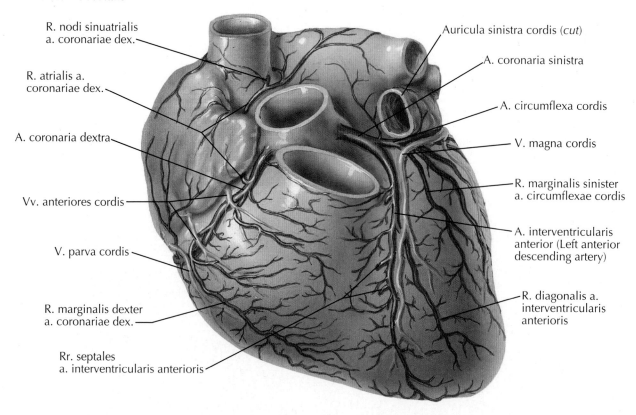

R. nodi sinuatrialis
a. coronariae dex.

R. atrialis a.
coronariae dex.

A. coronaria dextra

Vv. anteriores cordis

V. parva cordis

R. marginalis dexter
a. coronariae dex.

Rr. septales
a. interventricularis anterioris

Auricula sinistra cordis (*cut*)

A. coronaria sinistra

A. circumflexa cordis

V. magna cordis

R. marginalis sinister
a. circumflexae cordis

A. interventricularis
anterior (Left anterior
descending artery)

R. diagonalis a.
interventricularis
anterioris

Facies diaphragmatica

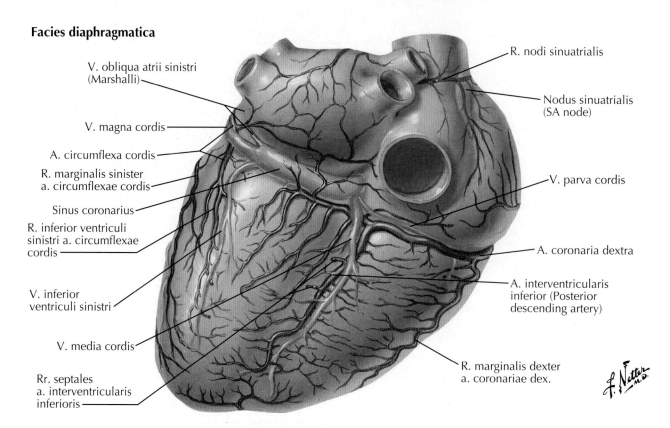

V. obliqua atrii sinistri
(Marshalli)

V. magna cordis

A. circumflexa cordis

R. marginalis sinister
a. circumflexae cordis

Sinus coronarius

R. inferior ventriculi
sinistri a. circumflexae
cordis

V. inferior
ventriculi sinistri

V. media cordis

Rr. septales
a. interventricularis
inferioris

R. nodi sinuatrialis

Nodus sinuatrialis
(SA node)

V. parva cordis

A. coronaria dextra

A. interventricularis
inferior (Posterior
descending artery)

R. marginalis dexter
a. coronariae dex.

Plate 239

Cor

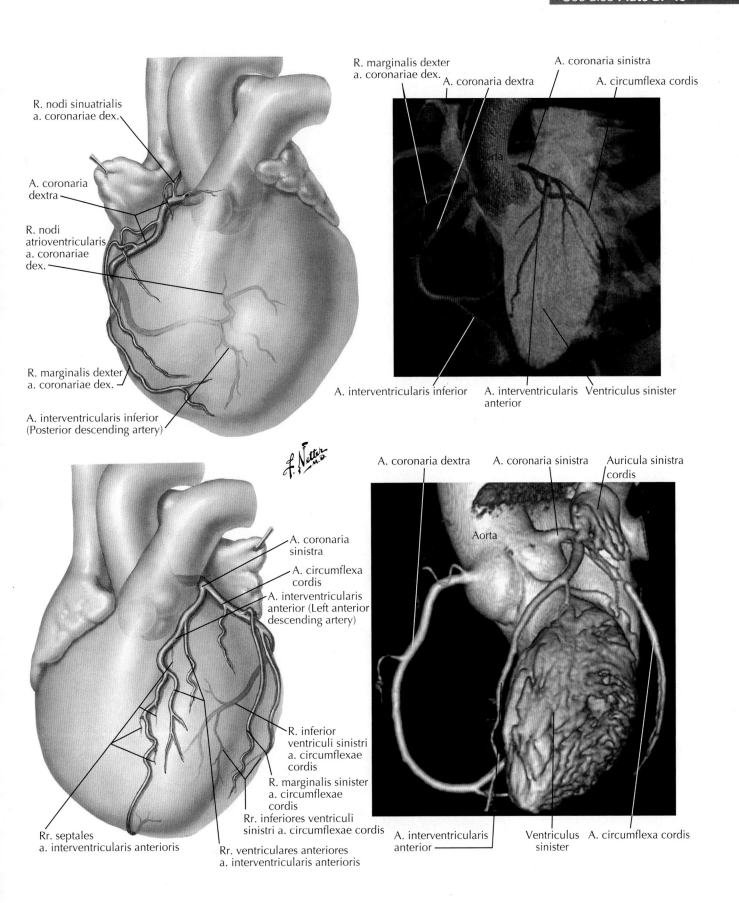

R. nodi sinuatrialis
a. coronariae dex.

A. coronaria
dextra

R. nodi
atrioventricularis
a. coronariae
dex.

R. marginalis dexter
a. coronariae dex.

A. interventricularis inferior
(Posterior descending artery)

R. marginalis dexter
a. coronariae dex.

A. coronaria dextra

A. coronaria sinistra

A. circumflexa cordis

Aorta

A. interventricularis inferior

A. interventricularis
anterior

Ventriculus sinister

A. coronaria
sinistra

A. circumflexa
cordis

A. interventricularis
anterior (Left anterior
descending artery)

R. inferior
ventriculi sinistri
a. circumflexae
cordis

R. marginalis sinister
a. circumflexae
cordis

Rr. inferiores ventriculi
sinistri a. circumflexae cordis

Rr. ventriculares anteriores
a. interventricularis anterioris

Rr. septales
a. interventricularis anterioris

A. coronaria dextra

A. coronaria sinistra

Auricula sinistra
cordis

Aorta

A. interventricularis
anterior

Ventriculus
sinister

A. circumflexa cordis

Cor

Plate 240

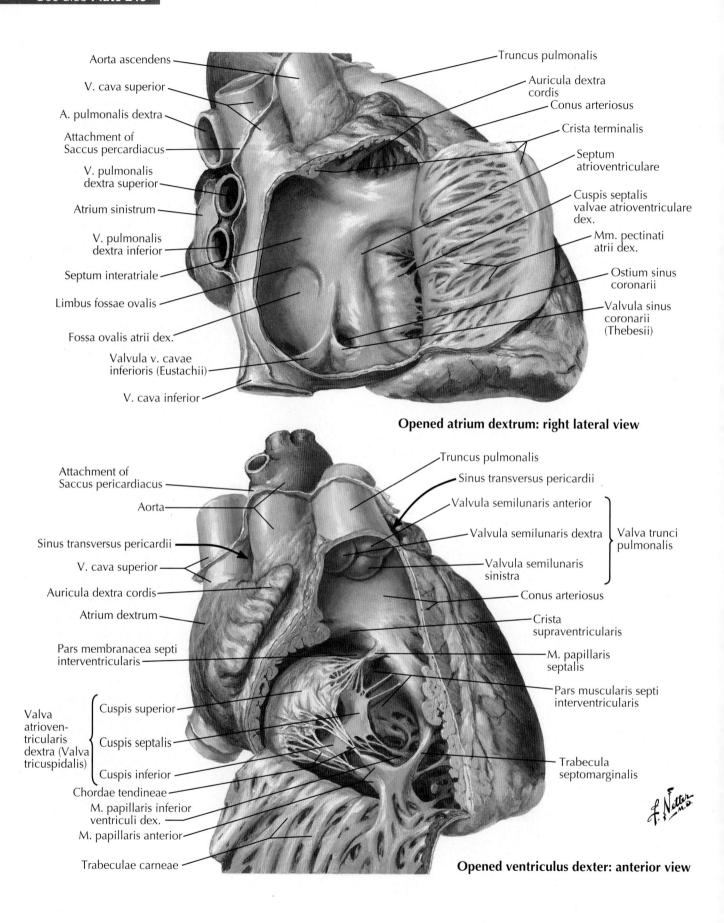

Aorta ascendens

V. cava superior

A. pulmonalis dextra

Attachment of
Saccus percardiacus

V. pulmonalis
dextra superior

Atrium sinistrum

V. pulmonalis
dextra inferior

Septum interatriale

Limbus fossae ovalis

Fossa ovalis atrii dex.

Valvula v. cavae
inferioris (Eustachii)

V. cava inferior

Truncus pulmonalis

Auricula dextra
cordis

Conus arteriosus

Crista terminalis

Septum
atrioventriculare

Cuspis septalis
valvae atrioventriculare
dex.

Mm. pectinati
atrii dex.

Ostium sinus
coronarii

Valvula sinus
coronarii
(Thebesii)

Opened atrium dextrum: right lateral view

Attachment of
Saccus pericardiacus

Aorta

Sinus transversus pericardii

V. cava superior

Auricula dextra cordis

Atrium dextrum

Pars membranacea septi
interventricularis

Valva
atrioven-
tricularis
dextra (Valva
tricuspidalis)

Cuspis superior

Cuspis septalis

Cuspis inferior

Chordae tendineae

M. papillaris inferior
ventriculi dex.

M. papillaris anterior

Trabeculae carneae

Truncus pulmonalis

Sinus transversus pericardii

Valvula semilunaris anterior

Valvula semilunaris dextra

Valvula semilunaris
sinistra

Valva trunci
pulmonalis

Conus arteriosus

Crista
supraventricularis

M. papillaris
septalis

Pars muscularis septi
interventricularis

Trabecula
septomarginalis

Opened ventriculus dexter: anterior view

Plate 241

Cor

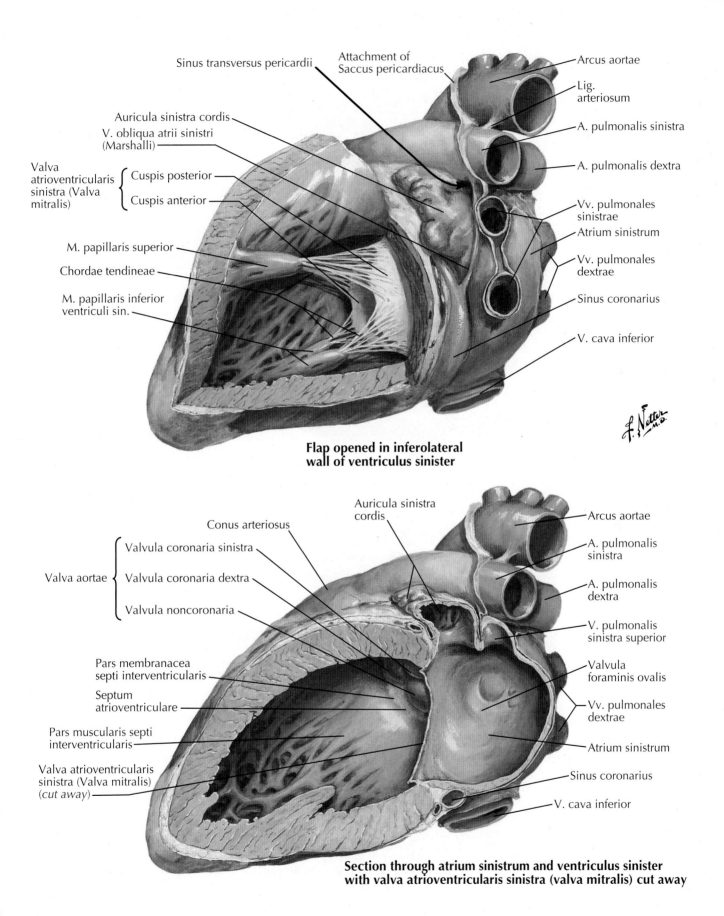

Sinus transversus pericardii

Attachment of Saccus pericardiacus

Arcus aortae

Lig. arteriosum

Auricula sinistra cordis

V. obliqua atrii sinistri (Marshalli)

A. pulmonalis sinistra

A. pulmonalis dextra

Valva atrioventricularis sinistra (Valva mitralis)
  { Cuspis posterior
    Cuspis anterior }

Vv. pulmonales sinistrae

Atrium sinistrum

Vv. pulmonales dextrae

M. papillaris superior

Chordae tendineae

Sinus coronarius

M. papillaris inferior ventriculi sin.

V. cava inferior

Flap opened in inferolateral wall of ventriculus sinister

Auricula sinistra cordis

Conus arteriosus

Arcus aortae

Valva aortae
  { Valvula coronaria sinistra
    Valvula coronaria dextra
    Valvula noncoronaria }

A. pulmonalis sinistra

A. pulmonalis dextra

Pars membranacea septi interventricularis

V. pulmonalis sinistra superior

Septum atrioventriculare

Valvula foraminis ovalis

Pars muscularis septi interventricularis

Vv. pulmonales dextrae

Valva atrioventricularis sinistra (Valva mitralis) (cut away)

Atrium sinistrum

Sinus coronarius

V. cava inferior

Section through atrium sinistrum and ventriculus sinister with valva atrioventricularis sinistra (valva mitralis) cut away

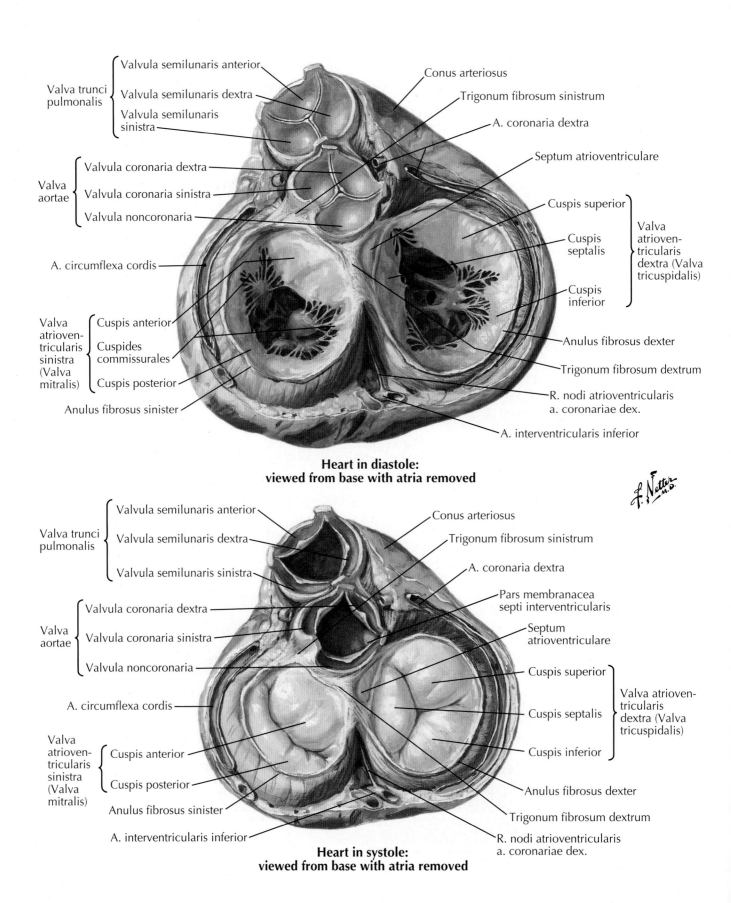

Valva trunci pulmonalis
- Valvula semilunaris anterior
- Valvula semilunaris dextra
- Valvula semilunaris sinistra

Valva aortae
- Valvula coronaria dextra
- Valvula coronaria sinistra
- Valvula noncoronaria

A. circumflexa cordis

Valva atrioventricularis sinistra (Valva mitralis)
- Cuspis anterior
- Cuspides commissurales
- Cuspis posterior

Anulus fibrosus sinister

Conus arteriosus

Trigonum fibrosum sinistrum

A. coronaria dextra

Septum atrioventriculare

Valva atrioventricularis dextra (Valva tricuspidalis)
- Cuspis superior
- Cuspis septalis
- Cuspis inferior

Anulus fibrosus dexter

Trigonum fibrosum dextrum

R. nodi atrioventricularis a. coronariae dex.

A. interventricularis inferior

Heart in diastole: viewed from base with atria removed

Valva trunci pulmonalis
- Valvula semilunaris anterior
- Valvula semilunaris dextra
- Valvula semilunaris sinistra

Valva aortae
- Valvula coronaria dextra
- Valvula coronaria sinistra
- Valvula noncoronaria

A. circumflexa cordis

Valva atrioventricularis sinistra (Valva mitralis)
- Cuspis anterior
- Cuspis posterior

Anulus fibrosus sinister

A. interventricularis inferior

Conus arteriosus

Trigonum fibrosum sinistrum

A. coronaria dextra

Pars membranacea septi interventricularis

Septum atrioventriculare

Valva atrioventricularis dextra (Valva tricuspidalis)
- Cuspis superior
- Cuspis septalis
- Cuspis inferior

Anulus fibrosus dexter

Trigonum fibrosum dextrum

R. nodi atrioventricularis a. coronariae dex.

Heart in systole: viewed from base with atria removed

Plate 243

Cor

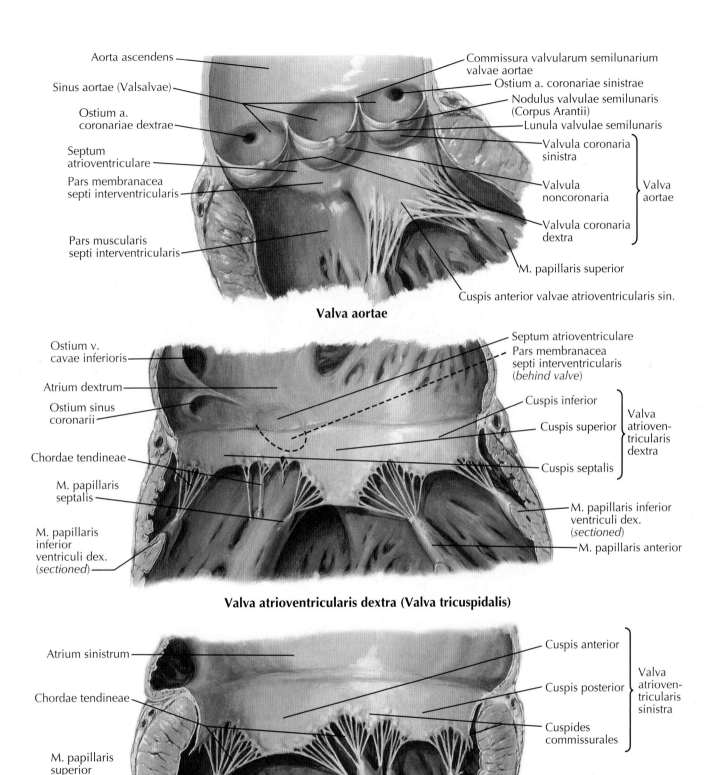

Aorta ascendens

Sinus aortae (Valsalvae)

Ostium a. coronariae dextrae

Septum atrioventriculare

Pars membranacea septi interventricularis

Pars muscularis septi interventricularis

Commissura valvularum semilunarium valvae aortae

Ostium a. coronariae sinistrae

Nodulus valvulae semilunaris (Corpus Arantii)

Lunula valvulae semilunaris

Valvula coronaria sinistra

Valvula noncoronaria

Valvula coronaria dextra

} Valva aortae

M. papillaris superior

Cuspis anterior valvae atrioventricularis sin.

Valva aortae

Ostium v. cavae inferioris

Atrium dextrum

Ostium sinus coronarii

Chordae tendineae

M. papillaris septalis

M. papillaris inferior ventriculi dex. (*sectioned*)

Septum atrioventriculare

Pars membranacea septi interventricularis (*behind valve*)

Cuspis inferior

Cuspis superior

Cuspis septalis

} Valva atrioventricularis dextra

M. papillaris inferior ventriculi dex. (*sectioned*)

M. papillaris anterior

Valva atrioventricularis dextra (Valva tricuspidalis)

Atrium sinistrum

Chordae tendineae

M. papillaris superior (*sectioned*)

M. papillaris inferior ventriculi sin.

Cuspis anterior

Cuspis posterior

Cuspides commissurales

} Valva atrioventricularis sinistra

M. papillaris superior (*sectioned*)

Valva atrioventricularis sinistra (Valva mitralis)

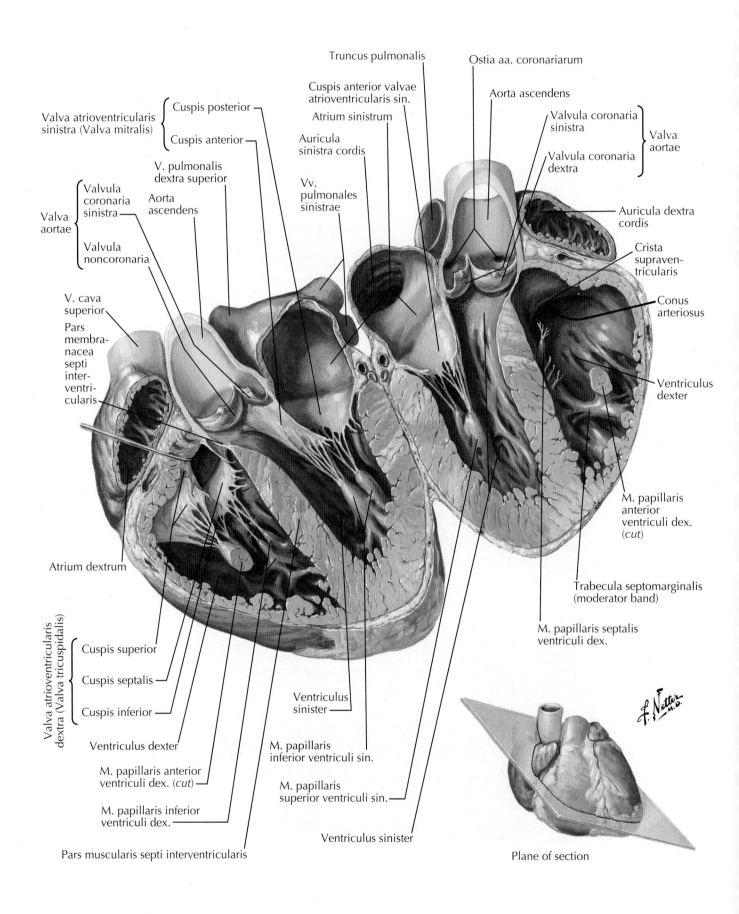

Truncus pulmonalis

Ostia aa. coronariarum

Cuspis anterior valvae atrioventricularis sin.

Aorta ascendens

Atrium sinistrum

Valva atrioventricularis sinistra (Valva mitralis)
{
Cuspis posterior
Cuspis anterior

Valvula coronaria sinistra

Valvula coronaria dextra
} Valva aortae

Auricula sinistra cordis

V. pulmonalis dextra superior

Vv. pulmonales sinistrae

Auricula dextra cordis

Valva aortae
{
Valvula coronaria sinistra

Aorta ascendens

Valvula noncoronaria
}

Crista supraventricularis

Conus arteriosus

V. cava superior

Ventriculus dexter

Pars membranacea septi interventricularis

M. papillaris anterior ventriculi dex. (cut)

Atrium dextrum

Trabecula septomarginalis (moderator band)

M. papillaris septalis ventriculi dex.

Valva atrioventricularis dextra (Valva tricuspidalis)
{
Cuspis superior
Cuspis septalis
Cuspis inferior
}

Ventriculus sinister

Ventriculus dexter

M. papillaris inferior ventriculi sin.

M. papillaris anterior ventriculi dex. (cut)

M. papillaris superior ventriculi sin.

M. papillaris inferior ventriculi dex.

Ventriculus sinister

Pars muscularis septi interventricularis

Plane of section

Plate 245

Cor

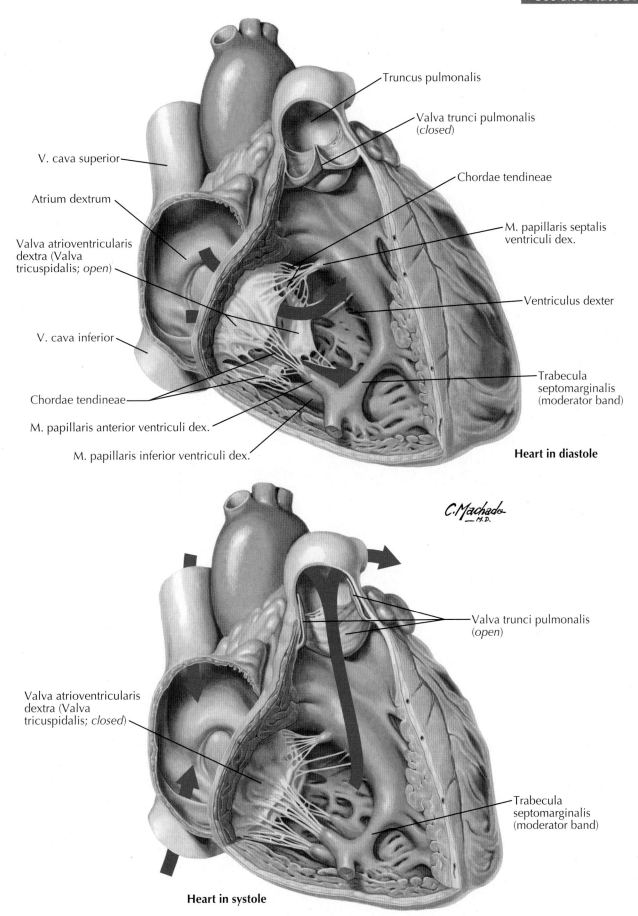

Truncus pulmonalis

Valva trunci pulmonalis (*closed*)

V. cava superior

Chordae tendineae

Atrium dextrum

M. papillaris septalis ventriculi dex.

Valva atrioventricularis dextra (Valva tricuspidalis; *open*)

Ventriculus dexter

V. cava inferior

Chordae tendineae

Trabecula septomarginalis (moderator band)

M. papillaris anterior ventriculi dex.

M. papillaris inferior ventriculi dex.

Heart in diastole

C. Machado M.D.

Valva trunci pulmonalis (*open*)

Valva atrioventricularis dextra (Valva tricuspidalis; *closed*)

Trabecula septomarginalis (moderator band)

Heart in systole

Prenatal circulation

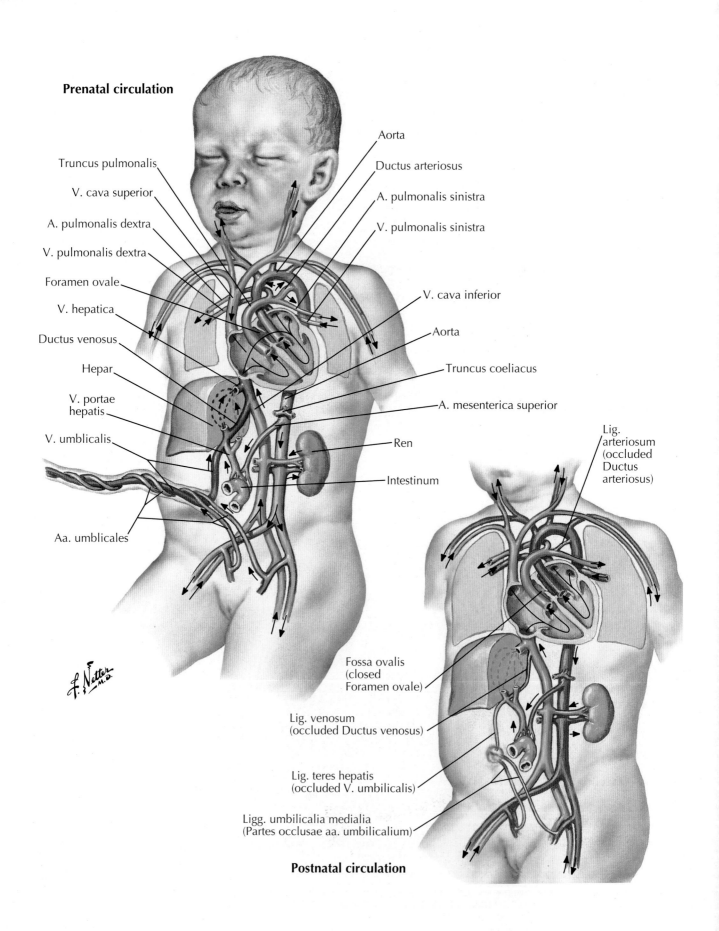

Truncus pulmonalis

V. cava superior

A. pulmonalis dextra

V. pulmonalis dextra

Foramen ovale

V. hepatica

Ductus venosus

Hepar

V. portae hepatis

V. umblicalis

Aa. umblicales

Aorta

Ductus arteriosus

A. pulmonalis sinistra

V. pulmonalis sinistra

V. cava inferior

Aorta

Truncus coeliacus

A. mesenterica superior

Ren

Intestinum

Lig. arteriosum (occluded Ductus arteriosus)

Fossa ovalis (closed Foramen ovale)

Lig. venosum (occluded Ductus venosus)

Lig. teres hepatis (occluded V. umbilicalis)

Ligg. umbilicalia medialia (Partes occlusae aa. umbilicalium)

Postnatal circulation

Plate 247

Cor

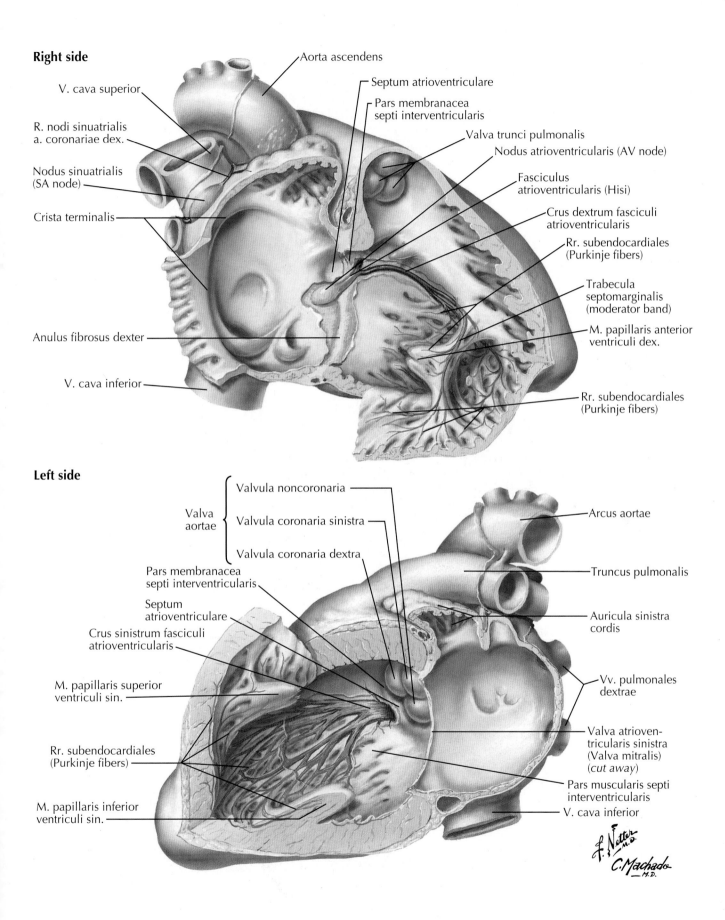

Right side

Aorta ascendens

V. cava superior

Septum atrioventriculare

Pars membranacea
septi interventricularis

R. nodi sinuatrialis
a. coronariae dex.

Valva trunci pulmonalis

Nodus atrioventricularis (AV node)

Nodus sinuatrialis
(SA node)

Fasciculus
atrioventricularis (Hisi)

Crista terminalis

Crus dextrum fasciculi
atrioventricularis

Rr. subendocardiales
(Purkinje fibers)

Trabecula
septomarginalis
(moderator band)

Anulus fibrosus dexter

M. papillaris anterior
ventriculi dex.

V. cava inferior

Rr. subendocardiales
(Purkinje fibers)

Left side

Valvula noncoronaria

Valva
aortae

Valvula coronaria sinistra

Valvula coronaria dextra

Arcus aortae

Truncus pulmonalis

Pars membranacea
septi interventricularis

Septum
atrioventriculare

Crus sinistrum fasciculi
atrioventricularis

Auricula sinistra
cordis

M. papillaris superior
ventriculi sin.

Vv. pulmonales
dextrae

Valva atrioven-
tricularis sinistra
(Valva mitralis)
(*cut away*)

Rr. subendocardiales
(Purkinje fibers)

Pars muscularis septi
interventricularis

M. papillaris inferior
ventriculi sin.

V. cava inferior

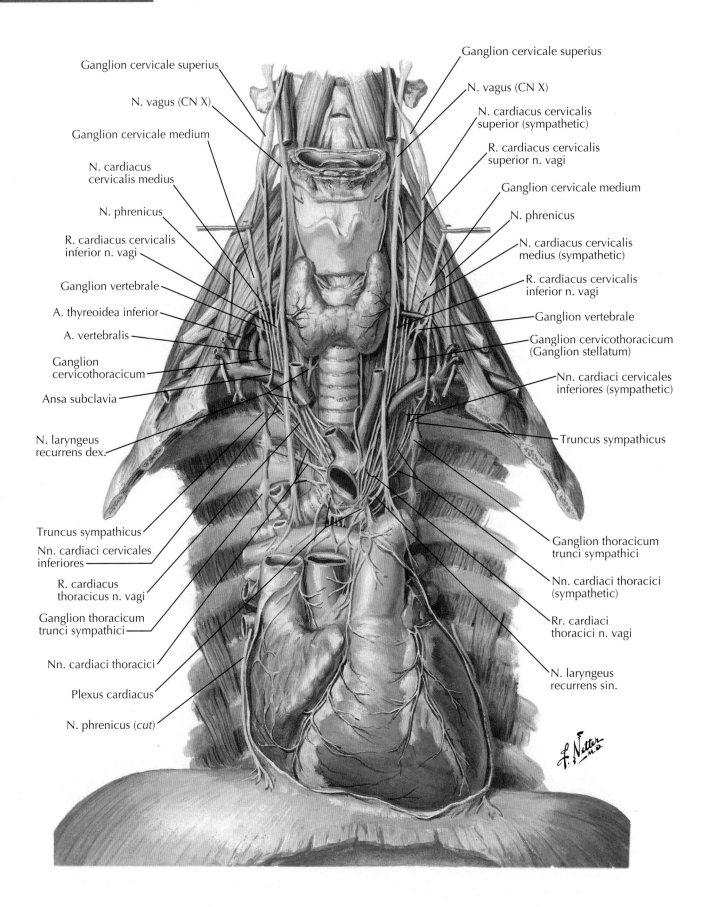

Ganglion cervicale superius

N. vagus (CN X)

Ganglion cervicale medium

N. cardiacus cervicalis medius

N. phrenicus

R. cardiacus cervicalis inferior n. vagi

Ganglion vertebrale

A. thyreoidea inferior

A. vertebralis

Ganglion cervicothoracicum

Ansa subclavia

N. laryngeus recurrens dex.

Truncus sympathicus

Nn. cardiaci cervicales inferiores

R. cardiacus thoracicus n. vagi

Ganglion thoracicum trunci sympathici

Nn. cardiaci thoracici

Plexus cardiacus

N. phrenicus (*cut*)

Ganglion cervicale superius

N. vagus (CN X)

N. cardiacus cervicalis superior (sympathetic)

R. cardiacus cervicalis superior n. vagi

Ganglion cervicale medium

N. phrenicus

N. cardiacus cervicalis medius (sympathetic)

R. cardiacus cervicalis inferior n. vagi

Ganglion vertebrale

Ganglion cervicothoracicum (Ganglion stellatum)

Nn. cardiaci cervicales inferiores (sympathetic)

Truncus sympathicus

Ganglion thoracicum trunci sympathici

Nn. cardiaci thoracici (sympathetic)

Rr. cardiaci thoracici n. vagi

N. laryngeus recurrens sin.

Plate 249

Cor

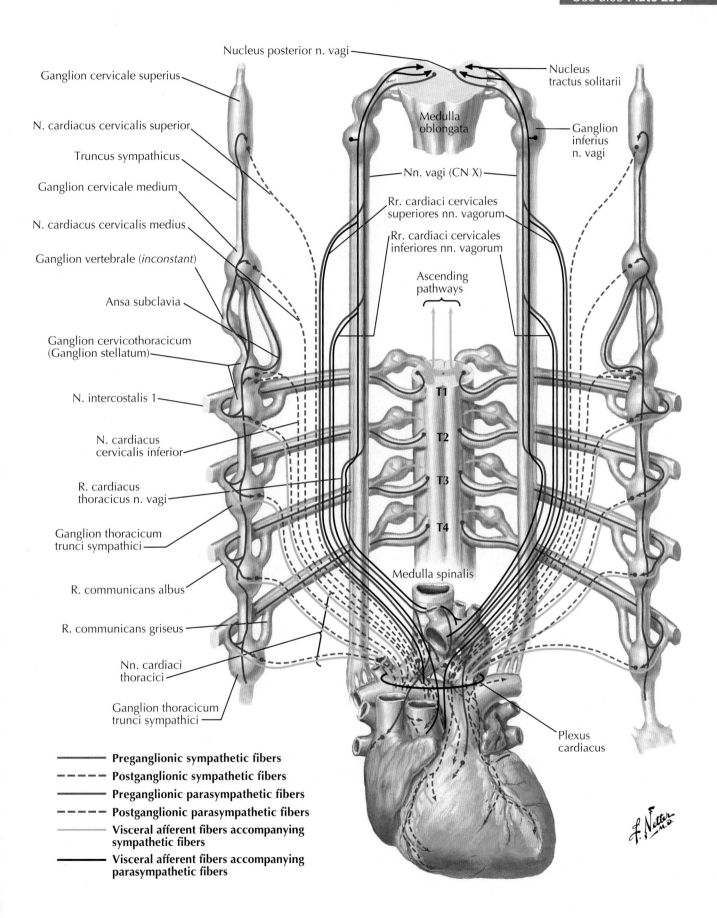

Nucleus posterior n. vagi

Ganglion cervicale superius

N. cardiacus cervicalis superior

Truncus sympathicus

Ganglion cervicale medium

N. cardiacus cervicalis medius

Ganglion vertebrale (*inconstant*)

Ansa subclavia

Ganglion cervicothoracicum
(Ganglion stellatum)

N. intercostalis 1

N. cardiacus
cervicalis inferior

R. cardiacus
thoracicus n. vagi

Ganglion thoracicum
trunci sympathici

R. communicans albus

R. communicans griseus

Nn. cardiaci
thoracici

Ganglion thoracicum
trunci sympathici

Nucleus
tractus solitarii

Medulla
oblongata

Ganglion
inferius
n. vagi

Nn. vagi (CN X)

Rr. cardiaci cervicales
superiores nn. vagorum

Rr. cardiaci cervicales
inferiores nn. vagorum

Ascending
pathways

T1

T2

T3

T4

Medulla spinalis

Plexus
cardiacus

——————— **Preganglionic sympathetic fibers**
– – – – – – – **Postganglionic sympathetic fibers**
——————— **Preganglionic parasympathetic fibers**
– – – – – – – **Postganglionic parasympathetic fibers**
——————— **Visceral afferent fibers accompanying
sympathetic fibers**
——————— **Visceral afferent fibers accompanying
parasympathetic fibers**

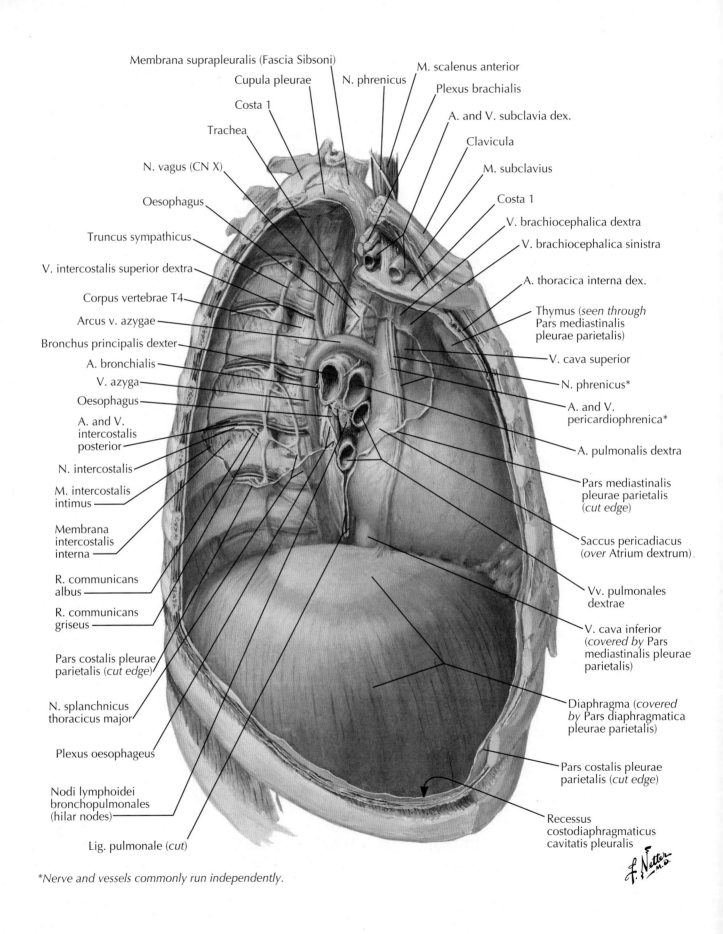

Membrana suprapleuralis (Fascia Sibsoni)

Cupula pleurae

N. phrenicus

M. scalenus anterior

Plexus brachialis

Costa 1

A. and V. subclavia dex.

Trachea

Clavicula

N. vagus (CN X)

M. subclavius

Oesophagus

Costa 1

Truncus sympathicus

V. brachiocephalica dextra

V. intercostalis superior dextra

V. brachiocephalica sinistra

Corpus vertebrae T4

A. thoracica interna dex.

Arcus v. azygae

Thymus (*seen through* Pars mediastinalis pleurae parietalis)

Bronchus principalis dexter

A. bronchialis

V. cava superior

V. azyga

N. phrenicus*

Oesophagus

A. and V. pericardiophrenica*

A. and V. intercostalis posterior

A. pulmonalis dextra

N. intercostalis

M. intercostalis intimus

Pars mediastinalis pleurae parietalis (*cut edge*)

Membrana intercostalis interna

Saccus pericadiacus (*over* Atrium dextrum)

R. communicans albus

Vv. pulmonales dextrae

R. communicans griseus

V. cava inferior (*covered by* Pars mediastinalis pleurae parietalis)

Pars costalis pleurae parietalis (*cut edge*)

N. splanchnicus thoracicus major

Diaphragma (*covered by* Pars diaphragmatica pleurae parietalis)

Plexus oesophageus

Pars costalis pleurae parietalis (*cut edge*)

Nodi lymphoidei bronchopulmonales (hilar nodes)

Recessus costodiaphragmaticus cavitatis pleuralis

Lig. pulmonale (*cut*)

Nerve and vessels commonly run independently.

Plate 251

Mediastinum

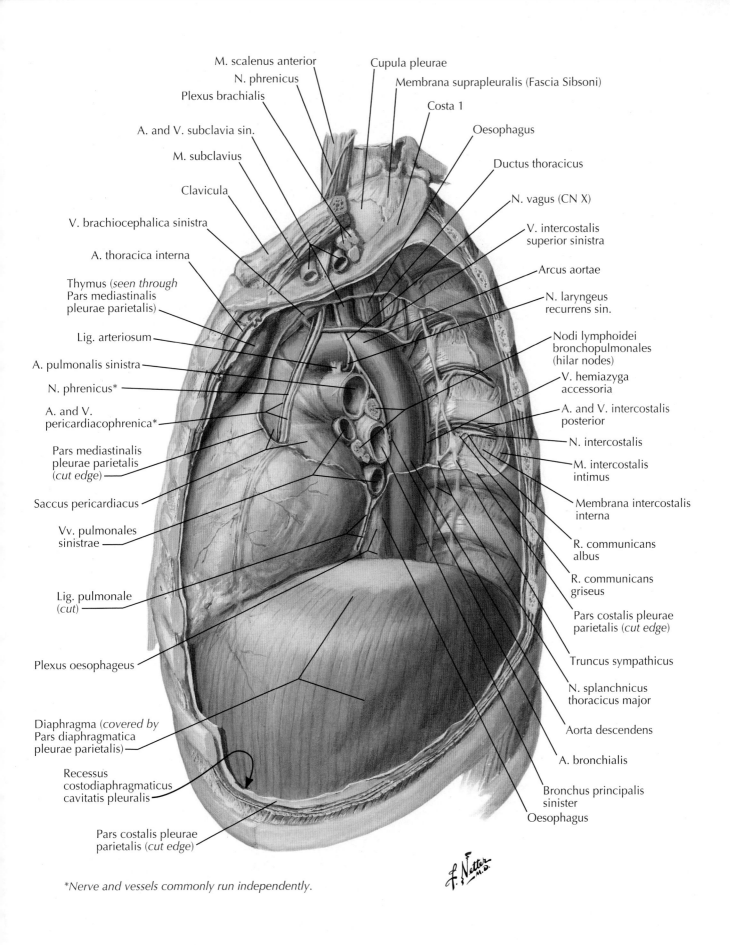

M. scalenus anterior

N. phrenicus

Plexus brachialis

A. and V. subclavia sin.

M. subclavius

Clavicula

V. brachiocephalica sinistra

A. thoracica interna

Thymus (*seen through Pars mediastinalis pleurae parietalis*)

Lig. arteriosum

A. pulmonalis sinistra

N. phrenicus*

A. and V. pericardiacophrenica*

Pars mediastinalis pleurae parietalis (*cut edge*)

Saccus pericardiacus

Vv. pulmonales sinistrae

Lig. pulmonale (*cut*)

Plexus oesophageus

Diaphragma (*covered by Pars diaphragmatica pleurae parietalis*)

Recessus costodiaphragmaticus cavitatis pleuralis

Pars costalis pleurae parietalis (*cut edge*)

Cupula pleurae

Membrana suprapleuralis (Fascia Sibsoni)

Costa 1

Oesophagus

Ductus thoracicus

N. vagus (CN X)

V. intercostalis superior sinistra

Arcus aortae

N. laryngeus recurrens sin.

Nodi lymphoidei bronchopulmonales (hilar nodes)

V. hemiazyga accessoria

A. and V. intercostalis posterior

N. intercostalis

M. intercostalis intimus

Membrana intercostalis interna

R. communicans albus

R. communicans griseus

Pars costalis pleurae parietalis (*cut edge*)

Truncus sympathicus

N. splanchnicus thoracicus major

Aorta descendens

A. bronchialis

Bronchus principalis sinister

Oesophagus

*Nerve and vessels commonly run independently.

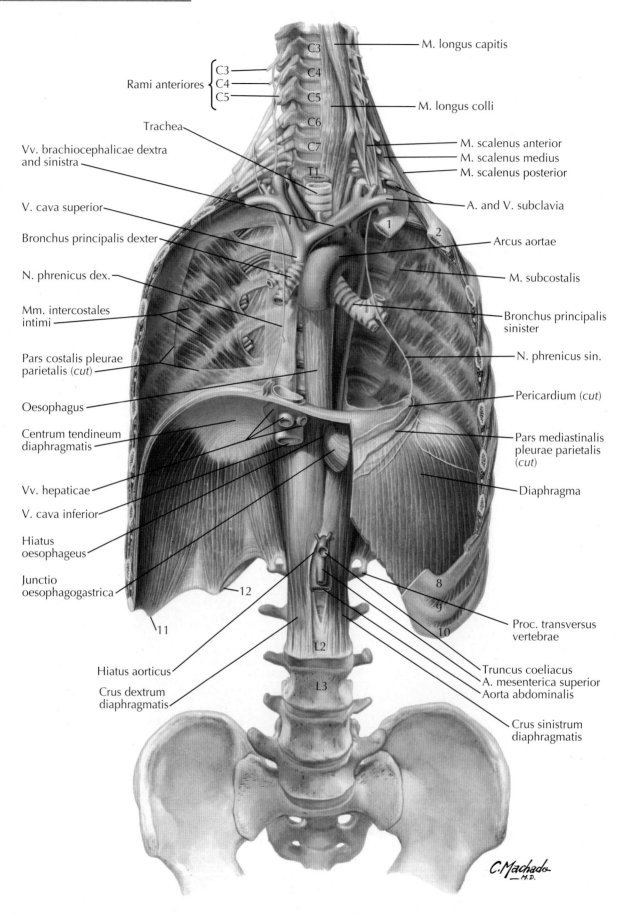

M. longus capitis

C3

Rami anteriores { C3 / C4 / C5

C4

C5

C6

C7

T1

M. longus colli

Trachea

M. scalenus anterior
M. scalenus medius
M. scalenus posterior

Vv. brachiocephalicae dextra and sinistra

A. and V. subclavia

1   2

Arcus aortae

V. cava superior

Bronchus principalis dexter

M. subcostalis

N. phrenicus dex.

Bronchus principalis sinister

Mm. intercostales intimi

N. phrenicus sin.

Pars costalis pleurae parietalis (cut)

Pericardium (cut)

Oesophagus

Centrum tendineum diaphragmatis

Pars mediastinalis pleurae parietalis (cut)

Diaphragma

Vv. hepaticae

V. cava inferior

Hiatus oesophageus

Junctio oesophagogastrica

12

8

9

11

10

Proc. transversus vertebrae

Truncus coeliacus

Hiatus aorticus

A. mesenterica superior
Aorta abdominalis

Crus dextrum diaphragmatis

Crus sinistrum diaphragmatis

L2

L3

Plate 253

Mediastinum

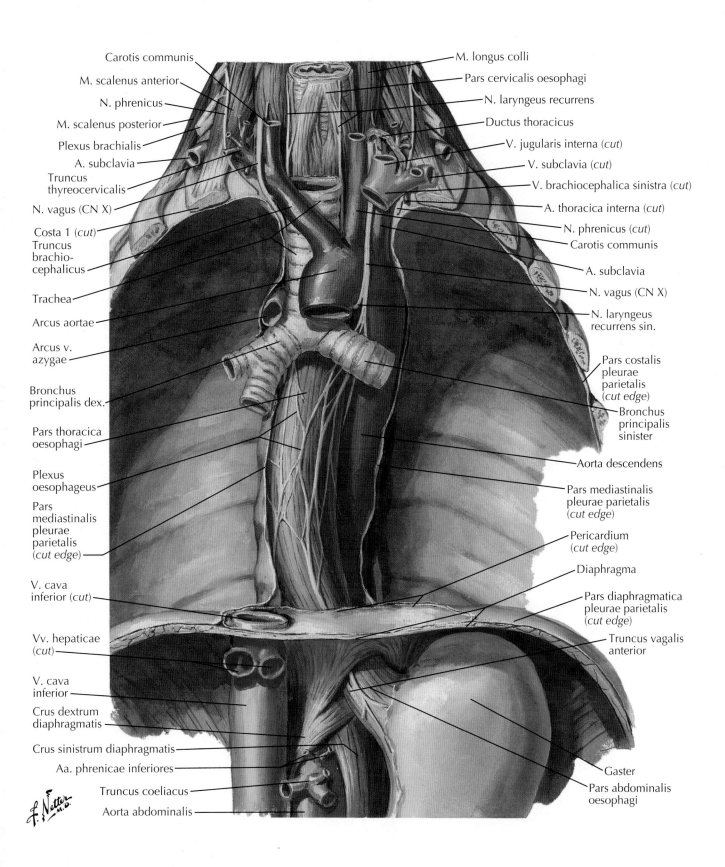

Carotis communis

M. scalenus anterior

N. phrenicus

M. scalenus posterior

Plexus brachialis

A. subclavia

Truncus thyreocervicalis

N. vagus (CN X)

Costa 1 (*cut*)

Truncus brachio-cephalicus

Trachea

Arcus aortae

Arcus v. azygae

Bronchus principalis dex.

Pars thoracica oesophagi

Plexus oesophageus

Pars mediastinalis pleurae parietalis (*cut edge*)

V. cava inferior (*cut*)

Vv. hepaticae (*cut*)

V. cava inferior

Crus dextrum diaphragmatis

Crus sinistrum diaphragmatis

Aa. phrenicae inferiores

Truncus coeliacus

Aorta abdominalis

M. longus colli

Pars cervicalis oesophagi

N. laryngeus recurrens

Ductus thoracicus

V. jugularis interna (*cut*)

V. subclavia (*cut*)

V. brachiocephalica sinistra (*cut*)

A. thoracica interna (*cut*)

N. phrenicus (*cut*)

Carotis communis

A. subclavia

N. vagus (CN X)

N. laryngeus recurrens sin.

Pars costalis pleurae parietalis (*cut edge*)

Bronchus principalis sinister

Aorta descendens

Pars mediastinalis pleurae parietalis (*cut edge*)

Pericardium (*cut edge*)

Diaphragma

Pars diaphragmatica pleurae parietalis (*cut edge*)

Truncus vagalis anterior

Gaster

Pars abdominalis oesophagi

f. Netter M.D.

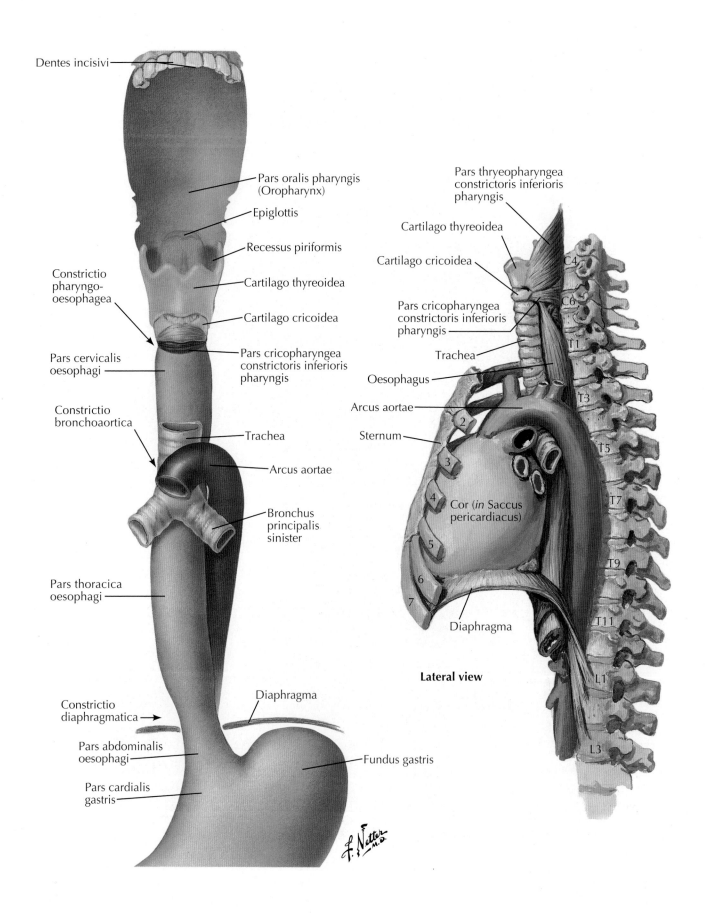

Dentes incisivi

Pars oralis pharyngis
(Oropharynx)

Epiglottis

Recessus piriformis

Constrictio
pharyngo-
oesophagea

Cartilago thyreoidea

Cartilago cricoidea

Pars cervicalis
oesophagi

Pars cricopharyngea
constrictoris inferioris
pharyngis

Constrictio
bronchoaortica

Trachea

Arcus aortae

Bronchus
principalis
sinister

Pars thoracica
oesophagi

Constrictio
diaphragmatica

Diaphragma

Pars abdominalis
oesophagi

Fundus gastris

Pars cardialis
gastris

Pars thryeopharyngea
constrictoris inferioris
pharyngis

Cartilago thyreoidea

Cartilago cricoidea

Pars cricopharyngea
constrictoris inferioris
pharyngis

Trachea

Oesophagus

Arcus aortae

Sternum

Cor (*in* Saccus
pericardiacus)

Diaphragma

C4

C6

T1

T3

T5

T7

T9

T11

L1

L3

2

3

4

5

6

7

Lateral view

Plate 255

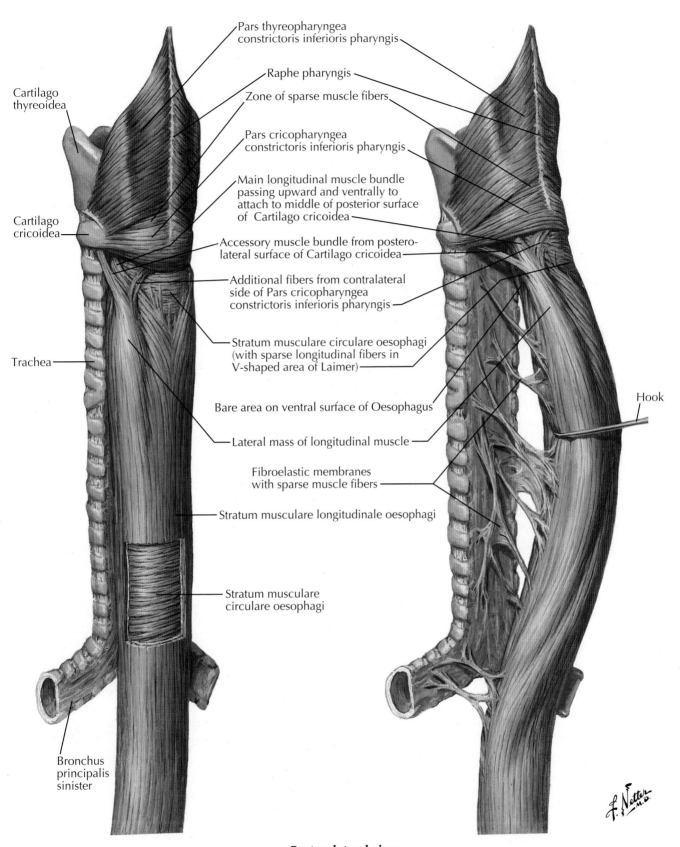

Pars thyreopharyngea
constrictoris inferioris pharyngis

Raphe pharyngis

Zone of sparse muscle fibers

Cartilago
thyreoidea

Pars cricopharyngea
constrictoris inferioris pharyngis

Main longitudinal muscle bundle
passing upward and ventrally to
attach to middle of posterior surface
of Cartilago cricoidea

Cartilago
cricoidea

Accessory muscle bundle from posterolateral surface of Cartilago cricoidea

Additional fibers from contralateral
side of Pars cricopharyngea
constrictoris inferioris pharyngis

Stratum musculare circulare oesophagi
(with sparse longitudinal fibers in
V-shaped area of Laimer)

Trachea

Bare area on ventral surface of Oesophagus

Hook

Lateral mass of longitudinal muscle

Fibroelastic membranes
with sparse muscle fibers

Stratum musculare longitudinale oesophagi

Stratum musculare
circulare oesophagi

Bronchus
principalis
sinister

Posterolateral view

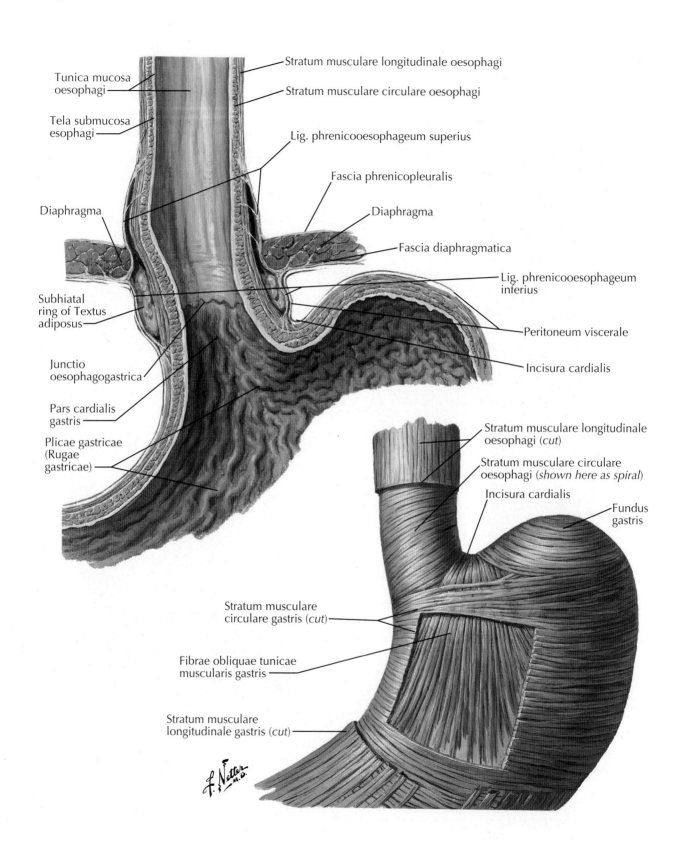

Tunica mucosa oesophagi

Tela submucosa esophagi

Diaphragma

Subhiatal ring of Textus adiposus

Junctio oesophagogastrica

Pars cardialis gastris

Plicae gastricae (Rugae gastricae)

Stratum musculare longitudinale oesophagi

Stratum musculare circulare oesophagi

Lig. phrenicooesophageum superius

Fascia phrenicopleuralis

Diaphragma

Fascia diaphragmatica

Lig. phrenicooesophageum inferius

Peritoneum viscerale

Incisura cardialis

Stratum musculare longitudinale oesophagi (*cut*)

Stratum musculare circulare oesophagi (*shown here as spiral*)

Incisura cardialis

Fundus gastris

Stratum musculare circulare gastris (*cut*)

Fibrae obliquae tunicae muscularis gastris

Stratum musculare longitudinale gastris (*cut*)

Plate 257

Mediastinum

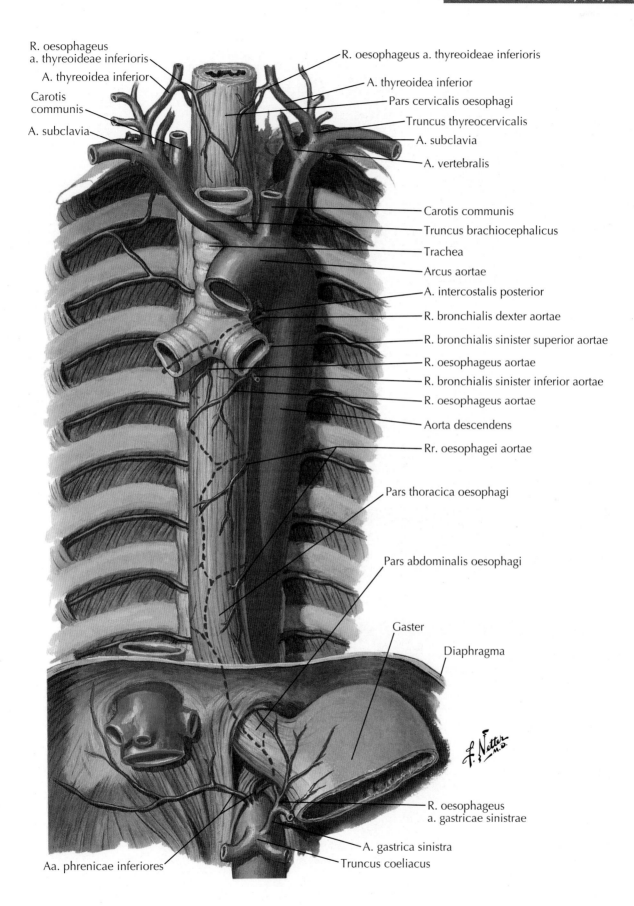

R. oesophageus
a. thyreoideae inferioris

A. thyreoidea inferior

Carotis
communis

A. subclavia

R. oesophageus a. thyreoideae inferioris

A. thyreoidea inferior

Pars cervicalis oesophagi

Truncus thyreocervicalis

A. subclavia

A. vertebralis

Carotis communis

Truncus brachiocephalicus

Trachea

Arcus aortae

A. intercostalis posterior

R. bronchialis dexter aortae

R. bronchialis sinister superior aortae

R. oesophageus aortae

R. bronchialis sinister inferior aortae

R. oesophageus aortae

Aorta descendens

Rr. oesophagei aortae

Pars thoracica oesophagi

Pars abdominalis oesophagi

Gaster

Diaphragma

R. oesophageus
a. gastricae sinistrae

A. gastrica sinistra

Truncus coeliacus

Aa. phrenicae inferiores

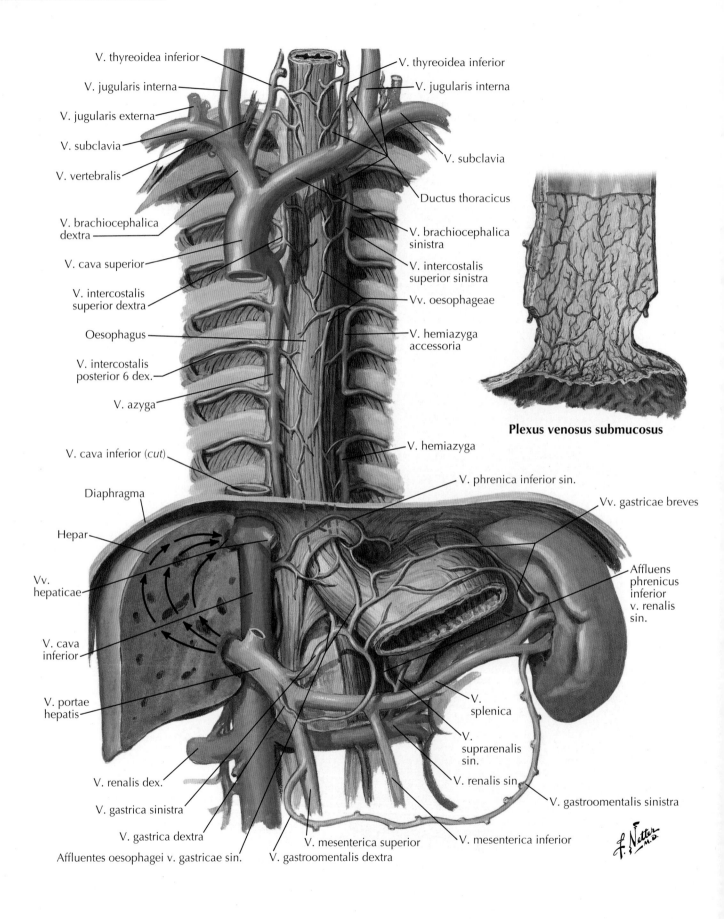

V. thyreoidea inferior

V. jugularis interna

V. jugularis externa

V. subclavia

V. vertebralis

V. brachiocephalica dextra

V. cava superior

V. intercostalis superior dextra

Oesophagus

V. intercostalis posterior 6 dex.

V. azyga

V. cava inferior (*cut*)

Diaphragma

Hepar

Vv. hepaticae

V. cava inferior

V. portae hepatis

V. renalis dex.

V. gastrica sinistra

V. gastrica dextra

Affluentes oesophagei v. gastricae sin.

V. gastroomentalis dextra

V. mesenterica superior

V. thyreoidea inferior

V. jugularis interna

V. subclavia

Ductus thoracicus

V. brachiocephalica sinistra

V. intercostalis superior sinistra

Vv. oesophageae

V. hemiazyga accessoria

V. hemiazyga

V. phrenica inferior sin.

Vv. gastricae breves

Affluens phrenicus inferior v. renalis sin.

V. splenica

V. suprarenalis sin.

V. renalis sin.

V. gastroomentalis sinistra

V. mesenterica inferior

Plexus venosus submucosus

Plate 259

Mediastinum

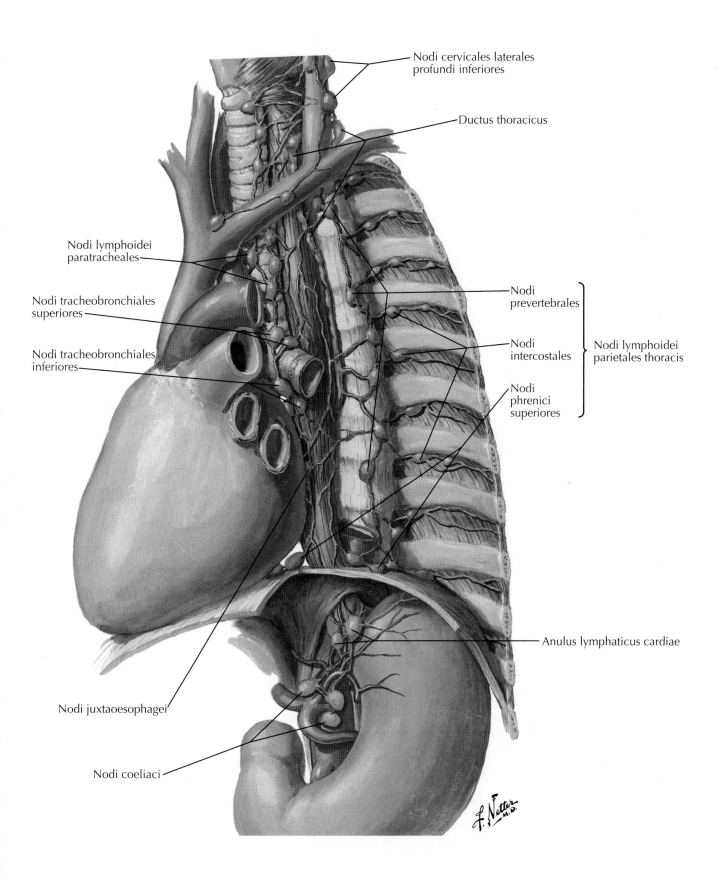

Nodi cervicales laterales
profundi inferiores

Ductus thoracicus

Nodi lymphoidei
paratracheales

Nodi tracheobronchiales
superiores

Nodi tracheobronchiales
inferiores

Nodi
prevertebrales

Nodi
intercostales

Nodi lymphoidei
parietales thoracis

Nodi
phrenici
superiores

Anulus lymphaticus cardiae

Nodi juxtaoesophagei

Nodi coeliaci

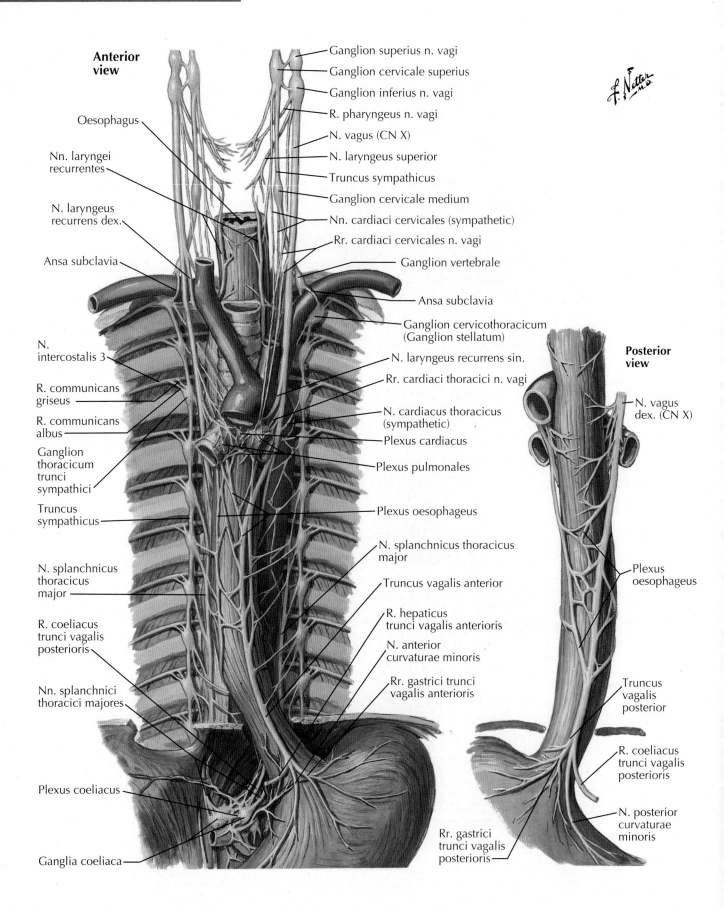

Anterior view

Ganglion superius n. vagi

Ganglion cervicale superius

Ganglion inferius n. vagi

R. pharyngeus n. vagi

N. vagus (CN X)

N. laryngeus superior

Truncus sympathicus

Ganglion cervicale medium

Nn. cardiaci cervicales (sympathetic)

Rr. cardiaci cervicales n. vagi

Ganglion vertebrale

Ansa subclavia

Ganglion cervicothoracicum (Ganglion stellatum)

N. laryngeus recurrens sin.

Rr. cardiaci thoracici n. vagi

N. cardiacus thoracicus (sympathetic)

Plexus cardiacus

Plexus pulmonales

Plexus oesophageus

N. splanchnicus thoracicus major

Truncus vagalis anterior

R. hepaticus trunci vagalis anterioris

N. anterior curvaturae minoris

Rr. gastrici trunci vagalis anterioris

Rr. gastrici trunci vagalis posterioris

Oesophagus

Nn. laryngei recurrentes

N. laryngeus recurrens dex.

Ansa subclavia

N. intercostalis 3

R. communicans griseus

R. communicans albus

Ganglion thoracicum trunci sympathici

Truncus sympathicus

N. splanchnicus thoracicus major

R. coeliacus trunci vagalis posterioris

Nn. splanchnici thoracici majores

Plexus coeliacus

Ganglia coeliaca

Posterior view

N. vagus dex. (CN X)

Plexus oesophageus

Truncus vagalis posterior

R. coeliacus trunci vagalis posterioris

N. posterior curvaturae minoris

Plate 261

Mediastinum

Axial CT images of the thorax from superior (A) to inferior (C)

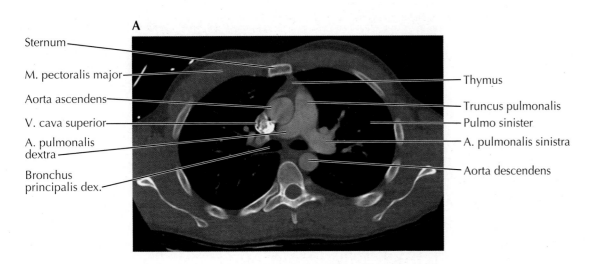

A

Sternum

M. pectoralis major

Aorta ascendens

V. cava superior

A. pulmonalis dextra

Bronchus principalis dex.

Thymus

Truncus pulmonalis

Pulmo sinister

A. pulmonalis sinistra

Aorta descendens

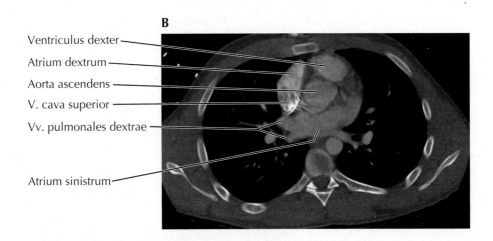

B

Ventriculus dexter

Atrium dextrum

Aorta ascendens

V. cava superior

Vv. pulmonales dextrae

Atrium sinistrum

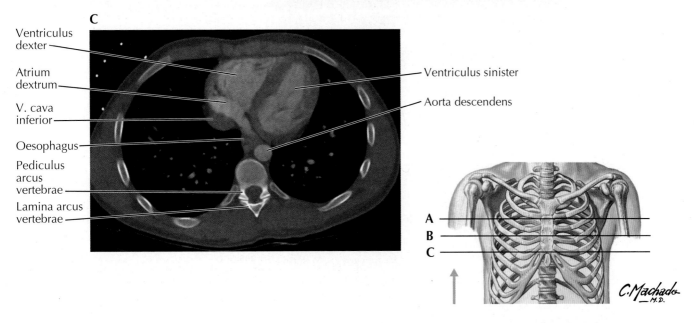

C

Ventriculus dexter

Atrium dextrum

V. cava inferior

Oesophagus

Pediculus arcus vertebrae

Lamina arcus vertebrae

Ventriculus sinister

Aorta descendens

A
B
C

C. Machado
— M.D.

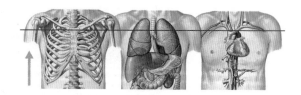

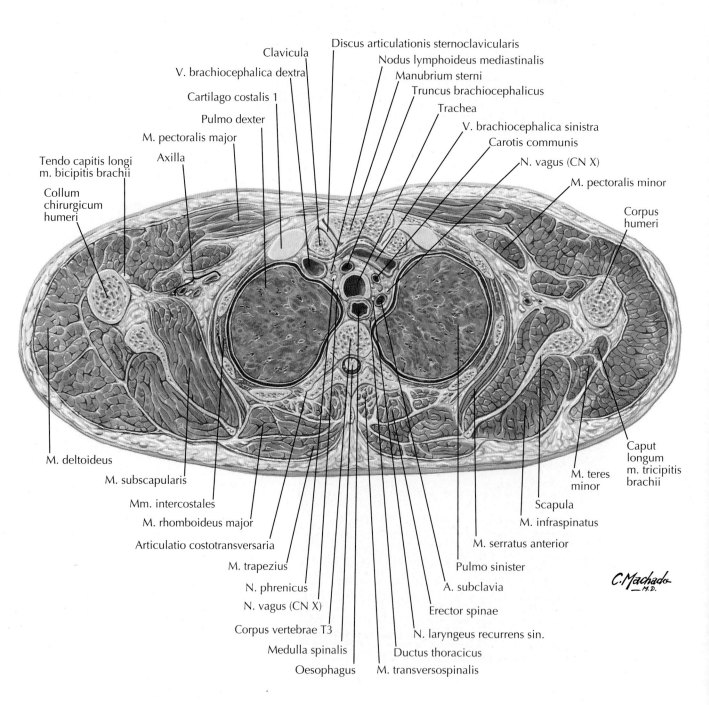

Clavicula

Discus articulationis sternoclavicularis

V. brachiocephalica dextra

Nodus lymphoideus mediastinalis

Manubrium sterni

Cartilago costalis 1

Truncus brachiocephalicus

Pulmo dexter

Trachea

M. pectoralis major

V. brachiocephalica sinistra

Axilla

Carotis communis

Tendo capitis longi
m. bicipitis brachii

N. vagus (CN X)

M. pectoralis minor

Collum
chirurgicum
humeri

Corpus
humeri

M. deltoideus

Caput
longum
m. tricipitis
brachii

M. subscapularis

M. teres
minor

Mm. intercostales

Scapula

M. rhomboideus major

M. infraspinatus

Articulatio costotransversaria

M. serratus anterior

M. trapezius

Pulmo sinister

N. phrenicus

A. subclavia

N. vagus (CN X)

Erector spinae

Corpus vertebrae T3

N. laryngeus recurrens sin.

Medulla spinalis

Ductus thoracicus

Oesophagus

M. transversospinalis

Plate 263

Cross-Sectional Anatomy

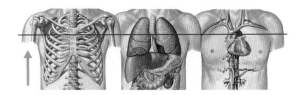

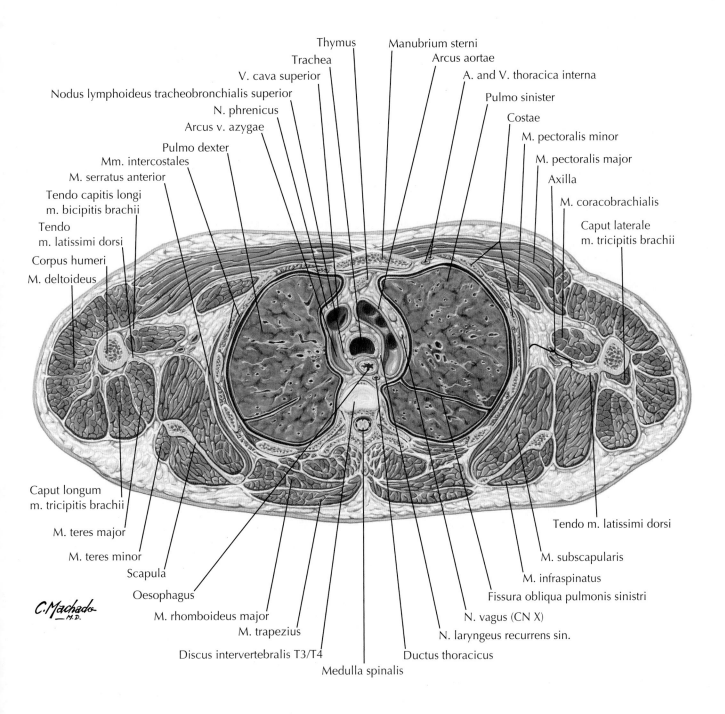

Thymus
Trachea
V. cava superior
Nodus lymphoideus tracheobronchialis superior
N. phrenicus
Arcus v. azygae
Pulmo dexter
Mm. intercostales
M. serratus anterior
Tendo capitis longi
m. bicipitis brachii
Tendo
m. latissimi dorsi
Corpus humeri
M. deltoideus

Manubrium sterni
Arcus aortae
A. and V. thoracica interna
Pulmo sinister
Costae
M. pectoralis minor
M. pectoralis major
Axilla
M. coracobrachialis
Caput laterale
m. tricipitis brachii

Caput laterale
m. tricipitis brachii

Caput longum
m. tricipitis brachii
M. teres major
M. teres minor
Scapula
Oesophagus
M. rhomboideus major
M. trapezius
Discus intervertebralis T3/T4
Medulla spinalis

Tendo m. latissimi dorsi
M. subscapularis
M. infraspinatus
Fissura obliqua pulmonis sinistri
N. vagus (CN X)
N. laryngeus recurrens sin.
Ductus thoracicus

C.Machado
_M.D._

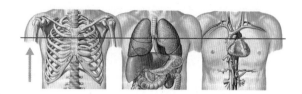

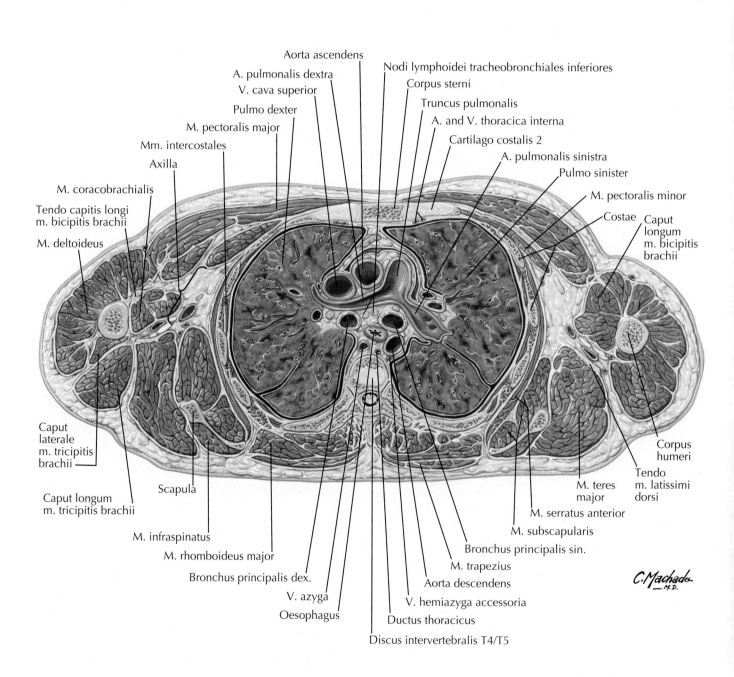

Aorta ascendens

A. pulmonalis dextra

V. cava superior

Pulmo dexter

M. pectoralis major

Mm. intercostales

Axilla

M. coracobrachialis

Tendo capitis longi
m. bicipitis brachii

M. deltoideus

Nodi lymphoidei tracheobronchiales inferiores

Corpus sterni

Truncus pulmonalis

A. and V. thoracica interna

Cartilago costalis 2

A. pulmonalis sinistra

Pulmo sinister

M. pectoralis minor

Costae

Caput
longum
m. bicipitis
brachii

Corpus
humeri

Tendo
m. latissimi
dorsi

M. teres
major

M. subscapularis

M. serratus anterior

Bronchus principalis sin.

M. trapezius

Aorta descendens

V. hemiazyga accessoria

Ductus thoracicus

Discus intervertebralis T4/T5

Caput
laterale
m. tricipitis
brachii

Caput longum
m. tricipitis brachii

Scapula

M. infraspinatus

M. rhomboideus major

Bronchus principalis dex.

V. azyga

Oesophagus

C.Machado
M.D.

Plate 265

Cross-Sectional Anatomy

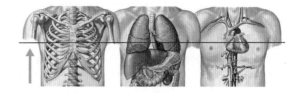

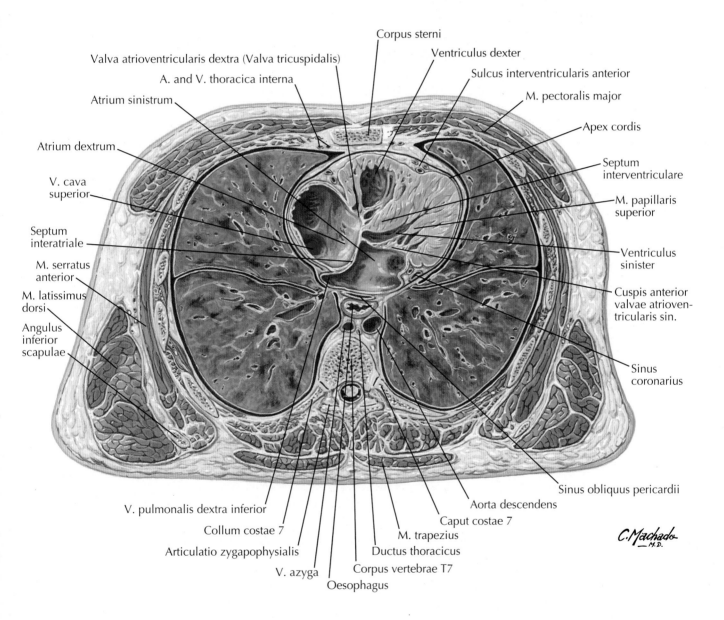

Corpus sterni

Ventriculus dexter

Valva atrioventricularis dextra (Valva tricuspidalis)

Sulcus interventricularis anterior

A. and V. thoracica interna

M. pectoralis major

Atrium sinistrum

Apex cordis

Atrium dextrum

Septum interventriculare

V. cava superior

M. papillaris superior

Septum interatriale

Ventriculus sinister

M. serratus anterior

Cuspis anterior valvae atrioventricularis sin.

M. latissimus dorsi

Angulus inferior scapulae

Sinus coronarius

Sinus obliquus pericardii

V. pulmonalis dextra inferior

Aorta descendens

Collum costae 7

Caput costae 7

Articulatio zygapophysialis

M. trapezius

V. azyga

Ductus thoracicus

Corpus vertebrae T7

Oesophagus

Structures with High* Clinical Significance

ANATOMICAL STRUCTURE	CLINICAL COMMENT	PLATE NUMBERS
Systema Nervosum		
N. thoracicus longus	May be damaged during chest tube placement or mastectomy, resulting in winged scapula (denervation of serratus anterior muscle)	206, 209
N. intercostalis	Site of local anesthetic nerve block for procedures such as thoracostomy or to alleviate pain caused by herpes zoster (shingles)	211, 212
Ganglion spinale (ganglion radicis posterioris)	Can house dormant varicella zoster virus, which, when activated, can result in herpes zoster (shingles)	212
N. phrenicus	Surgical injury to phrenic nerve may cause ipsilateral paralysis of diaphragm; diaphragmatic irritation may manifest as shoulder pain because of referral to C3–C5 spinal levels	214, 216, 232
N. laryngeus recurrens	The left nerve takes a circuitous path around aorta and may rarely become compressed by large thoracic aortic aneurysm or enlarged left atrium, producing hoarse voice (Ortner's syndrome); more often, these branches are affected by malignancies, such as those of thyroid gland	252, 254
Nn. cardiaci thoracici (sympathetic)	Pain of myocardial ischemia referred to upper thoracic dermatomes; may be perceived as somatic pain in thorax and medial upper limb	250
Systema Skeletale		
Costae	Rib fractures may cause respiratory dysfunction, predispose to pneumonia, and injure underlying structures (e.g., liver and spleen); severe fractures may breach pleural space and cause pneumothorax; flail chest occurs when multiple fractures in adjacent ribs create "floating" area of thorax with paradoxical motion during inspiration	203
Juncturae costochondrales; Articulationes sternochondrales (sternocostales)	Frequent sites of pain and tenderness after thoracic wall injury or excessive weightlifting (costochondritis); generally reproducible with palpation of joints	204
Claviculae	Common sites of fracture, often after falling onto outstretched limb or onto shoulder; fractures typically occur in middle third; supraclavicular nerve block relieves pain associated with fracture	203
Angulus sterni (Louisi)	Surface landmark for counting ribs (2nd pair of ribs articulate between manubrium and body of sternum) and intercostal spaces; divides superior from inferior mediastinum, and marks transition from aortic arch to descending thoracic aorta	203
Apertura superior thoracis	Compression of neurovascular structures (inferior trunk of brachial plexus and great vessels) that traverse superior thoracic aperture may produce thoracic outlet syndrome	213
Spatia intercostalia	Relationship of intercostal neurovascular bundle to ribs is crucial when placing chest tube to relieve pneumothorax or hemothorax, or needles to anesthetize nerves; tubes should be inserted along superior margin of ribs to avoid these bundles; of note, however, intercostal nerve may have collateral branch running along superior border of lower rib, which can result in pain	210, 238
Lig. cricothyreoideum medianum	Also known as cricothyroid membrane; site of cricothyrotomy, an emergency procedure to establish surgical airway	53, 103

Table 4.1 **Structures with High Clinical Significance**

ANATOMICAL STRUCTURE	CLINICAL COMMENT	PLATE NUMBERS
Systema Musculare		
Diaphragma	Widening of esophageal hiatus at T8 vertebral level or congenital defect allows for protrusion of stomach into thorax (hiatal hernia), which increases incidence of gastroesophageal reflux	216, 257
Systema Cardiovasculare		
A. thoracica interna	Commonly used for coronary artery bypass grafts, most often for anterior interventricular artery (left anterior descending artery)	211, 212
Aa. pulmonales	Thromboemboli, most often from pelvic and femoral sources, may obstruct pulmonary arteries (pulmonary embolus), leading to hypoxemia, hemodynamic compromise, and pulmonary infarction	220, 227
Pericardium	Pericardial space can contain small amounts of physiologic fluid (15–50 mL); effusion may compromise heart function (cardiac tamponade); pericardial sac can expand and become quite large with slow, progressive fluid accumulation	231, 236
Aa. coronariae	Fixed atherosclerotic disease may cause myocardial ischemia to manifest as thoracic pain; rupture and thrombosis of atherosclerotic plaque is main cause of acute myocardial infarction; severity and outcomes depend on amount of myocardium that vessel subtends, with proximal lesions of large vessels being most morbid	239
Venae pulmonales	Atrial fibrillation, a common arrhythmia, is believed to originate from within pulmonary veins; electrical ablation of this arrhythmia creates rings of fibrosis around pulmonary veins as they enter left atrium, thereby preventing propagation of electrical signals into heart	242, 247
Foramen ovale cordis	Provides channel for interatrial flow (right-to-left shunt) during fetal development; remains patent in approximately one in four adults and may provide route for venous microthromboses to enter left side of heart and cause ischemic stroke	242, 247
Septum interventriculare	Ventricular septal defect is common congenital cardiac defect, most often involving membranous portion of septum; myocardial infarction in territory of anterior interventricular artery (left anterior descending artery), especially if not promptly treated, may generate sufficient ischemia of septum to cause perforation	242, 245
Valvae cordis	Valvular disease (e.g., aortic stenosis, mitral insufficiency) is common, especially among older adults, and may cause progressive heart failure	243
Valva aortae	1% of population has bicuspid aortic valve (i.e., containing two rather than three leaflets), which predisposes to aortic stenosis and insufficiency and is also associated with aortic aneurysm	243, 244
Nodus sinuatrialis	Primary cardiac pacemaker, which generates action potentials that propagate through cardiac conduction system; aging, infiltrative diseases, and heart surgery may cause sinus node dysfunction, resulting in bradycardia	248
Nodus atrioventricularis	Conducts action potentials from atria to ventricles; intrinsic refractory period prevents rapid atrial rhythms from causing equivalent tachycardia of ventricles; dysfunction secondary to fibrosis, medications, cardiac surgery may result in heart block; when block is complete, atria and ventricles have independent rhythms	248
Ligamentum arteriosum	Remnant of ductus arteriosus, which connects pulmonary and systemic circulations during fetal development; lack of ductus closure after birth may cause exertional dyspnea, pulmonary vascular disease, or heart failure; acts as landmark to identify left recurrent laryngeal nerve looping inferior to ligament	232, 247

Structures with High Clinical Significance

Table 4.2

ANATOMICAL STRUCTURE	CLINICAL COMMENT	PLATE NUMBERS
Systema Cardiovasculare—Continued		
Aorta thoracica	Lies naturally to left of vertebral column in thorax and commences at T4 vertebral level, where aortic arch terminates; congenital coarctation (narrowing) of aorta may cause hypertension in children and young adults; significant difference in blood pressure between upper and lower extremities is suggestive	258
Aorta thoracica	Aneurysm (enlargement) may occur secondary to age and atherosclerotic risk factors (such as tobacco abuse and hypertension), connective tissue disorders, in association with bicuspid aortic valve, or from infection (e.g., syphilis). Large aneurysm can rupture or dissect; the latter occurs when a tear in intimal layer allows blood to propagate into a false lumen between intima and media	258
Vena azyga	Drains posterior thorax and provides important collateral channel between inferior vena cava and superior vena cava	259
Vasa Lymphatica and Organa Lymphoidea		
Vasa lymphatica mammae	Metastatic spread of cancer cells from mammary gland to axilla and thorax via lymphatics draining breast	208
Nodi lymphoidei axillares	Primary nodes that receive lymphatic drainage from upper limb, thoracic wall, and breast; commonly enlarged in patients with breast cancer	207, 208
Systema Respiratorium		
Pleura	Air or gas (spontaneous or traumatic) can leak into pleural space between visceral pleura and parietal pleura and compress lung, a condition known as pneumothorax; if severe enough to compromise venous return to heart, resulting in hypotension and dyspnea, condition is known as tension pneumothorax	217–220
Cupula pleurae	Extends into neck superior to anterior aspect of angled 1st rib or to level of 1st rib posteriorly; it may therefore be punctured during neck procedures, producing pneumothorax	69, 217
Bifurcatio tracheae	Important landmark when assessing position of endotracheal tube, which should terminate 4–5 cm above; often at T4/T5 vertebral level; right main bronchus is shorter, more vertical, and wider; therefore, aspirated objects more often enter right side; left main bronchus lies over esophagus and posterior to left atrium of heart	225
Apex pulmonis	Pancoast tumor (bronchogenic carcinoma of apex of lung) may compress sympathetic trunk, resulting in Horner's syndrome (ipsilateral miosis, ptosis, anhidrosis, facial flushing); apex is susceptible to pneumothorax from needles introduced in lower neck region	217, 251
Systemata Genitalia and Structurae Pertinentes		
Glandula mammaria	Breast cancer is most common malignancy in women; most common type originates in lactiferous duct and can either be localized within duct (ductal carcinoma in situ) or invasive into adjoining tissues (invasive ductal carcinoma)	205

*Selections were based largely on clinical data and commonly discussed clinical correlations in macroscopic ("gross") anatomy courses.

Table 4.3   **Structures with High Clinical Significance**

MUSCLE	MUSCLE GROUP	ORIGIN ATTACHMENT	INSERTION ATTACHMENT	INNERVATION	BLOOD SUPPLY	MAIN ACTIONS
Diaphragma	Diaphragma	Proc. xiphoideus; cartilagines costales 7–12; vertebrae L1–L3	Centrum tendineum diaphragmatis	N. phrenicus	Aa. pericardiacophrenica, musculophrenica, intercostales posteriores, and phrenicae superior and inferior	Draws central tendon down and forward during inspiration
Mm. intercostales externi	Paries thoracis	Margines inferiores costarum	Margines superiores costarum (below rib of origin)	Nn. intercostales	Aa. intercostales posteriores and suprema, thoracica interna, and musculophrenica	Support intercostal spaces in inspiration and expiration, elevate ribs in inspiration
Mm. intercostales intimi	Paries thoracis	Margines inferiores costarum	Margines superiores costarum (below rib of origin)	Nn. intercostales	Aa. intercostales posteriores and suprema, thoracica interna, and musculophrenica	Prevent pushing out or drawing in of intercostal spaces in inspiration and expiration, lower ribs in forced expiration
Mm. intercostales interni	Paries thoracis	Sulci costarum; margines inferiores cartilaginum costalium	Margines superiores costarum (below rib of origin)	Nn. intercostales	Aa. intercostales posteriores and suprema, thoracica interna, and musculophrenica	Prevent pushing out or drawing in of intercostal spaces in inspiration and expiration, lower ribs in forced expiration
Levatores costarum	Paries thoracis	Procc. transversi vertebrarum C7–T11	Costae (subjacent rib, between tuberculum costae and angulus costae)	Rami posteriores nn. spinalium thoracicorum	Aa. intercostales posteriores	Elevate ribs
M. pectoralis major	Pectus	*Pars clavicularis*: Pars medialis claviculae *Pars sternalis*: Facies anterior sterni; cartilagines costarum verarum *Pars abdominalis*: Aponeurosis m. obliqui externi abdominis	Labium laterale sulci intertubercularis humeri	Nn. pectorales medialis and lateralis	R. pectoralis a. thoracoacromialis; A. thoracica interna	Flexes, adducts, and medially rotates arm
M. pectoralis minor	Pectus	Facies externae marginum superiorum costarum 3–5	Proc. coracoideus scapulae	Nn. pectorales medialis and lateralis	R. pectoralis a. thoracoacromialis; Aa. thoracicae superior and lateralis	Lowers lateral angle of scapula and protracts scapula
M. serratus anterior	Omos	Facies laterales costarum 1–9	Facies costalis marginis medialis scapulae	N. thoracicus longus	A. thoracica lateralis	Protracts and rotates scapula and holds it against thoracic wall
M. subclavius	Omos	Facies superiores costae 1 and cartilaginis costalis 1	Facies inferior claviculae (middle third)	N. subclavius	R. clavicularis a. thoracoacromialis	Anchors and depresses clavicle
Mm. subcostales	Paries thoracis	Facies internae costarum inferiorum (near the angulus costae)	Margines superiores costarum (2nd or 3rd rib below the muscle origin)	Nn. intercostales	Aa. intercostales posteriores and musculophrenica	Depress ribs
M. transversus thoracis	Paries thoracis	Facies internae cartilaginum costalium 2–6	Facies posterior partis inferioris sterni	Nn. intercostales	A. thoracica interna	Depresses ribs and costal cartilages

Variations in spinal nerve contributions to the innervation of muscles, their arterial supply, their attachments, and their actions are common themes in human anatomy. Therefore, expect differences between texts and realize that anatomical variation is normal.

ABDOMEN 5

Surface Anatomy   267
Paries Abdominis   268–287
Cavitas Peritonealis   288–293
Gaster and Intestina   294–301
Hepar, Vesica Biliaris,
  Pancreas, and Splen   302–307
Vasa Sanguinea Visceralia   308–318
Nervi Viscerales and
  Plexus Viscerales   319–329

Renes and Glandulae
  Suprarenales   330–343
Vasa Lymphatica and
  Nodi Lymphoidei   344
Regional Imaging   345–346
Cross-Sectional Anatomy   347–351
Structures with High Clinical
  Significance   Tables 5.1–5.3
Musculi   Table 5.4
Electronic Bonus Plates   BP 53–BP 83

ELECTRONIC BONUS PLATES

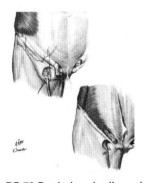

BP 53 Regio Inguinalis and Trigonum Femorale

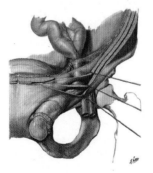

BP 54 Indirect Inguinal Hernia

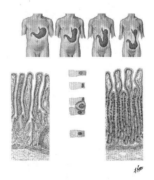

BP 55 Gaster: Variations in Position and Contour in Relation to Body Habitus

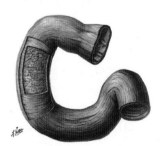

BP 56 Duodenum: Laminae

ELECTRONIC BONUS PLATES—*cont'd*

BP 57 Appendix Vermiformis in Coronal CT image and Vesica Biliaris in MRCP

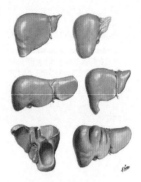

BP 58 Hepar: Topography

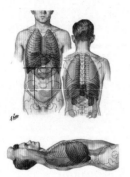

BP 59 Hepar: Variations in Form

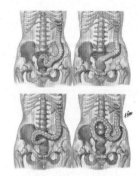

BP 60 Colon Sigmoideum: Variations in Position

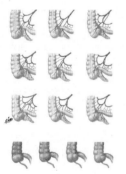

BP 61 Caecum: Variations in Arterial Supply and Posterior Peritoneal Attachment

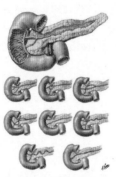

BP 62 Ductus Pancreaticus: Variations

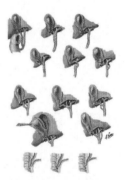

BP 63 Ductus Cysticus, Ductus Hepatici, and Ductus Pancreaticus: Variations

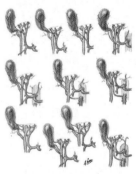

BP 64 Arteria Cystica: Variations

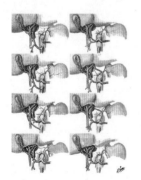

BP 65 Arteriae Hepaticae: Variations

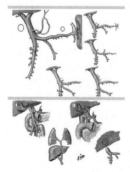

BP 66 Vena Portae Hepatis: Variations and Anomalies

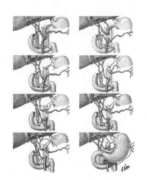

BP 67 Truncus Coeliacus: Variations

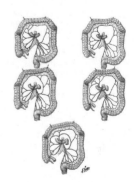

BP 68 Arteriae Colicae: Variations

ELECTRONIC BONUS PLATES—*cont'd*

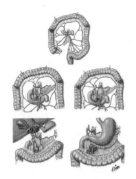

BP 69 Arteriae Colicae: Variations (Continued)

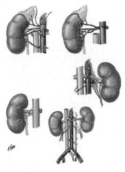

BP 70 Arteria Renalis and Vena Renalis: Variations

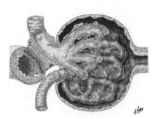

BP 71 Corpusculum renale: Histology

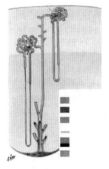

BP 72 Nephron and Tubulus Colligens: Schema

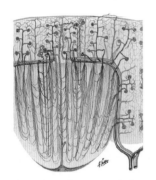

BP 73 Ren: Schema of Vasa Sanguinea Intrarenalia

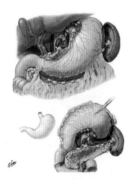

BP 74 Gaster: Vasa Lymphatica and Nodi Lymphoidei

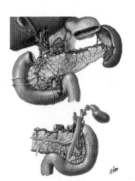

BP 75 Pancreas: Vasa Lymphatica and Nodi Lymphoidei

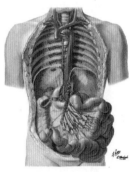

BP 76 Intestinum Tenue: Vasa Lymphatica and Nodi Lymphoidei

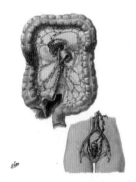

BP 77 Intestinum Crassum: Vasa Lymphatica and Nodi Lymphoidei

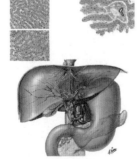

BP 78 Hepar: Vasa Lymphatica and Nodi Lymphoidei

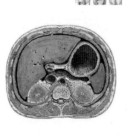

BP 79 Abdomen: Cross Section at T12 Vertebral Level

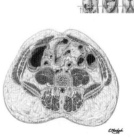

BP 80 Abdomen: Cross Section at L5 Vertebral Level, Near Planum Intertuberculare

ELECTRONIC BONUS PLATES—*cont'd*

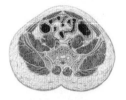

BP 81 Abdomen: Cross Section at S1 Vertebral Level, Near Spina Iliaca Anterior Superior

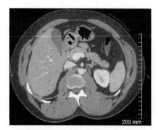

BP 82 Axial CT Image of Upper Abdomen

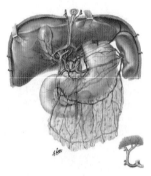

BP 83 Hepar and Vesica Biliaris: Variations in Arterial Blood Supply

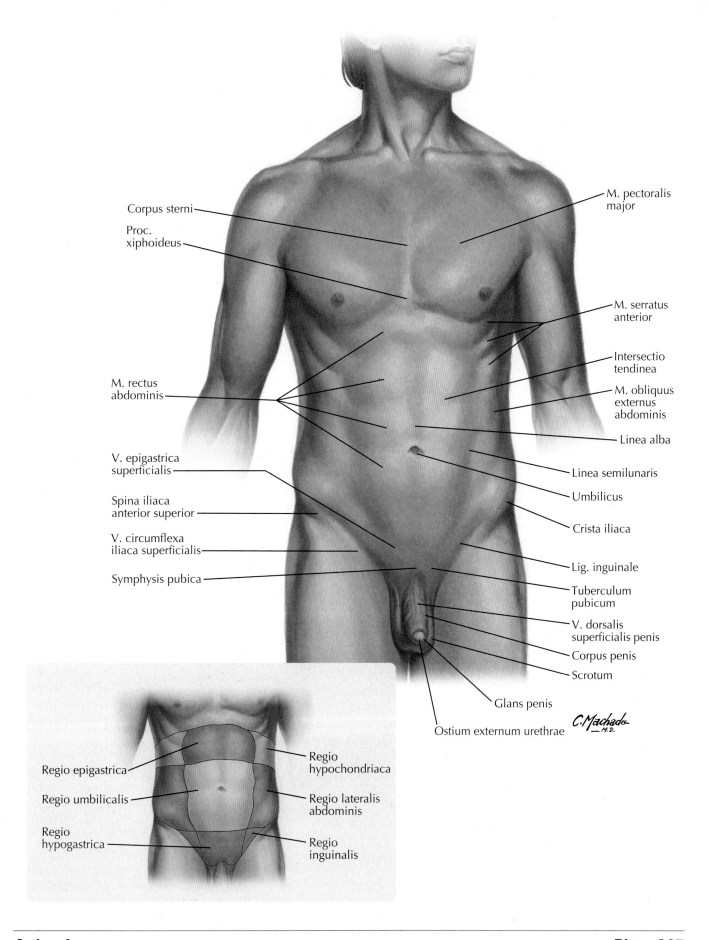

Corpus sterni

Proc. xiphoideus

M. rectus abdominis

V. epigastrica superficialis

Spina iliaca anterior superior

V. circumflexa iliaca superficialis

Symphysis pubica

M. pectoralis major

M. serratus anterior

Intersectio tendinea

M. obliquus externus abdominis

Linea alba

Linea semilunaris

Umbilicus

Crista iliaca

Lig. inguinale

Tuberculum pubicum

V. dorsalis superficialis penis

Corpus penis

Scrotum

Glans penis

Ostium externum urethrae

Regio epigastrica

Regio umbilicalis

Regio hypogastrica

Regio hypochondriaca

Regio lateralis abdominis

Regio inguinalis

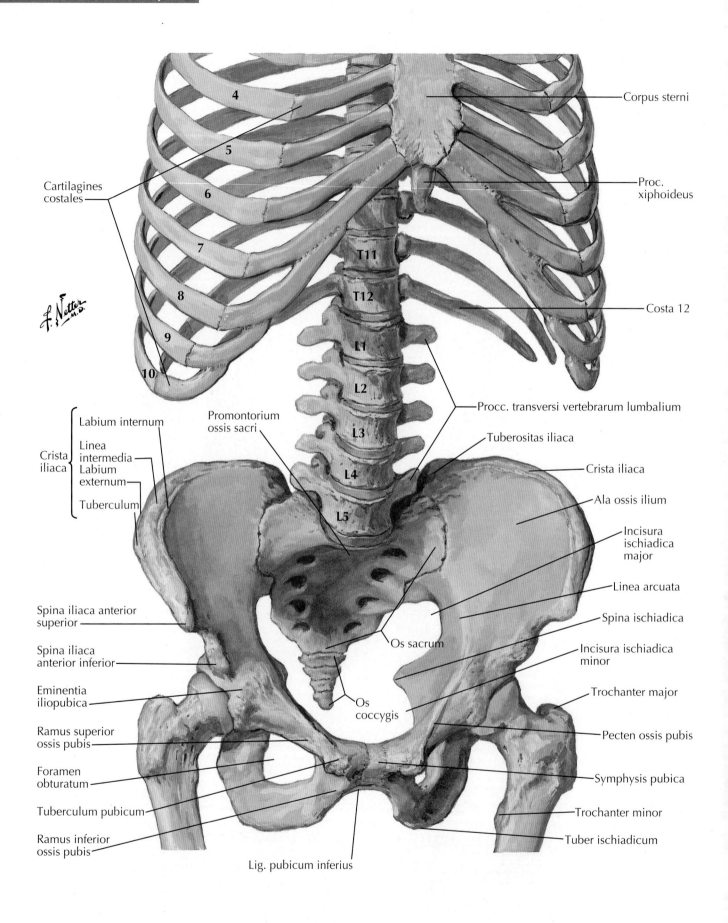

4

5

Cartilagines costales

6

7

8

9

10

Corpus sterni

Proc. xiphoideus

T11

T12

Costa 12

L1

L2

L3

L4

L5

Procc. transversi vertebrarum lumbalium

Promontorium ossis sacri

Tuberositas iliaca

Crista iliaca

Labium internum

Linea intermedia
Labium externum

Tuberculum

Crista iliaca

Ala ossis ilium

Incisura ischiadica major

Linea arcuata

Spina ischiadica

Incisura ischiadica minor

Trochanter major

Pecten ossis pubis

Symphysis pubica

Trochanter minor

Tuber ischiadicum

Os sacrum

Os coccygis

Spina iliaca anterior superior

Spina iliaca anterior inferior

Eminentia iliopubica

Ramus superior ossis pubis

Foramen obturatum

Tuberculum pubicum

Ramus inferior ossis pubis

Lig. pubicum inferius

Plate 268

Paries Abdominis

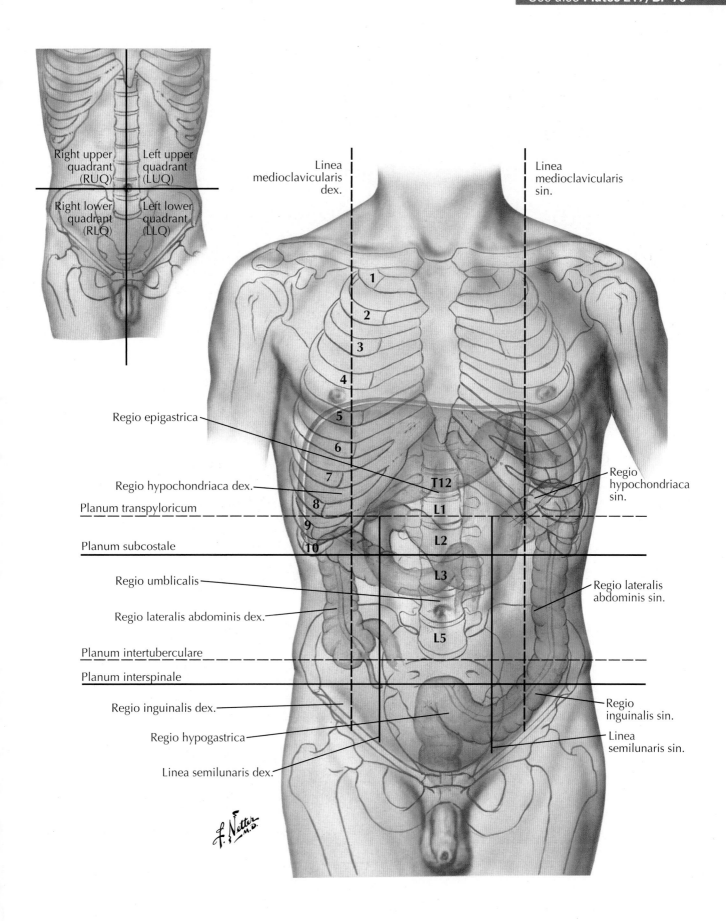

Right upper quadrant (RUQ)

Left upper quadrant (LUQ)

Right lower quadrant (RLQ)

Left lower quadrant (LLQ)

Linea medioclavicularis dex.

Linea medioclavicularis sin.

Regio epigastrica

Regio hypochondriaca dex.

Regio hypochondriaca sin.

Planum transpyloricum

Planum subcostale

Regio umblicalis

Regio lateralis abdominis dex.

Regio lateralis abdominis sin.

Planum intertuberculare

Planum interspinale

Regio inguinalis dex.

Regio inguinalis sin.

Regio hypogastrica

Linea semilunaris sin.

Linea semilunaris dex.

T12

L1

L2

L3

L5

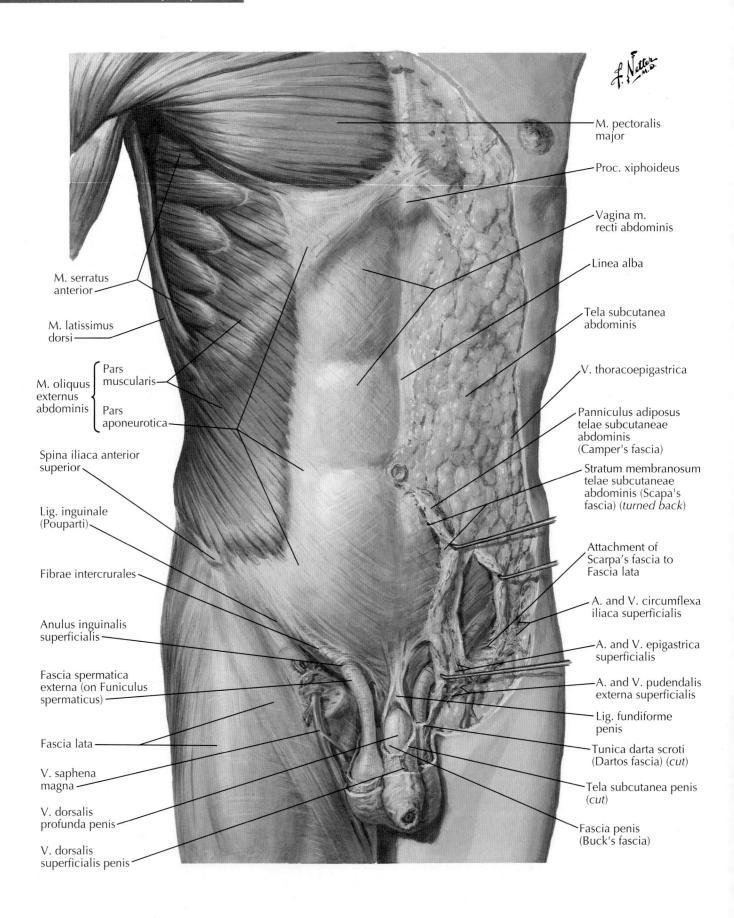

M. pectoralis
major

Proc. xiphoideus

Vagina m.
recti abdominis

Linea alba

Tela subcutanea
abdominis

V. thoracoepigastrica

Panniculus adiposus
telae subcutaneae
abdominis
(Camper's fascia)

Stratum membranosum
telae subcutaneae
abdominis (Scapa's
fascia) *(turned back)*

Attachment of
Scarpa's fascia to
Fascia lata

A. and V. circumflexa
iliaca superficialis

A. and V. epigastrica
superficialis

A. and V. pudendalis
externa superficialis

Lig. fundiforme
penis

Tunica darta scroti
(Dartos fascia) *(cut)*

Tela subcutanea penis
(cut)

Fascia penis
(Buck's fascia)

M. serratus
anterior

M. latissimus
dorsi

M. oliquus
externus
abdominis
{ Pars
muscularis

Pars
aponeurotica

Spina iliaca anterior
superior

Lig. inguinale
(Pouparti)

Fibrae intercrurales

Anulus inguinalis
superficialis

Fascia spermatica
externa (on Funiculus
spermaticus)

Fascia lata

V. saphena
magna

V. dorsalis
profunda penis

V. dorsalis
superficialis penis

Plate 270

Paries Abdominis

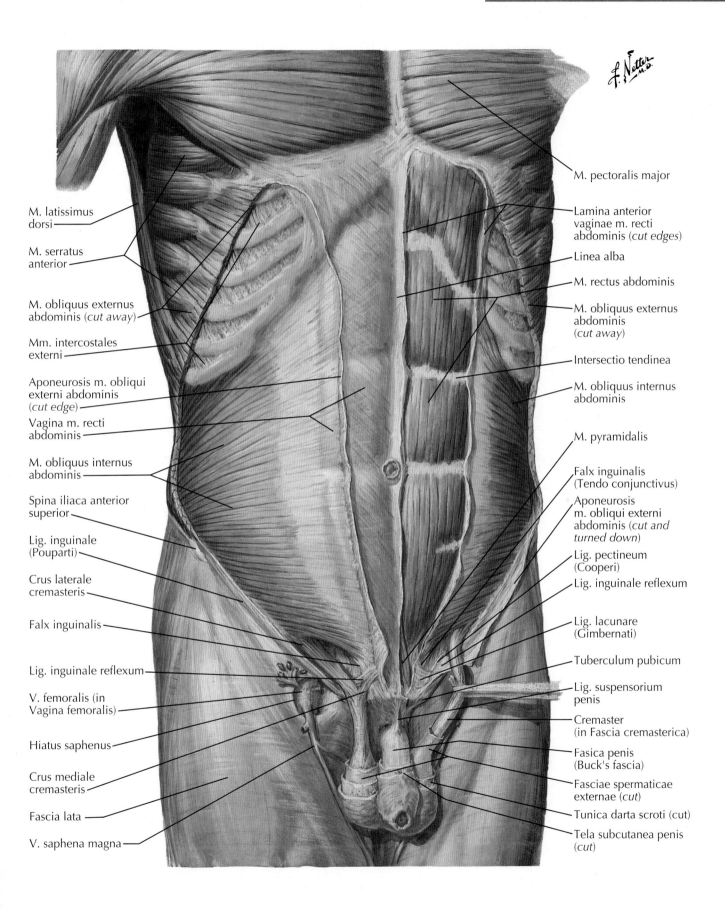

M. latissimus dorsi

M. serratus anterior

M. obliquus externus abdominis (*cut away*)

Mm. intercostales externi

Aponeurosis m. obliqui externi abdominis (*cut edge*)

Vagina m. recti abdominis

M. obliquus internus abdominis

Spina iliaca anterior superior

Lig. inguinale (Pouparti)

Crus laterale cremasteris

Falx inguinalis

Lig. inguinale reflexum

V. femoralis (in Vagina femoralis)

Hiatus saphenus

Crus mediale cremasteris

Fascia lata

V. saphena magna

M. pectoralis major

Lamina anterior vaginae m. recti abdominis (*cut edges*)

Linea alba

M. rectus abdominis

M. obliquus externus abdominis (*cut away*)

Intersectio tendinea

M. obliquus internus abdominis

M. pyramidalis

Falx inguinalis (Tendo conjunctivus)

Aponeurosis m. obliqui externi abdominis (*cut and turned down*)

Lig. pectineum (Cooperi)

Lig. inguinale reflexum

Lig. lacunare (Gimbernati)

Tuberculum pubicum

Lig. suspensorium penis

Cremaster (in Fascia cremasterica)

Fasica penis (Buck's fascia)

Fasciae spermaticae externae (*cut*)

Tunica darta scroti (cut)

Tela subcutanea penis (*cut*)

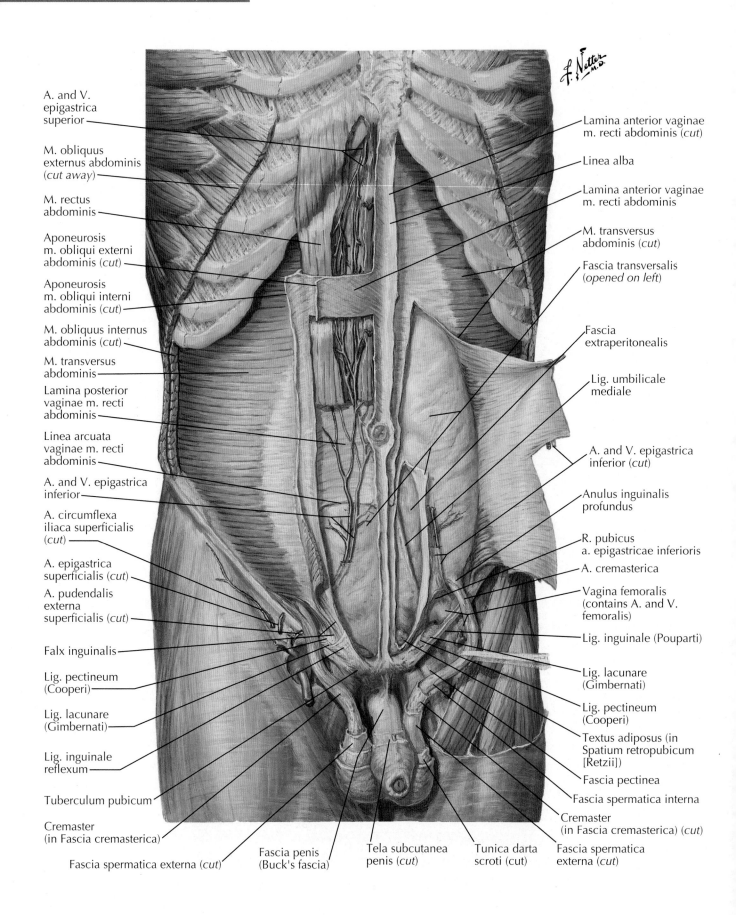

A. and V. epigastrica superior

M. obliquus externus abdominis (*cut away*)

M. rectus abdominis

Aponeurosis m. obliqui externi abdominis (*cut*)

Aponeurosis m. obliqui interni abdominis (*cut*)

M. obliquus internus abdominis (*cut*)

M. transversus abdominis

Lamina posterior vaginae m. recti abdominis

Linea arcuata vaginae m. recti abdominis

A. and V. epigastrica inferior

A. circumflexa iliaca superficialis (*cut*)

A. epigastrica superficialis (*cut*)

A. pudendalis externa superficialis (*cut*)

Falx inguinalis

Lig. pectineum (Cooperi)

Lig. lacunare (Gimbernati)

Lig. inguinale reflexum

Tuberculum pubicum

Cremaster (in Fascia cremasterica)

Fascia spermatica externa (*cut*)

Fascia penis (Buck's fascia)

Tela subcutanea penis (*cut*)

Tunica darta scroti (cut)

Lamina anterior vaginae m. recti abdominis (*cut*)

Linea alba

Lamina anterior vaginae m. recti abdominis

M. transversus abdominis (*cut*)

Fascia transversalis (*opened on left*)

Fascia extraperitonealis

Lig. umbilicale mediale

A. and V. epigastrica inferior (*cut*)

Anulus inguinalis profundus

R. pubicus a. epigastricae inferioris

A. cremasterica

Vagina femoralis (contains A. and V. femoralis)

Lig. inguinale (Pouparti)

Lig. lacunare (Gimbernati)

Lig. pectineum (Cooperi)

Textus adiposus (in Spatium retropubicum [Retzii])

Fascia pectinea

Fascia spermatica interna

Cremaster (in Fascia cremasterica) (*cut*)

Fascia spermatica externa (*cut*)

Plate 272

Paries Abdominis

Section superior to Linea arcuata vaginae m. recti abdominis

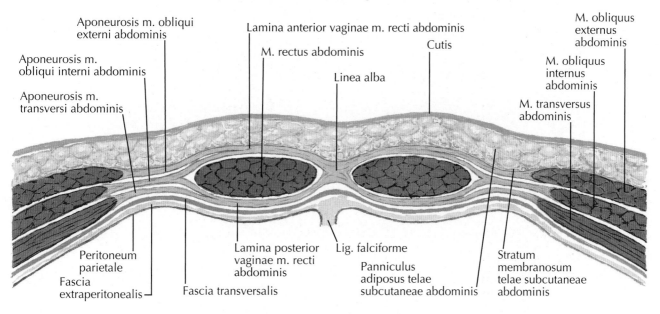

Aponeurosis m. obliqui interni abdominis — Aponeurosis m. obliqui externi abdominis — Aponeurosis m. transversi abdominis — Lamina anterior vaginae m. recti abdominis — M. rectus abdominis — Linea alba — Cutis — M. obliquus externus abdominis — M. obliquus internus abdominis — M. transversus abdominis — Peritoneum parietale — Fascia extraperitonealis — Fascia transversalis — Lamina posterior vaginae m. recti abdominis — Lig. falciforme — Panniculus adiposus telae subcutaneae abdominis — Stratum membranosum telae subcutaneae abdominis

Aponeurosis m. obliqui interni abdominis splits to form anterior and posterior laminae of Vagina m. recti abdominis. Aponeurosis m. obliqui externi abdominis joins anterior lamina; Aponeurosis m. transversi abdominis joins posterior lamina. Anterior and posterior laminae of Vagina m. recti abdominis unite medially to form Linea alba.

Section inferior to Linea arcuata vaginae m. recti abdominis

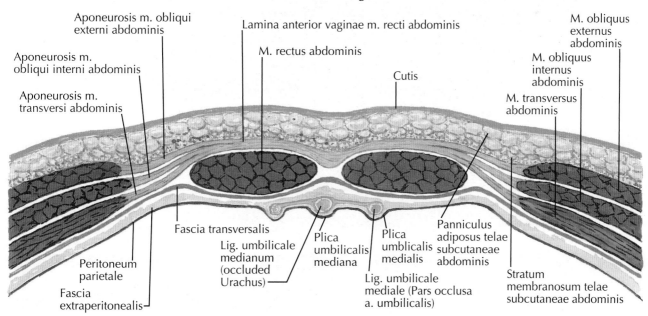

Aponeurosis m. obliqui interni abdominis — Aponeurosis m. obliqui externi abdominis — Aponeurosis m. transversi abdominis — Lamina anterior vaginae m. recti abdominis — M. rectus abdominis — Cutis — M. obliquus externus abdominis — M. obliquus internus abdominis — M. transversus abdominis — Peritoneum parietale — Fascia extraperitonealis — Fascia transversalis — Lig. umbilicale medianum (occluded Urachus) — Plica umbilicalis mediana — Plica umbilicalis medialis — Lig. umbilicale mediale (Pars occlusa a. umbilicalis) — Panniculus adiposus telae subcutaneae abdominis — Stratum membranosum telae subcutaneae abdominis

Aponeurosis m. obliqui interni abdominis does not split at this level but passes completely anterior to M. rectus abdominis and is fused there with both Aponeurosis m. obliqui externi abdominis and that of M. transversus abdominis. Thus, posterior lamina of Vagina m. recti abdominis is absent below Linea arcuata, leaving only Fascia transversalis.

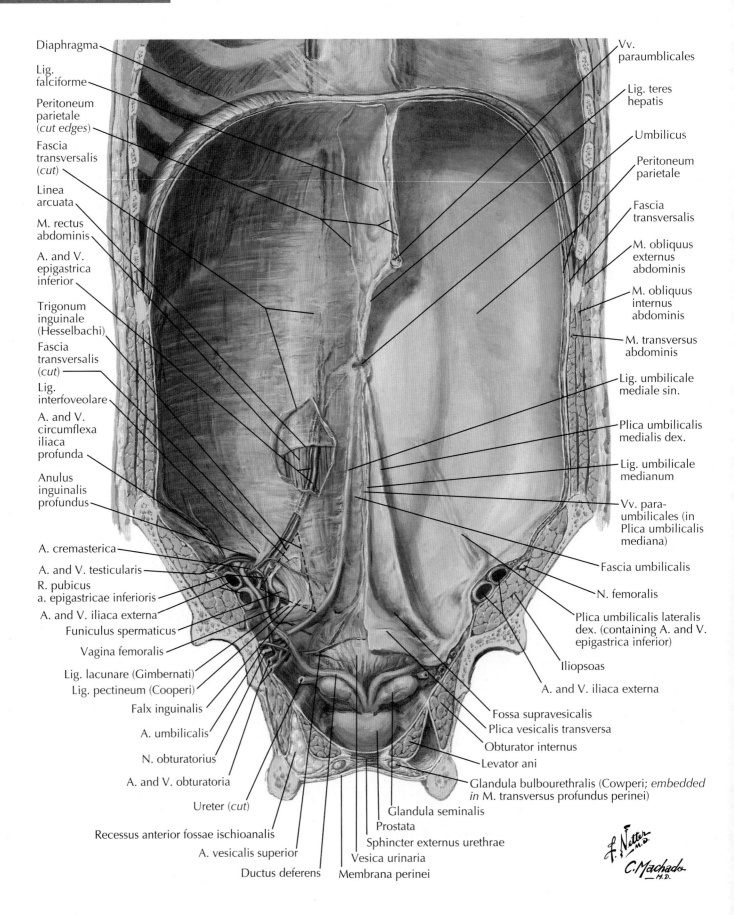

Diaphragma

Lig. falciforme

Peritoneum parietale (*cut edges*)

Fascia transversalis (*cut*)

Linea arcuata

M. rectus abdominis

A. and V. epigastrica inferior

Trigonum inguinale (Hesselbachi)

Fascia transversalis (*cut*)

Lig. interfoveolare

A. and V. circumflexa iliaca profunda

Anulus inguinalis profundus

A. cremasterica

A. and V. testicularis

R. pubicus a. epigastricae inferioris

A. and V. iliaca externa

Funiculus spermaticus

Vagina femoralis

Lig. lacunare (Gimbernati)

Lig. pectineum (Cooperi)

Falx inguinalis

A. umbilicalis

N. obturatorius

A. and V. obturatoria

Ureter (*cut*)

Recessus anterior fossae ischioanalis

A. vesicalis superior

Ductus deferens

Vv. paraumblicales

Lig. teres hepatis

Umbilicus

Peritoneum parietale

Fascia transversalis

M. obliquus externus abdominis

M. obliquus internus abdominis

M. transversus abdominis

Lig. umbilicale mediale sin.

Plica umbilicalis medialis dex.

Lig. umbilicale medianum

Vv. para-umbilicales (in Plica umbilicalis mediana)

Fascia umbilicalis

N. femoralis

Plica umbilicalis lateralis dex. (containing A. and V. epigastrica inferior)

Iliopsoas

A. and V. iliaca externa

Fossa supravesicalis

Plica vesicalis transversa

Obturator internus

Levator ani

Glandula bulbourethralis (Cowperi; *embedded in* M. transversus profundus perinei)

Glandula seminalis

Prostata

Sphincter externus urethrae

Vesica urinaria

Membrana perinei

Plate 274

Paries Abdominis

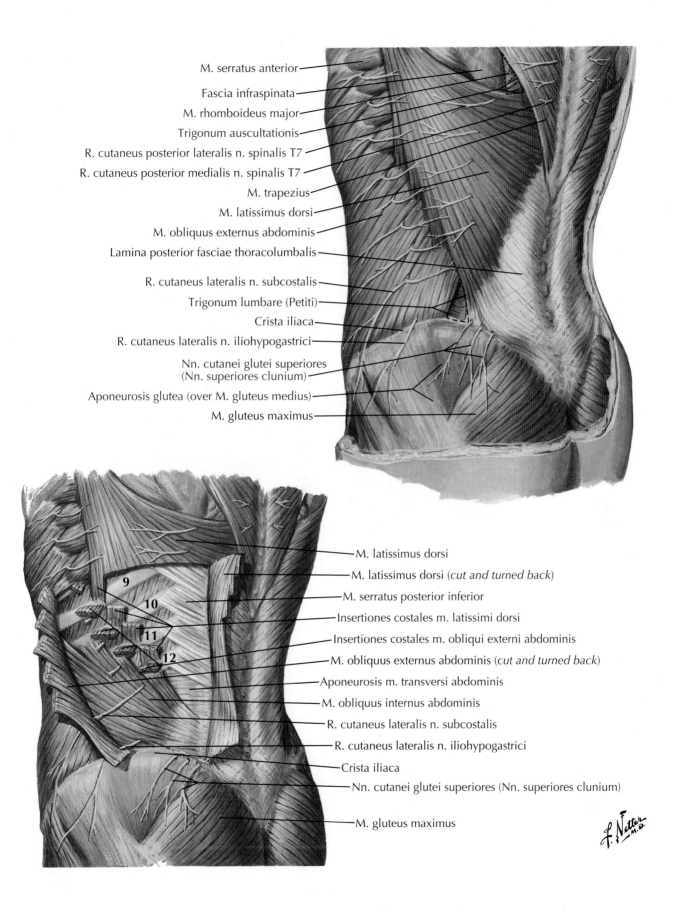

M. serratus anterior

Fascia infraspinata

M. rhomboideus major

Trigonum auscultationis

R. cutaneus posterior lateralis n. spinalis T7

R. cutaneus posterior medialis n. spinalis T7

M. trapezius

M. latissimus dorsi

M. obliquus externus abdominis

Lamina posterior fasciae thoracolumbalis

R. cutaneus lateralis n. subcostalis

Trigonum lumbare (Petiti)

Crista iliaca

R. cutaneus lateralis n. iliohypogastrici

Nn. cutanei glutei superiores
(Nn. superiores clunium)

Aponeurosis glutea (over M. gluteus medius)

M. gluteus maximus

9

10

11

12

M. latissimus dorsi

M. latissimus dorsi (*cut and turned back*)

M. serratus posterior inferior

Insertiones costales m. latissimi dorsi

Insertiones costales m. obliqui externi abdominis

M. obliquus externus abdominis (*cut and turned back*)

Aponeurosis m. transversi abdominis

M. obliquus internus abdominis

R. cutaneus lateralis n. subcostalis

R. cutaneus lateralis n. iliohypogastrici

Crista iliaca

Nn. cutanei glutei superiores (Nn. superiores clunium)

M. gluteus maximus

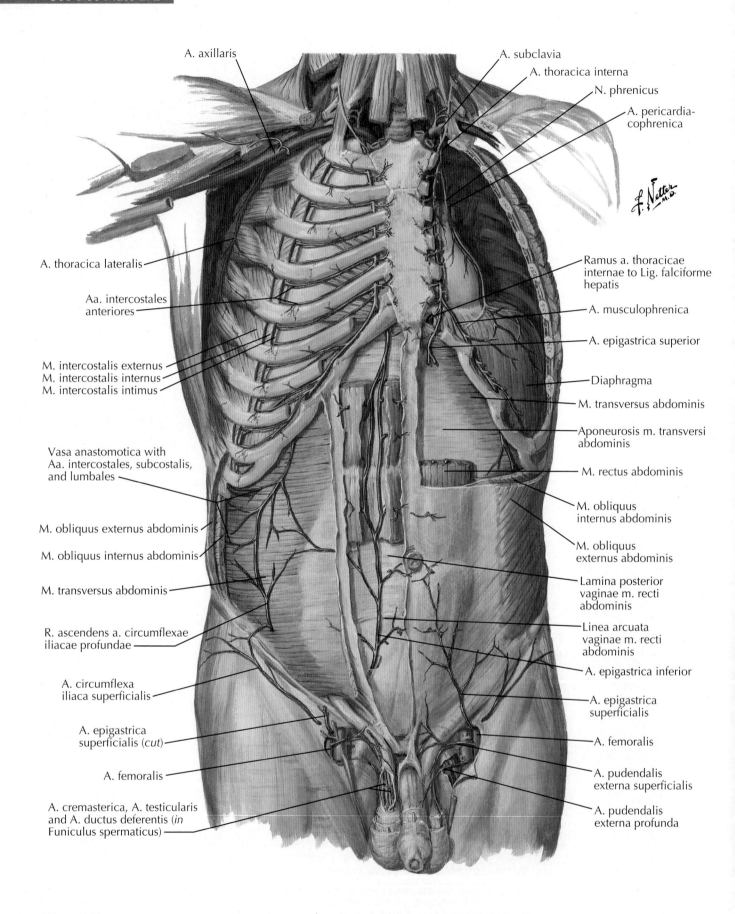

A. axillaris

A. subclavia

A. thoracica interna

N. phrenicus

A. pericardia-cophrenica

A. thoracica lateralis

Ramus a. thoracicae internae to Lig. falciforme hepatis

Aa. intercostales anteriores

A. musculophrenica

A. epigastrica superior

M. intercostalis externus
M. intercostalis internus
M. intercostalis intimus

Diaphragma

M. transversus abdominis

Aponeurosis m. transversi abdominis

M. rectus abdominis

Vasa anastomotica with Aa. intercostales, subcostalis, and lumbales

M. obliquus internus abdominis

M. obliquus externus abdominis

M. obliquus externus abdominis

M. obliquus internus abdominis

Lamina posterior vaginae m. recti abdominis

M. transversus abdominis

Linea arcuata vaginae m. recti abdominis

R. ascendens a. circumflexae iliacae profundae

A. epigastrica inferior

A. circumflexa iliaca superficialis

A. epigastrica superficialis

A. epigastrica superficialis (*cut*)

A. femoralis

A. femoralis

A. pudendalis externa superficialis

A. cremasterica, A. testicularis and A. ductus deferentis (*in* Funiculus spermaticus)

A. pudendalis externa profunda

Plate 276

Paries Abdominis

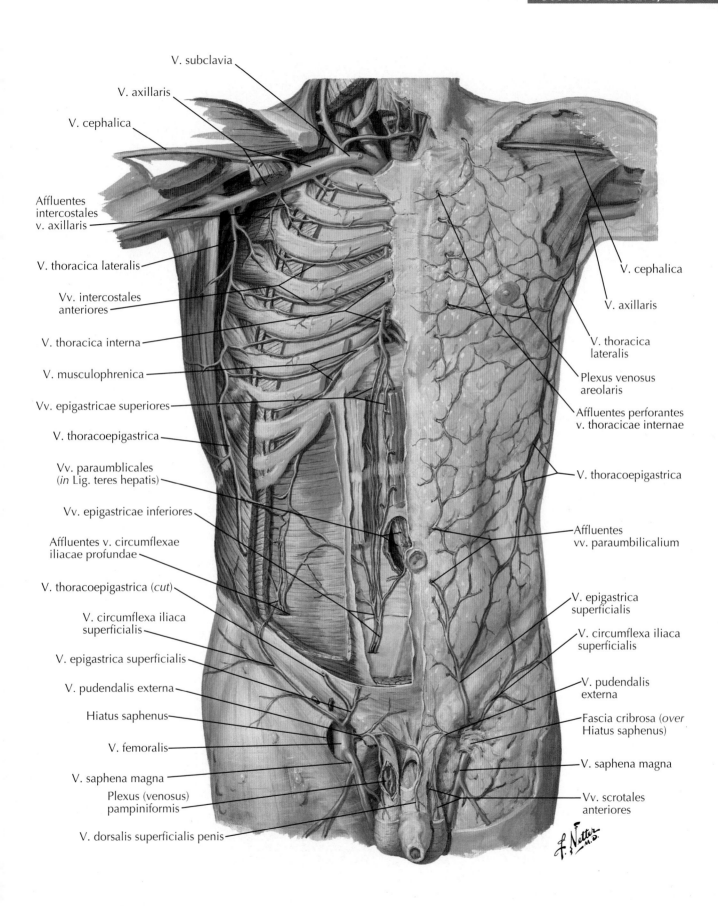

V. subclavia

V. axillaris

V. cephalica

Affluentes intercostales v. axillaris

V. thoracica lateralis

Vv. intercostales anteriores

V. thoracica interna

V. musculophrenica

Vv. epigastricae superiores

V. thoracoepigastrica

Vv. paraumblicales (*in* Lig. teres hepatis)

Vv. epigastricae inferiores

Affluentes v. circumflexae iliacae profundae

V. thoracoepigastrica (*cut*)

V. circumflexa iliaca superficialis

V. epigastrica superficialis

V. pudendalis externa

Hiatus saphenus

V. femoralis

V. saphena magna

Plexus (venosus) pampiniformis

V. dorsalis superficialis penis

V. cephalica

V. axillaris

V. thoracica lateralis

Plexus venosus areolaris

Affluentes perforantes v. thoracicae internae

V. thoracoepigastrica

Affluentes vv. paraumbilicalium

V. epigastrica superficialis

V. circumflexa iliaca superficialis

V. pudendalis externa

Fascia cribrosa (*over* Hiatus saphenus)

V. saphena magna

Vv. scrotales anteriores

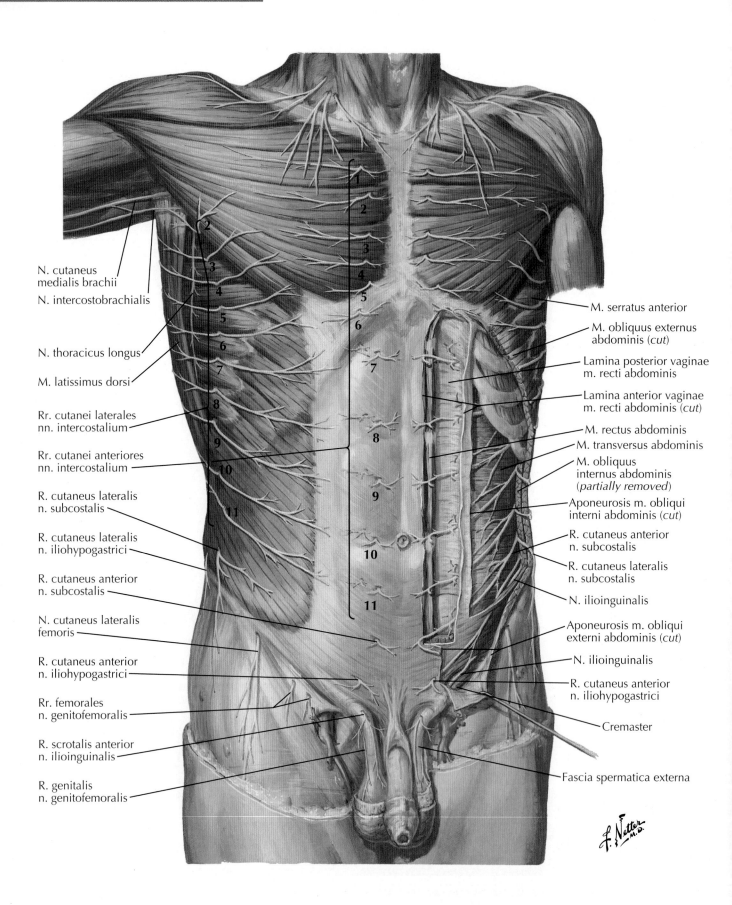

N. cutaneus
medialis brachii

N. intercostobrachialis

N. thoracicus longus

M. latissimus dorsi

Rr. cutanei laterales
nn. intercostalium

Rr. cutanei anteriores
nn. intercostalium

R. cutaneus lateralis
n. subcostalis

R. cutaneus lateralis
n. iliohypogastrici

R. cutaneus anterior
n. subcostalis

N. cutaneus lateralis
femoris

R. cutaneus anterior
n. iliohypogastrici

Rr. femorales
n. genitofemoralis

R. scrotalis anterior
n. ilioinguinalis

R. genitalis
n. genitofemoralis

M. serratus anterior

M. obliquus externus
abdominis (cut)

Lamina posterior vaginae
m. recti abdominis

Lamina anterior vaginae
m. recti abdominis (cut)

M. rectus abdominis

M. transversus abdominis

M. obliquus
internus abdominis
(partially removed)

Aponeurosis m. obliqui
interni abdominis (cut)

R. cutaneus anterior
n. subcostalis

R. cutaneus lateralis
n. subcostalis

N. ilioinguinalis

Aponeurosis m. obliqui
externi abdominis (cut)

N. ilioinguinalis

R. cutaneus anterior
n. iliohypogastrici

Cremaster

Fascia spermatica externa

Plate 278

Paries Abdominis

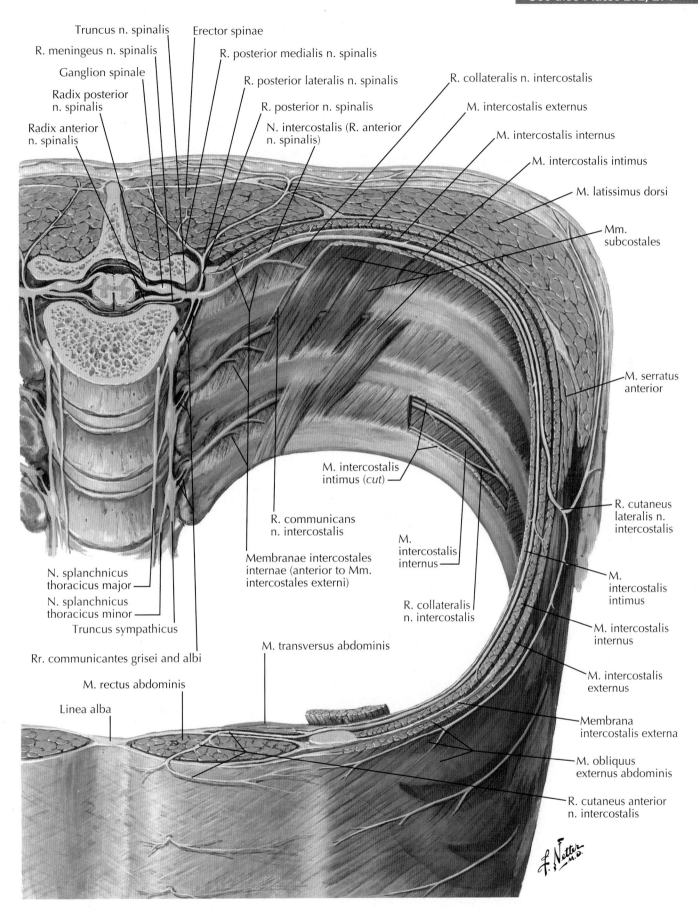

Truncus n. spinalis

R. meningeus n. spinalis

Ganglion spinale

Radix posterior n. spinalis

Radix anterior n. spinalis

Erector spinae

R. posterior medialis n. spinalis

R. posterior lateralis n. spinalis

R. posterior n. spinalis

N. intercostalis (R. anterior n. spinalis)

R. collateralis n. intercostalis

M. intercostalis externus

M. intercostalis internus

M. intercostalis intimus

M. latissimus dorsi

Mm. subcostales

M. serratus anterior

M. intercostalis intimus (cut)

R. communicans n. intercostalis

Membranae intercostales internae (anterior to Mm. intercostales externi)

M. intercostalis internus

R. collateralis n. intercostalis

N. splanchnicus thoracicus major

N. splanchnicus thoracicus minor

Truncus sympathicus

Rr. communicantes grisei and albi

M. rectus abdominis

Linea alba

M. transversus abdominis

R. cutaneus lateralis n. intercostalis

M. intercostalis intimus

M. intercostalis internus

M. intercostalis externus

Membrana intercostalis externa

M. obliquus externus abdominis

R. cutaneus anterior n. intercostalis

Anterior view

M. obliquus externus abdominis

Aponeurosis m. obliqui externi abdominis

Spina iliaca anterior superior

M. obliquus internus abdominis (*cut and reflected*)

M. transversus abdominis

Anulus inguinalis profundus

Caput laterale cremasteris

A. and V. epigastrica inferior (deep to Fascia transversalis)

Lig. inguinale (Pouparti)

Lig. lacunare (Gimbernati)

Caput mediale cremasteris

Anulus inguinalis superficalis

Crus laterale anuli inguinalis superficialis

Crus mediale anuli inguinalis superficialis

Crista pubica

Linea alba

Lamina anterior vaginae m. recti abdominis

Fascia transversalis (within Trigonum inguinale)

Falx inguinalis (conjoint tendon)

Lig. inguinale reflexum

Fibrae intercrurales

Fascia spermatica externa (on Funiculus spermaticus)

Anulus inguinalis superficalis

Lig. fundiforme penis

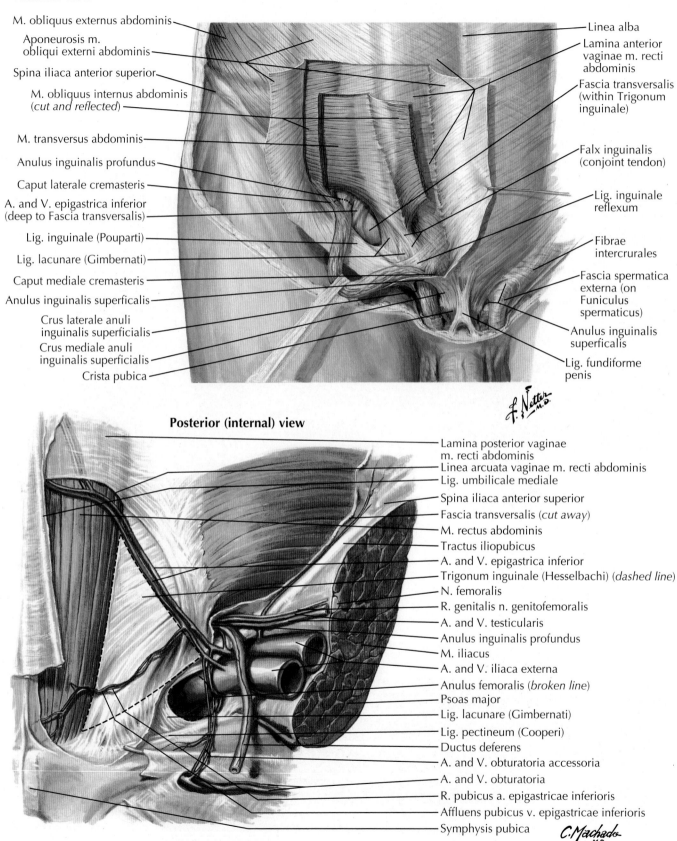

Posterior (internal) view

Lamina posterior vaginae m. recti abdominis

Linea arcuata vaginae m. recti abdominis

Lig. umbilicale mediale

Spina iliaca anterior superior

Fascia transversalis (*cut away*)

M. rectus abdominis

Tractus iliopubicus

A. and V. epigastrica inferior

Trigonum inguinale (Hesselbachi) (*dashed line*)

N. femoralis

R. genitalis n. genitofemoralis

A. and V. testicularis

Anulus inguinalis profundus

M. iliacus

A. and V. iliaca externa

Anulus femoralis (*broken line*)

Psoas major

Lig. lacunare (Gimbernati)

Lig. pectineum (Cooperi)

Ductus deferens

A. and V. obturatoria accessoria

A. and V. obturatoria

R. pubicus a. epigastricae inferioris

Affluens pubicus v. epigastricae inferioris

Symphysis pubica

Plate 280

Paries Abdominis

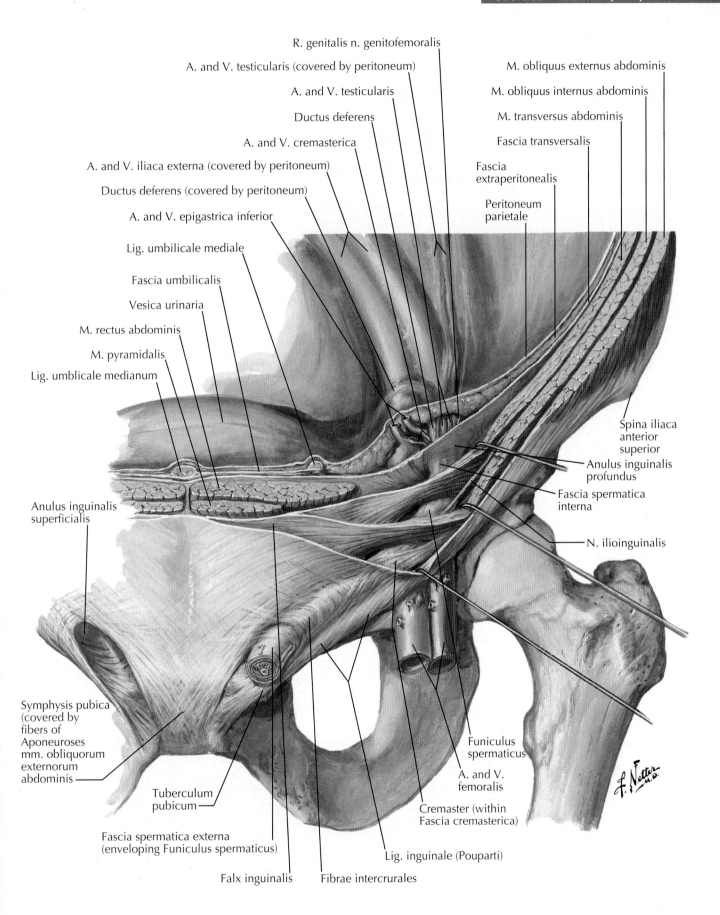

R. genitalis n. genitofemoralis

A. and V. testicularis (covered by peritoneum)

A. and V. testicularis

Ductus deferens

A. and V. cremasterica

A. and V. iliaca externa (covered by peritoneum)

Ductus deferens (covered by peritoneum)

A. and V. epigastrica inferior

Lig. umbilicale mediale

Fascia umbilicalis

Vesica urinaria

M. rectus abdominis

M. pyramidalis

Lig. umblicale medianum

M. obliquus externus abdominis

M. obliquus internus abdominis

M. transversus abdominis

Fascia transversalis

Fascia extraperitonealis

Peritoneum parietale

Spina iliaca anterior superior

Anulus inguinalis profundus

Fascia spermatica interna

N. ilioinguinalis

Anulus inguinalis superficialis

Symphysis pubica (covered by fibers of Aponeuroses mm. obliquorum externorum abdominis

Tuberculum pubicum

Fascia spermatica externa (enveloping Funiculus spermaticus)

Falx inguinalis

Fibrae intercrurales

Lig. inguinale (Pouparti)

Cremaster (within Fascia cremasterica)

A. and V. femoralis

Funiculus spermaticus

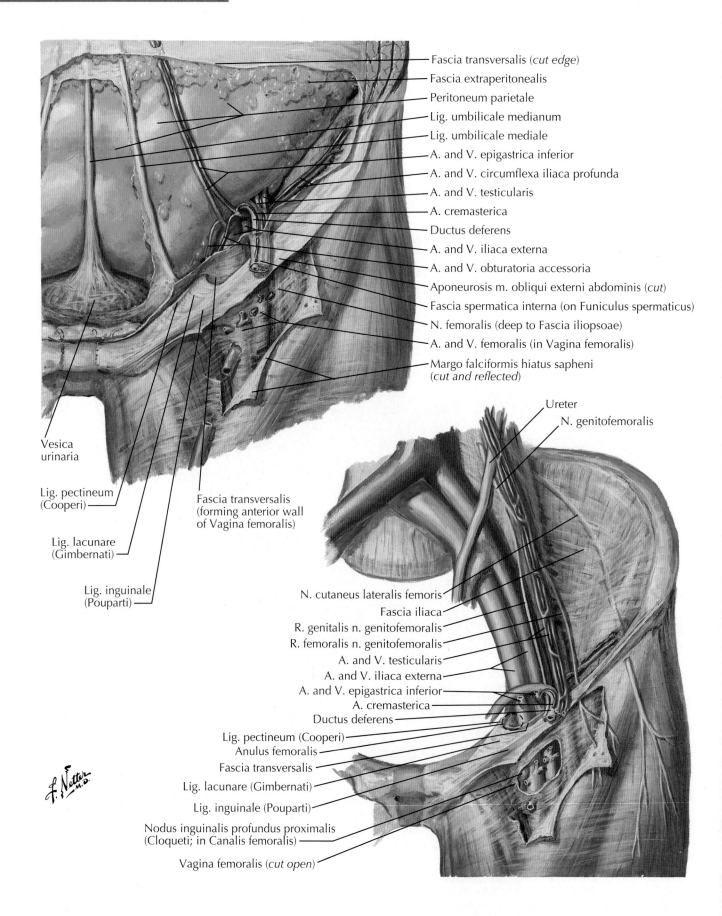

Fascia transversalis (*cut edge*)

Fascia extraperitonealis

Peritoneum parietale

Lig. umbilicale medianum

Lig. umbilicale mediale

A. and V. epigastrica inferior

A. and V. circumflexa iliaca profunda

A. and V. testicularis

A. cremasterica

Ductus deferens

A. and V. iliaca externa

A. and V. obturatoria accessoria

Aponeurosis m. obliqui externi abdominis (*cut*)

Fascia spermatica interna (on Funiculus spermaticus)

N. femoralis (deep to Fascia iliopsoae)

A. and V. femoralis (in Vagina femoralis)

Margo falciformis hiatus sapheni
(*cut and reflected*)

Ureter

N. genitofemoralis

Vesica
urinaria

Lig. pectineum
(Cooperi)

Fascia transversalis
(forming anterior wall
of Vagina femoralis)

Lig. lacunare
(Gimbernati)

Lig. inguinale
(Pouparti)

N. cutaneus lateralis femoris

Fascia iliaca

R. genitalis n. genitofemoralis

R. femoralis n. genitofemoralis

A. and V. testicularis

A. and V. iliaca externa

A. and V. epigastrica inferior

A. cremasterica

Ductus deferens

Lig. pectineum (Cooperi)

Anulus femoralis

Fascia transversalis

Lig. lacunare (Gimbernati)

Lig. inguinale (Pouparti)

Nodus inguinalis profundus proximalis
(Cloqueti; in Canalis femoralis)

Vagina femoralis (*cut open*)

Plate 282

Paries Abdominis

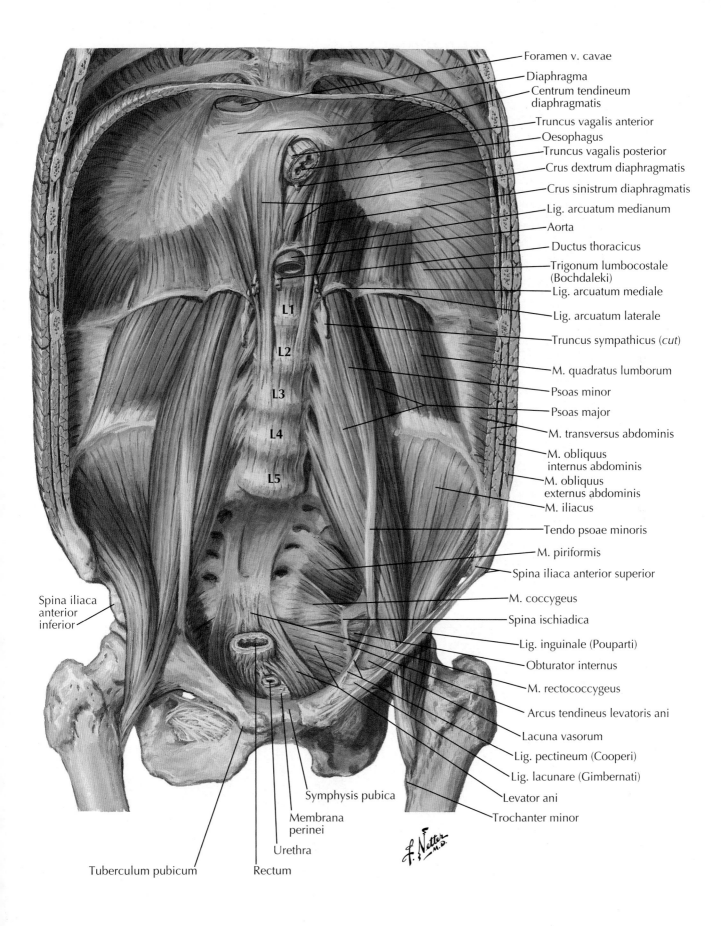

Foramen v. cavae

Diaphragma

Centrum tendineum diaphragmatis

Truncus vagalis anterior

Oesophagus

Truncus vagalis posterior

Crus dextrum diaphragmatis

Crus sinistrum diaphragmatis

Lig. arcuatum medianum

Aorta

Ductus thoracicus

Trigonum lumbocostale (Bochdaleki)

Lig. arcuatum mediale

Lig. arcuatum laterale

Truncus sympathicus (*cut*)

M. quadratus lumborum

Psoas minor

Psoas major

M. transversus abdominis

M. obliquus internus abdominis

M. obliquus externus abdominis

M. iliacus

Tendo psoae minoris

M. piriformis

Spina iliaca anterior superior

M. coccygeus

Spina ischiadica

Lig. inguinale (Pouparti)

Obturator internus

M. rectococcygeus

Arcus tendineus levatoris ani

Lacuna vasorum

Lig. pectineum (Cooperi)

Lig. lacunare (Gimbernati)

Levator ani

Trochanter minor

L1

L2

L3

L4

L5

Spina iliaca anterior inferior

Tuberculum pubicum

Rectum

Urethra

Membrana perinei

Symphysis pubica

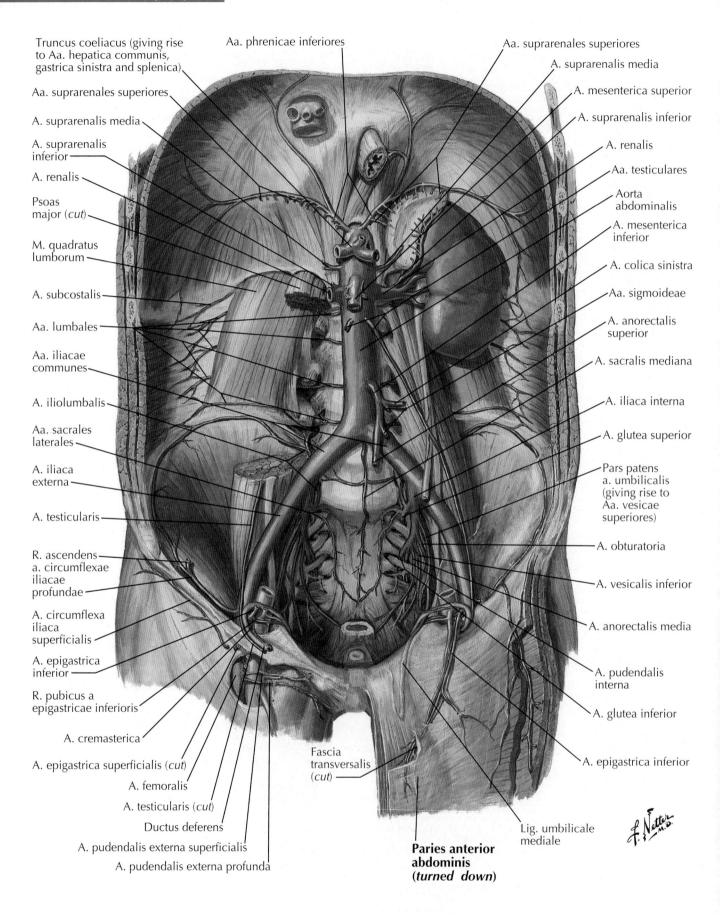

Truncus coeliacus (giving rise to Aa. hepatica communis, gastrica sinistra and splenica)

Aa. suprarenales superiores

A. suprarenalis media

A. suprarenalis inferior

A. renalis

Psoas major (*cut*)

M. quadratus lumborum

A. subcostalis

Aa. lumbales

Aa. iliacae communes

A. iliolumbalis

Aa. sacrales laterales

A. iliaca externa

A. testicularis

R. ascendens a. circumflexae iliacae profundae

A. circumflexa iliaca superficialis

A. epigastrica inferior

R. pubicus a epigastricae inferioris

A. cremasterica

A. epigastrica superficialis (*cut*)

A. femoralis

A. testicularis (*cut*)

Ductus deferens

A. pudendalis externa superficialis

A. pudendalis externa profunda

Aa. phrenicae inferiores

Aa. suprarenales superiores

A. suprarenalis media

A. mesenterica superior

A. suprarenalis inferior

A. renalis

Aa. testiculares

Aorta abdominalis

A. mesenterica inferior

A. colica sinistra

Aa. sigmoideae

A. anorectalis superior

A. sacralis mediana

A. iliaca interna

A. glutea superior

Pars patens a. umbilicalis (giving rise to Aa. vesicae superiores)

A. obturatoria

A. vesicalis inferior

A. anorectalis media

A. pudendalis interna

A. glutea inferior

A. epigastrica inferior

Fascia transversalis (*cut*)

Lig. umbilicale mediale

Paries anterior abdominis (*turned down*)

Plate 284

Paries Abdominis

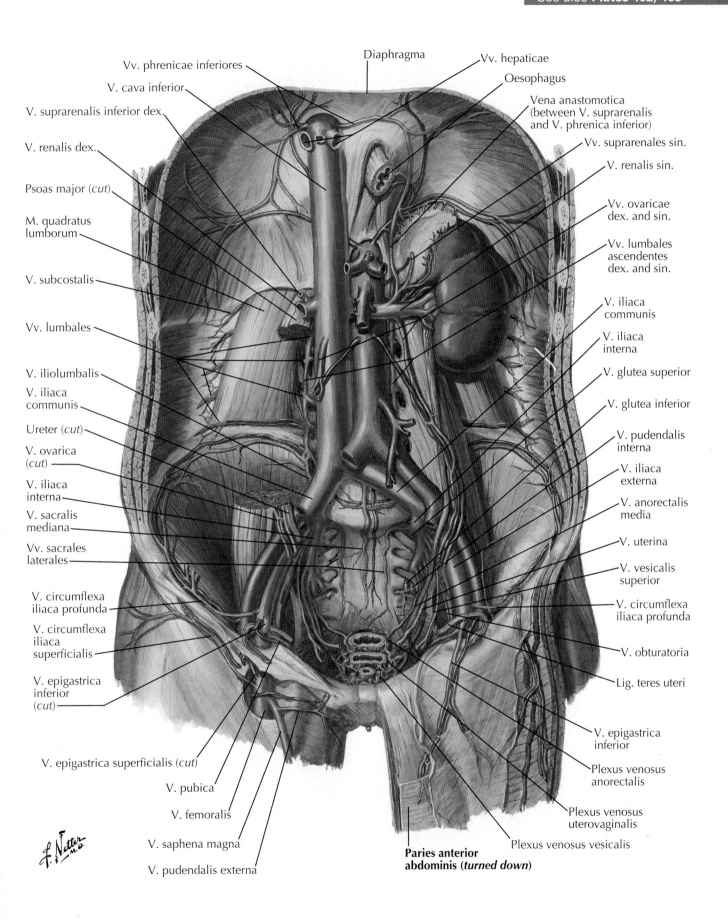

Vv. phrenicae inferiores

V. cava inferior

Diaphragma

Vv. hepaticae

Oesophagus

V. suprarenalis inferior dex.

V. renalis dex.

Psoas major (*cut*)

M. quadratus lumborum

V. subcostalis

Vv. lumbales

V. iliolumbalis

V. iliaca communis

Ureter (*cut*)

V. ovarica (*cut*)

V. iliaca interna

V. sacralis mediana

Vv. sacrales laterales

V. circumflexa iliaca profunda

V. circumflexa iliaca superficialis

V. epigastrica inferior (*cut*)

Vena anastomotica (between V. suprarenalis and V. phrenica inferior)

Vv. suprarenales sin.

V. renalis sin.

Vv. ovaricae dex. and sin.

Vv. lumbales ascendentes dex. and sin.

V. iliaca communis

V. iliaca interna

V. glutea superior

V. glutea inferior

V. pudendalis interna

V. iliaca externa

V. anorectalis media

V. uterina

V. vesicalis superior

V. circumflexa iliaca profunda

V. obturatoria

Lig. teres uteri

V. epigastrica inferior

Plexus venosus anorectalis

Plexus venosus uterovaginalis

V. epigastrica superficialis (*cut*)

V. pubica

V. femoralis

V. saphena magna

V. pudendalis externa

Plexus venosus vesicalis

Paries anterior abdominis (*turned down*)

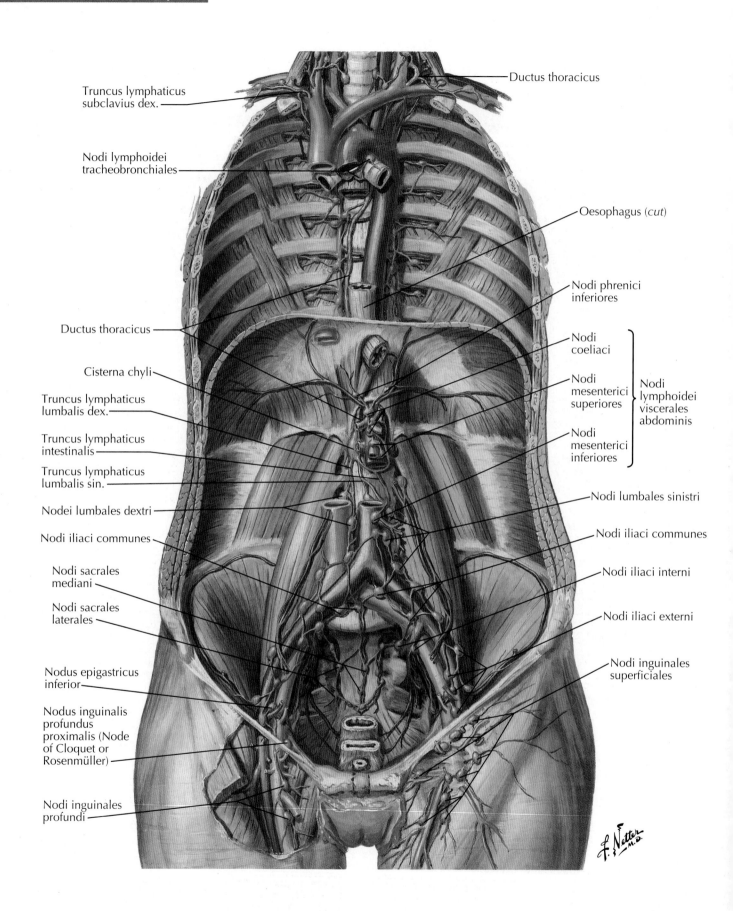

Truncus lymphaticus subclavius dex.

Nodi lymphoidei tracheobronchiales

Ductus thoracicus

Cisterna chyli

Truncus lymphaticus lumbalis dex.

Truncus lymphaticus intestinalis

Truncus lymphaticus lumbalis sin.

Nodei lumbales dextri

Nodi iliaci communes

Nodi sacrales mediani

Nodi sacrales laterales

Nodus epigastricus inferior

Nodus inguinalis profundus proximalis (Node of Cloquet or Rosenmüller)

Nodi inguinales profundi

Ductus thoracicus

Oesophagus (cut)

Nodi phrenici inferiores

Nodi coeliaci

Nodi mesenterici superiores

Nodi mesenterici inferiores

Nodi lymphoidei viscerales abdominis

Nodi lumbales sinistri

Nodi iliaci communes

Nodi iliaci interni

Nodi iliaci externi

Nodi inguinales superficiales

Plate 286

Paries Abdominis

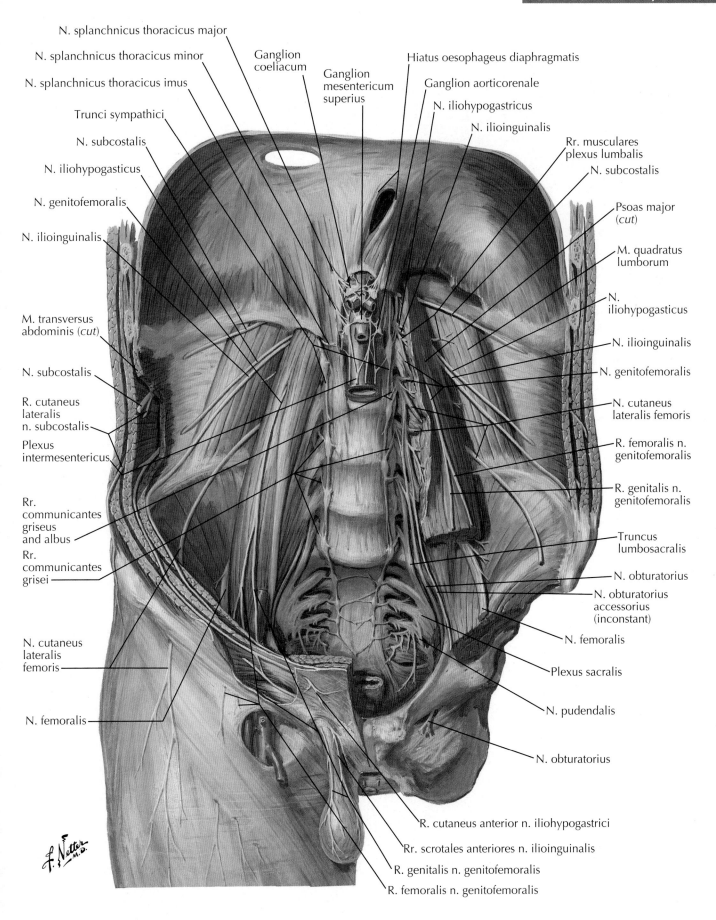

N. splanchnicus thoracicus major

N. splanchnicus thoracicus minor

N. splanchnicus thoracicus imus

Trunci sympathici

N. subcostalis

N. iliohypogasticus

N. genitofemoralis

N. ilioinguinalis

M. transversus abdominis (*cut*)

N. subcostalis

R. cutaneus lateralis n. subcostalis

Plexus intermesentericus

Rr. communicantes griseus and albus

Rr. communicantes grisei

N. cutaneus lateralis femoris

N. femoralis

Ganglion coeliacum

Ganglion mesentericum superius

Hiatus oesophageus diaphragmatis

Ganglion aorticorenale

N. iliohypogastricus

N. ilioinguinalis

Rr. musculares plexus lumbalis

N. subcostalis

Psoas major (*cut*)

M. quadratus lumborum

N. iliohypogasticus

N. ilioinguinalis

N. genitofemoralis

N. cutaneus lateralis femoris

R. femoralis n. genitofemoralis

R. genitalis n. genitofemoralis

Truncus lumbosacralis

N. obturatorius

N. obturatorius accessorius (inconstant)

N. femoralis

Plexus sacralis

N. pudendalis

N. obturatorius

R. cutaneus anterior n. iliohypogastrici

Rr. scrotales anteriores n. ilioinguinalis

R. genitalis n. genitofemoralis

R. femoralis n. genitofemoralis

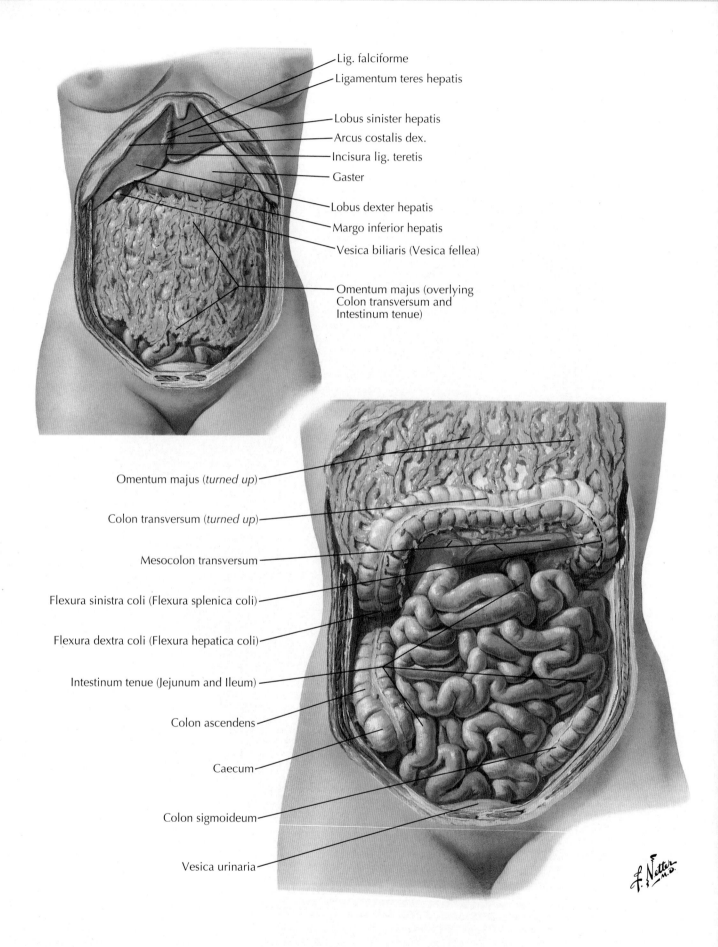

Lig. falciforme

Ligamentum teres hepatis

Lobus sinister hepatis

Arcus costalis dex.

Incisura lig. teretis

Gaster

Lobus dexter hepatis

Margo inferior hepatis

Vesica biliaris (Vesica fellea)

Omentum majus (overlying Colon transversum and Intestinum tenue)

Omentum majus (*turned up*)

Colon transversum (*turned up*)

Mesocolon transversum

Flexura sinistra coli (Flexura splenica coli)

Flexura dextra coli (Flexura hepatica coli)

Intestinum tenue (Jejunum and Ileum)

Colon ascendens

Caecum

Colon sigmoideum

Vesica urinaria

Plate 288

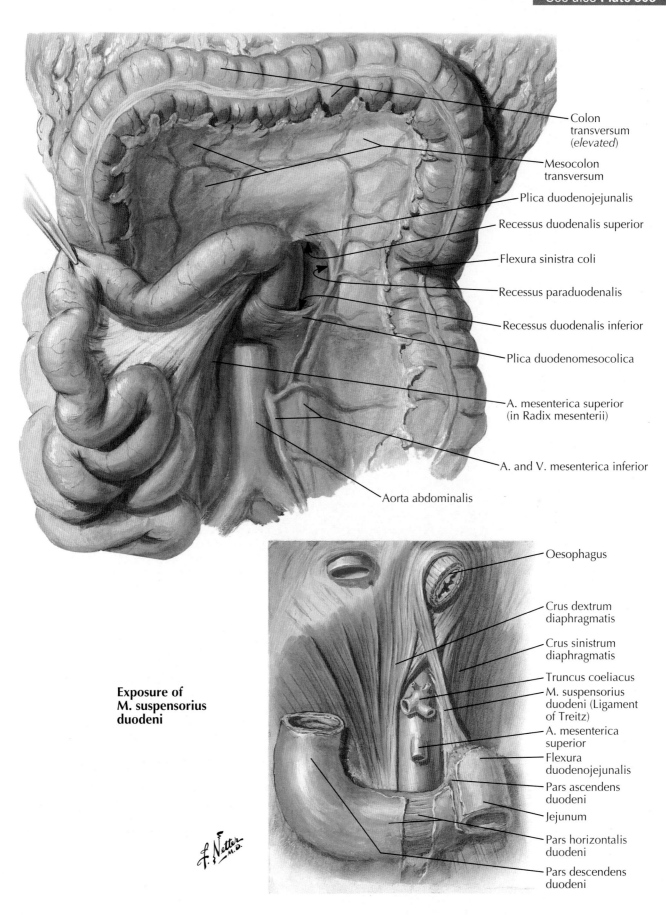

Colon
transversum
(*elevated*)

Mesocolon
transversum

Plica duodenojejunalis

Recessus duodenalis superior

Flexura sinistra coli

Recessus paraduodenalis

Recessus duodenalis inferior

Plica duodenomesocolica

A. mesenterica superior
(in Radix mesenterii)

A. and V. mesenterica inferior

Aorta abdominalis

Oesophagus

Crus dextrum
diaphragmatis

Crus sinistrum
diaphragmatis

Truncus coeliacus

M. suspensorius
duodeni (Ligament
of Treitz)

A. mesenterica
superior

Flexura
duodenojejunalis

Pars ascendens
duodeni

Jejunum

Pars horizontalis
duodeni

Pars descendens
duodeni

**Exposure of
M. suspensorius
duodeni**

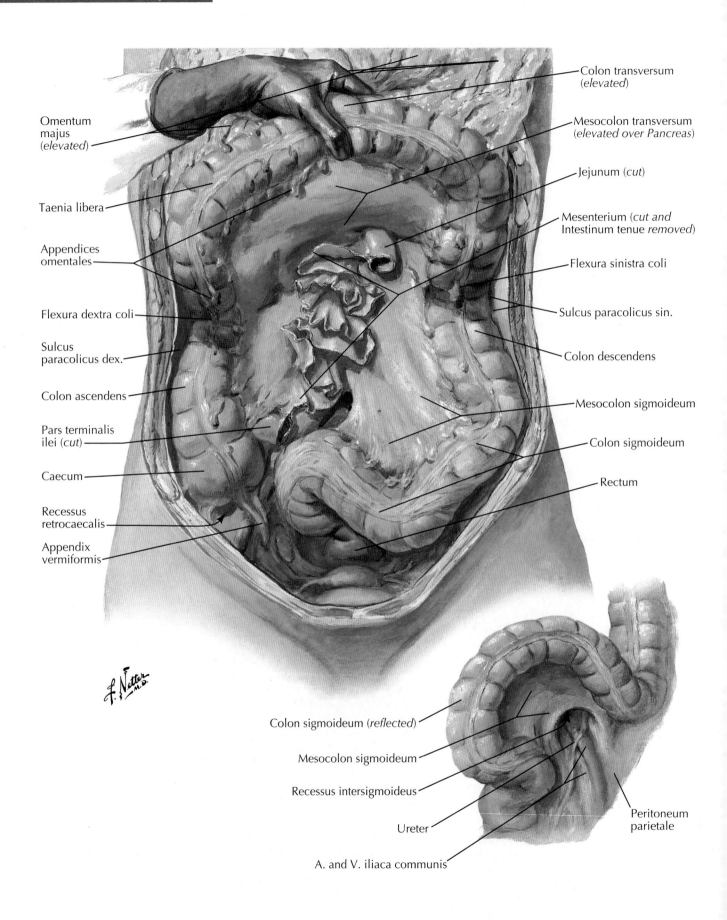

Omentum majus (*elevated*)

Taenia libera

Appendices omentales

Flexura dextra coli

Sulcus paracolicus dex.

Colon ascendens

Pars terminalis ilei (*cut*)

Caecum

Recessus retrocaecalis

Appendix vermiformis

Colon transversum (*elevated*)

Mesocolon transversum (*elevated over Pancreas*)

Jejunum (*cut*)

Mesenterium (*cut and Intestinum tenue removed*)

Flexura sinistra coli

Sulcus paracolicus sin.

Colon descendens

Mesocolon sigmoideum

Colon sigmoideum

Rectum

Colon sigmoideum (*reflected*)

Mesocolon sigmoideum

Recessus intersigmoideus

Ureter

A. and V. iliaca communis

Peritoneum parietale

Plate 290

Cavitas Peritonealis

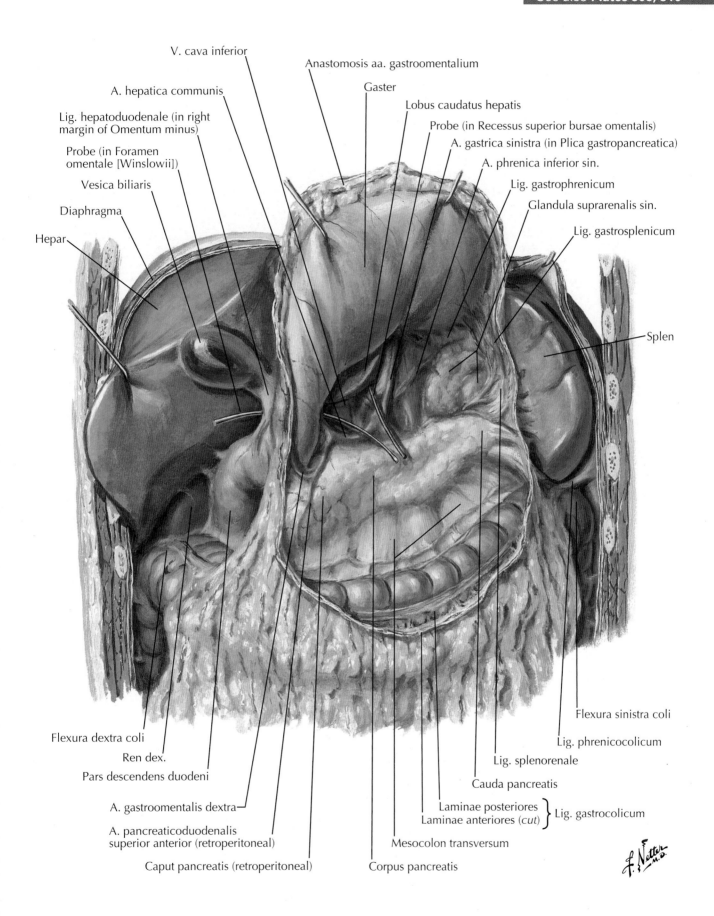

V. cava inferior

Anastomosis aa. gastroomentalium

A. hepatica communis

Gaster

Lig. hepatoduodenale (in right margin of Omentum minus)

Lobus caudatus hepatis

Probe (in Recessus superior bursae omentalis)

Probe (in Foramen omentale [Winslowii])

A. gastrica sinistra (in Plica gastropancreatica)

Vesica biliaris

A. phrenica inferior sin.

Lig. gastrophrenicum

Diaphragma

Glandula suprarenalis sin.

Hepar

Lig. gastrosplenicum

Splen

Flexura dextra coli

Flexura sinistra coli

Ren dex.

Lig. phrenicocolicum

Pars descendens duodeni

Lig. splenorenale

A. gastroomentalis dextra

Cauda pancreatis

A. pancreaticoduodenalis superior anterior (retroperitoneal)

Laminae posteriores

Laminae anteriores (*cut*) } Lig. gastrocolicum

Caput pancreatis (retroperitoneal)

Mesocolon transversum

Corpus pancreatis

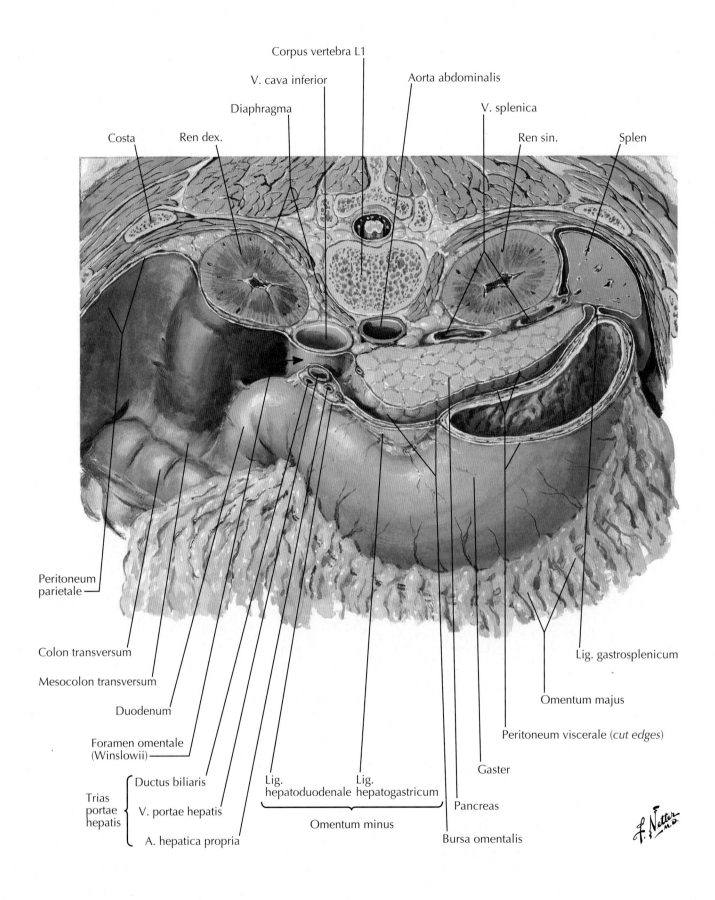

Corpus vertebra L1

V. cava inferior

Aorta abdominalis

Diaphragma

V. splenica

Costa

Ren dex.

Ren sin.

Splen

Peritoneum
parietale

Colon transversum

Mesocolon transversum

Duodenum

Foramen omentale
(Winslowii)

Ductus biliaris

Trias
portae
hepatis

V. portae hepatis

A. hepatica propria

Lig.
hepatoduodenale

Lig.
hepatogastricum

Omentum minus

Gaster

Pancreas

Bursa omentalis

Lig. gastrosplenicum

Omentum majus

Peritoneum viscerale (*cut edges*)

Plate 292

Cavitas Peritonealis

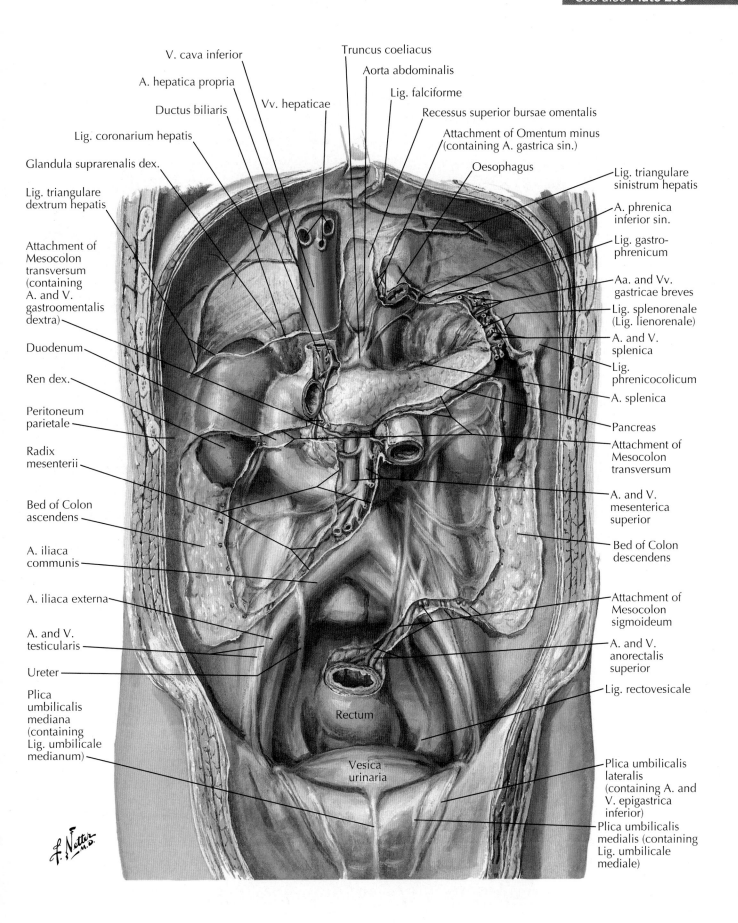

V. cava inferior

A. hepatica propria

Ductus biliaris

Lig. coronarium hepatis

Glandula suprarenalis dex.

Lig. triangulare
dextrum hepatis

Attachment of
Mesocolon
transversum
(containing
A. and V.
gastroomentalis
dextra)

Duodenum

Ren dex.

Peritoneum
parietale

Radix
mesenterii

Bed of Colon
ascendens

A. iliaca
communis

A. iliaca externa

A. and V.
testicularis

Ureter

Plica
umbilicalis
mediana
(containing
Lig. umbilicale
medianum)

Vv. hepaticae

Truncus coeliacus

Aorta abdominalis

Lig. falciforme

Recessus superior bursae omentalis

Attachment of Omentum minus
(containing A. gastrica sin.)

Oesophagus

Lig. triangulare
sinistrum hepatis

A. phrenica
inferior sin.

Lig. gastro-
phrenicum

Aa. and Vv.
gastricae breves

Lig. splenorenale
(Lig. lienorenale)

A. and V.
splenica

Lig.
phrenicocolicum

A. splenica

Pancreas

Attachment of
Mesocolon
transversum

A. and V.
mesenterica
superior

Bed of Colon
descendens

Attachment of
Mesocolon
sigmoideum

A. and V.
anorectalis
superior

Lig. rectovesicale

Rectum

Vesica
urinaria

Plica umbilicalis
lateralis
(containing A. and
V. epigastrica
inferior)

Plica umbilicalis
medialis (containing
Lig. umbilicale
mediale)

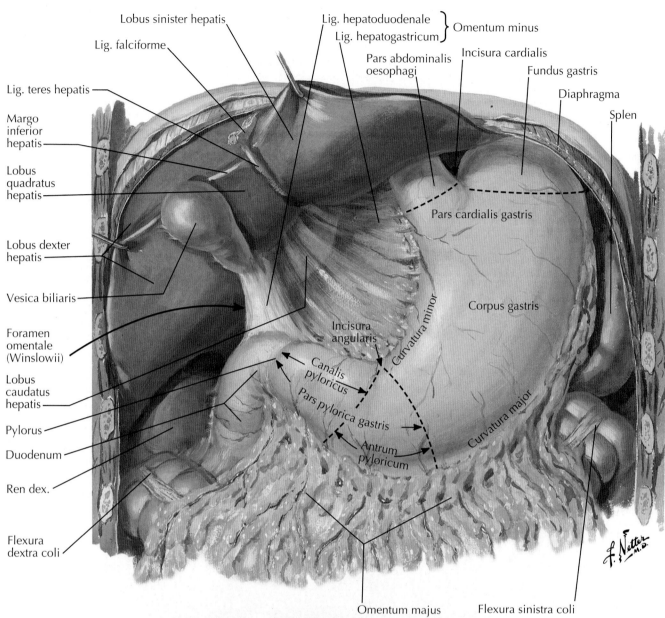

Lobus sinister hepatis

Lig. falciforme

Lig. teres hepatis

Margo inferior hepatis

Lobus quadratus hepatis

Lobus dexter hepatis

Vesica biliaris

Foramen omentale (Winslowii)

Lobus caudatus hepatis

Pylorus

Duodenum

Ren dex.

Flexura dextra coli

Lig. hepatoduodenale

Lig. hepatogastricum

} Omentum minus

Pars abdominalis oesophagi

Incisura cardialis

Fundus gastris

Diaphragma

Splen

Pars cardialis gastris

Corpus gastris

Curvatura minor

Incisura angularis

Canalis pyloricus

Pars pylorica gastris

Antrum pyloricum

Curvatura major

Omentum majus

Flexura sinistra coli

Transverse gray-scale ultrasound image of midabdomen

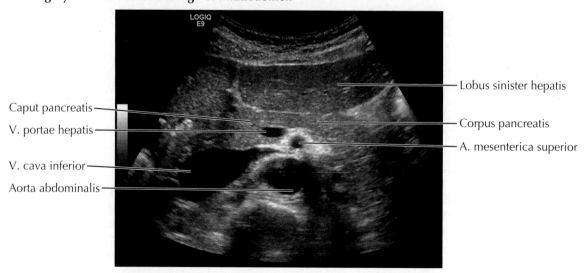

LOGIQ
E9

Caput pancreatis

V. portae hepatis

V. cava inferior

Aorta abdominalis

Lobus sinister hepatis

Corpus pancreatis

A. mesenterica superior

Plate 294

Gaster and Intestina

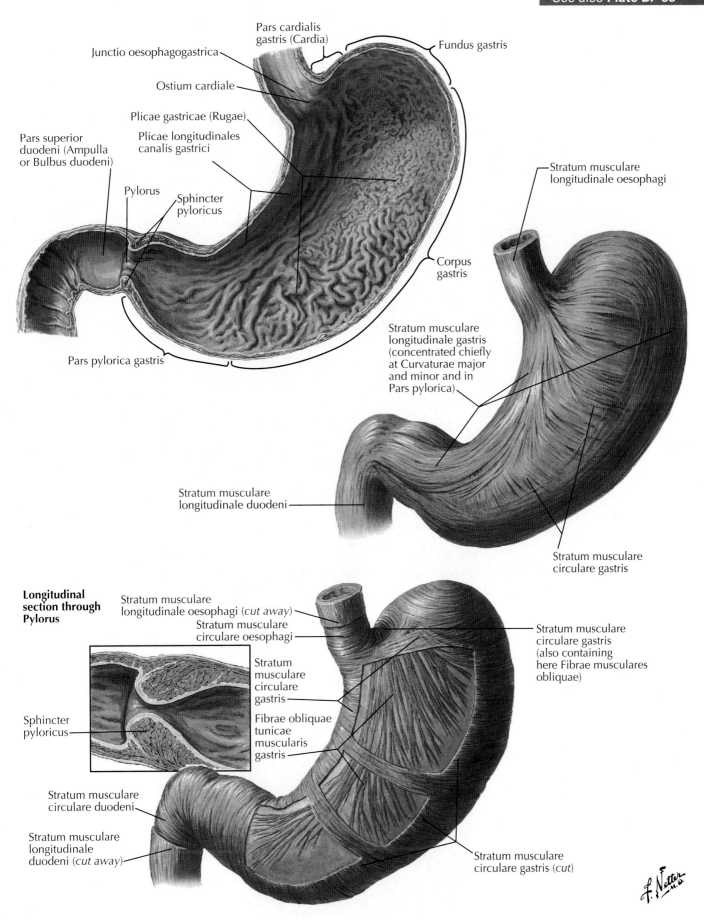

Junctio oesophagogastrica

Pars cardialis gastris (Cardia)

Fundus gastris

Ostium cardiale

Plicae gastricae (Rugae)

Pars superior duodeni (Ampulla or Bulbus duodeni)

Plicae longitudinales canalis gastrici

Stratum musculare longitudinale oesophagi

Pylorus

Sphincter pyloricus

Corpus gastris

Pars pylorica gastris

Stratum musculare longitudinale gastris (concentrated chiefly at Curvaturae major and minor and in Pars pylorica)

Stratum musculare longitudinale duodeni

Stratum musculare circulare gastris

Longitudinal section through Pylorus

Stratum musculare longitudinale oesophagi (cut away)

Stratum musculare circulare oesophagi

Stratum musculare circulare gastris

Stratum musculare circulare gastris (also containing here Fibrae musculares obliquae)

Sphincter pyloricus

Fibrae obliquae tunicae muscularis gastris

Stratum musculare circulare duodeni

Stratum musculare longitudinale duodeni (cut away)

Stratum musculare circulare gastris (cut)

Gaster and Intestina

Plate 295

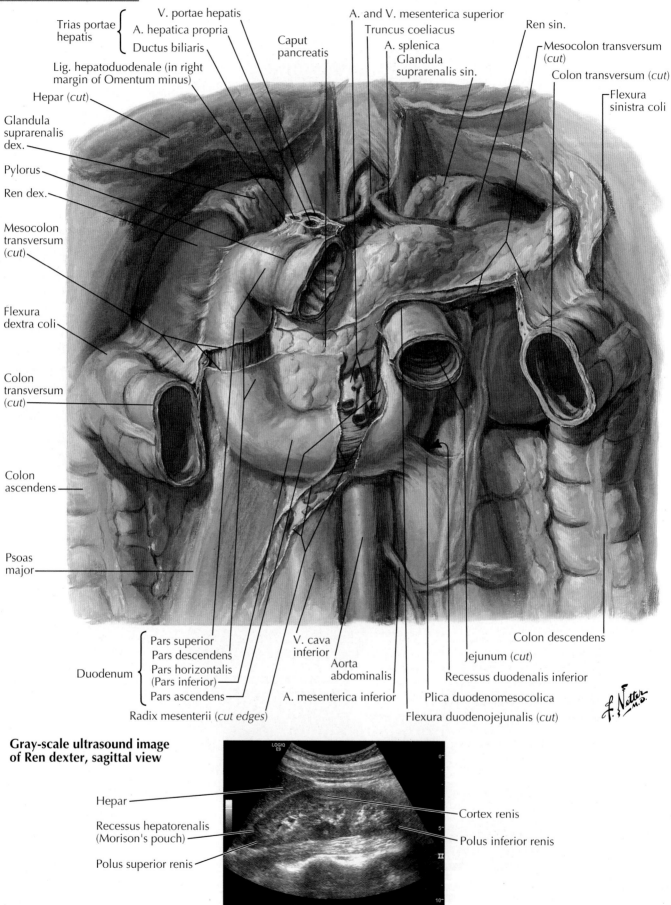

Trias portae hepatis {
V. portae hepatis
A. hepatica propria
Ductus biliaris

Caput pancreatis

A. and V. mesenterica superior
Truncus coeliacus
A. splenica
Glandula suprarenalis sin.

Ren sin.

Mesocolon transversum (*cut*)
Colon transversum (*cut*)
Flexura sinistra coli

Lig. hepatoduodenale (in right margin of Omentum minus)

Hepar (*cut*)

Glandula suprarenalis dex.

Pylorus

Ren dex.

Mesocolon transversum (*cut*)

Flexura dextra coli

Colon transversum (*cut*)

Colon ascendens

Psoas major

Duodenum {
Pars superior
Pars descendens
Pars horizontalis (Pars inferior)
Pars ascendens

Radix mesenterii (*cut edges*)

V. cava inferior

Aorta abdominalis

A. mesenterica inferior

Colon descendens

Jejunum (*cut*)

Recessus duodenalis inferior

Plica duodenomesocolica

Flexura duodenojejunalis (*cut*)

Gray-scale ultrasound image of Ren dexter, sagittal view

Hepar

Recessus hepatorenalis (Morison's pouch)

Polus superior renis

Cortex renis

Polus inferior renis

SAG RIGHT KIDNEY

Plate 296

Gaster and Intestina

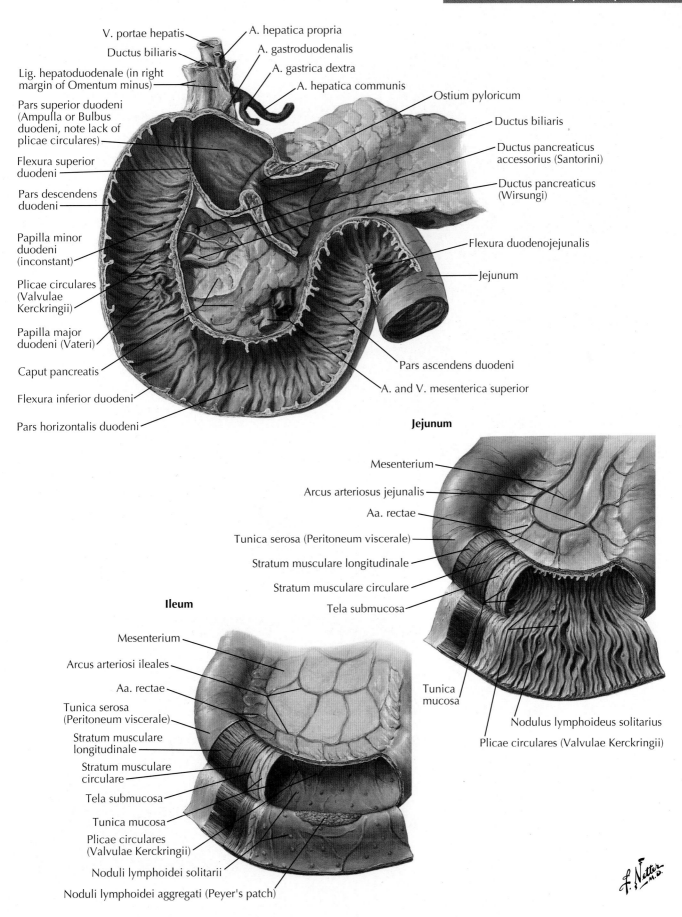

V. portae hepatis

Ductus biliaris

Lig. hepatoduodenale (in right margin of Omentum minus)

Pars superior duodeni (Ampulla or Bulbus duodeni, note lack of plicae circulares)

Flexura superior duodeni

Pars descendens duodeni

Papilla minor duodeni (inconstant)

Plicae circulares (Valvulae Kerckringii)

Papilla major duodeni (Vateri)

Caput pancreatis

Flexura inferior duodeni

Pars horizontalis duodeni

A. hepatica propria

A. gastroduodenalis

A. gastrica dextra

A. hepatica communis

Ostium pyloricum

Ductus biliaris

Ductus pancreaticus accessorius (Santorini)

Ductus pancreaticus (Wirsungi)

Flexura duodenojejunalis

Jejunum

Pars ascendens duodeni

A. and V. mesenterica superior

Jejunum

Mesenterium

Arcus arteriosus jejunalis

Aa. rectae

Tunica serosa (Peritoneum viscerale)

Stratum musculare longitudinale

Stratum musculare circulare

Tela submucosa

Tunica mucosa

Nodulus lymphoideus solitarius

Plicae circulares (Valvulae Kerckringii)

Ileum

Mesenterium

Arcus arteriosi ileales

Aa. rectae

Tunica serosa (Peritoneum viscerale)

Stratum musculare longitudinale

Stratum musculare circulare

Tela submucosa

Tunica mucosa

Plicae circulares (Valvulae Kerckringii)

Noduli lymphoidei solitarii

Noduli lymphoidei aggregati (Peyer's patch)

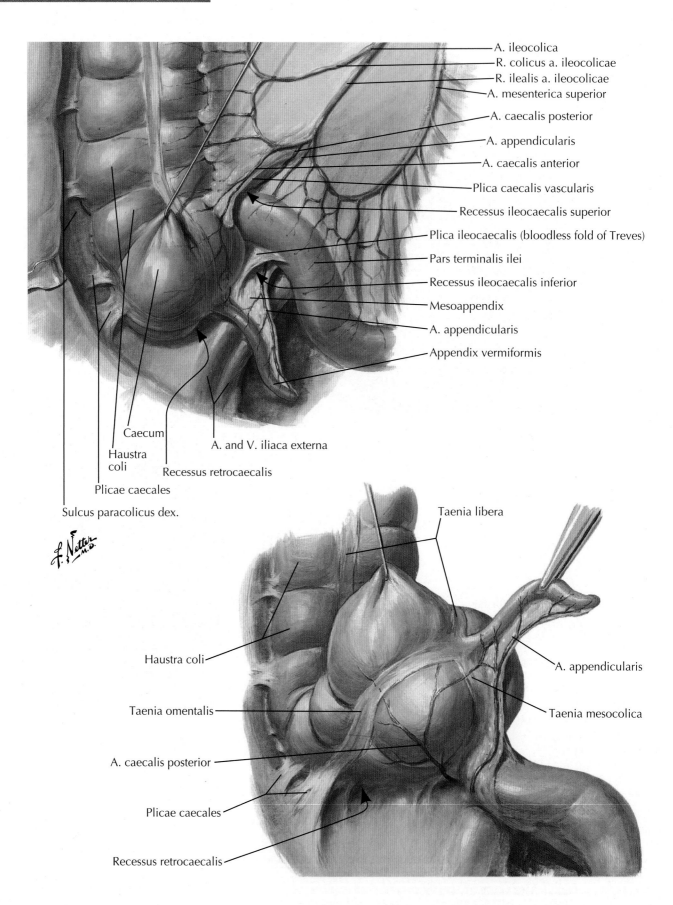

A. ileocolica

R. colicus a. ileocolicae

R. ilealis a. ileocolicae

A. mesenterica superior

A. caecalis posterior

A. appendicularis

A. caecalis anterior

Plica caecalis vascularis

Recessus ileocaecalis superior

Plica ileocaecalis (bloodless fold of Treves)

Pars terminalis ilei

Recessus ileocaecalis inferior

Mesoappendix

A. appendicularis

Appendix vermiformis

Caecum

Haustra coli

Recessus retrocaecalis

Plicae caecales

Sulcus paracolicus dex.

A. and V. iliaca externa

Taenia libera

Haustra coli

A. appendicularis

Taenia omentalis

Taenia mesocolica

A. caecalis posterior

Plicae caecales

Recessus retrocaecalis

Plate 298

Gaster and Intestina

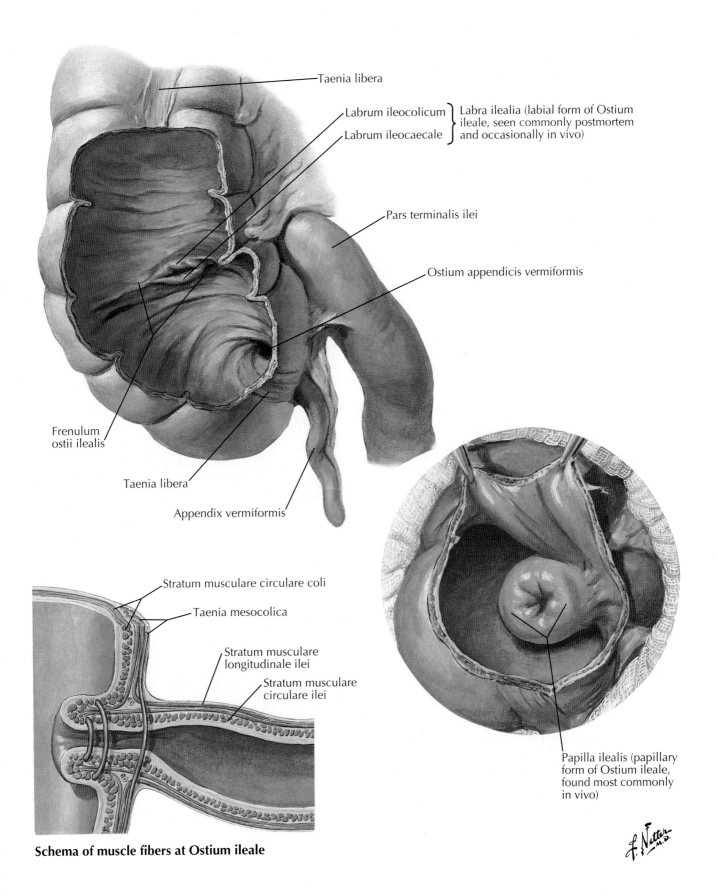

Taenia libera

Labrum ileocolicum ⎱
Labrum ileocaecale ⎰ Labra ilealia (labial form of Ostium ileale, seen commonly postmortem and occasionally in vivo)

Pars terminalis ilei

Ostium appendicis vermiformis

Frenulum ostii ilealis

Taenia libera

Appendix vermiformis

Stratum musculare circulare coli

Taenia mesocolica

Stratum musculare longitudinale ilei

Stratum musculare circulare ilei

Papilla ilealis (papillary form of Ostium ileale, found most commonly in vivo)

Schema of muscle fibers at Ostium ileale

McBurney's point (a third of the way along the ASIS umbilical line)

Spina iliaca anterior superior

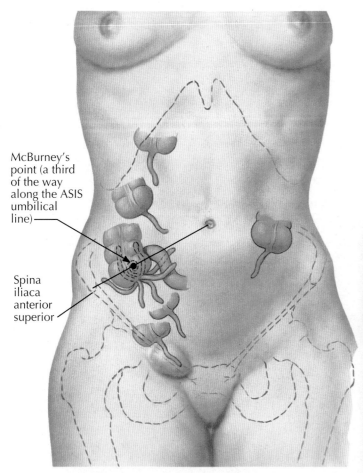

Variations in position of Appendix vermiformis

Coronal CT image with oral and intravenous contrast

Hepar   Vesica biliaris   Gaster   Flexura sinistra coli

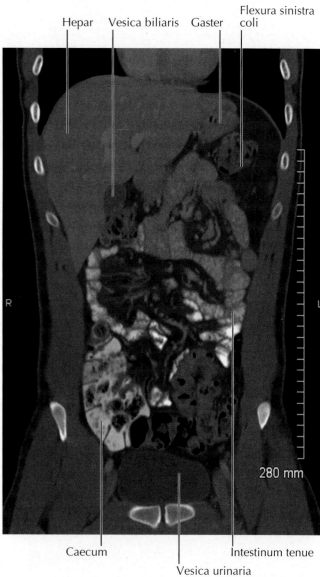

Caecum

Vesica urinaria

Intestinum tenue

280 mm

Fixed retrocecal Appendix vermiformis

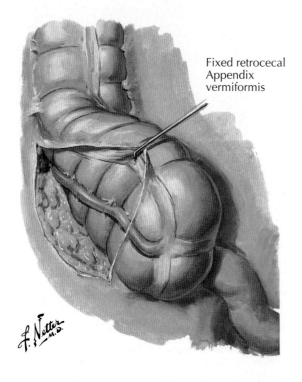

Plate 300   **Gaster and Intestina**

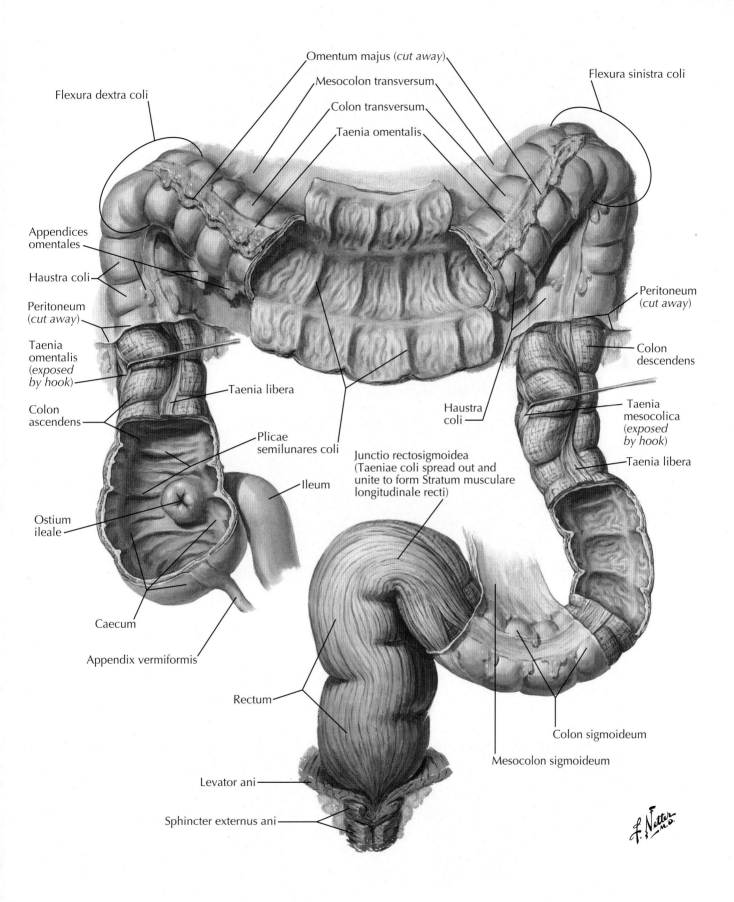

Omentum majus (*cut away*)

Mesocolon transversum

Colon transversum

Taenia omentalis

Flexura sinistra coli

Flexura dextra coli

Appendices omentales

Haustra coli

Peritoneum (*cut away*)

Taenia omentalis (*exposed by hook*)

Colon ascendens

Taenia libera

Plicae semilunares coli

Ileum

Ostium ileale

Caecum

Appendix vermiformis

Rectum

Levator ani

Sphincter externus ani

Peritoneum (*cut away*)

Colon descendens

Haustra coli

Taenia mesocolica (*exposed by hook*)

Taenia libera

Junctio rectosigmoidea (Taeniae coli spread out and unite to form Stratum musculare longitudinale recti)

Colon sigmoideum

Mesocolon sigmoideum

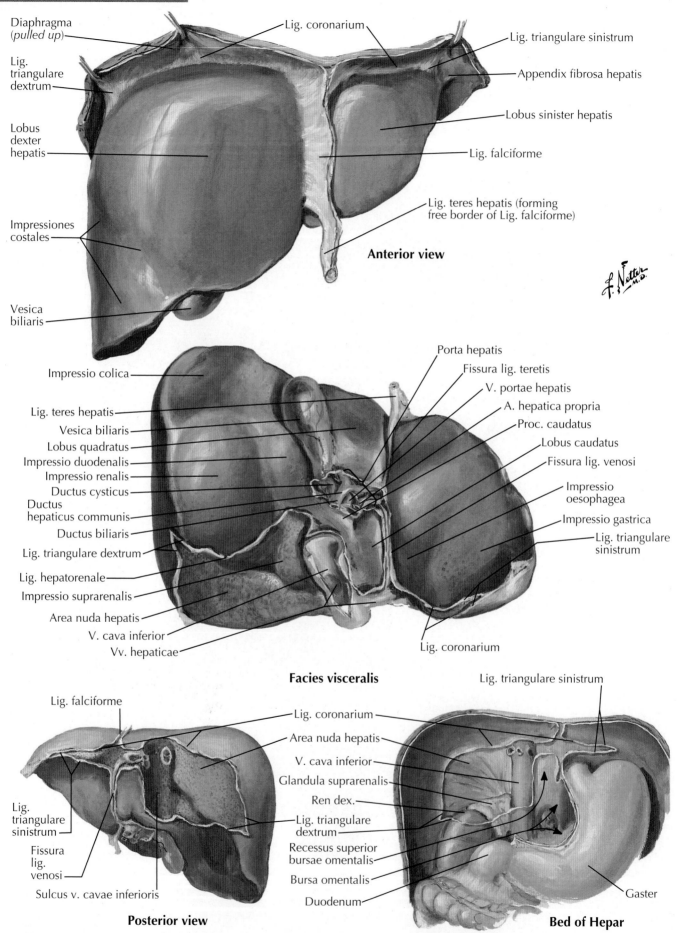

Diaphragma (*pulled up*)

Lig. coronarium

Lig. triangulare sinistrum

Lig. triangulare dextrum

Appendix fibrosa hepatis

Lobus dexter hepatis

Lobus sinister hepatis

Lig. falciforme

Impressiones costales

Lig. teres hepatis (forming free border of Lig. falciforme)

Anterior view

Vesica biliaris

Impressio colica

Porta hepatis

Fissura lig. teretis

V. portae hepatis

A. hepatica propria

Lig. teres hepatis

Proc. caudatus

Vesica biliaris

Lobus caudatus

Lobus quadratus

Fissura lig. venosi

Impressio duodenalis

Impressio renalis

Impressio oesophagea

Ductus cysticus

Ductus hepaticus communis

Impressio gastrica

Ductus biliaris

Lig. triangulare sinistrum

Lig. triangulare dextrum

Lig. hepatorenale

Impressio suprarenalis

Area nuda hepatis

V. cava inferior

Vv. hepaticae

Lig. coronarium

Facies visceralis

Lig. falciforme

Lig. triangulare sinistrum

Lig. coronarium

Area nuda hepatis

V. cava inferior

Glandula suprarenalis

Lig. triangulare sinistrum

Ren dex.

Fissura lig. venosi

Lig. triangulare dextrum

Recessus superior bursae omentalis

Sulcus v. cavae inferioris

Bursa omentalis

Duodenum

Gaster

Posterior view

Bed of Hepar

Plate 302

Hepar, Vesica Biliaris, Pancreas and Splen

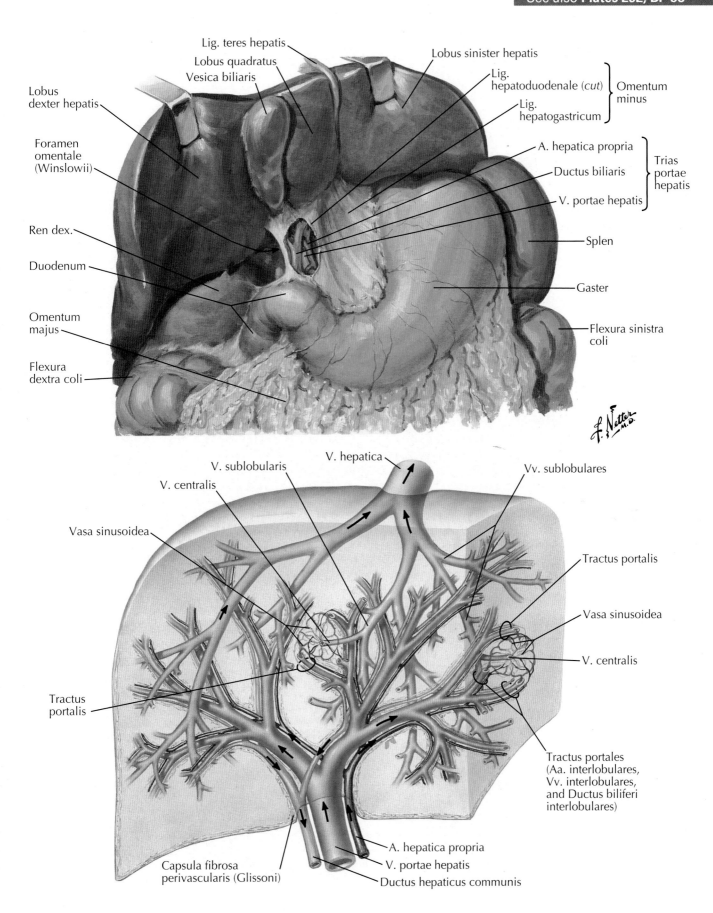

Lig. teres hepatis

Lobus quadratus

Vesica biliaris

Lobus sinister hepatis

Lig. hepatoduodenale (*cut*)

Lig. hepatogastricum

Omentum minus

Lobus dexter hepatis

Foramen omentale (Winslowii)

Ren dex.

Duodenum

Omentum majus

Flexura dextra coli

A. hepatica propria

Ductus biliaris

V. portae hepatis

Trias portae hepatis

Splen

Gaster

Flexura sinistra coli

V. hepatica

V. sublobularis

V. centralis

Vv. sublobulares

Vasa sinusoidea

Tractus portalis

Vasa sinusoidea

V. centralis

Tractus portalis

Tractus portales (Aa. interlobulares, Vv. interlobulares, and Ductus biliferi interlobulares)

Capsula fibrosa perivascularis (Glissoni)

A. hepatica propria

V. portae hepatis

Ductus hepaticus communis

Hepar, Vesica Biliaris, Pancreas and Splen

Plate 303

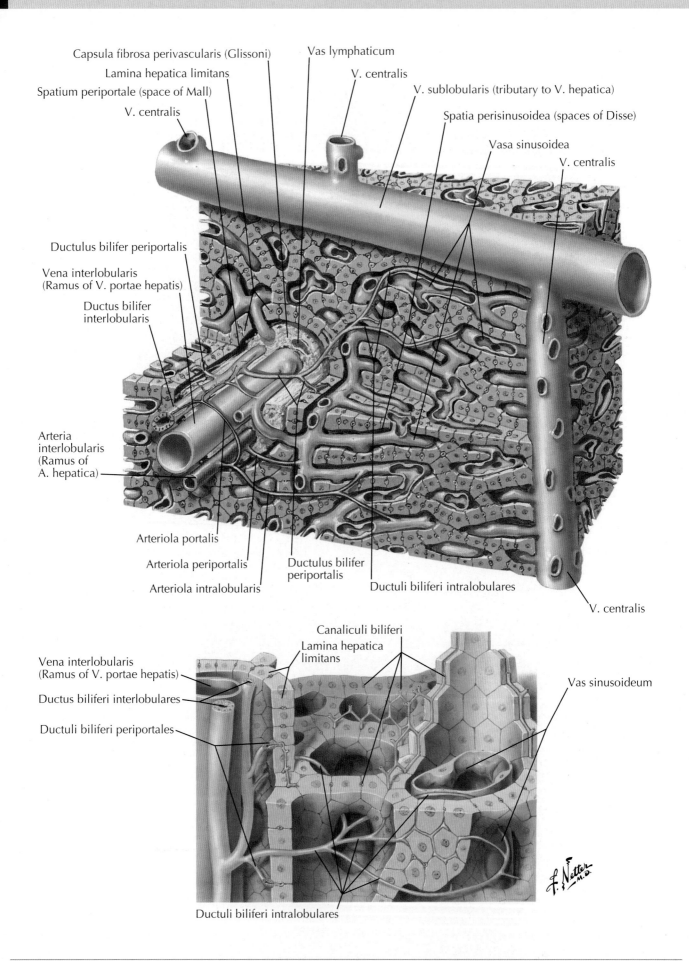

Capsula fibrosa perivascularis (Glissoni)

Lamina hepatica limitans

Spatium periportale (space of Mall)

V. centralis

Vas lymphaticum

V. centralis

V. sublobularis (tributary to V. hepatica)

Spatia perisinusoidea (spaces of Disse)

Vasa sinusoidea

V. centralis

Ductulus bilifer periportalis

Vena interlobularis
(Ramus of V. portae hepatis)

Ductus bilifer
interlobularis

Arteria
interlobularis
(Ramus of
A. hepatica)

Arteriola portalis

Arteriola periportalis

Arteriola intralobularis

Ductulus bilifer
periportalis

Ductuli biliferi intralobulares

V. centralis

Canaliculi biliferi

Lamina hepatica
limitans

Vena interlobularis
(Ramus of V. portae hepatis)

Ductus biliferi interlobulares

Ductuli biliferi periportales

Vas sinusoideum

Ductuli biliferi intralobulares

Plate 304

Hepar, Vesica Biliaris, Pancreas and Splen

See also **Plates BP 57, BP 62, BP 63**

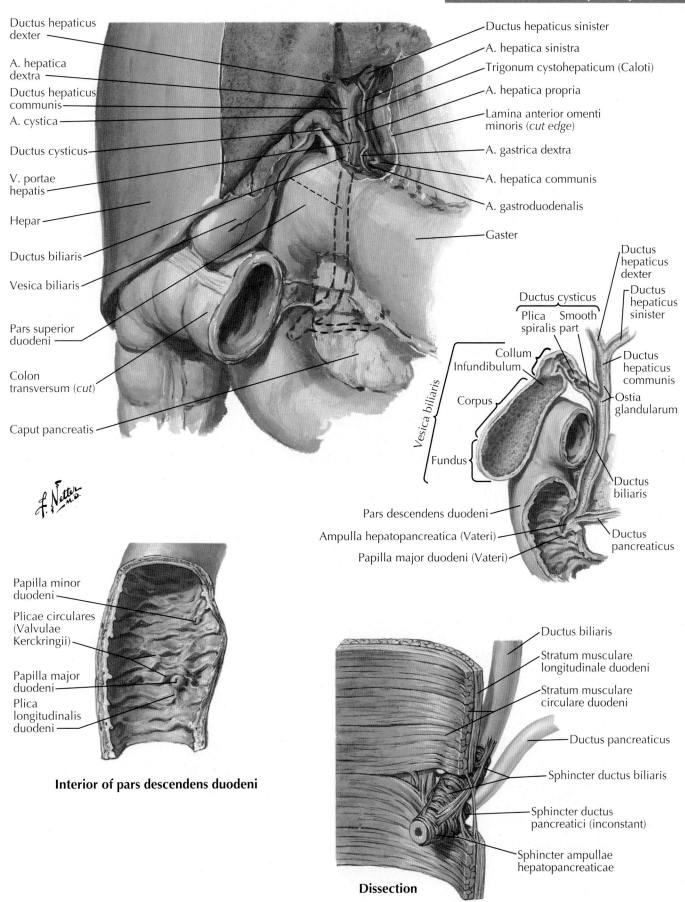

Ductus hepaticus dexter

A. hepatica dextra

Ductus hepaticus communis

A. cystica

Ductus cysticus

V. portae hepatis

Hepar

Ductus biliaris

Vesica biliaris

Pars superior duodeni

Colon transversum (cut)

Caput pancreatis

Ductus hepaticus sinister

A. hepatica sinistra

Trigonum cystohepaticum (Caloti)

A. hepatica propria

Lamina anterior omenti minoris (cut edge)

A. gastrica dextra

A. hepatica communis

A. gastroduodenalis

Gaster

Ductus cysticus
Plica spiralis   Smooth part

Collum
Infundibulum

Corpus

Vesica biliaris

Fundus

Ductus hepaticus dexter

Ductus hepaticus sinister

Ductus hepaticus communis

Ostia glandularum

Ductus biliaris

Ductus pancreaticus

Pars descendens duodeni

Ampulla hepatopancreatica (Vateri)

Papilla major duodeni (Vateri)

Papilla minor duodeni

Plicae circulares (Valvulae Kerckringii)

Papilla major duodeni

Plica longitudinalis duodeni

Interior of pars descendens duodeni

Ductus biliaris

Stratum musculare longitudinale duodeni

Stratum musculare circulare duodeni

Ductus pancreaticus

Sphincter ductus biliaris

Sphincter ductus pancreatici (inconstant)

Sphincter ampullae hepatopancreaticae

Dissection

Hepar, Vesica Biliaris, Pancreas and Splen

Plate 305

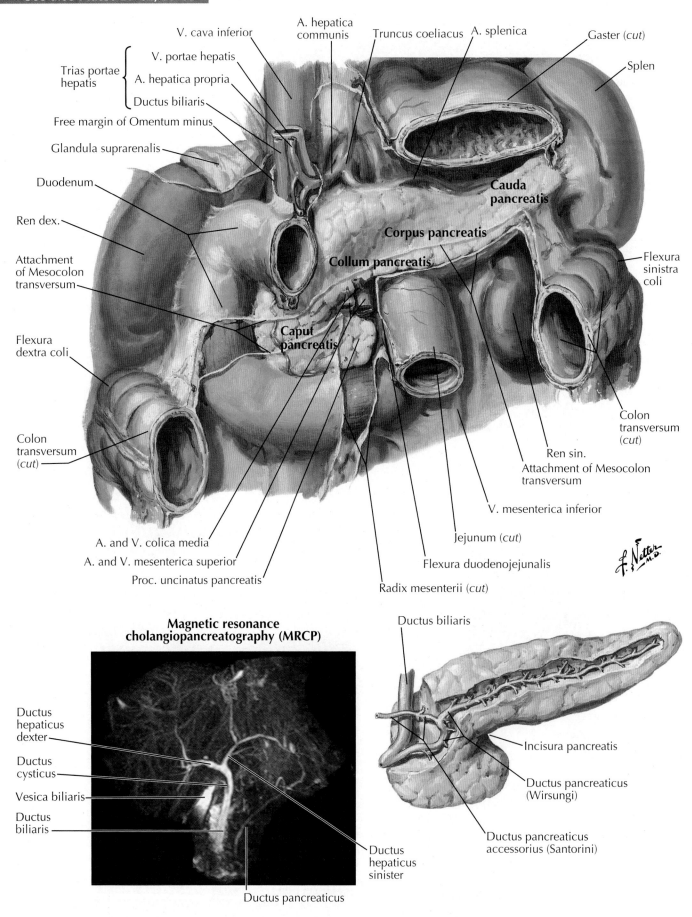

Trias portae hepatis
- V. portae hepatis
- A. hepatica propria
- Ductus biliaris

V. cava inferior

A. hepatica communis

Truncus coeliacus

A. splenica

Gaster (*cut*)

Splen

Free margin of Omentum minus

Glandula suprarenalis

Duodenum

Ren dex.

Attachment of Mesocolon transversum

Flexura dextra coli

Colon transversum (*cut*)

Cauda pancreatis

Corpus pancreatis

Collum pancreatis

Caput pancreatis

Flexura sinistra coli

Ren sin.

Attachment of Mesocolon transversum

Colon transversum (*cut*)

V. mesenterica inferior

Jejunum (*cut*)

Flexura duodenojejunalis

Radix mesenterii (*cut*)

A. and V. colica media

A. and V. mesenterica superior

Proc. uncinatus pancreatis

Magnetic resonance cholangiopancreatography (MRCP)

Ductus hepaticus dexter

Ductus cysticus

Vesica biliaris

Ductus biliaris

Ductus hepaticus sinister

Ductus pancreaticus

Ductus biliaris

Incisura pancreatis

Ductus pancreaticus (Wirsungi)

Ductus pancreaticus accessorius (Santorini)

Plate 306

Hepar, Vesica Biliaris, Pancreas and Splen

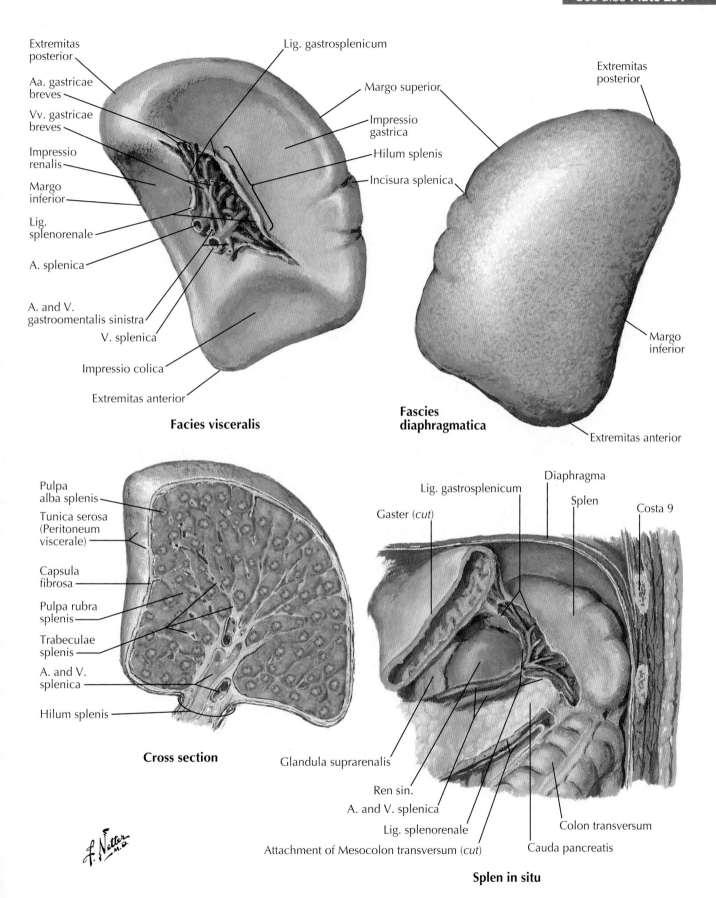

Extremitas posterior

Aa. gastricae breves

Vv. gastricae breves

Impressio renalis

Margo inferior

Lig. splenorenale

A. splenica

A. and V. gastroomentalis sinistra

V. splenica

Impressio colica

Extremitas anterior

Lig. gastrosplenicum

Margo superior

Impressio gastrica

Hilum splenis

Incisura splenica

Facies visceralis

Extremitas posterior

Margo inferior

Extremitas anterior

Fascies diaphragmatica

Pulpa alba splenis

Tunica serosa (Peritoneum viscerale)

Capsula fibrosa

Pulpa rubra splenis

Trabeculae splenis

A. and V. splenica

Hilum splenis

Cross section

Gaster (*cut*)

Lig. gastrosplenicum

Diaphragma

Splen

Costa 9

Glandula suprarenalis

Ren sin.

A. and V. splenica

Lig. splenorenale

Attachment of Mesocolon transversum (*cut*)

Colon transversum

Cauda pancreatis

Splen in situ

Hepar, Vesica Biliaris, Pancreas and Splen

Plate 307

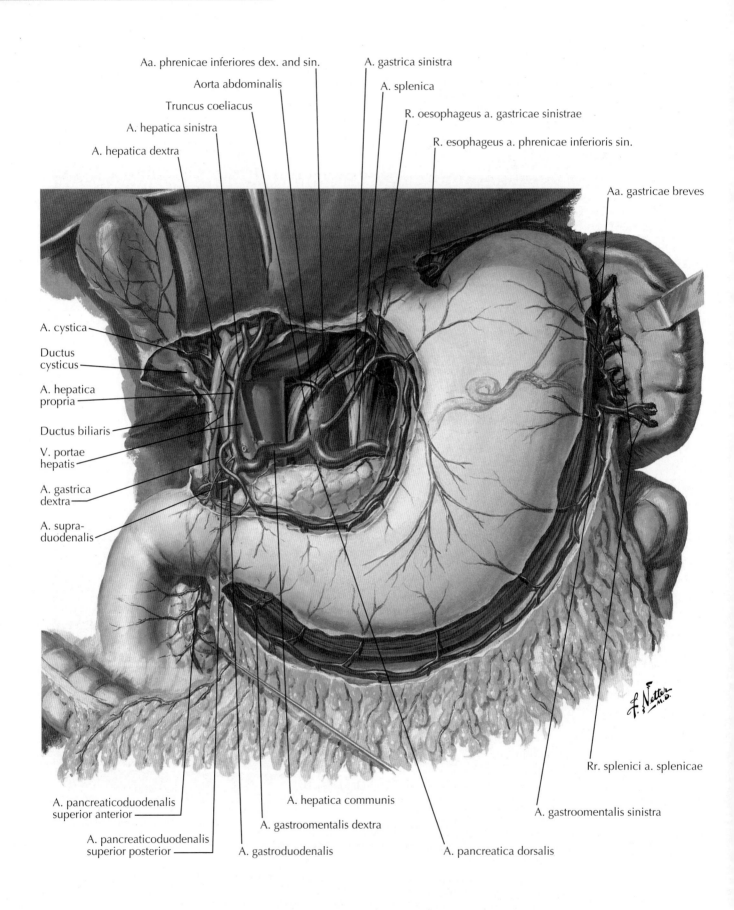

Aa. phrenicae inferiores dex. and sin.

Aorta abdominalis

Truncus coeliacus

A. hepatica sinistra

A. hepatica dextra

A. gastrica sinistra

A. splenica

R. oesophageus a. gastricae sinistrae

R. esophageus a. phrenicae inferioris sin.

Aa. gastricae breves

A. cystica

Ductus cysticus

A. hepatica propria

Ductus biliaris

V. portae hepatis

A. gastrica dextra

A. supra-duodenalis

Rr. splenici a. splenicae

A. gastroomentalis sinistra

A. pancreaticoduodenalis superior anterior

A. pancreaticoduodenalis superior posterior

A. gastroduodenalis

A. hepatica communis

A. gastroomentalis dextra

A. pancreatica dorsalis

Plate 308

Vasa Sanguinea Visceralia

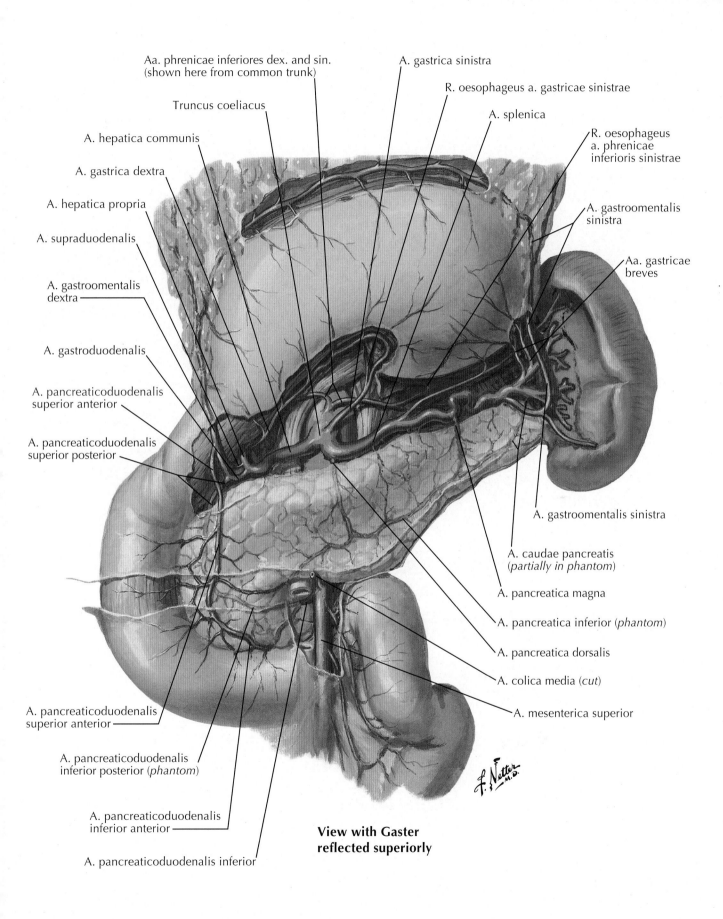

Aa. phrenicae inferiores dex. and sin.
(shown here from common trunk)

A. gastrica sinistra

Truncus coeliacus

R. oesophageus a. gastricae sinistrae

A. hepatica communis

A. splenica

A. gastrica dextra

R. oesophageus
a. phrenicae
inferioris sinistrae

A. hepatica propria

A. supraduodenalis

A. gastroomentalis
sinistra

A. gastroomentalis
dextra

Aa. gastricae
breves

A. gastroduodenalis

A. pancreaticoduodenalis
superior anterior

A. pancreaticoduodenalis
superior posterior

A. gastroomentalis sinistra

A. caudae pancreatis
(*partially in phantom*)

A. pancreatica magna

A. pancreatica inferior (*phantom*)

A. pancreatica dorsalis

A. colica media (*cut*)

A. pancreaticoduodenalis
superior anterior

A. mesenterica superior

A. pancreaticoduodenalis
inferior posterior (*phantom*)

A. pancreaticoduodenalis
inferior anterior

**View with Gaster
reflected superiorly**

A. pancreaticoduodenalis inferior

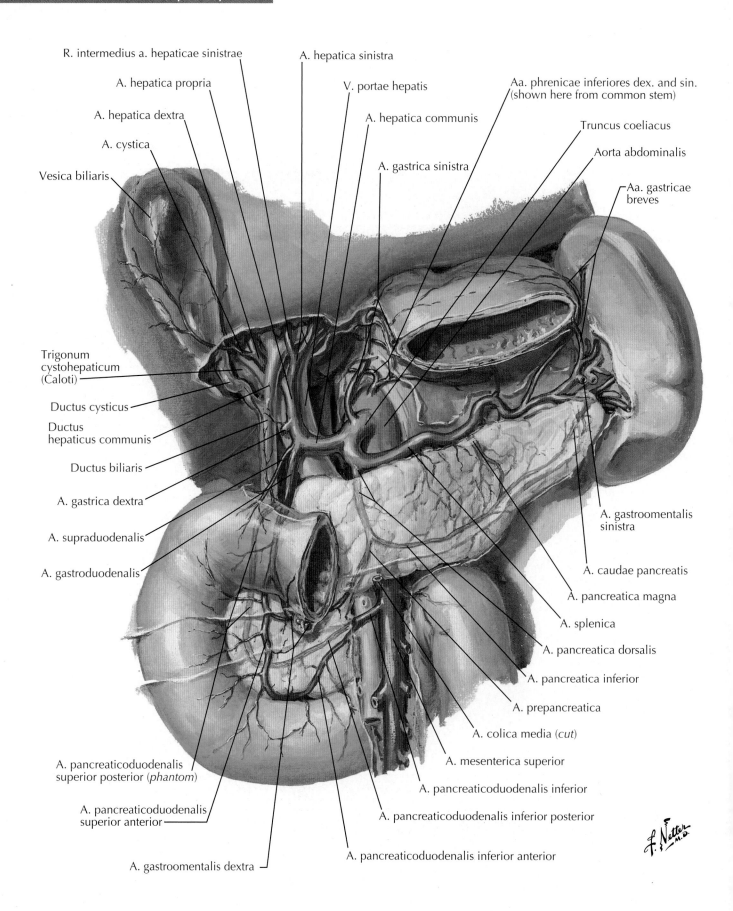

R. intermedius a. hepaticae sinistrae

A. hepatica propria

A. hepatica dextra

A. cystica

Vesica biliaris

A. hepatica sinistra

V. portae hepatis

A. hepatica communis

A. gastrica sinistra

Aa. phrenicae inferiores dex. and sin. (shown here from common stem)

Truncus coeliacus

Aorta abdominalis

Aa. gastricae breves

Trigonum cystohepaticum (Caloti)

Ductus cysticus

Ductus hepaticus communis

Ductus biliaris

A. gastrica dextra

A. supraduodenalis

A. gastroduodenalis

A. gastroomentalis sinistra

A. caudae pancreatis

A. pancreatica magna

A. splenica

A. pancreatica dorsalis

A. pancreatica inferior

A. prepancreatica

A. colica media (*cut*)

A. mesenterica superior

A. pancreaticoduodenalis superior posterior (*phantom*)

A. pancreaticoduodenalis superior anterior

A. gastroomentalis dextra

A. pancreaticoduodenalis inferior

A. pancreaticoduodenalis inferior posterior

A. pancreaticoduodenalis inferior anterior

Plate 310

Vasa Sanguinea Visceralia

3D volume-rendered CT image with intravenous contrast enhancement

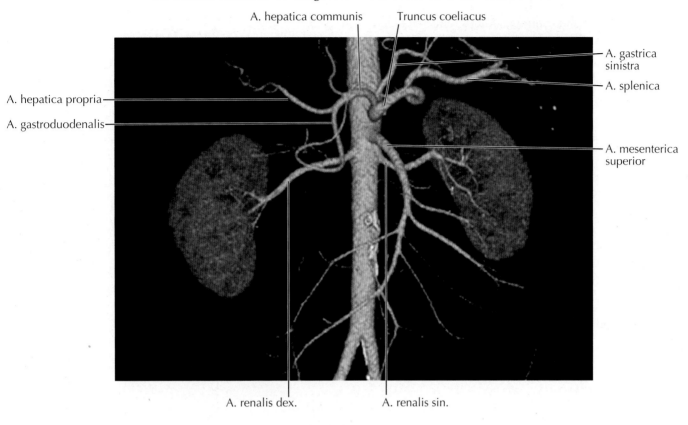

A. hepatica communis Truncus coeliacus

A. gastrica sinistra

A. splenica

A. hepatica propria

A. gastroduodenalis

A. mesenterica superior

A. renalis dex. A. renalis sin.

Selective digital subtraction angiogram, Truncus coeliacus

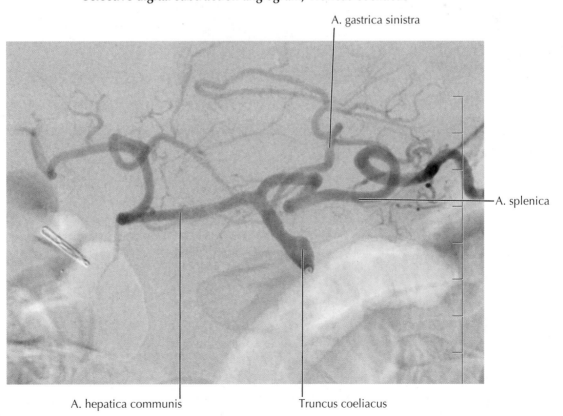

A. gastrica sinistra

A. splenica

A. hepatica communis Truncus coeliacus

Duodenum and caput pancreatis reflected to left

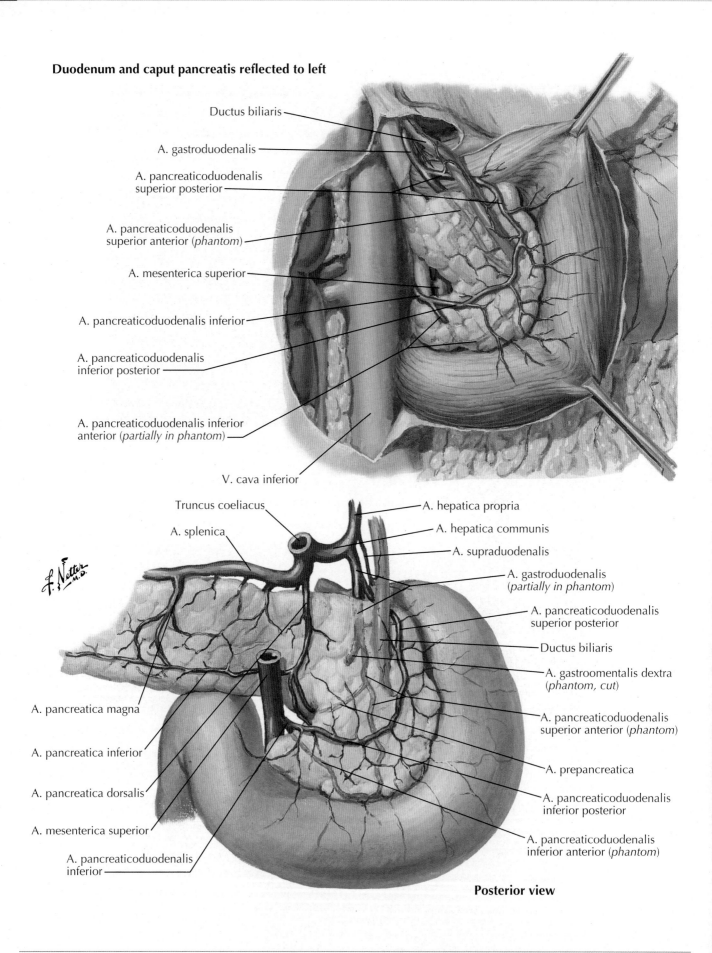

Ductus biliaris

A. gastroduodenalis

A. pancreaticoduodenalis
superior posterior

A. pancreaticoduodenalis
superior anterior (*phantom*)

A. mesenterica superior

A. pancreaticoduodenalis inferior

A. pancreaticoduodenalis
inferior posterior

A. pancreaticoduodenalis inferior
anterior (*partially in phantom*)

V. cava inferior

Truncus coeliacus

A. splenica

A. pancreatica magna

A. pancreatica inferior

A. pancreatica dorsalis

A. mesenterica superior

A. pancreaticoduodenalis
inferior

A. hepatica propria

A. hepatica communis

A. supraduodenalis

A. gastroduodenalis
(*partially in phantom*)

A. pancreaticoduodenalis
superior posterior

Ductus biliaris

A. gastroomentalis dextra
(*phantom, cut*)

A. pancreaticoduodenalis
superior anterior (*phantom*)

A. prepancreatica

A. pancreaticoduodenalis
inferior posterior

A. pancreaticoduodenalis
inferior anterior (*phantom*)

Posterior view

Plate 312   **Vasa Sanguinea Visceralia**

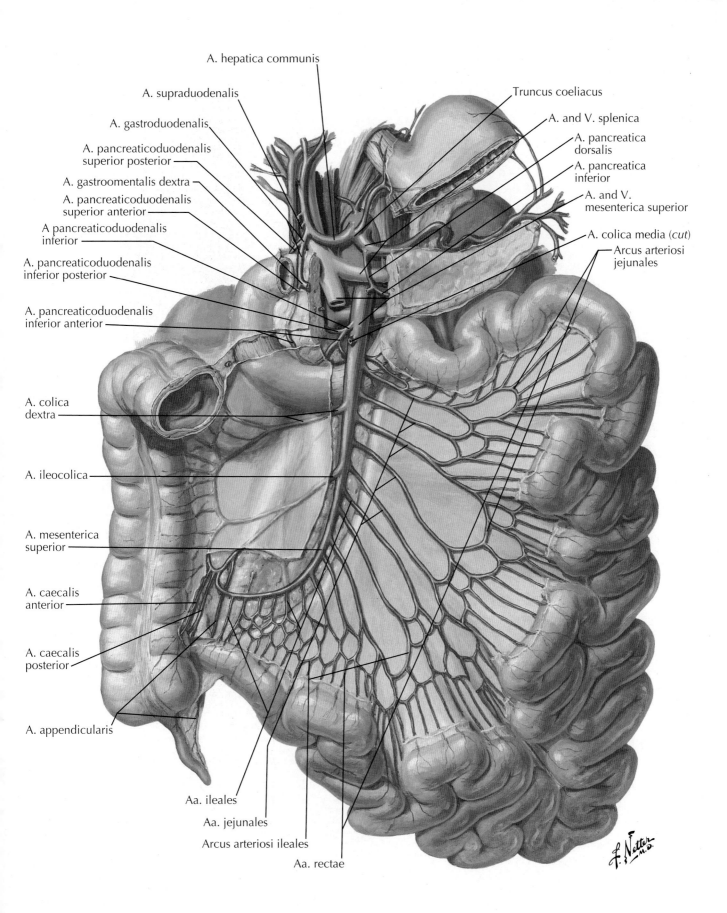

A. hepatica communis

A. supraduodenalis

A. gastroduodenalis

A. pancreaticoduodenalis
superior posterior

A. gastroomentalis dextra

A. pancreaticoduodenalis
superior anterior

A pancreaticoduodenalis
inferior

A. pancreaticoduodenalis
inferior posterior

A. pancreaticoduodenalis
inferior anterior

A. colica
dextra

A. ileocolica

A. mesenterica
superior

A. caecalis
anterior

A. caecalis
posterior

A. appendicularis

Aa. ileales

Aa. jejunales

Arcus arteriosi ileales

Aa. rectae

Truncus coeliacus

A. and V. splenica

A. pancreatica
dorsalis

A. pancreatica
inferior

A. and V.
mesenterica superior

A. colica media (*cut*)

Arcus arteriosi
jejunales

f. Netter
m.d.

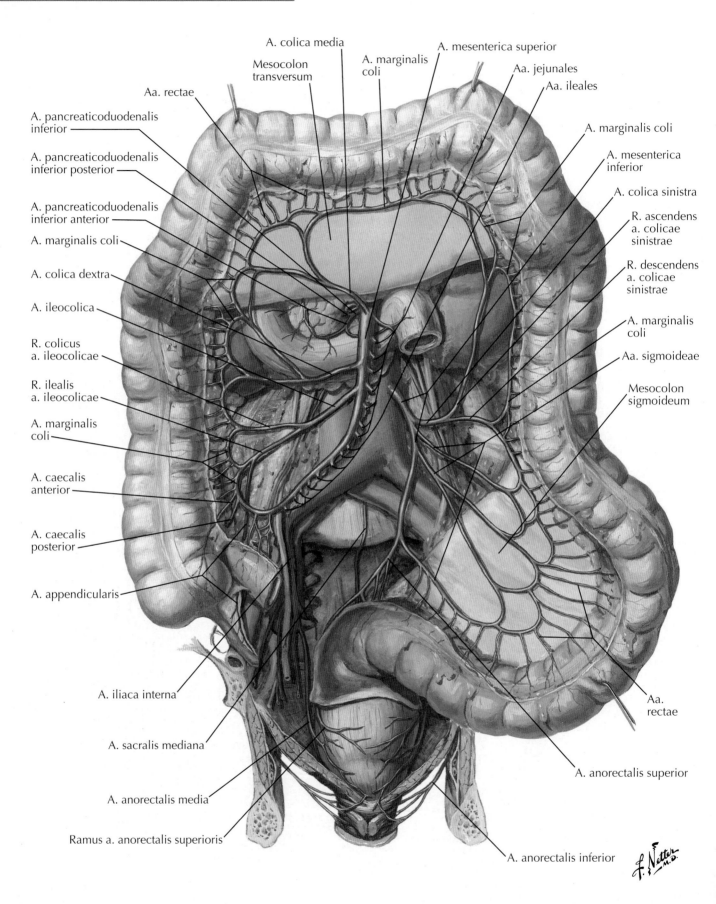

A. colica media

Mesocolon transversum

A. marginalis coli

A. mesenterica superior

Aa. jejunales

Aa. ileales

Aa. rectae

A. pancreaticoduodenalis inferior

A. pancreaticoduodenalis inferior posterior

A. pancreaticoduodenalis inferior anterior

A. marginalis coli

A. colica dextra

A. ileocolica

R. colicus a. ileocolicae

R. ilealis a. ileocolicae

A. marginalis coli

A. caecalis anterior

A. caecalis posterior

A. appendicularis

A. iliaca interna

A. sacralis mediana

A. anorectalis media

Ramus a. anorectalis superioris

A. marginalis coli

A. mesenterica inferior

A. colica sinistra

R. ascendens a. colicae sinistrae

R. descendens a. colicae sinistrae

A. marginalis coli

Aa. sigmoideae

Mesocolon sigmoideum

Aa. rectae

A. anorectalis superior

A. anorectalis inferior

Plate 314

Vasa Sanguinea Visceralia

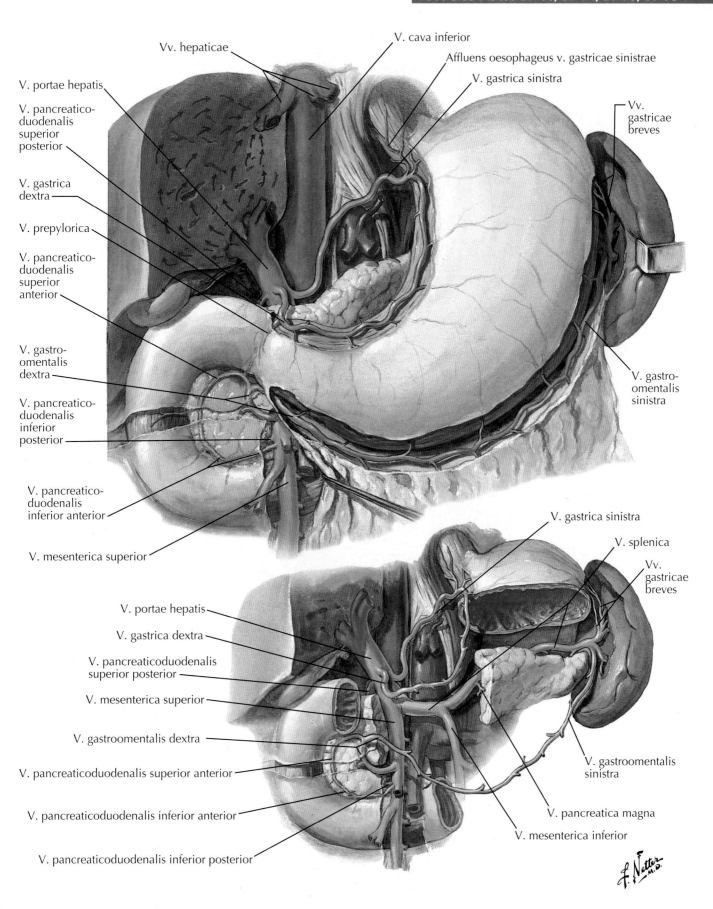

Vv. hepaticae

V. cava inferior

Affluens oesophageus v. gastricae sinistrae

V. gastrica sinistra

V. portae hepatis

V. pancreatico-duodenalis superior posterior

V. gastrica dextra

V. prepylorica

V. pancreatico-duodenalis superior anterior

V. gastro-omentalis dextra

V. pancreatico-duodenalis inferior posterior

V. pancreatico-duodenalis inferior anterior

V. mesenterica superior

Vv. gastricae breves

V. gastro-omentalis sinistra

V. gastrica sinistra

V. splenica

Vv. gastricae breves

V. portae hepatis

V. gastrica dextra

V. pancreaticoduodenalis superior posterior

V. mesenterica superior

V. gastroomentalis dextra

V. pancreaticoduodenalis superior anterior

V. pancreaticoduodenalis inferior anterior

V. pancreaticoduodenalis inferior posterior

V. gastroomentalis sinistra

V. pancreatica magna

V. mesenterica inferior

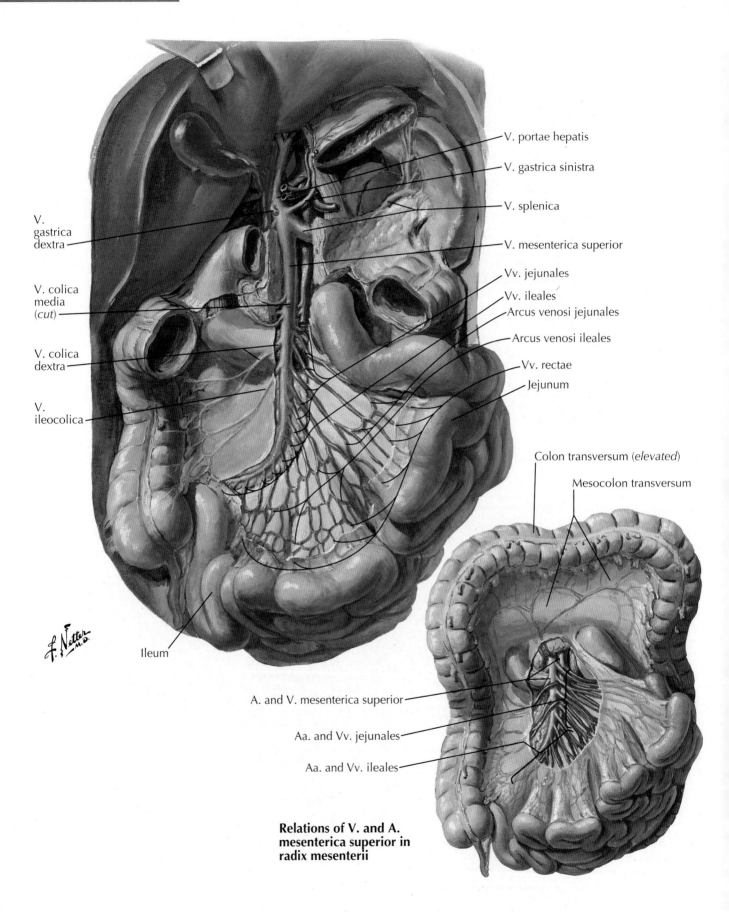

V. portae hepatis

V. gastrica sinistra

V. splenica

V. mesenterica superior

Vv. jejunales

Vv. ileales

Arcus venosi jejunales

Arcus venosi ileales

Vv. rectae

Jejunum

V. gastrica dextra

V. colica media (*cut*)

V. colica dextra

V. ileocolica

Ileum

Colon transversum (*elevated*)

Mesocolon transversum

A. and V. mesenterica superior

Aa. and Vv. jejunales

Aa. and Vv. ileales

Relations of V. and A. mesenterica superior in radix mesenterii

Plate 316   **Vasa Sanguinea Visceralia**

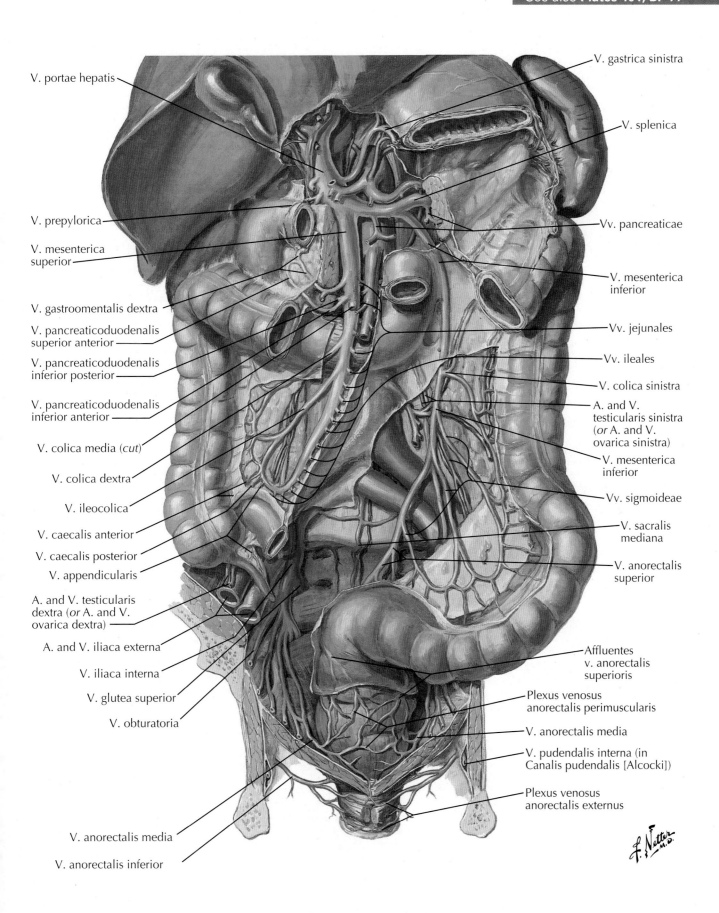

V. portae hepatis

V. gastrica sinistra

V. splenica

V. prepylorica

Vv. pancreaticae

V. mesenterica superior

V. mesenterica inferior

V. gastroomentalis dextra

Vv. jejunales

V. pancreaticoduodenalis superior anterior

Vv. ileales

V. pancreaticoduodenalis inferior posterior

V. colica sinistra

A. and V. testicularis sinistra (or A. and V. ovarica sinistra)

V. pancreaticoduodenalis inferior anterior

V. mesenterica inferior

V. colica media (cut)

Vv. sigmoideae

V. colica dextra

V. ileocolica

V. sacralis mediana

V. caecalis anterior

V. caecalis posterior

V. anorectalis superior

V. appendicularis

A. and V. testicularis dextra (or A. and V. ovarica dextra)

Affluentes v. anorectalis superioris

A. and V. iliaca externa

V. iliaca interna

Plexus venosus anorectalis perimuscularis

V. glutea superior

V. anorectalis media

V. obturatoria

V. pudendalis interna (in Canalis pudendalis [Alcocki])

Plexus venosus anorectalis externus

V. anorectalis media

V. anorectalis inferior

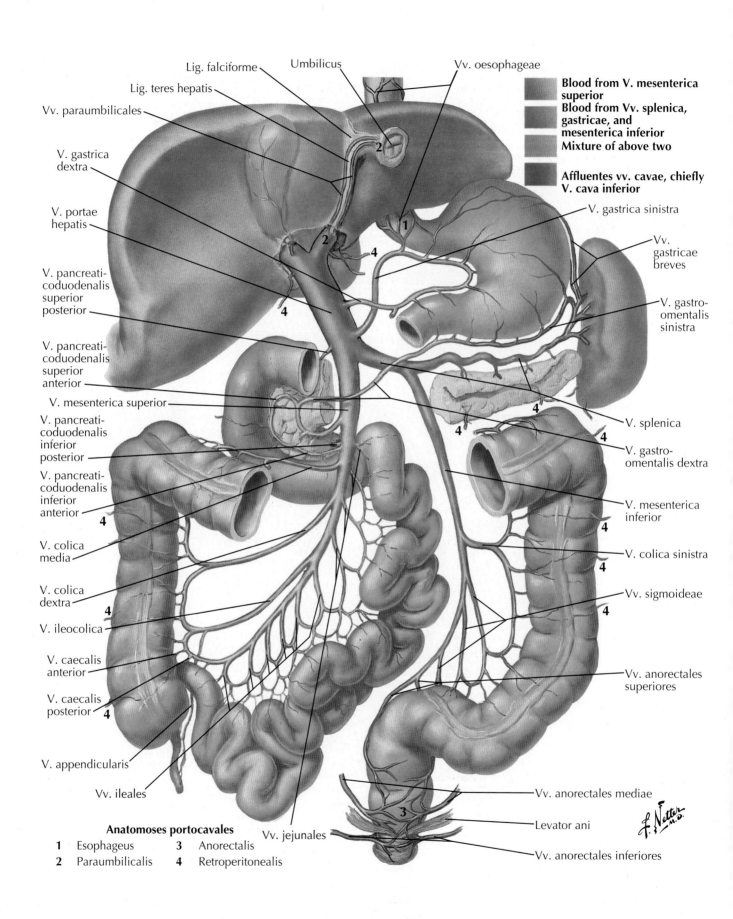

Lig. falciforme

Umbilicus

Vv. oesophageae

Lig. teres hepatis

Vv. paraumbilicales

Blood from V. mesenterica superior

Blood from Vv. splenica, gastricae, and mesenterica inferior

Mixture of above two

Affluentes vv. cavae, chiefly V. cava inferior

V. gastrica dextra

V. gastrica sinistra

Vv. gastricae breves

V. portae hepatis

V. gastro-omentalis sinistra

V. pancreati-coduodenalis superior posterior

V. pancreati-coduodenalis superior anterior

V. splenica

V. mesenterica superior

V. gastro-omentalis dextra

V. pancreati-coduodenalis inferior posterior

V. pancreati-coduodenalis inferior anterior

V. mesenterica inferior

V. colica media

V. colica sinistra

V. colica dextra

Vv. sigmoideae

V. ileocolica

V. caecalis anterior

Vv. anorectales superiores

V. caecalis posterior

V. appendicularis

Vv. ileales

Vv. anorectales mediae

Levator ani

Vv. anorectales inferiores

Anastomoses portocavales

1   Esophageus   3   Anorectalis
2   Paraumbilicalis   4   Retroperitonealis

Vv. jejunales

Plate 318   **Vasa Sanguinea Visceralia**

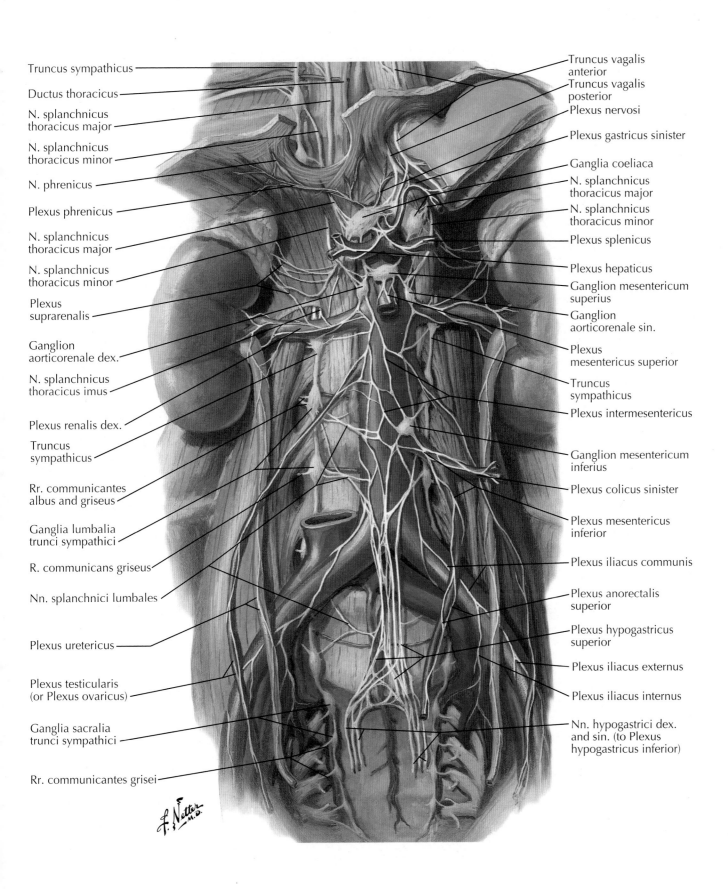

Truncus sympathicus

Ductus thoracicus

N. splanchnicus thoracicus major

N. splanchnicus thoracicus minor

N. phrenicus

Plexus phrenicus

N. splanchnicus thoracicus major

N. splanchnicus thoracicus minor

Plexus suprarenalis

Ganglion aorticorenale dex.

N. splanchnicus thoracicus imus

Plexus renalis dex.

Truncus sympathicus

Rr. communicantes albus and griseus

Ganglia lumbalia trunci sympathici

R. communicans griseus

Nn. splanchnici lumbales

Plexus uretericus

Plexus testicularis (or Plexus ovaricus)

Ganglia sacralia trunci sympathici

Rr. communicantes grisei

Truncus vagalis anterior

Truncus vagalis posterior

Plexus nervosi

Plexus gastricus sinister

Ganglia coeliaca

N. splanchnicus thoracicus major

N. splanchnicus thoracicus minor

Plexus splenicus

Plexus hepaticus

Ganglion mesentericum superius

Ganglion aorticorenale sin.

Plexus mesentericus superior

Truncus sympathicus

Plexus intermesentericus

Ganglion mesentericum inferius

Plexus colicus sinister

Plexus mesentericus inferior

Plexus iliacus communis

Plexus anorectalis superior

Plexus hypogastricus superior

Plexus iliacus externus

Plexus iliacus internus

Nn. hypogastrici dex. and sin. (to Plexus hypogastricus inferior)

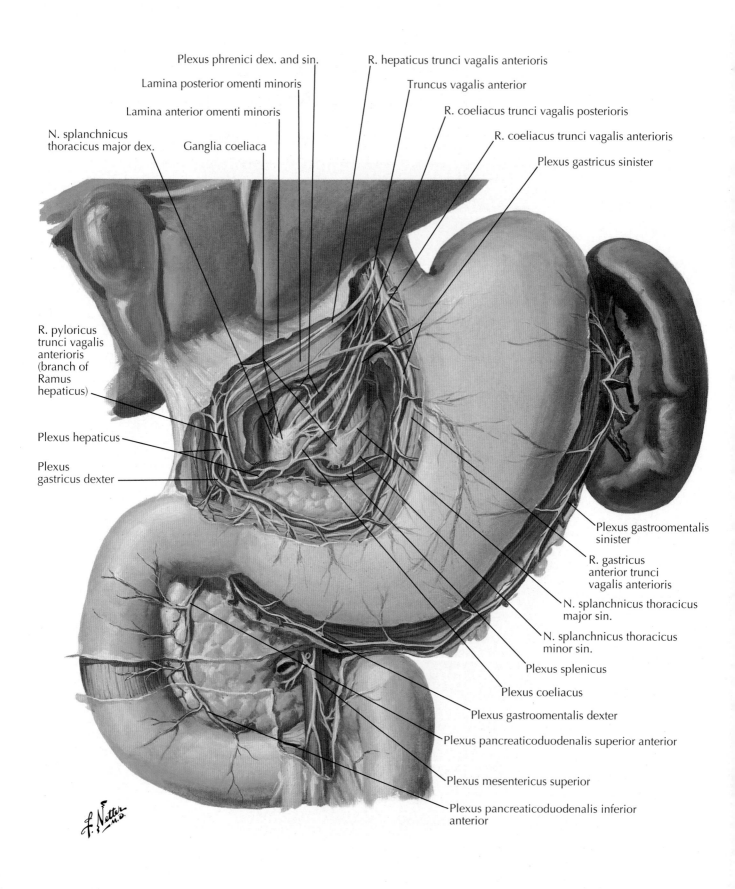

Plexus phrenici dex. and sin.

Lamina posterior omenti minoris

Lamina anterior omenti minoris

N. splanchnicus thoracicus major dex.

Ganglia coeliaca

R. hepaticus trunci vagalis anterioris

Truncus vagalis anterior

R. coeliacus trunci vagalis posterioris

R. coeliacus trunci vagalis anterioris

Plexus gastricus sinister

R. pyloricus trunci vagalis anterioris (branch of Ramus hepaticus)

Plexus hepaticus

Plexus gastricus dexter

Plexus gastroomentalis sinister

R. gastricus anterior trunci vagalis anterioris

N. splanchnicus thoracicus major sin.

N. splanchnicus thoracicus minor sin.

Plexus splenicus

Plexus coeliacus

Plexus gastroomentalis dexter

Plexus pancreaticoduodenalis superior anterior

Plexus mesentericus superior

Plexus pancreaticoduodenalis inferior anterior

Plate 320

Nervi Viscerales and Plexus Viscerales

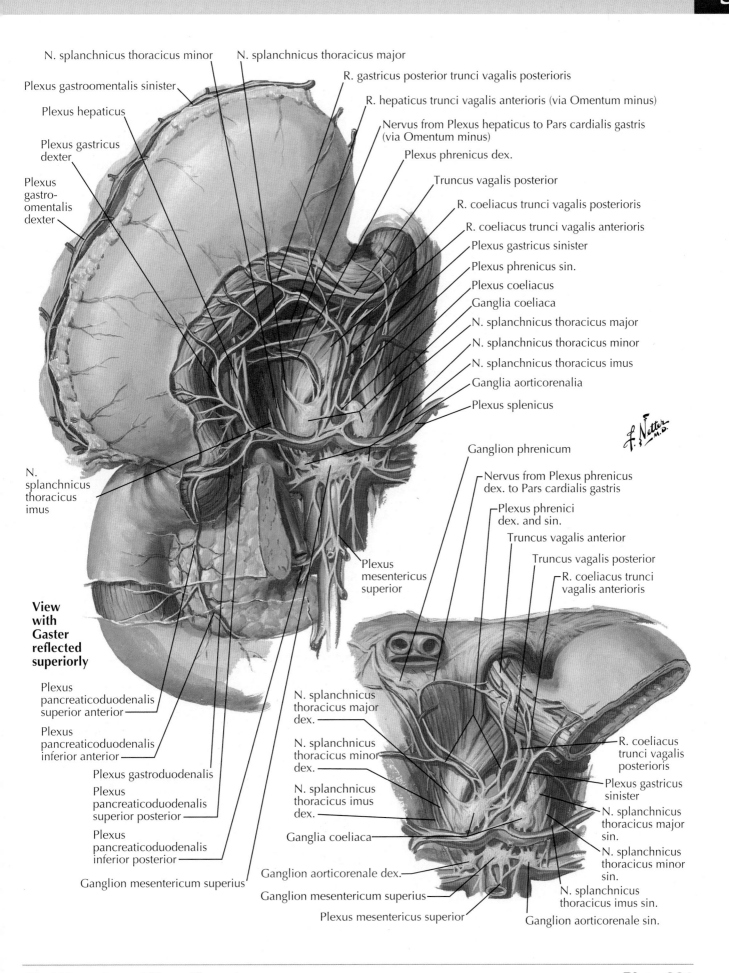

N. splanchnicus thoracicus minor

N. splanchnicus thoracicus major

R. gastricus posterior trunci vagalis posterioris

Plexus gastroomentalis sinister

R. hepaticus trunci vagalis anterioris (via Omentum minus)

Plexus hepaticus

Nervus from Plexus hepaticus to Pars cardialis gastris (via Omentum minus)

Plexus gastricus dexter

Plexus phrenicus dex.

Plexus gastro-omentalis dexter

Truncus vagalis posterior

R. coeliacus trunci vagalis posterioris

R. coeliacus trunci vagalis anterioris

Plexus gastricus sinister

Plexus phrenicus sin.

Plexus coeliacus

Ganglia coeliaca

N. splanchnicus thoracicus major

N. splanchnicus thoracicus minor

N. splanchnicus thoracicus imus

Ganglia aorticorenalia

Plexus splenicus

N. splanchnicus thoracicus imus

Ganglion phrenicum

Nervus from Plexus phrenicus dex. to Pars cardialis gastris

Plexus phrenici dex. and sin.

Truncus vagalis anterior

Truncus vagalis posterior

R. coeliacus trunci vagalis anterioris

Plexus mesentericus superior

View with Gaster reflected superiorly

Plexus pancreaticoduodenalis superior anterior

Plexus pancreaticoduodenalis inferior anterior

Plexus gastroduodenalis

Plexus pancreaticoduodenalis superior posterior

Plexus pancreaticoduodenalis inferior posterior

Ganglion mesentericum superius

N. splanchnicus thoracicus major dex.

N. splanchnicus thoracicus minor dex.

N. splanchnicus thoracicus imus dex.

Ganglia coeliaca

Ganglion aorticorenale dex.

Ganglion mesentericum superius

Plexus mesentericus superior

R. coeliacus trunci vagalis posterioris

Plexus gastricus sinister

N. splanchnicus thoracicus major sin.

N. splanchnicus thoracicus minor sin.

N. splanchnicus thoracicus imus sin.

Ganglion aorticorenale sin.

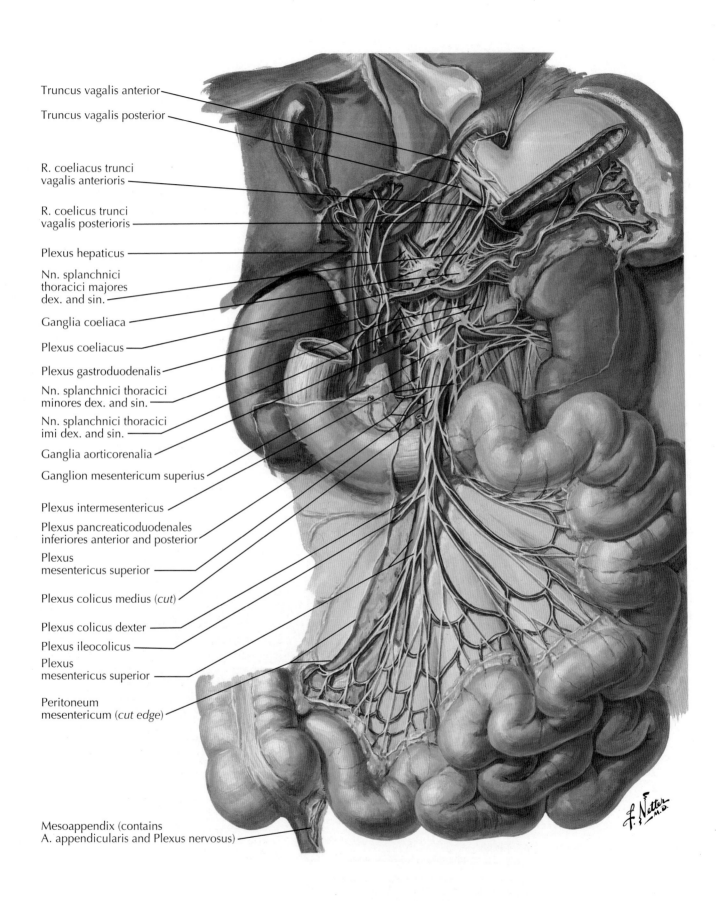

Truncus vagalis anterior

Truncus vagalis posterior

R. coeliacus trunci vagalis anterioris

R. coelicus trunci vagalis posterioris

Plexus hepaticus

Nn. splanchnici thoracici majores dex. and sin.

Ganglia coeliaca

Plexus coeliacus

Plexus gastroduodenalis

Nn. splanchnici thoracici minores dex. and sin.

Nn. splanchnici thoracici imi dex. and sin.

Ganglia aorticorenalia

Ganglion mesentericum superius

Plexus intermesentericus

Plexus pancreaticoduodenales inferiores anterior and posterior

Plexus mesentericus superior

Plexus colicus medius (cut)

Plexus colicus dexter

Plexus ileocolicus

Plexus mesentericus superior

Peritoneum mesentericum (cut edge)

Mesoappendix (contains A. appendicularis and Plexus nervosus)

Plate 322

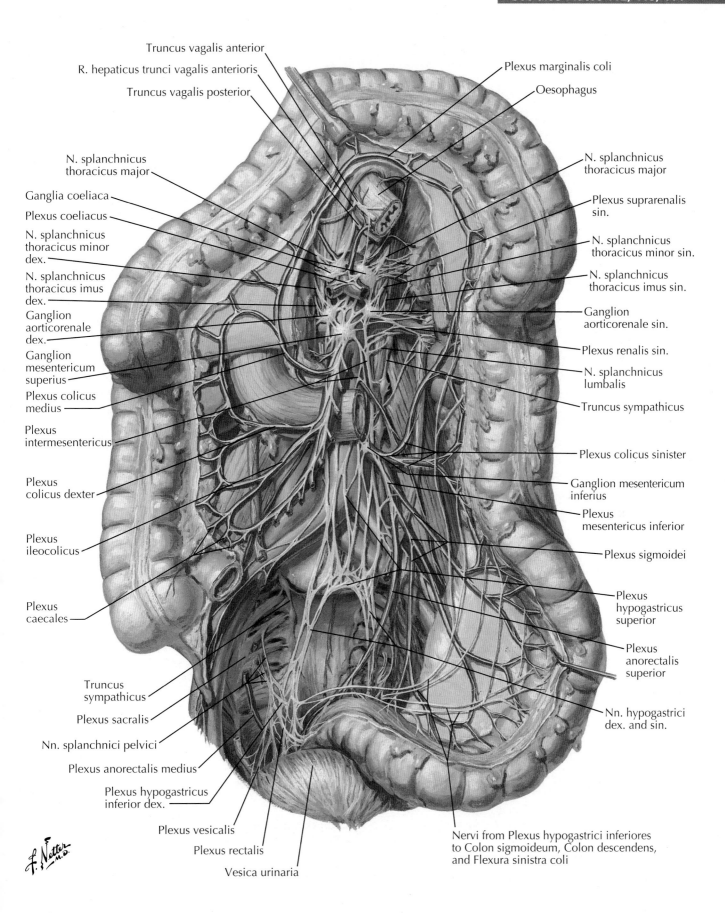

Truncus vagalis anterior

R. hepaticus trunci vagalis anterioris

Truncus vagalis posterior

N. splanchnicus thoracicus major

Ganglia coeliaca

Plexus coeliacus

N. splanchnicus thoracicus minor dex.

N. splanchnicus thoracicus imus dex.

Ganglion aorticorenale dex.

Ganglion mesentericum superius

Plexus colicus medius

Plexus intermesentericus

Plexus colicus dexter

Plexus ileocolicus

Plexus caecales

Truncus sympathicus

Plexus sacralis

Nn. splanchnici pelvici

Plexus anorectalis medius

Plexus hypogastricus inferior dex.

Plexus vesicalis

Plexus rectalis

Vesica urinaria

Plexus marginalis coli

Oesophagus

N. splanchnicus thoracicus major

Plexus suprarenalis sin.

N. splanchnicus thoracicus minor sin.

N. splanchnicus thoracicus imus sin.

Ganglion aorticorenale sin.

Plexus renalis sin.

N. splanchnicus lumbalis

Truncus sympathicus

Plexus colicus sinister

Ganglion mesentericum inferius

Plexus mesentericus inferior

Plexus sigmoidei

Plexus hypogastricus superior

Plexus anorectalis superior

Nn. hypogastrici dex. and sin.

Nervi from Plexus hypogastrici inferiores to Colon sigmoideum, Colon descendens, and Flexura sinistra coli

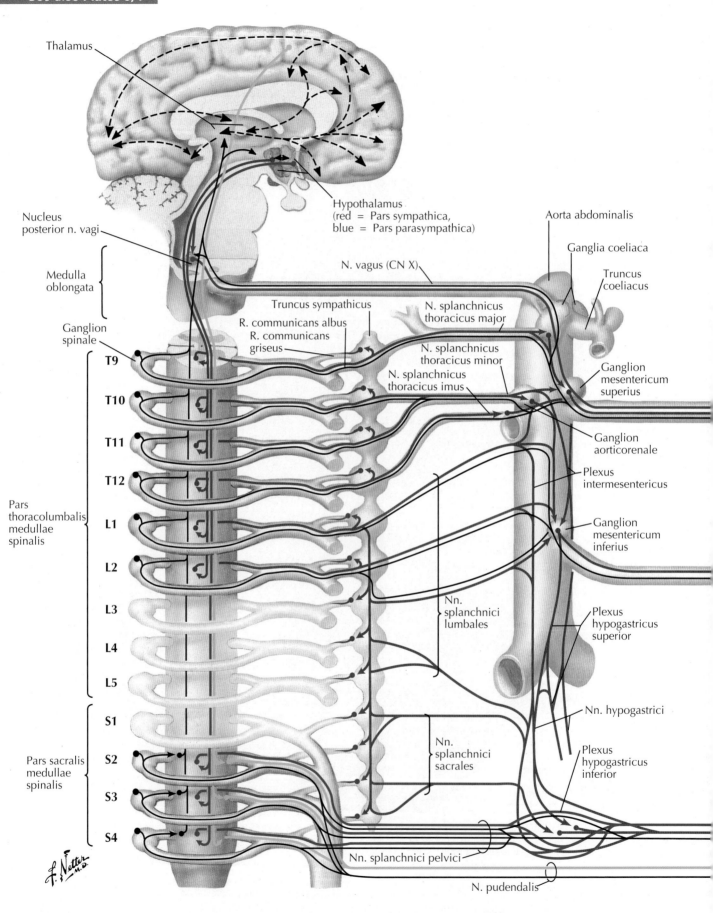

Thalamus

Hypothalamus
(red = Pars sympathica,
blue = Pars parasympathica)

Aorta abdominalis

Ganglia coeliaca

Truncus coeliacus

Nucleus posterior n. vagi

N. vagus (CN X)

Medulla oblongata

Truncus sympathicus

N. splanchnicus thoracicus major

Ganglion spinale

R. communicans albus
R. communicans griseus

N. splanchnicus thoracicus minor

N. splanchnicus thoracicus imus

Ganglion mesentericum superius

T9

T10

Ganglion aorticorenale

T11

Plexus intermesentericus

T12

Pars thoracolumbalis medullae spinalis

L1

Ganglion mesentericum inferius

L2

L3

Nn. splanchnici lumbales

L4

Plexus hypogastricus superior

L5

S1

Nn. hypogastrici

Nn. splanchnici sacrales

Pars sacralis medullae spinalis

S2

Plexus hypogastricus inferior

S3

S4

Nn. splanchnici pelvici

N. pudendalis

Plate 324

Nervi Viscerales and Plexus Viscerales

Sympathetic fibers ▬▬▬
Parasympathetic fibers ▬▬▬
Somatic efferent fibers ▬▬▬
Afferents and CNS connections ▬▬▬
Indefinite paths ▬ ▬ ▬ ▬

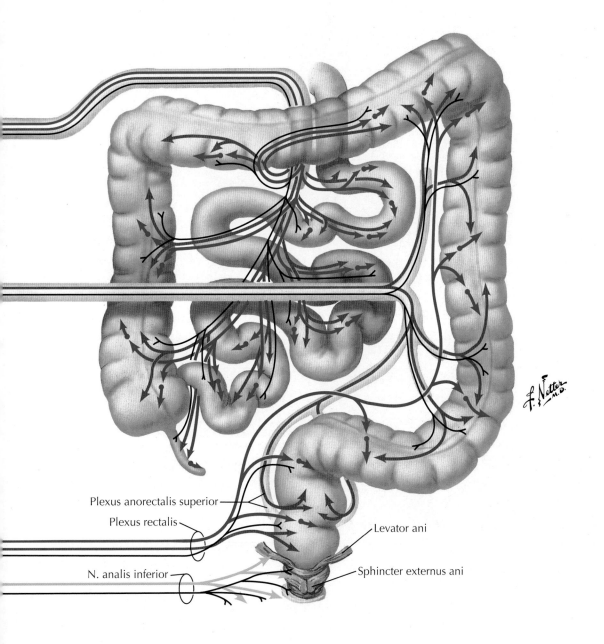

Plexus anorectalis superior
Plexus rectalis
Levator ani
N. analis inferior
Sphincter externus ani

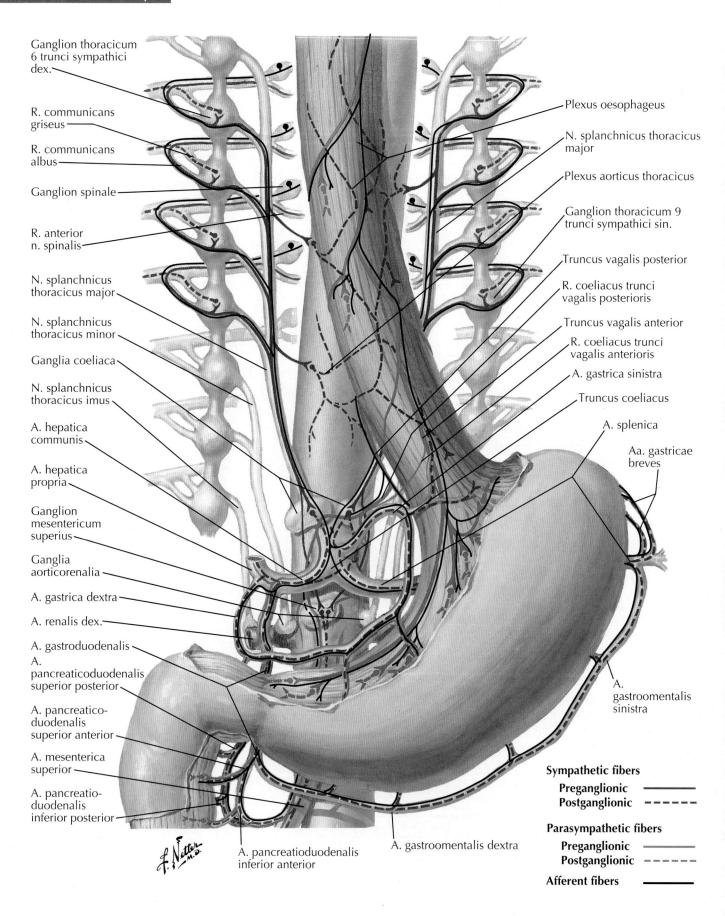

Ganglion thoracicum 6 trunci sympathici dex.

R. communicans griseus

R. communicans albus

Ganglion spinale

R. anterior n. spinalis

N. splanchnicus thoracicus major

N. splanchnicus thoracicus minor

Ganglia coeliaca

N. splanchnicus thoracicus imus

A. hepatica communis

A. hepatica propria

Ganglion mesentericum superius

Ganglia aorticorenalia

A. gastrica dextra

A. renalis dex.

A. gastroduodenalis

A. pancreaticoduodenalis superior posterior

A. pancreatico-duodenalis superior anterior

A. mesenterica superior

A. pancreatio-duodenalis inferior posterior

A. pancreatioduodenalis inferior anterior

A. gastroomentalis dextra

Plexus oesophagus

N. splanchnicus thoracicus major

Plexus aorticus thoracicus

Ganglion thoracicum 9 trunci sympathici sin.

Truncus vagalis posterior

R. coeliacus trunci vagalis posterioris

Truncus vagalis anterior

R. coeliacus trunci vagalis anterioris

A. gastrica sinistra

Truncus coeliacus

A. splenica

Aa. gastricae breves

A. gastroomentalis sinistra

Sympathetic fibers

Preganglionic ——————
Postganglionic – – – – –

Parasympathetic fibers

Preganglionic ——————
Postganglionic – – – – –

Afferent fibers ——————

Plate 325

Nervi Viscerales and Plexus Viscerales

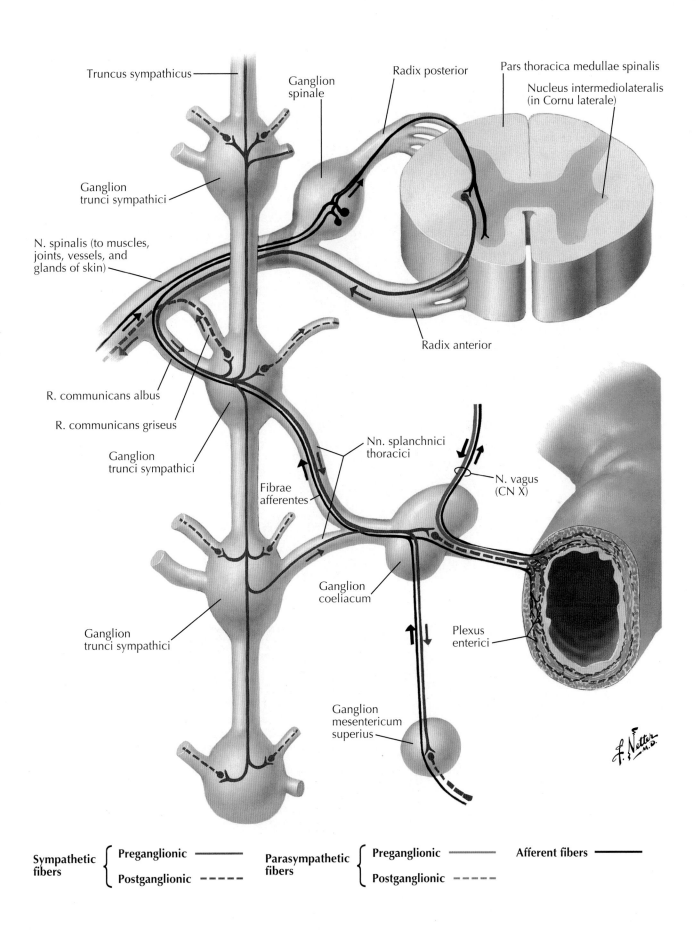

Truncus sympathicus

Ganglion spinale

Radix posterior

Pars thoracica medullae spinalis

Nucleus intermediolateralis (in Cornu laterale)

Ganglion trunci sympathici

N. spinalis (to muscles, joints, vessels, and glands of skin)

Radix anterior

R. communicans albus

R. communicans griseus

Ganglion trunci sympathici

Nn. splanchnici thoracici

N. vagus (CN X)

Fibrae afferentes

Ganglion coeliacum

Plexus enterici

Ganglion trunci sympathici

Ganglion mesentericum superius

Sympathetic fibers { Preganglionic ——— Postganglionic – – –

Parasympathetic fibers { Preganglionic ——— Postganglionic – – – – –

Afferent fibers ———

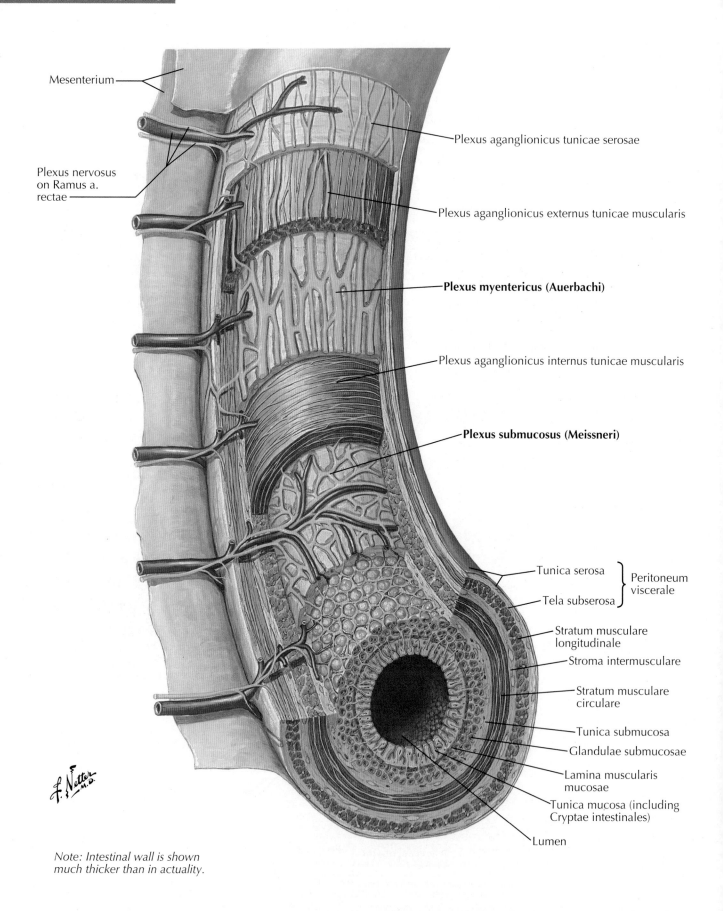

Mesenterium

Plexus nervosus on Ramus a. rectae

Plexus aganglionicus tunicae serosae

Plexus aganglionicus externus tunicae muscularis

Plexus myentericus (Auerbachi)

Plexus aganglionicus internus tunicae muscularis

Plexus submucosus (Meissneri)

Tunica serosa ⎫ Peritoneum
Tela subserosa ⎭ viscerale

Stratum musculare longitudinale

Stroma intermusculare

Stratum musculare circulare

Tunica submucosa

Glandulae submucosae

Lamina muscularis mucosae

Tunica mucosa (including Cryptae intestinales)

Lumen

Note: Intestinal wall is shown much thicker than in actuality.

Plate 327

Nervi Viscerales and Plexus Viscerales

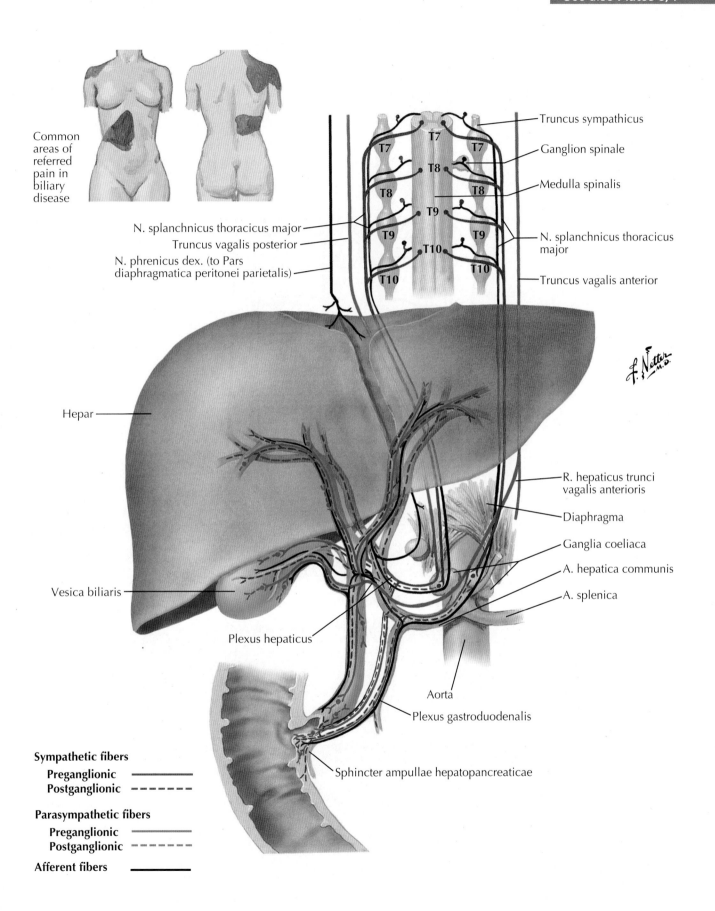

Common areas of referred pain in biliary disease

Truncus sympathicus

Ganglion spinale

Medulla spinalis

N. splanchnicus thoracicus major

Truncus vagalis anterior

N. splanchnicus thoracicus major
Truncus vagalis posterior
N. phrenicus dex. (to Pars diaphragmatica peritonei parietalis)

T7
T8
T9
T10

Hepar

R. hepaticus trunci vagalis anterioris

Diaphragma

Ganglia coeliaca

A. hepatica communis

A. splenica

Vesica biliaris

Plexus hepaticus

Aorta

Plexus gastroduodenalis

Sphincter ampullae hepatopancreaticae

Sympathetic fibers
   Preganglionic ───────
   Postganglionic ─ ─ ─ ─

Parasympathetic fibers
   Preganglionic ───────
   Postganglionic ─ ─ ─ ─

Afferent fibers ───────

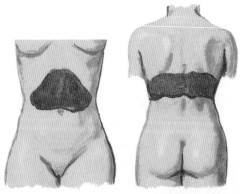

Common areas
of referred pain
in pancreatic
disease

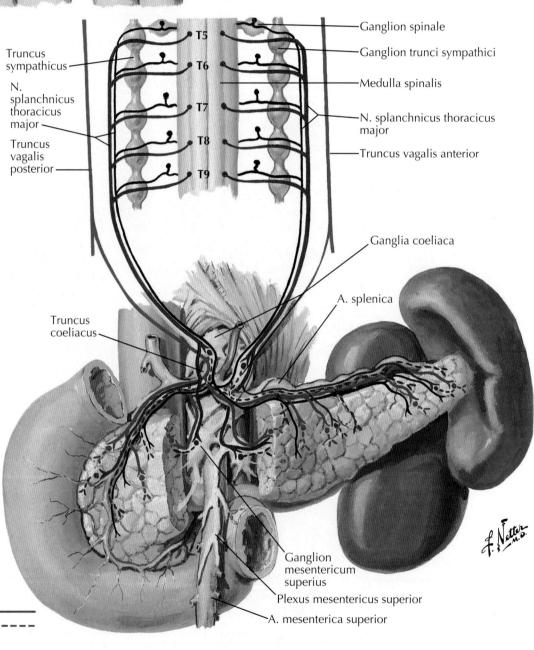

Truncus
symphaticus

N.
splanchnicus
thoracicus
major

Truncus
vagalis
posterior

Ganglion spinale

Ganglion trunci sympathici

Medulla spinalis

N. splanchnicus thoracicus
major

Truncus vagalis anterior

T5
T6
T7
T8
T9

Ganglia coeliaca

A. splenica

Truncus
coeliacus

Ganglion
mesentericum
superius

Plexus mesentericus superior

A. mesenterica superior

Sympathetic fibers

Preganglionic

Postganglionic ---------

Parasympathetic fibers

Preganglionic

Postganglionic ---------

Afferent fibers

Plate 329

Nervi Viscerales and Plexus Viscerales

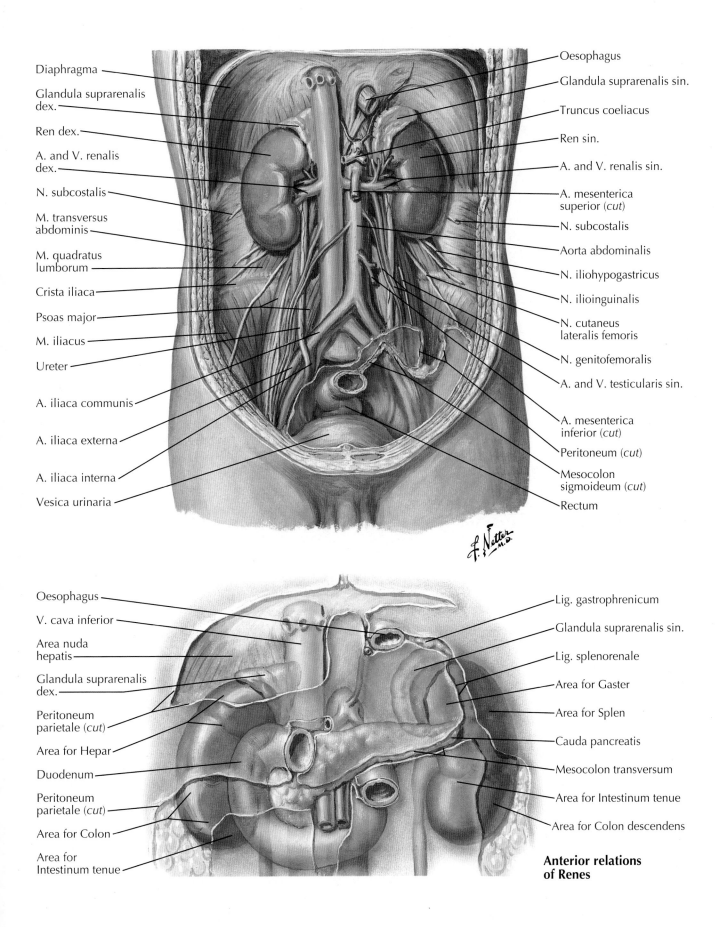

Diaphragma

Glandula suprarenalis dex.

Ren dex.

A. and V. renalis dex.

N. subcostalis

M. transversus abdominis

M. quadratus lumborum

Crista iliaca

Psoas major

M. iliacus

Ureter

A. iliaca communis

A. iliaca externa

A. iliaca interna

Vesica urinaria

Oesophagus

Glandula suprarenalis sin.

Truncus coeliacus

Ren sin.

A. and V. renalis sin.

A. mesenterica superior (*cut*)

N. subcostalis

Aorta abdominalis

N. iliohypogastricus

N. ilioinguinalis

N. cutaneus lateralis femoris

N. genitofemoralis

A. and V. testicularis sin.

A. mesenterica inferior (*cut*)

Peritoneum (*cut*)

Mesocolon sigmoideum (*cut*)

Rectum

Oesophagus

V. cava inferior

Area nuda hepatis

Glandula suprarenalis dex.

Peritoneum parietale (*cut*)

Area for Hepar

Duodenum

Peritoneum parietale (*cut*)

Area for Colon

Area for Intestinum tenue

Lig. gastrophrenicum

Glandula suprarenalis sin.

Lig. splenorenale

Area for Gaster

Area for Splen

Cauda pancreatis

Mesocolon transversum

Area for Intestinum tenue

Area for Colon descendens

Anterior relations of Renes

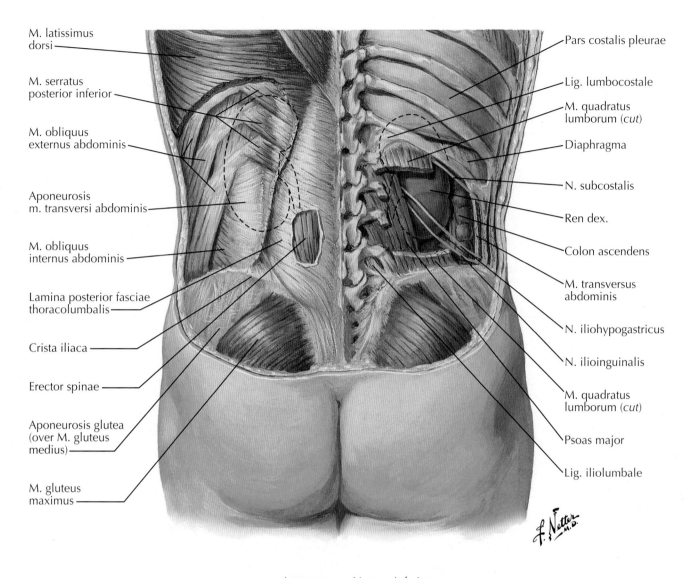

M. latissimus dorsi

M. serratus posterior inferior

M. obliquus externus abdominis

Aponeurosis m. transversi abdominis

M. obliquus internus abdominis

Lamina posterior fasciae thoracolumbalis

Crista iliaca

Erector spinae

Aponeurosis glutea (over M. gluteus medius)

M. gluteus maximus

Pars costalis pleurae

Lig. lumbocostale

M. quadratus lumborum (cut)

Diaphragma

N. subcostalis

Ren dex.

Colon ascendens

M. transversus abdominis

N. iliohypogastricus

N. ilioinguinalis

M. quadratus lumborum (cut)

Psoas major

Lig. iliolumbale

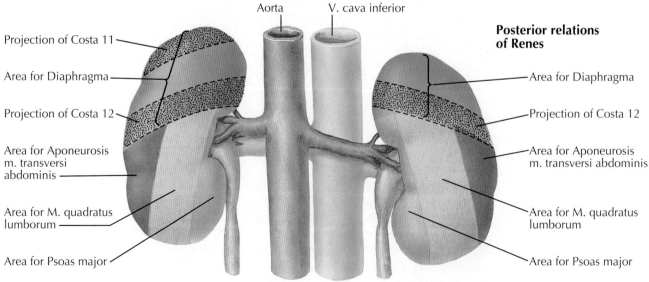

Aorta   V. cava inferior

Posterior relations of Renes

Projection of Costa 11

Area for Diaphragma

Projection of Costa 12

Area for Aponeurosis m. transversi abdominis

Area for M. quadratus lumborum

Area for Psoas major

Area for Diaphragma

Projection of Costa 12

Area for Aponeurosis m. transversi abdominis

Area for M. quadratus lumborum

Area for Psoas major

Plate 331   **Renes and Glandulae Suprarenales**

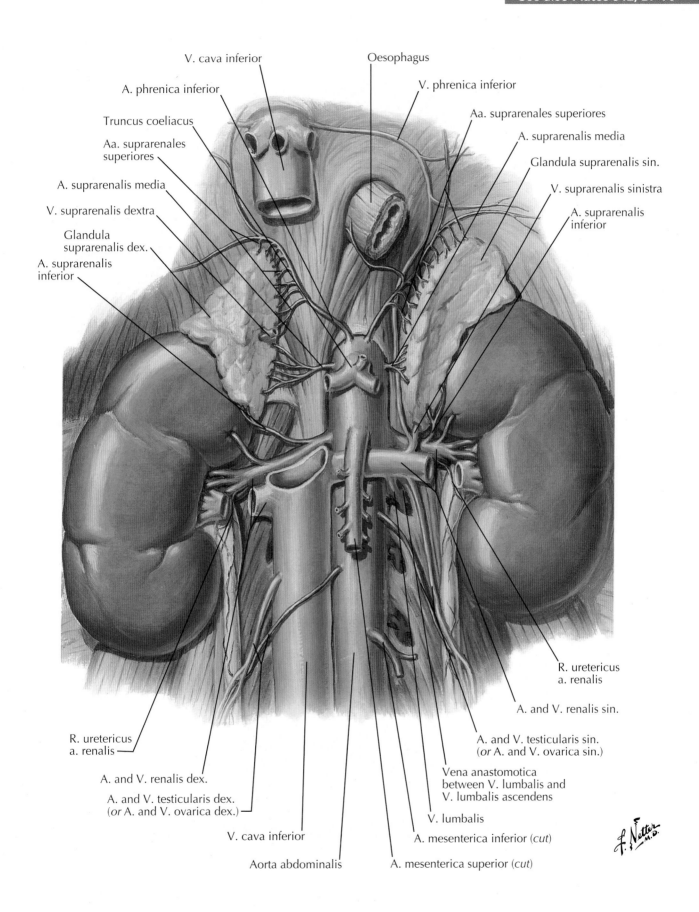

V. cava inferior

Oesophagus

A. phrenica inferior

V. phrenica inferior

Truncus coeliacus

Aa. suprarenales superiores

Aa. suprarenales superiores

A. suprarenalis media

A. suprarenalis media

Glandula suprarenalis sin.

V. suprarenalis dextra

V. suprarenalis sinistra

Glandula suprarenalis dex.

A. suprarenalis inferior

A. suprarenalis inferior

R. uretericus a. renalis

A. and V. renalis sin.

R. uretericus a. renalis

A. and V. testicularis sin. (*or* A. and V. ovarica sin.)

A. and V. renalis dex.

Vena anastomotica between V. lumbalis and V. lumbalis ascendens

A. and V. testicularis dex. (*or* A. and V. ovarica dex.)

V. lumbalis

V. cava inferior

A. mesenterica inferior (*cut*)

Aorta abdominalis

A. mesenterica superior (*cut*)

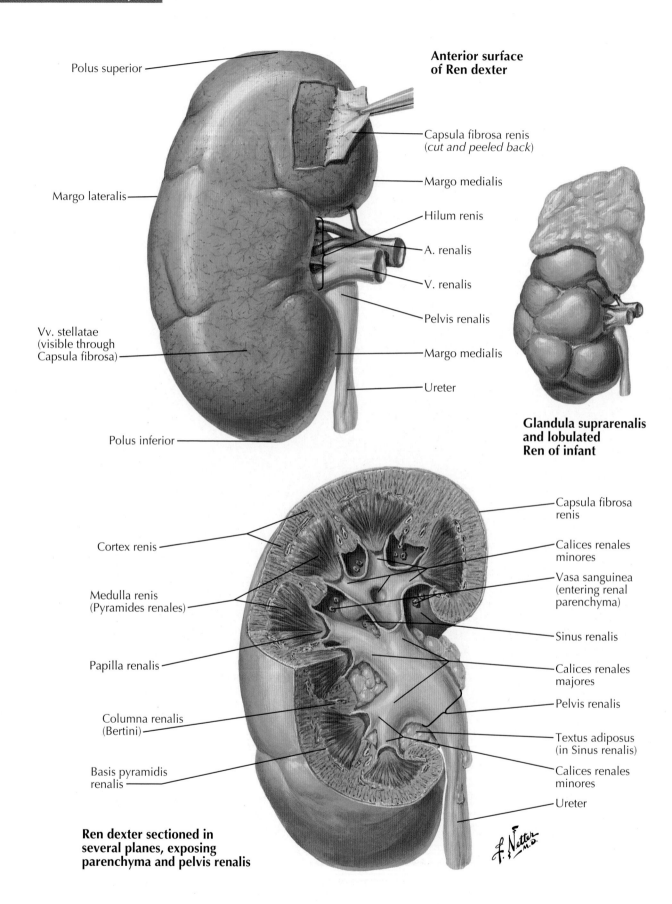

Polus superior

**Anterior surface
of Ren dexter**

Capsula fibrosa renis
(*cut and peeled back*)

Margo medialis

Margo lateralis

Hilum renis

A. renalis

V. renalis

Pelvis renalis

Vv. stellatae
(visible through
Capsula fibrosa)

Margo medialis

Ureter

Polus inferior

**Glandula suprarenalis
and lobulated
Ren of infant**

Cortex renis

Capsula fibrosa
renis

Calices renales
minores

Vasa sanguinea
(entering renal
parenchyma)

Medulla renis
(Pyramides renales)

Sinus renalis

Papilla renalis

Calices renales
majores

Pelvis renalis

Columna renalis
(Bertini)

Textus adiposus
(in Sinus renalis)

Calices renales
minores

Basis pyramidis
renalis

Ureter

**Ren dexter sectioned in
several planes, exposing
parenchyma and pelvis renalis**

Plate 333

Renes and Glandulae Suprarenales

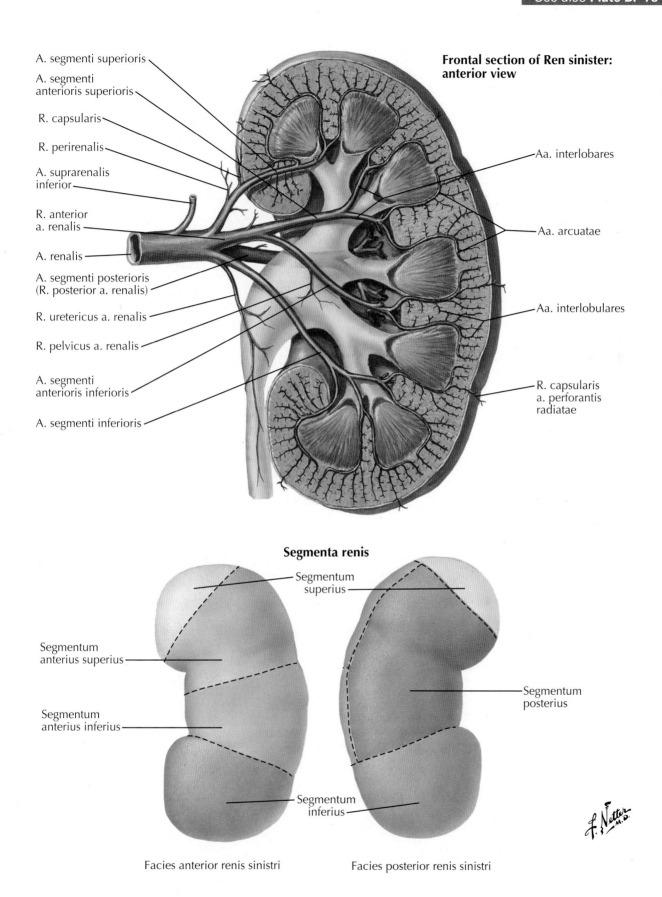

A. segmenti superioris

A. segmenti anterioris superioris

R. capsularis

R. perirenalis

A. suprarenalis inferior

R. anterior a. renalis

A. renalis

A. segmenti posterioris (R. posterior a. renalis)

R. uretericus a. renalis

R. pelvicus a. renalis

A. segmenti anterioris inferioris

A. segmenti inferioris

Frontal section of Ren sinister: anterior view

Aa. interlobares

Aa. arcuatae

Aa. interlobulares

R. capsularis a. perforantis radiatae

Segmenta renis

Segmentum superius

Segmentum anterius superius

Segmentum anterius inferius

Segmentum posterius

Segmentum inferius

Facies anterior renis sinistri

Facies posterior renis sinistri

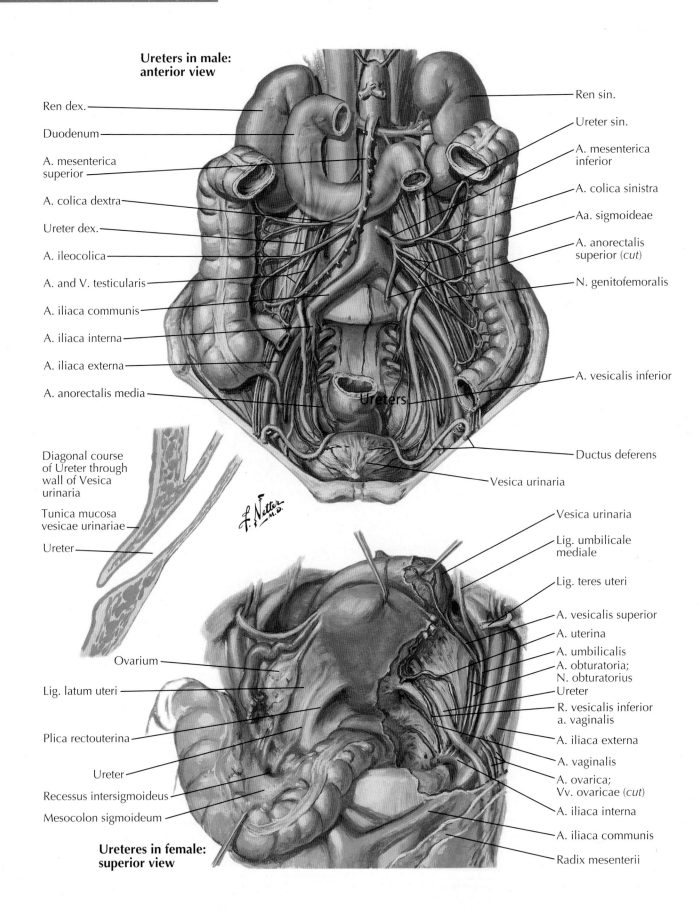

Ureters in male: anterior view

Ren dex.
Duodenum
A. mesenterica superior
A. colica dextra
Ureter dex.
A. ileocolica
A. and V. testicularis
A. iliaca communis
A. iliaca interna
A. iliaca externa
A. anorectalis media

Ren sin.
Ureter sin.
A. mesenterica inferior
A. colica sinistra
Aa. sigmoideae
A. anorectalis superior (cut)
N. genitofemoralis
A. vesicalis inferior

Ureters

Ductus deferens
Vesica urinaria

Diagonal course of Ureter through wall of Vesica urinaria
Tunica mucosa vesicae urinariae
Ureter

Vesica urinaria
Lig. umbilicale mediale
Lig. teres uteri
A. vesicalis superior
A. uterina
A. umbilicalis
A. obturatoria; N. obturatorius
Ureter
R. vesicalis inferior a. vaginalis
A. iliaca externa
A. vaginalis
A. ovarica; Vv. ovaricae (cut)
A. iliaca interna
A. iliaca communis
Radix mesenterii

Ovarium
Lig. latum uteri
Plica rectouterina
Ureter
Recessus intersigmoideus
Mesocolon sigmoideum

Ureteres in female: superior view

Plate 335

Renes and Glandulae Suprarenales

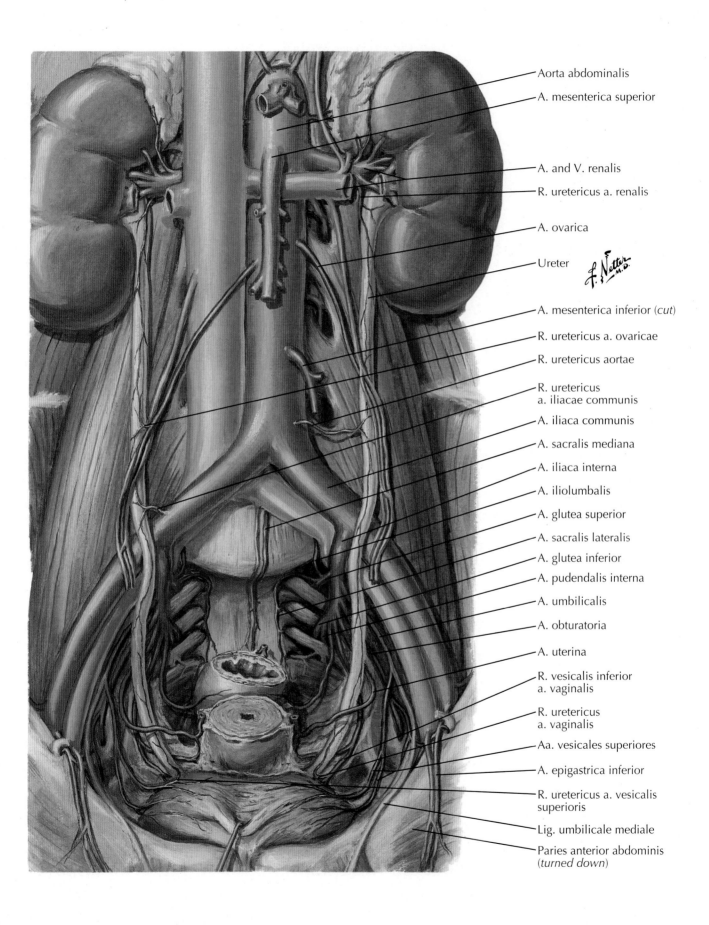

Aorta abdominalis

A. mesenterica superior

A. and V. renalis

R. uretericus a. renalis

A. ovarica

Ureter

A. mesenterica inferior (*cut*)

R. uretericus a. ovaricae

R. uretericus aortae

R. uretericus
a. iliacae communis

A. iliaca communis

A. sacralis mediana

A. iliaca interna

A. iliolumbalis

A. glutea superior

A. sacralis lateralis

A. glutea inferior

A. pudendalis interna

A. umbilicalis

A. obturatoria

A. uterina

R. vesicalis inferior
a. vaginalis

R. uretericus
a. vaginalis

Aa. vesicales superiores

A. epigastrica inferior

R. uretericus a. vesicalis
superioris

Lig. umbilicale mediale

Paries anterior abdominis
(*turned down*)

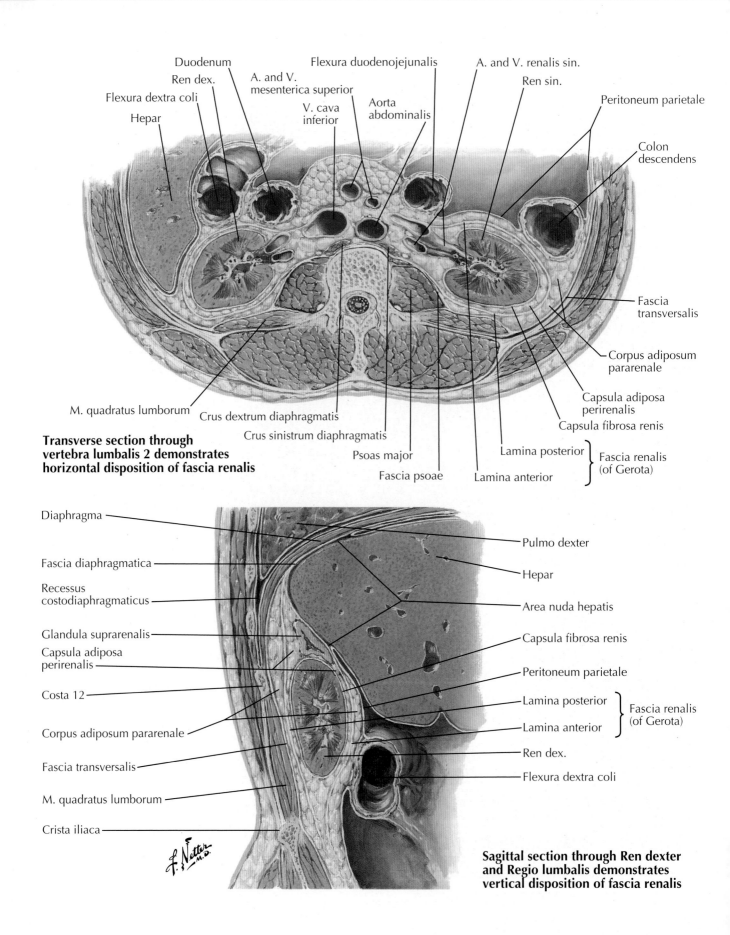

Duodenum
Ren dex.
Flexura dextra coli
Hepar
A. and V. mesenterica superior
V. cava inferior
Flexura duodenojejunalis
Aorta abdominalis
A. and V. renalis sin.
Ren sin.
Peritoneum parietale
Colon descendens
Fascia transversalis
Corpus adiposum pararenale
Capsula adiposa perirenalis
Capsula fibrosa renis
M. quadratus lumborum
Crus dextrum diaphragmatis
Crus sinistrum diaphragmatis
Psoas major
Fascia psoae
Lamina posterior
Lamina anterior
} Fascia renalis (of Gerota)

Transverse section through vertebra lumbalis 2 demonstrates horizontal disposition of fascia renalis

Diaphragma
Fascia diaphragmatica
Recessus costodiaphragmaticus
Glandula suprarenalis
Capsula adiposa perirenalis
Costa 12
Corpus adiposum pararenale
Fascia transversalis
M. quadratus lumborum
Crista iliaca
Pulmo dexter
Hepar
Area nuda hepatis
Capsula fibrosa renis
Peritoneum parietale
Lamina posterior
Lamina anterior
} Fascia renalis (of Gerota)
Ren dex.
Flexura dextra coli

Sagittal section through Ren dexter and Regio lumbalis demonstrates vertical disposition of fascia renalis

Plate 337

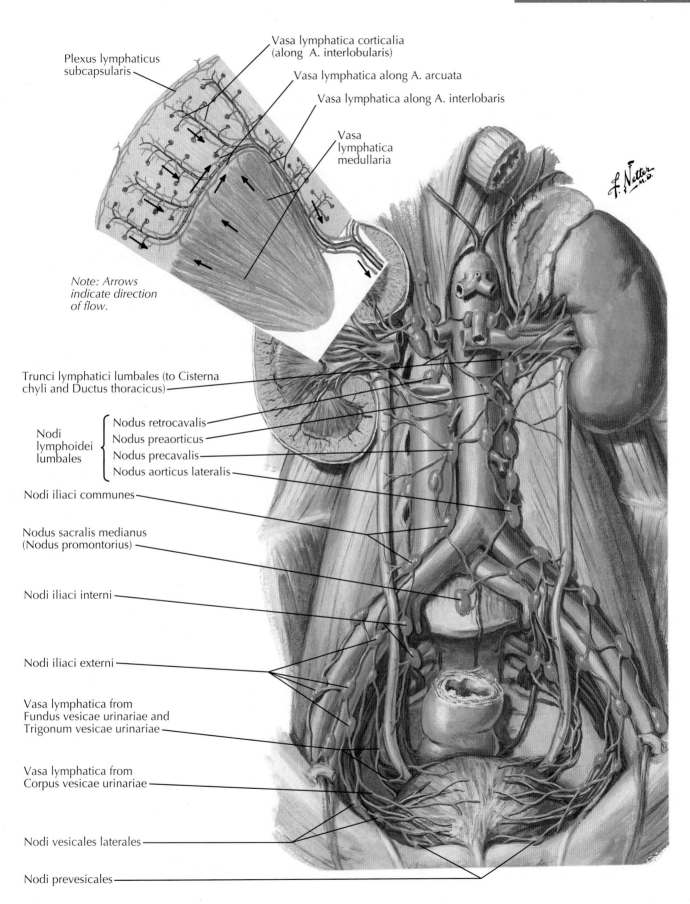

Plexus lymphaticus subcapsularis

Vasa lymphatica corticalia (along A. interlobularis)

Vasa lymphatica along A. arcuata

Vasa lymphatica along A. interlobaris

Vasa lymphatica medullaria

Note: Arrows indicate direction of flow.

Trunci lymphatici lumbales (to Cisterna chyli and Ductus thoracicus)

Nodi lymphoidei lumbales
- Nodus retrocavalis
- Nodus preaorticus
- Nodus precavalis
- Nodus aorticus lateralis

Nodi iliaci communes

Nodus sacralis medianus (Nodus promontorius)

Nodi iliaci interni

Nodi iliaci externi

Vasa lymphatica from Fundus vesicae urinariae and Trigonum vesicae urinariae

Vasa lymphatica from Corpus vesicae urinariae

Nodi vesicales laterales

Nodi prevesicales

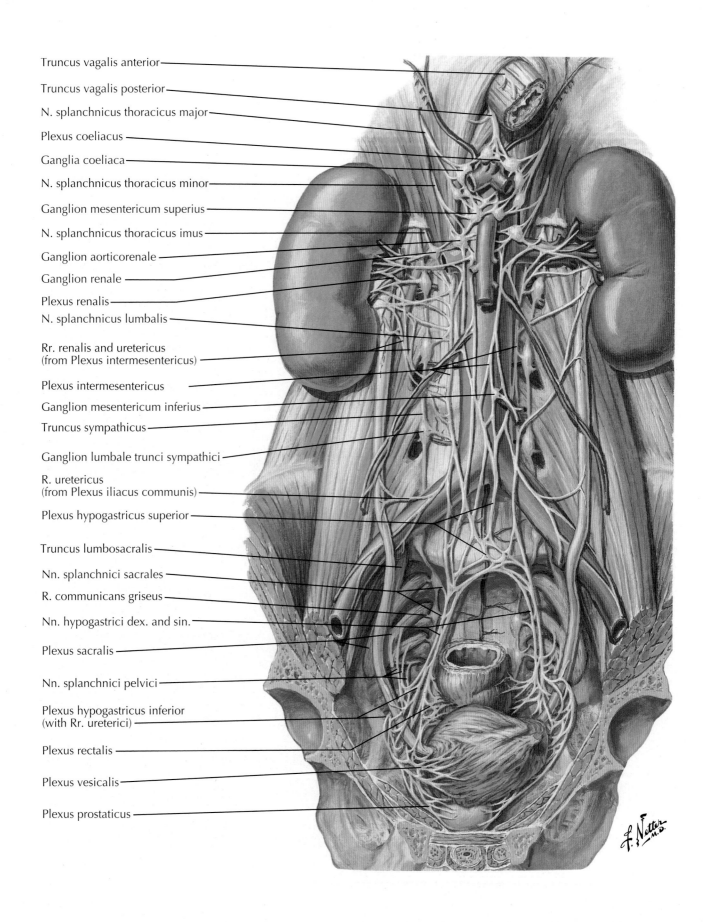

Truncus vagalis anterior

Truncus vagalis posterior

N. splanchnicus thoracicus major

Plexus coeliacus

Ganglia coeliaca

N. splanchnicus thoracicus minor

Ganglion mesentericum superius

N. splanchnicus thoracicus imus

Ganglion aorticorenale

Ganglion renale

Plexus renalis

N. splanchnicus lumbalis

Rr. renalis and uretericus
(from Plexus intermesentericus)

Plexus intermesentericus

Ganglion mesentericum inferius

Truncus sympathicus

Ganglion lumbale trunci sympathici

R. uretericus
(from Plexus iliacus communis)

Plexus hypogastricus superior

Truncus lumbosacralis

Nn. splanchnici sacrales

R. communicans griseus

Nn. hypogastrici dex. and sin.

Plexus sacralis

Nn. splanchnici pelvici

Plexus hypogastricus inferior
(with Rr. ureterici)

Plexus rectalis

Plexus vesicalis

Plexus prostaticus

Plate 339

Renes and Glandulae Suprarenales

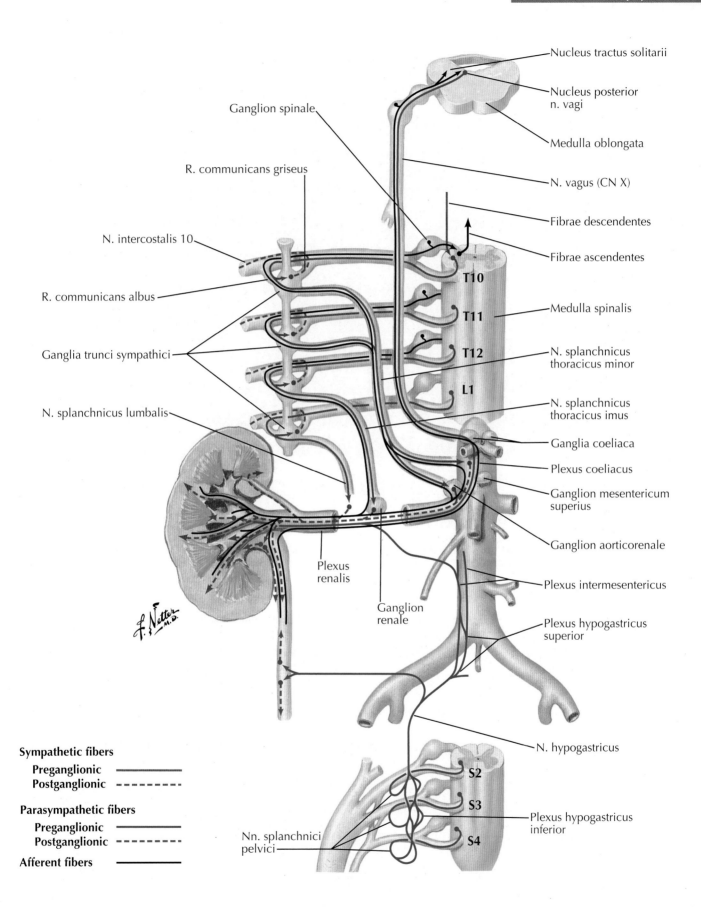

Nucleus tractus solitarii

Nucleus posterior n. vagi

Medulla oblongata

N. vagus (CN X)

Fibrae descendentes

Fibrae ascendentes

Ganglion spinale

R. communicans griseus

N. intercostalis 10

R. communicans albus

Ganglia trunci sympathici

N. splanchnicus lumbalis

T10

T11

T12

L1

Medulla spinalis

N. splanchnicus thoracicus minor

N. splanchnicus thoracicus imus

Ganglia coeliaca

Plexus coeliacus

Ganglion mesentericum superius

Ganglion aorticorenale

Plexus intermesentericus

Plexus hypogastricus superior

Plexus renalis

Ganglion renale

N. hypogastricus

S2

S3

S4

Plexus hypogastricus inferior

Nn. splanchnici pelvici

Sympathetic fibers
  Preganglionic ————
  Postganglionic - - - - -

Parasympathetic fibers
  Preganglionic ————
  Postganglionic - - - - -

Afferent fibers ————

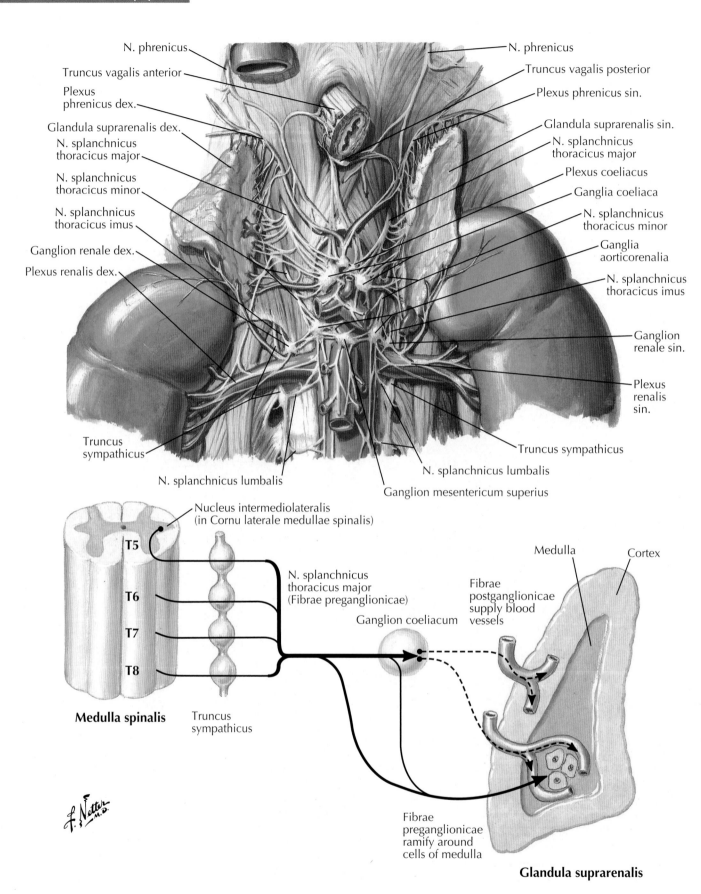

N. phrenicus

Truncus vagalis anterior

Plexus phrenicus dex.

Glandula suprarenalis dex.

N. splanchnicus thoracicus major

N. splanchnicus thoracicus minor

N. splanchnicus thoracicus imus

Ganglion renale dex.

Plexus renalis dex.

Truncus sympathicus

N. splanchnicus lumbalis

N. phrenicus

Truncus vagalis posterior

Plexus phrenicus sin.

Glandula suprarenalis sin.

N. splanchnicus thoracicus major

Plexus coeliacus

Ganglia coeliaca

N. splanchnicus thoracicus minor

Ganglia aorticorenalia

N. splanchnicus thoracicus imus

Ganglion renale sin.

Plexus renalis sin.

Truncus sympathicus

N. splanchnicus lumbalis

Ganglion mesentericum superius

Nucleus intermediolateralis (in Cornu laterale medullae spinalis)

T5

T6

T7

T8

Medulla spinalis

Truncus sympathicus

N. splanchnicus thoracicus major (Fibrae preganglionicae)

Ganglion coeliacum

Fibrae postganglionicae supply blood vessels

Medulla

Cortex

Fibrae preganglionicae ramify around cells of medulla

Glandula suprarenalis

Plate 341

Renes and Glandulae Suprarenales

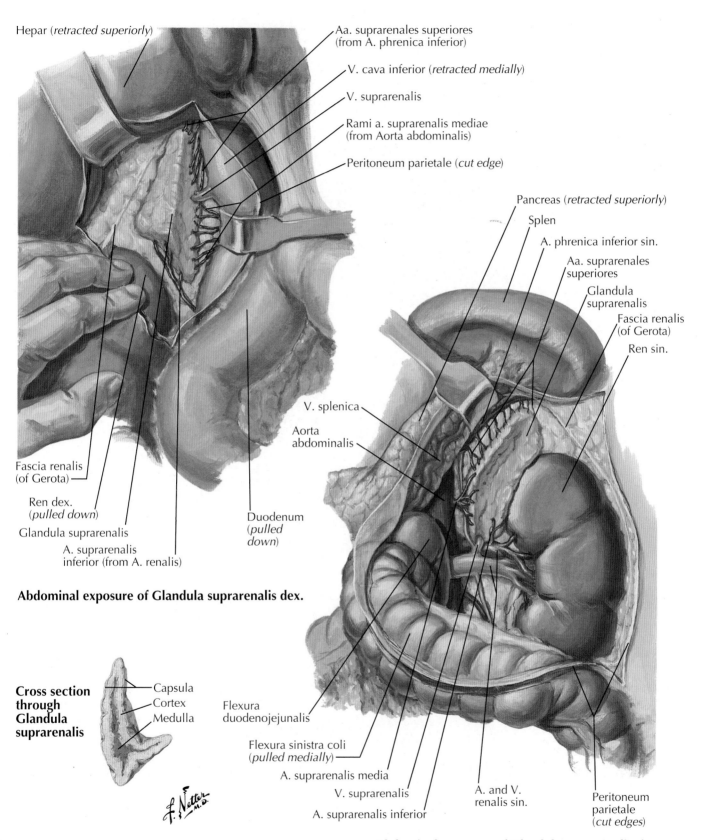

Hepar (*retracted superiorly*)

Aa. suprarenales superiores
(from A. phrenica inferior)

V. cava inferior (*retracted medially*)

V. suprarenalis

Rami a. suprarenalis mediae
(from Aorta abdominalis)

Peritoneum parietale (*cut edge*)

Pancreas (*retracted superiorly*)

Splen

A. phrenica inferior sin.

Aa. suprarenales
superiores

Glandula
suprarenalis

Fascia renalis
(of Gerota)

Ren sin.

V. splenica

Aorta
abdominalis

Fascia renalis
(of Gerota)

Ren dex.
(*pulled down*)

Glandula suprarenalis

A. suprarenalis
inferior (from A. renalis)

Duodenum
(*pulled
down*)

Abdominal exposure of Glandula suprarenalis dex.

**Cross section
through
Glandula
suprarenalis**

Capsula

Cortex

Medulla

Flexura
duodenojejunalis

Flexura sinistra coli
(*pulled medially*)

A. suprarenalis media

V. suprarenalis

A. suprarenalis inferior

A. and V.
renalis sin.

Peritoneum
parietale
(*cut edges*)

Abdominal exposure of Glandula suprarenalis sin.

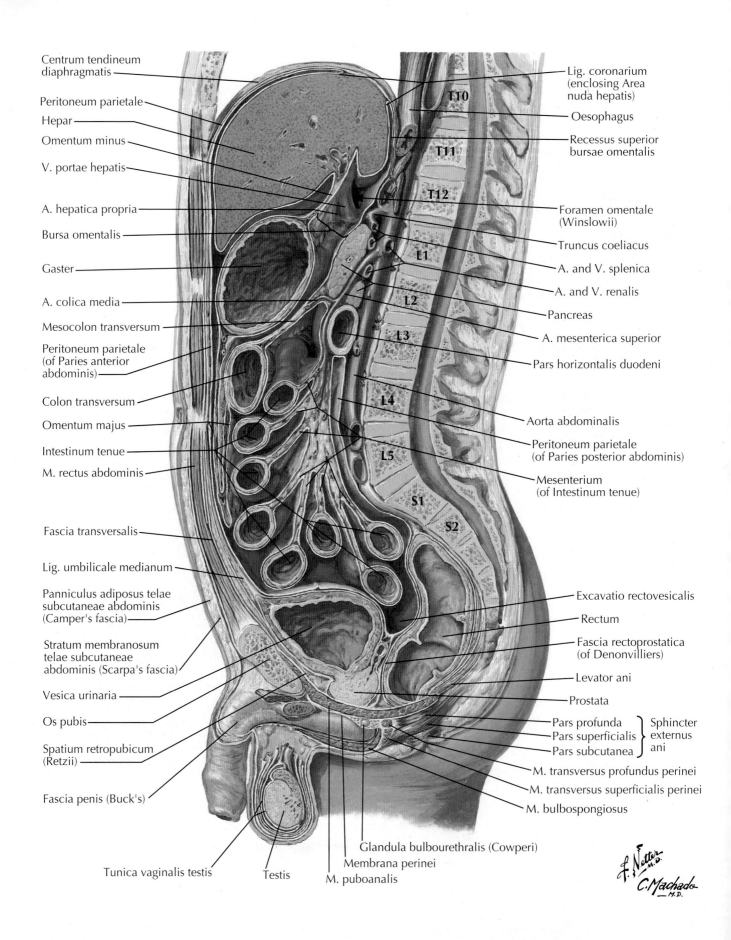

Centrum tendineum diaphragmatis

Peritoneum parietale

Hepar

Omentum minus

V. portae hepatis

A. hepatica propria

Bursa omentalis

Gaster

A. colica media

Mesocolon transversum

Peritoneum parietale (of Paries anterior abdominis)

Colon transversum

Omentum majus

Intestinum tenue

M. rectus abdominis

Fascia transversalis

Lig. umbilicale medianum

Panniculus adiposus telae subcutaneae abdominis (Camper's fascia)

Stratum membranosum telae subcutaneae abdominis (Scarpa's fascia)

Vesica urinaria

Os pubis

Spatium retropubicum (Retzii)

Fascia penis (Buck's)

Tunica vaginalis testis

Testis

M. puboanalis

Membrana perinei

Glandula bulbourethralis (Cowperi)

T10

T11

T12

L1

L2

L3

L4

L5

S1

S2

Lig. coronarium (enclosing Area nuda hepatis)

Oesophagus

Recessus superior bursae omentalis

Foramen omentale (Winslowii)

Truncus coeliacus

A. and V. splenica

A. and V. renalis

Pancreas

A. mesenterica superior

Pars horizontalis duodeni

Aorta abdominalis

Peritoneum parietale (of Paries posterior abdominis)

Mesenterium (of Intestinum tenue)

Excavatio rectovesicalis

Rectum

Fascia rectoprostatica (of Denonvilliers)

Levator ani

Prostata

Pars profunda ⎫
Pars superficialis ⎬ Sphincter externus ani
Pars subcutanea ⎭

M. transversus profundus perinei

M. transversus superficialis perinei

M. bulbospongiosus

Plate 343

Renes and Glandulae Suprarenales

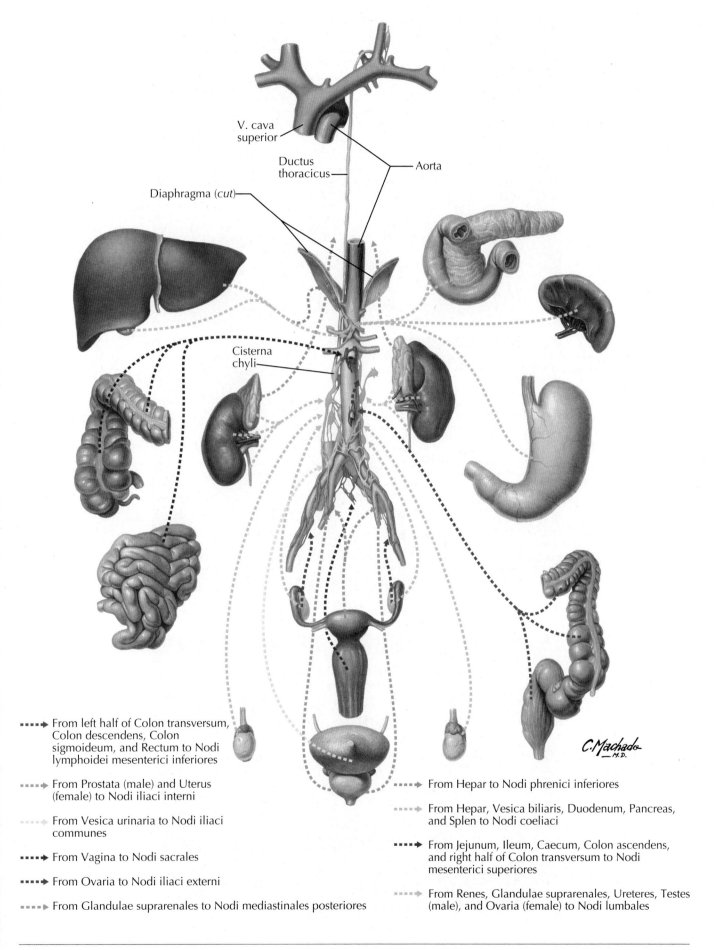

V. cava superior

Ductus thoracicus

Aorta

Diaphragma (*cut*)

Cisterna chyli

C. Machado
_M.D._

▪▪▪▶ From left half of Colon transversum, Colon descendens, Colon sigmoideum, and Rectum to Nodi lymphoidei mesenterici inferiores

▪▪▪▶ From Prostata (male) and Uterus (female) to Nodi iliaci interni

▪▪▪▶ From Vesica urinaria to Nodi iliaci communes

▪▪▪▶ From Vagina to Nodi sacrales

▪▪▪▶ From Ovaria to Nodi iliaci externi

▪▪▪▶ From Glandulae suprarenales to Nodi mediastinales posteriores

▪▪▪▶ From Hepar to Nodi phrenici inferiores

▪▪▪▶ From Hepar, Vesica biliaris, Duodenum, Pancreas, and Splen to Nodi coeliaci

▪▪▪▶ From Jejunum, Ileum, Caecum, Colon ascendens, and right half of Colon transversum to Nodi mesenterici superiores

▪▪▪▶ From Renes, Glandulae suprarenales, Ureteres, Testes (male), and Ovaria (female) to Nodi lumbales

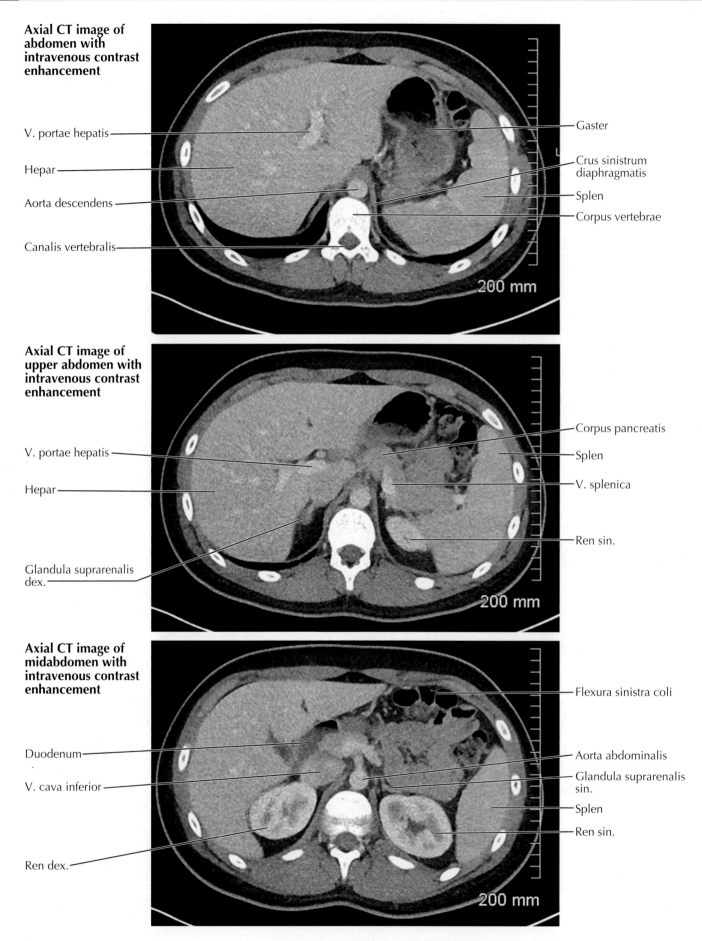

Axial CT image of abdomen with intravenous contrast enhancement

V. portae hepatis

Hepar

Aorta descendens

Canalis vertebralis

Gaster

Crus sinistrum diaphragmatis

Splen

Corpus vertebrae

200 mm

Axial CT image of upper abdomen with intravenous contrast enhancement

V. portae hepatis

Hepar

Glandula suprarenalis dex.

Corpus pancreatis

Splen

V. splenica

Ren sin.

200 mm

Axial CT image of midabdomen with intravenous contrast enhancement

Duodenum

V. cava inferior

Ren dex.

Flexura sinistra coli

Aorta abdominalis

Glandula suprarenalis sin.

Splen

Ren sin.

200 mm

Plate 345   **Regional Imaging**

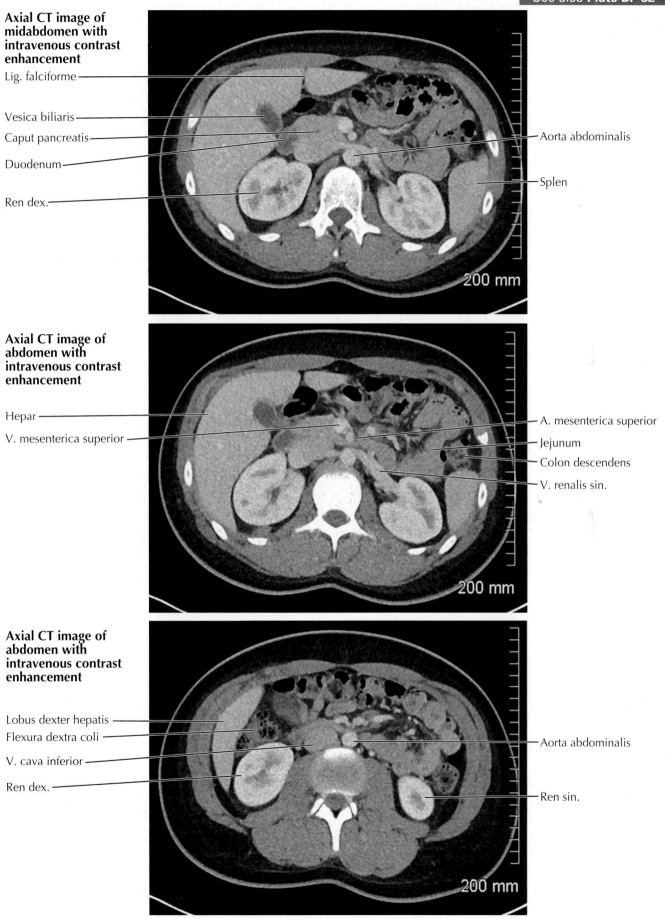

Axial CT image of midabdomen with intravenous contrast enhancement

Lig. falciforme

Vesica biliaris

Caput pancreatis

Duodenum

Ren dex.

Aorta abdominalis

Splen

200 mm

Axial CT image of abdomen with intravenous contrast enhancement

Hepar

V. mesenterica superior

A. mesenterica superior

Jejunum

Colon descendens

V. renalis sin.

200 mm

Axial CT image of abdomen with intravenous contrast enhancement

Lobus dexter hepatis

Flexura dextra coli

V. cava inferior

Ren dex.

Aorta abdominalis

Ren sin.

200 mm

Regional Imaging

Plate 346

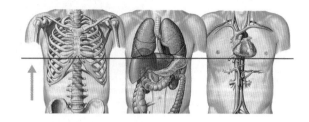

Diaphragma

Proc. xiphoideus

Cartilagines costales

Junctio oesophagogastrica

M. rectus abdominis

Crus sinistrum diaphragmatis (forming left boundary of Hiatus oesophageus)

Hepar

Crus dextrum diaphragmatis (forming right boundary of Hiatus oesophageus)

Plicae gastricae (Rugae)

V. cava inferior

M. serratus anterior

Fundus gastris

V. azyga

Aorta descendens

Crus sinistrum diaphragmatis

Splen

Diaphragma

M. latissimus dorsi

Lobus inferior pulmonis dextri (in Recessus costodiaphragmaticus)

Lobus inferior pulmonis sinistri (in Recessus costodiaphragmaticus)

Corpus vertebrae T10

Ductus thoracicus

Erector spinae

C. Machado
—M.D.

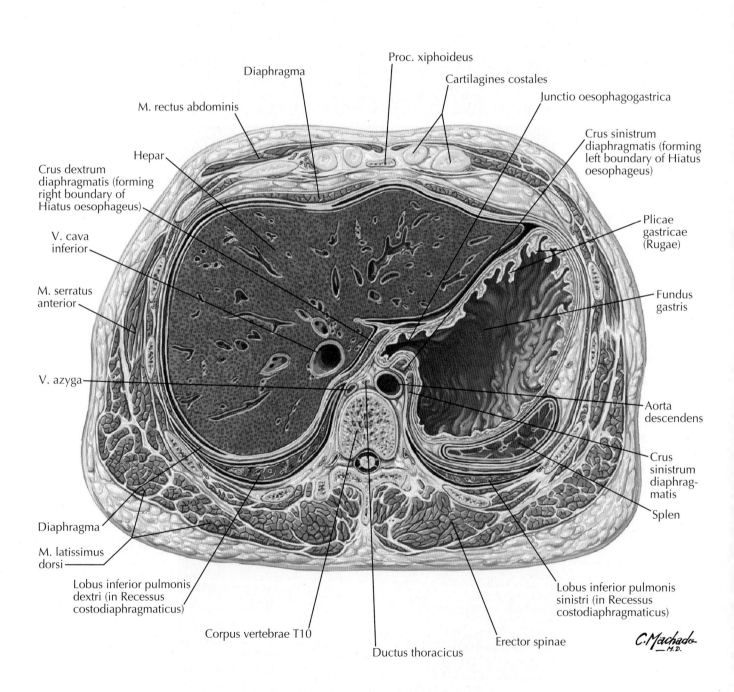

Plate 347

Cross-Sectional Anatomy

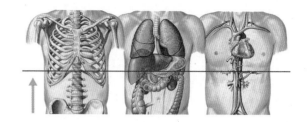

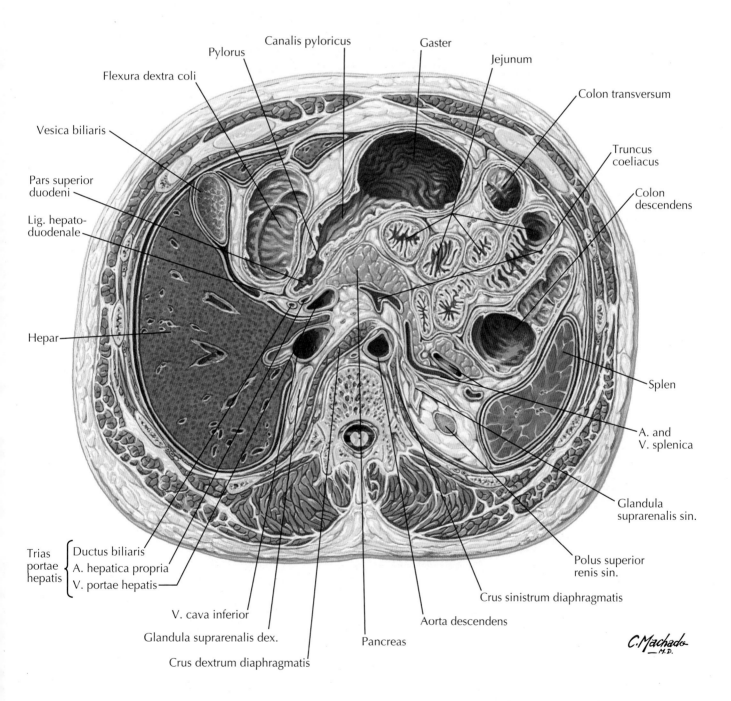

Pylorus

Canalis pyloricus

Gaster

Jejunum

Flexura dextra coli

Colon transversum

Vesica biliaris

Truncus coeliacus

Pars superior duodeni

Colon descendens

Lig. hepato-duodenale

Hepar

Splen

A. and V. splenica

Glandula suprarenalis sin.

Polus superior renis sin.

Trias portae hepatis { Ductus biliaris / A. hepatica propria / V. portae hepatis

Crus sinistrum diaphragmatis

V. cava inferior

Glandula suprarenalis dex.

Aorta descendens

Crus dextrum diaphragmatis

Pancreas

C. Machado
—M.D.

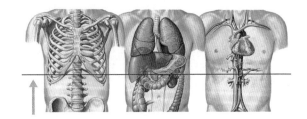

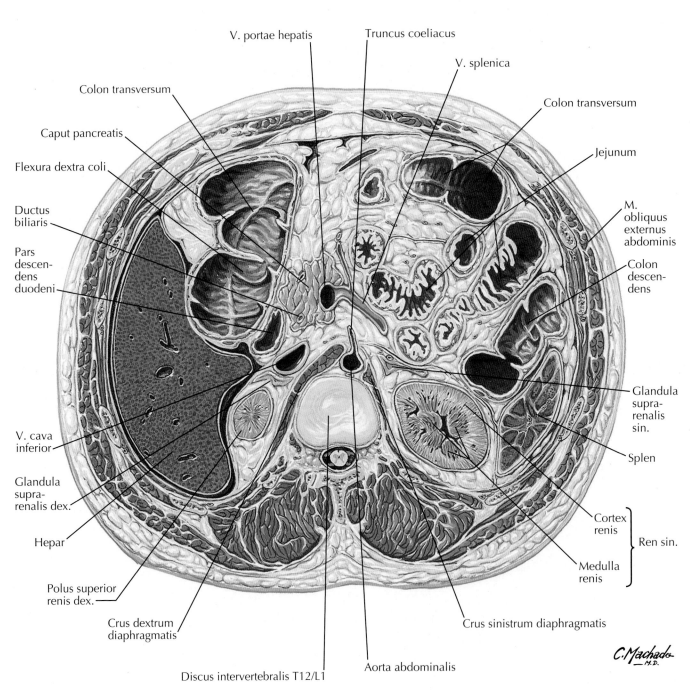

V. portae hepatis

Truncus coeliacus

V. splenica

Colon transversum

Colon transversum

Caput pancreatis

Jejunum

Flexura dextra coli

M. obliquus externus abdominis

Ductus biliaris

Colon descendens

Pars descendens duodeni

Glandula suprarenalis sin.

V. cava inferior

Splen

Glandula suprarenalis dex.

Cortex renis

Hepar

Ren sin.

Medulla renis

Polus superior renis dex.

Crus dextrum diaphragmatis

Crus sinistrum diaphragmatis

Discus intervertebralis T12/L1

Aorta abdominalis

C. Machado M.D.

Plate 349

Cross-Sectional Anatomy

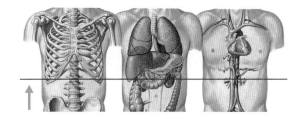

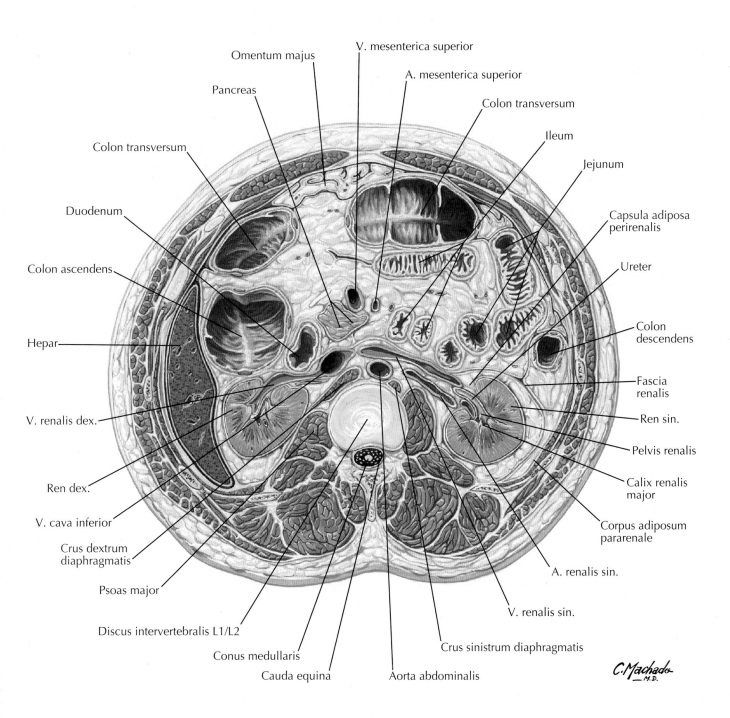

Omentum majus

V. mesenterica superior

A. mesenterica superior

Pancreas

Colon transversum

Colon transversum

Ileum

Jejunum

Duodenum

Capsula adiposa perirenalis

Colon ascendens

Ureter

Colon descendens

Hepar

Fascia renalis

Ren sin.

V. renalis dex.

Pelvis renalis

Calix renalis major

Ren dex.

Corpus adiposum pararenale

V. cava inferior

A. renalis sin.

Crus dextrum diaphragmatis

Psoas major

V. renalis sin.

Discus intervertebralis L1/L2

Crus sinistrum diaphragmatis

Conus medullaris

Cauda equina

Aorta abdominalis

C. Machado
_M.D._

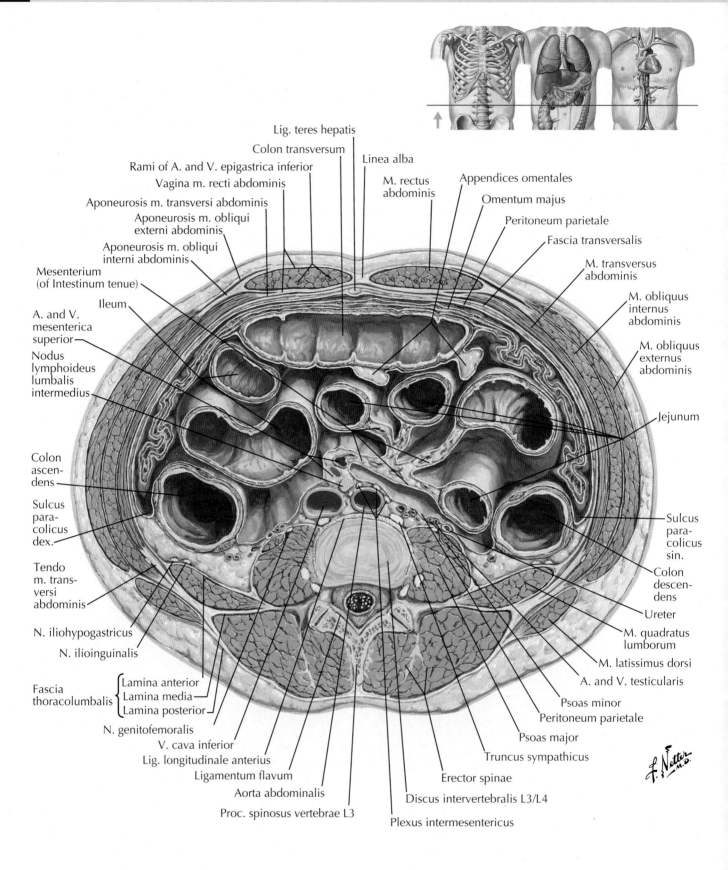

Lig. teres hepatis

Colon transversum

Rami of A. and V. epigastrica inferior

Vagina m. recti abdominis

Aponeurosis m. transversi abdominis

Aponeurosis m. obliqui externi abdominis

Aponeurosis m. obliqui interni abdominis

Mesenterium (of Intestinum tenue)

Ileum

A. and V. mesenterica superior

Nodus lymphoideus lumbalis intermedius

Colon ascendens

Sulcus paracolicus dex.

Tendo m. transversi abdominis

N. iliohypogastricus

N. ilioinguinalis

Fascia thoracolumbalis { Lamina anterior / Lamina media / Lamina posterior

N. genitofemoralis

V. cava inferior

Lig. longitudinale anterius

Ligamentum flavum

Aorta abdominalis

Proc. spinosus vertebrae L3

Linea alba

M. rectus abdominis

Appendices omentales

Omentum majus

Peritoneum parietale

Fascia transversalis

M. transversus abdominis

M. obliquus internus abdominis

M. obliquus externus abdominis

Jejunum

Sulcus paracolicus sin.

Colon descendens

Ureter

M. quadratus lumborum

M. latissimus dorsi

A. and V. testicularis

Psoas minor

Peritoneum parietale

Psoas major

Truncus sympathicus

Erector spinae

Discus intervertebralis L3/L4

Plexus intermesentericus

Plate 351

ANATOMICAL STRUCTURE	CLINICAL COMMENT	PLATE NUMBERS
Systema Nervosum		
Nn. ilioinguinalis and genitofemoralis	Mediate cremasteric reflex; femoral branch of genitofemoral nerve provides cutaneous innervation to skin over femoral triangle	287
Nn. intercostales, subcostalis, and iliohypogastricus	Convey well-localized pain sensations from abdominal wall and parietal peritoneum; pain in dermatomal distribution indicates problem with spinal nerves (e.g., herpes zoster infection)	278
Ganglion coeliacum	Some patients with medically intractable pain from chronic pancreatitis or advanced pancreatic malignancy undergo celiac ganglion block; located typically at upper or lower L1 vertebral level	320, 329
Nn. splanchnici thoracici and lumbales (sympathetic)	Convey pain sensations from abdominal viscera that are often referred to other sites; quadrant in which pain is located and site of radiation provide clues to source of pain	324, 325
N. iliohypogastricus	Nephrectomy through quadratus lumborum muscle can damage iliohypogastric nerve, with resultant anesthesia superior to the pubic symphysis	331
Systema Skeletale		
Processus xiphoideus; symphysis pubica	Palpable landmarks used to locate transpyloric plane (of Addison; L1 plane), located halfway between these structures; plane may contain pylorus of stomach, horizontal portion of duodenum, head and neck of pancreas, superior mesenteric artery, and hilum of spleen	267
Spina iliaca anterior superior (ASIS)	Palpable landmark used to locate McBurney's point; tenderness over McBurney's point is indication of appendicitis	268, 300
Systema Musculare		
Linea alba	Site used for abdominal wall incisions because this location provides access to many organs during exploratory surgery and is unlikely to have significant vessels crossing it	267, 272
Ligamentum inguinale	Surface landmark from ASIS to pubic tubercle that marks division between abdomen and lower limb; formed from external abdominal oblique aponeurosis	267, 271
Trigonum inguinale (Hesselbachi)	Important region on interior surface of anterior abdominal wall, bounded by inferior epigastric vessels, inguinal ligament, and rectus abdominis muscle, through which abdominal contents may herniate to produce direct inguinal hernias	274, 280
Anulus inguinalis profundus	Slit-like opening in transversalis fascia just above midpoint of inguinal ligament and lateral to inferior epigastric artery, through which abdominal contents may herniate to produce indirect inguinal hernias	280, 281
Anulus inguinalis superficialis	Triangular opening in external abdominal oblique aponeurosis superior and lateral to pubic tubercle and medial to inferior epigastric artery, through which abdominal contents may herniate to produce indirect inguinal hernias	270, 280, 281
Anulus femoralis	Superior opening of femoral canal bounded by medial part of inguinal ligament, femoral vein, and lacunar ligament; abdominal contents may herniate through femoral ring into upper femoral triangle situated inferolateral to pubic tubercle, producing femoral hernia	282
Hiatus oesophageus	Widening of opening through diaphragm allows stomach to protrude into mediastinum, which can increase incidence of gastroesophageal reflux disease (GERD)	287, 289
M. rectus abdominis	Separation (abdominal diastasis) commonly caused from multiple pregnancies, abdominal surgeries, and excessive weight gain; bleeding of inferior epigastric artery may cause blood to accumulate in rectus abdominis muscle (rectus sheath hematoma), which may be mistaken for acute abdominal pathologies, such as appendicitis	271

Structures with High Clinical Significance

Table 5.1

ANATOMICAL STRUCTURE	CLINICAL COMMENT	PLATE NUMBERS
Systema Cardiovasculare		
Venae paraumbilacales	May become dilated in patients with portal hypertension and in late-term pregnancy	277, 318
A. cystica	Ligated during cholecystectomy; can have multiple origins; found classically in cystohepatic triangle (of Calot)	310
A. mesenterica superior	May compress horizontal (third) part of duodenum in thin patient or patient who has recently lost large amount of weight; can shear or tear in sudden deceleration injuries	310, 313
Aa. intestinales	Areas without significant collateral circulation between major vessels (watershed areas) are at risk for ischemia, which can occur secondary to atherosclerosis or thromboembolism of mesenteric arteries	313, 314
A. marginalis coli	Marginal artery connects right, middle, and left colic arteries, providing important anastomosis for collateral circulation	314
Venae oesophageae	May become dilated in portal hypertension, resulting in esophageal varices; variceal hemorrhage can be life-threatening and often requires emergent endoscopic intervention	315, 318
Vena portae hepatis	Increased resistance to blood flow through liver (e.g., due to cirrhosis) may produce portal hypertension and dilation of tributaries of hepatic portal vein; blood may return to heart at sites of portosystemic anastomosis	317, 318
Vena anorectalis superior	Anastomoses with systemic middle and inferior anorectal veins may become dilated in portal hypertension	317, 318
Aorta abdominalis	Common site for aneurysm in abdomen, especially inferior to renal arteries; assessed routinely with ultrasound to exclude aneurysms	336
A. renalis	Stenosis may occur secondary to atherosclerosis or fibromuscular dysplasia, resulting in difficult-to-control hypertension; can be affected in abdominal aortic aneurysms	334, 336
Vasa Lymphatica and Organa Lymphoidea		
Splen	May be ruptured by fracture of ribs 10 to 12; enlargement (splenomegaly) may occur in cirrhosis, viral infections, and hematologic malignancies; if palpable, the spleen is enlarged	291, 307
Systema Digestorium		
Hepar	Palpable inferior to right costal margin; hepatomegaly may occur in conditions such as hepatitis, heart failure, and infiltrative diseases; shrunken, nodular appearance of liver on imaging indicates cirrhosis; common site of metastasis	269, 294
Junctio oesophagogastrica	Transient relaxations or decreased tone of lower esophageal sphincter can cause gastroesophageal reflux disease (GERD), a common cause of epigastric pain; common site of esophageal cancer	257, 295, 347
Gaster; Duodenum	Primary sites of peptic ulcers; nonsteroidal anti-inflammatory drug (NSAID) overuse and/or *Helicobacter pylori* infection may cause ulceration	292, 294, 295
Pylorus	Infantile hypertrophic pyloric stenosis causes postprandial projectile vomiting among newborns	295
Papilla major duodeni (Vateri)	Catheterized and injected with contrast during endoscopic retrograde cholangiopancreatography (ERCP), a common diagnostic procedure; sphincter of hepatopancreatic ampulla (sphincter of Oddi) dysfunction may obstruct biliary flow through major duodenal papilla, resulting in right upper quadrant pain	297, 305
Appendix vermiformis	Prone to inflammation and rupture (appendicitis); may have retrocecal position, in which case appendicitis causes inflammation of adjacent psoas fascia and atypical location of pain	298, 300

Table 5.2

ANATOMICAL STRUCTURE	CLINICAL COMMENT	PLATE NUMBERS
Colon	Common site of diverticula and malignancies; colonoscopy is performed to screen for colon cancer	301
Vesica biliaris	May become inflamed (cholecystitis) and cause pain secondary to gallstones blocking cystic duct	302, 305, 308, 328
Ductus biliaris	Gallstones may become impacted in bile duct (choledocholithiasis), resulting in hepatitis and jaundice; some cases may be complicated by pancreatitis and/or infection of obstructed biliary ducts (cholangitis); small stones can be problematic, whereas large stones usually remain in gallbladder and are more typically asymptomatic; ERCP is performed to locate and relieve obstruction	302, 303, 305
Umbilicus	Remnant of umbilical cord insertion into fetal umbilical vessels; landmark for locating transumbilical plane, which is used to divide abdomen into quadrants; marks position of T10 dermatome; used to locate McBurney's point; common site for hernias in abdominal wall	267, 269
Pancreas	Lies primarily retroperitoneal and deep to stomach; thus, inflamed pancreas may be compressed by stomach and cause intense pain referred to the back; inflamed pancreas, most often caused by biliary obstruction or alcohol abuse, may cause severe life-threatening complications; cancer of head/neck of pancreas can compress biliary tree	292, 306, 329
Systema Urinarium		
Ren	Right kidney is lower or more inferior than left kidney due to position inferior to liver; renal arteries are generally located at L2 vertebral level and may be involved in abdominal aortic aneurysms; renal calculi (kidney stones) cause significant pain when impacted in ureter	333
Pelvis renalis	May become dilated secondary to ureteral or urinary bladder outlet obstruction, a condition known as hydronephrosis, which is readily visualized using ultrasound	333
Glandulae Endocrinae		
Glandula suprarenalis	Produces hormones in its cortex (e.g., cortisol, aldosterone) and medulla (e.g., epinephrine, norepinephrine); small masses are frequently incidentally discovered on axial abdominal imaging; need for further workup depends in part on size	330

*Selections were based largely on clinical data and commonly discussed clinical correlations in macroscopic ("gross") anatomy courses.

MUSCLE	MUSCLE GROUP	ORIGIN ATTACHMENT	INSERTION ATTACHMENT	INNERVATION	BLOOD SUPPLY	MAIN ACTIONS
M. obliquus externus abdominis	Paries anterolateralis abdominis	Facies externae costarum 5–12	Linea alba; tuberculum pubicum; crista iliaca (anterior half)	Rr. anteriores nn. spinalium T7–T12	Aa. epigastricae superior and inferior, and lumbales	Compresses and supports abdominal viscera, flexes and rotates trunk
M. obliquus internus abdominis	Paries anterolateralis abdominis	Fascia thoracolumalis; crista iliaca (anterior two-thirds)	Margines inferiores costarum 10–12; linea alba (via vagina m. recti abdominis); crista pubica and Pecten ossis pubis (via falx inguinalis)	Rr. anteriores nn. spinalium T7–L1	Aa. epigastricae superior and inferior, circumflexa iliaca profunda, and lumbales	Compresses and supports abdominal viscera, flexes and rotates trunk
M. pyramidalis	Paries anterolateralis abdominis	Corpus ossis pubis and symphysis pubica (anterior to m. rectus abdominis)	Linea alba (inferior to umbilicus)	R. anterior n. spinalis T12 (via n. subcostalis or n. iliohypogastricus)	A. epigastrica inferior	Tenses linea alba
M. quadratus lumborum	Paries posterior abdominis	Margo inferior costae 12 (medial half); tips of procc. transversi vertebrarum L1–L4	Labium internum cristae iliacae; lig. iliolumbale	Rr. anteriores nn. spinalium T12–L1	A. iliolumbalis	Extends and laterally flexes vertebral column, fixes 12th rib during inspiration
M. rectus abdominis	Paries anterolateralis abdominis	Crista pubica; Symphysis pubica	Cartilagines costales 5–7; proc. xiphoideus	Rr. anteriores nn. spinalium T7–T12	Aa. epigastricae superior and inferior	Flexes trunk, compresses abdominal viscera
M. transversus abdominis	Paries anterolateralis abdominis	Facies internae cartilaginum costalium 7–12; fascia thoracolumbalis; crista iliaca	Linea alba (via vagina m. rectus abdominis), crista pubica and Pecten ossis pubis (via falx inguinalis)	Rr. anteriores nn. spinalium T7–L1	A. circumflexa iliaca profunda, epigastrica inferior, and lumbales	Compresses and supports abdominal viscera

Variations in spinal nerve contributions to the innervation of muscles, their arterial supply, their attachments, and their actions are common themes in human anatomy. Therefore, expect differences between texts and realize that anatomical variation is normal.

Table 5.4   **Musculi**

PELVIS 6

Surface Anatomy   352
Pelvis Ossea   353–357
Diaphragma Pelvis and
   Organa Visceralia Pelvis   358–368
Vesica Urinaria   369–371
Organa Genitalia Feminina
   Interna   372–376
Perineum Femininum and
   Organa Genitalia
   Feminina Externa   377–380
Perineum Masculinum and
   Organa Genitalia
   Masculina Externa   381–388
Homologies of Organa
   Genitalia Masculina and
   Organa Genitalis Feminina   389–390

Organa Genitalia
   Masculina Interna   391–392
Rectum and Canalis
   Analis   393–399
Vasa Sanguinea, Vasa
   Lymphatica, and Nodi
   Lymphoidei   400–410
Nervi Perinei and Nervi
   Viscerales Pelvis   411–419
Cross-Sectional Anatomy   420–421
Structures with High
   Clinical Significance   Tables 6.1–6.2
Musculi   Table 6.3
Electronic Bonus Plates   BP 84–BP 95

ELECTRONIC BONUS PLATES

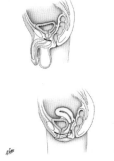

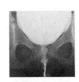

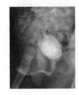

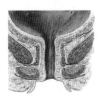

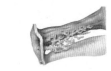

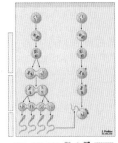

BP 84 Fasciae of Pelvis and Perineum: Male and Female

BP 85 Cystourethrograms: Male and Female

BP 86 Urethra Feminina

BP 87 Genetics of Reproduction

ELECTRONIC BONUS PLATES—*cont'd*

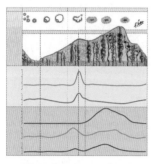

BP 88 Menstrual Cycle

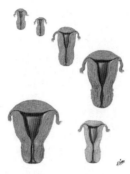

BP 89 Development of Uterus

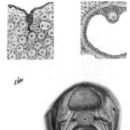

BP 90 Ovarium, Oocytia, and Folliculi

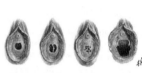

BP 91 Variations in Hymen

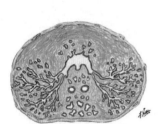

BP 92 Cross Section of Pelvis Through Prostata

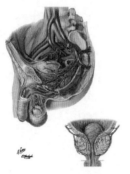

BP 93 Arteriae and Venae of Pelvis: Male (Featuring Prostata)

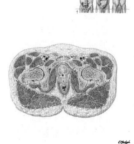

BP 94 Cross Section of Lower Pelvis

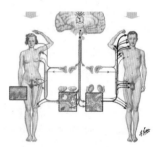

BP 95 Endocrine Glands, Hormones, and Puberty

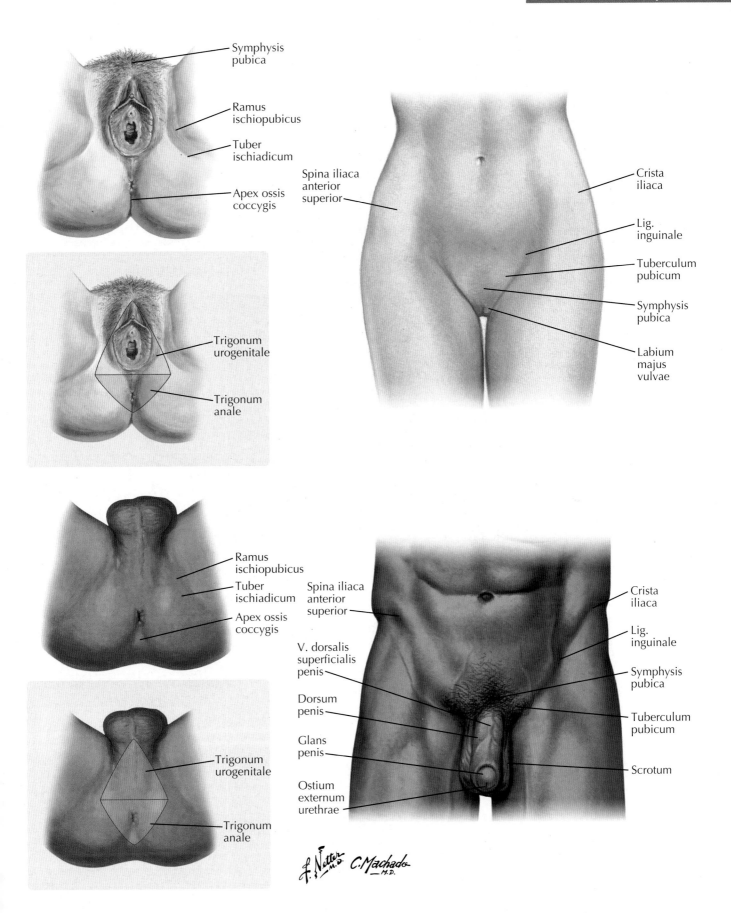

Symphysis pubica

Ramus ischiopubicus

Tuber ischiadicum

Apex ossis coccygis

Trigonum urogenitale

Trigonum anale

Spina iliaca anterior superior

Crista iliaca

Lig. inguinale

Tuberculum pubicum

Symphysis pubica

Labium majus vulvae

Ramus ischiopubicus

Tuber ischiadicum

Apex ossis coccygis

Trigonum urogenitale

Trigonum anale

Spina iliaca anterior superior

V. dorsalis superficialis penis

Dorsum penis

Glans penis

Ostium externum urethrae

Crista iliaca

Lig. inguinale

Symphysis pubica

Tuberculum pubicum

Scrotum

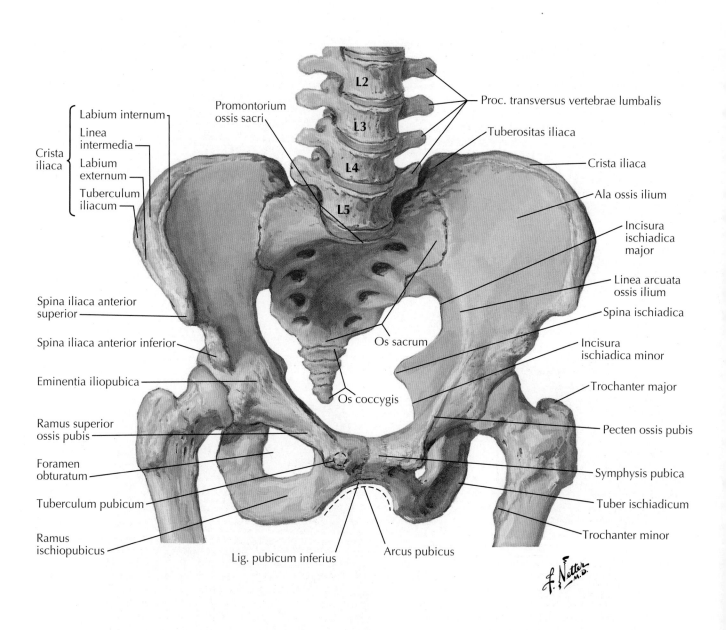

Labium internum

Linea intermedia

Crista iliaca

Labium externum

Tuberculum iliacum

Promontorium ossis sacri

L2

L3

L4

L5

Proc. transversus vertebrae lumbalis

Tuberositas iliaca

Crista iliaca

Ala ossis ilium

Incisura ischiadica major

Linea arcuata ossis ilium

Spina iliaca anterior superior

Spina iliaca anterior inferior

Eminentia iliopubica

Ramus superior ossis pubis

Foramen obturatum

Tuberculum pubicum

Ramus ischiopubicus

Os sacrum

Os coccygis

Lig. pubicum inferius

Arcus pubicus

Spina ischiadica

Incisura ischiadica minor

Trochanter major

Pecten ossis pubis

Symphysis pubica

Tuber ischiadicum

Trochanter minor

Plate 353

Pelvis Ossea

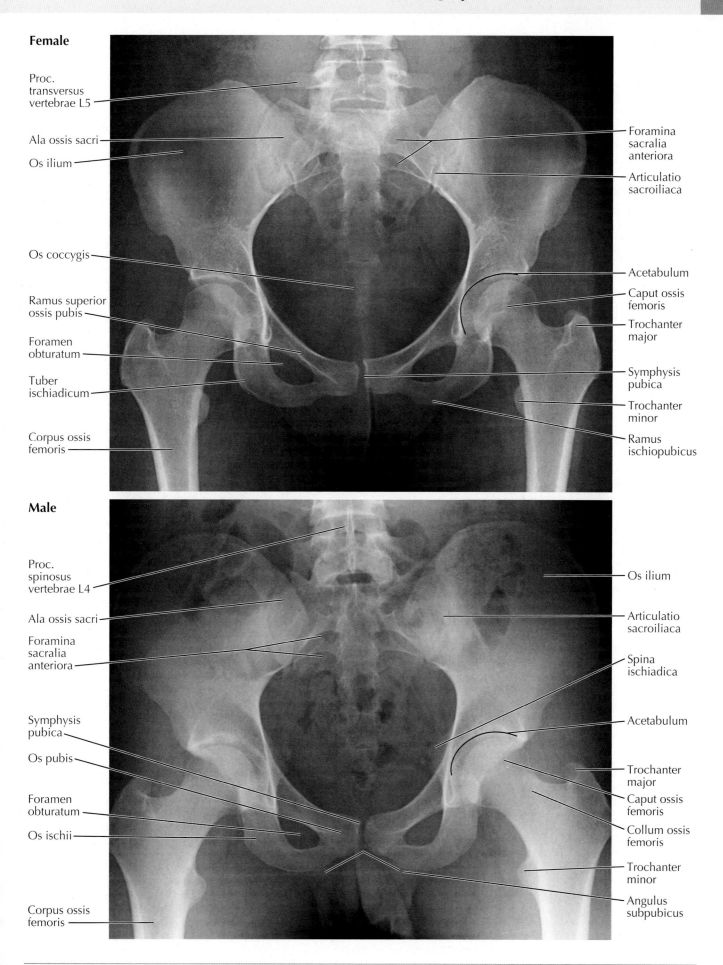

Female

Proc. transversus vertebrae L5

Ala ossis sacri

Os ilium

Os coccygis

Ramus superior ossis pubis

Foramen obturatum

Tuber ischiadicum

Corpus ossis femoris

Foramina sacralia anteriora

Articulatio sacroiliaca

Acetabulum

Caput ossis femoris

Trochanter major

Symphysis pubica

Trochanter minor

Ramus ischiopubicus

Male

Proc. spinosus vertebrae L4

Ala ossis sacri

Foramina sacralia anteriora

Symphysis pubica

Os pubis

Foramen obturatum

Os ischii

Corpus ossis femoris

Os ilium

Articulatio sacroiliaca

Spina ischiadica

Acetabulum

Trochanter major

Caput ossis femoris

Collum ossis femoris

Trochanter minor

Angulus subpubicus

Pelvis Ossea

Plate 354

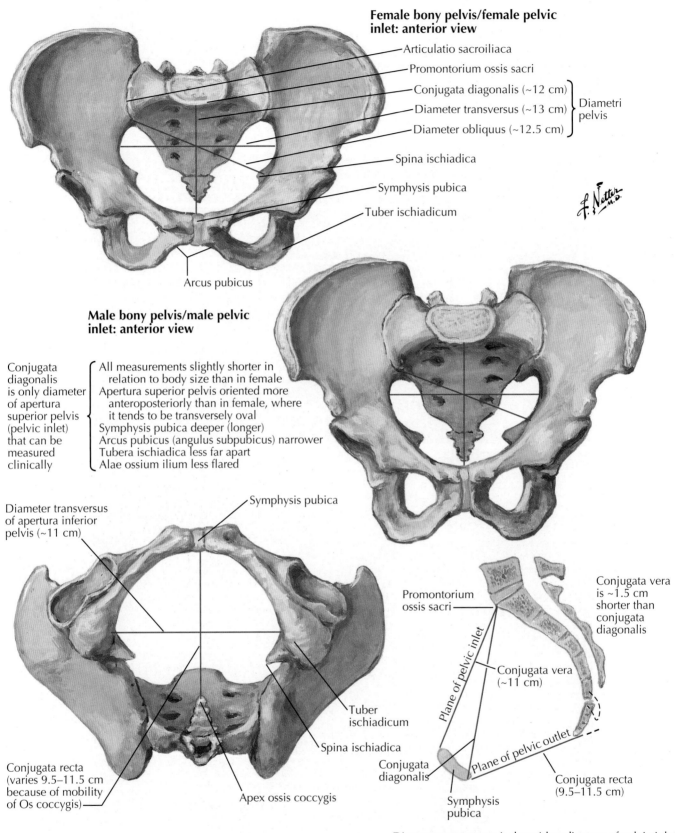

Female bony pelvis/female pelvic inlet: anterior view

Articulatio sacroiliaca

Promontorium ossis sacri

Conjugata diagonalis (~12 cm)

Diameter transversus (~13 cm) — Diametri pelvis

Diameter obliquus (~12.5 cm)

Spina ischiadica

Symphysis pubica

Tuber ischiadicum

Arcus pubicus

Male bony pelvis/male pelvic inlet: anterior view

Conjugata diagonalis is only diameter of apertura superior pelvis (pelvic inlet) that can be measured clinically
- All measurements slightly shorter in relation to body size than in female
- Apertura superior pelvis oriented more anteroposteriorly than in female, where it tends to be transversely oval
- Symphysis pubica deeper (longer)
- Arcus pubicus (angulus subpubicus) narrower
- Tubera ischiadica less far apart
- Alae ossium ilium less flared

Diameter transversus of apertura inferior pelvis (~11 cm)

Symphysis pubica

Conjugata recta (varies 9.5–11.5 cm because of mobility of Os coccygis)

Apex ossis coccygis

Tuber ischiadicum

Spina ischiadica

Promontorium ossis sacri

Conjugata vera is ~1.5 cm shorter than conjugata diagonalis

Plane of pelvic inlet

Conjugata vera (~11 cm)

Plane of pelvic outlet

Conjugata diagonalis

Symphysis pubica

Conjugata recta (9.5–11.5 cm)

Diameter transversus is the widest distance of pelvic inlet

Female bony pelvis/female pelvic outlet: inferior view

Female: sagittal section

Plate 355

Pelvis Ossea

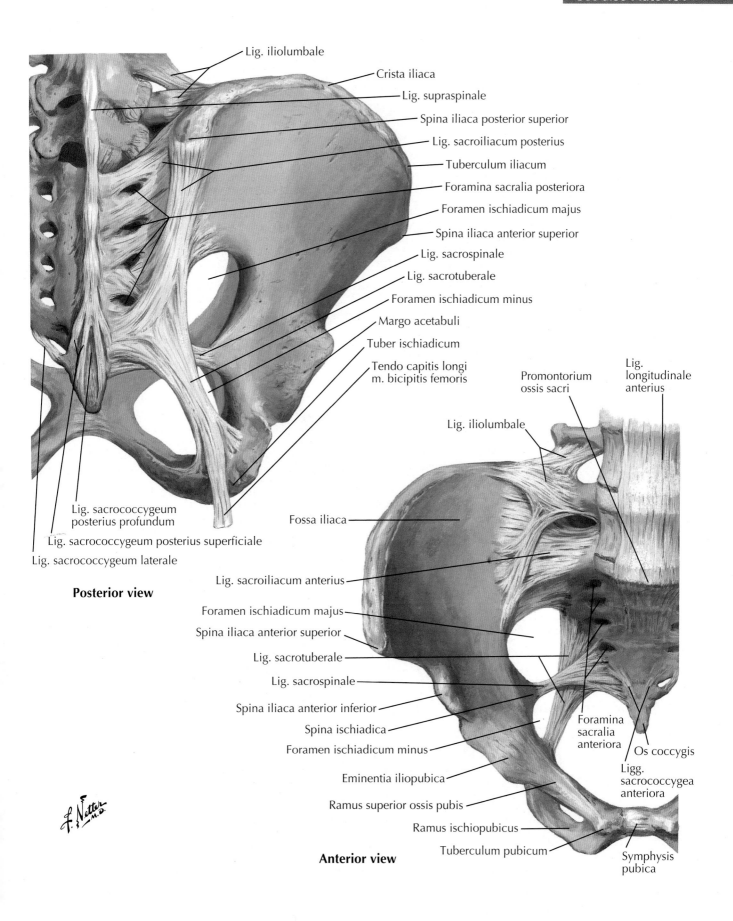

Lig. iliolumbale

Crista iliaca

Lig. supraspinale

Spina iliaca posterior superior

Lig. sacroiliacum posterius

Tuberculum iliacum

Foramina sacralia posteriora

Foramen ischiadicum majus

Spina iliaca anterior superior

Lig. sacrospinale

Lig. sacrotuberale

Foramen ischiadicum minus

Margo acetabuli

Tuber ischiadicum

Tendo capitis longi m. bicipitis femoris

Lig. sacrococcygeum posterius profundum

Lig. sacrococcygeum posterius superficiale

Lig. sacrococcygeum laterale

Posterior view

Promontorium ossis sacri

Lig. longitudinale anterius

Lig. iliolumbale

Fossa iliaca

Lig. sacroiliacum anterius

Foramen ischiadicum majus

Spina iliaca anterior superior

Lig. sacrotuberale

Lig. sacrospinale

Spina iliaca anterior inferior

Spina ischiadica

Foramen ischiadicum minus

Eminentia iliopubica

Ramus superior ossis pubis

Ramus ischiopubicus

Tuberculum pubicum

Foramina sacralia anteriora

Os coccygis

Ligg. sacrococcygea anteriora

Symphysis pubica

Anterior view

f. Netter M.D.

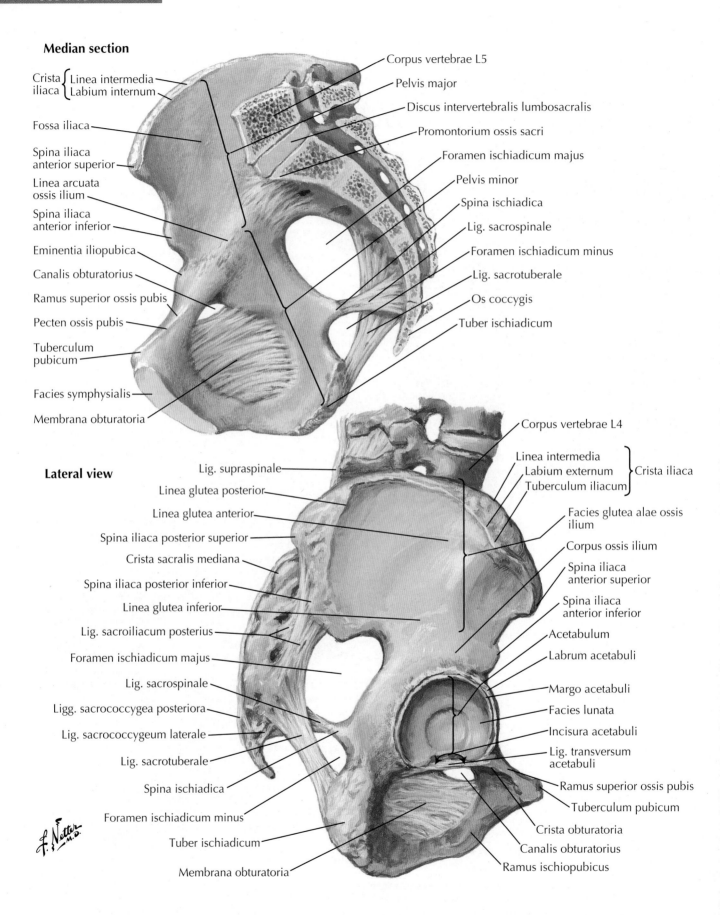

Median section

Crista iliaca { Linea intermedia / Labium internum

Fossa iliaca

Spina iliaca anterior superior

Linea arcuata ossis ilium

Spina iliaca anterior inferior

Eminentia iliopubica

Canalis obturatorius

Ramus superior ossis pubis

Pecten ossis pubis

Tuberculum pubicum

Facies symphysialis

Membrana obturatoria

Corpus vertebrae L5

Pelvis major

Discus intervertebralis lumbosacralis

Promontorium ossis sacri

Foramen ischiadicum majus

Pelvis minor

Spina ischiadica

Lig. sacrospinale

Foramen ischiadicum minus

Lig. sacrotuberale

Os coccygis

Tuber ischiadicum

Lateral view

Lig. supraspinale

Linea glutea posterior

Linea glutea anterior

Spina iliaca posterior superior

Crista sacralis mediana

Spina iliaca posterior inferior

Linea glutea inferior

Lig. sacroiliacum posterius

Foramen ischiadicum majus

Lig. sacrospinale

Ligg. sacrococcygea posteriora

Lig. sacrococcygeum laterale

Lig. sacrotuberale

Spina ischiadica

Foramen ischiadicum minus

Tuber ischiadicum

Membrana obturatoria

Corpus vertebrae L4

Linea intermedia / Labium externum / Tuberculum iliacum } Crista iliaca

Facies glutea alae ossis ilium

Corpus ossis ilium

Spina iliaca anterior superior

Spina iliaca anterior inferior

Acetabulum

Labrum acetabuli

Margo acetabuli

Facies lunata

Incisura acetabuli

Lig. transversum acetabuli

Ramus superior ossis pubis

Tuberculum pubicum

Crista obturatoria

Canalis obturatorius

Ramus ischiopubicus

Plate 357

Pelvis Ossea

Medial view

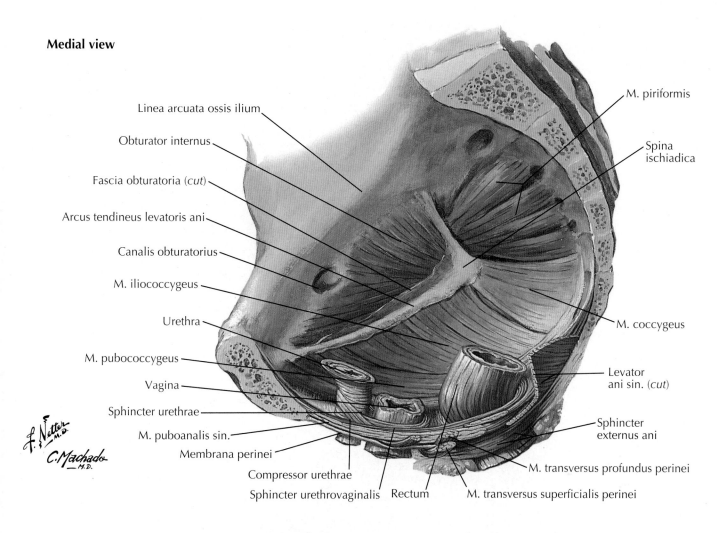

Linea arcuata ossis ilium

Obturator internus

Fascia obturatoria (*cut*)

Arcus tendineus levatoris ani

Canalis obturatorius

M. iliococcygeus

Urethra

M. pubococcygeus

Vagina

Sphincter urethrae

M. puboanalis sin.

Membrana perinei

Compressor urethrae

Sphincter urethrovaginalis

Rectum

M. transversus superficialis perinei

M. transversus profundus perinei

Sphincter externus ani

Levator ani sin. (*cut*)

M. coccygeus

Spina ischiadica

M. piriformis

Lateral view

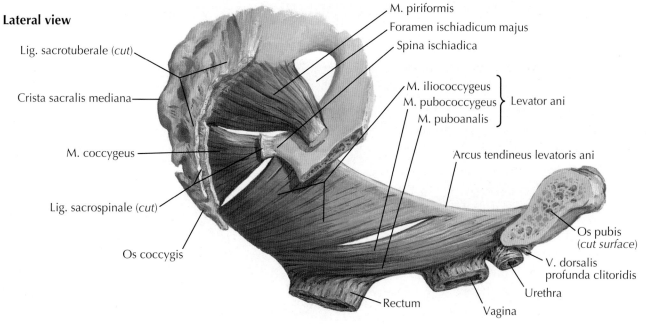

Lig. sacrotuberale (*cut*)

Crista sacralis mediana

M. coccygeus

Lig. sacrospinale (*cut*)

Os coccygis

M. piriformis

Foramen ischiadicum majus

Spina ischiadica

M. iliococcygeus

M. pubococcygeus } Levator ani

M. puboanalis

Arcus tendineus levatoris ani

Os pubis (*cut surface*)

V. dorsalis profunda clitoridis

Urethra

Vagina

Rectum

Medial view

Os pubis (*cut surface*)

Fascia obturatoria (*cut*)

Canalis obturatorius

Urethra

Linea arcuata ossis ilium

Vagina

Obturator internus

M. pubococcygeus

Arcus tendineus
levatoris ani

Spina ischiadica

M. iliococcygeus

Rectum

M. piriformis

M. coccygeus

Os coccygis

Superior view

Lig. pubicum inferius

Symphysis pubica

V. dorsalis profunda clitoridis

Lig. transversum perinei

Lig. inguinale
(Pouparti)

Fascia mm. profundorum perinei

Urethra

Vagina

Canalis obturatorius

Fascia obturatoria
(*over* Obturator
internus)

M. pubococcygeus
(*part of* Levator ani)

Arcus tendineus
levatoris ani

Rectum

M. iliococcygeus
(*part of* Levator ani)

Spina ischiadica

Raphe diaphragmatis pelvis

M. coccygeus

M. piriformis

Os coccygis

Lig. sacro-
coccygeum anterius

Promontorium ossis sacri

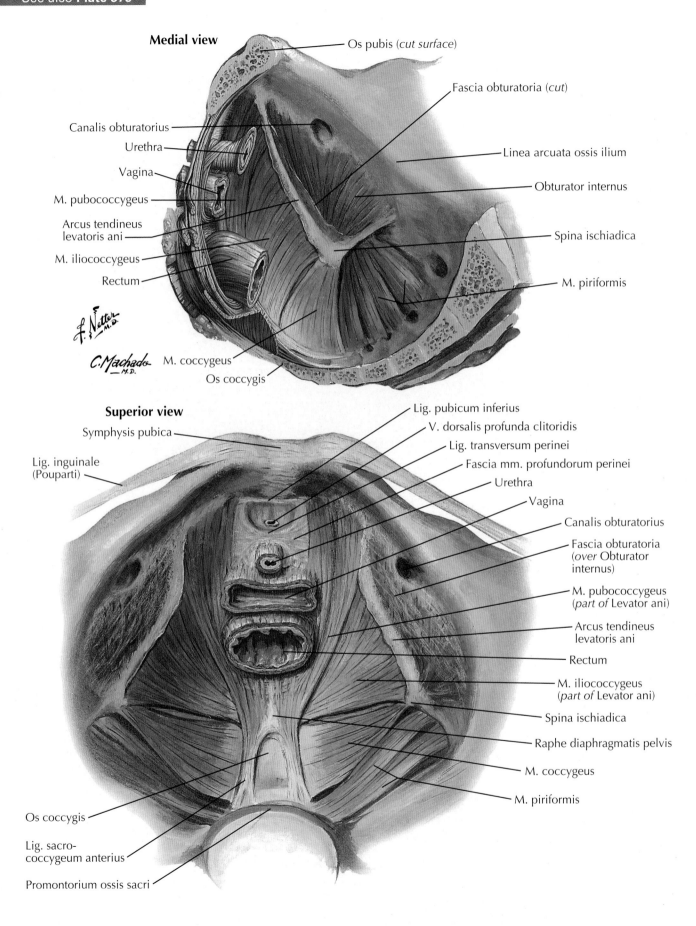

Plate 359

Diaphragma Pelvis and Organa Visceralia Pelvis

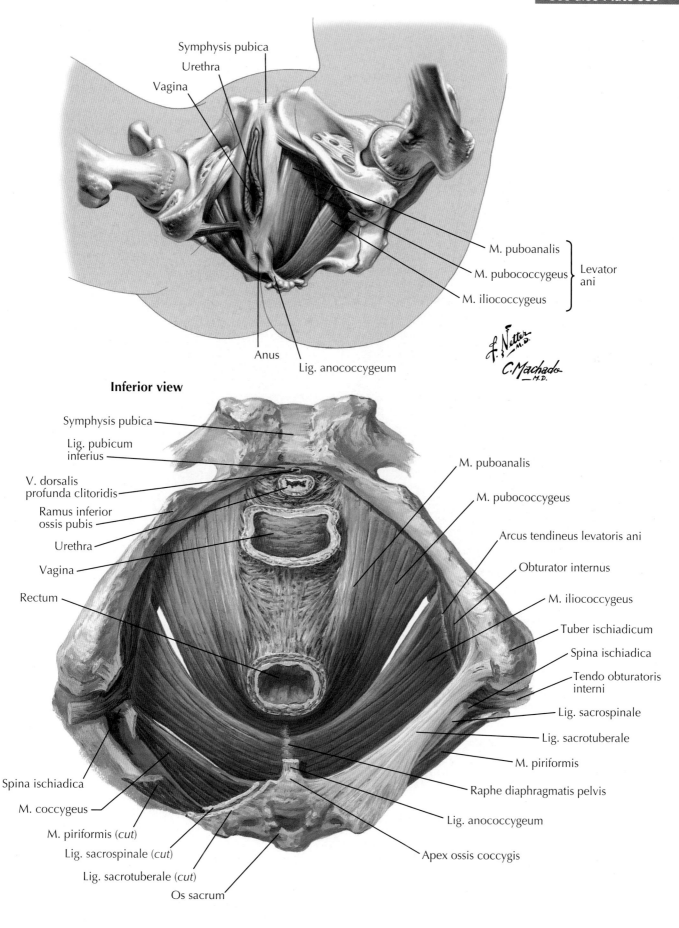

Symphysis pubica

Urethra

Vagina

M. puboanalis ⎫
M. pubococcygeus ⎬ Levator ani
M. iliococcygeus ⎭

Anus

Lig. anococcygeum

Inferior view

Symphysis pubica

Lig. pubicum inferius

V. dorsalis profunda clitoridis

Ramus inferior ossis pubis

Urethra

Vagina

Rectum

M. puboanalis

M. pubococcygeus

Arcus tendineus levatoris ani

Obturator internus

M. iliococcygeus

Tuber ischiadicum

Spina ischiadica

Tendo obturatoris interni

Lig. sacrospinale

Lig. sacrotuberale

M. piriformis

Raphe diaphragmatis pelvis

Lig. anococcygeum

Apex ossis coccygis

Spina ischiadica

M. coccygeus

M. piriformis (*cut*)

Lig. sacrospinale (*cut*)

Lig. sacrotuberale (*cut*)

Os sacrum

Superior view
(*viscera removed*)

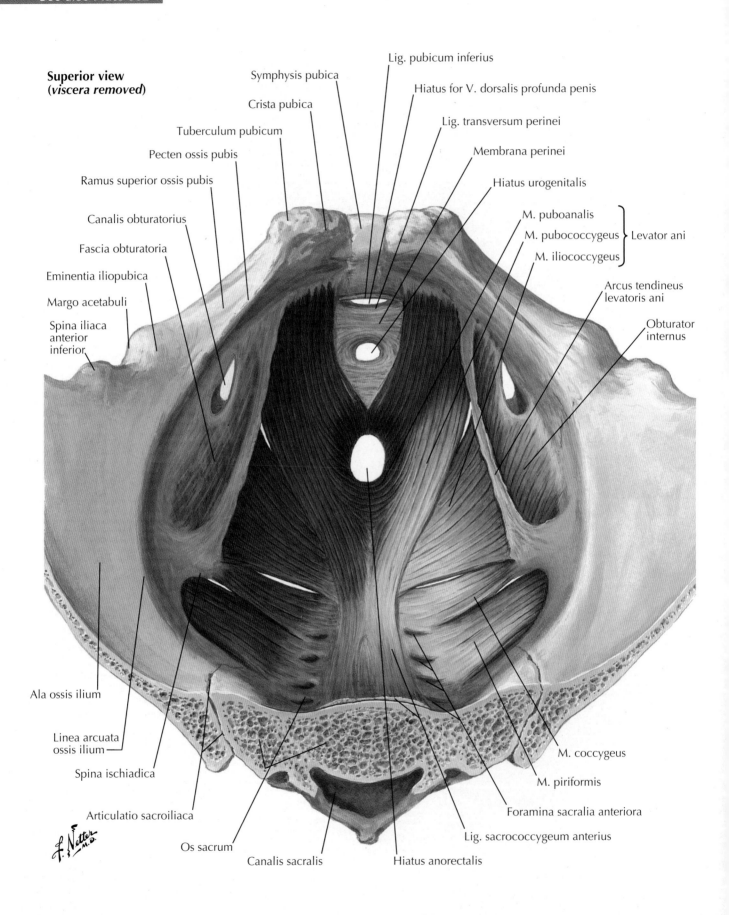

Lig. pubicum inferius

Symphysis pubica

Hiatus for V. dorsalis profunda penis

Crista pubica

Lig. transversum perinei

Tuberculum pubicum

Membrana perinei

Pecten ossis pubis

Hiatus urogenitalis

Ramus superior ossis pubis

M. puboanalis

Canalis obturatorius

M. pubococcygeus ⎱ Levator ani

Fascia obturatoria

M. iliococcygeus ⎰

Eminentia iliopubica

Arcus tendineus
levatoris ani

Margo acetabuli

Obturator
internus

Spina iliaca
anterior
inferior

Ala ossis ilium

Linea arcuata
ossis ilium

M. coccygeus

Spina ischiadica

M. piriformis

Articulatio sacroiliaca

Foramina sacralia anteriora

Lig. sacrococcygeum anterius

Os sacrum

Canalis sacralis

Hiatus anorectalis

Plate 361

Diaphragma Pelvis and Organa Visceralia Pelvis

Inferior view

Rr. sinister et dexter v. dorsalis profundae penis

Symphysis pubica

Textus adiposus in Spatium retropubicum (Retzii)

Lig. pubicum inferius

Sphincter externus urethrae

Tuberculum pubicum

Urethra

Corpus perineale

Fascia rectoprostatica

Margo medialis levatoris ani

M. rectoperinealis

Membrana perinei (cut away)

Ramus ischiopubicus

Tendo obturatoris interni

Tuber ischiadicum

Lig. sacrotuberale (cut)

Lig. sacrospinale (cut)

M. coccygeus

Lig. sacrospinale (cut)

Lig. sacrotuberale (cut)

Apex ossis coccygis

M. gluteus maximus

Obturator internus

Arcus tendineus levatoris ani

M. iliococcygeus ⎫
M. pubococcygeus ⎬ Levator ani
M. puboanalis ⎭

Stratum circulare ⎫ Tunica muscularis
Stratum longitudinale ⎭ junctionis anorectalis

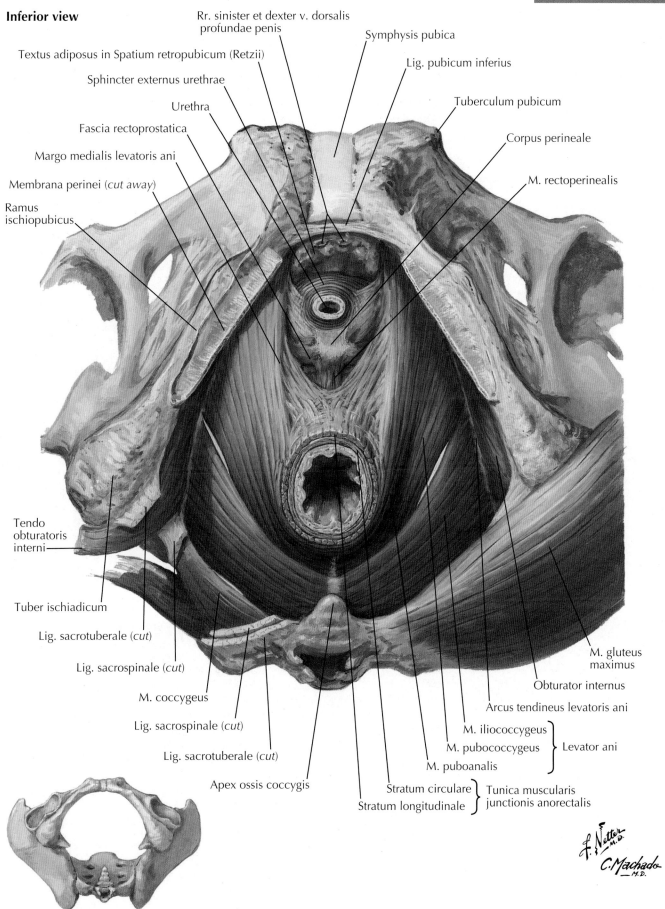

Superior view

Lig. umbilicale medianum
Linea alba
Fundus uteri
Lig. proprium ovarii
Ovarium
Tuba uterina (Fallopii)
Lig. teres uteri
Lig. latum uteri
Anulus femoralis
Anulus inguinalis profundus
Tractus iliopubicus (*covered by* peritoneum)
A. and V. iliaca externa
Fossa iliaca
Recessus paracolicus sin.

Plica umbilicalis mediana
Vesica urinaria
M. rectus abdominis
Lig. umbilicale mediale
Plica umbilicalis medialis
Plica vesicalis transversa
Rectum
A. and V. epigastrica inferior
Plica umbilicalis lateralis
Plica rectouterina
Ureter (*covered by* peritoneum)
Lig. suspensorium ovarii (*contains* A. and V. ovarica)
Caecum
Plicae caecales
Recessus paracolicus dex.

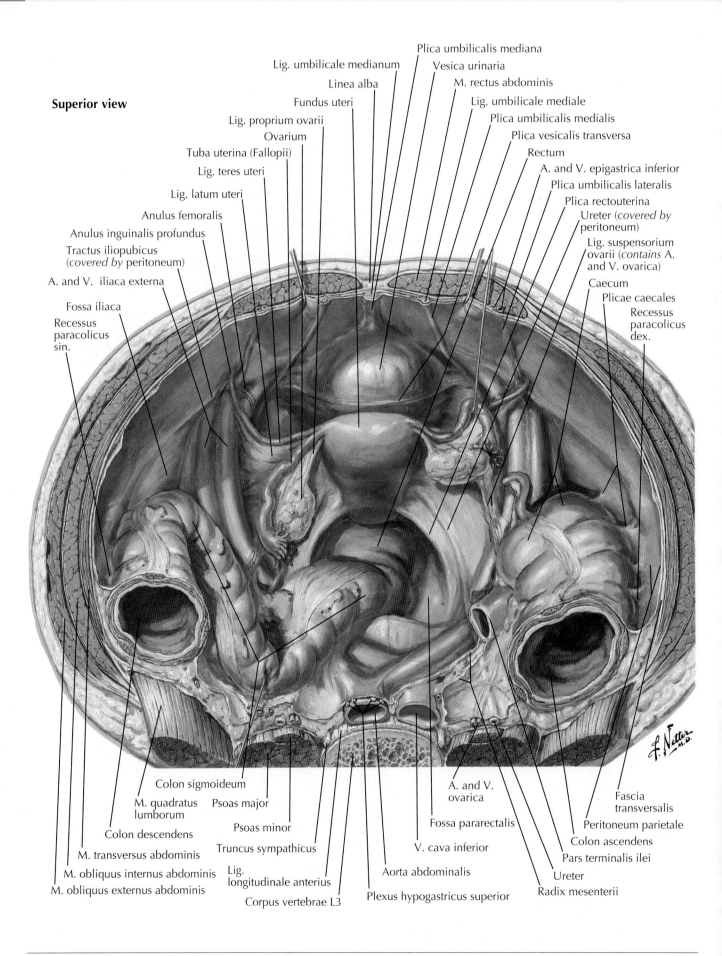

Colon sigmoideum
M. quadratus lumborum
Colon descendens
M. transversus abdominis
M. obliquus internus abdominis
M. obliquus externus abdominis

Psoas major
Psoas minor
Truncus sympathicus
Lig. longitudinale anterius
Corpus vertebrae L3

A. and V. ovarica
Fossa pararectalis
V. cava inferior
Aorta abdominalis
Plexus hypogastricus superior

Fascia transversalis
Peritoneum parietale
Colon ascendens
Pars terminalis ilei
Ureter
Radix mesenterii

Plate 363

Diaphragma Pelvis and Organa Visceralia Pelvis

Paramedian (sagittal) dissection

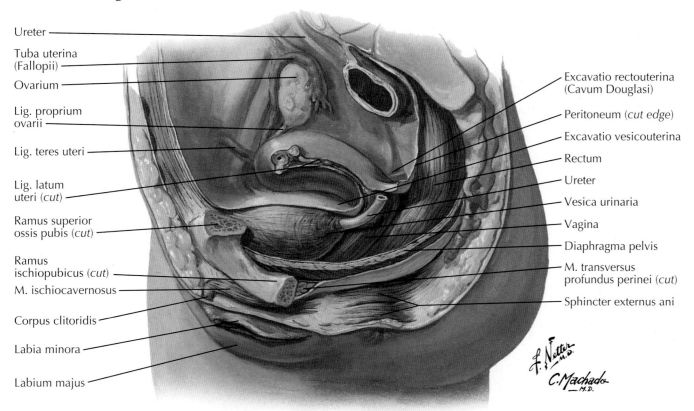

Ureter

Tuba uterina (Fallopii)

Ovarium

Lig. proprium ovarii

Lig. teres uteri

Lig. latum uteri (*cut*)

Ramus superior ossis pubis (*cut*)

Ramus ischiopubicus (*cut*)

M. ischiocavernosus

Corpus clitoridis

Labia minora

Labium majus

Excavatio rectouterina (Cavum Douglasi)

Peritoneum (*cut edge*)

Excavatio vesicouterina

Rectum

Ureter

Vesica urinaria

Vagina

Diaphragma pelvis

M. transversus profundus perinei (*cut*)

Sphincter externus ani

Median (sagittal) section

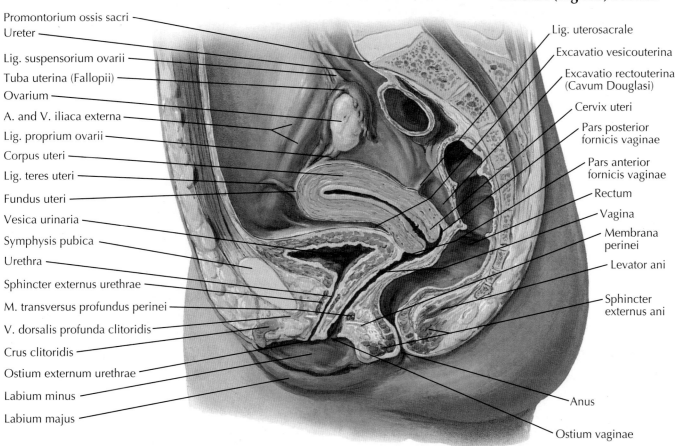

Promontorium ossis sacri

Ureter

Lig. suspensorium ovarii

Tuba uterina (Fallopii)

Ovarium

A. and V. iliaca externa

Lig. proprium ovarii

Corpus uteri

Lig. teres uteri

Fundus uteri

Vesica urinaria

Symphysis pubica

Urethra

Sphincter externus urethrae

M. transversus profundus perinei

V. dorsalis profunda clitoridis

Crus clitoridis

Ostium externum urethrae

Labium minus

Labium majus

Lig. uterosacrale

Excavatio vesicouterina

Excavatio rectouterina (Cavum Douglasi)

Cervix uteri

Pars posterior fornicis vaginae

Pars anterior fornicis vaginae

Rectum

Vagina

Membrana perinei

Levator ani

Sphincter externus ani

Anus

Ostium vaginae

Diaphragma Pelvis and Organa Visceralia Pelvis

Plate 364

Superior view with peritoneum intact

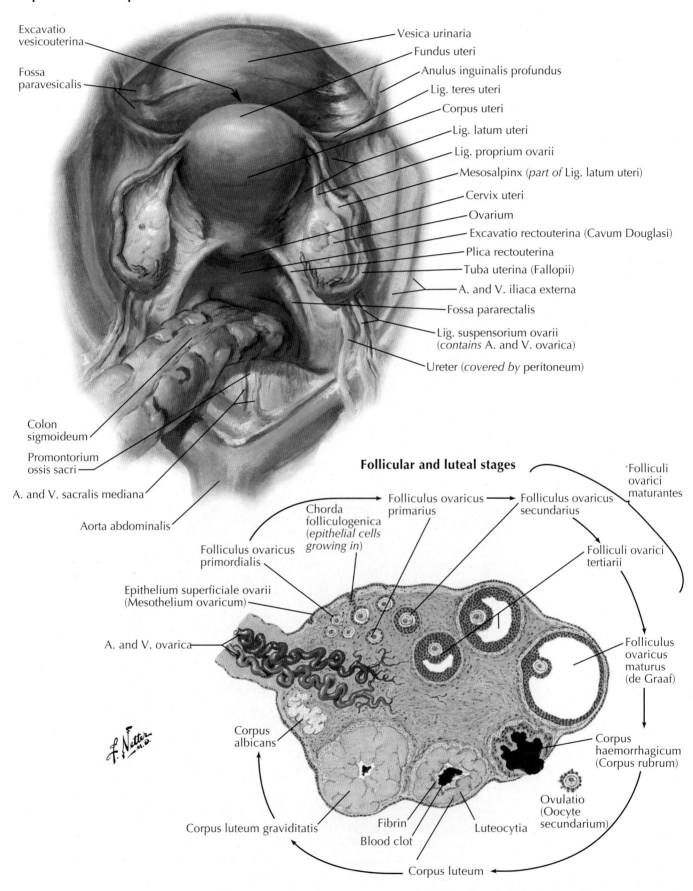

Excavatio vesicouterina

Fossa paravesicalis

Vesica urinaria

Fundus uteri

Anulus inguinalis profundus

Lig. teres uteri

Corpus uteri

Lig. latum uteri

Lig. proprium ovarii

Mesosalpinx (*part of* Lig. latum uteri)

Cervix uteri

Ovarium

Excavatio rectouterina (Cavum Douglasi)

Plica rectouterina

Tuba uterina (Fallopii)

A. and V. iliaca externa

Fossa pararectalis

Lig. suspensorium ovarii (*contains* A. and V. ovarica)

Ureter (*covered by* peritoneum)

Colon sigmoideum

Promontorium ossis sacri

A. and V. sacralis mediana

Aorta abdominalis

Follicular and luteal stages

Folliculi ovarici maturantes

Chorda folliculogenica (*epithelial cells growing in*)

Folliculus ovaricus primarius

Folliculus ovaricus secundarius

Folliculi ovarici tertiarii

Folliculus ovaricus primordialis

Epithelium superficiale ovarii (Mesothelium ovaricum)

A. and V. ovarica

Folliculus ovaricus maturus (de Graaf)

Corpus albicans

Corpus haemorrhagicum (Corpus rubrum)

Ovulatio (Oocyte secundarium)

Corpus luteum graviditatis

Fibrin

Blood clot

Luteocytia

Corpus luteum

Plate 365

Diaphragma Pelvis and Organa Visceralia Pelvis

Female: superior view (peritoneum and loose connective tissue removed)

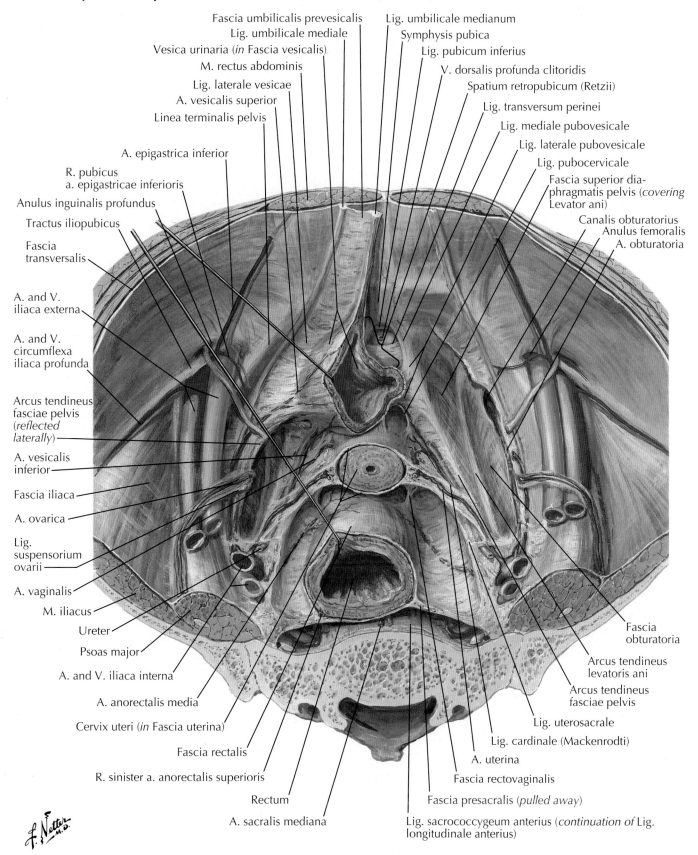

Fascia umbilicalis prevesicalis
Lig. umbilicale mediale
Vesica urinaria (*in Fascia vesicalis*)
M. rectus abdominis
Lig. laterale vesicae
A. vesicalis superior
Linea terminalis pelvis

Lig. umbilicale medianum
Symphysis pubica
Lig. pubicum inferius
V. dorsalis profunda clitoridis
Spatium retropubicum (Retzii)
Lig. transversum perinei
Lig. mediale pubovesicale
Lig. laterale pubovesicale
Lig. pubocervicale
Fascia superior dia-
phragmatis pelvis (*covering*
Levator ani)
Canalis obturatorius
Anulus femoralis
A. obturatoria

A. epigastrica inferior

R. pubicus
a. epigastricae inferioris
Anulus inguinalis profundus
Tractus iliopubicus
Fascia
transversalis

A. and V.
iliaca externa

A. and V.
circumflexa
iliaca profunda

Arcus tendineus
fasciae pelvis
(*reflected
laterally*)

A. vesicalis
inferior

Fascia iliaca

A. ovarica

Lig.
suspensorium
ovarii

A. vaginalis

M. iliacus

Ureter

Psoas major

A. and V. iliaca interna

A. anorectalis media

Cervix uteri (*in Fascia uterina*)

Fascia rectalis

R. sinister a. anorectalis superioris

Rectum

A. sacralis mediana

Fascia obturatoria

Arcus tendineus
levatoris ani

Arcus tendineus
fasciae pelvis

Lig. uterosacrale

Lig. cardinale (Mackenrodti)

A. uterina

Fascia rectovaginalis

Fascia presacralis (*pulled away*)

Lig. sacrococcygeum anterius (*continuation of* Lig.
longitudinale anterius)

Diaphragma Pelvis and Organa Visceralia Pelvis

Plate 366

Superior view

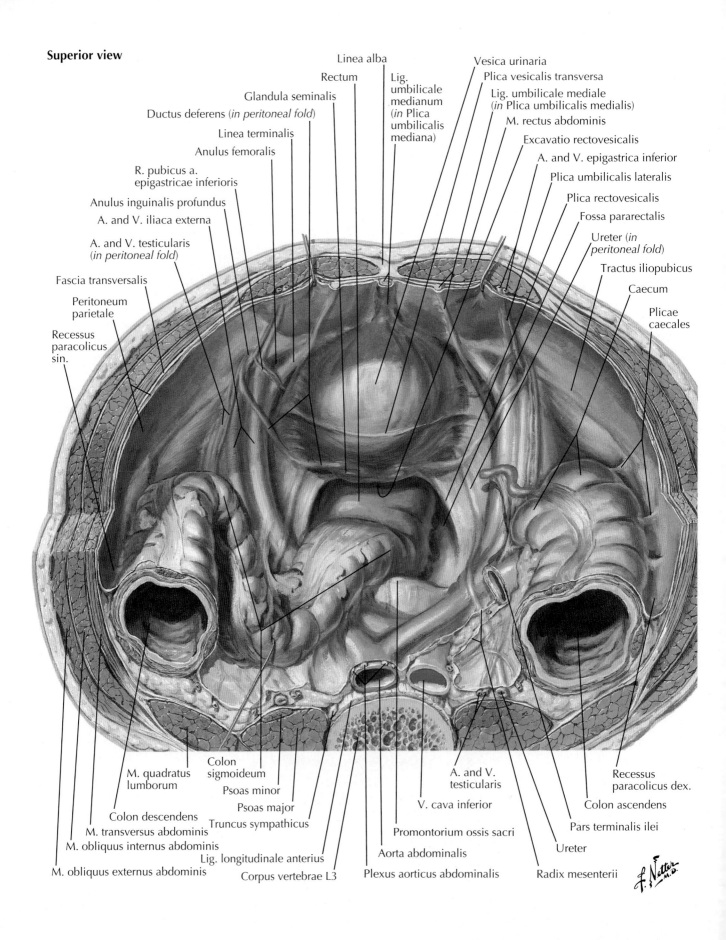

Linea alba

Rectum

Glandula seminalis

Ductus deferens (*in peritoneal fold*)

Linea terminalis

Anulus femoralis

R. pubicus a. epigastricae inferioris

Anulus inguinalis profundus

A. and V. iliaca externa

A. and V. testicularis (*in peritoneal fold*)

Fascia transversalis

Peritoneum parietale

Recessus paracolicus sin.

Lig. umbilicale medianum (*in* Plica umbilicalis mediana)

Vesica urinaria

Plica vesicalis transversa

Lig. umbilicale mediale (*in* Plica umbilicalis medialis)

M. rectus abdominis

Excavatio rectovesicalis

A. and V. epigastrica inferior

Plica umbilicalis lateralis

Plica rectovesicalis

Fossa pararectalis

Ureter (*in peritoneal fold*)

Tractus iliopubicus

Caecum

Plicae caecales

M. quadratus lumborum

Colon sigmoideum

Psoas minor

Colon descendens

Psoas major

M. transversus abdominis

Truncus sympathicus

M. obliquus internus abdominis

Lig. longitudinale anterius

M. obliquus externus abdominis

Corpus vertebrae L3

A. and V. testicularis

V. cava inferior

Promontorium ossis sacri

Aorta abdominalis

Plexus aorticus abdominalis

Recessus paracolicus dex.

Colon ascendens

Pars terminalis ilei

Ureter

Radix mesenterii

Plate 367

Diaphragma Pelvis and Organa Visceralia Pelvis

Parasagittal view

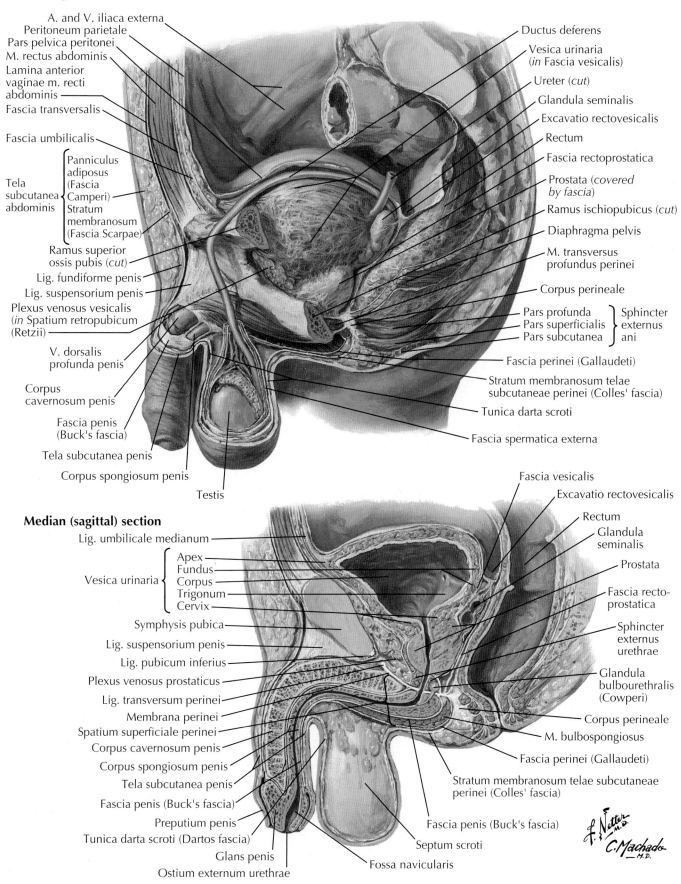

A. and V. iliaca externa
Peritoneum parietale
Pars pelvica peritonei
M. rectus abdominis
Lamina anterior vaginae m. recti abdominis
Fascia transversalis

Fascia umbilicalis

Tela subcutanea abdominis
{ Panniculus adiposus (Fascia Camperi)
Stratum membranosum (Fascia Scarpae) }

Ramus superior ossis pubis (cut)
Lig. fundiforme penis
Lig. suspensorium penis
Plexus venosus vesicalis (in Spatium retropubicum (Retzii)
V. dorsalis profunda penis

Corpus cavernosum penis

Fascia penis (Buck's fascia)

Tela subcutanea penis

Corpus spongiosum penis

Testis

Ductus deferens
Vesica urinaria (in Fascia vesicalis)
Ureter (cut)
Glandula seminalis
Excavatio rectovesicalis
Rectum
Fascia rectoprostatica
Prostata (covered by fascia)
Ramus ischiopubicus (cut)
Diaphragma pelvis
M. transversus profundus perinei
Corpus perineale
Pars profunda
Pars superficialis } Sphincter externus ani
Pars subcutanea
Fascia perinei (Gallaudeti)
Stratum membranosum telae subcutaneae perinei (Colles' fascia)
Tunica darta scroti
Fascia spermatica externa

Median (sagittal) section

Lig. umbilicale medianum

Vesica urinaria {
Apex
Fundus
Corpus
Trigonum
Cervix
}

Symphysis pubica
Lig. suspensorium penis
Lig. pubicum inferius
Plexus venosus prostaticus
Lig. transversum perinei
Membrana perinei
Spatium superficiale perinei
Corpus cavernosum penis
Corpus spongiosum penis
Tela subcutanea penis
Fascia penis (Buck's fascia)
Preputium penis
Tunica darta scroti (Dartos fascia)
Glans penis
Ostium externum urethrae

Fascia vesicalis
Excavatio rectovesicalis
Rectum
Glandula seminalis
Prostata
Fascia recto-prostatica
Sphincter externus urethrae
Glandula bulbourethralis (Cowperi)
Corpus perineale
M. bulbospongiosus
Fascia perinei (Gallaudeti)
Stratum membranosum telae subcutaneae perinei (Colles' fascia)
Fascia penis (Buck's fascia)
Septum scroti
Fossa navicularis

F. Netter M.D.
C. Machado M.D.

Diaphragma Pelvis and Organa Visceralia Pelvis

Plate 368

Female: median section

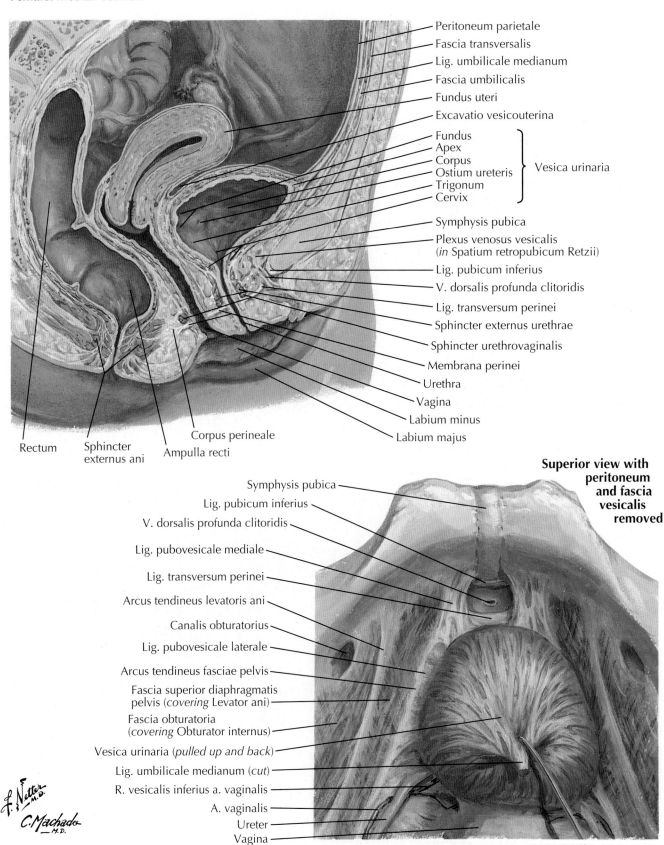

Peritoneum parietale
Fascia transversalis
Lig. umbilicale medianum
Fascia umbilicalis
Fundus uteri
Excavatio vesicouterina

Fundus
Apex
Corpus
Ostium ureteris
Trigonum
Cervix
} Vesica urinaria

Symphysis pubica
Plexus venosus vesicalis
(*in* Spatium retropubicum Retzii)
Lig. pubicum inferius
V. dorsalis profunda clitoridis
Lig. transversum perinei
Sphincter externus urethrae
Sphincter urethrovaginalis
Membrana perinei
Urethra
Vagina
Labium minus
Labium majus

Rectum
Sphincter externus ani
Ampulla recti
Corpus perineale

Superior view with peritoneum and fascia vesicalis removed

Symphysis pubica
Lig. pubicum inferius
V. dorsalis profunda clitoridis
Lig. pubovesicale mediale
Lig. transversum perinei
Arcus tendineus levatoris ani
Canalis obturatorius
Lig. pubovesicale laterale
Arcus tendineus fasciae pelvis
Fascia superior diaphragmatis pelvis (*covering* Levator ani)
Fascia obturatoria (*covering* Obturator internus)
Vesica urinaria (*pulled up and back*)
Lig. umbilicale medianum (*cut*)
R. vesicalis inferius a. vaginalis
A. vaginalis
Ureter
Vagina

Plate 369

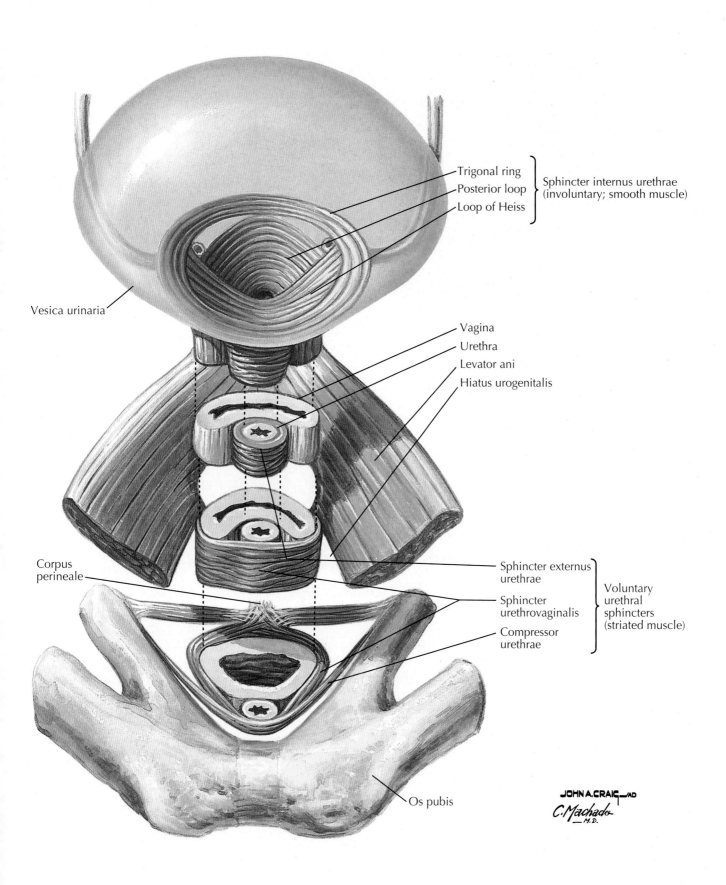

Trigonal ring
Posterior loop
Loop of Heiss
} Sphincter internus urethrae
(involuntary; smooth muscle)

Vesica urinaria

Vagina
Urethra
Levator ani
Hiatus urogenitalis

Corpus
perineale

Sphincter externus
urethrae
}
Sphincter
urethrovaginalis
Voluntary
urethral
sphincters
(striated muscle)
Compressor
urethrae

Os pubis

JOHN A. CRAIG—AD
C. Machado
—M.D.

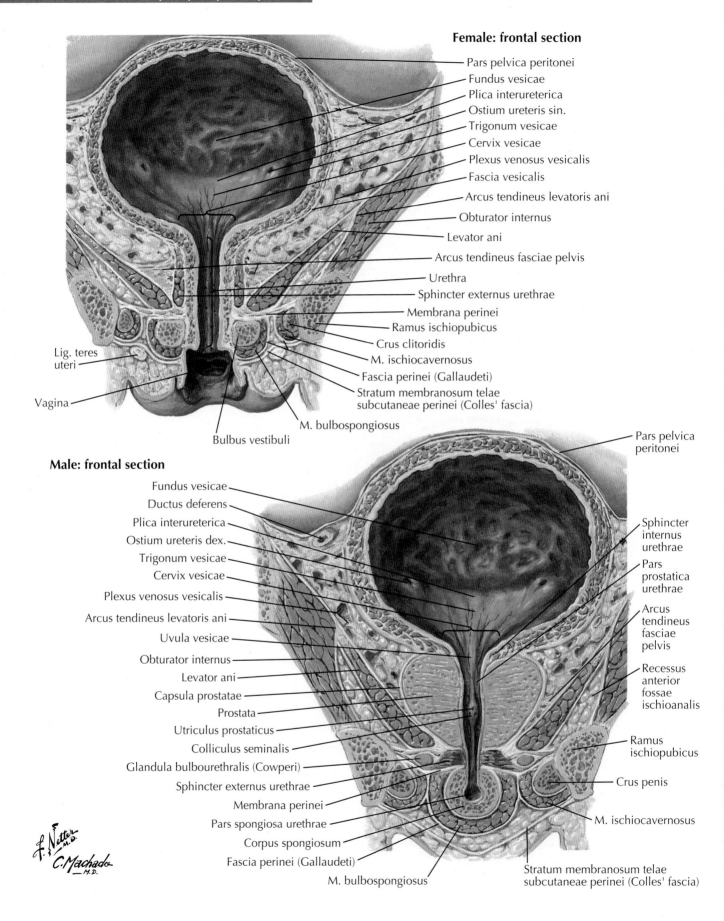

Female: frontal section

- Pars pelvica peritonei
- Fundus vesicae
- Plica interureterica
- Ostium ureteris sin.
- Trigonum vesicae
- Cervix vesicae
- Plexus venosus vesicalis
- Fascia vesicalis
- Arcus tendineus levatoris ani
- Obturator internus
- Levator ani
- Arcus tendineus fasciae pelvis
- Urethra
- Sphincter externus urethrae
- Membrana perinei
- Ramus ischiopubicus
- Crus clitoridis
- M. ischiocavernosus
- Fascia perinei (Gallaudeti)
- Stratum membranosum telae subcutaneae perinei (Colles' fascia)

- Lig. teres uteri
- Vagina
- Bulbus vestibuli
- M. bulbospongiosus

Male: frontal section

- Fundus vesicae
- Ductus deferens
- Plica interureterica
- Ostium ureteris dex.
- Trigonum vesicae
- Cervix vesicae
- Plexus venosus vesicalis
- Arcus tendineus levatoris ani
- Uvula vesicae
- Obturator internus
- Levator ani
- Capsula prostatae
- Prostata
- Utriculus prostaticus
- Colliculus seminalis
- Glandula bulbourethralis (Cowperi)
- Sphincter externus urethrae
- Membrana perinei
- Pars spongiosa urethrae
- Corpus spongiosum
- Fascia perinei (Gallaudeti)
- M. bulbospongiosus

- Pars pelvica peritonei
- Sphincter internus urethrae
- Pars prostatica urethrae
- Arcus tendineus fasciae pelvis
- Recessus anterior fossae ischioanalis
- Ramus ischiopubicus
- Crus penis
- M. ischiocavernosus
- Stratum membranosum telae subcutaneae perinei (Colles' fascia)

Plate 371

Vesica Urinaria

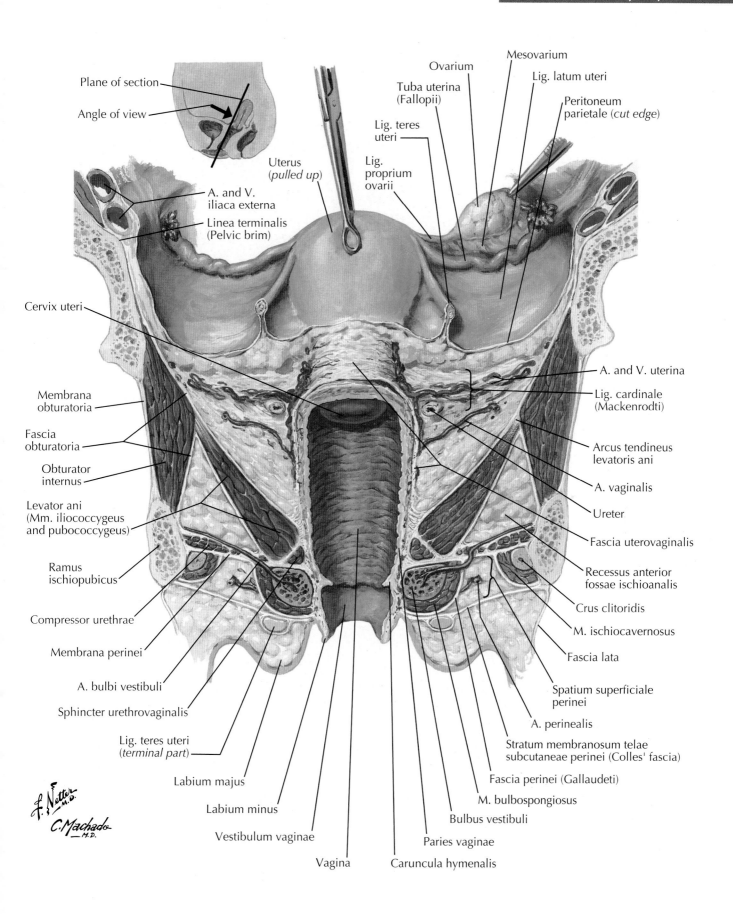

Plane of section

Angle of view

Uterus (*pulled up*)

A. and V. iliaca externa

Linea terminalis (Pelvic brim)

Ovarium

Mesovarium

Lig. latum uteri

Tuba uterina (Fallopii)

Peritoneum parietale (*cut edge*)

Lig. teres uteri

Lig. proprium ovarii

Cervix uteri

Membrana obturatoria

Fascia obturatoria

Obturator internus

Levator ani (Mm. iliococcygeus and pubococcygeus)

Ramus ischiopubicus

Compressor urethrae

Membrana perinei

A. bulbi vestibuli

Sphincter urethrovaginalis

Lig. teres uteri (*terminal part*)

Labium majus

Labium minus

Vestibulum vaginae

Vagina

A. and V. uterina

Lig. cardinale (Mackenrodti)

Arcus tendineus levatoris ani

A. vaginalis

Ureter

Fascia uterovaginalis

Recessus anterior fossae ischioanalis

Crus clitoridis

M. ischiocavernosus

Fascia lata

Spatium superficiale perinei

A. perinealis

Stratum membranosum telae subcutaneae perinei (Colles' fascia)

Fascia perinei (Gallaudeti)

M. bulbospongiosus

Bulbus vestibuli

Paries vaginae

Caruncula hymenalis

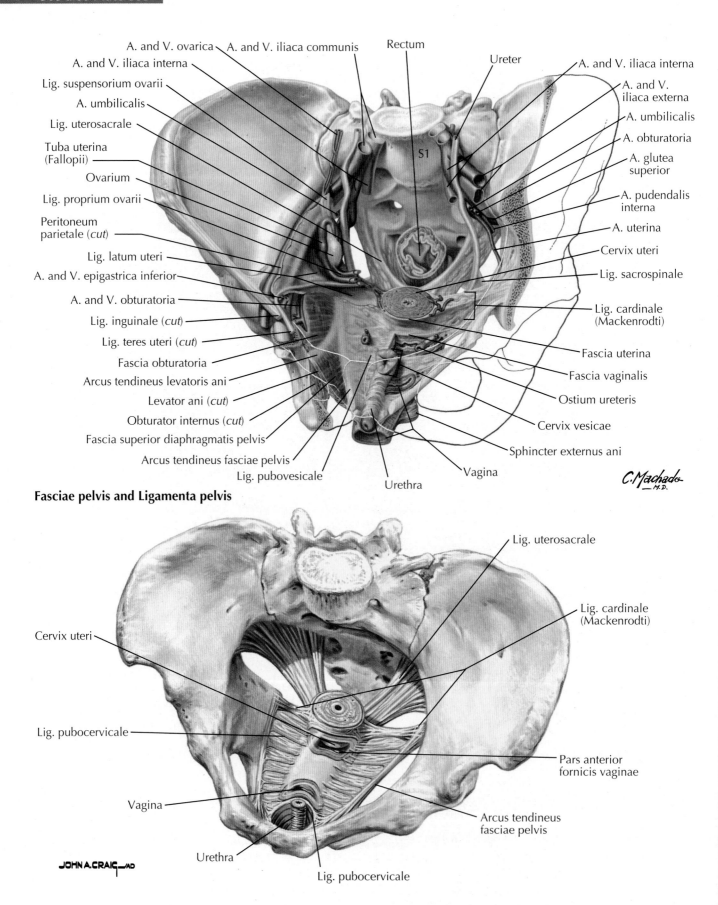

A. and V. ovarica

A. and V. iliaca communis

Rectum

Ureter

A. and V. iliaca interna

A. and V. iliaca interna

Lig. suspensorium ovarii

A. and V. iliaca externa

A. umbilicalis

A. umbilicalis

Lig. uterosacrale

A. obturatoria

Tuba uterina (Fallopii)

A. glutea superior

Ovarium

A. pudendalis interna

Lig. proprium ovarii

A. uterina

Peritoneum parietale (*cut*)

Cervix uteri

Lig. latum uteri

Lig. sacrospinale

A. and V. epigastrica inferior

Lig. cardinale (Mackenrodti)

A. and V. obturatoria

Fascia uterina

Lig. inguinale (*cut*)

Fascia vaginalis

Lig. teres uteri (*cut*)

Ostium ureteris

Fascia obturatoria

Cervix vesicae

Arcus tendineus levatoris ani

Sphincter externus ani

Levator ani (*cut*)

Obturator internus (*cut*)

Fascia superior diaphragmatis pelvis

Vagina

Arcus tendineus fasciae pelvis

Lig. pubovesicale

Urethra

S1

Fasciae pelvis and Ligamenta pelvis

Lig. uterosacrale

Lig. cardinale (Mackenrodti)

Cervix uteri

Lig. pubocervicale

Pars anterior fornicis vaginae

Vagina

Arcus tendineus fasciae pelvis

Urethra

Lig. pubocervicale

Plate 373

Organa Genitalia Feminina Interna

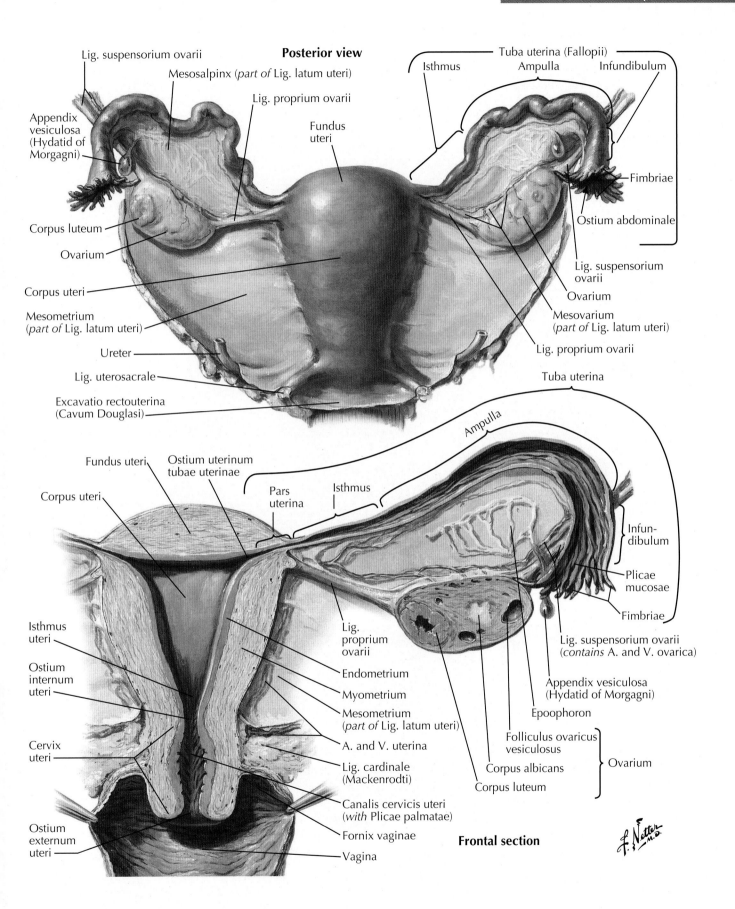

Posterior view

Lig. suspensorium ovarii

Mesosalpinx (*part of* Lig. latum uteri)

Lig. proprium ovarii

Fundus uteri

Appendix vesiculosa (Hydatid of Morgagni)

Corpus luteum

Ovarium

Corpus uteri

Mesometrium (*part of* Lig. latum uteri)

Ureter

Lig. uterosacrale

Excavatio rectouterina (Cavum Douglasi)

Tuba uterina (Fallopii)

Isthmus

Ampulla

Infundibulum

Fimbriae

Ostium abdominale

Lig. suspensorium ovarii

Ovarium

Mesovarium (*part of* Lig. latum uteri)

Lig. proprium ovarii

Tuba uterina

Ampulla

Fundus uteri

Corpus uteri

Ostium uterinum tubae uterinae

Pars uterina

Isthmus

Infundibulum

Plicae mucosae

Fimbriae

Lig. suspensorium ovarii (*contains* A. and V. ovarica)

Lig. proprium ovarii

Endometrium

Myometrium

Mesometrium (*part of* Lig. latum uteri)

A. and V. uterina

Lig. cardinale (Mackenrodti)

Canalis cervicis uteri (*with* Plicae palmatae)

Fornix vaginae

Vagina

Isthmus uteri

Ostium internum uteri

Cervix uteri

Ostium externum uteri

Appendix vesiculosa (Hydatid of Morgagni)

Epoophoron

Folliculus ovaricus vesiculosus

Corpus albicans

Corpus luteum

Ovarium

Frontal section

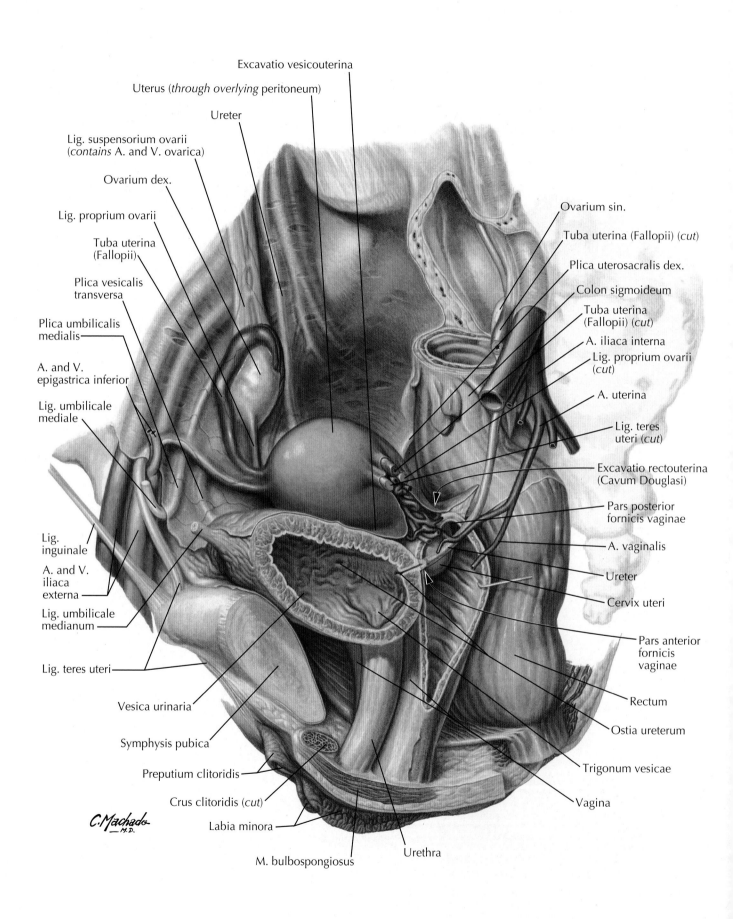

Excavatio vesicouterina

Uterus (*through overlying* peritoneum)

Ureter

Lig. suspensorium ovarii (*contains* A. and V. ovarica)

Ovarium dex.

Lig. proprium ovarii

Tuba uterina (Fallopii)

Plica vesicalis transversa

Plica umbilicalis medialis

A. and V. epigastrica inferior

Lig. umbilicale mediale

Lig. inguinale

A. and V. iliaca externa

Lig. umbilicale medianum

Lig. teres uteri

Vesica urinaria

Symphysis pubica

Preputium clitoridis

Crus clitoridis (*cut*)

Labia minora

M. bulbospongiosus

Urethra

Ovarium sin.

Tuba uterina (Fallopii) (*cut*)

Plica uterosacralis dex.

Colon sigmoideum

Tuba uterina (Fallopii) (*cut*)

A. iliaca interna

Lig. proprium ovarii (*cut*)

A. uterina

Lig. teres uteri (*cut*)

Excavatio rectouterina (Cavum Douglasi)

Pars posterior fornicis vaginae

A. vaginalis

Ureter

Cervix uteri

Pars anterior fornicis vaginae

Rectum

Ostia ureterum

Trigonum vesicae

Vagina

Plate 375

Anterior   Posterior

Lig. suspensorium ovarii
(*containing* A. and V. ovarica)

**Subdivisions and
contents of
Lig. latum uteri**

Infundibulum tubae uterinae

A. and V. iliaca externa

Fimbriae tubae uterinae

Ampulla tubae uterinae

Lig. teres uteri

Ovarium

Ureter

Laminae mesosalpingis

Lig. umbilicale mediale

Laminae mesovarii

R. ovaricus a. uterinae

Lamina posterior lig. lati uteri

Lig. teres uteri

Lamina anterior lig. lati uteri

Plica vesicalis transversa

Plexus venosus uterinus

Excavatio vesicouterina

A. uterina

C. Machado
_M.D._

A. vaginalis

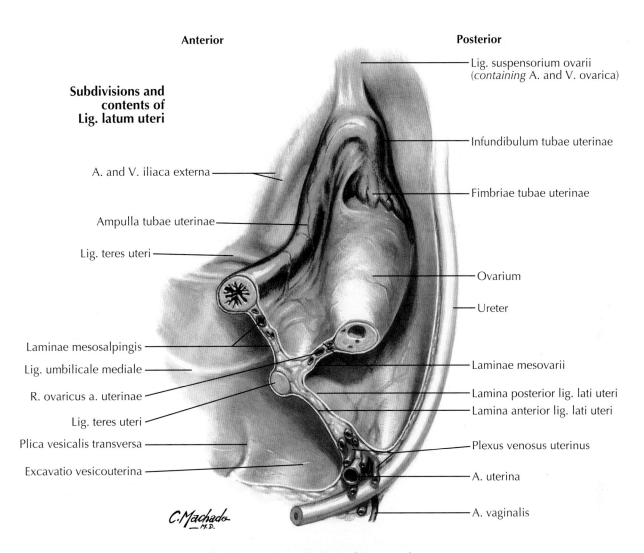

Anteroposterior fluoroscopic image obtained during hysterosalpingography

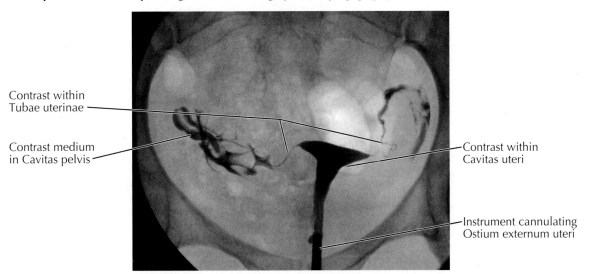

Contrast within
Tubae uterinae

Contrast within
Cavitas uteri

Contrast medium
in Cavitas pelvis

Instrument cannulating
Ostium externum uteri

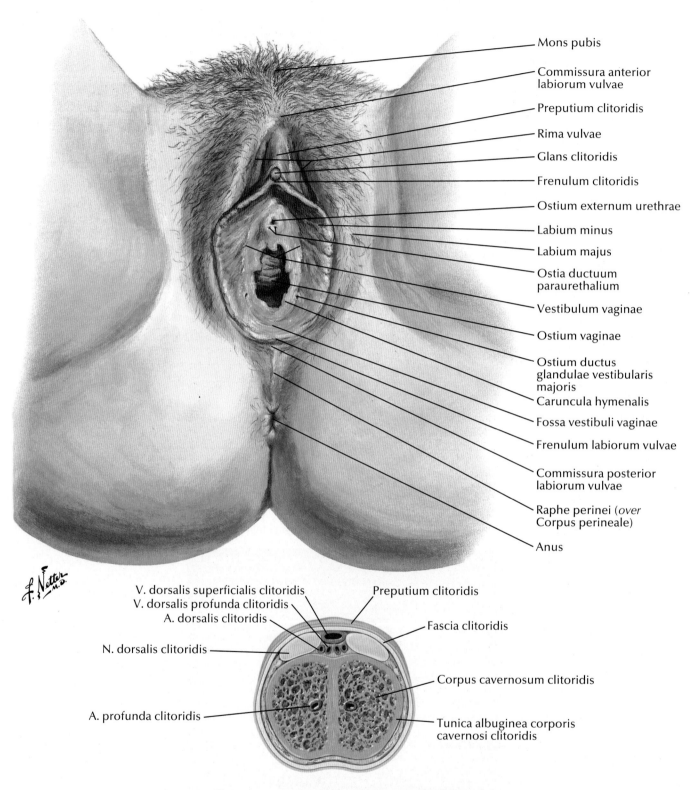

Mons pubis

Commissura anterior labiorum vulvae

Preputium clitoridis

Rima vulvae

Glans clitoridis

Frenulum clitoridis

Ostium externum urethrae

Labium minus

Labium majus

Ostia ductuum paraurethalium

Vestibulum vaginae

Ostium vaginae

Ostium ductus glandulae vestibularis majoris

Caruncula hymenalis

Fossa vestibuli vaginae

Frenulum labiorum vulvae

Commissura posterior labiorum vulvae

Raphe perinei (*over* Corpus perineale)

Anus

V. dorsalis superficialis clitoridis
V. dorsalis profunda clitoridis
A. dorsalis clitoridis

Preputium clitoridis

N. dorsalis clitoridis

Fascia clitoridis

Corpus cavernosum clitoridis

A. profunda clitoridis

Tunica albuginea corporis cavernosi clitoridis

Transverse section through corpus clitoridis

Plate 377

Perineum Femininum and Organa Genitalia Feminina Externa

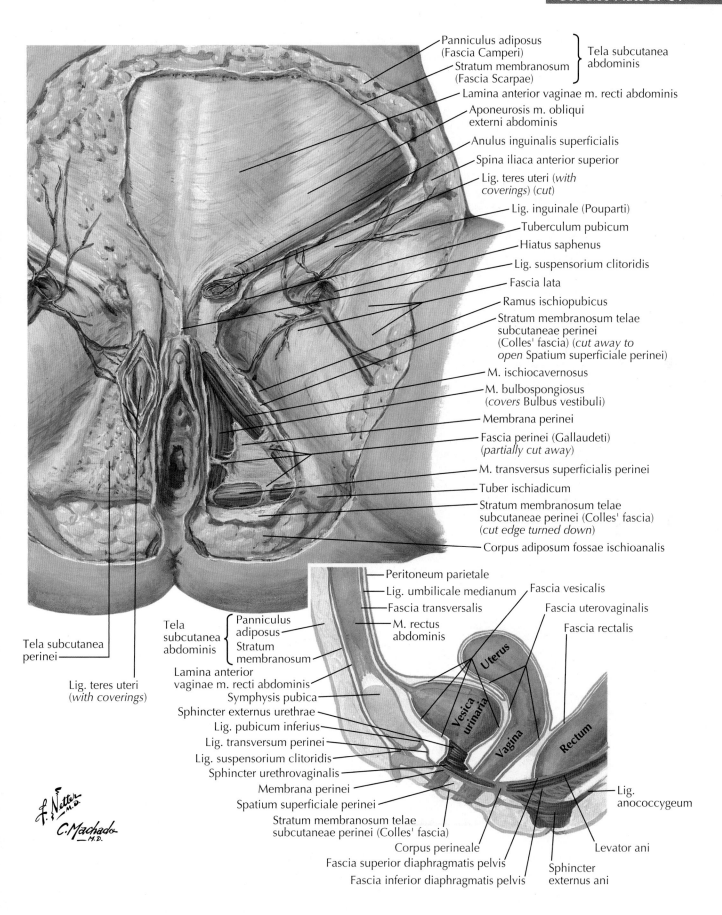

Panniculus adiposus
(Fascia Camperi)

Stratum membranosum
(Fascia Scarpae)

Tela subcutanea
abdominis

Lamina anterior vaginae m. recti abdominis

Aponeurosis m. obliqui
externi abdominis

Anulus inguinalis superficialis

Spina iliaca anterior superior

Lig. teres uteri (with
coverings) (cut)

Lig. inguinale (Pouparti)

Tuberculum pubicum

Hiatus saphenus

Lig. suspensorium clitoridis

Fascia lata

Ramus ischiopubicus

Stratum membranosum telae
subcutaneae perinei
(Colles' fascia) (cut away to
open Spatium superficiale perinei)

M. ischiocavernosus

M. bulbospongiosus
(covers Bulbus vestibuli)

Membrana perinei

Fascia perinei (Gallaudeti)
(partially cut away)

M. transversus superficialis perinei

Tuber ischiadicum

Stratum membranosum telae
subcutaneae perinei (Colles' fascia)
(cut edge turned down)

Corpus adiposum fossae ischioanalis

Tela subcutanea
perinei

Lig. teres uteri
(with coverings)

Tela
subcutanea
abdominis

Panniculus
adiposus

Stratum
membranosum

Lamina anterior
vaginae m. recti abdominis

Symphysis pubica

Sphincter externus urethrae

Lig. pubicum inferius

Lig. transversum perinei

Lig. suspensorium clitoridis

Sphincter urethrovaginalis

Membrana perinei

Spatium superficiale perinei

Stratum membranosum telae
subcutaneae perinei (Colles' fascia)

Corpus perineale

Fascia superior diaphragmatis pelvis

Fascia inferior diaphragmatis pelvis

Peritoneum parietale

Lig. umbilicale medianum

Fascia transversalis

M. rectus
abdominis

Fascia vesicalis

Fascia uterovaginalis

Fascia rectalis

Uterus

Vesica
urinaria

Vagina

Rectum

Lig.
anococcygeum

Levator ani

Sphincter
externus ani

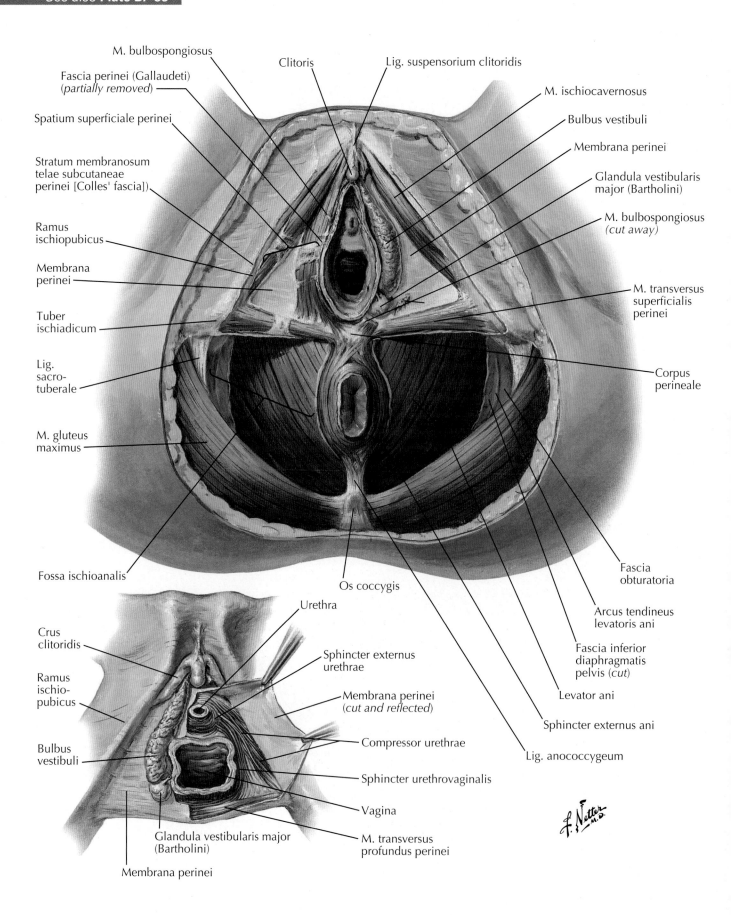

M. bulbospongiosus

Fascia perinei (Gallaudeti) (*partially removed*)

Spatium superficiale perinei

Stratum membranosum telae subcutaneae perinei [Colles' fascia]

Ramus ischiopubicus

Membrana perinei

Tuber ischiadicum

Lig. sacro- tuberale

M. gluteus maximus

Fossa ischioanalis

Clitoris

Lig. suspensorium clitoridis

M. ischiocavernosus

Bulbus vestibuli

Membrana perinei

Glandula vestibularis major (Bartholini)

M. bulbospongiosus (*cut away*)

M. transversus superficialis perinei

Corpus perineale

Fascia obturatoria

Arcus tendineus levatoris ani

Fascia inferior diaphragmatis pelvis (*cut*)

Levator ani

Sphincter externus ani

Lig. anococcygeum

Os coccygis

Urethra

Crus clitoridis

Ramus ischio- pubicus

Bulbus vestibuli

Sphincter externus urethrae

Membrana perinei (*cut and reflected*)

Compressor urethrae

Sphincter urethrovaginalis

Vagina

M. transversus profundus perinei

Glandula vestibularis major (Bartholini)

Membrana perinei

Plate 379

Perineum Femininum and Organa Genitalia Feminina Externa

Spatium superficiale perinei

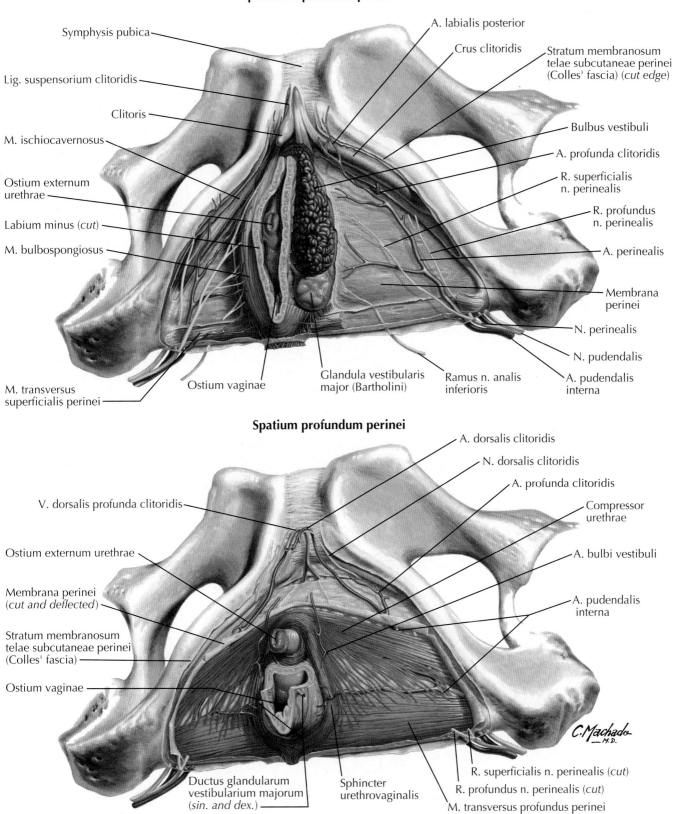

Symphysis pubica

A. labialis posterior

Crus clitoridis

Stratum membranosum telae subcutaneae perinei (Colles' fascia) (cut edge)

Lig. suspensorium clitoridis

Clitoris

Bulbus vestibuli

M. ischiocavernosus

A. profunda clitoridis

R. superficialis n. perinealis

Ostium externum urethrae

R. profundus n. perinealis

Labium minus (cut)

A. perinealis

M. bulbospongiosus

Membrana perinei

N. perinealis

N. pudendalis

M. transversus superficialis perinei

Ostium vaginae

Glandula vestibularis major (Bartholini)

Ramus n. analis inferioris

A. pudendalis interna

Spatium profundum perinei

A. dorsalis clitoridis

N. dorsalis clitoridis

A. profunda clitoridis

V. dorsalis profunda clitoridis

Compressor urethrae

Ostium externum urethrae

A. bulbi vestibuli

Membrana perinei (cut and deflected)

A. pudendalis interna

Stratum membranosum telae subcutaneae perinei (Colles' fascia)

Ostium vaginae

Ductus glandularum vestibularium majorum (sin. and dex.)

Sphincter urethrovaginalis

R. superficialis n. perinealis (cut)

R. profundus n. perinealis (cut)

M. transversus profundus perinei

C. Machado
_M.D._

Perineum Femininum and Organa Genitalia Feminina Externa

Plate 380

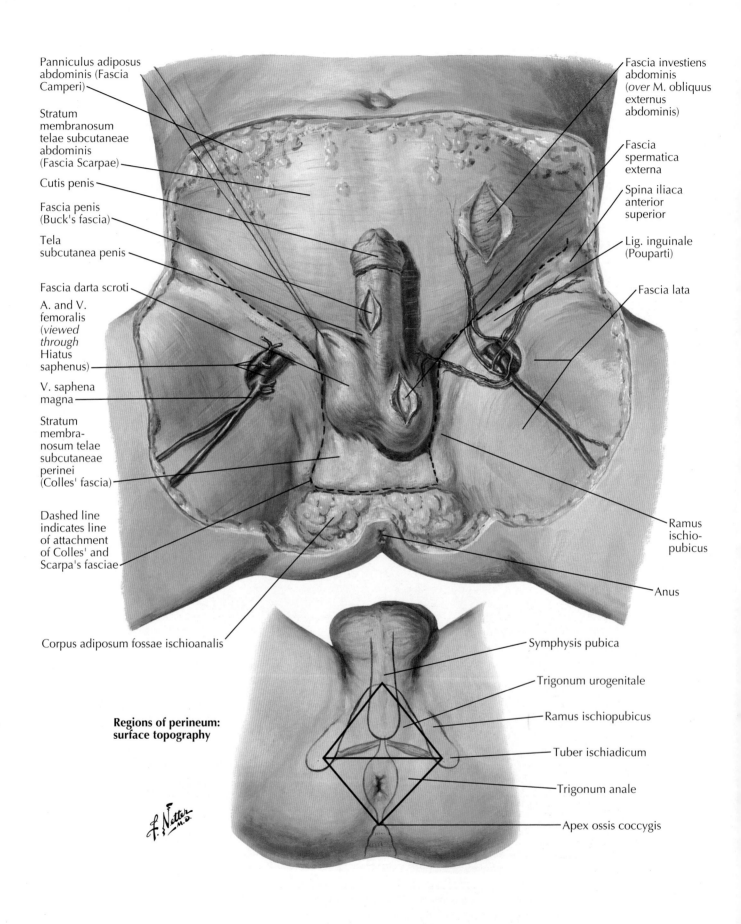

Panniculus adiposus abdominis (Fascia Camperi)

Stratum membranosum telae subcutaneae abdominis (Fascia Scarpae)

Cutis penis

Fascia penis (Buck's fascia)

Tela subcutanea penis

Fascia darta scroti

A. and V. femoralis (viewed through Hiatus saphenus)

V. saphena magna

Stratum membranosum telae subcutaneae perinei (Colles' fascia)

Dashed line indicates line of attachment of Colles' and Scarpa's fasciae

Corpus adiposum fossae ischioanalis

Fascia investiens abdominis (over M. obliquus externus abdominis)

Fascia spermatica externa

Spina iliaca anterior superior

Lig. inguinale (Pouparti)

Fascia lata

Ramus ischiopubicus

Anus

Regions of perineum: surface topography

Symphysis pubica

Trigonum urogenitale

Ramus ischiopubicus

Tuber ischiadicum

Trigonum anale

Apex ossis coccygis

Plate 381

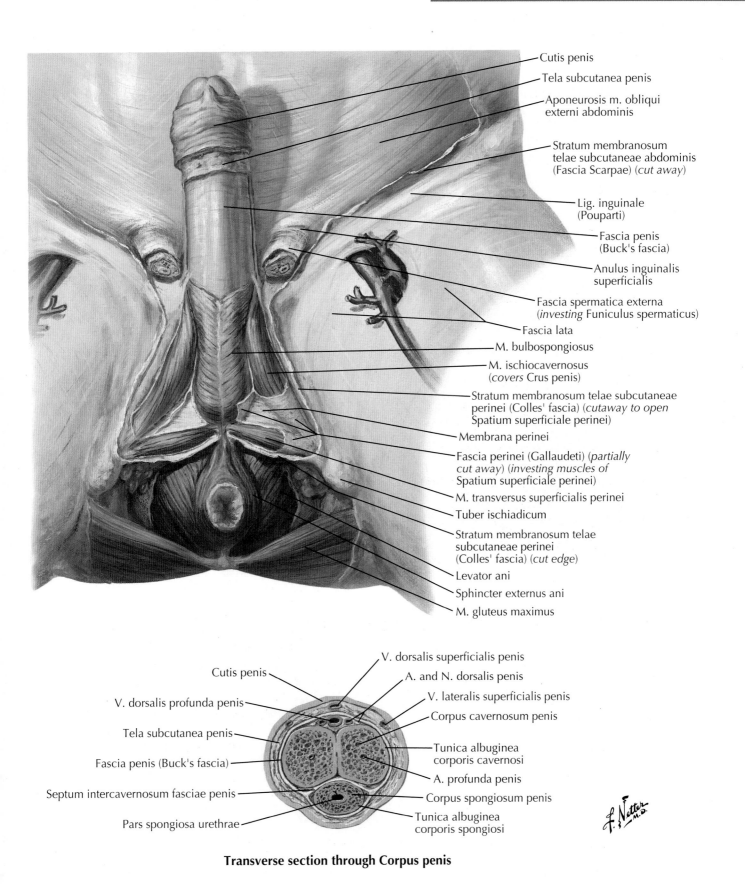

Cutis penis

Tela subcutanea penis

Aponeurosis m. obliqui externi abdominis

Stratum membranosum telae subcutaneae abdominis (Fascia Scarpae) (*cut away*)

Lig. inguinale (Pouparti)

Fascia penis (Buck's fascia)

Anulus inguinalis superficialis

Fascia spermatica externa (*investing* Funiculus spermaticus)

Fascia lata

M. bulbospongiosus

M. ischiocavernosus (*covers* Crus penis)

Stratum membranosum telae subcutaneae perinei (Colles' fascia) (*cutaway to open* Spatium superficiale perinei)

Membrana perinei

Fascia perinei (Gallaudeti) (*partially cut away*) (*investing muscles of* Spatium superficiale perinei)

M. transversus superficialis perinei

Tuber ischiadicum

Stratum membranosum telae subcutaneae perinei (Colles' fascia) (*cut edge*)

Levator ani

Sphincter externus ani

M. gluteus maximus

V. dorsalis superficialis penis

A. and N. dorsalis penis

V. lateralis superficialis penis

Corpus cavernosum penis

Tunica albuginea corporis cavernosi

A. profunda penis

Corpus spongiosum penis

Tunica albuginea corporis spongiosi

Cutis penis

V. dorsalis profunda penis

Tela subcutanea penis

Fascia penis (Buck's fascia)

Septum intercavernosum fasciae penis

Pars spongiosa urethrae

Transverse section through Corpus penis

f. Netter.
M.D.

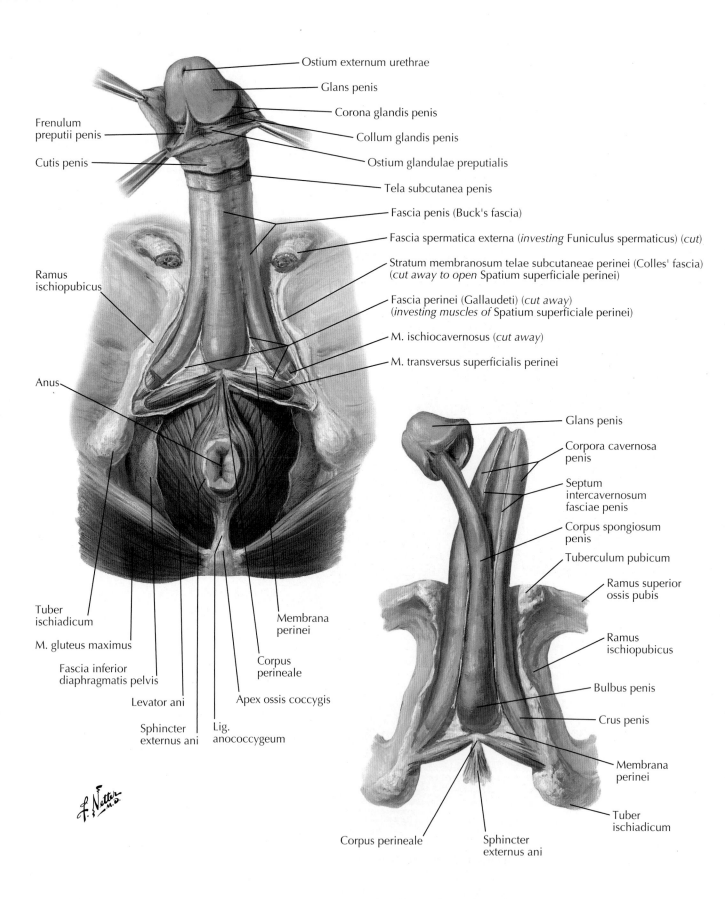

Ostium externum urethrae

Glans penis

Corona glandis penis

Collum glandis penis

Ostium glandulae preputialis

Frenulum preputii penis

Cutis penis

Tela subcutanea penis

Fascia penis (Buck's fascia)

Fascia spermatica externa (*investing* Funiculus spermaticus) (*cut*)

Stratum membranosum telae subcutaneae perinei (Colles' fascia) (*cut away to open* Spatium superficiale perinei)

Fascia perinei (Gallaudeti) (*cut away*) (*investing muscles of* Spatium superficiale perinei)

Ramus ischiopubicus

M. ischiocavernosus (*cut away*)

M. transversus superficialis perinei

Anus

Tuber ischiadicum

M. gluteus maximus

Fascia inferior diaphragmatis pelvis

Levator ani

Sphincter externus ani

Lig. anococcygeum

Apex ossis coccygis

Corpus perineale

Membrana perinei

Glans penis

Corpora cavernosa penis

Septum intercavernosum fasciae penis

Corpus spongiosum penis

Tuberculum pubicum

Ramus superior ossis pubis

Ramus ischiopubicus

Bulbus penis

Crus penis

Membrana perinei

Tuber ischiadicum

Corpus perineale

Sphincter externus ani

Plate 383

Perineum Masculinum and Organa Genitalia Masculina Externa

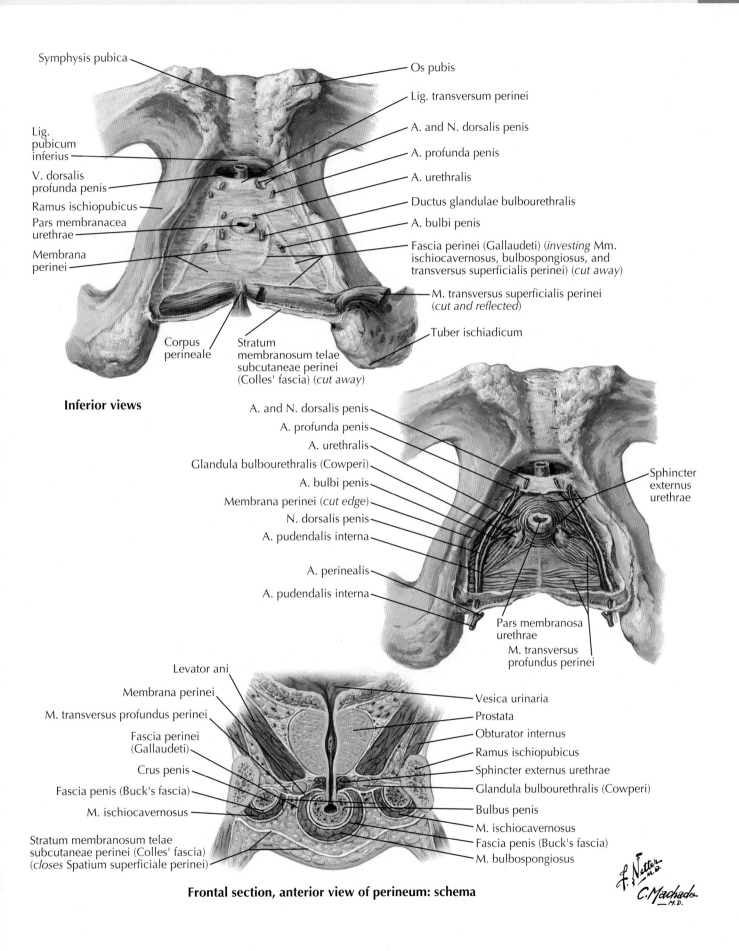

Symphysis pubica

Os pubis

Lig. transversum perinei

A. and N. dorsalis penis

A. profunda penis

A. urethralis

Lig. pubicum inferius

V. dorsalis profunda penis

Ductus glandulae bulbourethralis

Ramus ischiopubicus

A. bulbi penis

Pars membranacea urethrae

Fascia perinei (Gallaudeti) (*investing* Mm. ischiocavernosus, bulbospongiosus, and transversus superficialis perinei) (*cut away*)

Membrana perinei

M. transversus superficialis perinei (*cut and reflected*)

Corpus perineale

Stratum membranosum telae subcutaneae perinei (Colles' fascia) (*cut away*)

Tuber ischiadicum

Inferior views

A. and N. dorsalis penis

A. profunda penis

A. urethralis

Glandula bulbourethralis (Cowperi)

A. bulbi penis

Membrana perinei (*cut edge*)

N. dorsalis penis

A. pudendalis interna

Sphincter externus urethrae

A. perinealis

A. pudendalis interna

Pars membranosa urethrae

M. transversus profundus perinei

Levator ani

Membrana perinei

M. transversus profundus perinei

Fascia perinei (Gallaudeti)

Crus penis

Fascia penis (Buck's fascia)

M. ischiocavernosus

Stratum membranosum telae subcutaneae perinei (Colles' fascia) (*closes* Spatium superficiale perinei)

Vesica urinaria

Prostata

Obturator internus

Ramus ischiopubicus

Sphincter externus urethrae

Glandula bulbourethralis (Cowperi)

Bulbus penis

M. ischiocavernosus

Fascia penis (Buck's fascia)

M. bulbospongiosus

Frontal section, anterior view of perineum: schema

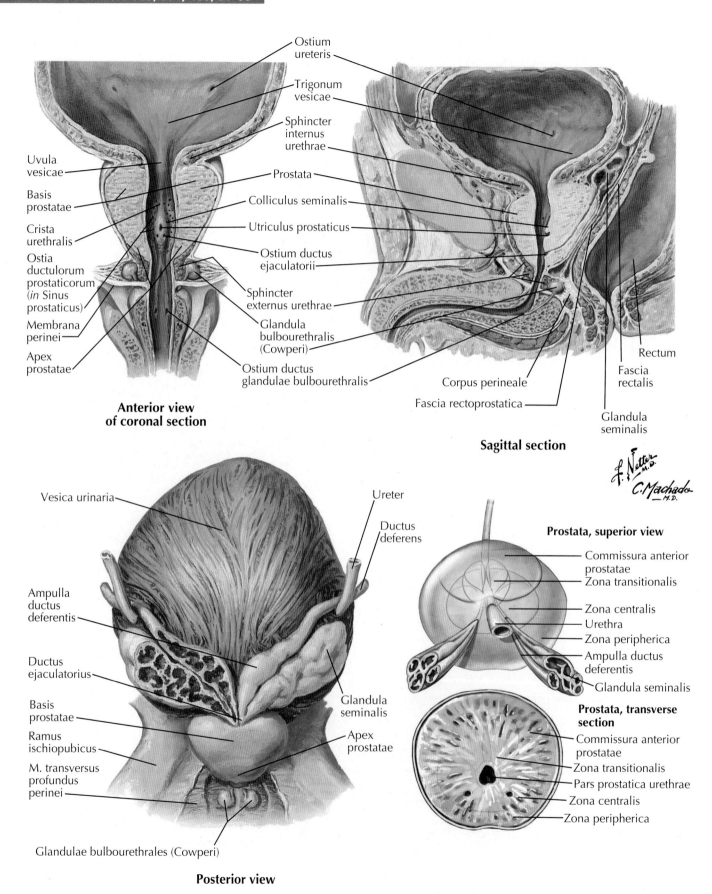

Ostium ureteris

Trigonum vesicae

Sphincter internus urethrae

Uvula vesicae

Basis prostatae

Crista urethralis

Ostia ductulorum prostaticorum (*in Sinus prostaticus*)

Membrana perinei

Apex prostatae

Prostata

Colliculus seminalis

Utriculus prostaticus

Ostium ductus ejaculatorii

Sphincter externus urethrae

Glandula bulbourethralis (Cowperi)

Ostium ductus glandulae bulbourethralis

Anterior view of coronal section

Rectum

Fascia rectalis

Corpus perineale

Fascia rectoprostatica

Glandula seminalis

Sagittal section

Vesica urinaria

Ureter

Ductus deferens

Ampulla ductus deferentis

Ductus ejaculatorius

Basis prostatae

Ramus ischiopubicus

M. transversus profundus perinei

Glandula seminalis

Apex prostatae

Glandulae bulbourethrales (Cowperi)

Posterior view

Prostata, superior view

Commissura anterior prostatae

Zona transitionalis

Zona centralis

Urethra

Zona peripherica

Ampulla ductus deferentis

Glandula seminalis

Prostata, transverse section

Commissura anterior prostatae

Zona transitionalis

Pars prostatica urethrae

Zona centralis

Zona peripherica

Plate 385

Perineum Masculinum and Organa Genitalia Masculina Externa

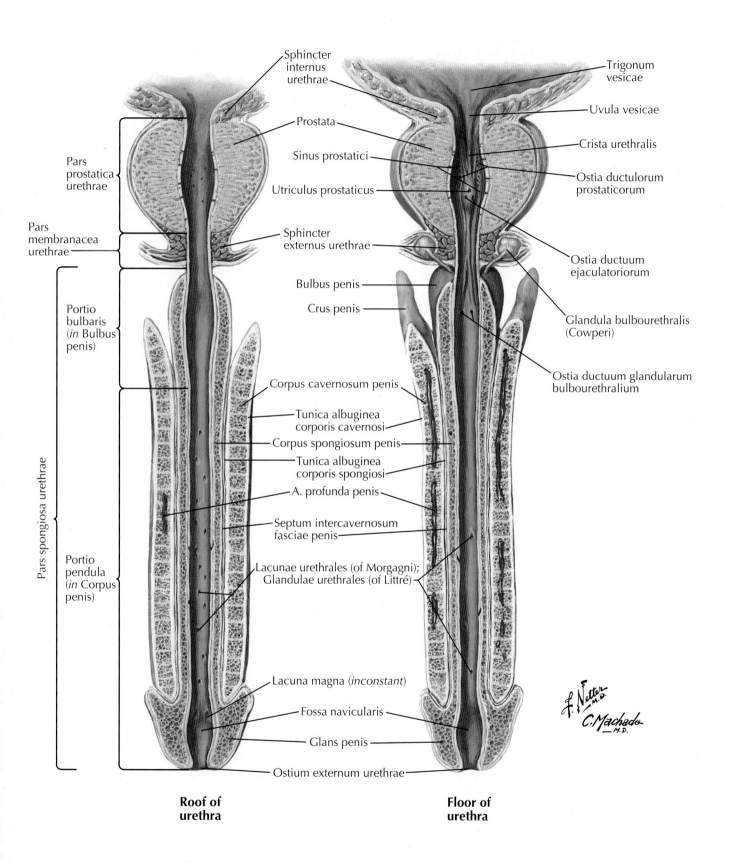

Sphincter internus urethrae

Prostata

Sinus prostatici

Utriculus prostaticus

Sphincter externus urethrae

Bulbus penis

Crus penis

Corpus cavernosum penis

Tunica albuginea corporis cavernosi

Corpus spongiosum penis

Tunica albuginea corporis spongiosi

A. profunda penis

Septum intercavernosum fasciae penis

Lacunae urethrales (of Morgagni); Glandulae urethrales (of Littré)

Lacuna magna (*inconstant*)

Fossa navicularis

Glans penis

Ostium externum urethrae

Trigonum vesicae

Uvula vesicae

Crista urethralis

Ostia ductulorum prostaticorum

Ostia ductuum ejaculatoriorum

Glandula bulbourethralis (Cowperi)

Ostia ductuum glandularum bulbourethralium

Pars prostatica urethrae

Pars membranacea urethrae

Portio bulbaris (*in* Bulbus penis)

Pars spongiosa urethrae

Portio pendula (*in* Corpus penis)

Roof of urethra

Floor of urethra

Perineum Masculinum and Organa Genitalia Masculina Externa

Plate 386

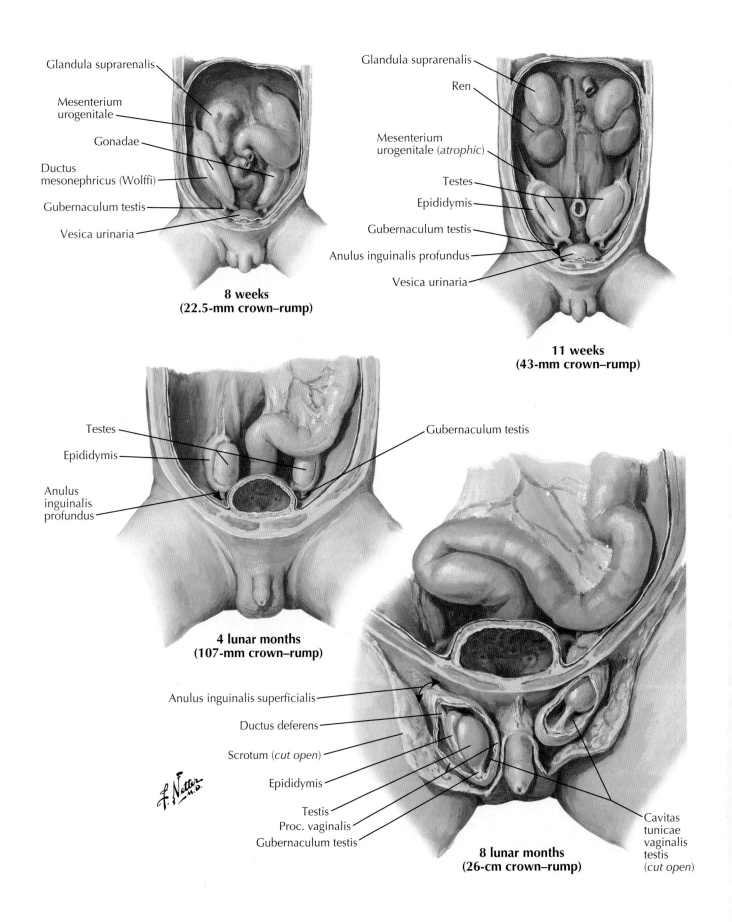

Glandula suprarenalis

Mesenterium urogenitale

Gonadae

Ductus mesonephricus (Wolffi)

Gubernaculum testis

Vesica urinaria

8 weeks
(22.5-mm crown–rump)

Glandula suprarenalis

Ren

Mesenterium urogenitale (*atrophic*)

Testes

Epididymis

Gubernaculum testis

Anulus inguinalis profundus

Vesica urinaria

11 weeks
(43-mm crown–rump)

Testes

Epididymis

Anulus inguinalis profundus

Gubernaculum testis

4 lunar months
(107-mm crown–rump)

Anulus inguinalis superficialis

Ductus deferens

Scrotum (*cut open*)

Epididymis

Testis

Proc. vaginalis

Gubernaculum testis

Cavitas tunicae vaginalis testis (*cut open*)

8 lunar months
(26-cm crown–rump)

Plate 387   **Perineum Masculinum and Organa Genitalia Masculina Externa**

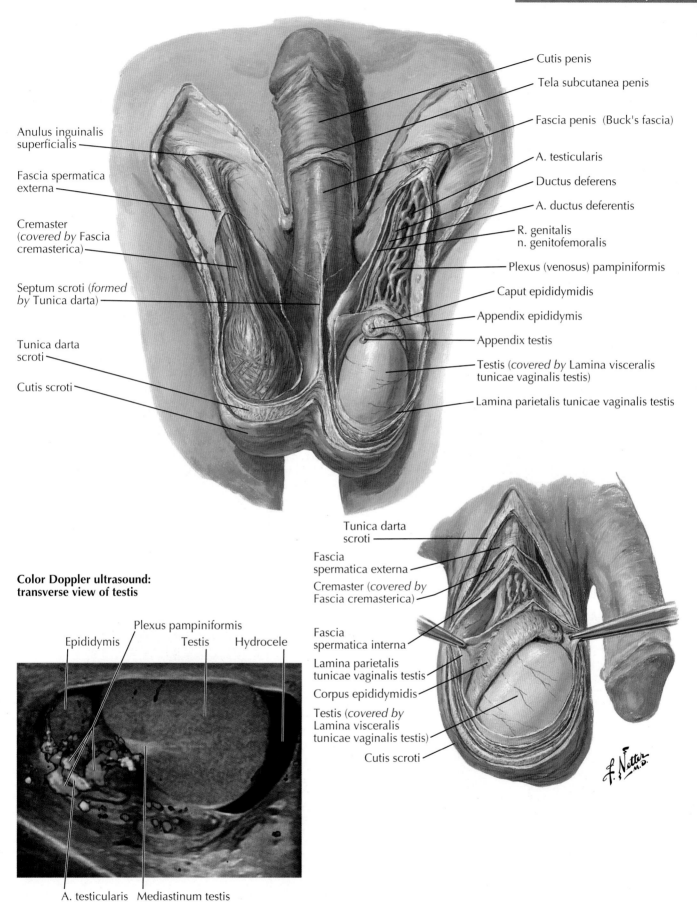

Cutis penis

Tela subcutanea penis

Fascia penis (Buck's fascia)

A. testicularis

Ductus deferens

A. ductus deferentis

R. genitalis
n. genitofemoralis

Plexus (venosus) pampiniformis

Caput epididymidis

Appendix epididymis

Appendix testis

Testis (*covered by* Lamina visceralis
tunicae vaginalis testis)

Lamina parietalis tunicae vaginalis testis

Anulus inguinalis
superficialis

Fascia spermatica
externa

Cremaster
(*covered by* Fascia
cremasterica)

Septum scroti (*formed
by* Tunica darta)

Tunica darta
scroti

Cutis scroti

**Color Doppler ultrasound:
transverse view of testis**

Plexus pampiniformis

Epididymis   Testis   Hydrocele

A. testicularis   Mediastinum testis

Tunica darta
scroti

Fascia
spermatica externa

Cremaster (*covered by*
Fascia cremasterica)

Fascia
spermatica interna

Lamina parietalis
tunicae vaginalis testis

Corpus epididymidis

Testis (*covered by*
Lamina visceralis
tunicae vaginalis testis)

Cutis scroti

F. Netter M.D.

Perineum Masculinum and Organa Genitalia Masculina Externa

Plate 388

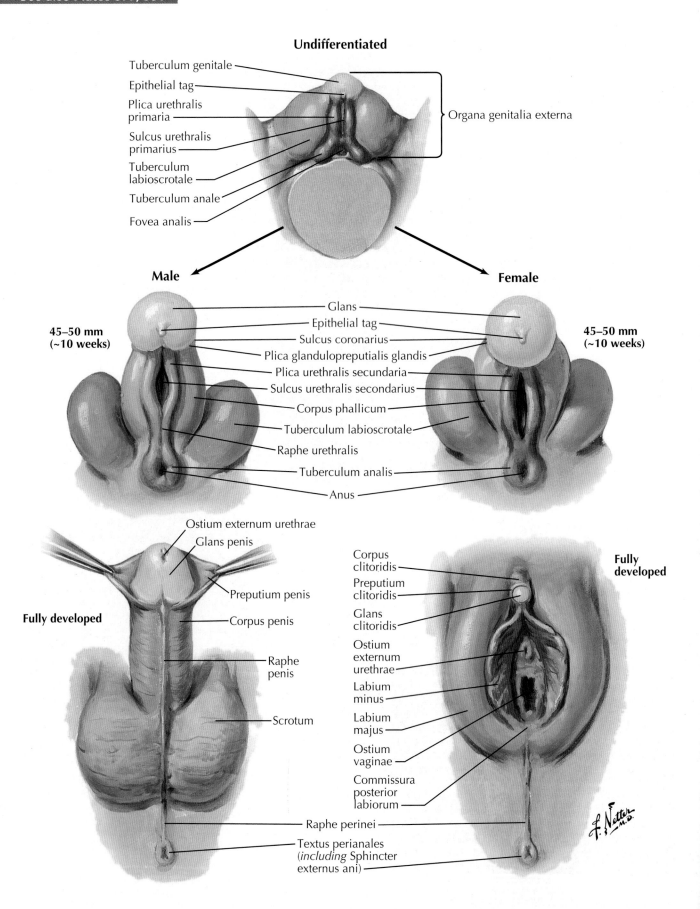

Undifferentiated

Tuberculum genitale

Epithelial tag

Plica urethralis primaria

Sulcus urethralis primarius

Tuberculum labioscrotale

Tuberculum anale

Fovea analis

Organa genitalia externa

Male

45–50 mm (~10 weeks)

Female

45–50 mm (~10 weeks)

Glans

Epithelial tag

Sulcus coronarius

Plica glandulopreputialis glandis

Plica urethralis secundaria

Sulcus urethralis secundarius

Corpus phallicum

Tuberculum labioscrotale

Raphe urethralis

Tuberculum analis

Anus

Ostium externum urethrae

Glans penis

Preputium penis

Fully developed

Corpus penis

Raphe penis

Scrotum

Corpus clitoridis

Preputium clitoridis

Glans clitoridis

Ostium externum urethrae

Labium minus

Labium majus

Ostium vaginae

Commissura posterior labiorum

Fully developed

Raphe perinei

Textus perianales (*including* Sphincter externus ani)

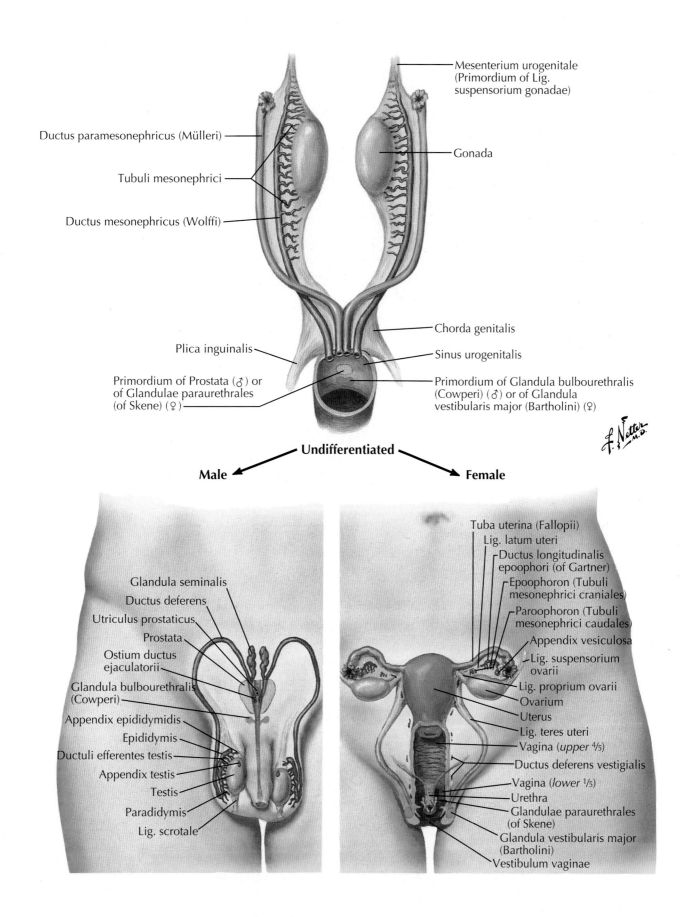

Mesenterium urogenitale (Primordium of Lig. suspensorium gonadae)

Ductus paramesonephricus (Mülleri)

Gonada

Tubuli mesonephrici

Ductus mesonephricus (Wolffi)

Chorda genitalis

Plica inguinalis

Sinus urogenitalis

Primordium of Prostata (♂) or of Glandulae paraurethrales (of Skene) (♀)

Primordium of Glandula bulbourethralis (Cowperi) (♂) or of Glandula vestibularis major (Bartholini) (♀)

Undifferentiated

Male

Female

Glandula seminalis

Ductus deferens

Utriculus prostaticus

Prostata

Ostium ductus ejaculatorii

Glandula bulbourethralis (Cowperi)

Appendix epididymidis

Epididymis

Ductuli efferentes testis

Appendix testis

Testis

Paradidymis

Lig. scrotale

Tuba uterina (Fallopii)

Lig. latum uteri

Ductus longitudinalis epoophori (of Gartner)

Epoophoron (Tubuli mesonephrici craniales)

Paroophoron (Tubuli mesonephrici caudales)

Appendix vesiculosa

Lig. suspensorium ovarii

Lig. proprium ovarii

Ovarium

Uterus

Lig. teres uteri

Vagina (upper 4/5)

Ductus deferens vestigialis

Vagina (lower 1/5)

Urethra

Glandulae paraurethrales (of Skene)

Glandula vestibularis major (Bartholini)

Vestibulum vaginae

Epithelium spermatogenicum: spermatogenesis

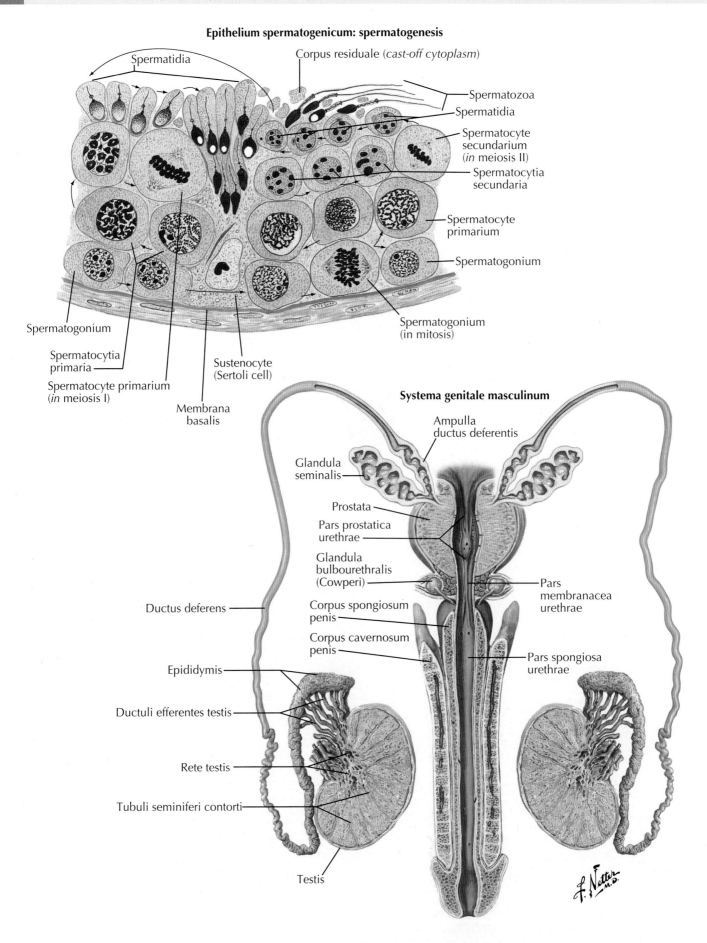

Spermatidia

Corpus residuale (*cast-off cytoplasm*)

Spermatozoa

Spermatidia

Spermatocyte secundarium (*in meiosis II*)

Spermatocytia secundaria

Spermatocyte primarium

Spermatogonium

Spermatogonium (in mitosis)

Spermatogonium

Spermatocytia primaria

Spermatocyte primarium (*in meiosis I*)

Sustenocyte (Sertoli cell)

Membrana basalis

Systema genitale masculinum

Ampulla ductus deferentis

Glandula seminalis

Prostata

Pars prostatica urethrae

Glandula bulbourethralis (Cowperi)

Corpus spongiosum penis

Corpus cavernosum penis

Pars membranacea urethrae

Pars spongiosa urethrae

Ductus deferens

Epididymis

Ductuli efferentes testis

Rete testis

Tubuli seminiferi contorti

Testis

Plate 391

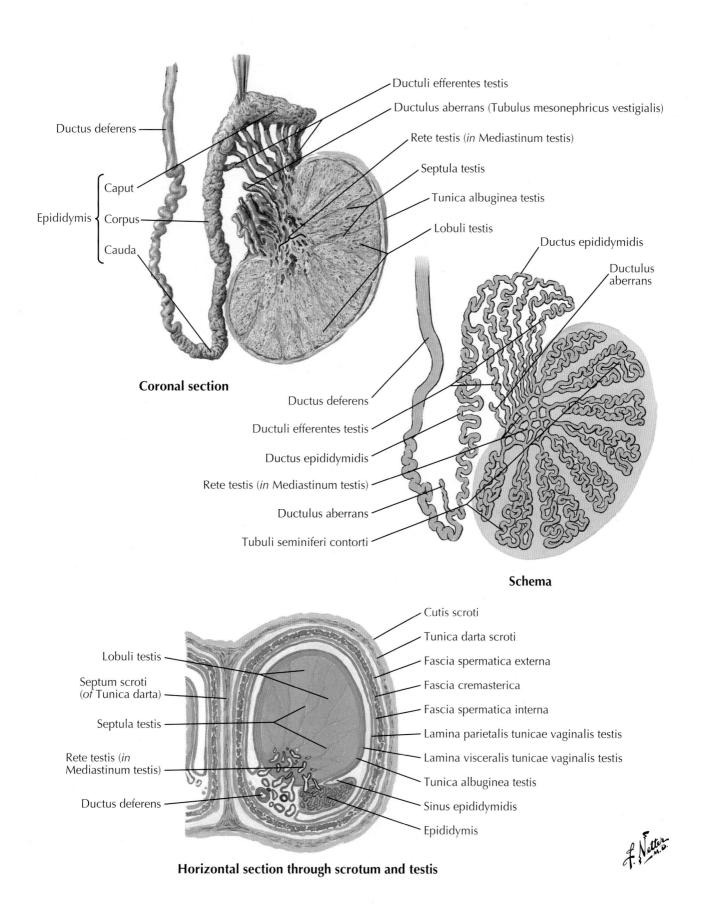

Ductus deferens

Ductuli efferentes testis

Ductulus aberrans (Tubulus mesonephricus vestigialis)

Rete testis (*in* Mediastinum testis)

Septula testis

Tunica albuginea testis

Lobuli testis

Caput

Corpus

Cauda

Epididymis

Coronal section

Ductus epididymidis

Ductulus aberrans

Ductus deferens

Ductuli efferentes testis

Ductus epididymidis

Rete testis (*in* Mediastinum testis)

Ductulus aberrans

Tubuli seminiferi contorti

Schema

Lobuli testis

Septum scroti (*of* Tunica darta)

Septula testis

Rete testis (*in* Mediastinum testis)

Ductus deferens

Cutis scroti

Tunica darta scroti

Fascia spermatica externa

Fascia cremasterica

Fascia spermatica interna

Lamina parietalis tunicae vaginalis testis

Lamina visceralis tunicae vaginalis testis

Tunica albuginea testis

Sinus epididymidis

Epididymis

Horizontal section through scrotum and testis

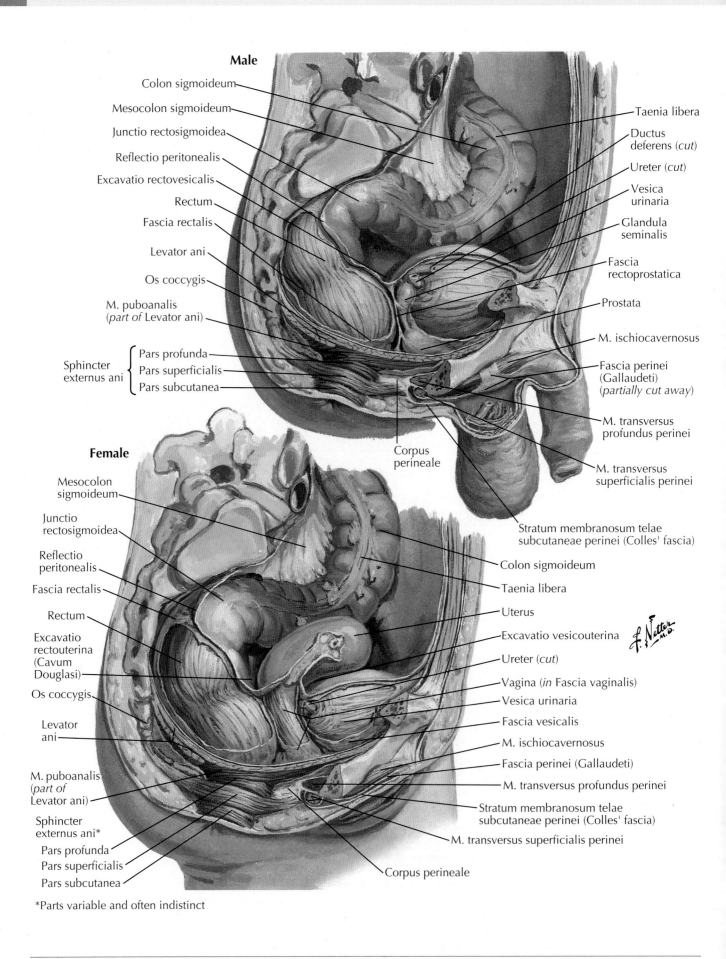

Male

Colon sigmoideum

Mesocolon sigmoideum

Junctio rectosigmoidea

Reflectio peritonealis

Excavatio rectovesicalis

Rectum

Fascia rectalis

Levator ani

Os coccygis

M. puboanalis
(*part of* Levator ani)

Sphincter
externus ani { Pars profunda
Pars superficialis
Pars subcutanea

Taenia libera

Ductus
deferens (*cut*)

Ureter (*cut*)

Vesica
urinaria

Glandula
seminalis

Fascia
rectoprostatica

Prostata

M. ischiocavernosus

Fascia perinei
(Gallaudeti)
(*partially cut away*)

M. transversus
profundus perinei

Corpus
perineale

M. transversus
superficialis perinei

Stratum membranosum telae
subcutaneae perinei (Colles' fascia)

Female

Mesocolon
sigmoideum

Junctio
rectosigmoidea

Reflectio
peritonealis

Fascia rectalis

Rectum

Excavatio
rectouterina
(Cavum
Douglasi)

Os coccygis

Levator
ani

M. puboanalis
(*part of*
Levator ani)

Sphincter
externus ani*

Pars profunda

Pars superficialis

Pars subcutanea

*Parts variable and often indistinct

Colon sigmoideum

Taenia libera

Uterus

Excavatio vesicouterina

Ureter (*cut*)

Vagina (*in* Fascia vaginalis)

Vesica urinaria

Fascia vesicalis

M. ischiocavernosus

Fascia perinei (Gallaudeti)

M. transversus profundus perinei

Stratum membranosum telae
subcutaneae perinei (Colles' fascia)

M. transversus superficialis perinei

Corpus perineale

Plate 393

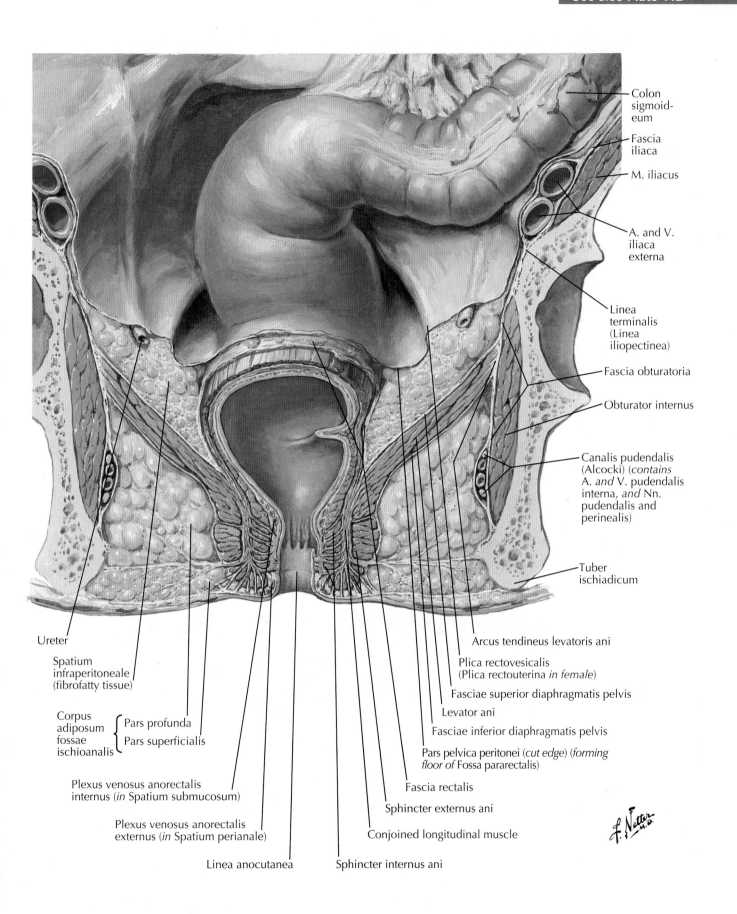

Colon sigmoid-eum

Fascia iliaca

M. iliacus

A. and V. iliaca externa

Linea terminalis (Linea iliopectinea)

Fascia obturatoria

Obturator internus

Canalis pudendalis (Alcocki) (*contains* A. *and* V. pudendalis interna, *and* Nn. pudendalis and perinealis)

Tuber ischiadicum

Arcus tendineus levatoris ani

Plica rectovesicalis (Plica rectouterina *in female*)

Fasciae superior diaphragmatis pelvis

Levator ani

Fasciae inferior diaphragmatis pelvis

Pars pelvica peritonei (*cut edge*) (*forming floor of* Fossa pararectalis)

Fascia rectalis

Sphincter externus ani

Conjoined longitudinal muscle

Ureter

Spatium infraperitoneale (fibrofatty tissue)

Corpus adiposum fossae ischioanalis { Pars profunda / Pars superficialis

Plexus venosus anorectalis internus (*in Spatium submucosum*)

Plexus venosus anorectalis externus (*in Spatium perianale*)

Linea anocutanea

Sphincter internus ani

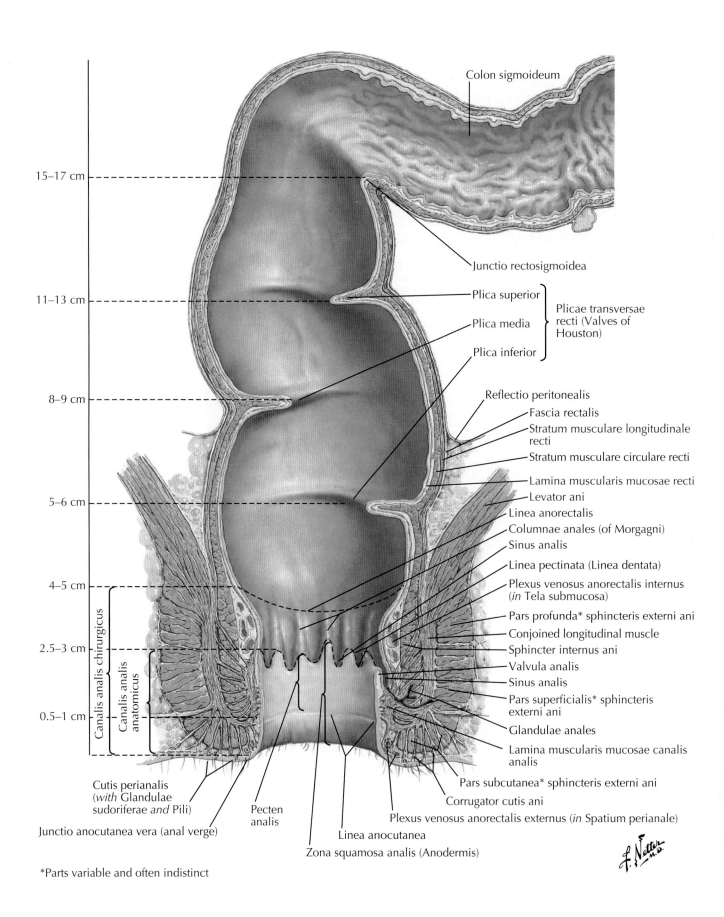

Colon sigmoideum

15–17 cm

11–13 cm

8–9 cm

5–6 cm

4–5 cm

2.5–3 cm

0.5–1 cm

Canalis analis chirurgicus

Canalis analis anatomicus

Junctio rectosigmoidea

Plica superior
Plica media
Plica inferior

Plicae transversae recti (Valves of Houston)

Reflectio peritonealis

Fascia rectalis

Stratum musculare longitudinale recti

Stratum musculare circulare recti

Lamina muscularis mucosae recti

Levator ani

Linea anorectalis

Columnae anales (of Morgagni)

Sinus analis

Linea pectinata (Linea dentata)

Plexus venosus anorectalis internus (in Tela submucosa)

Pars profunda* sphincteris externi ani

Conjoined longitudinal muscle

Sphincter internus ani

Valvula analis

Sinus analis

Pars superficialis* sphincteris externi ani

Glandulae anales

Lamina muscularis mucosae canalis analis

Pars subcutanea* sphincteris externi ani

Corrugator cutis ani

Plexus venosus anorectalis externus (in Spatium perianale)

Cutis perianalis (*with* Glandulae sudoriferae *and* Pili)

Pecten analis

Junctio anocutanea vera (anal verge)

Linea anocutanea

Zona squamosa analis (Anodermis)

*Parts variable and often indistinct

Plate 395

Rectum and Canalis Analis

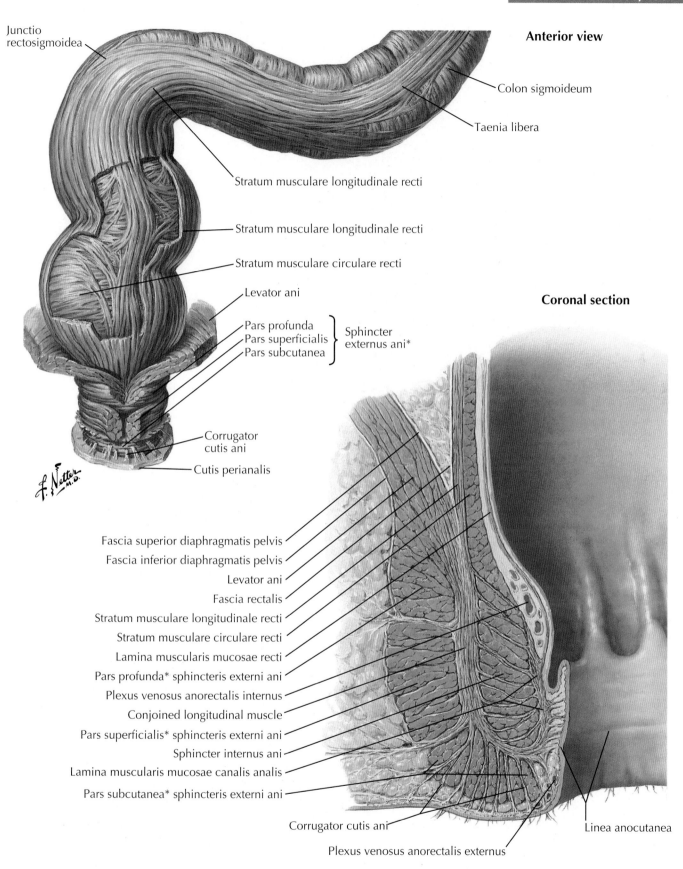

Anterior view

Junctio rectosigmoidea

Colon sigmoideum

Taenia libera

Stratum musculare longitudinale recti

Stratum musculare longitudinale recti

Stratum musculare circulare recti

Levator ani

Pars profunda
Pars superficialis
Pars subcutanea
} Sphincter externus ani*

Coronal section

Corrugator cutis ani

Cutis perianalis

Fascia superior diaphragmatis pelvis
Fascia inferior diaphragmatis pelvis
Levator ani
Fascia rectalis
Stratum musculare longitudinale recti
Stratum musculare circulare recti
Lamina muscularis mucosae recti
Pars profunda* sphincteris externi ani
Plexus venosus anorectalis internus
Conjoined longitudinal muscle
Pars superficialis* sphincteris externi ani
Sphincter internus ani
Lamina muscularis mucosae canalis analis
Pars subcutanea* sphincteris externi ani

Corrugator cutis ani

Plexus venosus anorectalis externus

Linea anocutanea

*Parts variable and often indistinct

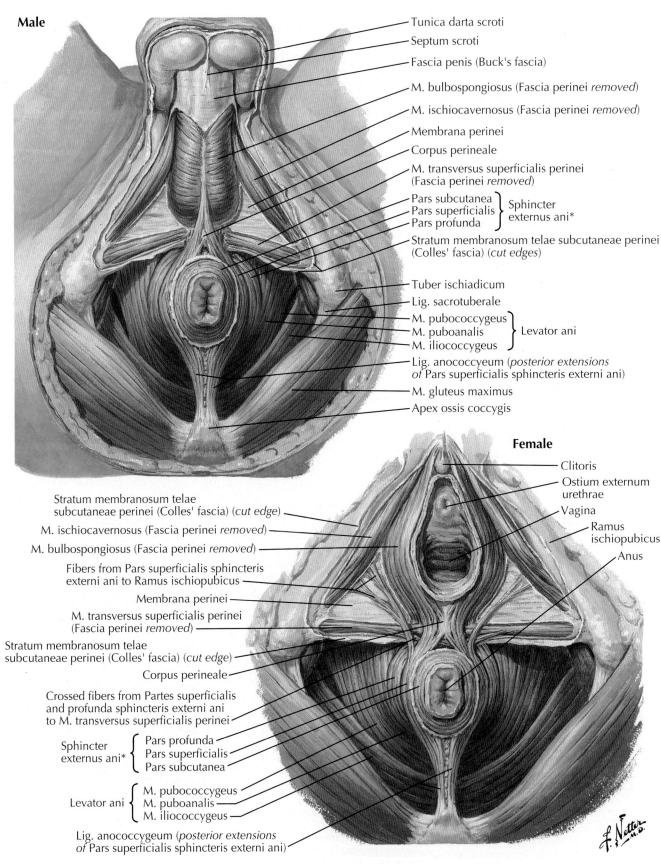

Male

Tunica darta scroti

Septum scroti

Fascia penis (Buck's fascia)

M. bulbospongiosus (Fascia perinei *removed*)

M. ischiocavernosus (Fascia perinei *removed*)

Membrana perinei

Corpus perineale

M. transversus superficialis perinei (Fascia perinei *removed*)

Pars subcutanea
Pars superficialis
Pars profunda
} Sphincter externus ani*

Stratum membranosum telae subcutaneae perinei (Colles' fascia) (*cut edges*)

Tuber ischiadicum

Lig. sacrotuberale

M. pubococcygeus
M. puboanalis
M. iliococcygeus
} Levator ani

Lig. anococcyeum (*posterior extensions of* Pars superficialis sphincteris externi ani)

M. gluteus maximus

Apex ossis coccygis

Female

Clitoris

Ostium externum urethrae

Vagina

Ramus ischiopubicus

Anus

Stratum membranosum telae subcutaneae perinei (Colles' fascia) (*cut edge*)

M. ischiocavernosus (Fascia perinei *removed*)

M. bulbospongiosus (Fascia perinei *removed*)

Fibers from Pars superficialis sphincteris externi ani to Ramus ischiopubicus

Membrana perinei

M. transversus superficialis perinei (Fascia perinei *removed*)

Stratum membranosum telae subcutaneae perinei (Colles' fascia) (*cut edge*)

Corpus perineale

Crossed fibers from Partes superficialis and profunda sphincteris externi ani to M. transversus superficialis perinei

Sphincter externus ani* {
Pars profunda
Pars superficialis
Pars subcutanea

Levator ani {
M. pubococcygeus
M. puboanalis
M. iliococcygeus

Lig. anococcygeum (*posterior extensions of* Pars superficialis sphincteris externi ani)

*Parts variable and often indistinct

Plate 397

Rectum and Canalis Analis

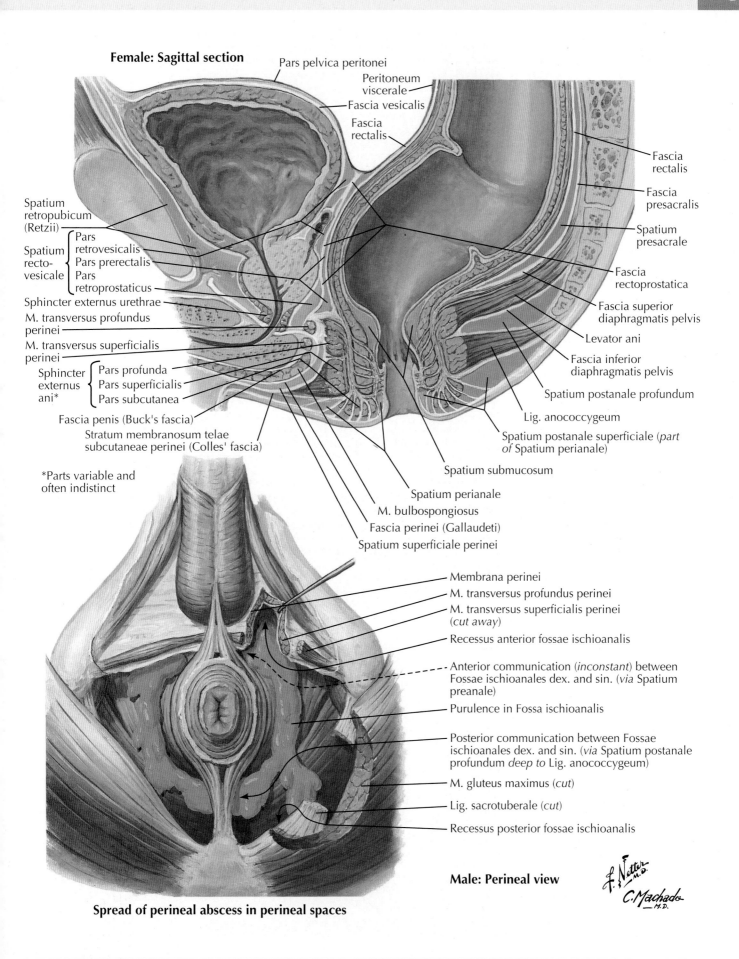

Female: Sagittal section

Pars pelvica peritonei

Peritoneum viscerale

Fascia vesicalis

Fascia rectalis

Fascia rectalis

Fascia presacralis

Spatium presacrale

Fascia rectoprostatica

Fascia superior diaphragmatis pelvis

Levator ani

Fascia inferior diaphragmatis pelvis

Spatium postanale profundum

Lig. anococcygeum

Spatium postanale superficiale (*part of* Spatium perianale)

Spatium retropubicum (Retzii)

Spatium recto-vesicale
- Pars retrovesicalis
- Pars prerectalis
- Pars retroprostaticus

Sphincter externus urethrae

M. transversus profundus perinei

M. transversus superficialis perinei

Sphincter externus ani*
- Pars profunda
- Pars superficialis
- Pars subcutanea

Fascia penis (Buck's fascia)

Stratum membranosum telae subcutaneae perinei (Colles' fascia)

*Parts variable and often indistinct

Spatium submucosum

Spatium perianale

M. bulbospongiosus

Fascia perinei (Gallaudeti)

Spatium superficiale perinei

Membrana perinei

M. transversus profundus perinei

M. transversus superficialis perinei (*cut away*)

Recessus anterior fossae ischioanalis

Anterior communication (*inconstant*) between Fossae ischioanales dex. and sin. (*via* Spatium preanale)

Purulence in Fossa ischioanalis

Posterior communication between Fossae ischioanales dex. and sin. (*via* Spatium postanale profundum *deep to* Lig. anococcygeum)

M. gluteus maximus (*cut*)

Lig. sacrotuberale (*cut*)

Recessus posterior fossae ischioanalis

Male: Perineal view

Spread of perineal abscess in perineal spaces

Rectum and Canalis Analis

Plate 398

MRI of female pelvis (without intravenous contrast medium)

Corpus vertebrae L5

Os sacrum (segmentum S1)

M. rectus abdominis

Myometrium

Endometrium

Fundus uteri

Rectum

Vesica urinaria

Os pubis

Vagina

MRI of male pelvis (without intravenous contrast medium)

Umbilicus

Vertebra L4

Discus intervertebralis L4/L5

Os sacrum (segmentum S1)

M. rectus abdominis

Vesica urinaria

Rectum

Os pubis

Prostata

Penis

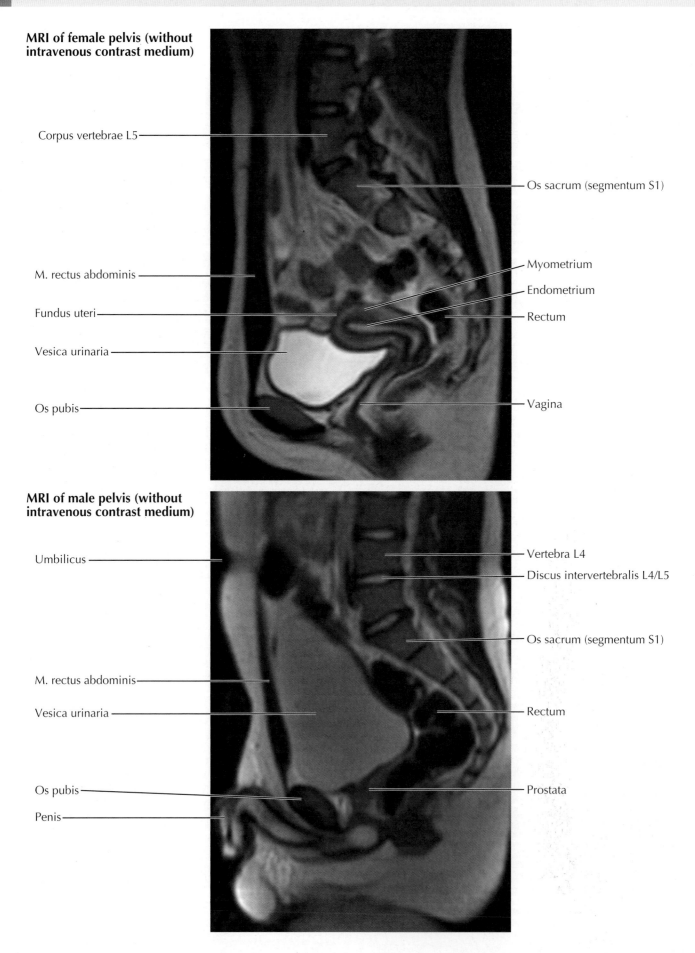

Plate 399

Rectum and Canalis Analis

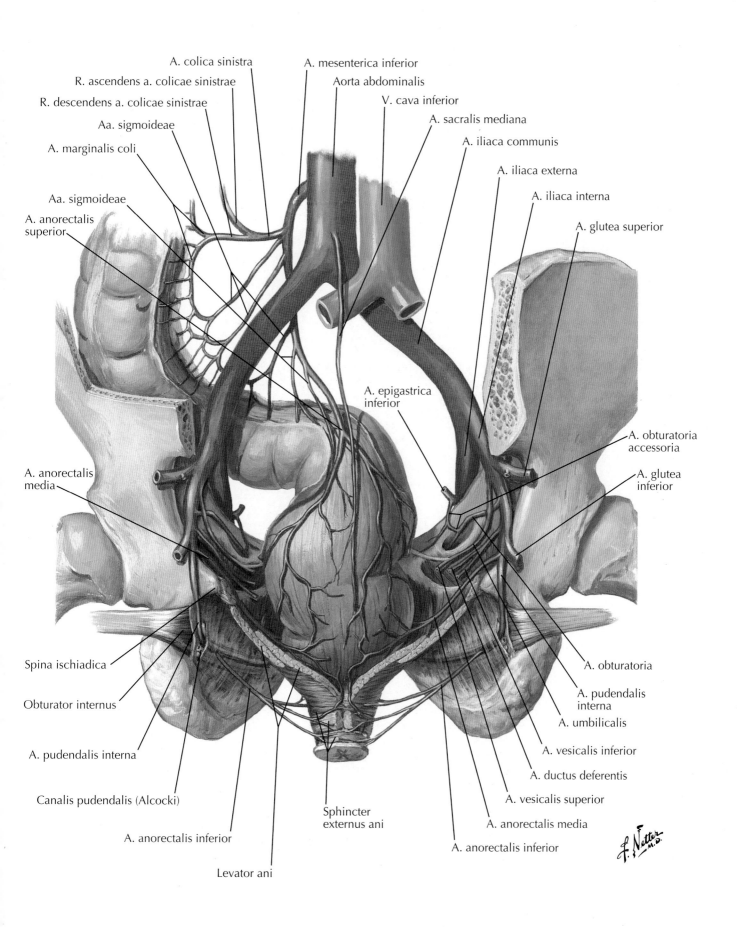

A. colica sinistra
R. ascendens a. colicae sinistrae
R. descendens a. colicae sinistrae
Aa. sigmoideae
A. marginalis coli
Aa. sigmoideae
A. anorectalis superior
A. mesenterica inferior
Aorta abdominalis
V. cava inferior
A. sacralis mediana
A. iliaca communis
A. iliaca externa
A. iliaca interna
A. glutea superior
A. epigastrica inferior
A. obturatoria accessoria
A. anorectalis media
A. glutea inferior
Spina ischiadica
Obturator internus
A. pudendalis interna
Canalis pudendalis (Alcocki)
A. anorectalis inferior
Levator ani
Sphincter externus ani
A. obturatoria
A. pudendalis interna
A. umbilicalis
A. vesicalis inferior
A. ductus deferentis
A. vesicalis superior
A. anorectalis media
A. anorectalis inferior

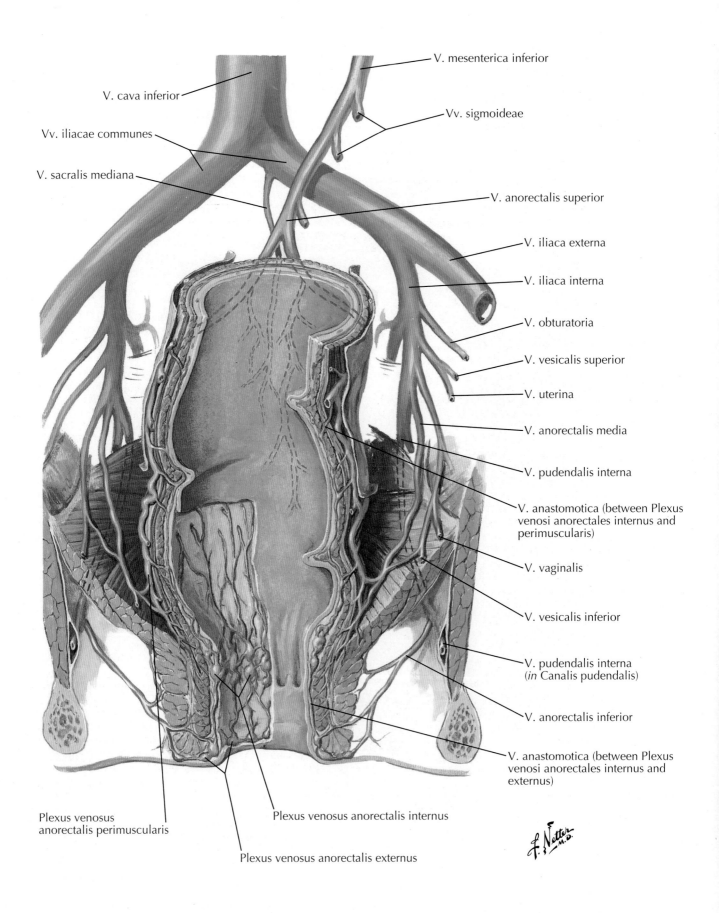

V. mesenterica inferior

V. cava inferior

Vv. sigmoideae

Vv. iliacae communes

V. sacralis mediana

V. anorectalis superior

V. iliaca externa

V. iliaca interna

V. obturatoria

V. vesicalis superior

V. uterina

V. anorectalis media

V. pudendalis interna

V. anastomotica (between Plexus venosi anorectales internus and perimuscularis)

V. vaginalis

V. vesicalis inferior

V. pudendalis interna (*in* Canalis pudendalis)

V. anorectalis inferior

V. anastomotica (between Plexus venosi anorectales internus and externus)

Plexus venosus anorectalis perimuscularis

Plexus venosus anorectalis internus

Plexus venosus anorectalis externus

Plate 401

Vasa Sanguinea, Vasa Lymphatica, and Nodi Lymphoidei

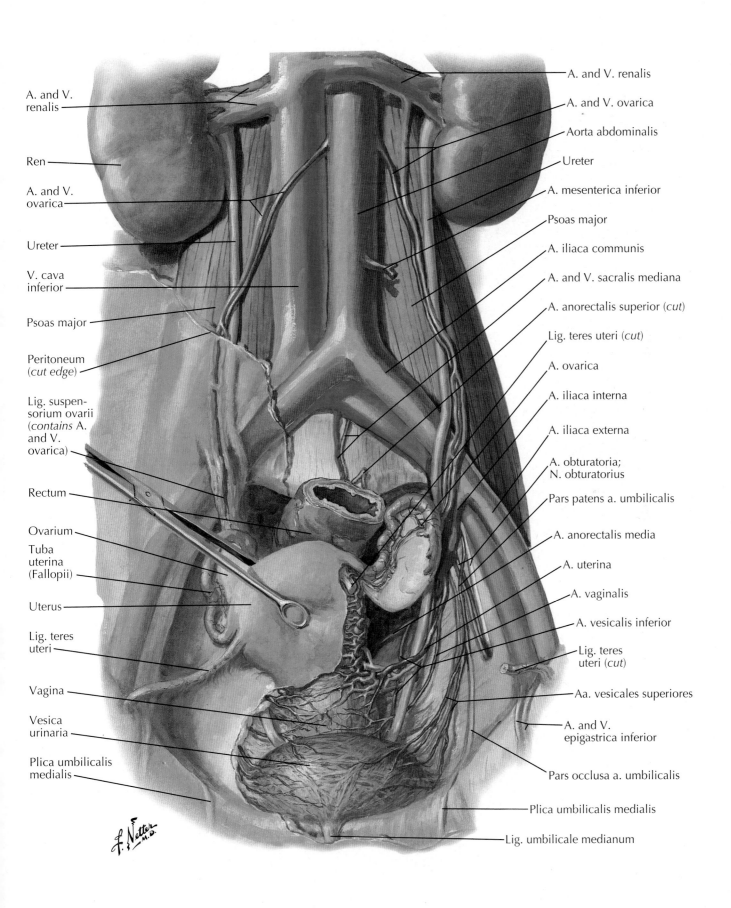

A. and V. renalis

A. and V. ovarica

Aorta abdominalis

Ureter

A. mesenterica inferior

Psoas major

A. iliaca communis

A. and V. sacralis mediana

A. anorectalis superior (*cut*)

Lig. teres uteri (*cut*)

A. ovarica

A. iliaca interna

A. iliaca externa

A. obturatoria; N. obturatorius

Pars patens a. umbilicalis

A. anorectalis media

A. uterina

A. vaginalis

A. vesicalis inferior

Lig. teres uteri (*cut*)

Aa. vesicales superiores

A. and V. epigastrica inferior

Pars occlusa a. umbilicalis

Plica umbilicalis medialis

Lig. umbilicale medianum

A. and V. renalis

Ren

A. and V. ovarica

Ureter

V. cava inferior

Psoas major

Peritoneum (*cut edge*)

Lig. suspensorium ovarii (*contains* A. and V. ovarica)

Rectum

Ovarium

Tuba uterina (Fallopii)

Uterus

Lig. teres uteri

Vagina

Vesica urinaria

Plica umbilicalis medialis

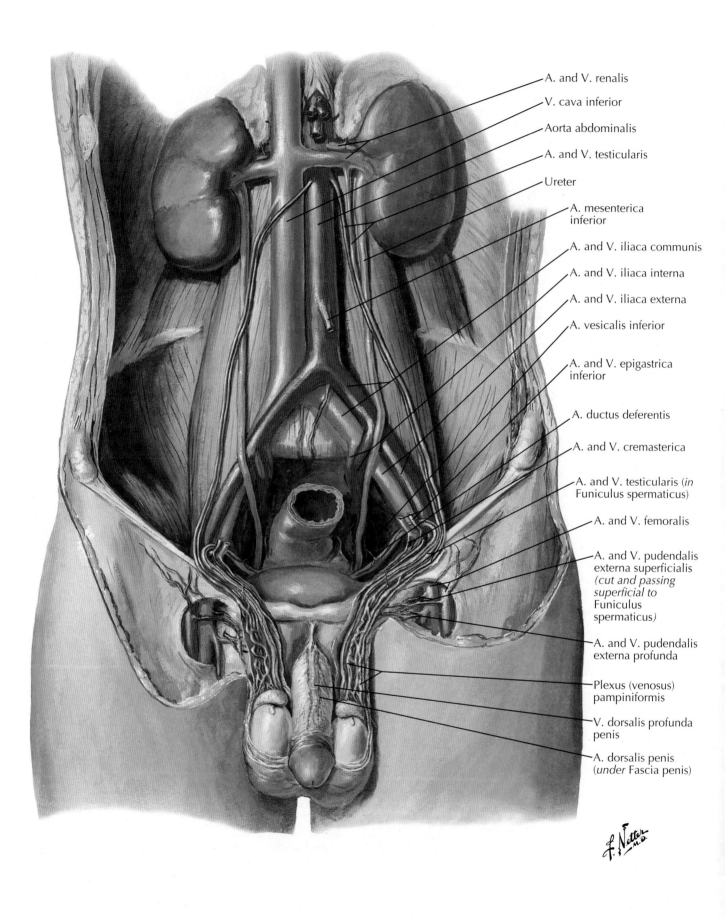

A. and V. renalis

V. cava inferior

Aorta abdominalis

A. and V. testicularis

Ureter

A. mesenterica inferior

A. and V. iliaca communis

A. and V. iliaca interna

A. and V. iliaca externa

A. vesicalis inferior

A. and V. epigastrica inferior

A. ductus deferentis

A. and V. cremasterica

A. and V. testicularis (*in* Funiculus spermaticus)

A. and V. femoralis

A. and V. pudendalis externa superficialis (*cut and passing superficial to* Funiculus spermaticus)

A. and V. pudendalis externa profunda

Plexus (venosus) pampiniformis

V. dorsalis profunda penis

A. dorsalis penis (*under* Fascia penis)

Plate 403   **Vasa Sanguinea, Vasa Lymphatica, and Nodi Lymphoidei**

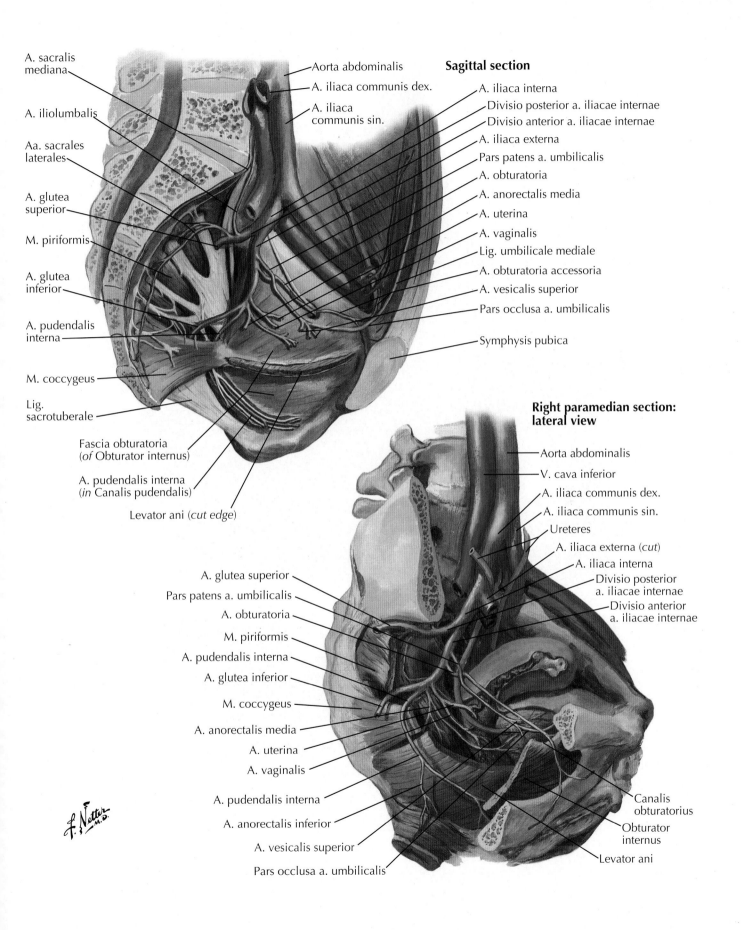

A. sacralis mediana

A. iliolumbalis

Aa. sacrales laterales

A. glutea superior

M. piriformis

A. glutea inferior

A. pudendalis interna

M. coccygeus

Lig. sacrotuberale

Fascia obturatoria (*of* Obturator internus)

A. pudendalis interna (*in* Canalis pudendalis)

Levator ani (*cut edge*)

Aorta abdominalis

A. iliaca communis dex.

A. iliaca communis sin.

Sagittal section

A. iliaca interna

Divisio posterior a. iliacae internae

Divisio anterior a. iliacae internae

A. iliaca externa

Pars patens a. umbilicalis

A. obturatoria

A. anorectalis media

A. uterina

A. vaginalis

Lig. umbilicale mediale

A. obturatoria accessoria

A. vesicalis superior

Pars occlusa a. umbilicalis

Symphysis pubica

Right paramedian section: lateral view

Aorta abdominalis

V. cava inferior

A. iliaca communis dex.

A. iliaca communis sin.

Ureteres

A. iliaca externa (*cut*)

A. iliaca interna

Divisio posterior a. iliacae internae

Divisio anterior a. iliacae internae

A. glutea superior

Pars patens a. umbilicalis

A. obturatoria

M. piriformis

A. pudendalis interna

A. glutea inferior

M. coccygeus

A. anorectalis media

A. uterina

A. vaginalis

A. pudendalis interna

A. anorectalis inferior

A. vesicalis superior

Pars occlusa a. umbilicalis

Canalis obturatorius

Obturator internus

Levator ani

f. Netter M.D.

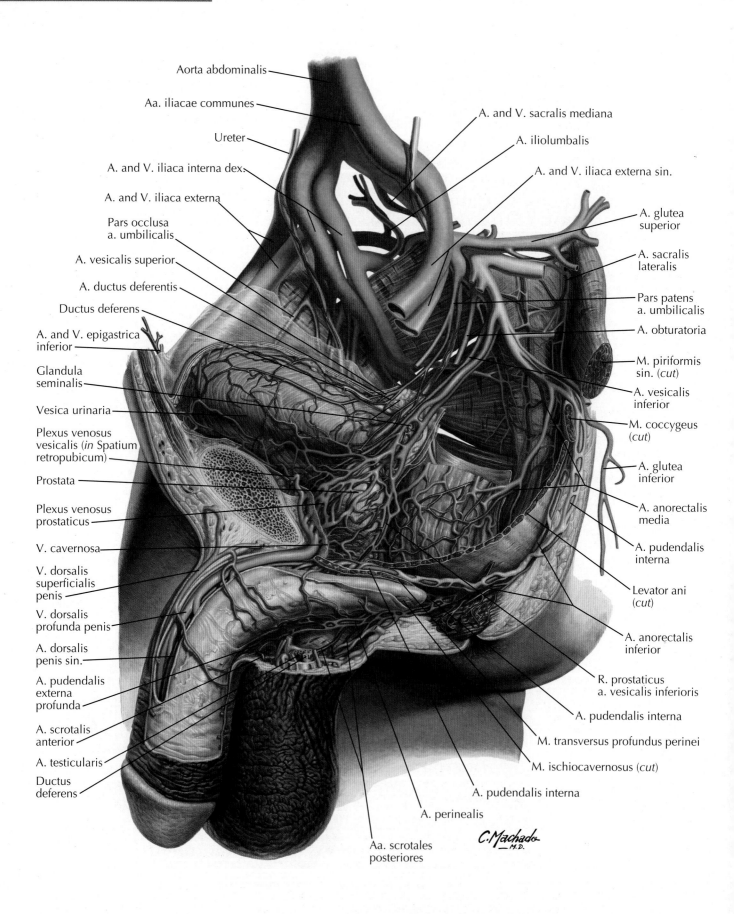

Aorta abdominalis

Aa. iliacae communes

Ureter

A. and V. iliaca interna dex.

A. and V. iliaca externa

Pars occlusa
a. umbilicalis

A. vesicalis superior

A. ductus deferentis

Ductus deferens

A. and V. epigastrica
inferior

Glandula
seminalis

Vesica urinaria

Plexus venosus
vesicalis (in Spatium
retropubicum)

Prostata

Plexus venosus
prostaticus

V. cavernosa

V. dorsalis
superficialis
penis

V. dorsalis
profunda penis

A. dorsalis
penis sin.

A. pudendalis
externa
profunda

A. scrotalis
anterior

A. testicularis

Ductus
deferens

A. and V. sacralis mediana

A. iliolumbalis

A. and V. iliaca externa sin.

A. glutea
superior

A. sacralis
lateralis

Pars patens
a. umbilicalis

A. obturatoria

M. piriformis
sin. (cut)

A. vesicalis
inferior

M. coccygeus
(cut)

A. glutea
inferior

A. anorectalis
media

A. pudendalis
interna

Levator ani
(cut)

A. anorectalis
inferior

R. prostaticus
a. vesicalis inferioris

A. pudendalis interna

M. transversus profundus perinei

M. ischiocavernosus (cut)

A. pudendalis interna

A. perinealis

Aa. scrotales
posteriores

C. Machado
_M.D.

Plate 405

Vasa Sanguinea, Vasa Lymphatica, and Nodi Lymphoidei

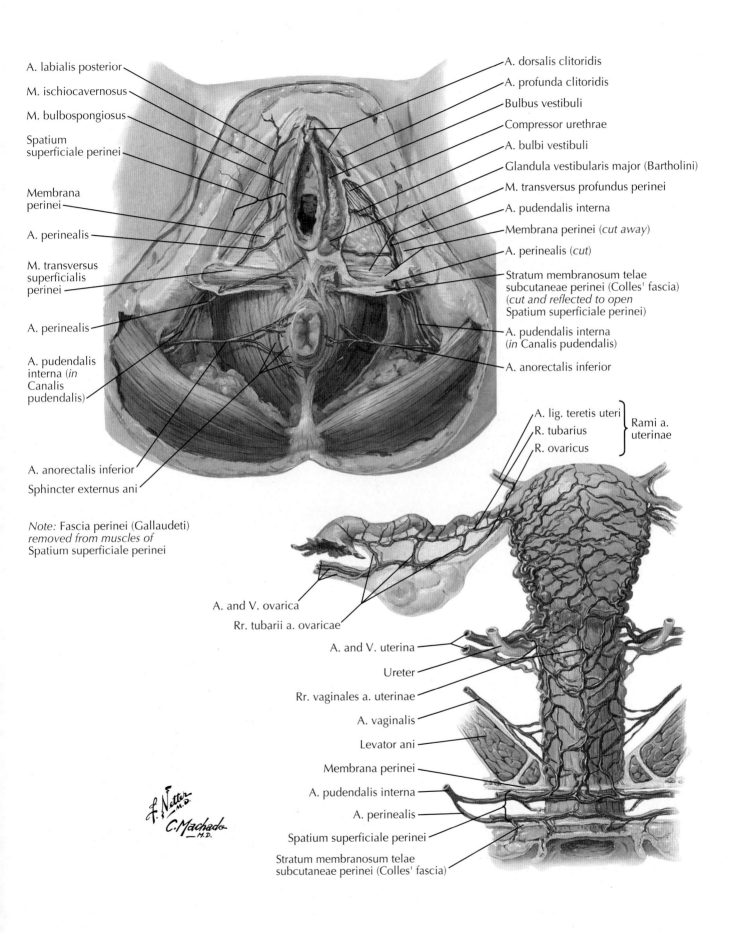

A. labialis posterior

M. ischiocavernosus

M. bulbospongiosus

Spatium
superficiale perinei

Membrana
perinei

A. perinealis

M. transversus
superficialis
perinei

A. perinealis

A. pudendalis
interna (*in
Canalis
pudendalis*)

A. anorectalis inferior

Sphincter externus ani

Note: Fascia perinei (Gallaudeti)
removed from muscles of
Spatium superficiale perinei

A. dorsalis clitoridis

A. profunda clitoridis

Bulbus vestibuli

Compressor urethrae

A. bulbi vestibuli

Glandula vestibularis major (Bartholini)

M. transversus profundus perinei

A. pudendalis interna

Membrana perinei (*cut away*)

A. perinealis (*cut*)

Stratum membranosum telae
subcutaneae perinei (Colles' fascia)
(*cut and reflected to open*
Spatium superficiale perinei)

A. pudendalis interna
(*in Canalis pudendalis*)

A. anorectalis inferior

A. lig. teretis uteri ⎫
R. tubarius   ⎬ Rami a.
R. ovaricus   ⎭ uterinae

A. and V. ovarica

Rr. tubarii a. ovaricae

A. and V. uterina

Ureter

Rr. vaginales a. uterinae

A. vaginalis

Levator ani

Membrana perinei

A. pudendalis interna

A. perinealis

Spatium superficiale perinei

Stratum membranosum telae
subcutaneae perinei (Colles' fascia)

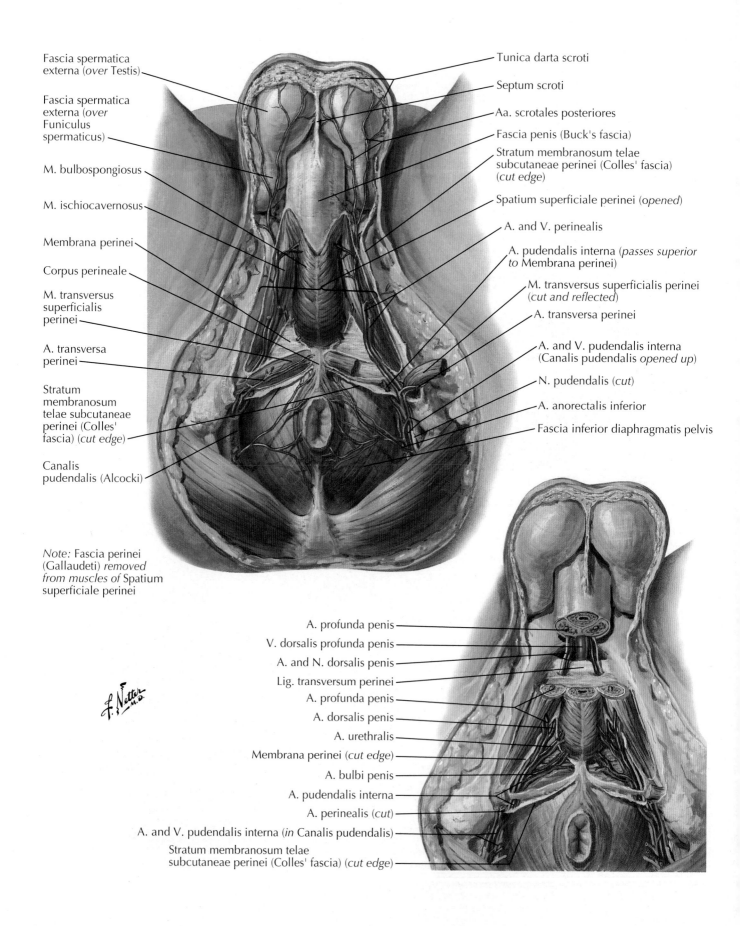

Fascia spermatica externa (*over* Testis)

Fascia spermatica externa (*over* Funiculus spermaticus)

M. bulbospongiosus

M. ischiocavernosus

Membrana perinei

Corpus perineale

M. transversus superficialis perinei

A. transversa perinei

Stratum membranosum telae subcutaneae perinei (Colles' fascia) (*cut edge*)

Canalis pudendalis (Alcocki)

Note: Fascia perinei (Gallaudeti) *removed from muscles of* Spatium superficiale perinei

Tunica darta scroti

Septum scroti

Aa. scrotales posteriores

Fascia penis (Buck's fascia)

Stratum membranosum telae subcutaneae perinei (Colles' fascia) (*cut edge*)

Spatium superficiale perinei (*opened*)

A. and V. perinealis

A. pudendalis interna (*passes superior to* Membrana perinei)

M. transversus superficialis perinei (*cut and reflected*)

A. transversa perinei

A. and V. pudendalis interna (Canalis pudendalis *opened up*)

N. pudendalis (*cut*)

A. anorectalis inferior

Fascia inferior diaphragmatis pelvis

A. profunda penis

V. dorsalis profunda penis

A. and N. dorsalis penis

Lig. transversum perinei

A. profunda penis

A. dorsalis penis

A. urethralis

Membrana perinei (*cut edge*)

A. bulbi penis

A. pudendalis interna

A. perinealis (*cut*)

A. and V. pudendalis interna (*in* Canalis pudendalis)

Stratum membranosum telae subcutaneae perinei (Colles' fascia) (*cut edge*)

Plate 407

Vasa Sanguinea, Vasa Lymphatica, and Nodi Lymphoidei

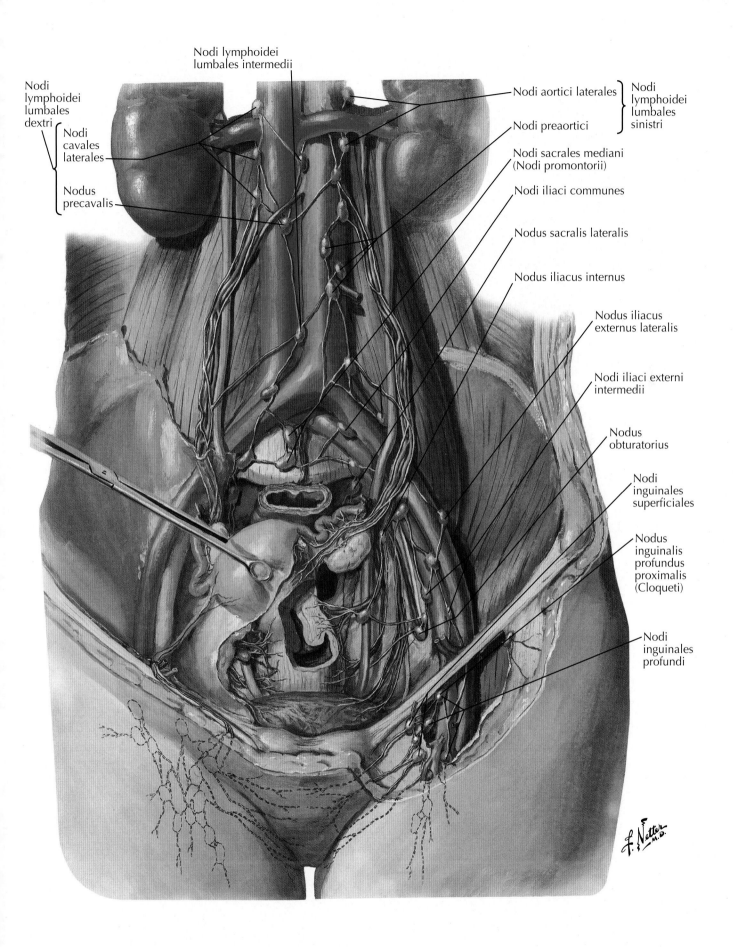

Nodi lymphoidei lumbales intermedii

Nodi lymphoidei lumbales dextri

Nodi cavales laterales

Nodus precavalis

Nodi aortici laterales

Nodi preaortici

Nodi lymphoidei lumbales sinistri

Nodi sacrales mediani (Nodi promontorii)

Nodi iliaci communes

Nodus sacralis lateralis

Nodus iliacus internus

Nodus iliacus externus lateralis

Nodi iliaci externi intermedii

Nodus obturatorius

Nodi inguinales superficiales

Nodus inguinalis profundus proximalis (Cloqueti)

Nodi inguinales profundi

Vasa Sanguinea, Vasa Lymphatica, and Nodi Lymphoidei

Plate 408

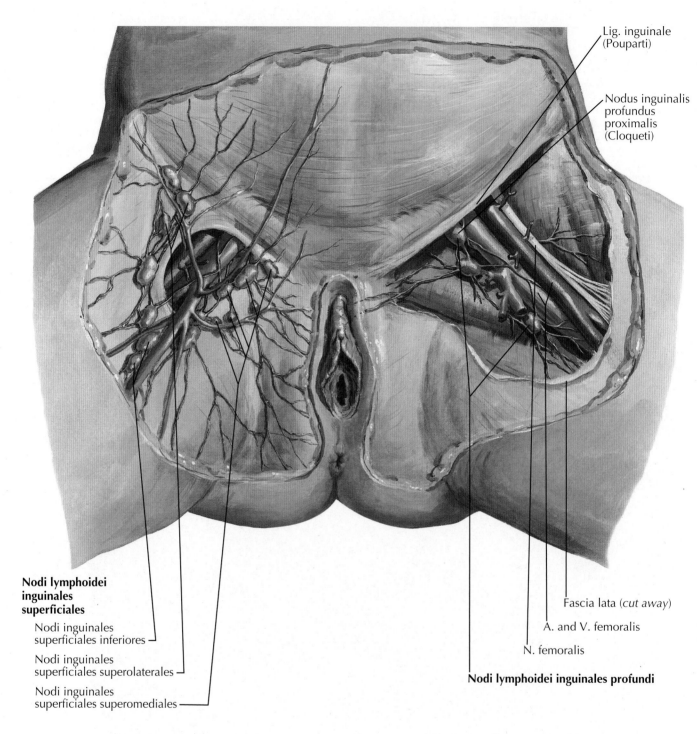

Lig. inguinale
(Pouparti)

Nodus inguinalis
profundus
proximalis
(Cloqueti)

**Nodi lymphoidei
inguinales
superficiales**

Nodi inguinales
superficiales inferiores ⌐

Nodi inguinales
superficiales superolaterales ⌐

Nodi inguinales
superficiales superomediales ⌐

Fascia lata (*cut away*)

A. and V. femoralis

N. femoralis

Nodi lymphoidei inguinales profundi

Plate 409

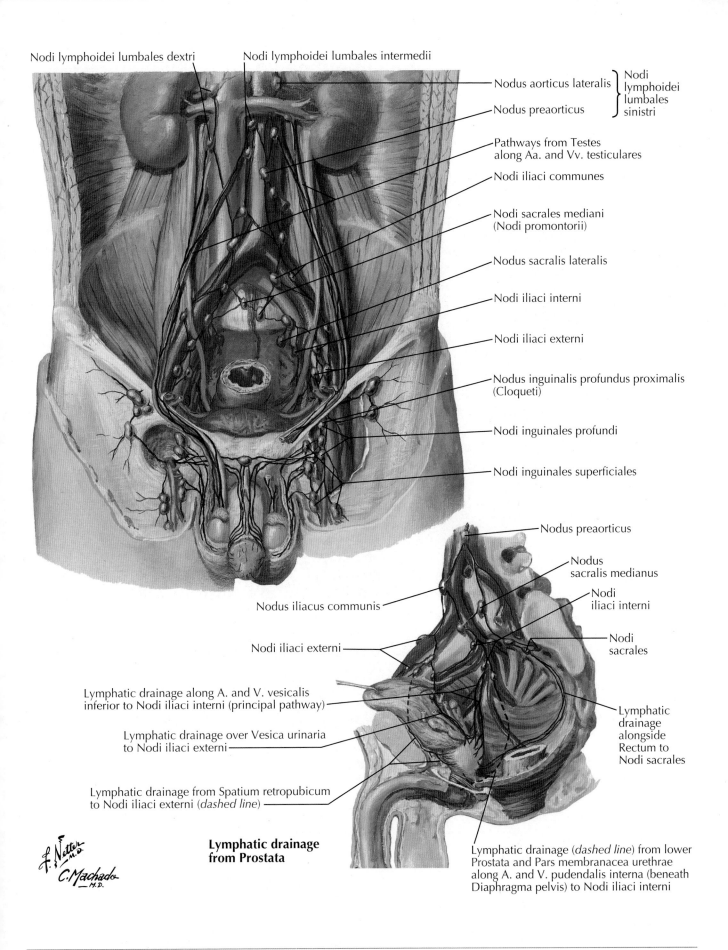

Nodi lymphoidei lumbales dextri

Nodi lymphoidei lumbales intermedii

Nodus aorticus lateralis } Nodi lymphoidei lumbales sinistri

Nodus preaorticus

Pathways from Testes along Aa. and Vv. testiculares

Nodi iliaci communes

Nodi sacrales mediani (Nodi promontorii)

Nodus sacralis lateralis

Nodi iliaci interni

Nodi iliaci externi

Nodus inguinalis profundus proximalis (Cloqueti)

Nodi inguinales profundi

Nodi inguinales superficiales

Nodus preaorticus

Nodus sacralis medianus

Nodi iliaci interni

Nodi sacrales

Nodus iliacus communis

Nodi iliaci externi

Lymphatic drainage along A. and V. vesicalis inferior to Nodi iliaci interni (principal pathway)

Lymphatic drainage over Vesica urinaria to Nodi iliaci externi

Lymphatic drainage alongside Rectum to Nodi sacrales

Lymphatic drainage from Spatium retropubicum to Nodi iliaci externi (dashed line)

Lymphatic drainage from Prostata

Lymphatic drainage (dashed line) from lower Prostata and Pars membranacea urethrae along A. and V. pudendalis interna (beneath Diaphragma pelvis) to Nodi iliaci interni

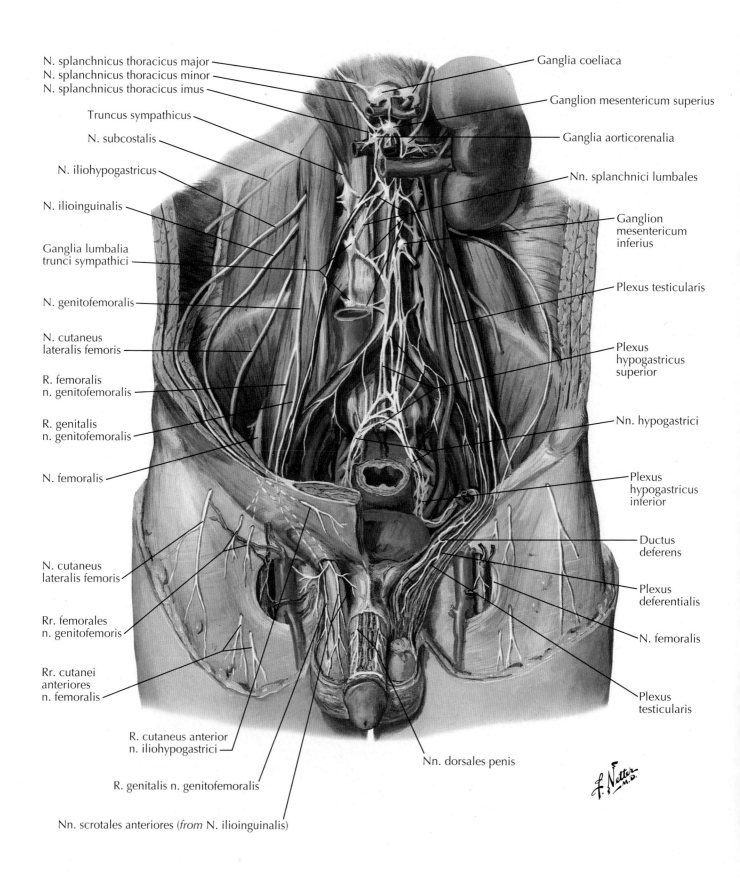

N. splanchnicus thoracicus major
N. splanchnicus thoracicus minor
N. splanchnicus thoracicus imus

Truncus sympathicus

N. subcostalis

N. iliohypogastricus

N. ilioinguinalis

Ganglia lumbalia
trunci sympathici

N. genitofemoralis

N. cutaneus
lateralis femoris

R. femoralis
n. genitofemoralis

R. genitalis
n. genitofemoralis

N. femoralis

N. cutaneus
lateralis femoris

Rr. femorales
n. genitofemoris

Rr. cutanei
anteriores
n. femoralis

R. cutaneus anterior
n. iliohypogastrici

R. genitalis n. genitofemoralis

Nn. scrotales anteriores (*from* N. ilioinguinalis)

Ganglia coeliaca

Ganglion mesentericum superius

Ganglia aorticorenalia

Nn. splanchnici lumbales

Ganglion
mesentericum
inferius

Plexus testicularis

Plexus
hypogastricus
superior

Nn. hypogastrici

Plexus
hypogastricus
inferior

Ductus
deferens

Plexus
deferentialis

N. femoralis

Plexus
testicularis

Nn. dorsales penis

Plate 411

Nervi Perinei and Nervi Viscerales Pelvis

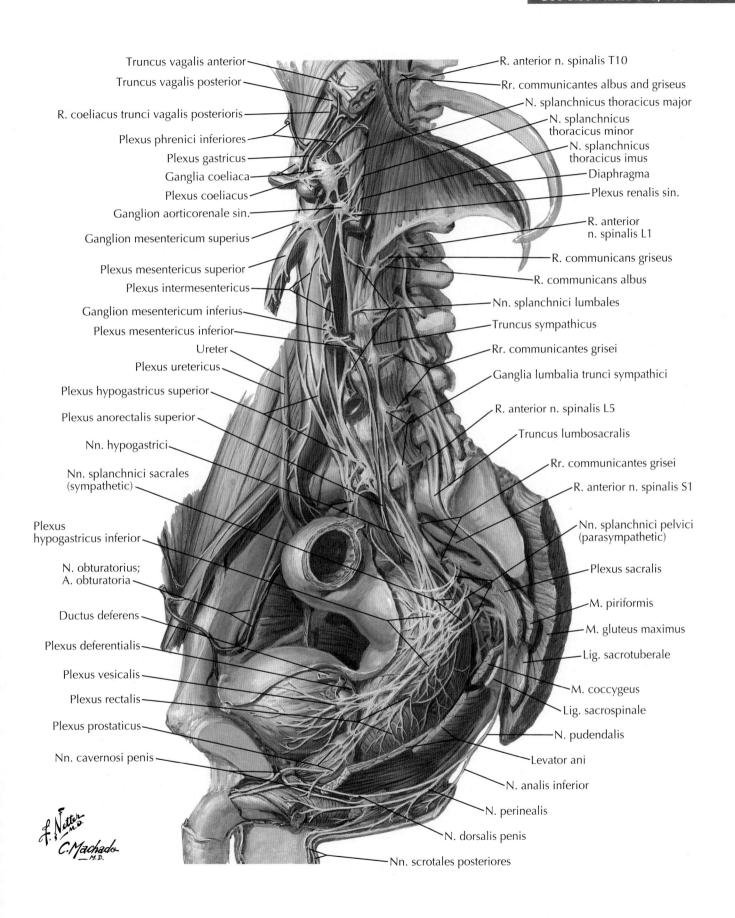

Truncus vagalis anterior
Truncus vagalis posterior
R. coeliacus trunci vagalis posterioris
Plexus phrenici inferiores
Plexus gastricus
Ganglia coeliaca
Plexus coeliacus
Ganglion aorticorenale sin.
Ganglion mesentericum superius
Plexus mesentericus superior
Plexus intermesentericus
Ganglion mesentericum inferius
Plexus mesentericus inferior
Ureter
Plexus uretericus
Plexus hypogastricus superior
Plexus anorectalis superior
Nn. hypogastrici
Nn. splanchnici sacrales (sympathetic)
Plexus hypogastricus inferior
N. obturatorius; A. obturatoria
Ductus deferens
Plexus deferentialis
Plexus vesicalis
Plexus rectalis
Plexus prostaticus
Nn. cavernosi penis

R. anterior n. spinalis T10
Rr. communicantes albus and griseus
N. splanchnicus thoracicus major
N. splanchnicus thoracicus minor
N. splanchnicus thoracicus imus
Diaphragma
Plexus renalis sin.
R. anterior n. spinalis L1
R. communicans griseus
R. communicans albus
Nn. splanchnici lumbales
Truncus sympathicus
Rr. communicantes grisei
Ganglia lumbalia trunci sympathici
R. anterior n. spinalis L5
Truncus lumbosacralis
Rr. communicantes grisei
R. anterior n. spinalis S1
Nn. splanchnici pelvici (parasympathetic)
Plexus sacralis
M. piriformis
M. gluteus maximus
Lig. sacrotuberale
M. coccygeus
Lig. sacrospinale
N. pudendalis
Levator ani
N. analis inferior
N. perinealis
N. dorsalis penis
Nn. scrotales posteriores

Nervi Perinei and Nervi Viscerales Pelvis

Plate 412

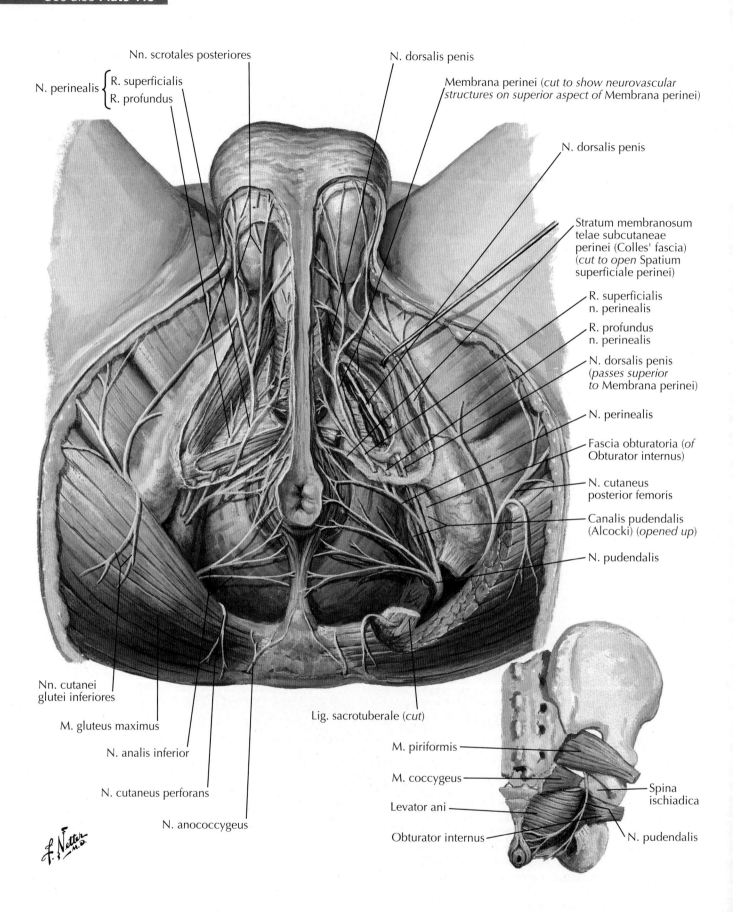

Nn. scrotales posteriores

N. dorsalis penis

N. perinealis { R. superficialis / R. profundus

Membrana perinei (*cut to show neurovascular structures on superior aspect of* Membrana perinei)

N. dorsalis penis

Stratum membranosum telae subcutaneae perinei (Colles' fascia) (*cut to open* Spatium superficiale perinei)

R. superficialis n. perinealis

R. profundus n. perinealis

N. dorsalis penis (*passes superior to* Membrana perinei)

N. perinealis

Fascia obturatoria (*of* Obturator internus)

N. cutaneus posterior femoris

Canalis pudendalis (Alcocki) (*opened up*)

N. pudendalis

Nn. cutanei glutei inferiores

M. gluteus maximus

N. analis inferior

N. cutaneus perforans

N. anococcygeus

Lig. sacrotuberale (*cut*)

M. piriformis

M. coccygeus

Levator ani

Obturator internus

Spina ischiadica

N. pudendalis

Plate 413

Nervi Perinei and Nervi Viscerales Pelvis

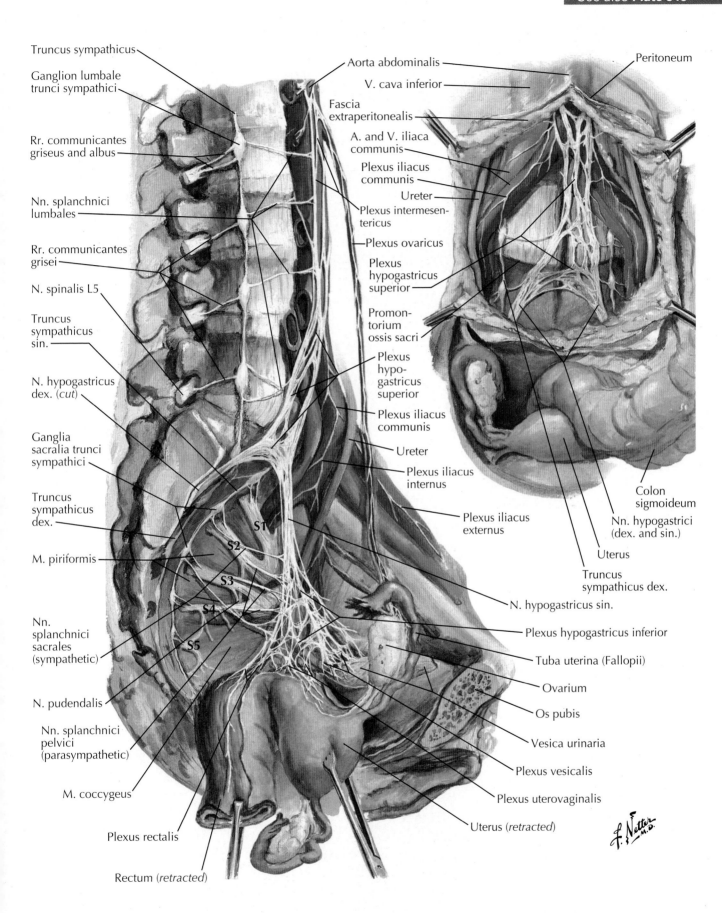

Truncus sympathicus

Ganglion lumbale trunci sympathici

Rr. communicantes griseus and albus

Nn. splanchnici lumbales

Rr. communicantes grisei

N. spinalis L5

Truncus sympathicus sin.

N. hypogastricus dex. (cut)

Ganglia sacralia trunci sympathici

Truncus sympathicus dex.

M. piriformis

Nn. splanchnici sacrales (sympathetic)

N. pudendalis

Nn. splanchnici pelvici (parasympathetic)

M. coccygeus

Plexus rectalis

Rectum (retracted)

Aorta abdominalis

V. cava inferior

Fascia extraperitonealis

A. and V. iliaca communis

Plexus iliacus communis

Ureter

Plexus intermesentericus

Plexus ovaricus

Plexus hypogastricus superior

Promontorium ossis sacri

Plexus hypogastricus superior

Plexus iliacus communis

Ureter

Plexus iliacus internus

Plexus iliacus externus

Peritoneum

Colon sigmoideum

Nn. hypogastrici (dex. and sin.)

Uterus

Truncus sympathicus dex.

N. hypogastricus sin.

Plexus hypogastricus inferior

Tuba uterina (Fallopii)

Ovarium

Os pubis

Vesica urinaria

Plexus vesicalis

Plexus uterovaginalis

Uterus (retracted)

S1
S2
S3
S4
S5

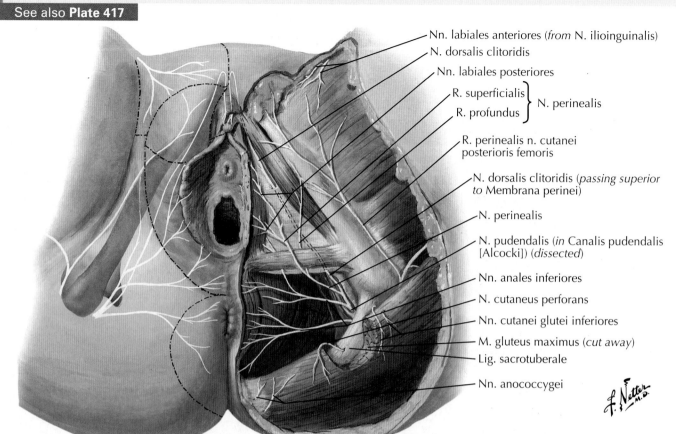

Nn. labiales anteriores (*from* N. ilioinguinalis)

N. dorsalis clitoridis

Nn. labiales posteriores

R. superficialis
R. profundus } N. perinealis

R. perinealis n. cutanei posterioris femoris

N. dorsalis clitoridis (*passing superior to* Membrana perinei)

N. perinealis

N. pudendalis (*in* Canalis pudendalis [Alcocki]) (*dissected*)

Nn. anales inferiores

N. cutaneus perforans

Nn. cutanei glutei inferiores

M. gluteus maximus (*cut away*)

Lig. sacrotuberale

Nn. anococcygei

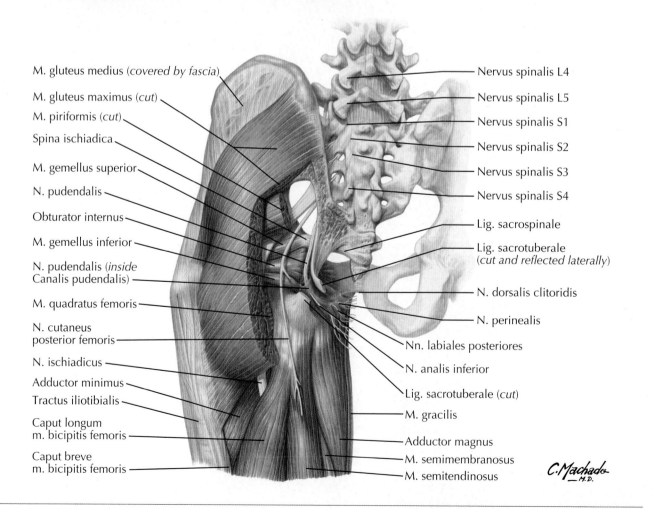

M. gluteus medius (*covered by fascia*)

M. gluteus maximus (*cut*)

M. piriformis (*cut*)

Spina ischiadica

M. gemellus superior

N. pudendalis

Obturator internus

M. gemellus inferior

N. pudendalis (*inside* Canalis pudendalis)

M. quadratus femoris

N. cutaneus posterior femoris

N. ischiadicus

Adductor minimus

Tractus iliotibialis

Caput longum m. bicipitis femoris

Caput breve m. bicipitis femoris

Nervus spinalis L4

Nervus spinalis L5

Nervus spinalis S1

Nervus spinalis S2

Nervus spinalis S3

Nervus spinalis S4

Lig. sacrospinale

Lig. sacrotuberale (*cut and reflected laterally*)

N. dorsalis clitoridis

N. perinealis

Nn. labiales posteriores

N. analis inferior

Lig. sacrotuberale (*cut*)

M. gracilis

Adductor magnus

M. semimembranosus

M. semitendinosus

Plate 415

Nervi Perinei and Nervi Viscerales Pelvis

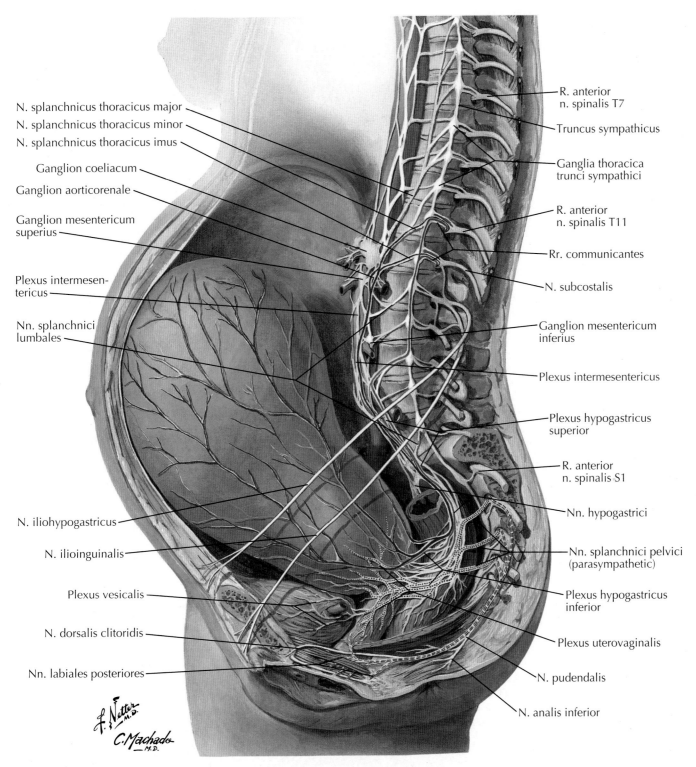

N. splanchnicus thoracicus major
N. splanchnicus thoracicus minor
N. splanchnicus thoracicus imus
Ganglion coeliacum
Ganglion aorticorenale
Ganglion mesentericum superius
Plexus intermesentericus
Nn. splanchnici lumbales
N. iliohypogastricus
N. ilioinguinalis
Plexus vesicalis
N. dorsalis clitoridis
Nn. labiales posteriores

R. anterior n. spinalis T7
Truncus sympathicus
Ganglia thoracica trunci sympathici
R. anterior n. spinalis T11
Rr. communicantes
N. subcostalis
Ganglion mesentericum inferius
Plexus intermesentericus
Plexus hypogastricus superior
R. anterior n. spinalis S1
Nn. hypogastrici
Nn. splanchnici pelvici (parasympathetic)
Plexus hypogastricus inferior
Plexus uterovaginalis
N. pudendalis
N. analis inferior

——— Sensory fibers from Corpus and Fundus uteri accompany sympathetic fibers to lower thoracic part of spinal cord via Plexus hypogastrici

——— Sympathetic fibers to Corpus and Fundus uteri

·········· Sensory fibers from Cervix uteri and upper Vagina accompany parasympathetic fibers to sacral part of spinal cord via Nn. splanchnici pelvici

·········· Parasympathetic fibers to lower Uterus, Cervix uteri, and upper Vagina

– – – – Sensory fibers from lower Vagina and Perineum accompany somatic motor fibers to sacral part of spinal cord via N. pudendalis

– – – – – Somatic motor fibers to lower Vagina and Perineum via N. pudendalis

Nervi Perinei and Nervi Viscerales Pelvis

Plate 416

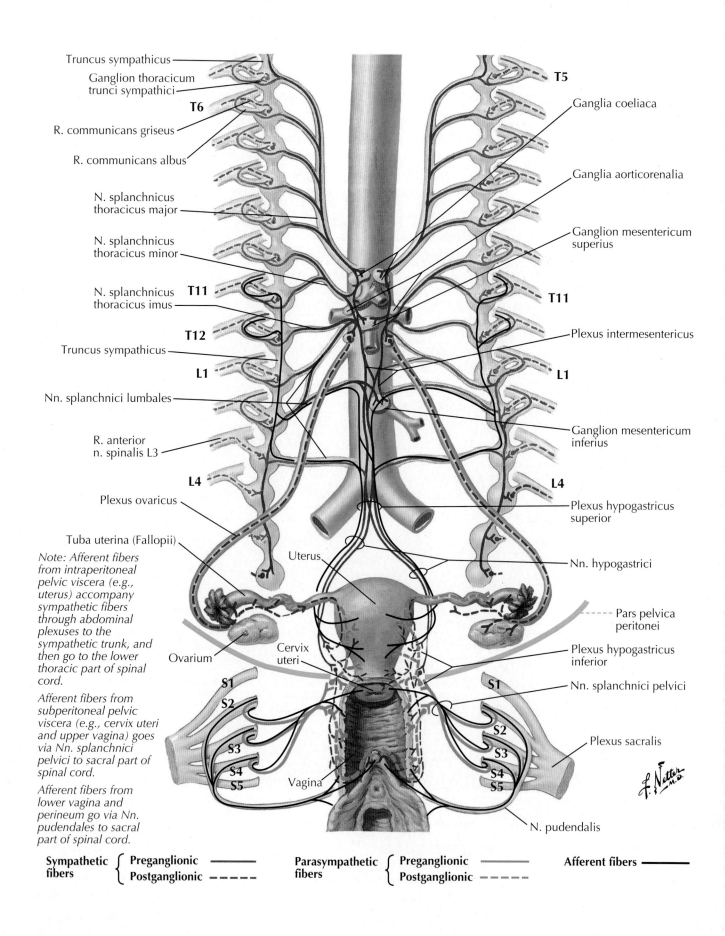

Truncus sympathicus

Ganglion thoracicum
trunci sympathici

T6

R. communicans griseus

R. communicans albus

N. splanchnicus
thoracicus major

N. splanchnicus
thoracicus minor

N. splanchnicus **T11**
thoracicus imus

T12

Truncus sympathicus

L1

Nn. splanchnici lumbales

R. anterior
n. spinalis L3

L4

Plexus ovaricus

Tuba uterina (Fallopii)

*Note: Afferent fibers
from intraperitoneal
pelvic viscera (e.g.,
uterus) accompany
sympathetic fibers
through abdominal
plexuses to the
sympathetic trunk, and
then go to the lower
thoracic part of spinal
cord.*

*Afferent fibers from
subperitoneal pelvic
viscera (e.g., cervix uteri
and upper vagina) goes
via Nn. splanchnici
pelvici to sacral part of
spinal cord.*

*Afferent fibers from
lower vagina and
perineum go via Nn.
pudendales to sacral
part of spinal cord.*

T5

Ganglia coeliaca

Ganglia aorticorenalia

Ganglion mesentericum
superius

T11

Plexus intermesentericus

L1

Ganglion mesentericum
inferius

L4

Plexus hypogastricus
superior

Nn. hypogastrici

Pars pelvica
peritonei

Plexus hypogastricus
inferior

Nn. splanchnici pelvici

Plexus sacralis

Uterus

Cervix
uteri

Ovarium

S1

S2

S3

S4
S5

Vagina

S1

S2

S3

S4
S5

N. pudendalis

| Sympathetic fibers | Preganglionic ——— | Parasympathetic fibers | Preganglionic ——— | Afferent fibers ——— |
| | Postganglionic - - - | | Postganglionic - - - | |

Plate 417

Nervi Perinei and Nervi Viscerales Pelvis

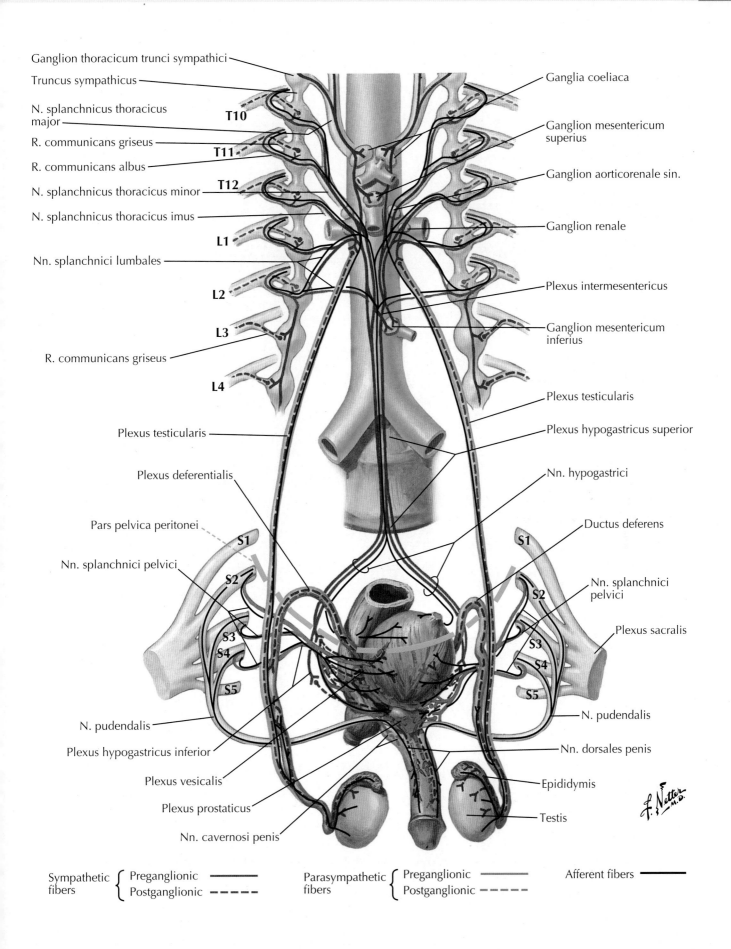

Ganglion thoracicum trunci sympathici

Truncus sympathicus

N. splanchnicus thoracicus major

R. communicans griseus

R. communicans albus

N. splanchnicus thoracicus minor

N. splanchnicus thoracicus imus

Nn. splanchnici lumbales

R. communicans griseus

Plexus testicularis

Plexus deferentialis

Pars pelvica peritonei

Nn. splanchnici pelvici

N. pudendalis

Plexus hypogastricus inferior

Plexus vesicalis

Plexus prostaticus

Nn. cavernosi penis

T10
T11
T12
L1
L2
L3
L4

S1
S2
S3
S4
S5

Ganglia coeliaca

Ganglion mesentericum superius

Ganglion aorticorenale sin.

Ganglion renale

Plexus intermesentericus

Ganglion mesentericum inferius

Plexus testicularis

Plexus hypogastricus superior

Nn. hypogastrici

Ductus deferens

Nn. splanchnici pelvici

Plexus sacralis

N. pudendalis

Nn. dorsales penis

Epididymis

Testis

S1
S2
S3
S4
S5

| Sympathetic fibers | Preganglionic ———— | | Parasympathetic fibers | Preganglionic ———— | Afferent fibers ———— |
| | Postganglionic – – – – | | | Postganglionic – – – – | |

F. Netter M.D.

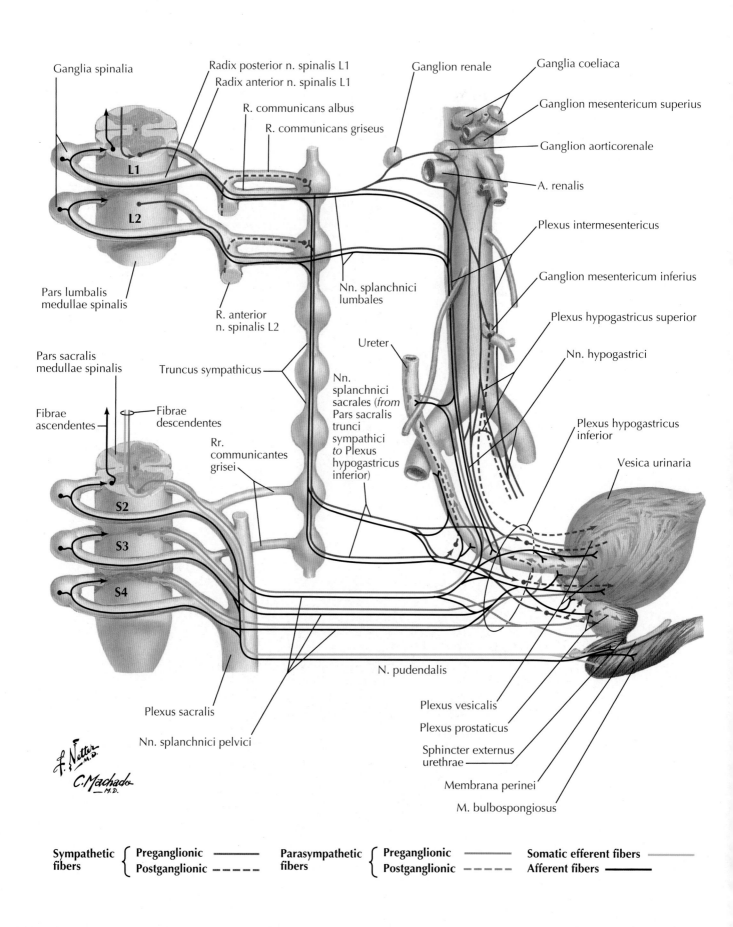

Ganglia spinalia

Radix posterior n. spinalis L1

Radix anterior n. spinalis L1

R. communicans albus

R. communicans griseus

Ganglion renale

Ganglia coeliaca

Ganglion mesentericum superius

Ganglion aorticorenale

A. renalis

Plexus intermesentericus

Ganglion mesentericum inferius

L1

L2

Pars lumbalis medullae spinalis

R. anterior n. spinalis L2

Nn. splanchnici lumbales

Truncus sympathicus

Pars sacralis medullae spinalis

Fibrae ascendentes

Fibrae descendentes

Rr. communicantes grisei

Ureter

Nn. splanchnici sacrales (from Pars sacralis trunci sympathici to Plexus hypogastricus inferior)

Plexus hypogastricus superior

Nn. hypogastrici

Plexus hypogastricus inferior

Vesica urinaria

S2

S3

S4

N. pudendalis

Plexus sacralis

Nn. splanchnici pelvici

Plexus vesicalis

Plexus prostaticus

Sphincter externus urethrae

Membrana perinei

M. bulbospongiosus

| Sympathetic fibers | { Preganglionic ——— Postganglionic - - - - - | Parasympathetic fibers | { Preganglionic ——— Postganglionic - - - - - | Somatic efferent fibers ——— Afferent fibers ——— |

Plate 419

Nervi Perinei and Nervi Viscerales Pelvis

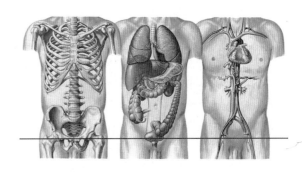

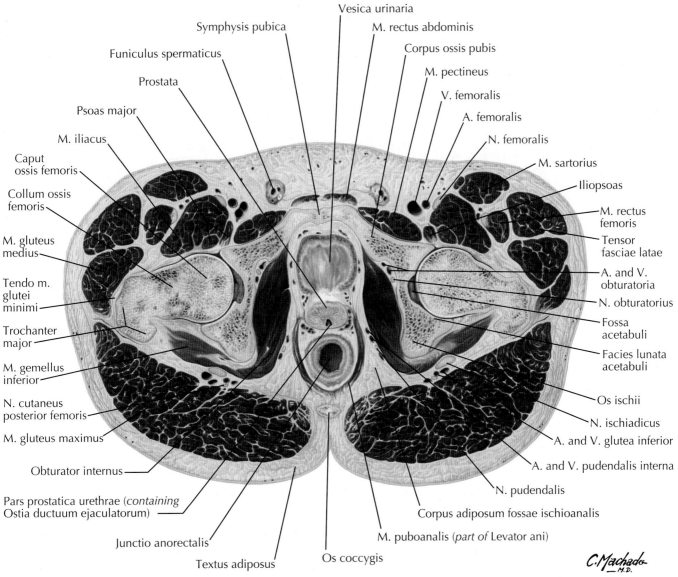

Vesica urinaria

Symphysis pubica

M. rectus abdominis

Funiculus spermaticus

Corpus ossis pubis

Prostata

M. pectineus

Psoas major

V. femoralis

M. iliacus

A. femoralis

Caput ossis femoris

N. femoralis

Collum ossis femoris

M. sartorius

Iliopsoas

M. gluteus medius

M. rectus femoris

Tendo m. glutei minimi

Tensor fasciae latae

Trochanter major

A. and V. obturatoria

M. gemellus inferior

N. obturatorius

N. cutaneus posterior femoris

Fossa acetabuli

M. gluteus maximus

Facies lunata acetabuli

Obturator internus

Os ischii

Pars prostatica urethrae (*containing* Ostia ductuum ejaculatorum)

N. ischiadicus

A. and V. glutea inferior

A. and V. pudendalis interna

Junctio anorectalis

N. pudendalis

Textus adiposus

Corpus adiposum fossae ischioanalis

Os coccygis

M. puboanalis (*part of* Levator ani)

C. Machado
—M.D.

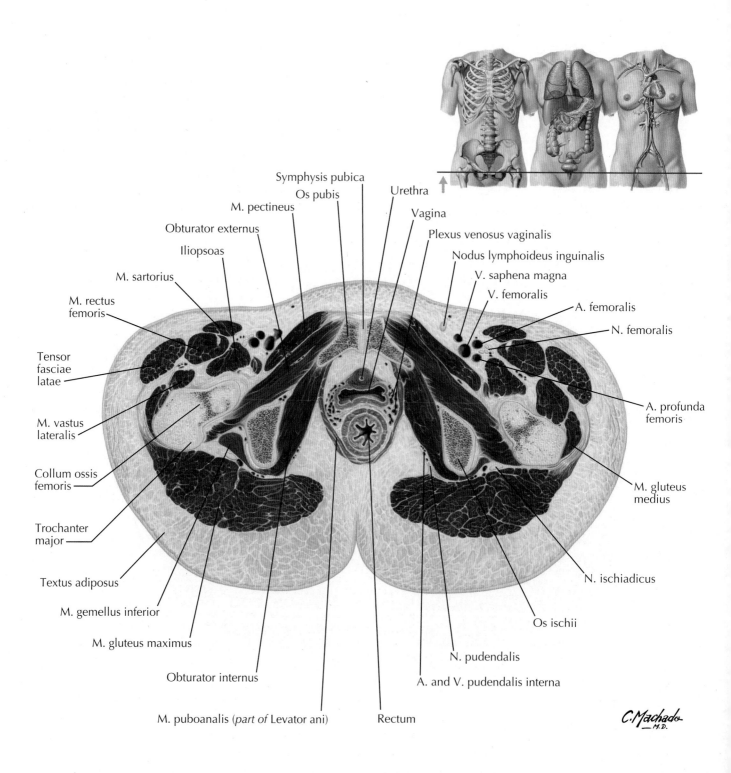

Symphysis pubica

Os pubis

Urethra

M. pectineus

Vagina

Obturator externus

Plexus venosus vaginalis

Iliopsoas

Nodus lymphoideus inguinalis

M. sartorius

V. saphena magna

M. rectus femoris

V. femoralis

A. femoralis

Tensor fasciae latae

N. femoralis

M. vastus lateralis

A. profunda femoris

Collum ossis femoris

M. gluteus medius

Trochanter major

N. ischiadicus

Textus adiposus

Os ischii

M. gemellus inferior

M. gluteus maximus

N. pudendalis

Obturator internus

A. and V. pudendalis interna

M. puboanalis (*part of* Levator ani)

Rectum

Plate 421

Cross-Sectional Anatomy

ANATOMICAL STRUCTURE	CLINICAL COMMENT	PLATE NUMBERS
Systema Nervosum		
N. pudendalis	Pudendal block is performed to anesthetize the perineum for childbirth or minor surgical procedures in the perineum	415
N. analis inferior	Anesthetized in ischioanal fossa for surgical excision of external hemorrhoids	413
Plexus prostaticus; Nn. cavernosi penis	Disruption of these nerves during procedures (e.g., prostate surgery) can produce inability to achieve erection	412
Systema Skeletale		
Symphysis pubica	Palpable landmark used to obtain pelvic measurements (e.g., diagonal conjugate) that may be used to assess adequacy of pelvis for childbirth; during prenatal examinations, used for estimating fetal growth (symphysis–fundal height measurement); injury may result in widening on x-ray	355
Spina ischiadica	Palpable landmark used to estimate interspinous diameter for childbirth and to locate pudendal nerve for pudendal nerve block	355
Tuber ischiadicum	Palpable landmark used to estimate width of pelvic outlet for childbirth; proximal attachment site of hamstring muscles	355
Ramus superior ossis pubis	Often fractured by lateral compression injury of pelvis in anteroposterior plane by crush injury or falls in elderly with osteoporosis	353
Articulatio sacroiliaca	Stiffening, sclerosis, and fusion occur in autoimmune disease known as ankylosing spondylitis; difficult diagnosis to make and known to refer pain to adjacent joints	355
Systema Musculare		
Diaphragma pelvis (levator ani and m. coccygeus)	Provides support to urethrovesical angle, helping to maintain urinary continence; weakness or injury during childbirth can lead to stress urinary incontinence in women	359, 370
Fasciae extraperitoneales pelvis (fasciae endopelvicae)	Weakness or tearing of endopelvic fascial ligaments (e.g., pubovesical or cardinal ligaments) may result in prolapse of pelvic organs	366, 373
Corpus perineale	Tearing of perineal body may occur during childbirth; prophylactic incision into or lateral to perineal body, known as episiotomy, may be performed to facilitate vaginal delivery in some circumstances	379
Systema Cardiovasculare		
Plexus pampiniformis	Dilation of these veins can cause testicular varicocele, affecting testicular temperature regulation and potentially contributing to infertility; most commonly occurs on left side due to longer course of left gonadal vein and angle of drainage into renal vein	403
A. uterina	Ligated or cauterized during hysterectomy; selective embolization of branches may be performed to treat uterine fibroids	402, 406
Aa. profunda penis and dorsalis penis; Corpus cavernosum penis	Blockage or loss of vascular smooth muscle function can lead to erectile dysfunction, treated with vasodilators	407
Venae iliacae internae	Provide communication between prostatic venous plexus and veins draining vertebral column, which is route of spread for prostate cancer	405
Venae anorectales	Portal hypertension may cause dilated anorectal veins if portosystemic anastomoses develop between superior anorectal veins (portal drainage) and middle and/or inferior anorectal veins (systemic drainage)	318, 401
Plexus venosi anorectales internus and externus	Enlargement may result in painful condition known as hemorrhoids	395, 401

Structures with High Clinical Significance   Table 6.1

Vasa Lymphatica and Organa Lymphoidea

Nodi lymphoidei pelvis and lumbales	Spread of ovarian cancer cells via venous drainage to inferior vena cava and lungs or via lymphatics	408
Nodi lymphoidei lumbales and tracheobronchiales	Prostate cancer cells may spread via lymphatics to retroperitoneum and mediastinum	260. 410
Nodi lymphoidei lumbales (e.g., nodi aortici laterales, preaortici and cavales laterales)	Receive lymphatic drainage from ovary, uterine tube, and fundus of uterus in women and from testis in men; cancers in these organs may therefore spread to retroperitoneum	408, 410
Nodi lymphoidei pelvis	Sampling or dissection is performed to assess spread of gynecological malignancies	408

Systema Digestorium

Rectum; canalis analis	Examined by digital rectal examination to detect internal hemorrhoids, fecal impaction, and rectal cancer	301, 393, 395
Peritoneum	Common site for metastatic spread of ovarian cancer via fluid in peritoneal cavity	363, 364

Systema Urinarium

Vesica urinaria	Degree of filling is readily assessed with ultrasound; in patients with poor urine output, this can establish diagnosis of bladder outlet obstruction	368, 369
Ostium ureteris	Abnormal reflux of urine from urinary bladder to ureters (vesicoureteral reflux) may occur in children, contributing to recurrent urinary infections and progressive renal fibrosis	371
Ureter	Enlargement indicates obstruction of ureter or urinary bladder; impaction of renal stone in ureter causes severe pain and, in some cases, hematuria; ureter may be injured during hysterectomy because of its close relationship to uterine artery	335, 336, 402

Systemata Genitalia

Excavatio rectouterina (cavum Douglasi)	Region examined with ultrasound to detect presence of abdominopelvic fluid; common site of ectopic pregnancy; may be accessed via posterior vaginal fornix; normally contains small, physiologic amount of peritoneal fluid	364, 365
Uterus	Site of fetal gestation; palpated during prenatal examinations to assess fetal growth; can also contain large, sometimes painful growths known as leiomyomas (fibroids)	364, 374
Tuba uterina (Fallopii)	Common site of ectopic pregnancy; inflammation (salpingitis) may occur in pelvic inflammatory disease (PID), the result of sexually transmitted infection, possibly leading to fibrosis and infertility; surgical occlusion (tubal ligation) is performed when women desire permanent contraception	363, 364, 375
Cervix uteri	Epithelium of transformation zone of cervix is prone to dysplasia and malignancy; cells are sampled from this region during Pap smear examination and tested for infection with human papillomavirus, the leading risk factor for cervical malignancy	372, 374
Vagina	Posterior part of vaginal fornix allows access to rectouterine pouch (of Douglas)	364
Ovarium	Examined with ultrasound to identify cysts, or for oocyte collection; torsion is painful condition that occurs when ovary twists on axis of suspensory ligament of ovary, occluding ovarian vessels and causing engorgement and ischemia	363, 374, 375
Testis	Torsion is painful condition that occurs when testis twists on axis of testicular vasculature, causing engorgement and ischemia	388
Prostata	Prone to benign hypertrophy with aging, which results in urinary outflow obstruction; prostate cancer is second most common cancer in men	368, 385
Ductus deferens (vas deferens)	Ligation (vasectomy) performed when men desire permanent contraception	368, 388

*Selections were based largely on clinical data and commonly discussed clinical correlations in macroscopic ("gross") anatomy courses.

Table 6.2   **Structures with High Clinical Significance**

MUSCLE	MUSCLE GROUP	ORIGIN ATTACHMENT	INSERTION ATTACHMENT	INNERVATION	BLOOD SUPPLY	MAIN ACTIONS
M. bulbospongiosus	Mm. perinei	*Male*: Corpus perineale *Female*: Corpus perineale	*Male*: Membrana perinei; corpus cavernosum penis; bulbus penis *Female*: Dorsum clitoridis; membrana perinei; bulbus vestibuli; arcus pubicus	N. perinealis	A. perinealis	*Male*: compresses bulb of penis, forces blood into body of penis during erection, propels urine and semen through urethra *Female*: constricts vaginal orifice, assists in expressing secretions of greater vestibular gland, forces blood into body of clitoris
M. coccygeus	Diaphragma pelvis	Spina ischiadica	Pars inferior ossis sacri; os coccygis	N. musculi coccygei	A. glutea inferior	Supports pelvic viscera
Compressor urethrae (female only)	Mm. perinei	Ramus ischiopubicus	Merges with contralateral partner anterior to urethra	N. perinealis	A. perinealis	Sphincter of urethra
Cremaster	Funiculus spermaticus	M. obliquus internus abdominis (inferior edge); lig. inguinale (middle portion)	Tuberculum pubicum; crista pubica	R. genitalis n. genitofemoralis	A. cremasterica	Retracts testis
M. ischiocavernosus	Mm. perinei	Ramus ossis ischii (inferior internal surface); tuber ischiadicum	*Male*: Crus penis (anterior end) *Female*: Crus clitoridis (anterior end)	N. perinealis	A. perinealis	Forces blood into body of penis and clitoris during erection
Levator ani (Mm. iliococcygeus, pubococcygeus, and puboanalis)	Diaphragma pelvis	Corpus ossis pubis; arcus tendineus levatoris ani (on fascia obturatoria); spina ischiadica	Corpus perineale; os coccygis; Raphe diaphragmatis pelvis; prostata or vagina; junctio anorectalis	Nn. levatoris ani and perinealis	A. glutea inferior; A. pudendalis interna and its branches (Aa. anorectalis inferior and perinealis)	Supports pelvic viscera, elevates pelvic floor
Sphincter externus ani	Mm. perinei	Lig. anococcygeum	Corpus perineale	Nn. perinealis and analis inferior	Aa. anorectalis inferior and perinealis	Closes anal orifice
Sphincter externus urethrae	Mm. perinei	Ramus ischiopubicus	*Male*: Median raphe in front and behind urethra *Female*: encloses urethra, attaches to sides of vagina	N. perinealis	A. perinealis	Compresses urethra at end of micturition; in female also compresses distal vagina
Sphincter urethrovaginalis (female only)	Mm. perinei	Corpus perineale	Passes anteriorly around urethra and merges with its contralateral partner	N. perinealis	A. perinealis	Sphincter of urethra and vagina
M. transversus profundus perinei	Mm. perinei	Ramus ossis ischii (internal surface); tuber ischiadicum	Corpus perineale	N. perinealis	A. perinealis	Stabilizes perineal body, supports prostate/vagina
M. transversus superficialis perinei	Mm. perinei	Ramus ossis ischii; tuber ischiadicum	Corpus perineale	N. perinealis	A. perinealis	Stabilizes perineal body

Variations in spinal nerve contributions to the innervation of muscles, their arterial supply, their attachments, and their actions are common themes in human anatomy. Therefore, expect differences between texts and realize that anatomical variation is normal.

MEMBRUM SUPERIUS 7

Surface Anatomy	422–426	**Regional Imaging**	490
Omos and Axilla	427–439	**Structures with High**	
Brachium	440–445	**Clinical Significance**	Tables 7.1–7.2
Cubitus and Antebrachium	446–461	**Nervi Plexus Brachialis**	Tables 7.3–7.5
Carpus and Manus	462–481	**Musculi**	Tables 7.6–7.8
Nervi	482–489	**Electronic Bonus Plates**	BP 96–BP 102

ELECTRONIC BONUS PLATES

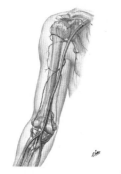

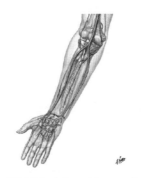

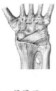

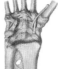

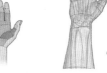

BP 96 Brachium: Arteriae

BP 97 Antebrachium and Manus: Arteriae

BP 98 Ligamenta Carpi: Posterior and Anterior Views

BP 99 Flexor and Extensor Zones of Hand

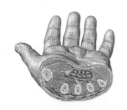

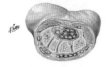

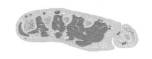

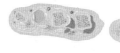

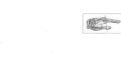

BP 100 Cross Sections Through Ossa Metacarpi and Carpi

BP 101 Cross Section of Manus: Axial View

BP 102 Cross Section of Manus: Axial View (Continued)

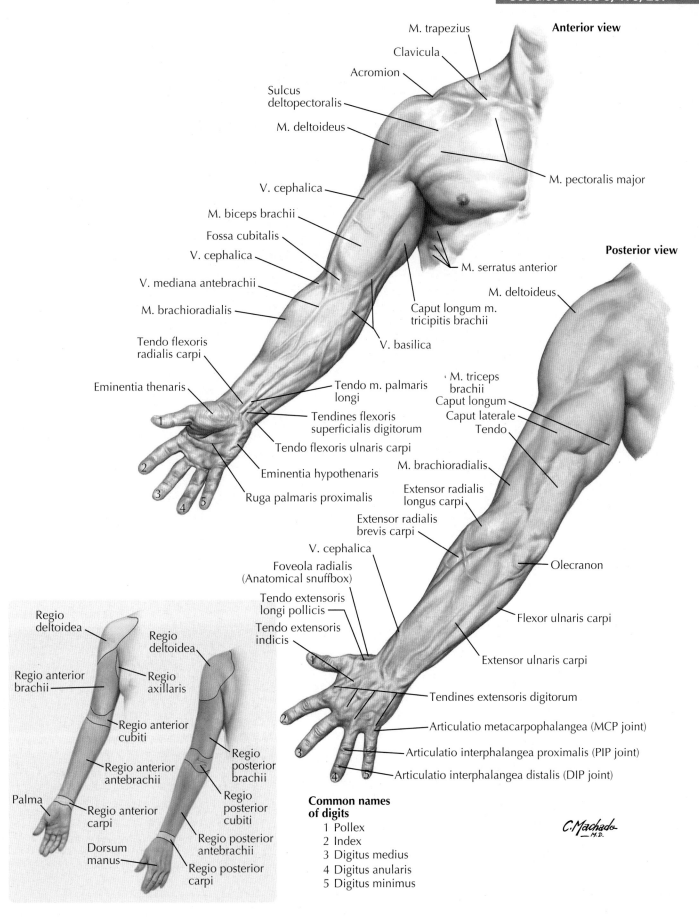

Anterior view

M. trapezius

Clavicula

Acromion

Sulcus deltopectoralis

M. deltoideus

V. cephalica

M. biceps brachii

Fossa cubitalis

V. cephalica

V. mediana antebrachii

M. brachioradialis

Tendo flexoris radialis carpi

Eminentia thenaris

Tendo m. palmaris longi

Tendines flexoris superficialis digitorum

Tendo flexoris ulnaris carpi

Eminentia hypothenaris

Ruga palmaris proximalis

1
2
3
4 5

M. pectoralis major

M. serratus anterior

Caput longum m. tricipitis brachii

V. basilica

Posterior view

M. deltoideus

M. triceps brachii

Caput longum

Caput laterale

Tendo

M. brachioradialis

Extensor radialis longus carpi

Extensor radialis brevis carpi

V. cephalica

Foveola radialis (Anatomical snuffbox)

Tendo extensoris longi pollicis

Tendo extensoris indicis

Olecranon

Flexor ulnaris carpi

Extensor ulnaris carpi

Tendines extensoris digitorum

Articulatio metacarpophalangea (MCP joint)

Articulatio interphalangea proximalis (PIP joint)

Articulatio interphalangea distalis (DIP joint)

1
2
3
4 5

Common names of digits
1 Pollex
2 Index
3 Digitus medius
4 Digitus anularis
5 Digitus minimus

Regio deltoidea

Regio deltoidea

Regio anterior brachii

Regio axillaris

Regio anterior cubiti

Regio anterior antebrachii

Regio posterior brachii

Regio posterior cubiti

Palma

Regio anterior carpi

Dorsum manus

Regio posterior antebrachii

Regio posterior carpi

C. Machado
M.D.

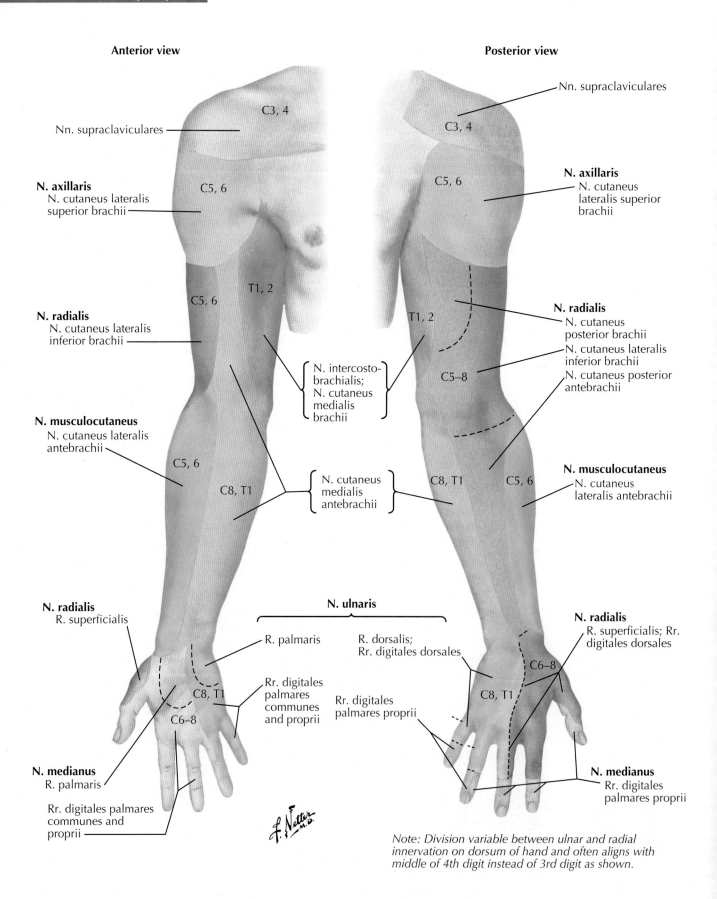

Anterior view

Nn. supraclaviculares

C3, 4

N. axillaris
N. cutaneus lateralis superior brachii

C5, 6

C5, 6

T1, 2

N. radialis
N. cutaneus lateralis inferior brachii

N. intercosto-brachialis;
N. cutaneus medialis brachii

N. musculocutaneus
N. cutaneus lateralis antebrachii

C5, 6

C8, T1

N. cutaneus medialis antebrachii

N. radialis
R. superficialis

N. ulnaris

R. palmaris

R. dorsalis;
Rr. digitales dorsales

C8, T1

C6–8

Rr. digitales palmares communes and proprii

N. medianus
R. palmaris

Rr. digitales palmares communes and proprii

Posterior view

Nn. supraclaviculares

C3, 4

N. axillaris
N. cutaneus lateralis superior brachii

C5, 6

T1, 2

N. radialis
N. cutaneus posterior brachii
N. cutaneus lateralis inferior brachii
N. cutaneus posterior antebrachii

C5–8

N. musculocutaneus
N. cutaneus lateralis antebrachii

C8, T1

C5, 6

N. radialis
R. superficialis; Rr. digitales dorsales

C6–8

C8, T1

Rr. digitales palmares proprii

N. medianus
Rr. digitales palmares proprii

Note: Division variable between ulnar and radial innervation on dorsum of hand and often aligns with middle of 4th digit instead of 3rd digit as shown.

Plate 423

Surface Anatomy

Anterior view

Posterior view

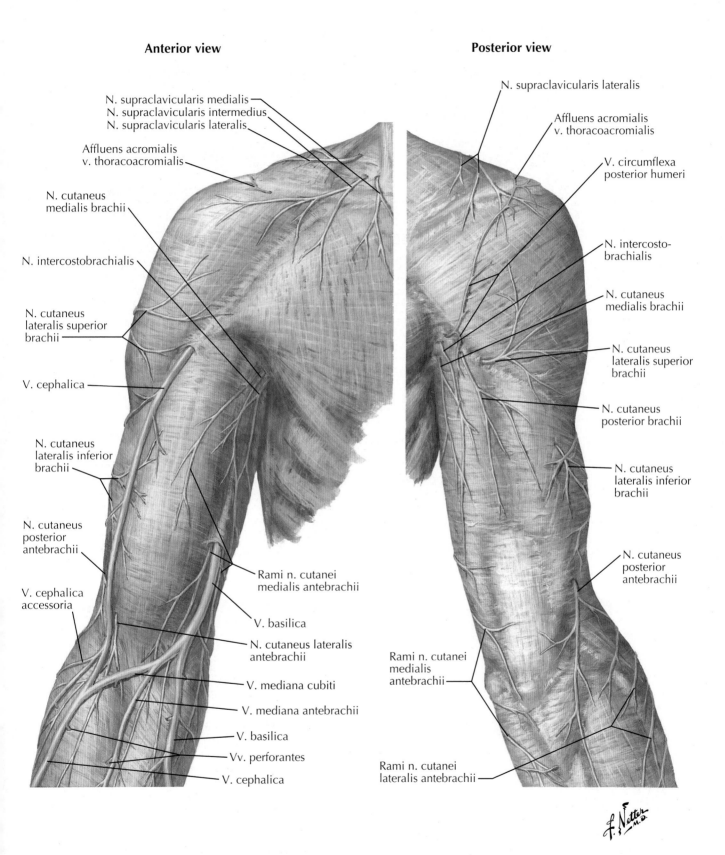

N. supraclavicularis medialis
N. supraclavicularis intermedius
N. supraclavicularis lateralis

Affluens acromialis
v. thoracoacromialis

N. cutaneus
medialis brachii

N. intercostobrachialis

N. cutaneus
lateralis superior
brachii

V. cephalica

N. cutaneus
lateralis inferior
brachii

N. cutaneus
posterior
antebrachii

V. cephalica
accessoria

Rami n. cutanei
medialis antebrachii

V. basilica

N. cutaneus lateralis
antebrachii

V. mediana cubiti

V. mediana antebrachii

V. basilica

Vv. perforantes

V. cephalica

N. supraclavicularis lateralis

Affluens acromialis
v. thoracoacromialis

V. circumflexa
posterior humeri

N. intercosto-
brachialis

N. cutaneus
medialis brachii

N. cutaneus
lateralis superior
brachii

N. cutaneus
posterior brachii

N. cutaneus
lateralis inferior
brachii

N. cutaneus
posterior
antebrachii

Rami n. cutanei
medialis
antebrachii

Rami n. cutanei
lateralis antebrachii

Surface Anatomy

Plate 424

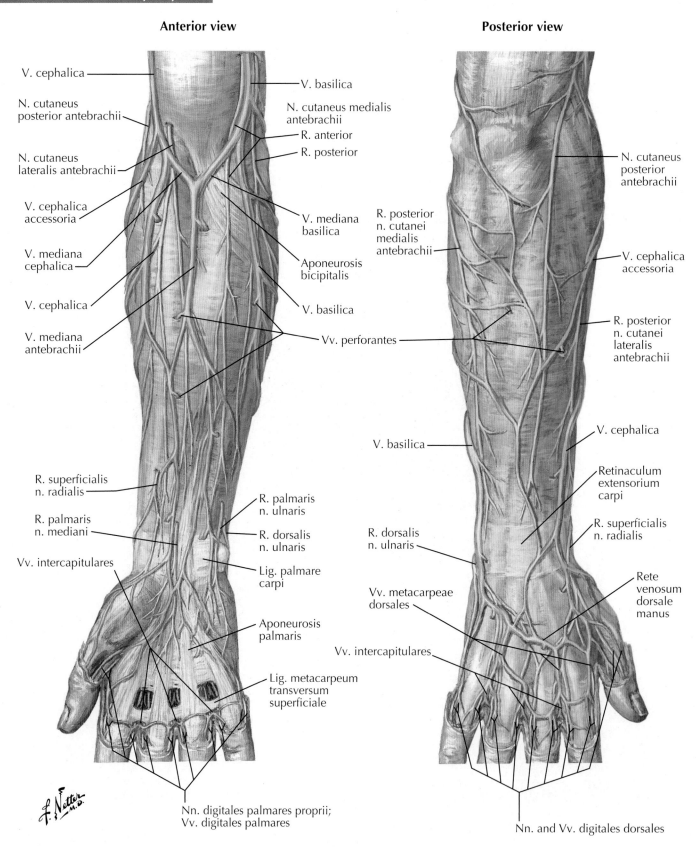

Anterior view

Posterior view

V. cephalica

N. cutaneus posterior antebrachii

N. cutaneus lateralis antebrachii

V. cephalica accessoria

V. mediana cephalica

V. cephalica

V. mediana antebrachii

R. superficialis n. radialis

R. palmaris n. mediani

Vv. intercapitulares

V. basilica

N. cutaneus medialis antebrachii

R. anterior

R. posterior

V. mediana basilica

Aponeurosis bicipitalis

V. basilica

Vv. perforantes

R. palmaris n. ulnaris

R. dorsalis n. ulnaris

Lig. palmare carpi

Aponeurosis palmaris

Lig. metacarpeum transversum superficiale

Nn. digitales palmares proprii; Vv. digitales palmares

N. cutaneus posterior antebrachii

R. posterior n. cutanei medialis antebrachii

V. cephalica accessoria

R. posterior n. cutanei lateralis antebrachii

V. basilica

V. cephalica

Retinaculum extensorium carpi

R. superficialis n. radialis

R. dorsalis n. ulnaris

Vv. metacarpeae dorsales

Vv. intercapitulares

Rete venosum dorsale manus

Nn. and Vv. digitales dorsales

Note: In 70% of cases, a median cubital vein (a tributary to the basilic vein) replaces the median cephalic and median basilic veins (see Plate 424).

Plate 425

Surface Anatomy

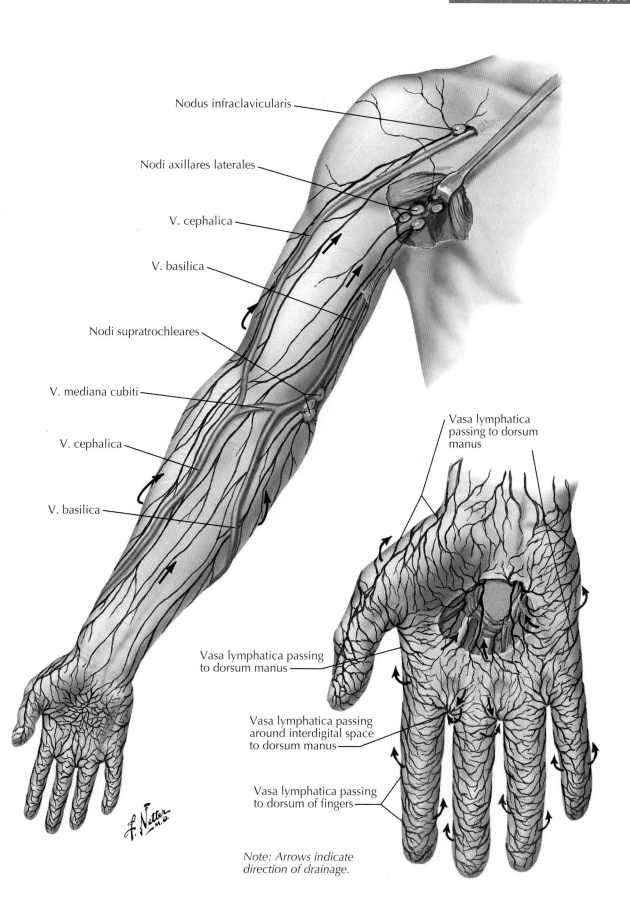

Nodus infraclavicularis

Nodi axillares laterales

V. cephalica

V. basilica

Nodi supratrochleares

V. mediana cubiti

V. cephalica

V. basilica

Vasa lymphatica passing to dorsum manus

Vasa lymphatica passing to dorsum manus

Vasa lymphatica passing around interdigital space to dorsum manus

Vasa lymphatica passing to dorsum of fingers

Note: Arrows indicate direction of drainage.

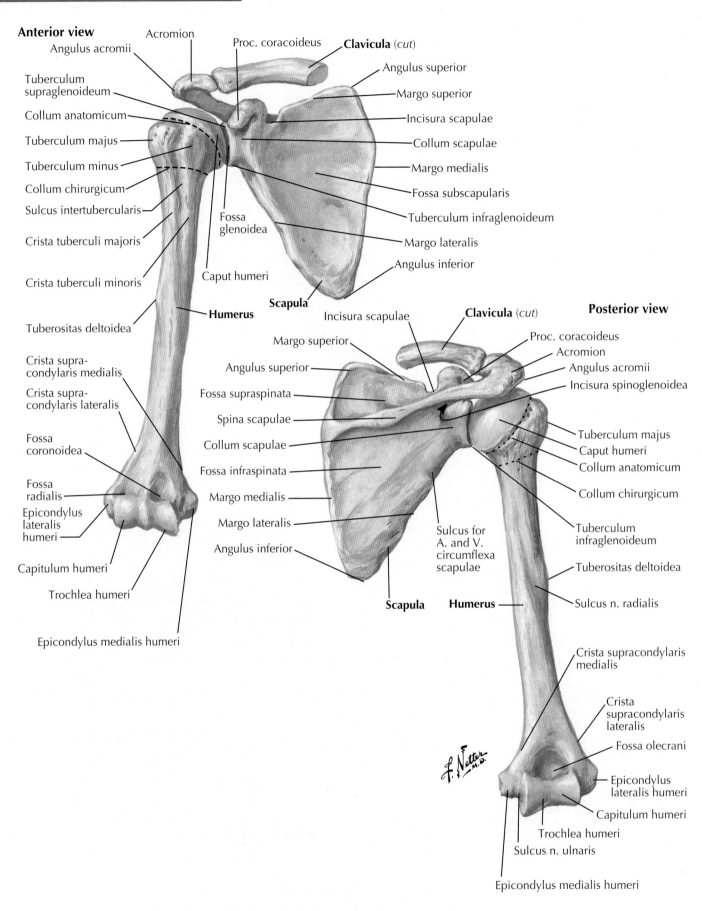

Anterior view

Angulus acromii

Acromion

Tuberculum supraglenoideum

Collum anatomicum

Tuberculum majus

Tuberculum minus

Collum chirurgicum

Sulcus intertubercularis

Crista tuberculi majoris

Crista tuberculi minoris

Tuberositas deltoidea

Crista supra-condylaris medialis

Crista supra-condylaris lateralis

Fossa coronoidea

Fossa radialis

Epicondylus lateralis humeri

Capitulum humeri

Trochlea humeri

Epicondylus medialis humeri

Proc. coracoideus

Clavicula (*cut*)

Angulus superior

Margo superior

Incisura scapulae

Collum scapulae

Margo medialis

Fossa subscapularis

Tuberculum infraglenoideum

Margo lateralis

Angulus inferior

Fossa glenoidea

Caput humeri

Humerus

Scapula

Incisura scapulae

Margo superior

Angulus superior

Fossa supraspinata

Spina scapulae

Collum scapulae

Fossa infraspinata

Margo medialis

Margo lateralis

Angulus inferior

Clavicula (*cut*)

Posterior view

Proc. coracoideus

Acromion

Angulus acromii

Incisura spinoglenoidea

Tuberculum majus

Caput humeri

Collum anatomicum

Collum chirurgicum

Tuberculum infraglenoideum

Tuberositas deltoidea

Sulcus n. radialis

Sulcus for A. and V. circumflexa scapulae

Scapula

Humerus

Crista supracondylaris medialis

Crista supracondylaris lateralis

Fossa olecrani

Epicondylus lateralis humeri

Capitulum humeri

Trochlea humeri

Sulcus n. ulnaris

Epicondylus medialis humeri

Plate 427

Omos and Axilla

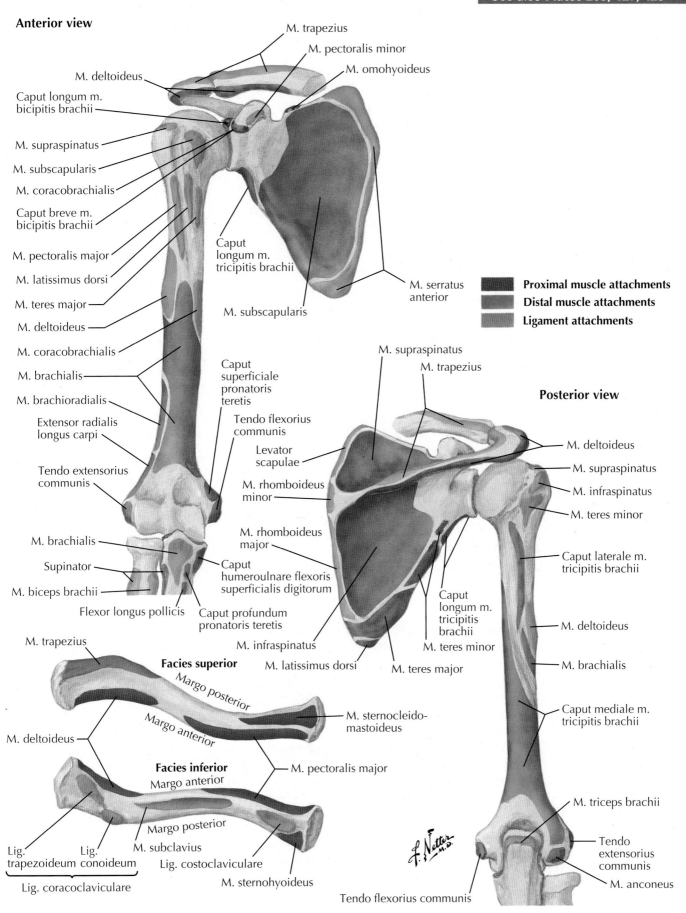

Anterior view

M. trapezius
M. pectoralis minor
M. omohyoideus
M. deltoideus
Caput longum m. bicipitis brachii
M. supraspinatus
M. subscapularis
M. coracobrachialis
Caput breve m. bicipitis brachii
M. pectoralis major
M. latissimus dorsi
M. teres major
M. deltoideus
M. coracobrachialis
M. brachialis
M. brachioradialis
Extensor radialis longus carpi
Tendo extensorius communis
M. brachialis
Supinator
M. biceps brachii
Flexor longus pollicis

Caput longum m. tricipitis brachii
M. subscapularis
M. serratus anterior

Caput superficiale pronatoris teretis
Tendo flexorius communis
Levator scapulae
M. rhomboideus minor
M. rhomboideus major
Caput humeroulnare flexoris superficialis digitorum
Caput profundum pronatoris teretis
M. infraspinatus
M. latissimus dorsi

Proximal muscle attachments
Distal muscle attachments
Ligament attachments

M. supraspinatus
M. trapezius

Posterior view

M. deltoideus
M. supraspinatus
M. infraspinatus
M. teres minor
Caput laterale m. tricipitis brachii
Caput longum m. tricipitis brachii
M. teres minor
M. teres major
M. deltoideus
M. brachialis
Caput mediale m. tricipitis brachii
M. triceps brachii
Tendo extensorius communis
M. anconeus

M. trapezius
Facies superior
Margo posterior
Margo anterior
M. deltoideus
Facies inferior
Margo anterior
Margo posterior
M. subclavius
Lig. trapezoideum
Lig. conoideum
Lig. coracoclaviculare
Lig. costoclaviculare
M. sternohyoideus
M. sternocleido-mastoideus
M. pectoralis major
Tendo flexorius communis

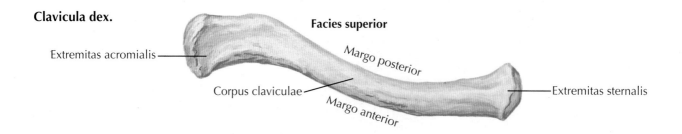

Clavicula dex.

Facies superior

Extremitas acromialis

Margo posterior

Corpus claviculae

Extremitas sternalis

Margo anterior

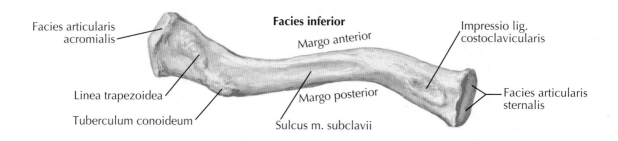

Facies inferior

Facies articularis acromialis

Margo anterior

Impressio lig. costoclavicularis

Linea trapezoidea

Margo posterior

Facies articularis sternalis

Tuberculum conoideum

Sulcus m. subclavii

Articulatio sternoclavicularis

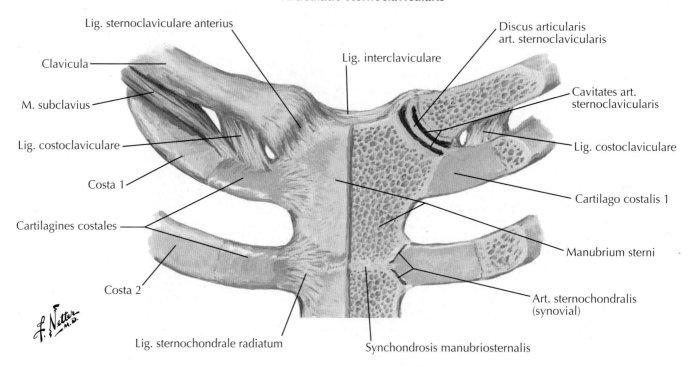

Lig. sternoclaviculare anterius

Lig. interclaviculare

Discus articularis art. sternoclavicularis

Clavicula

Cavitates art. sternoclavicularis

M. subclavius

Lig. costoclaviculare

Lig. costoclaviculare

Costa 1

Cartilago costalis 1

Cartilagines costales

Manubrium sterni

Costa 2

Art. sternochondralis (synovial)

Lig. sternochondrale radiatum

Synchondrosis manubriosternalis

Plate 429

Omos and Axilla

Anteroposterior radiograph of right shoulder

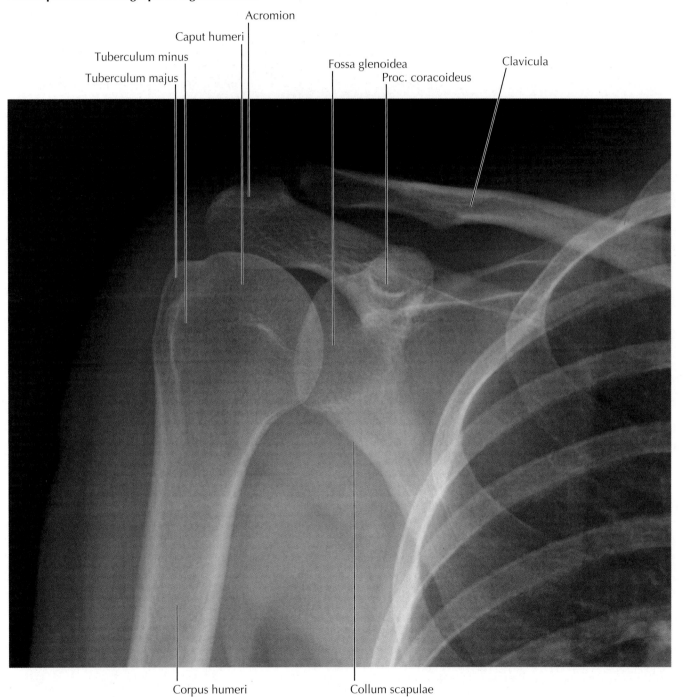

Acromion

Caput humeri

Tuberculum minus

Tuberculum majus

Fossa glenoidea

Proc. coracoideus

Clavicula

Corpus humeri

Collum scapulae

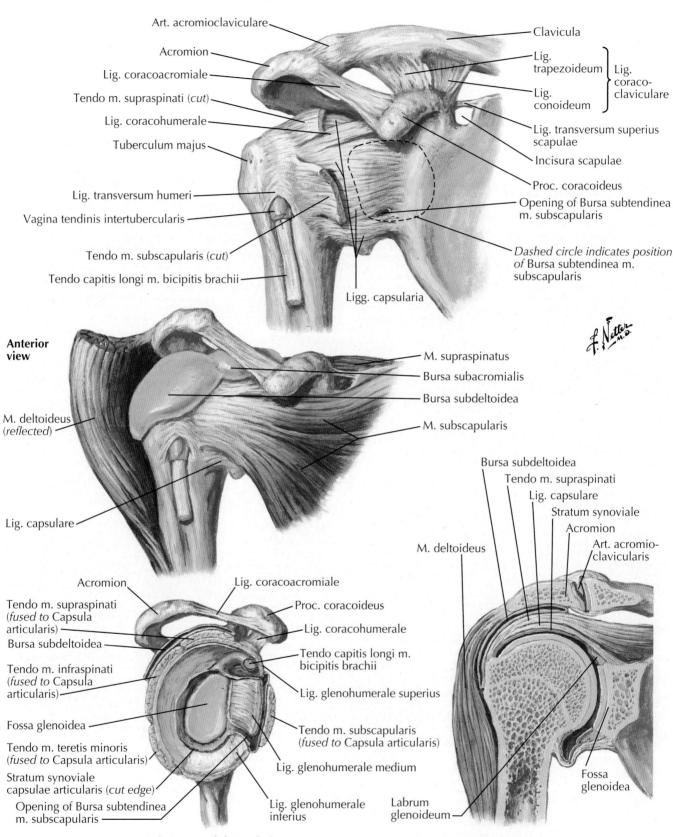

Anterior view

Art. acromioclaviculare

Acromion

Lig. coracoacromiale

Tendo m. supraspinati (*cut*)

Lig. coracohumerale

Tuberculum majus

Lig. transversum humeri

Vagina tendinis intertubercularis

Tendo m. subscapularis (*cut*)

Tendo capitis longi m. bicipitis brachii

Clavicula

Lig. trapezoideum

Lig. coraco-claviculare

Lig. conoideum

Lig. transversum superius scapulae

Incisura scapulae

Proc. coracoideus

Opening of Bursa subtendinea m. subscapularis

Dashed circle indicates position of Bursa subtendinea m. subscapularis

Ligg. capsularia

Anterior view

M. deltoideus (*reflected*)

Lig. capsulare

M. supraspinatus

Bursa subacromialis

Bursa subdeltoidea

M. subscapularis

Bursa subdeltoidea

Tendo m. supraspinati

Lig. capsulare

Stratum synoviale

Acromion

Art. acromio-clavicularis

M. deltoideus

Fossa glenoidea

Labrum glenoideum

Acromion

Tendo m. supraspinati (*fused to* Capsula articularis)

Bursa subdeltoidea

Tendo m. infraspinati (*fused to* Capsula articularis)

Fossa glenoidea

Tendo m. teretis minoris (*fused to* Capsula articularis)

Stratum synoviale capsulae articularis (*cut edge*)

Opening of Bursa subtendinea m. subscapularis

Lig. coracoacromiale

Proc. coracoideus

Lig. coracohumerale

Tendo capitis longi m. bicipitis brachii

Lig. glenohumerale superius

Tendo m. subscapularis (*fused to* Capsula articularis)

Lig. glenohumerale medium

Lig. glenohumerale inferius

Joint opened: lateral view

Coronal section through shoulder girdle

Plate 431

Omos and Axilla

See also **Plates 195, 209**

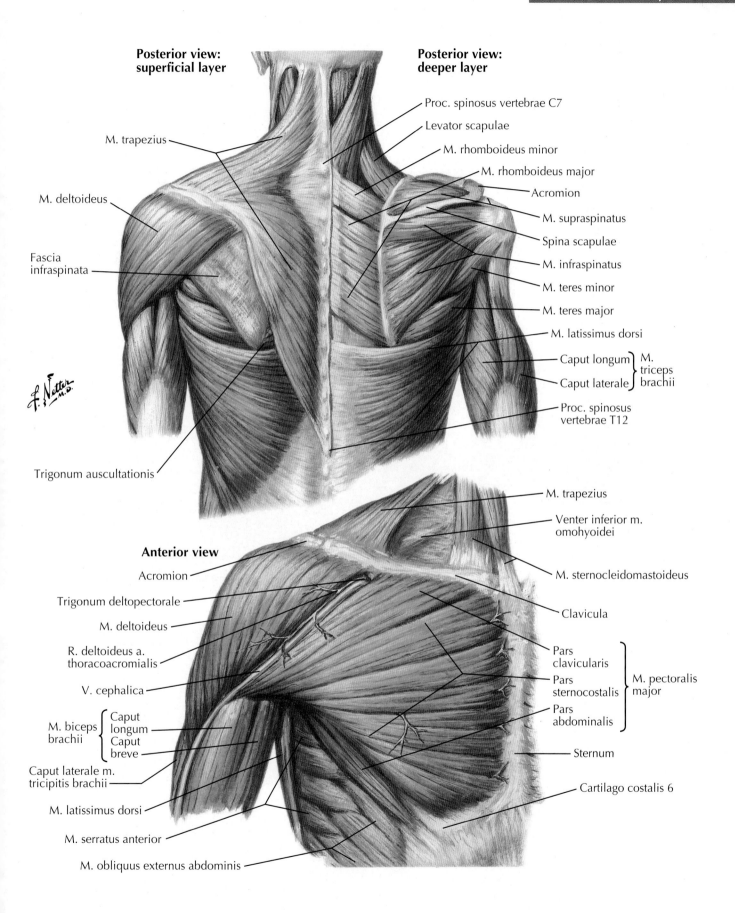

Posterior view: superficial layer

M. trapezius

M. deltoideus

Fascia infraspinata

Trigonum auscultationis

Posterior view: deeper layer

Proc. spinosus vertebrae C7

Levator scapulae

M. rhomboideus minor

M. rhomboideus major

Acromion

M. supraspinatus

Spina scapulae

M. infraspinatus

M. teres minor

M. teres major

M. latissimus dorsi

Caput longum ⎫ M.
Caput laterale ⎬ triceps
               ⎭ brachii

Proc. spinosus vertebrae T12

M. trapezius

Venter inferior m. omohyoidei

M. sternocleidomastoideus

Anterior view

Acromion

Trigonum deltopectorale

M. deltoideus

R. deltoideus a. thoracoacromialis

V. cephalica

M. biceps brachii ⎰ Caput longum
                   ⎱ Caput breve

Caput laterale m. tricipitis brachii

M. latissimus dorsi

M. serratus anterior

M. obliquus externus abdominis

Clavicula

Pars clavicularis ⎫
Pars sternocostalis ⎬ M. pectoralis major
Pars abdominalis ⎭

Sternum

Cartilago costalis 6

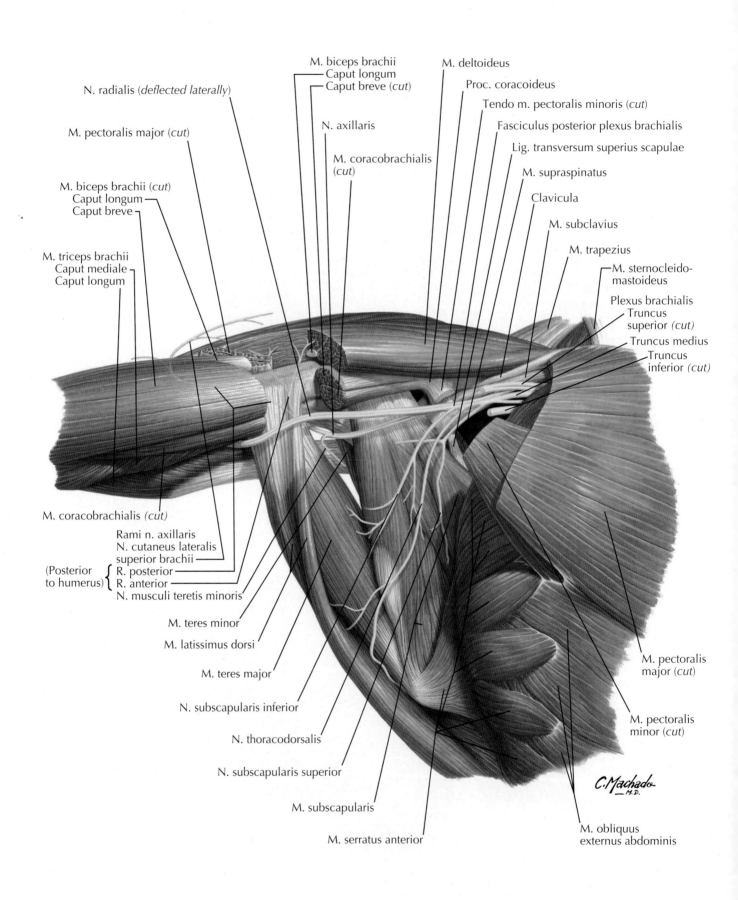

N. radialis (*deflected laterally*)

M. pectoralis major (*cut*)

M. biceps brachii (*cut*)
Caput longum
Caput breve

M. triceps brachii
Caput mediale
Caput longum

M. biceps brachii
Caput longum
Caput breve (*cut*)

N. axillaris

M. coracobrachialis
(*cut*)

M. deltoideus

Proc. coracoideus

Tendo m. pectoralis minoris (*cut*)

Fasciculus posterior plexus brachialis

Lig. transversum superius scapulae

M. supraspinatus

Clavicula

M. subclavius

M. trapezius

M. sternocleido-
mastoideus

Plexus brachialis
Truncus
superior (*cut*)

Truncus medius

Truncus
inferior (*cut*)

M. coracobrachialis (*cut*)

Rami n. axillaris
N. cutaneus lateralis
superior brachii

(Posterior
to humerus) { R. posterior
R. anterior
N. musculi teretis minoris

M. teres minor

M. latissimus dorsi

M. teres major

N. subscapularis inferior

N. thoracodorsalis

N. subscapularis superior

M. subscapularis

M. serratus anterior

M. pectoralis
major (*cut*)

M. pectoralis
minor (*cut*)

M. obliquus
externus abdominis

C. Machado
M.D.

Plate 433

Omos and Axilla

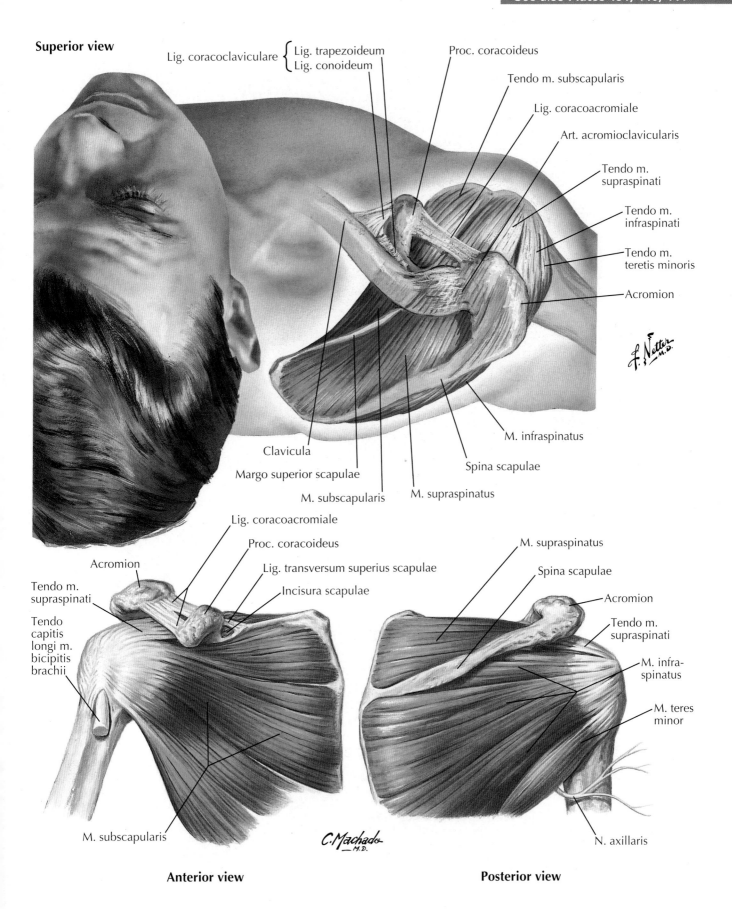

Superior view

Lig. coracoclaviculare { Lig. trapezoideum / Lig. conoideum

Proc. coracoideus

Tendo m. subscapularis

Lig. coracoacromiale

Art. acromioclavicularis

Tendo m. supraspinati

Tendo m. infraspinati

Tendo m. teretis minoris

Acromion

M. infraspinatus

Spina scapulae

M. supraspinatus

M. subscapularis

Margo superior scapulae

Clavicula

Acromion

Tendo m. supraspinati

Tendo capitis longi m. bicipitis brachii

Lig. coracoacromiale

Proc. coracoideus

Lig. transversum superius scapulae

Incisura scapulae

M. subscapularis

Anterior view

M. supraspinatus

Spina scapulae

Acromion

Tendo m. supraspinati

M. infra-spinatus

M. teres minor

N. axillaris

Posterior view

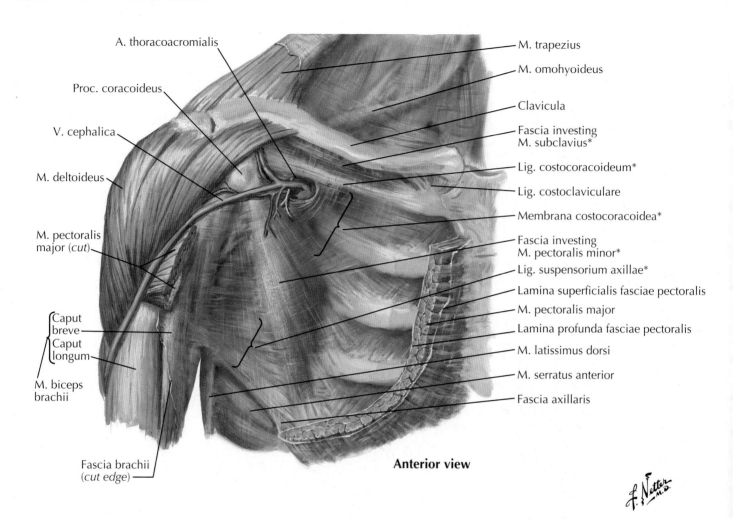

A. thoracoacromialis

Proc. coracoideus

V. cephalica

M. deltoideus

M. pectoralis major (*cut*)

Caput breve
Caput longum
M. biceps brachii

Fascia brachii (*cut edge*)

M. trapezius

M. omohyoideus

Clavicula

Fascia investing M. subclavius*

Lig. costocoracoideum*

Lig. costoclaviculare

Membrana costocoracoidea*

Fascia investing M. pectoralis minor*

Lig. suspensorium axillae*

Lamina superficialis fasciae pectoralis

M. pectoralis major

Lamina profunda fasciae pectoralis

M. latissimus dorsi

M. serratus anterior

Fascia axillaris

Anterior view

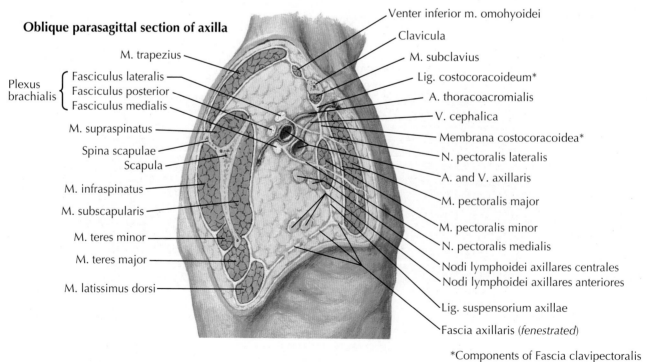

Oblique parasagittal section of axilla

M. trapezius

Plexus brachialis
Fasciculus lateralis
Fasciculus posterior
Fasciculus medialis

M. supraspinatus

Spina scapulae

Scapula

M. infraspinatus

M. subscapularis

M. teres minor

M. teres major

M. latissimus dorsi

Venter inferior m. omohyoidei

Clavicula

M. subclavius

Lig. costocoracoideum*

A. thoracoacromialis

V. cephalica

Membrana costocoracoidea*

N. pectoralis lateralis

A. and V. axillaris

M. pectoralis major

M. pectoralis minor

N. pectoralis medialis

Nodi lymphoidei axillares centrales

Nodi lymphoidei axillares anteriores

Lig. suspensorium axillae

Fascia axillaris (*fenestrated*)

*Components of Fascia clavipectoralis

Plate 435

Omos and Axilla

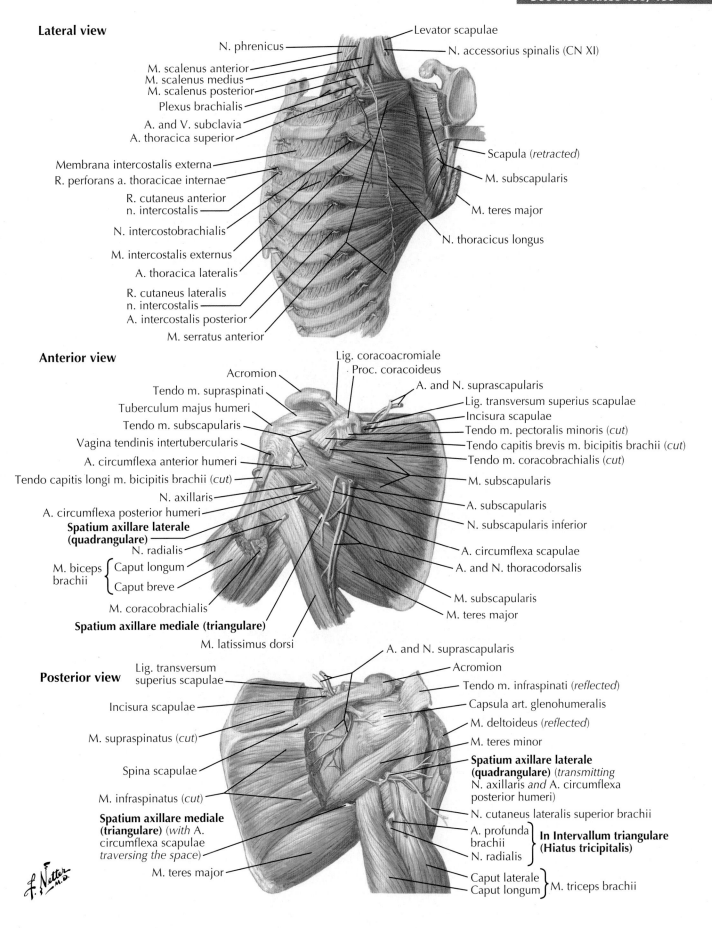

Lateral view

Levator scapulae

N. phrenicus

N. accessorius spinalis (CN XI)

M. scalenus anterior
M. scalenus medius
M. scalenus posterior
Plexus brachialis
A. and V. subclavia
A. thoracica superior

Scapula (*retracted*)

M. subscapularis

Membrana intercostalis externa
R. perforans a. thoracicae internae
R. cutaneus anterior
n. intercostalis
N. intercostobrachialis
M. intercostalis externus
A. thoracica lateralis
R. cutaneus lateralis
n. intercostalis
A. intercostalis posterior
M. serratus anterior

M. teres major

N. thoracicus longus

Anterior view

Lig. coracoacromiale
Proc. coracoideus

Acromion
Tendo m. supraspinati
Tuberculum majus humeri
Tendo m. subscapularis
Vagina tendinis intertubercularis
A. circumflexa anterior humeri
Tendo capitis longi m. bicipitis brachii (*cut*)
N. axillaris
A. circumflexa posterior humeri
**Spatium axillare laterale
(quadrangulare)**
N. radialis

M. biceps { Caput longum
brachii { Caput breve

M. coracobrachialis

Spatium axillare mediale (triangulare)

M. latissimus dorsi

A. and N. suprascapularis
Lig. transversum superius scapulae
Incisura scapulae
Tendo m. pectoralis minoris (*cut*)
Tendo capitis brevis m. bicipitis brachii (*cut*)
Tendo m. coracobrachialis (*cut*)
M. subscapularis
A. subscapularis
N. subscapularis inferior
A. circumflexa scapulae
A. and N. thoracodorsalis
M. subscapularis
M. teres major

Posterior view

Lig. transversum
superius scapulae
Incisura scapulae
M. supraspinatus (*cut*)
Spina scapulae
M. infraspinatus (*cut*)
**Spatium axillare mediale
(triangulare)** (*with* A.
circumflexa scapulae
traversing the space)
M. teres major

A. and N. suprascapularis
Acromion
Tendo m. infraspinati (*reflected*)
Capsula art. glenohumeralis
M. deltoideus (*reflected*)
M. teres minor
**Spatium axillare laterale
(quadrangulare)** (*transmitting*
N. axillaris *and* A. circumflexa
posterior humeri)
N. cutaneus lateralis superior brachii
A. profunda } **In Intervallum triangulare
brachii** } **(Hiatus tricipitalis)**
N. radialis }
Caput laterale }
Caput longum } M. triceps brachii

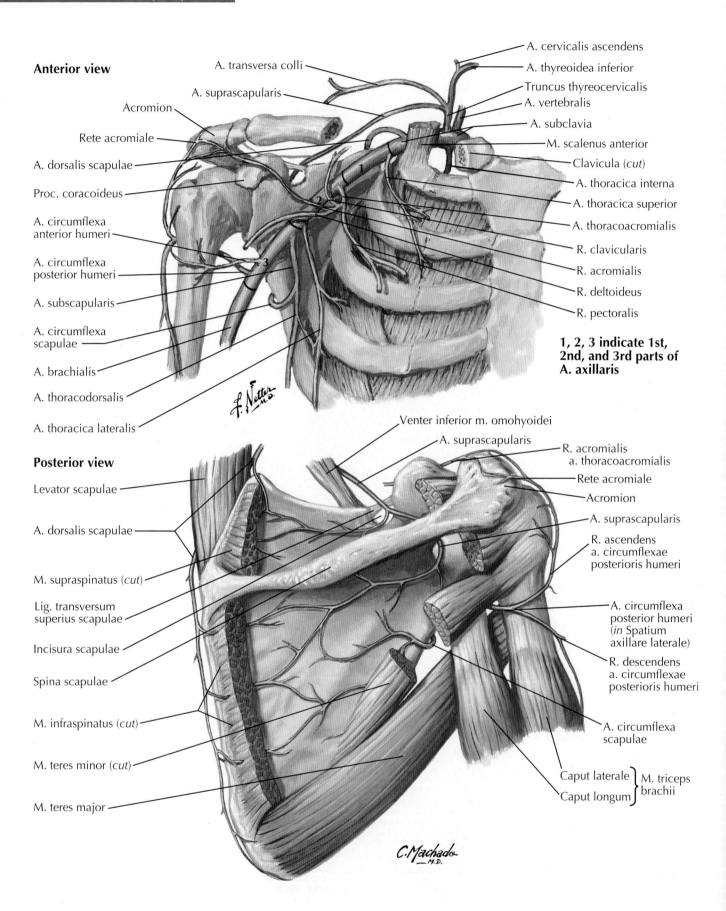

Anterior view

A. transversa colli

A. suprascapularis

Acromion

Rete acromiale

A. dorsalis scapulae

Proc. coracoideus

A. circumflexa anterior humeri

A. circumflexa posterior humeri

A. subscapularis

A. circumflexa scapulae

A. brachialis

A. thoracodorsalis

A. thoracica lateralis

A. cervicalis ascendens

A. thyreoidea inferior

Truncus thyreocervicalis

A. vertebralis

A. subclavia

M. scalenus anterior

Clavicula (cut)

A. thoracica interna

A. thoracica superior

A. thoracoacromialis

R. clavicularis

R. acromialis

R. deltoideus

R. pectoralis

1, 2, 3 indicate 1st, 2nd, and 3rd parts of A. axillaris

Posterior view

Levator scapulae

A. dorsalis scapulae

M. supraspinatus (cut)

Lig. transversum superius scapulae

Incisura scapulae

Spina scapulae

M. infraspinatus (cut)

M. teres minor (cut)

M. teres major

Venter inferior m. omohyoidei

A. suprascapularis

R. acromialis a. thoracoacromialis

Rete acromiale

Acromion

A. suprascapularis

R. ascendens a. circumflexae posterioris humeri

A. circumflexa posterior humeri (in Spatium axillare laterale)

R. descendens a. circumflexae posterioris humeri

A. circumflexa scapulae

Caput laterale } M. triceps
Caput longum } brachii

Plate 437

Omos and Axilla

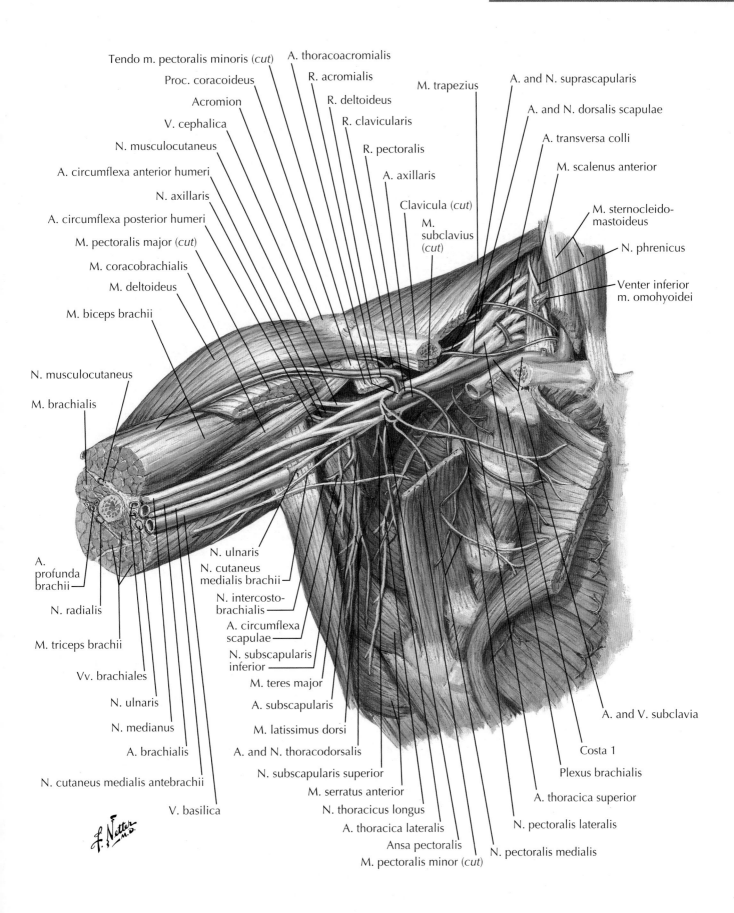

Tendo m. pectoralis minoris (*cut*)

Proc. coracoideus

Acromion

V. cephalica

N. musculocutaneus

A. circumflexa anterior humeri

N. axillaris

A. circumflexa posterior humeri

M. pectoralis major (*cut*)

M. coracobrachialis

M. deltoideus

M. biceps brachii

N. musculocutaneus

M. brachialis

A. thoracoacromialis

R. acromialis

R. deltoideus

R. clavicularis

R. pectoralis

A. axillaris

M. trapezius

Clavicula (*cut*)

M. subclavius (*cut*)

A. and N. suprascapularis

A. and N. dorsalis scapulae

A. transversa colli

M. scalenus anterior

M. sternocleido-mastoideus

N. phrenicus

Venter inferior m. omohyoidei

A. profunda brachii

N. radialis

M. triceps brachii

Vv. brachiales

N. ulnaris

N. medianus

A. brachialis

N. cutaneus medialis antebrachii

V. basilica

N. ulnaris

N. cutaneus medialis brachii

N. intercosto-brachialis

A. circumflexa scapulae

N. subscapularis inferior

M. teres major

A. subscapularis

M. latissimus dorsi

A. and N. thoracodorsalis

N. subscapularis superior

M. serratus anterior

N. thoracicus longus

A. thoracica lateralis

Ansa pectoralis

M. pectoralis minor (*cut*)

A. and V. subclavia

Costa 1

Plexus brachialis

A. thoracica superior

N. pectoralis lateralis

N. pectoralis medialis

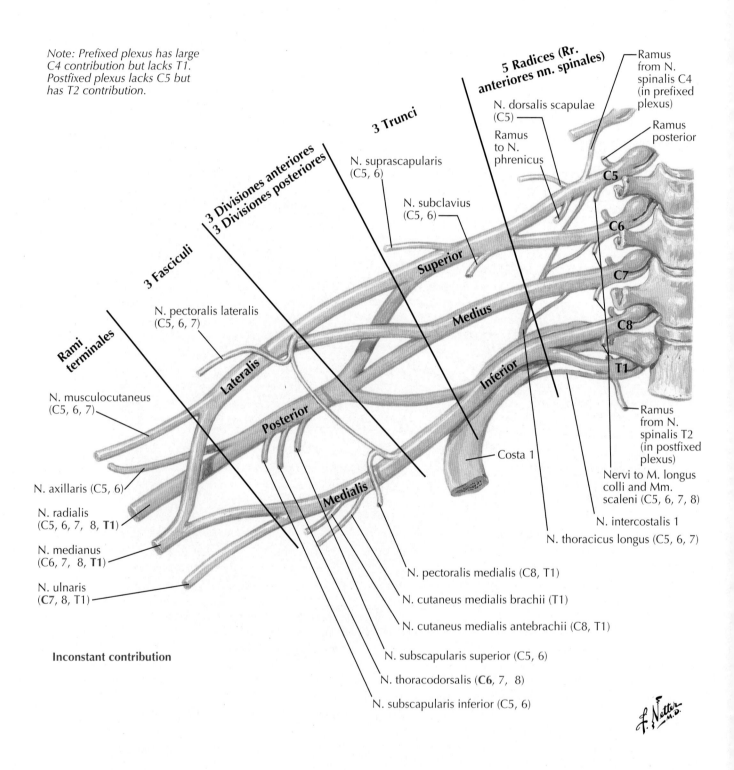

Note: Prefixed plexus has large
C4 contribution but lacks T1.
Postfixed plexus lacks C5 but
has T2 contribution.

5 Radices (Rr. anteriores nn. spinales)

3 Trunci

3 Divisiones anteriores
3 Divisiones posteriores

3 Fasciculi

Rami terminales

N. dorsalis scapulae (C5)

Ramus to N. phrenicus

Ramus from N. spinalis C4 (in prefixed plexus)

Ramus posterior

C5

C6

C7

C8

T1

N. suprascapularis (C5, 6)

N. subclavius (C5, 6)

Superior

Medius

Inferior

N. pectoralis lateralis (C5, 6, 7)

Lateralis

Posterior

N. musculocutaneus (C5, 6, 7)

Costa 1

Ramus from N. spinalis T2 (in postfixed plexus)

Nervi to M. longus colli and Mm. scaleni (C5, 6, 7, 8)

N. intercostalis 1

N. thoracicus longus (C5, 6, 7)

N. axillaris (C5, 6)

N. radialis (C5, 6, 7, 8, **T1**)

N. medianus (C6, 7, 8, **T1**)

N. ulnaris (**C7**, 8, T1)

Medialis

N. pectoralis medialis (C8, T1)

N. cutaneus medialis brachii (T1)

N. cutaneus medialis antebrachii (C8, T1)

Inconstant contribution

N. subscapularis superior (C5, 6)

N. thoracodorsalis (**C6**, 7, 8)

N. subscapularis inferior (C5, 6)

Plate 439

Omos and Axilla

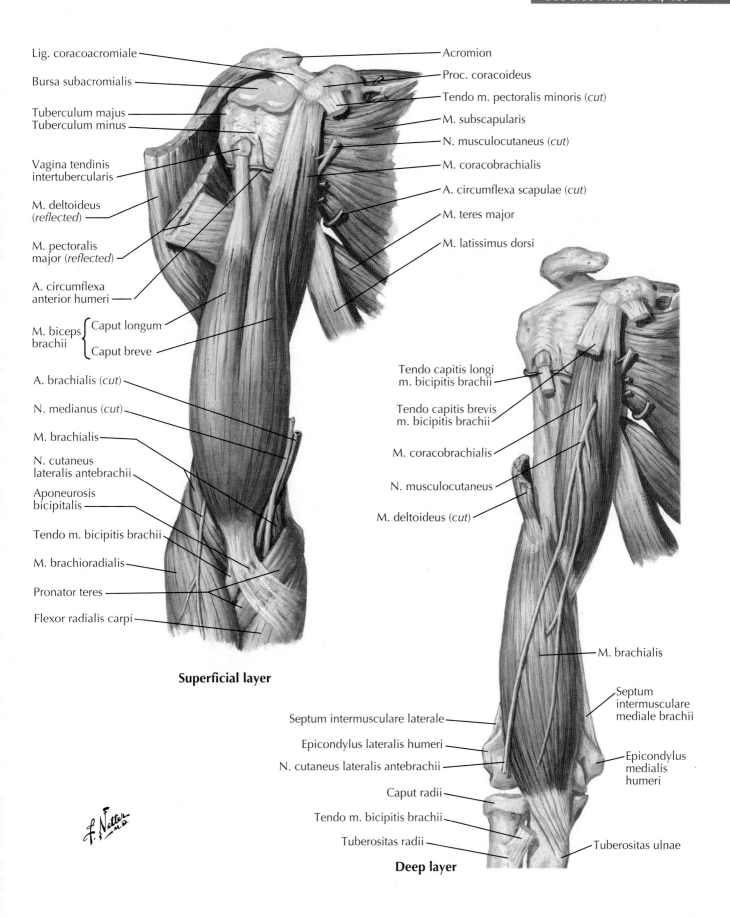

Lig. coracoacromiale

Bursa subacromialis

Tuberculum majus
Tuberculum minus

Vagina tendinis
intertubercularis

M. deltoideus
(*reflected*)

M. pectoralis
major (*reflected*)

A. circumflexa
anterior humeri

M. biceps { Caput longum
brachii { Caput breve

A. brachialis (*cut*)

N. medianus (*cut*)

M. brachialis

N. cutaneus
lateralis antebrachii

Aponeurosis
bicipitalis

Tendo m. bicipitis brachii

M. brachioradialis

Pronator teres

Flexor radialis carpi

Acromion

Proc. coracoideus

Tendo m. pectoralis minoris (*cut*)

M. subscapularis

N. musculocutaneus (*cut*)

M. coracobrachialis

A. circumflexa scapulae (*cut*)

M. teres major

M. latissimus dorsi

Superficial layer

Tendo capitis longi
m. bicipitis brachii

Tendo capitis brevis
m. bicipitis brachii

M. coracobrachialis

N. musculocutaneus

M. deltoideus (*cut*)

M. brachialis

Septum
intermusculare
mediale brachii

Septum intermusculare laterale

Epicondylus lateralis humeri

N. cutaneus lateralis antebrachii

Caput radii

Tendo m. bicipitis brachii

Tuberositas radii

Epicondylus
medialis
humeri

Tuberositas ulnae

Deep layer

Superficial layer

M. supraspinatus

M. infraspinatus

M. teres minor

N. axillaris

M. deltoideus (*cut and reflected*)

A. circumflexa posterior humeri

N. cutaneus lateralis superior brachii

Caput longum
Caput laterale } M. triceps brachii
Tendo

M. brachioradialis

Capsula
art. glenohumeralis

Tendo m. supraspinati

Tendo m. infraspinati (cut)

Tendo m. teretis minoris (*cut*)

N. axillaris

A. circumflexa posterior humeri

N. cutaneus lateralis superior brachii

M. teres major

N. cutaneus posterior brachii

Septum intermusculare mediale brachii

N. ulnaris

Epicondylus medialis humeri

Olecranon

Flexor ulnaris carpi

M. anconeus

Extensor radialis longus carpi

Extensor ulnaris carpi

N. cutaneus posterior antebrachii

Extensor digitorum

Extensor radialis brevis carpi

M. teres major; Tendo

A. profunda brachii

N. radialis

A. collateralis media

A. collateralis radialis

N. cutaneus lateralis inferior brachii

Septum intermusculare laterale brachii

Caput longum m. tricipitis brachii

Caput laterale m. tricipitis brachii (*cut*)

Caput mediale m. tricipitis brachii

Epicondylus medialis humeri

N. ulnaris

Olecranon

Deep layer

M. anconeus

N. cutaneus posterior antebrachii

Epicondylus lateralis humeri

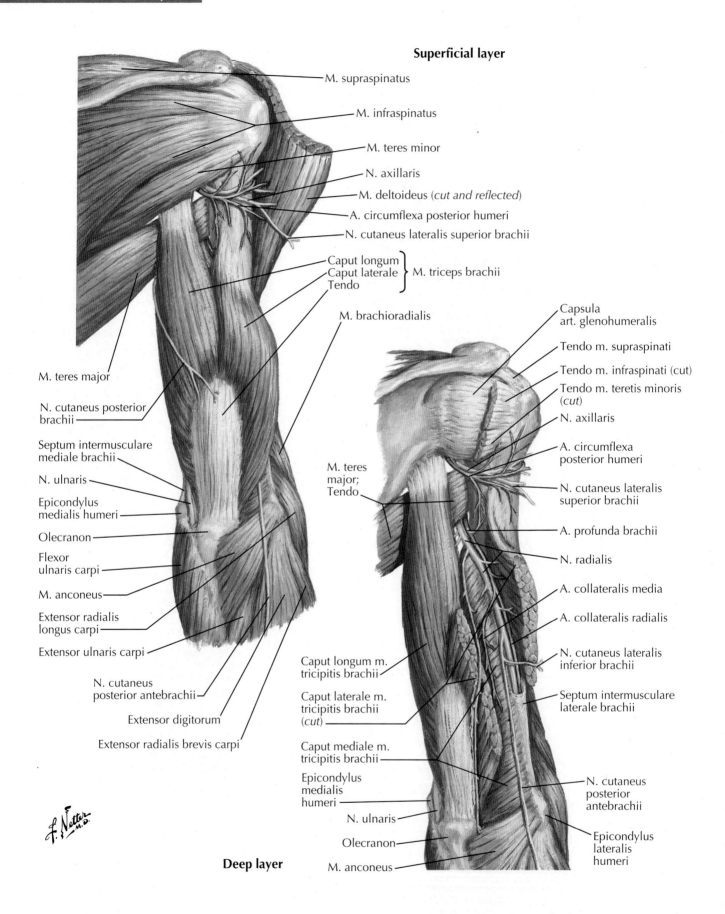

Plate 441

Brachium

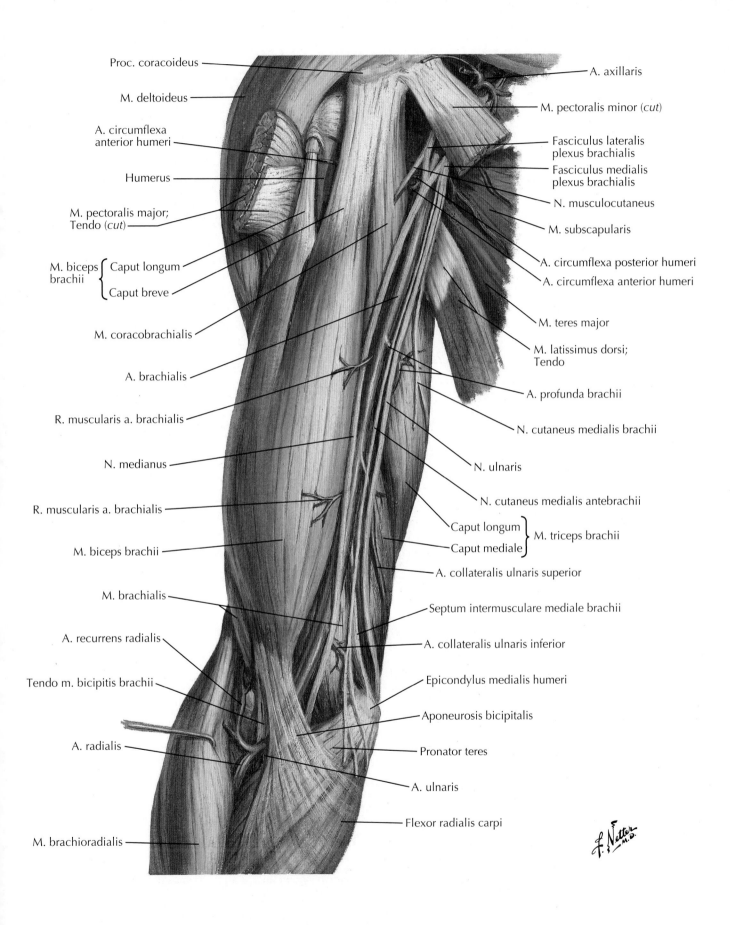

Proc. coracoideus

M. deltoideus

A. circumflexa anterior humeri

Humerus

M. pectoralis major; Tendo (*cut*)

M. biceps brachii { Caput longum

Caput breve

M. coracobrachialis

A. brachialis

R. muscularis a. brachialis

N. medianus

R. muscularis a. brachialis

M. biceps brachii

M. brachialis

A. recurrens radialis

Tendo m. bicipitis brachii

A. radialis

M. brachioradialis

A. axillaris

M. pectoralis minor (*cut*)

Fasciculus lateralis plexus brachialis

Fasciculus medialis plexus brachialis

N. musculocutaneus

M. subscapularis

A. circumflexa posterior humeri

A. circumflexa anterior humeri

M. teres major

M. latissimus dorsi; Tendo

A. profunda brachii

N. cutaneus medialis brachii

N. ulnaris

N. cutaneus medialis antebrachii

Caput longum } M. triceps brachii

Caput mediale

A. collateralis ulnaris superior

Septum intermusculare mediale brachii

A. collateralis ulnaris inferior

Epicondylus medialis humeri

Aponeurosis bicipitalis

Pronator teres

A. ulnaris

Flexor radialis carpi

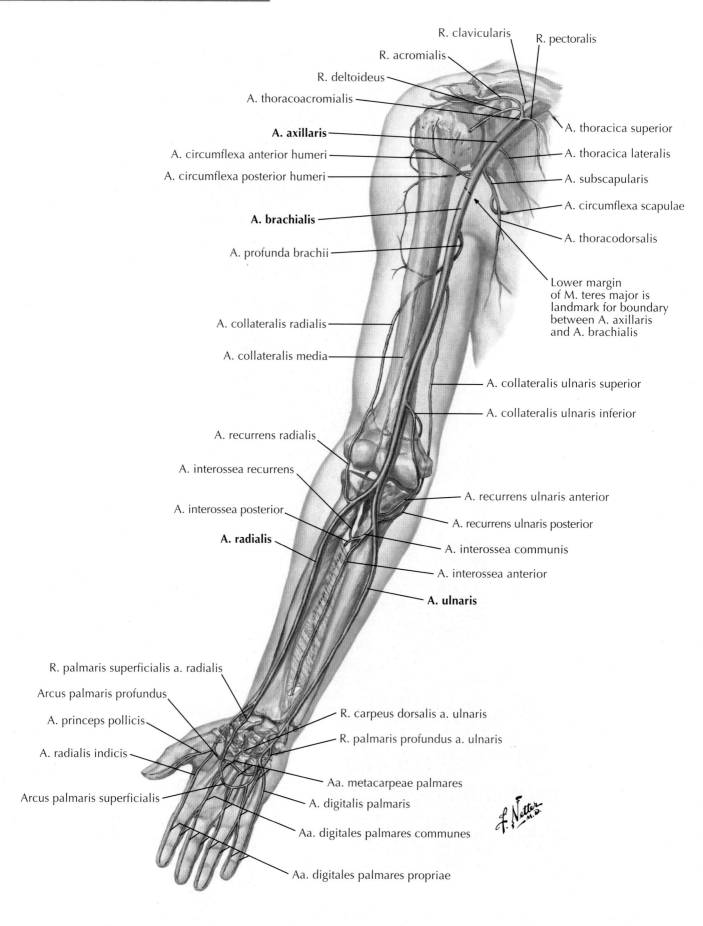

R. clavicularis

R. pectoralis

R. acromialis

R. deltoideus

A. thoracoacromialis

A. axillaris

A. circumflexa anterior humeri

A. circumflexa posterior humeri

A. brachialis

A. profunda brachii

A. collateralis radialis

A. collateralis media

A. recurrens radialis

A. interossea recurrens

A. interossea posterior

A. radialis

R. palmaris superficialis a. radialis

Arcus palmaris profundus

A. princeps pollicis

A. radialis indicis

Arcus palmaris superficialis

A. thoracica superior

A. thoracica lateralis

A. subscapularis

A. circumflexa scapulae

A. thoracodorsalis

Lower margin
of M. teres major is
landmark for boundary
between A. axillaris
and A. brachialis

A. collateralis ulnaris superior

A. collateralis ulnaris inferior

A. recurrens ulnaris anterior

A. recurrens ulnaris posterior

A. interossea communis

A. interossea anterior

A. ulnaris

R. carpeus dorsalis a. ulnaris

R. palmaris profundus a. ulnaris

Aa. metacarpeae palmares

A. digitalis palmaris

Aa. digitales palmares communes

Aa. digitales palmares propriae

Plate 443

Brachium

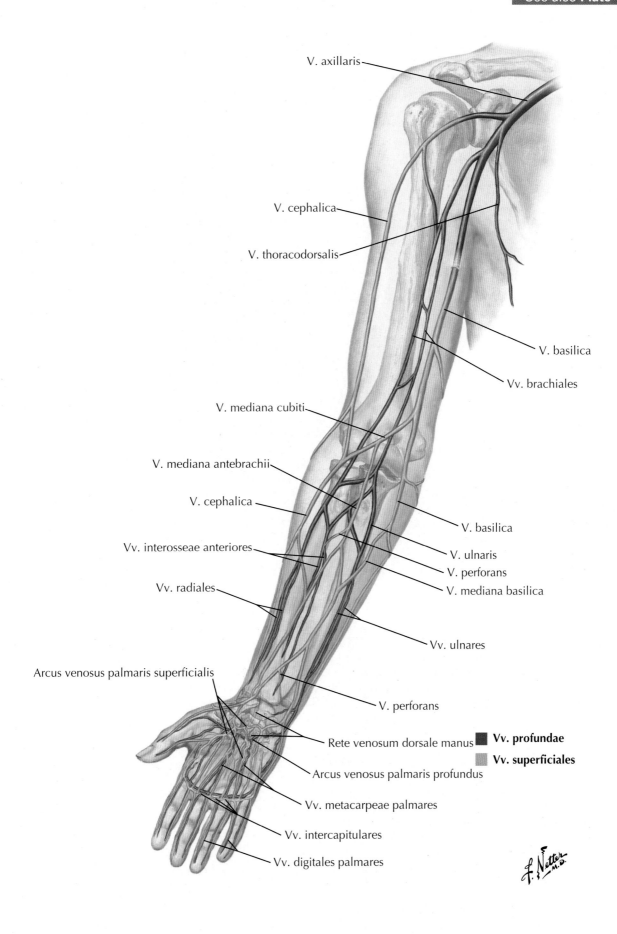

V. axillaris

V. cephalica

V. thoracodorsalis

V. basilica

Vv. brachiales

V. mediana cubiti

V. mediana antebrachii

V. cephalica

V. basilica

V. ulnaris

Vv. interosseae anteriores

V. perforans

V. mediana basilica

Vv. radiales

Vv. ulnares

Arcus venosus palmaris superficialis

V. perforans

Rete venosum dorsale manus

Vv. profundae

Vv. superficiales

Arcus venosus palmaris profundus

Vv. metacarpeae palmares

Vv. intercapitulares

Vv. digitales palmares

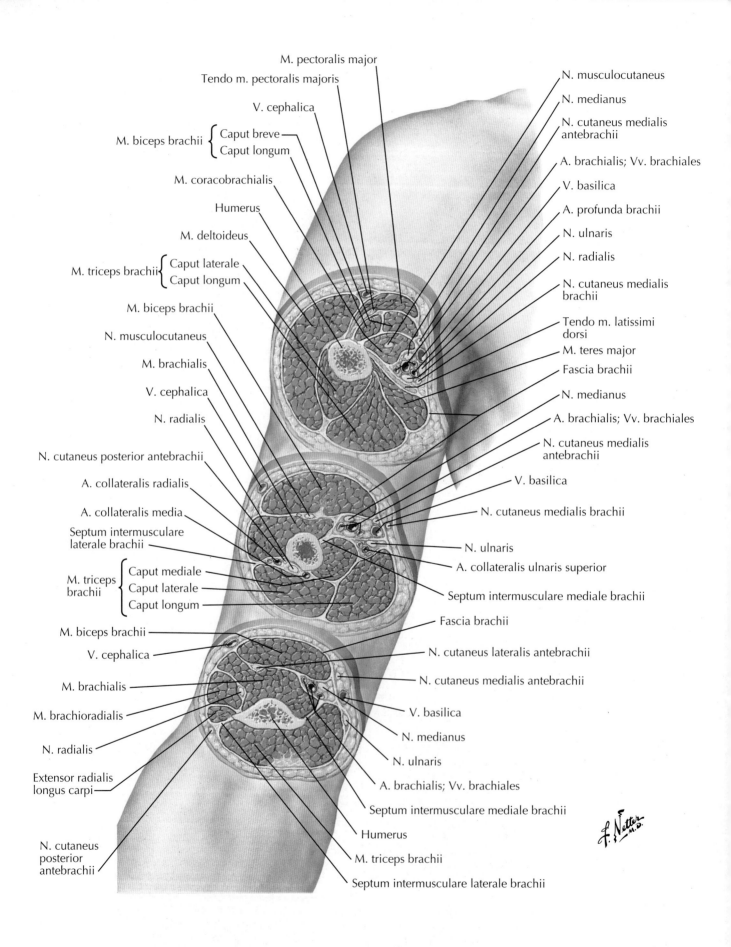

M. pectoralis major

Tendo m. pectoralis majoris

V. cephalica

M. biceps brachii { Caput breve
Caput longum

M. coracobrachialis

Humerus

M. deltoideus

M. triceps brachii { Caput laterale
Caput longum

M. biceps brachii

N. musculocutaneus

M. brachialis

V. cephalica

N. radialis

N. cutaneus posterior antebrachii

A. collateralis radialis

A. collateralis media

Septum intermusculare
laterale brachii

M. triceps
brachii { Caput mediale
Caput laterale
Caput longum

M. biceps brachii

V. cephalica

M. brachialis

M. brachioradialis

N. radialis

Extensor radialis
longus carpi

N. cutaneus
posterior
antebrachii

N. musculocutaneus

N. medianus

N. cutaneus medialis
antebrachii

A. brachialis; Vv. brachiales

V. basilica

A. profunda brachii

N. ulnaris

N. radialis

N. cutaneus medialis
brachii

Tendo m. latissimi
dorsi

M. teres major

Fascia brachii

N. medianus

A. brachialis; Vv. brachiales

N. cutaneus medialis
antebrachii

V. basilica

N. cutaneus medialis brachii

N. ulnaris

A. collateralis ulnaris superior

Septum intermusculare mediale brachii

Fascia brachii

N. cutaneus lateralis antebrachii

N. cutaneus medialis antebrachii

V. basilica

N. medianus

N. ulnaris

A. brachialis; Vv. brachiales

Septum intermusculare mediale brachii

Humerus

M. triceps brachii

Septum intermusculare laterale brachii

Plate 445

Brachium

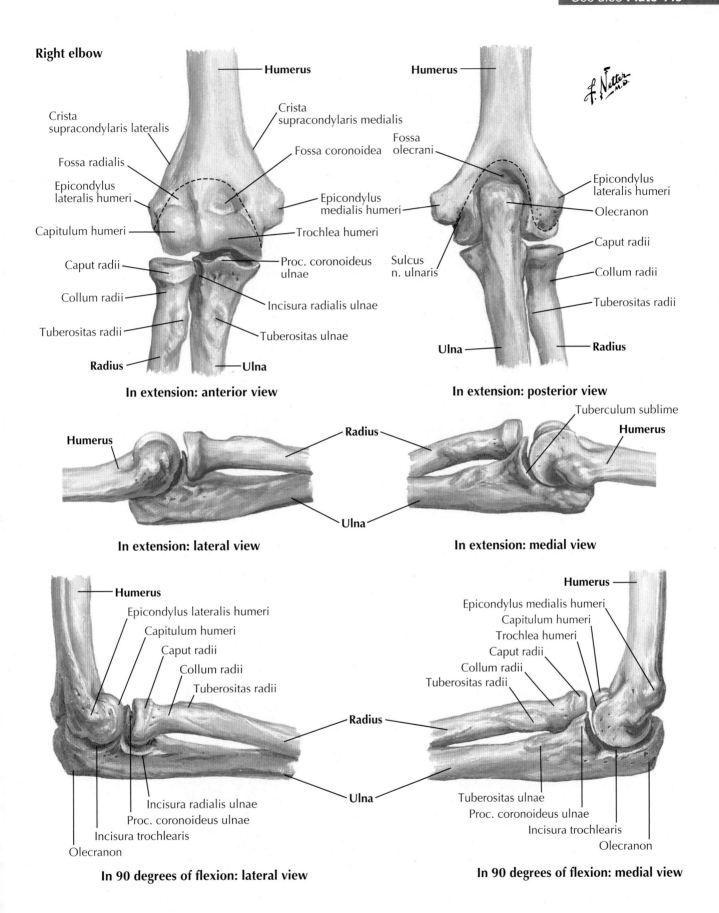

Right elbow

In extension: anterior view

- Humerus
- Crista supracondylaris lateralis
- Crista supracondylaris medialis
- Fossa radialis
- Fossa coronoidea
- Epicondylus lateralis humeri
- Epicondylus medialis humeri
- Capitulum humeri
- Trochlea humeri
- Caput radii
- Proc. coronoideus ulnae
- Collum radii
- Incisura radialis ulnae
- Tuberositas radii
- Tuberositas ulnae
- Radius
- Ulna

In extension: posterior view

- Humerus
- Fossa olecrani
- Epicondylus lateralis humeri
- Olecranon
- Caput radii
- Collum radii
- Sulcus n. ulnaris
- Tuberositas radii
- Ulna
- Radius

In extension: lateral view

- Humerus
- Radius
- Ulna

In extension: medial view

- Tuberculum sublime
- Humerus
- Radius
- Ulna

In 90 degrees of flexion: lateral view

- Humerus
- Epicondylus lateralis humeri
- Capitulum humeri
- Caput radii
- Collum radii
- Tuberositas radii
- Radius
- Incisura radialis ulnae
- Proc. coronoideus ulnae
- Incisura trochlearis
- Olecranon
- Ulna

In 90 degrees of flexion: medial view

- Humerus
- Epicondylus medialis humeri
- Capitulum humeri
- Trochlea humeri
- Caput radii
- Collum radii
- Tuberositas radii
- Radius
- Tuberositas ulnae
- Proc. coronoideus ulnae
- Incisura trochlearis
- Olecranon
- Ulna

Anteroposterior view

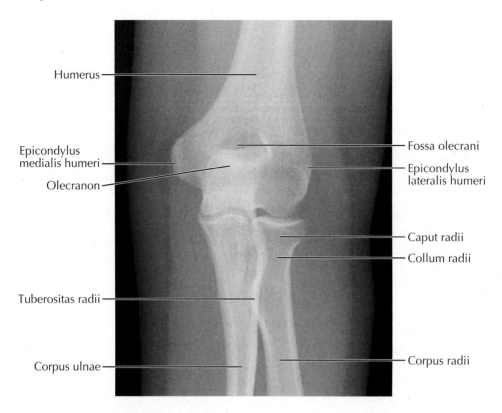

Humerus

Epicondylus medialis humeri

Olecranon

Fossa olecrani

Epicondylus lateralis humeri

Caput radii

Collum radii

Tuberositas radii

Corpus ulnae

Corpus radii

Lateral view

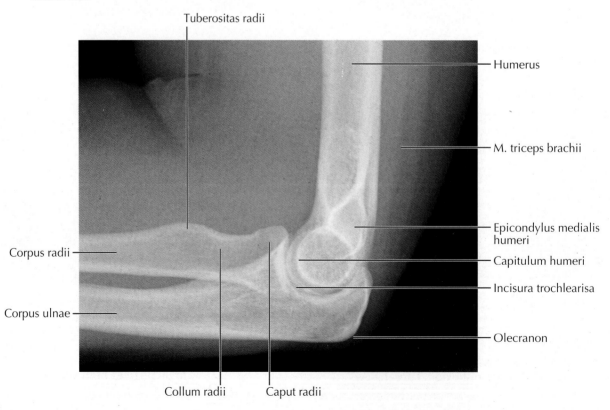

Tuberositas radii

Humerus

M. triceps brachii

Epicondylus medialis humeri

Capitulum humeri

Incisura trochlearisa

Olecranon

Corpus radii

Corpus ulnae

Collum radii

Caput radii

Plate 447   **Cubitus and Antebrachium**

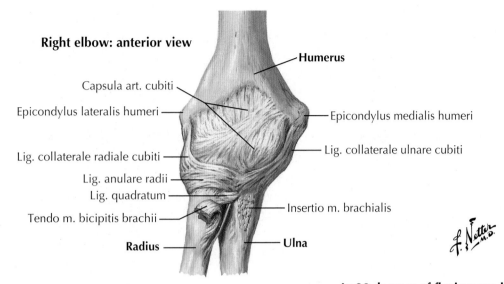

Right elbow: anterior view

Capsula art. cubiti

Epicondylus lateralis humeri

Lig. collaterale radiale cubiti

Lig. anulare radii

Lig. quadratum

Tendo m. bicipitis brachii

Radius

Humerus

Epicondylus medialis humeri

Lig. collaterale ulnare cubiti

Insertio m. brachialis

Ulna

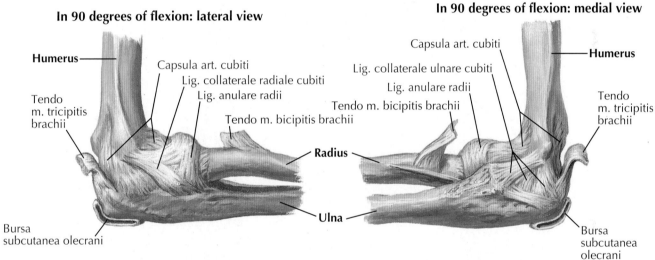

In 90 degrees of flexion: lateral view

Humerus

Tendo
m. tricipitis
brachii

Capsula art. cubiti

Lig. collaterale radiale cubiti

Lig. anulare radii

Tendo m. bicipitis brachii

Radius

Bursa
subcutanea olecrani

Ulna

In 90 degrees of flexion: medial view

Capsula art. cubiti

Lig. collaterale ulnare cubiti

Lig. anulare radii

Tendo m. bicipitis brachii

Humerus

Tendo
m. tricipitis
brachii

Bursa
subcutanea
olecrani

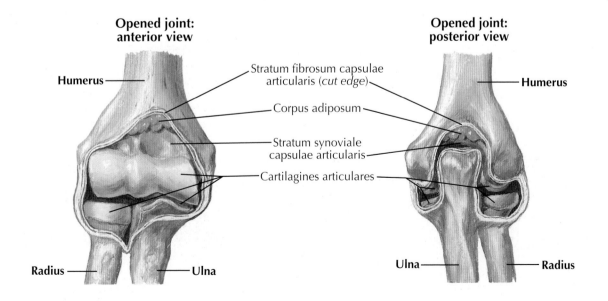

**Opened joint:
anterior view**

Humerus

Radius   **Ulna**

Stratum fibrosum capsulae
articularis (*cut edge*)

Corpus adiposum

Stratum synoviale
capsulae articularis

Cartilagines articulares

**Opened joint:
posterior view**

Humerus

Ulna   **Radius**

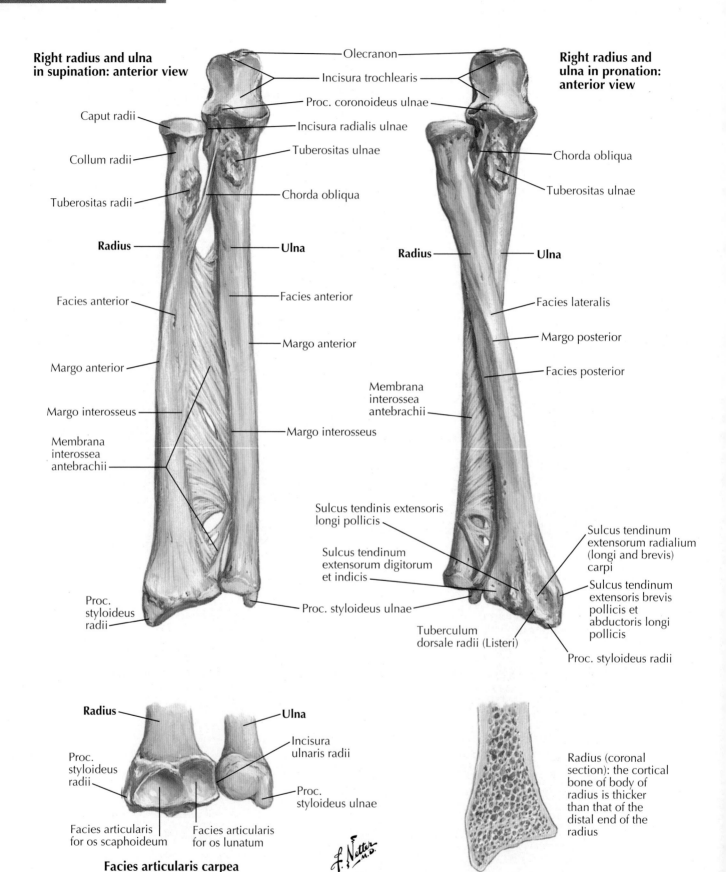

Right radius and ulna
in supination: anterior view

Olecranon

Incisura trochlearis

Proc. coronoideus ulnae

Caput radii

Incisura radialis ulnae

Collum radii

Tuberositas ulnae

Chorda obliqua

Tuberositas radii

Radius

Ulna

Facies anterior

Facies anterior

Margo anterior

Margo anterior

Margo interosseus

Margo interosseus

Membrana
interossea
antebrachii

Right radius and
ulna in pronation:
anterior view

Chorda obliqua

Tuberositas ulnae

Radius

Ulna

Facies lateralis

Margo posterior

Facies posterior

Membrana
interossea
antebrachii

Sulcus tendinis extensoris
longi pollicis

Sulcus tendinum
extensorum digitorum
et indicis

Proc. styloideus ulnae

Sulcus tendinum
extensorum radialium
(longi and brevis)
carpi

Sulcus tendinum
extensoris brevis
pollicis et
abductoris longi
pollicis

Tuberculum
dorsale radii (Listeri)

Proc. styloideus radii

Proc.
styloideus
radii

Radius

Ulna

Proc.
styloideus
radii

Incisura
ulnaris radii

Proc.
styloideus ulnae

Facies articularis
for os scaphoideum

Facies articularis
for os lunatum

Facies articularis carpea

Radius (coronal
section): the cortical
bone of body of
radius is thicker
than that of the
distal end of the
radius

Plate 449

Cubitus and Antebrachium

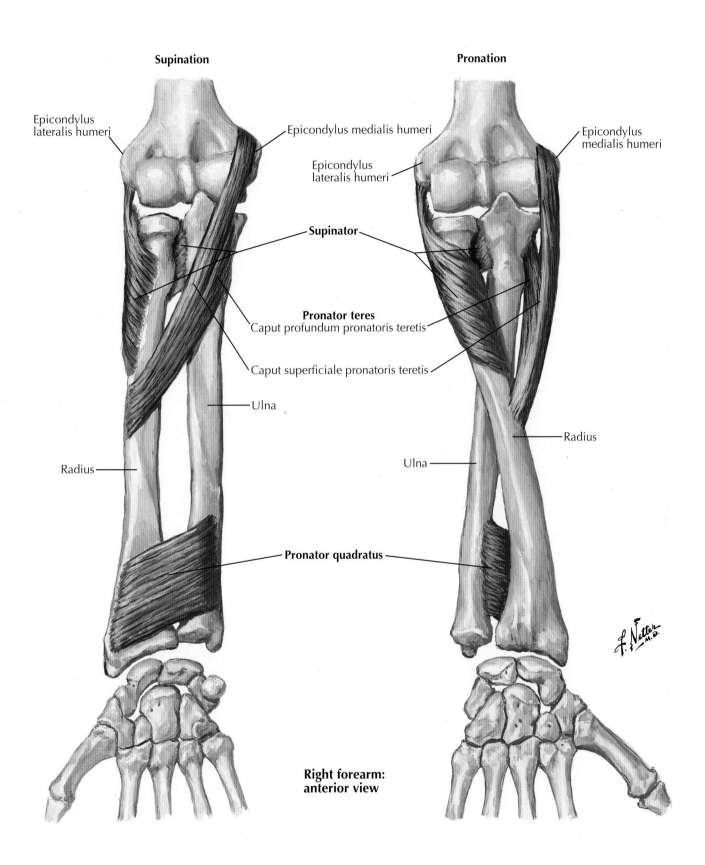

Supination

Pronation

Epicondylus lateralis humeri

Epicondylus medialis humeri

Epicondylus medialis humeri

Epicondylus lateralis humeri

Epicondylus medialis humeri

Supinator

Pronator teres
Caput profundum pronatoris teretis

Caput superficiale pronatoris teretis

Ulna

Radius

Radius

Ulna

Pronator quadratus

Right forearm: anterior view

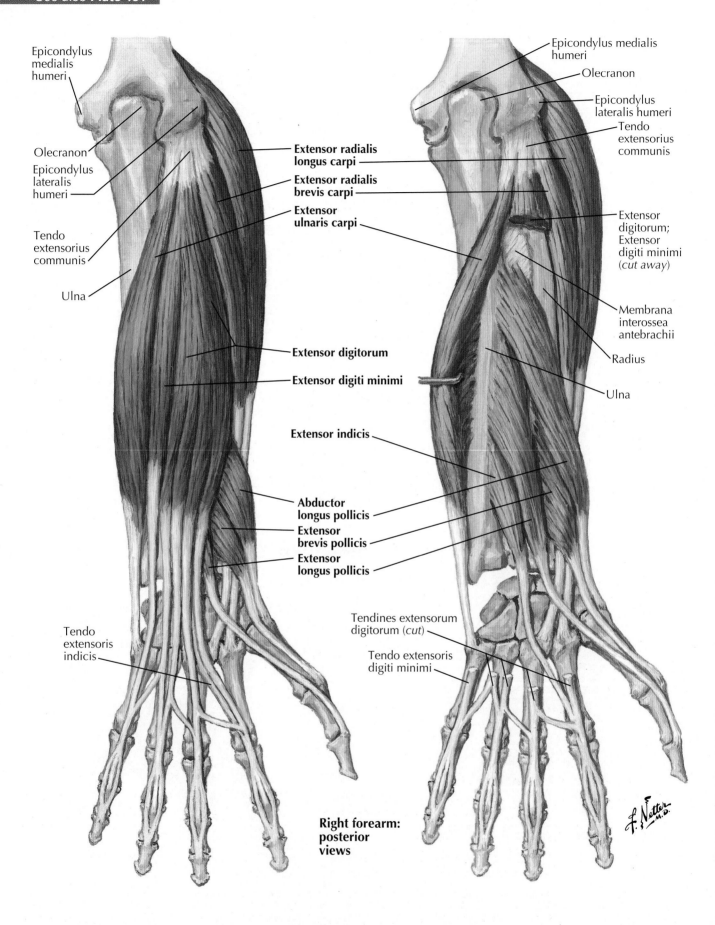

Epicondylus
medialis
humeri

Olecranon

Epicondylus
lateralis
humeri

Tendo
extensorius
communis

Ulna

**Extensor radialis
longus carpi**

**Extensor radialis
brevis carpi**

**Extensor
ulnaris carpi**

Extensor digitorum

Extensor digiti minimi

Extensor indicis

**Abductor
longus pollicis**

**Extensor
brevis pollicis**

**Extensor
longus pollicis**

Tendo
extensoris
indicis

Epicondylus medialis
humeri

Olecranon

Epicondylus
lateralis humeri

Tendo
extensorius
communis

Extensor
digitorum;
Extensor
digiti minimi
(*cut away*)

Membrana
interossea
antebrachii

Radius

Ulna

Tendines extensorum
digitorum (*cut*)

Tendo extensoris
digiti minimi

**Right forearm:
posterior
views**

Plate 451

Cubitus and Antebrachium

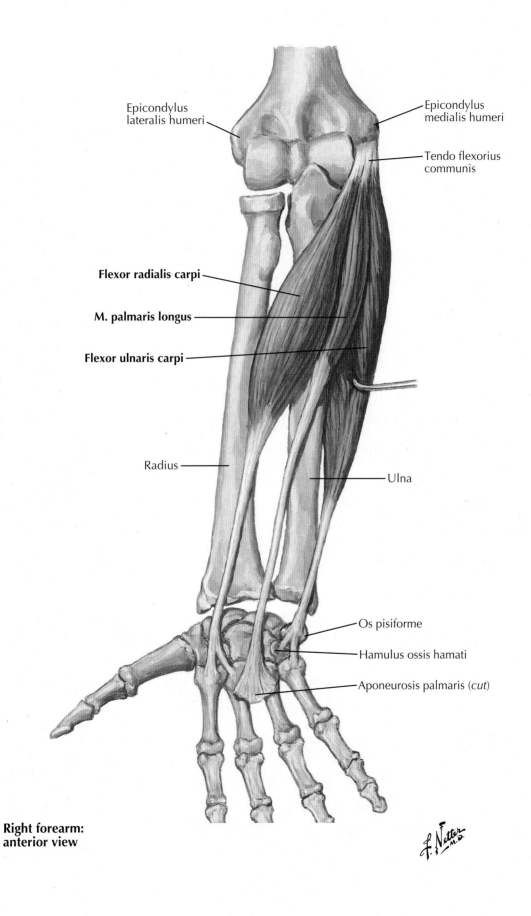

Epicondylus
lateralis humeri

Epicondylus
medialis humeri

Tendo flexorius
communis

Flexor radialis carpi

M. palmaris longus

Flexor ulnaris carpi

Radius

Ulna

Os pisiforme

Hamulus ossis hamati

Aponeurosis palmaris (*cut*)

**Right forearm:
anterior view**

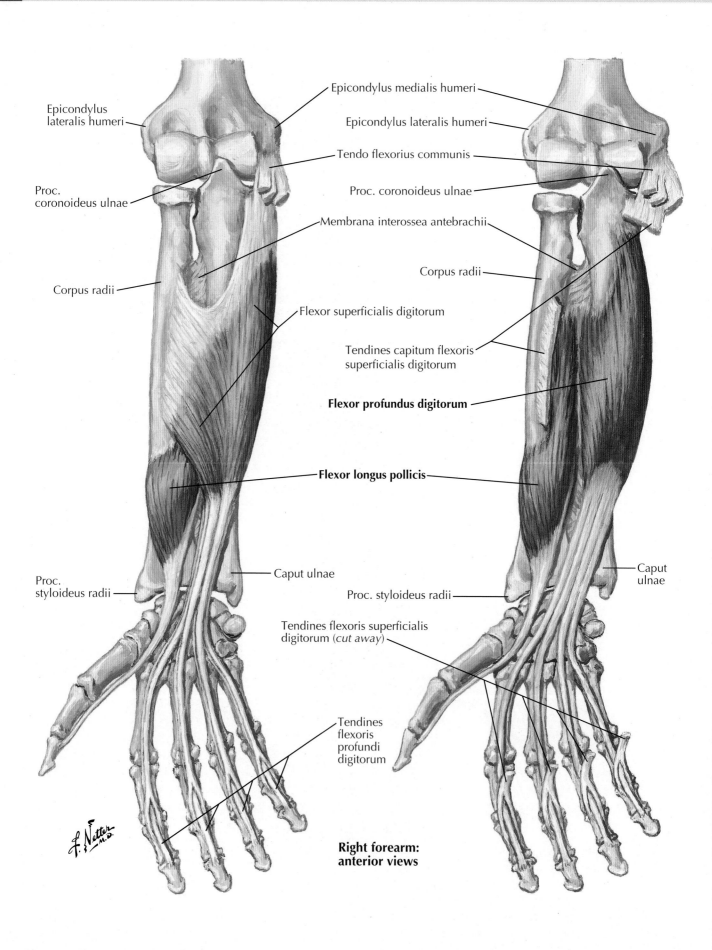

Epicondylus lateralis humeri

Proc. coronoideus ulnae

Corpus radii

Proc. styloideus radii

Tendines flexoris profundi digitorum

Epicondylus medialis humeri

Epicondylus lateralis humeri

Tendo flexorius communis

Proc. coronoideus ulnae

Membrana interossea antebrachii

Corpus radii

Flexor superficialis digitorum

Tendines capitum flexoris superficialis digitorum

Flexor profundus digitorum

Flexor longus pollicis

Caput ulnae

Proc. styloideus radii

Tendines flexoris superficialis digitorum (*cut away*)

Caput ulnae

Right forearm: anterior views

Plate 453

Cubitus and Antebrachium

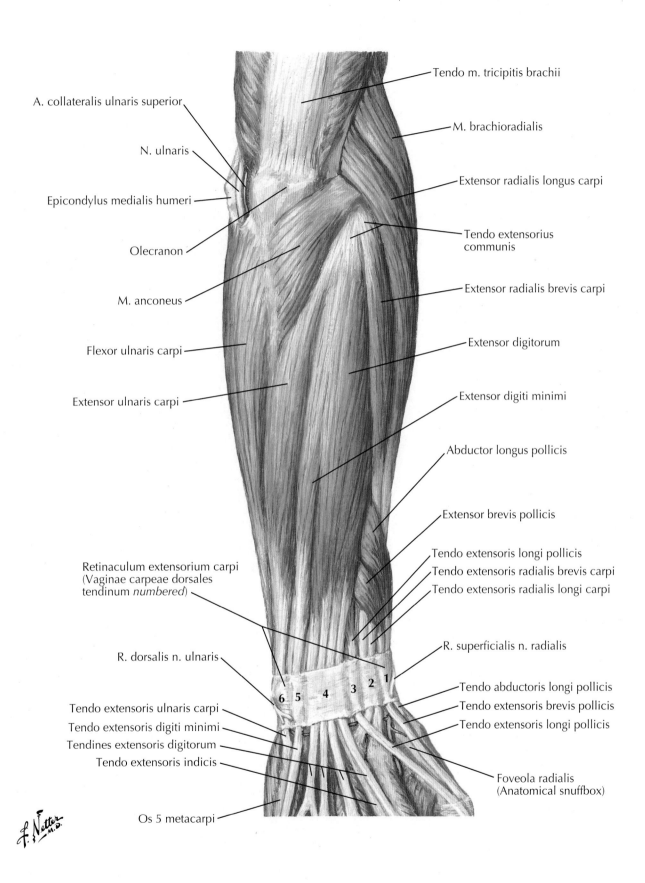

A. collateralis ulnaris superior

N. ulnaris

Epicondylus medialis humeri

Olecranon

M. anconeus

Flexor ulnaris carpi

Extensor ulnaris carpi

Retinaculum extensorium carpi
(Vaginae carpeae dorsales
tendinum *numbered*)

R. dorsalis n. ulnaris

Tendo extensoris ulnaris carpi
Tendo extensoris digiti minimi
Tendines extensoris digitorum
Tendo extensoris indicis

Os 5 metacarpi

Tendo m. tricipitis brachii

M. brachioradialis

Extensor radialis longus carpi

Tendo extensorius
communis

Extensor radialis brevis carpi

Extensor digitorum

Extensor digiti minimi

Abductor longus pollicis

Extensor brevis pollicis

Tendo extensoris longi pollicis
Tendo extensoris radialis brevis carpi
Tendo extensoris radialis longi carpi

R. superficialis n. radialis

Tendo abductoris longi pollicis
Tendo extensoris brevis pollicis
Tendo extensoris longi pollicis

Foveola radialis
(Anatomical snuffbox)

6 5 4 3 2 1

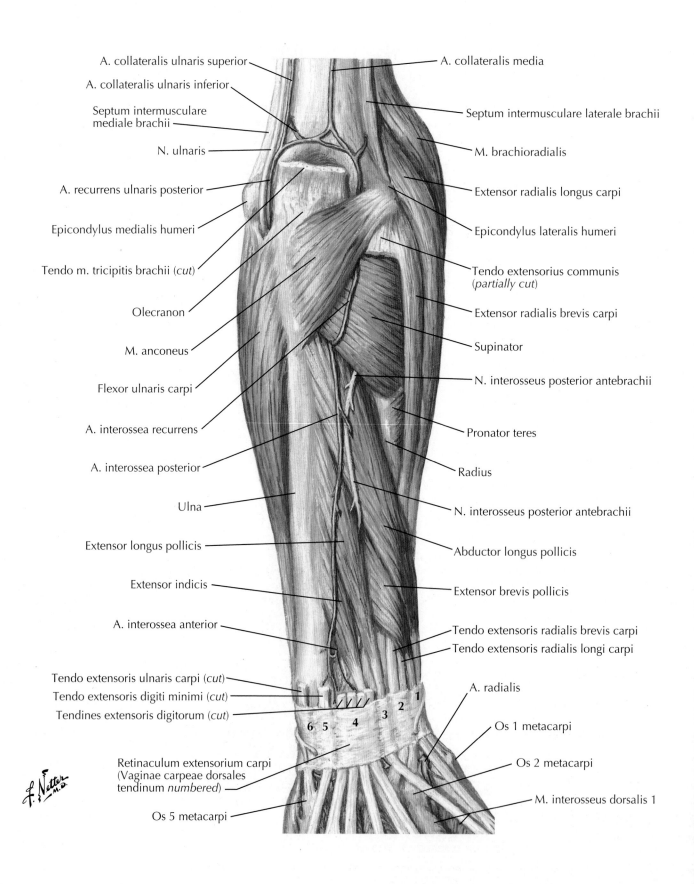

A. collateralis ulnaris superior

A. collateralis ulnaris inferior

Septum intermusculare
mediale brachii

N. ulnaris

A. recurrens ulnaris posterior

Epicondylus medialis humeri

Tendo m. tricipitis brachii (*cut*)

Olecranon

M. anconeus

Flexor ulnaris carpi

A. interossea recurrens

A. interossea posterior

Ulna

Extensor longus pollicis

Extensor indicis

A. interossea anterior

Tendo extensoris ulnaris carpi (*cut*)

Tendo extensoris digiti minimi (*cut*)

Tendines extensoris digitorum (*cut*)

Retinaculum extensorium carpi
(Vaginae carpeae dorsales
tendinum *numbered*)

Os 5 metacarpi

A. collateralis media

Septum intermusculare laterale brachii

M. brachioradialis

Extensor radialis longus carpi

Epicondylus lateralis humeri

Tendo extensorius communis
(*partially cut*)

Extensor radialis brevis carpi

Supinator

N. interosseus posterior antebrachii

Pronator teres

Radius

N. interosseus posterior antebrachii

Abductor longus pollicis

Extensor brevis pollicis

Tendo extensoris radialis brevis carpi

Tendo extensoris radialis longi carpi

A. radialis

Os 1 metacarpi

Os 2 metacarpi

M. interosseus dorsalis 1

Plate 455

Cubitus and Antebrachium

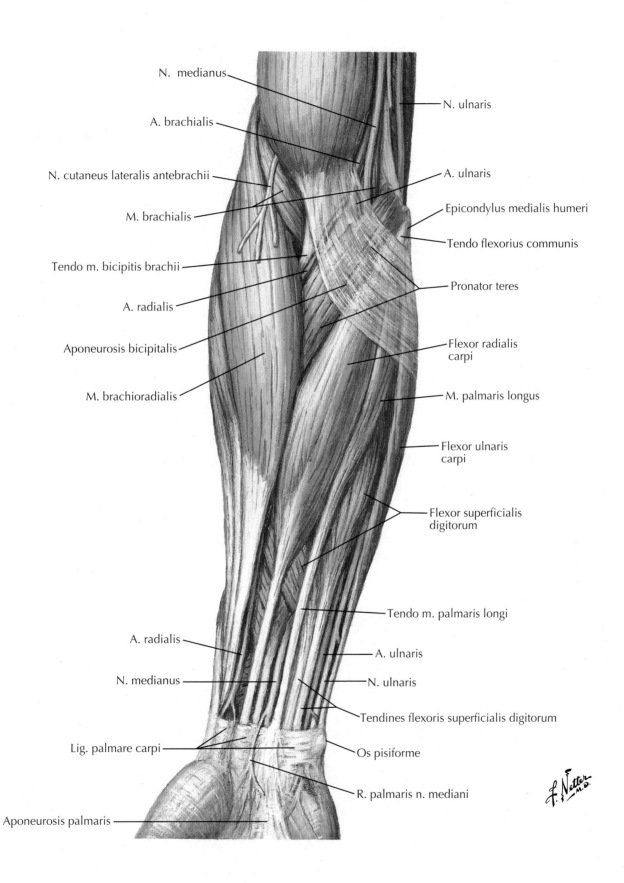

N. medianus

N. ulnaris

A. brachialis

N. cutaneus lateralis antebrachii

A. ulnaris

M. brachialis

Epicondylus medialis humeri

Tendo flexorius communis

Tendo m. bicipitis brachii

Pronator teres

A. radialis

Aponeurosis bicipitalis

Flexor radialis carpi

M. brachioradialis

M. palmaris longus

Flexor ulnaris carpi

Flexor superficialis digitorum

Tendo m. palmaris longi

A. radialis

A. ulnaris

N. medianus

N. ulnaris

Tendines flexoris superficialis digitorum

Lig. palmare carpi

Os pisiforme

R. palmaris n. mediani

Aponeurosis palmaris

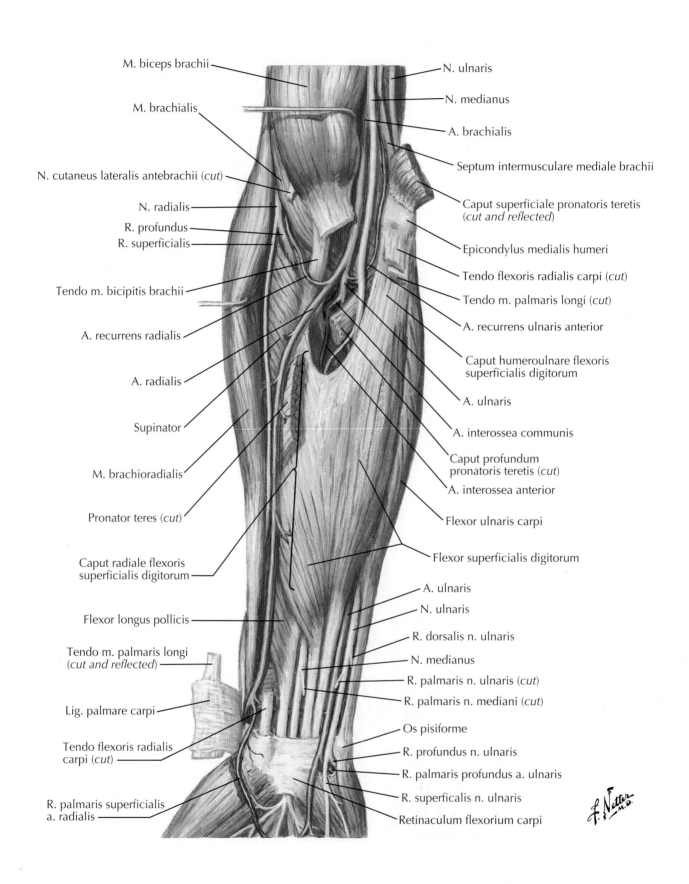

M. biceps brachii

M. brachialis

N. cutaneus lateralis antebrachii (*cut*)

N. radialis

R. profundus

R. superficialis

Tendo m. bicipitis brachii

A. recurrens radialis

A. radialis

Supinator

M. brachioradialis

Pronator teres (*cut*)

Caput radiale flexoris superficialis digitorum

Flexor longus pollicis

Tendo m. palmaris longi (*cut and reflected*)

Lig. palmare carpi

Tendo flexoris radialis carpi (*cut*)

R. palmaris superficialis a. radialis

N. ulnaris

N. medianus

A. brachialis

Septum intermusculare mediale brachii

Caput superficiale pronatoris teretis (*cut and reflected*)

Epicondylus medialis humeri

Tendo flexoris radialis carpi (*cut*)

Tendo m. palmaris longi (*cut*)

A. recurrens ulnaris anterior

Caput humeroulnare flexoris superficialis digitorum

A. ulnaris

A. interossea communis

Caput profundum pronatoris teretis (*cut*)

A. interossea anterior

Flexor ulnaris carpi

Flexor superficialis digitorum

A. ulnaris

N. ulnaris

R. dorsalis n. ulnaris

N. medianus

R. palmaris n. ulnaris (*cut*)

R. palmaris n. mediani (*cut*)

Os pisiforme

R. profundus n. ulnaris

R. palmaris profundus a. ulnaris

R. superficalis n. ulnaris

Retinaculum flexorium carpi

Plate 457

Cubitus and Antebrachium

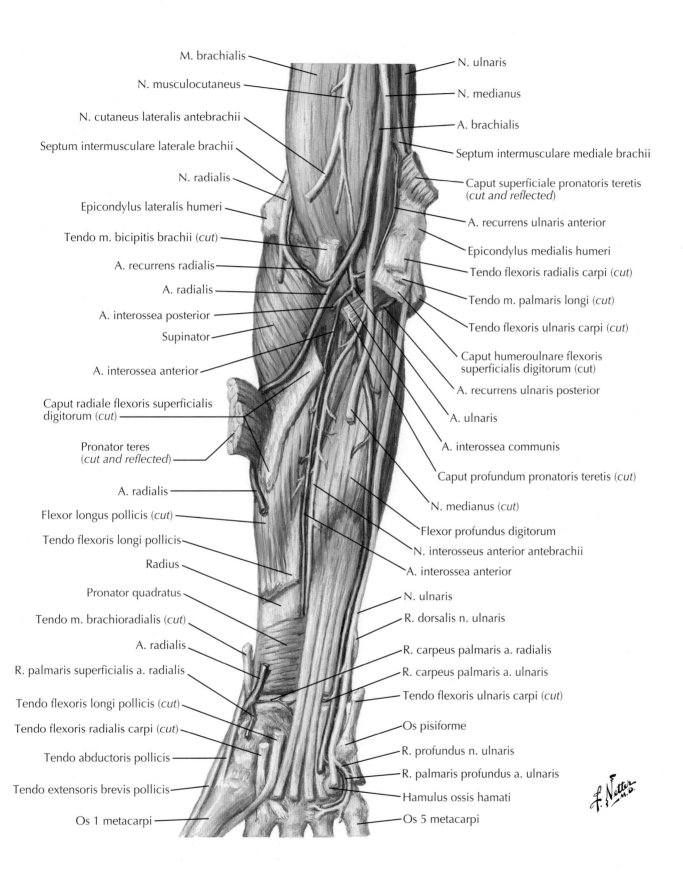

M. brachialis

N. musculocutaneus

N. cutaneus lateralis antebrachii

Septum intermusculare laterale brachii

N. radialis

Epicondylus lateralis humeri

Tendo m. bicipitis brachii (*cut*)

A. recurrens radialis

A. radialis

A. interossea posterior

Supinator

A. interossea anterior

Caput radiale flexoris superficialis
digitorum (*cut*)

Pronator teres
(*cut and reflected*)

A. radialis

Flexor longus pollicis (*cut*)

Tendo flexoris longi pollicis

Radius

Pronator quadratus

Tendo m. brachioradialis (*cut*)

A. radialis

R. palmaris superficialis a. radialis

Tendo flexoris longi pollicis (*cut*)

Tendo flexoris radialis carpi (*cut*)

Tendo abductoris pollicis

Tendo extensoris brevis pollicis

Os 1 metacarpi

N. ulnaris

N. medianus

A. brachialis

Septum intermusculare mediale brachii

Caput superficiale pronatoris teretis
(*cut and reflected*)

A. recurrens ulnaris anterior

Epicondylus medialis humeri

Tendo flexoris radialis carpi (*cut*)

Tendo m. palmaris longi (*cut*)

Tendo flexoris ulnaris carpi (*cut*)

Caput humeroulnare flexoris
superficialis digitorum (cut)

A. recurrens ulnaris posterior

A. ulnaris

A. interossea communis

Caput profundum pronatoris teretis (*cut*)

N. medianus (*cut*)

Flexor profundus digitorum

N. interosseus anterior antebrachii

A. interossea anterior

N. ulnaris

R. dorsalis n. ulnaris

R. carpeus palmaris a. radialis

R. carpeus palmaris a. ulnaris

Tendo flexoris ulnaris carpi (*cut*)

Os pisiforme

R. profundus n. ulnaris

R. palmaris profundus a. ulnaris

Hamulus ossis hamati

Os 5 metacarpi

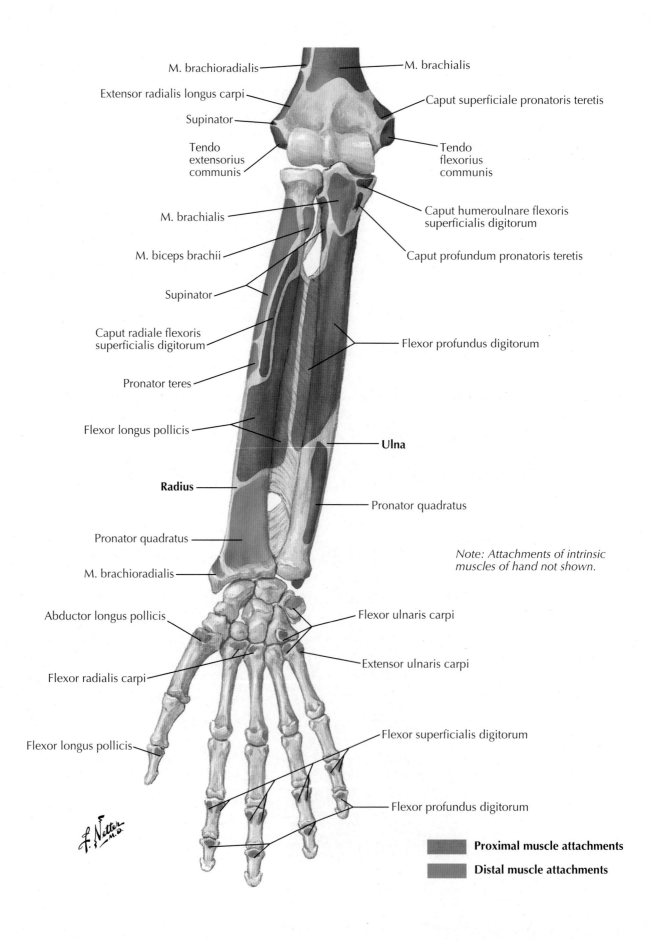

M. brachioradialis

Extensor radialis longus carpi

Supinator

Tendo extensorius communis

M. brachialis

M. biceps brachii

Supinator

Caput radiale flexoris superficialis digitorum

Pronator teres

Flexor longus pollicis

Radius

Pronator quadratus

M. brachioradialis

Abductor longus pollicis

Flexor radialis carpi

Flexor longus pollicis

M. brachialis

Caput superficiale pronatoris teretis

Tendo flexorius communis

Caput humeroulnare flexoris superficialis digitorum

Caput profundum pronatoris teretis

Flexor profundus digitorum

Ulna

Pronator quadratus

Note: Attachments of intrinsic muscles of hand not shown.

Flexor ulnaris carpi

Extensor ulnaris carpi

Flexor superficialis digitorum

Flexor profundus digitorum

Proximal muscle attachments

Distal muscle attachments

Plate 459   **Cubitus and Antebrachium**

Note: Attachments of intrinsic muscles of hand not shown.

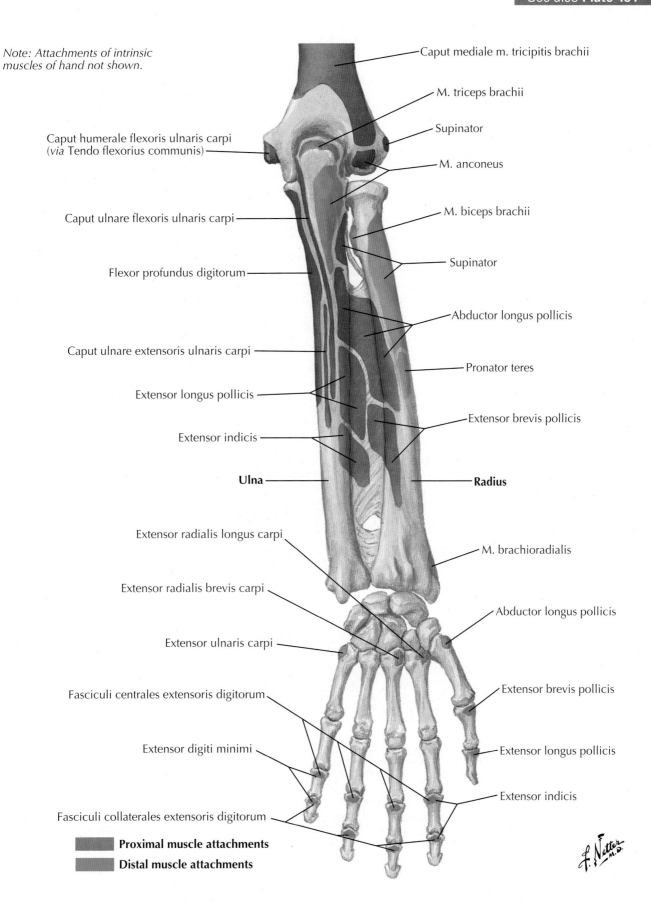

Caput mediale m. tricipitis brachii

M. triceps brachii

Supinator

M. anconeus

M. biceps brachii

Supinator

Abductor longus pollicis

Pronator teres

Extensor brevis pollicis

Radius

M. brachioradialis

Abductor longus pollicis

Extensor brevis pollicis

Extensor longus pollicis

Extensor indicis

Caput humerale flexoris ulnaris carpi (*via* Tendo flexorius communis)

Caput ulnare flexoris ulnaris carpi

Flexor profundus digitorum

Caput ulnare extensoris ulnaris carpi

Extensor longus pollicis

Extensor indicis

Ulna

Extensor radialis longus carpi

Extensor radialis brevis carpi

Extensor ulnaris carpi

Fasciculi centrales extensoris digitorum

Extensor digiti minimi

Fasciculi collaterales extensoris digitorum

	Proximal muscle attachments
	Distal muscle attachments

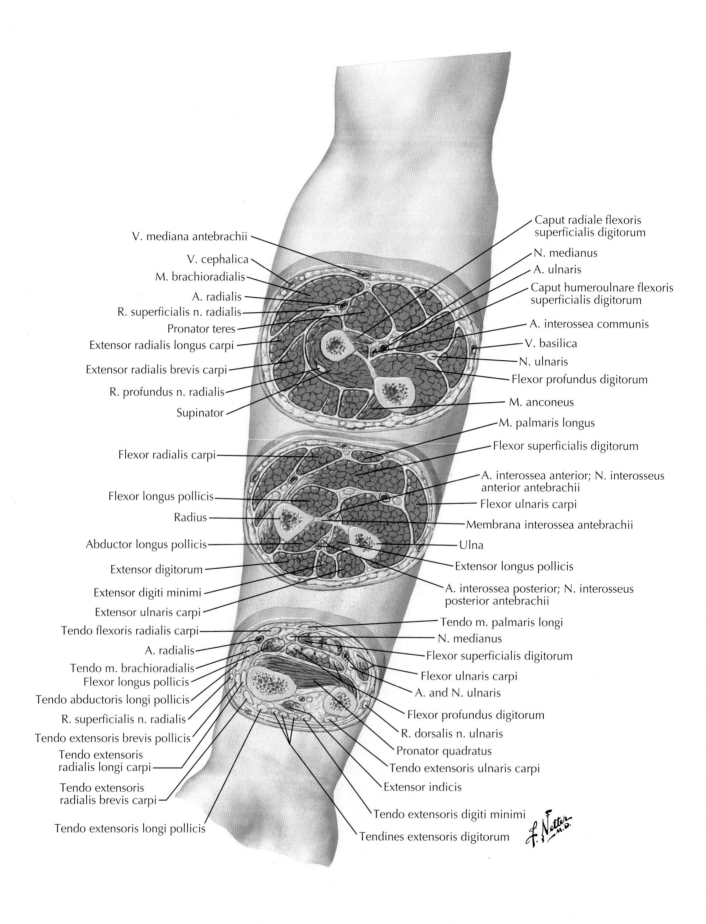

V. mediana antebrachii
V. cephalica
M. brachioradialis
A. radialis
R. superficialis n. radialis
Pronator teres
Extensor radialis longus carpi
Extensor radialis brevis carpi
R. profundus n. radialis
Supinator

Caput radiale flexoris superficialis digitorum
N. medianus
A. ulnaris
Caput humeroulnare flexoris superficialis digitorum
A. interossea communis
V. basilica
N. ulnaris
Flexor profundus digitorum
M. anconeus
M. palmaris longus
Flexor superficialis digitorum

Flexor radialis carpi

Flexor longus pollicis
Radius
Abductor longus pollicis
Extensor digitorum
Extensor digiti minimi
Extensor ulnaris carpi
Tendo flexoris radialis carpi
A. radialis
Tendo m. brachioradialis
Flexor longus pollicis
Tendo abductoris longi pollicis
R. superficialis n. radialis
Tendo extensoris brevis pollicis
Tendo extensoris radialis longi carpi
Tendo extensoris radialis brevis carpi
Tendo extensoris longi pollicis

A. interossea anterior; N. interosseus anterior antebrachii
Flexor ulnaris carpi
Membrana interossea antebrachii
Ulna
Extensor longus pollicis
A. interossea posterior; N. interosseus posterior antebrachii
Tendo m. palmaris longi
N. medianus
Flexor superficialis digitorum
Flexor ulnaris carpi
A. and N. ulnaris
Flexor profundus digitorum
R. dorsalis n. ulnaris
Pronator quadratus
Tendo extensoris ulnaris carpi
Extensor indicis
Tendo extensoris digiti minimi
Tendines extensoris digitorum

Plate 461

Cubitus and Antebrachium

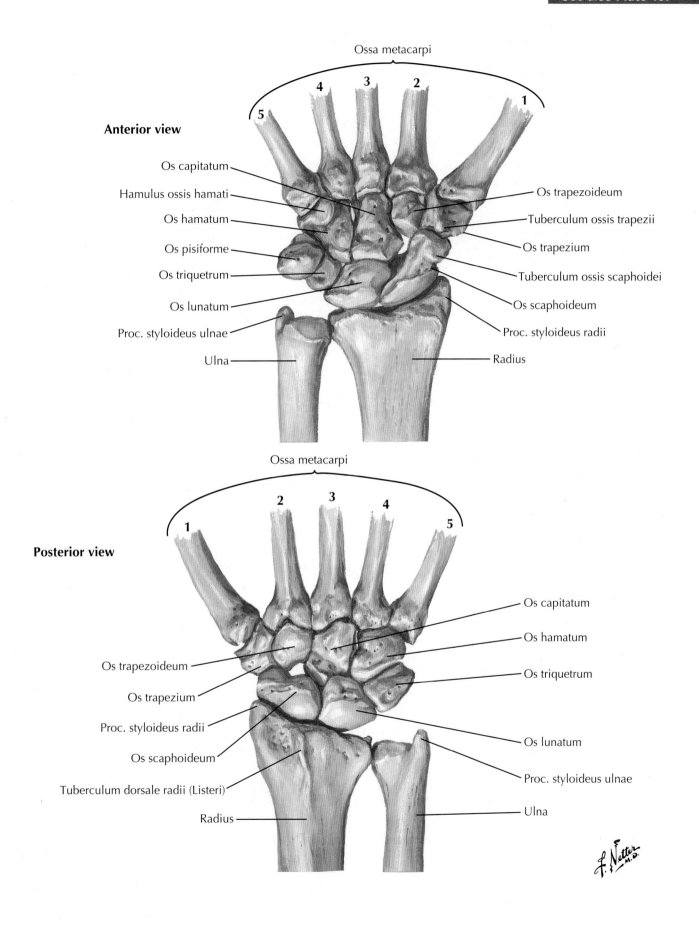

Ossa metacarpi

Anterior view

Os capitatum
Hamulus ossis hamati
Os hamatum
Os pisiforme
Os triquetrum
Os lunatum
Proc. styloideus ulnae
Ulna

Os trapezoideum
Tuberculum ossis trapezii
Os trapezium
Tuberculum ossis scaphoidei
Os scaphoideum
Proc. styloideus radii
Radius

Ossa metacarpi

Posterior view

Os trapezoideum
Os trapezium
Proc. styloideus radii
Os scaphoideum
Tuberculum dorsale radii (Listeri)
Radius

Os capitatum
Os hamatum
Os triquetrum
Os lunatum
Proc. styloideus ulnae
Ulna

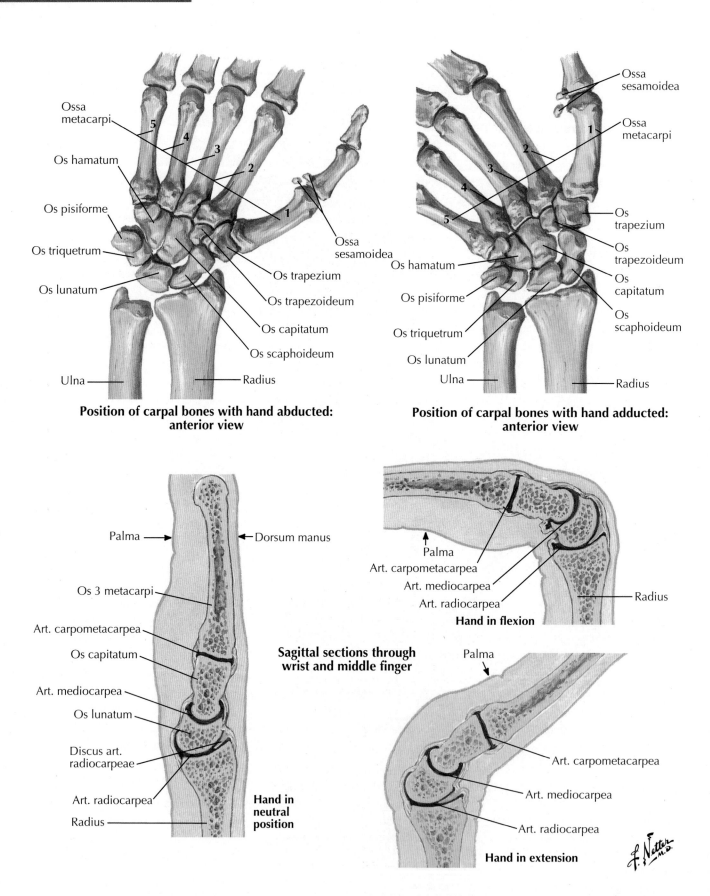

Ossa metacarpi

Os hamatum

Os pisiforme

Os triquetrum

Os lunatum

Ulna

5 4 3 2 1

Ossa sesamoidea

Os trapezium

Os trapezoideum

Os capitatum

Os scaphoideum

Radius

Position of carpal bones with hand abducted: anterior view

Ossa sesamoidea

Ossa metacarpi

2 1

3

4

5

Os hamatum

Os pisiforme

Os triquetrum

Os lunatum

Ulna

Os trapezium

Os trapezoideum

Os capitatum

Os scaphoideum

Radius

Position of carpal bones with hand adducted: anterior view

Palma

Dorsum manus

Os 3 metacarpi

Art. carpometacarpea

Os capitatum

Art. mediocarpea

Os lunatum

Discus art. radiocarpeae

Art. radiocarpea

Radius

Hand in neutral position

Sagittal sections through wrist and middle finger

Palma

Art. carpometacarpea

Art. mediocarpea

Art. radiocarpea

Radius

Hand in flexion

Palma

Art. carpometacarpea

Art. mediocarpea

Art. radiocarpea

Hand in extension

Plate 463

Carpus and Manus

Deep palm

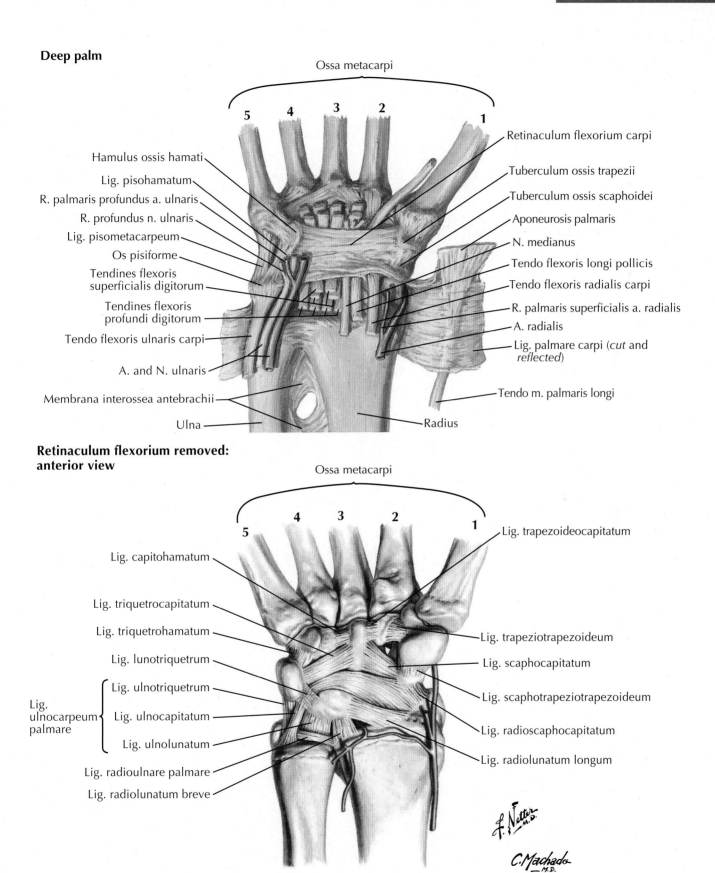

Ossa metacarpi

5   4   3   2   1

Hamulus ossis hamati

Lig. pisohamatum

R. palmaris profundus a. ulnaris

R. profundus n. ulnaris

Lig. pisometacarpeum

Os pisiforme

Tendines flexoris superficialis digitorum

Tendines flexoris profundi digitorum

Tendo flexoris ulnaris carpi

A. and N. ulnaris

Membrana interossea antebrachii

Ulna

Retinaculum flexorium carpi

Tuberculum ossis trapezii

Tuberculum ossis scaphoidei

Aponeurosis palmaris

N. medianus

Tendo flexoris longi pollicis

Tendo flexoris radialis carpi

R. palmaris superficialis a. radialis

A. radialis

Lig. palmare carpi (cut and reflected)

Tendo m. palmaris longi

Radius

Retinaculum flexorium removed: anterior view

Ossa metacarpi

5   4   3   2   1

Lig. capitohamatum

Lig. triquetrocapitatum

Lig. triquetrohamatum

Lig. lunotriquetrum

Lig. ulnocarpeum palmare
 { Lig. ulnotriquetrum

Lig. ulnocapitatum

Lig. ulnolunatum }

Lig. radioulnare palmare

Lig. radiolunatum breve

Lig. trapezoideocapitatum

Lig. trapeziotrapezoideum

Lig. scaphocapitatum

Lig. scaphotrapeziotrapezoideum

Lig. radioscaphocapitatum

Lig. radiolunatum longum

F. Netter M.D.

C. Machado M.D.

Carpus and Manus   **Plate 464**

Posterior view

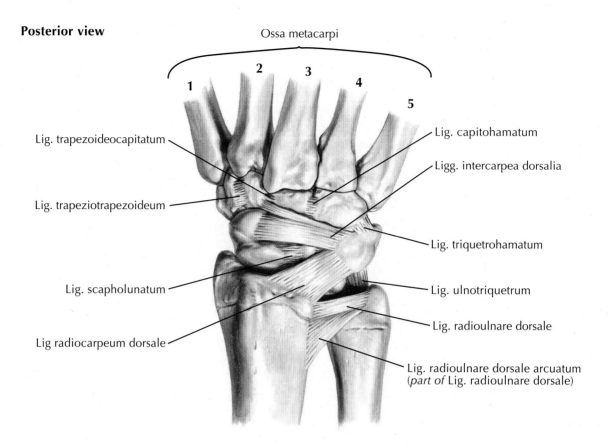

Ossa metacarpi

1   2   3   4   5

Lig. trapezoideocapitatum

Lig. trapeziotrapezoideum

Lig. scapholunatum

Lig radiocarpeum dorsale

Lig. capitohamatum

Ligg. intercarpea dorsalia

Lig. triquetrohamatum

Lig. ulnotriquetrum

Lig. radioulnare dorsale

Lig. radioulnare dorsale arcuatum
(*part of* Lig. radioulnare dorsale)

Coronal section: posterior view

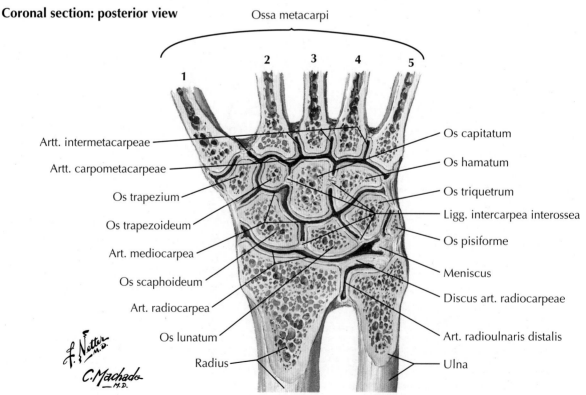

Ossa metacarpi

1   2   3   4   5

Artt. intermetacarpeae

Artt. carpometacarpeae

Os trapezium

Os trapezoideum

Art. mediocarpea

Os scaphoideum

Art. radiocarpea

Os lunatum

Radius

Os capitatum

Os hamatum

Os triquetrum

Ligg. intercarpea interossea

Os pisiforme

Meniscus

Discus art. radiocarpeae

Art. radioulnaris distalis

Ulna

Plate 465

Carpus and Manus

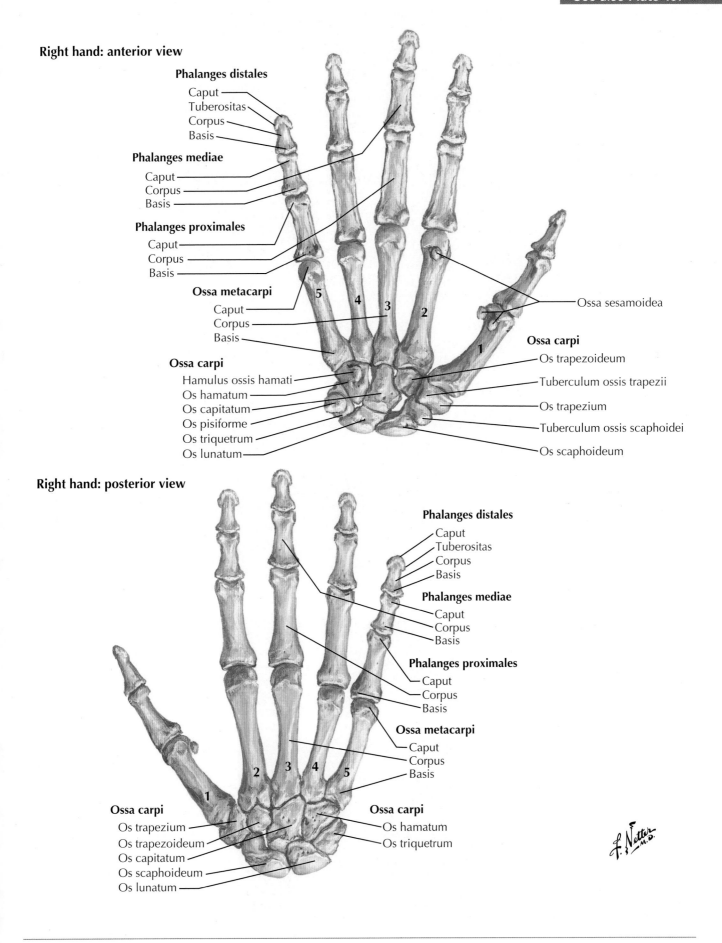

Right hand: anterior view

Phalanges distales
Caput
Tuberositas
Corpus
Basis

Phalanges mediae
Caput
Corpus
Basis

Phalanges proximales
Caput
Corpus
Basis

Ossa metacarpi
Caput
Corpus
Basis

Ossa carpi
Hamulus ossis hamati
Os hamatum
Os capitatum
Os pisiforme
Os triquetrum
Os lunatum

Ossa sesamoidea

Ossa carpi
Os trapezoideum
Tuberculum ossis trapezii
Os trapezium
Tuberculum ossis scaphoidei
Os scaphoideum

Right hand: posterior view

Phalanges distales
Caput
Tuberositas
Corpus
Basis

Phalanges mediae
Caput
Corpus
Basis

Phalanges proximales
Caput
Corpus
Basis

Ossa metacarpi
Caput
Corpus
Basis

Ossa carpi
Os trapezium
Os trapezoideum
Os capitatum
Os scaphoideum
Os lunatum

Ossa carpi
Os hamatum
Os triquetrum

Anteroposterior view

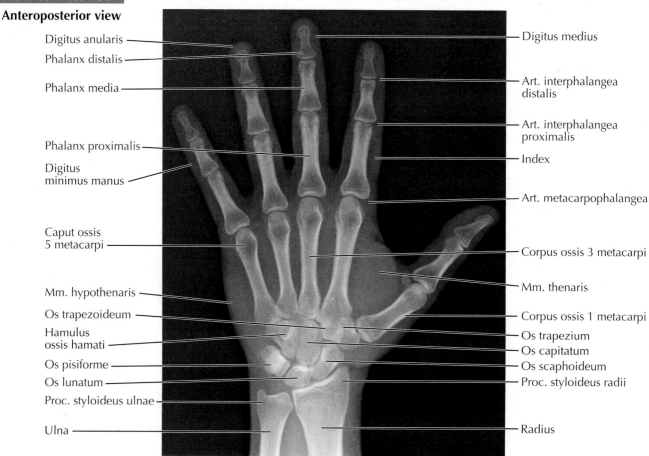

Digitus anularis

Phalanx distalis

Phalanx media

Phalanx proximalis

Digitus minimus manus

Caput ossis 5 metacarpi

Mm. hypothenaris

Os trapezoideum

Hamulus ossis hamati

Os pisiforme

Os lunatum

Proc. styloideus ulnae

Ulna

Digitus medius

Art. interphalangea distalis

Art. interphalangea proximalis

Index

Art. metacarpophalangea

Corpus ossis 3 metacarpi

Mm. thenaris

Corpus ossis 1 metacarpi

Os trapezium

Os capitatum

Os scaphoideum

Proc. styloideus radii

Radius

Lateral view

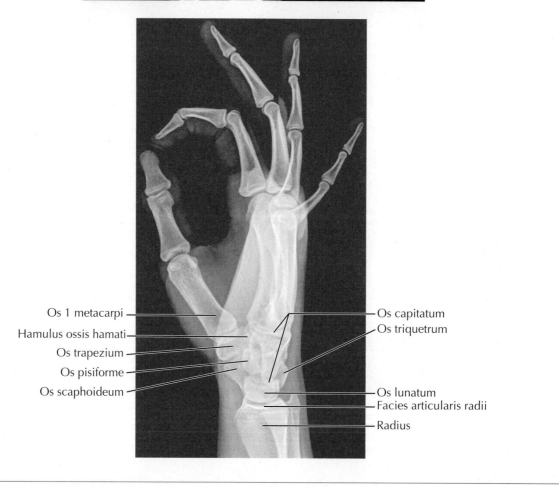

Os 1 metacarpi

Hamulus ossis hamati

Os trapezium

Os pisiforme

Os scaphoideum

Os capitatum

Os triquetrum

Os lunatum

Facies articularis radii

Radius

Plate 467

Carpus and Manus

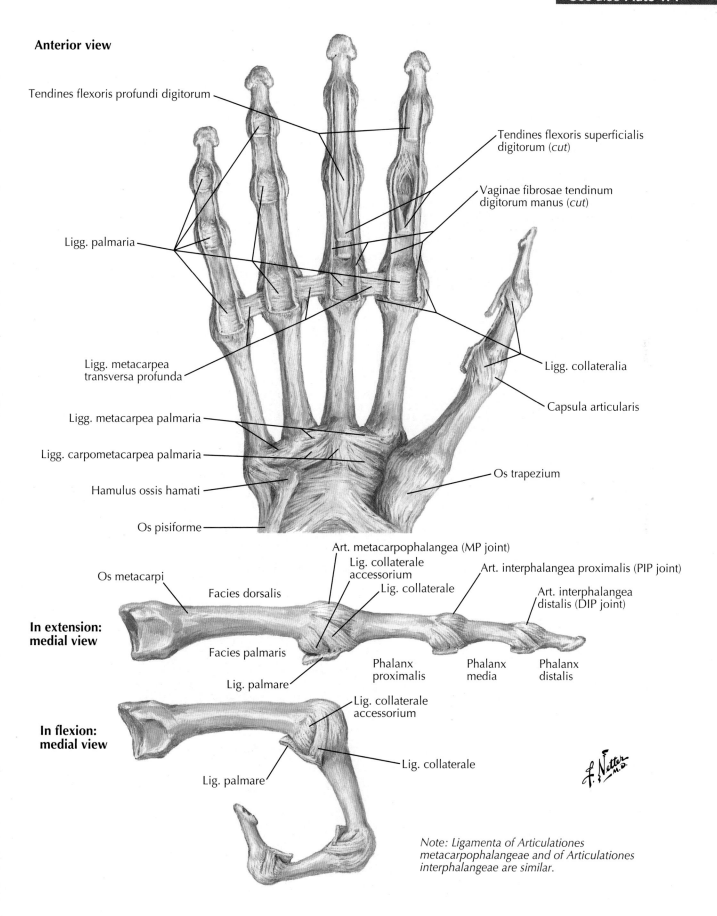

Anterior view

Tendines flexoris profundi digitorum

Tendines flexoris superficialis digitorum (*cut*)

Vaginae fibrosae tendinum digitorum manus (*cut*)

Ligg. palmaria

Ligg. collateralia

Capsula articularis

Ligg. metacarpea transversa profunda

Ligg. metacarpea palmaria

Ligg. carpometacarpea palmaria

Hamulus ossis hamati

Os pisiforme

Os trapezium

Art. metacarpophalangea (MP joint)

Lig. collaterale accessorium

Lig. collaterale

Art. interphalangea proximalis (PIP joint)

Art. interphalangea distalis (DIP joint)

Os metacarpi

Facies dorsalis

In extension: medial view

Facies palmaris

Lig. palmare

Phalanx proximalis

Phalanx media

Phalanx distalis

In flexion: medial view

Lig. collaterale accessorium

Lig. collaterale

Lig. palmare

Note: Ligamenta of Articulationes metacarpophalangeae and of Articulationes interphalangeae are similar.

Carpus and Manus

Plate 468

Anterior views

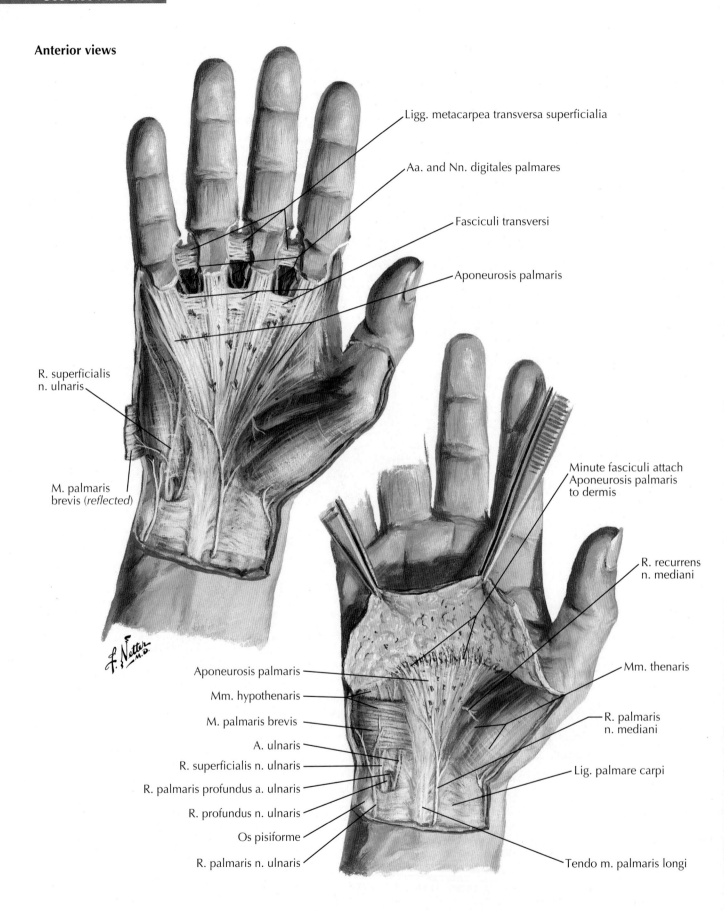

Ligg. metacarpea transversa superficialia

Aa. and Nn. digitales palmares

Fasciculi transversi

Aponeurosis palmaris

R. superficialis
n. ulnaris

M. palmaris
brevis (*reflected*)

Minute fasciculi attach
Aponeurosis palmaris
to dermis

R. recurrens
n. mediani

Mm. thenaris

R. palmaris
n. mediani

Lig. palmare carpi

Tendo m. palmaris longi

Aponeurosis palmaris

Mm. hypothenaris

M. palmaris brevis

A. ulnaris

R. superficialis n. ulnaris

R. palmaris profundus a. ulnaris

R. profundus n. ulnaris

Os pisiforme

R. palmaris n. ulnaris

Plate 469

Carpus and Manus

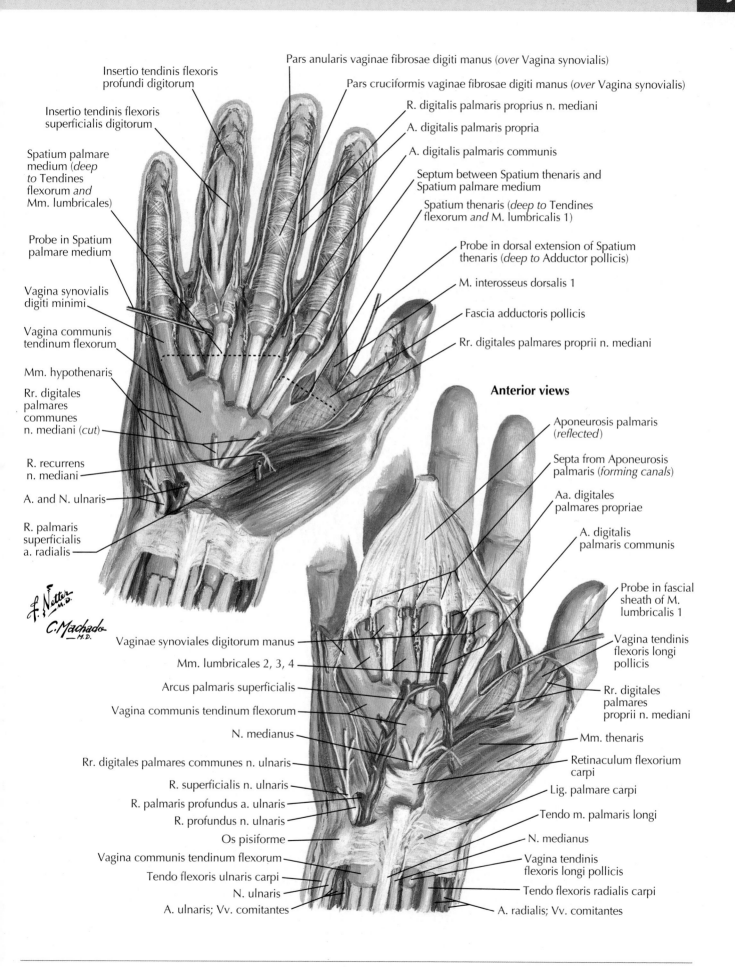

Insertio tendinis flexoris profundi digitorum

Insertio tendinis flexoris superficialis digitorum

Spatium palmare medium (*deep to* Tendines flexorum *and* Mm. lumbricales)

Probe in Spatium palmare medium

Vagina synovialis digiti minimi

Vagina communis tendinum flexorum

Mm. hypothenaris

Rr. digitales palmares communes n. mediani (*cut*)

R. recurrens n. mediani

A. and N. ulnaris

R. palmaris superficialis a. radialis

Pars anularis vaginae fibrosae digiti manus (*over* Vagina synovialis)

Pars cruciformis vaginae fibrosae digiti manus (*over* Vagina synovialis)

R. digitalis palmaris proprius n. mediani

A. digitalis palmaris propria

A. digitalis palmaris communis

Septum between Spatium thenaris and Spatium palmare medium

Spatium thenaris (*deep to* Tendines flexorum *and* M. lumbricalis 1)

Probe in dorsal extension of Spatium thenaris (*deep to* Adductor pollicis)

M. interosseus dorsalis 1

Fascia adductoris pollicis

Rr. digitales palmares proprii n. mediani

Anterior views

Aponeurosis palmaris (*reflected*)

Septa from Aponeurosis palmaris (*forming canals*)

Aa. digitales palmares propriae

A. digitalis palmaris communis

Probe in fascial sheath of M. lumbricalis 1

Vagina tendinis flexoris longi pollicis

Rr. digitales palmares proprii n. mediani

Mm. thenaris

Retinaculum flexorium carpi

Lig. palmare carpi

Tendo m. palmaris longi

N. medianus

Vagina tendinis flexoris longi pollicis

Tendo flexoris radialis carpi

A. radialis; Vv. comitantes

Vaginae synoviales digitorum manus

Mm. lumbricales 2, 3, 4

Arcus palmaris superficialis

Vagina communis tendinum flexorum

N. medianus

Rr. digitales palmares communes n. ulnaris

R. superficialis n. ulnaris

R. palmaris profundus a. ulnaris

R. profundus n. ulnaris

Os pisiforme

Vagina communis tendinum flexorum

Tendo flexoris ulnaris carpi

N. ulnaris

A. ulnaris; Vv. comitantes

Common variation

Usual arrangement

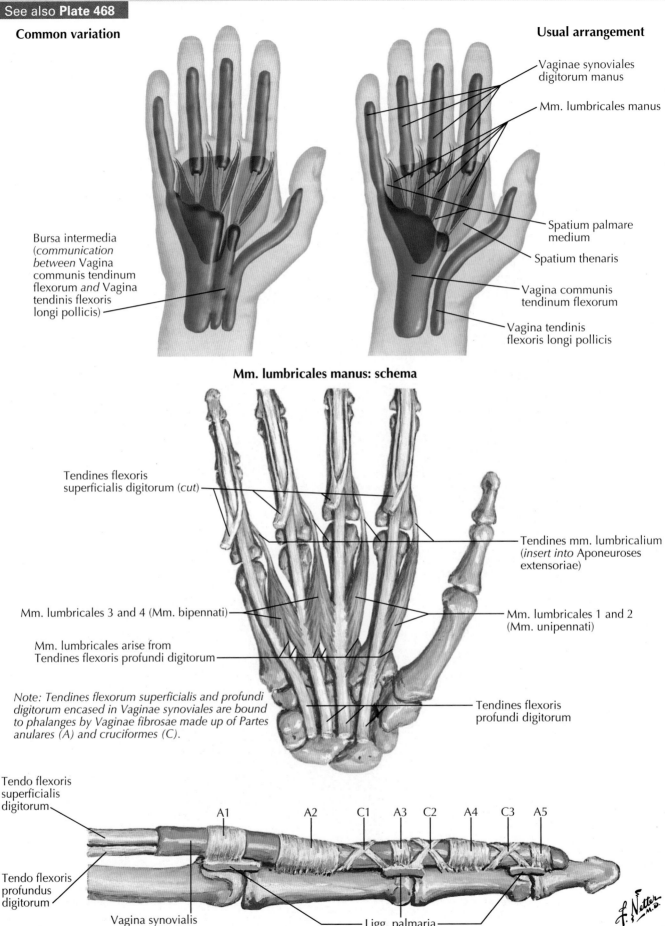

Vaginae synoviales
digitorum manus

Mm. lumbricales manus

Bursa intermedia
(*communication
between* Vagina
communis tendinum
flexorum *and* Vagina
tendinis flexoris
longi pollicis)

Spatium palmare
medium

Spatium thenaris

Vagina communis
tendinum flexorum

Vagina tendinis
flexoris longi pollicis

Mm. lumbricales manus: schema

Tendines flexoris
superficialis digitorum (*cut*)

Tendines mm. lumbricalium
(*insert into* Aponeuroses
extensoriae)

Mm. lumbricales 3 and 4 (Mm. bipennati)

Mm. lumbricales 1 and 2
(Mm. unipennati)

Mm. lumbricales arise from
Tendines flexoris profundi digitorum

Tendines flexoris
profundi digitorum

Note: *Tendines flexorum superficialis and profundi
digitorum encased in Vaginae synoviales are bound
to phalanges by Vaginae fibrosae made up of Partes
anulares (A) and cruciformes (C).*

Tendo flexoris
superficialis
digitorum

A1   A2   C1   A3   C2   A4   C3   A5

Tendo flexoris
profundus
digitorum

Vagina synovialis

Ligg. palmaria

Plate 471

Carpus and Manus

Palmar view

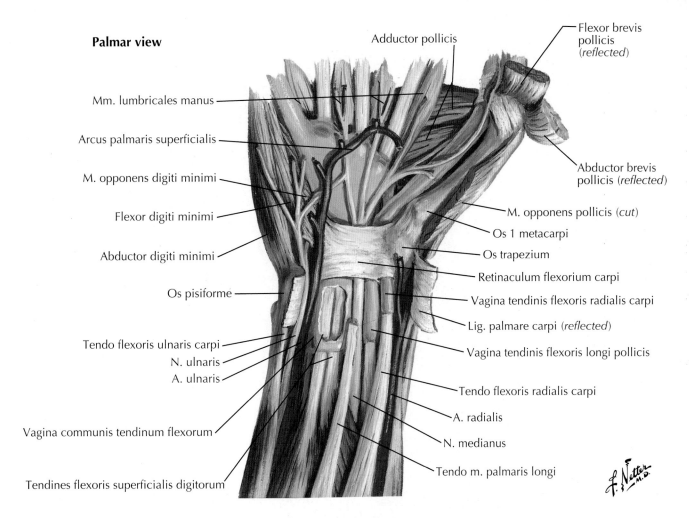

Adductor pollicis

Flexor brevis pollicis (*reflected*)

Mm. lumbricales manus

Arcus palmaris superficialis

M. opponens digiti minimi

Flexor digiti minimi

Abductor digiti minimi

Os pisiforme

Tendo flexoris ulnaris carpi

N. ulnaris

A. ulnaris

Vagina communis tendinum flexorum

Tendines flexoris superficialis digitorum

Abductor brevis pollicis (*reflected*)

M. opponens pollicis (*cut*)

Os 1 metacarpi

Os trapezium

Retinaculum flexorium carpi

Vagina tendinis flexoris radialis carpi

Lig. palmare carpi (*reflected*)

Vagina tendinis flexoris longi pollicis

Tendo flexoris radialis carpi

A. radialis

N. medianus

Tendo m. palmaris longi

Cross section of wrist demonstrating carpal tunnel

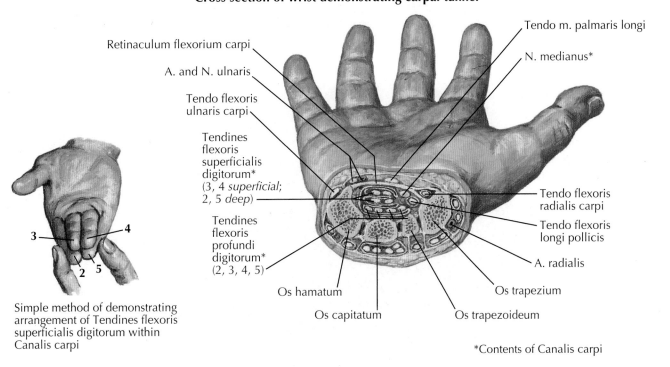

Retinaculum flexorium carpi

A. and N. ulnaris

Tendo flexoris ulnaris carpi

Tendines flexoris superficialis digitorum* (3, 4 *superficial*; 2, 5 *deep*)

Tendines flexoris profundi digitorum* (2, 3, 4, 5)

Os hamatum

Os capitatum

Tendo m. palmaris longi

N. medianus*

Tendo flexoris radialis carpi

Tendo flexoris longi pollicis

A. radialis

Os trapezium

Os trapezoideum

*Contents of Canalis carpi

Simple method of demonstrating arrangement of Tendines flexoris superficialis digitorum within Canalis carpi

3 4
2 5

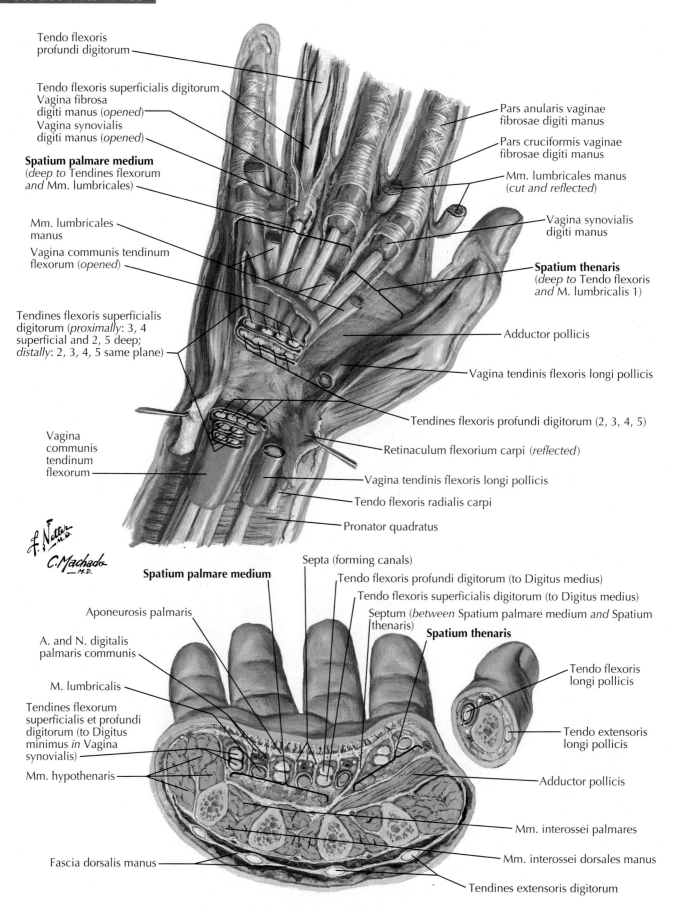

Tendo flexoris profundi digitorum

Tendo flexoris superficialis digitorum
Vagina fibrosa digiti manus (*opened*)
Vagina synovialis digiti manus (*opened*)

Spatium palmare medium
(*deep to* Tendines flexorum *and* Mm. lumbricales)

Mm. lumbricales manus

Vagina communis tendinum flexorum (*opened*)

Tendines flexoris superficialis digitorum (*proximally*: 3, 4 superficial and 2, 5 deep; *distally*: 2, 3, 4, 5 same plane)

Vagina communis tendinum flexorum

Pars anularis vaginae fibrosae digiti manus

Pars cruciformis vaginae fibrosae digiti manus

Mm. lumbricales manus (*cut and reflected*)

Vagina synovialis digiti manus

Spatium thenaris
(*deep to* Tendo flexoris *and* M. lumbricalis 1)

Adductor pollicis

Vagina tendinis flexoris longi pollicis

Tendines flexoris profundi digitorum (2, 3, 4, 5)

Retinaculum flexorium carpi (*reflected*)

Vagina tendinis flexoris longi pollicis

Tendo flexoris radialis carpi

Pronator quadratus

Septa (forming canals)

Tendo flexoris profundi digitorum (to Digitus medius)

Tendo flexoris superficialis digitorum (to Digitus medius)

Septum (*between* Spatium palmare medium *and* Spatium thenaris)

Spatium thenaris

Spatium palmare medium

Aponeurosis palmaris

A. and N. digitalis palmaris communis

M. lumbricalis

Tendines flexorum superficialis et profundi digitorum (to Digitus minimus *in* Vagina synovialis)

Mm. hypothenaris

Fascia dorsalis manus

Tendo flexoris longi pollicis

Tendo extensoris longi pollicis

Adductor pollicis

Mm. interossei palmares

Mm. interossei dorsales manus

Tendines extensoris digitorum

Plate 473

Carpus and Manus

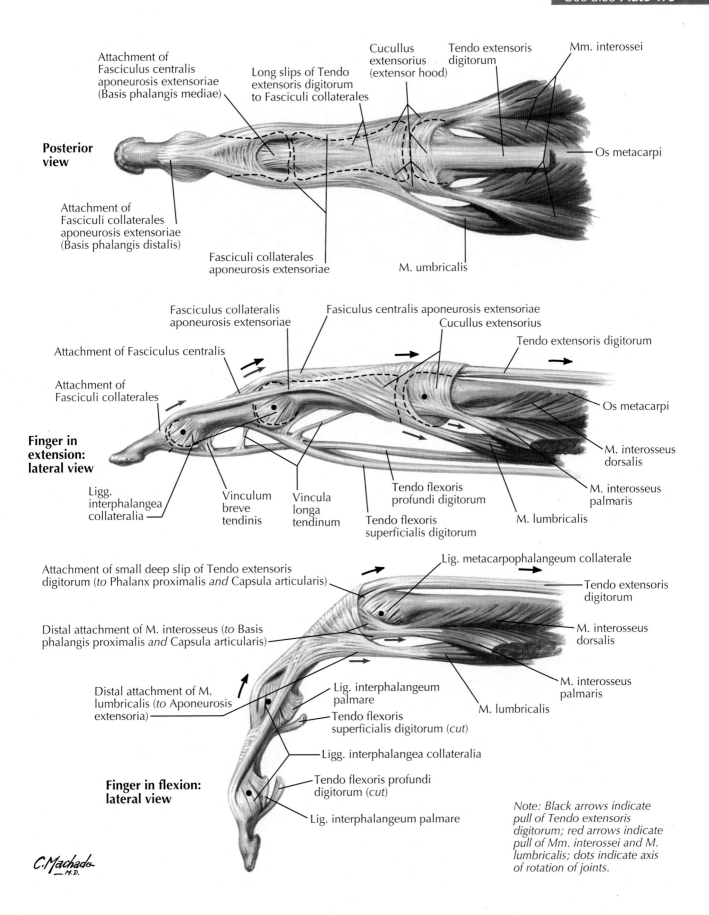

Posterior view

Attachment of Fasciculus centralis aponeurosis extensoriae (Basis phalangis mediae)

Long slips of Tendo extensoris digitorum to Fasciculi collaterales

Cucullus extensorius (extensor hood)

Tendo extensoris digitorum

Mm. interossei

Os metacarpi

Attachment of Fasciculi collaterales aponeurosis extensoriae (Basis phalangis distalis)

Fasciculi collaterales aponeurosis extensoriae

M. umbricalis

Finger in extension: lateral view

Fasciculus collateralis aponeurosis extensoriae

Fasiculus centralis aponeurosis extensoriae

Cucullus extensorius

Tendo extensoris digitorum

Attachment of Fasciculus centralis

Attachment of Fasciculi collaterales

Os metacarpi

M. interosseus dorsalis

M. interosseus palmaris

Ligg. interphalangea collateralia

Vinculum breve tendinis

Vincula longa tendinum

Tendo flexoris profundi digitorum

Tendo flexoris superficialis digitorum

M. lumbricalis

Finger in flexion: lateral view

Attachment of small deep slip of Tendo extensoris digitorum (*to* Phalanx proximalis *and* Capsula articularis)

Lig. metacarpophalangeum collaterale

Tendo extensoris digitorum

Distal attachment of M. interosseus (*to* Basis phalangis proximalis *and* Capsula articularis)

M. interosseus dorsalis

Distal attachment of M. lumbricalis (*to* Aponeurosis extensoria)

Lig. interphalangeum palmare

Tendo flexoris superficialis digitorum (*cut*)

Ligg. interphalangea collateralia

Tendo flexoris profundi digitorum (*cut*)

Lig. interphalangeum palmare

M. interosseus palmaris

M. lumbricalis

Note: Black arrows indicate pull of Tendo extensoris digitorum; red arrows indicate pull of Mm. interossei and M. lumbricalis; dots indicate axis of rotation of joints.

C. Machado M.D.

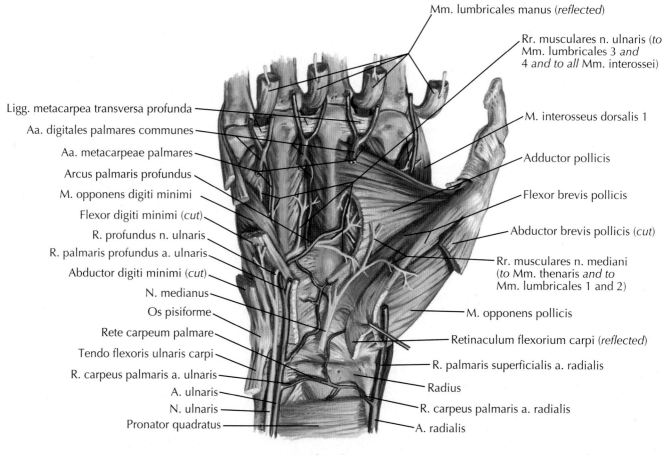

Mm. lumbricales manus (*reflected*)

Rr. musculares n. ulnaris (*to* Mm. lumbricales 3 *and* 4 *and to all* Mm. interossei)

Ligg. metacarpea transversa profunda

Aa. digitales palmares communes

Aa. metacarpeae palmares

Arcus palmaris profundus

M. opponens digiti minimi

Flexor digiti minimi (*cut*)

R. profundus n. ulnaris

R. palmaris profundus a. ulnaris

Abductor digiti minimi (*cut*)

N. medianus

Os pisiforme

Rete carpeum palmare

Tendo flexoris ulnaris carpi

R. carpeus palmaris a. ulnaris

A. ulnaris

N. ulnaris

Pronator quadratus

M. interosseus dorsalis 1

Adductor pollicis

Flexor brevis pollicis

Abductor brevis pollicis (*cut*)

Rr. musculares n. mediani (*to* Mm. thenaris *and to* Mm. lumbricales 1 and 2)

M. opponens pollicis

Retinaculum flexorium carpi (*reflected*)

R. palmaris superficialis a. radialis

Radius

R. carpeus palmaris a. radialis

A. radialis

Anterior view

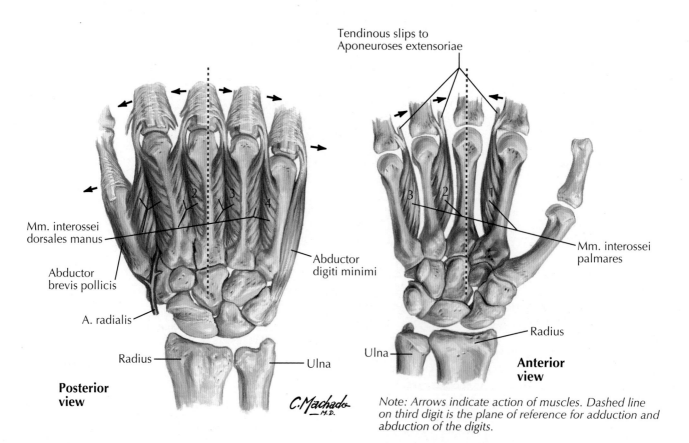

Tendinous slips to Aponeuroses extensoriae

Mm. interossei dorsales manus

Abductor brevis pollicis

A. radialis

Radius

Posterior view

Abductor digiti minimi

Ulna

Mm. interossei palmares

Radius

Ulna

Anterior view

Note: Arrows indicate action of muscles. Dashed line on third digit is the plane of reference for adduction and abduction of the digits.

C.Machado
M.D.

Plate 475

Carpus and Manus

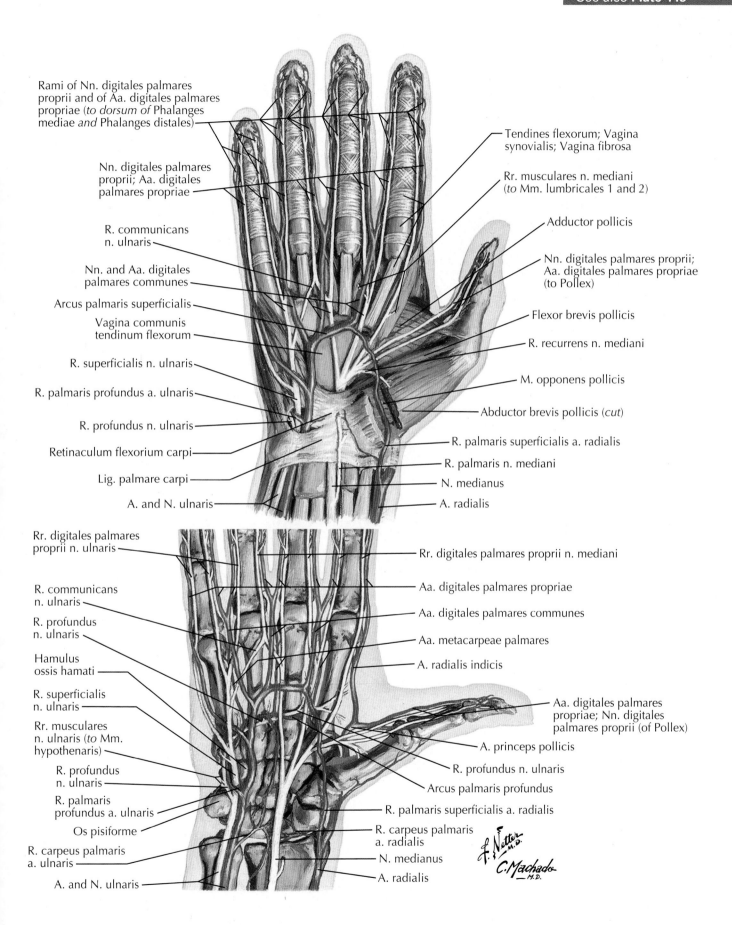

Rami of Nn. digitales palmares proprii and of Aa. digitales palmares propriae (*to dorsum of* Phalanges mediae *and* Phalanges distales)

Nn. digitales palmares proprii; Aa. digitales palmares propriae

R. communicans n. ulnaris

Nn. and Aa. digitales palmares communes

Arcus palmaris superficialis

Vagina communis tendinum flexorum

R. superficialis n. ulnaris

R. palmaris profundus a. ulnaris

R. profundus n. ulnaris

Retinaculum flexorium carpi

Lig. palmare carpi

A. and N. ulnaris

Tendines flexorum; Vagina synovialis; Vagina fibrosa

Rr. musculares n. mediani (*to* Mm. lumbricales 1 and 2)

Adductor pollicis

Nn. digitales palmares proprii; Aa. digitales palmares propriae (to Pollex)

Flexor brevis pollicis

R. recurrens n. mediani

M. opponens pollicis

Abductor brevis pollicis (*cut*)

R. palmaris superficialis a. radialis

R. palmaris n. mediani

N. medianus

A. radialis

Rr. digitales palmares proprii n. ulnaris

R. communicans n. ulnaris

R. profundus n. ulnaris

Hamulus ossis hamati

R. superficialis n. ulnaris

Rr. musculares n. ulnaris (*to* Mm. hypothenaris)

R. profundus n. ulnaris

R. palmaris profundus a. ulnaris

Os pisiforme

R. carpeus palmaris a. ulnaris

A. and N. ulnaris

Rr. digitales palmares proprii n. mediani

Aa. digitales palmares propriae

Aa. digitales palmares communes

Aa. metacarpeae palmares

A. radialis indicis

Aa. digitales palmares propriae; Nn. digitales palmares proprii (of Pollex)

A. princeps pollicis

R. profundus n. ulnaris

Arcus palmaris profundus

R. palmaris superficialis a. radialis

R. carpeus palmaris a. radialis

N. medianus

A. radialis

f. Netter M.D.

C. Machado M.D.

Foveola radialis (anatomical snuffbox) boundaries
Roof: Cutis
Floor: Os scaphoideum and Os trapezium
Anterior border: Tendo extensoris brevis pollicis and
  Tendo abductoris longi pollicis
Posterior border: Tendo extensoris longi pollicis
Proximal border: Proc. styloideus radii
Distal border: Basis ossis 1 metacarpi

Foveola radialis contents (superficial to deep)
R. digitalis dorsalis n. radialis
Tributaries of V. cephalica (*cut away*)
A. radialis and branches

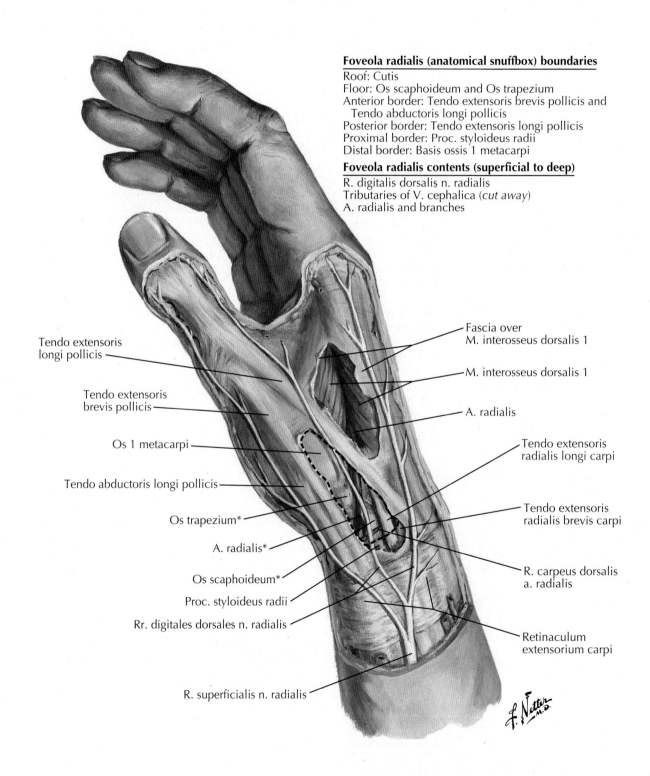

Tendo extensoris
longi pollicis

Tendo extensoris
brevis pollicis

Os 1 metacarpi

Tendo abductoris longi pollicis

Os trapezium*

A. radialis*

Os scaphoideum*

Proc. styloideus radii

Rr. digitales dorsales n. radialis

R. superficialis n. radialis

Fascia over
M. interosseus dorsalis 1

M. interosseus dorsalis 1

A. radialis

Tendo extensoris
radialis longi carpi

Tendo extensoris
radialis brevis carpi

R. carpeus dorsalis
a. radialis

Retinaculum
extensorium carpi

Plate 477

Carpus and Manus

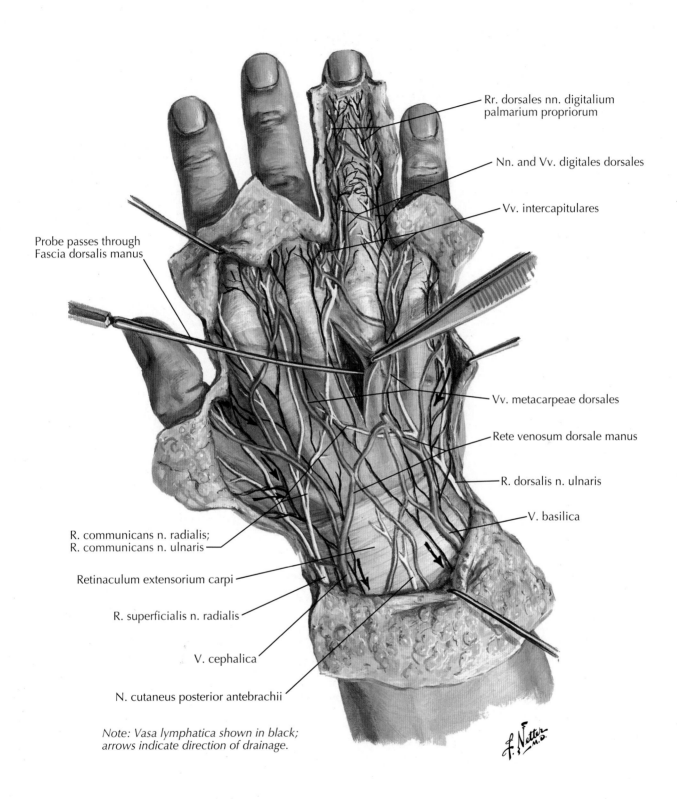

Rr. dorsales nn. digitalium palmarium propriorum

Nn. and Vv. digitales dorsales

Vv. intercapitulares

Probe passes through Fascia dorsalis manus

Vv. metacarpeae dorsales

Rete venosum dorsale manus

R. dorsalis n. ulnaris

V. basilica

R. communicans n. radialis; R. communicans n. ulnaris

Retinaculum extensorium carpi

R. superficialis n. radialis

V. cephalica

N. cutaneus posterior antebrachii

Note: Vasa lymphatica shown in black; arrows indicate direction of drainage.

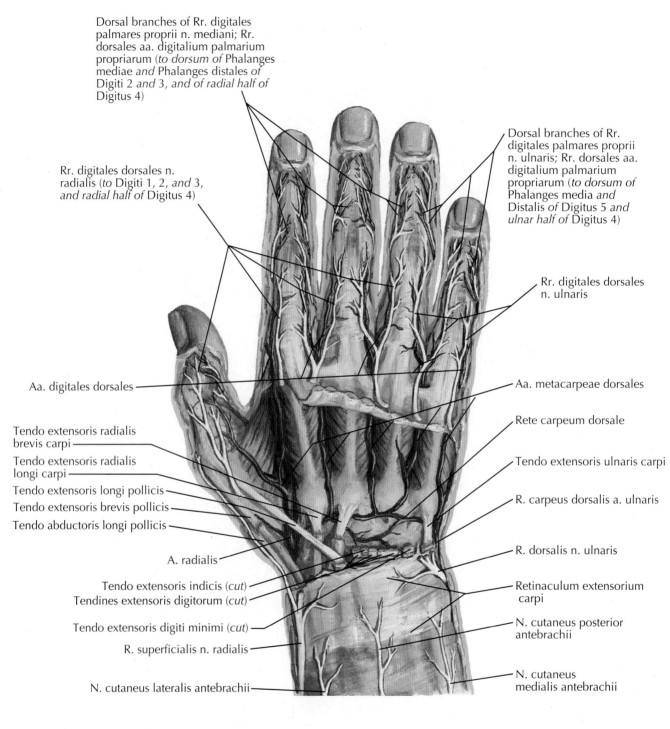

Dorsal branches of Rr. digitales palmares proprii n. mediani; Rr. dorsales aa. digitalium palmarium propriarum (*to dorsum of* Phalanges mediae *and* Phalanges distales *of* Digiti 2 *and* 3, *and of radial half of* Digitus 4)

Rr. digitales dorsales n. radialis (*to* Digiti 1, 2, *and* 3, *and radial half of* Digitus 4)

Dorsal branches of Rr. digitales palmares proprii n. ulnaris; Rr. dorsales aa. digitalium palmarium propriarum (*to dorsum of* Phalanges media *and* Distalis *of* Digitus 5 *and* ulnar half *of* Digitus 4)

Rr. digitales dorsales n. ulnaris

Aa. digitales dorsales

Aa. metacarpeae dorsales

Rete carpeum dorsale

Tendo extensoris radialis brevis carpi

Tendo extensoris radialis longi carpi

Tendo extensoris longi pollicis

Tendo extensoris brevis pollicis

Tendo abductoris longi pollicis

A. radialis

Tendo extensoris indicis (*cut*)

Tendines extensoris digitorum (*cut*)

Tendo extensoris digiti minimi (*cut*)

R. superficialis n. radialis

N. cutaneus lateralis antebrachii

Tendo extensoris ulnaris carpi

R. carpeus dorsalis a. ulnaris

R. dorsalis n. ulnaris

Retinaculum extensorium carpi

N. cutaneus posterior antebrachii

N. cutaneus medialis antebrachii

Plate 479

Carpus and Manus

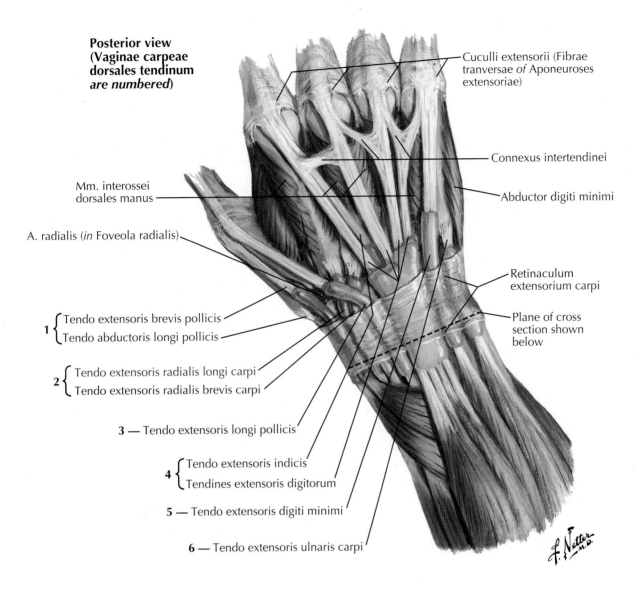

**Posterior view
(Vaginae carpeae
dorsales tendinum
are numbered)**

Cuculi extensorii (Fibrae
tranversae *of* Aponeuroses
extensoriae)

Connexus intertendinei

Abductor digiti minimi

Mm. interossei
dorsales manus

A. radialis (*in* Foveola radialis)

Retinaculum
extensorium carpi

Plane of cross
section shown
below

1 { Tendo extensoris brevis pollicis
    Tendo abductoris longi pollicis

2 { Tendo extensoris radialis longi carpi
    Tendo extensoris radialis brevis carpi

3 — Tendo extensoris longi pollicis

4 { Tendo extensoris indicis
    Tendines extensoris digitorum

5 — Tendo extensoris digiti minimi

6 — Tendo extensoris ulnaris carpi

Cross section of distal forearm

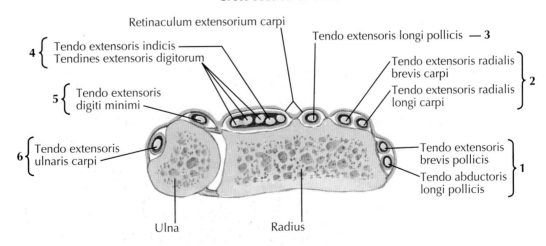

Retinaculum extensorium carpi

Tendo extensoris longi pollicis — 3

4 { Tendo extensoris indicis
    Tendines extensoris digitorum

Tendo extensoris radialis
brevis carpi

Tendo extensoris radialis
longi carpi   } 2

5 { Tendo extensoris
    digiti minimi

6 { Tendo extensoris
    ulnaris carpi

Tendo extensoris
brevis pollicis

Tendo abductoris
longi pollicis   } 1

Ulna

Radius

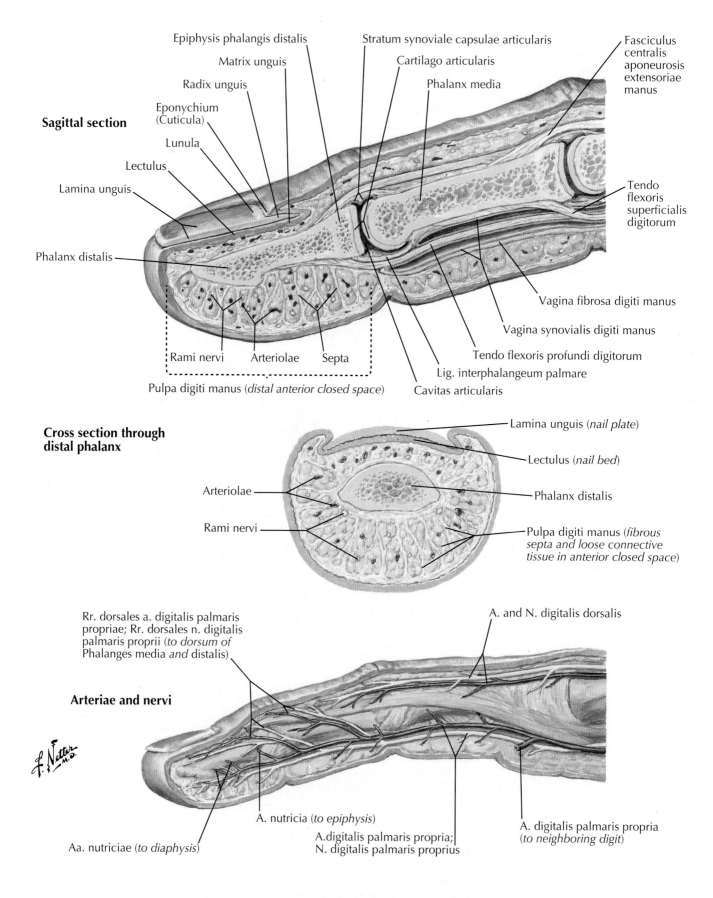

Sagittal section

Epiphysis phalangis distalis

Matrix unguis

Radix unguis

Eponychium (Cuticula)

Lunula

Lectulus

Lamina unguis

Phalanx distalis

Stratum synoviale capsulae articularis

Cartilago articularis

Phalanx media

Fasciculus centralis aponeurosis extensoriae manus

Tendo flexoris superficialis digitorum

Vagina fibrosa digiti manus

Vagina synovialis digiti manus

Tendo flexoris profundi digitorum

Lig. interphalangeum palmare

Cavitas articularis

Rami nervi   Arteriolae   Septa

Pulpa digiti manus (*distal anterior closed space*)

Cross section through distal phalanx

Lamina unguis (*nail plate*)

Lectulus (*nail bed*)

Arteriolae

Phalanx distalis

Rami nervi

Pulpa digiti manus (*fibrous septa and loose connective tissue in anterior closed space*)

Rr. dorsales a. digitalis palmaris propriae; Rr. dorsales n. digitalis palmaris proprii (*to dorsum of Phalanges media and distalis*)

A. and N. digitalis dorsalis

Arteriae and nervi

A. nutricia (*to epiphysis*)

A.digitalis palmaris propria; N. digitalis palmaris proprius

A. digitalis palmaris propria (*to neighboring digit*)

Aa. nutriciae (*to diaphysis*)

Plate 481

Carpus and Manus

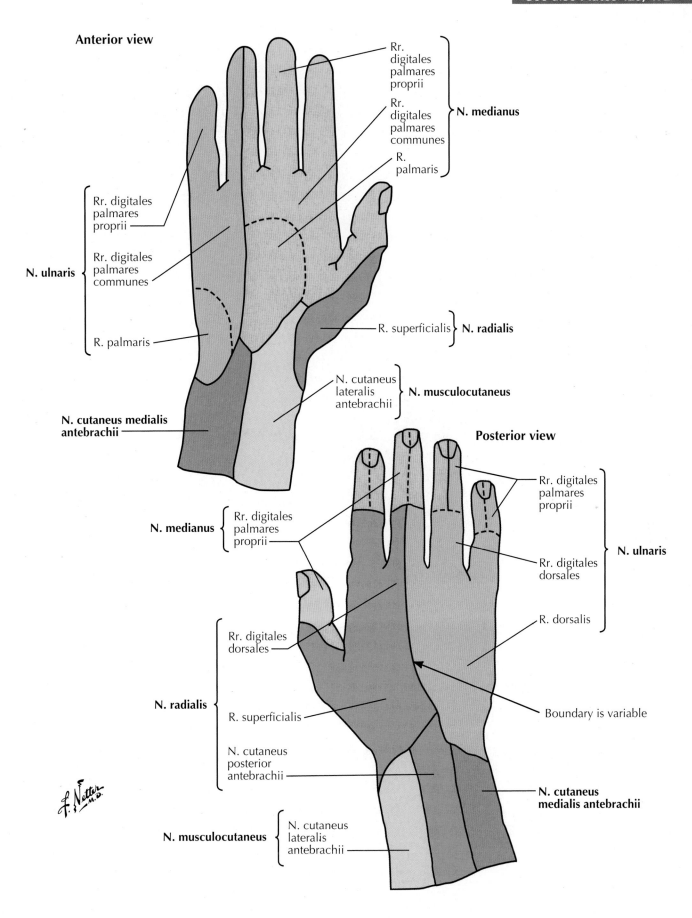

Anterior view

Rr. digitales palmares proprii

Rr. digitales palmares communes

R. palmaris

N. medianus

Rr. digitales palmares proprii

Rr. digitales palmares communes

N. ulnaris

R. palmaris

R. superficialis **N. radialis**

N. cutaneus lateralis antebrachii **N. musculocutaneus**

N. cutaneus medialis antebrachii

Posterior view

N. medianus Rr. digitales palmares proprii

Rr. digitales palmares proprii

Rr. digitales dorsales

N. ulnaris

R. dorsalis

Rr. digitales dorsales

Boundary is variable

N. radialis

R. superficialis

N. cutaneus posterior antebrachii

N. cutaneus medialis antebrachii

N. musculocutaneus N. cutaneus lateralis antebrachii

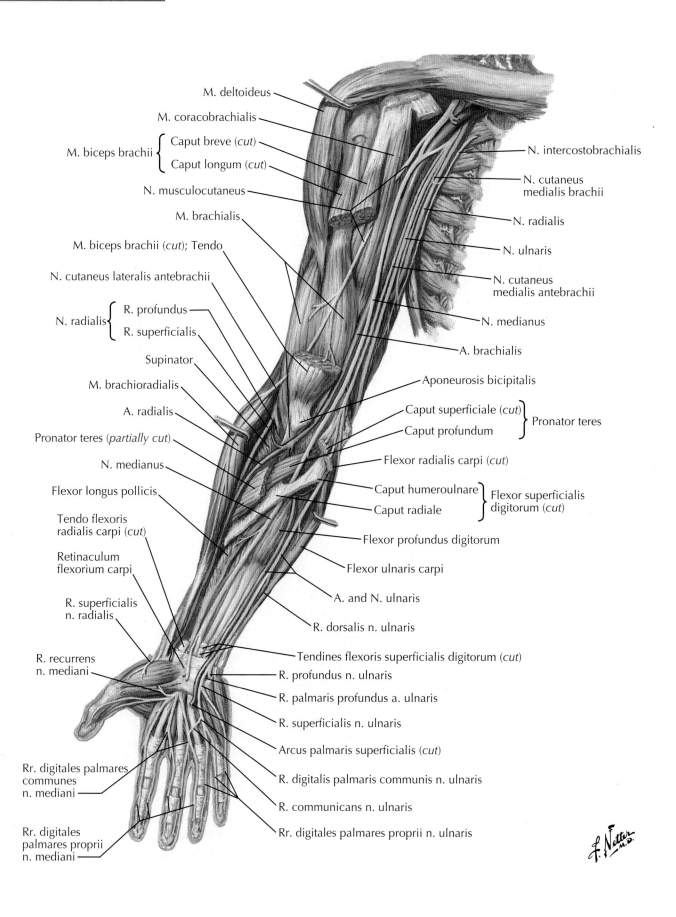

M. deltoideus

M. coracobrachialis

M. biceps brachii { Caput breve (*cut*)

Caput longum (*cut*)

N. musculocutaneus

M. brachialis

M. biceps brachii (*cut*); Tendo

N. cutaneus lateralis antebrachii

N. radialis { R. profundus

R. superficialis

Supinator

M. brachioradialis

A. radialis

Pronator teres (*partially cut*)

N. medianus

Flexor longus pollicis

Tendo flexoris
radialis carpi (*cut*)

Retinaculum
flexorium carpi

R. superficialis
n. radialis

R. recurrens
n. mediani

Rr. digitales palmares
communes
n. mediani

Rr. digitales
palmares proprii
n. mediani

N. intercostobrachialis

N. cutaneus
medialis brachii

N. radialis

N. ulnaris

N. cutaneus
medialis antebrachii

N. medianus

A. brachialis

Aponeurosis bicipitalis

Caput superficiale (*cut*) }
Pronator teres
Caput profundum

Flexor radialis carpi (*cut*)

Caput humeroulnare } Flexor superficialis
digitorum (*cut*)
Caput radiale

Flexor profundus digitorum

Flexor ulnaris carpi

A. and N. ulnaris

R. dorsalis n. ulnaris

Tendines flexoris superficialis digitorum (*cut*)

R. profundus n. ulnaris

R. palmaris profundus a. ulnaris

R. superficialis n. ulnaris

Arcus palmaris superficialis (*cut*)

R. digitalis palmaris communis n. ulnaris

R. communicans n. ulnaris

Rr. digitales palmares proprii n. ulnaris

Plate 483

Nervi

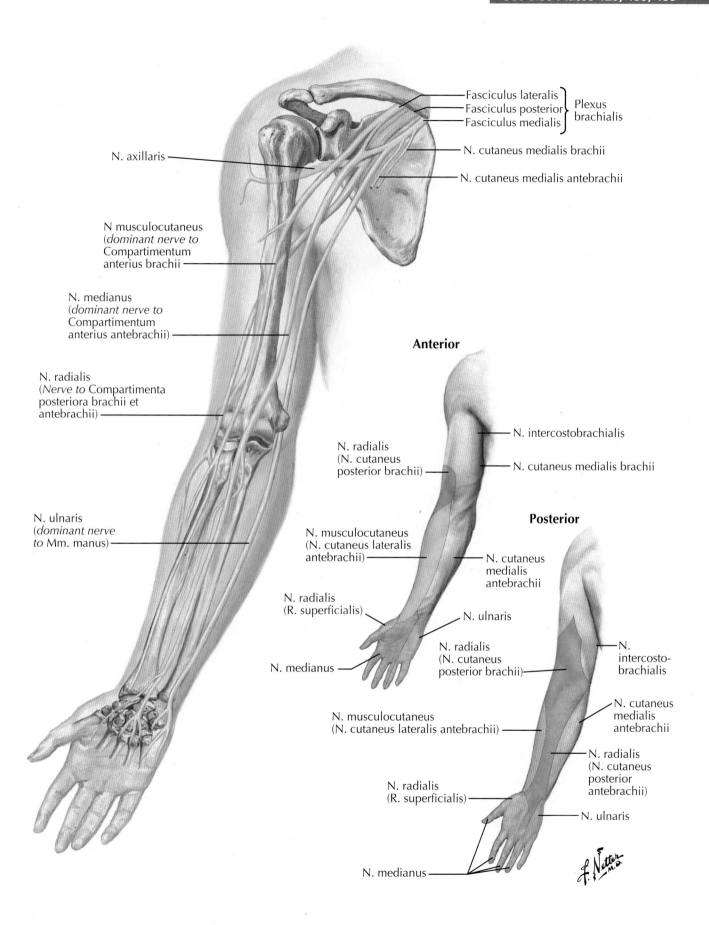

Fasciculus lateralis
Fasciculus posterior   } Plexus brachialis
Fasciculus medialis

N. cutaneus medialis brachii

N. cutaneus medialis antebrachii

N. axillaris

N musculocutaneus
(*dominant nerve to* Compartimentum anterius brachii)

N. medianus
(*dominant nerve to* Compartimentum anterius antebrachii)

N. radialis
(*Nerve to* Compartimenta posteriora brachii et antebrachii)

N. ulnaris
(*dominant nerve to* Mm. manus)

Anterior

N. intercostobrachialis

N. cutaneus medialis brachii

N. radialis
(N. cutaneus posterior brachii)

Posterior

N. musculocutaneus
(N. cutaneus lateralis antebrachii)

N. cutaneus medialis antebrachii

N. radialis
(R. superficialis)

N. ulnaris

N. radialis
(N. cutaneus posterior brachii)

N. medianus

N.
intercosto-
brachialis

N. musculocutaneus
(N. cutaneus lateralis antebrachii)

N. cutaneus medialis antebrachii

N. radialis
(N. cutaneus posterior antebrachii)

N. radialis
(R. superficialis)

N. ulnaris

N. medianus

Nervi

Plate 484

Note: Only muscles innervated
by N. musculocutaneus are shown.

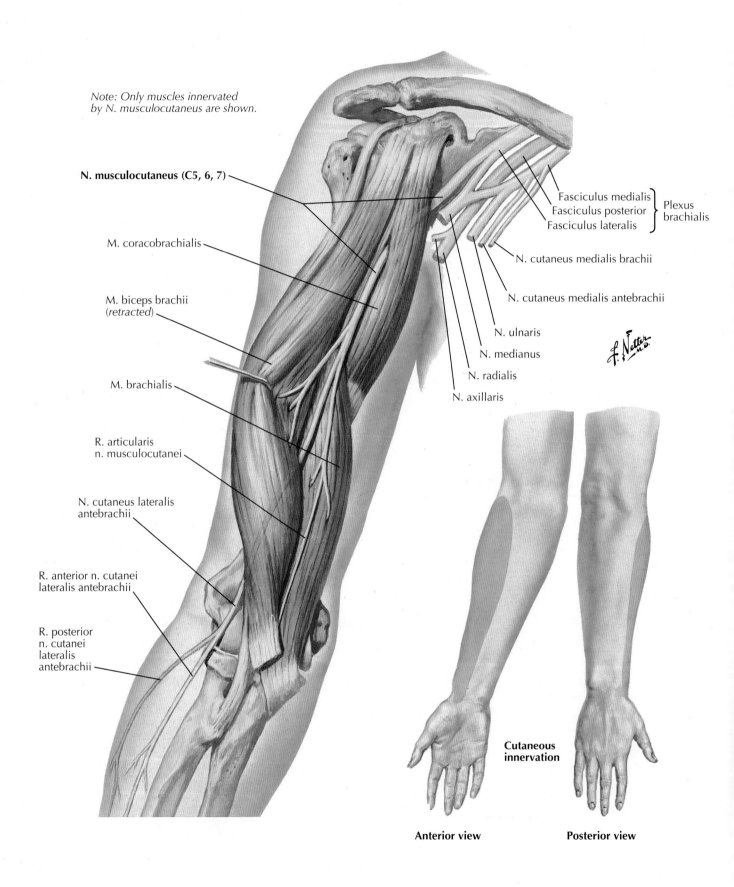

N. musculocutaneus (C5, 6, 7)

Fasciculus medialis
Fasciculus posterior } Plexus
Fasciculus lateralis   brachialis

M. coracobrachialis

N. cutaneus medialis brachii

M. biceps brachii
(*retracted*)

N. cutaneus medialis antebrachii

N. ulnaris

N. medianus

M. brachialis

N. radialis

R. articularis
n. musculocutanei

N. axillaris

N. cutaneus lateralis
antebrachii

R. anterior n. cutanei
lateralis antebrachii

R. posterior
n. cutanei
lateralis
antebrachii

**Cutaneous
innervation**

Anterior view   Posterior view

Plate 485   **Nervi**

Note: Only muscles innervated by N. medianus are shown.

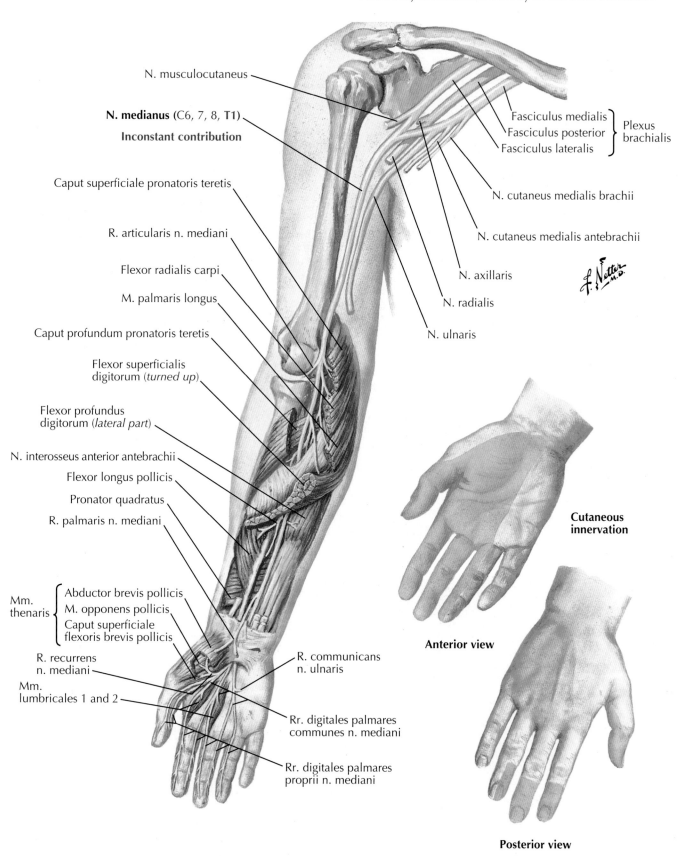

N. musculocutaneus

N. medianus (C6, 7, 8, T1)
Inconstant contribution

Caput superficiale pronatoris teretis

R. articularis n. mediani

Flexor radialis carpi

M. palmaris longus

Caput profundum pronatoris teretis

Flexor superficialis digitorum (*turned up*)

Flexor profundus digitorum (*lateral part*)

N. interosseus anterior antebrachii

Flexor longus pollicis

Pronator quadratus

R. palmaris n. mediani

Mm. thenaris {
Abductor brevis pollicis
M. opponens pollicis
Caput superficiale flexoris brevis pollicis

R. recurrens n. mediani

Mm. lumbricales 1 and 2

Fasciculus medialis
Fasciculus posterior
Fasciculus lateralis
} Plexus brachialis

N. cutaneus medialis brachii

N. cutaneus medialis antebrachii

N. axillaris

N. radialis

N. ulnaris

R. communicans n. ulnaris

Rr. digitales palmares communes n. mediani

Rr. digitales palmares proprii n. mediani

Cutaneous innervation

Anterior view

Posterior view

Note: *Only muscles innervated by N. ulnaris are shown.*

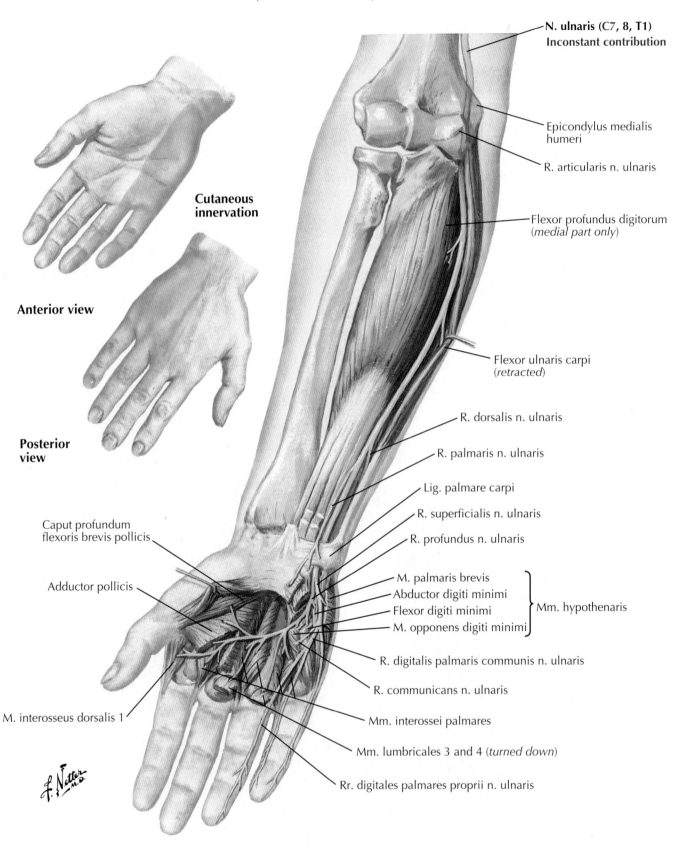

Cutaneous innervation

Anterior view

Posterior view

N. ulnaris (C7, 8, T1)
Inconstant contribution

Epicondylus medialis humeri

R. articularis n. ulnaris

Flexor profundus digitorum (*medial part only*)

Flexor ulnaris carpi (*retracted*)

R. dorsalis n. ulnaris

R. palmaris n. ulnaris

Lig. palmare carpi

R. superficialis n. ulnaris

R. profundus n. ulnaris

Caput profundum flexoris brevis pollicis

Adductor pollicis

M. palmaris brevis
Abductor digiti minimi
Flexor digiti minimi
M. opponens digiti minimi

Mm. hypothenaris

R. digitalis palmaris communis n. ulnaris

R. communicans n. ulnaris

M. interosseus dorsalis 1

Mm. interossei palmares

Mm. lumbricales 3 and 4 (*turned down*)

Rr. digitales palmares proprii n. ulnaris

Plate 487

Nervi

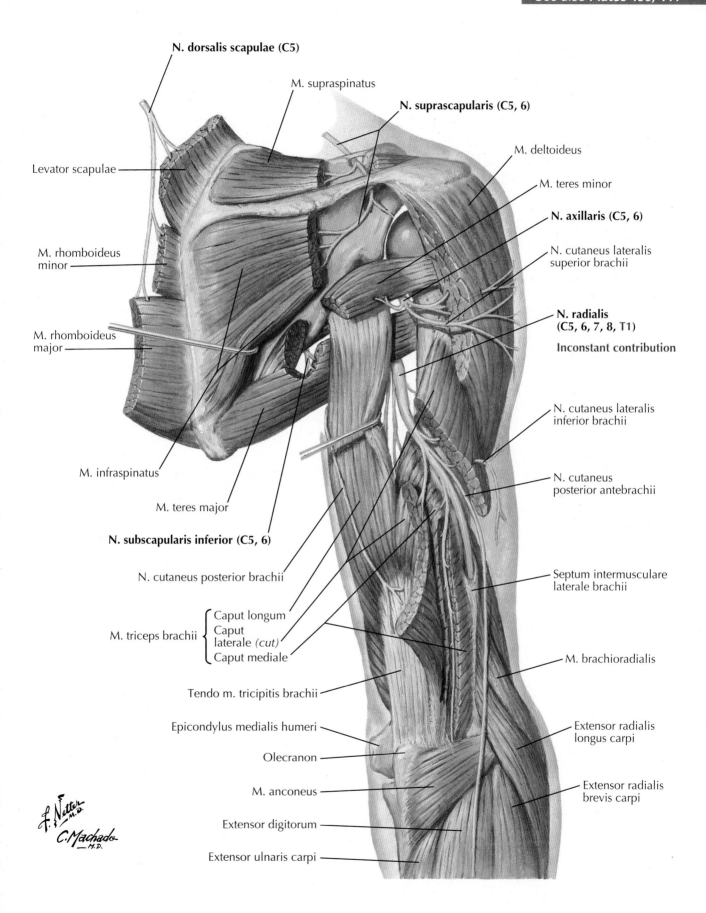

N. dorsalis scapulae (C5)

M. supraspinatus

N. suprascapularis (C5, 6)

M. deltoideus

M. teres minor

N. axillaris (C5, 6)

N. cutaneus lateralis superior brachii

N. radialis (C5, 6, 7, 8, T1)

Inconstant contribution

N. cutaneus lateralis inferior brachii

N. cutaneus posterior antebrachii

Septum intermusculare laterale brachii

M. brachioradialis

Extensor radialis longus carpi

Extensor radialis brevis carpi

Levator scapulae

M. rhomboideus minor

M. rhomboideus major

M. infraspinatus

M. teres major

N. subscapularis inferior (C5, 6)

N. cutaneus posterior brachii

M. triceps brachii { Caput longum
Caput laterale (cut)
Caput mediale

Tendo m. tricipitis brachii

Epicondylus medialis humeri

Olecranon

M. anconeus

Extensor digitorum

Extensor ulnaris carpi

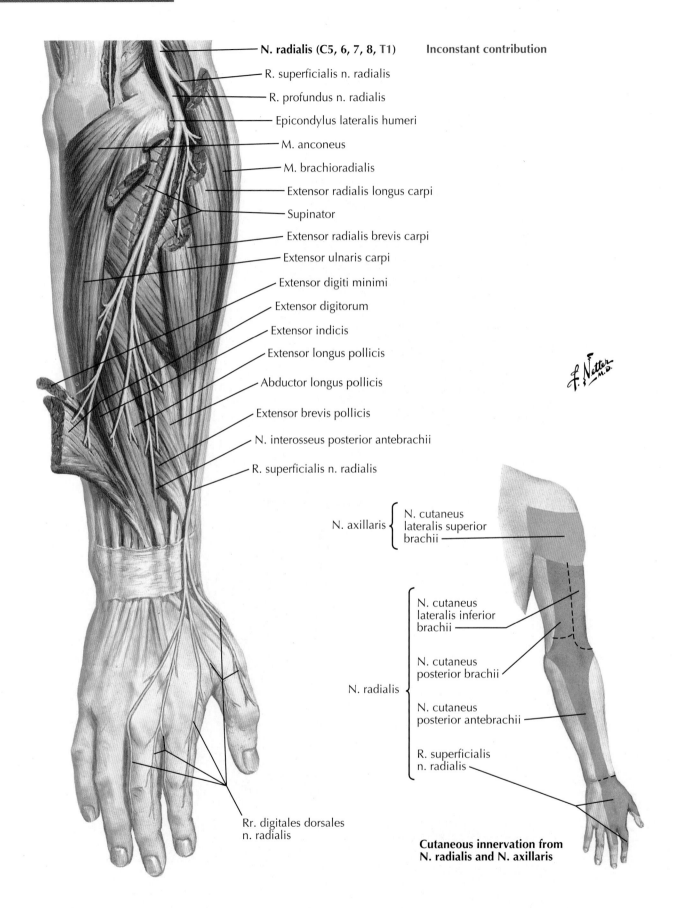

N. radialis (C5, 6, 7, 8, T1)   Inconstant contribution

R. superficialis n. radialis

R. profundus n. radialis

Epicondylus lateralis humeri

M. anconeus

M. brachioradialis

Extensor radialis longus carpi

Supinator

Extensor radialis brevis carpi

Extensor ulnaris carpi

Extensor digiti minimi

Extensor digitorum

Extensor indicis

Extensor longus pollicis

Abductor longus pollicis

Extensor brevis pollicis

N. interosseus posterior antebrachii

R. superficialis n. radialis

N. axillaris { N. cutaneus lateralis superior brachii

N. cutaneus lateralis inferior brachii

N. cutaneus posterior brachii

N. radialis {

N. cutaneus posterior antebrachii

R. superficialis n. radialis

Rr. digitales dorsales n. radialis

Cutaneous innervation from N. radialis and N. axillaris

Plate 489   **Nervi**

See also **Plates 263, 431**

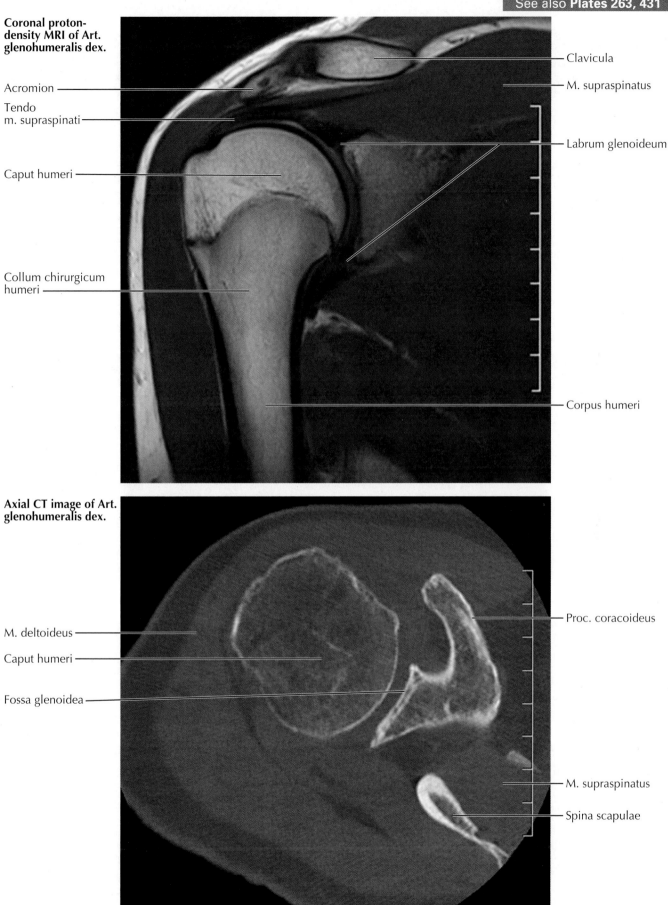

**Coronal proton-
density MRI of Art.
glenohumeralis dex.**

Acromion

Tendo
m. supraspinati

Caput humeri

Collum chirurgicum
humeri

Clavicula

M. supraspinatus

Labrum glenoideum

Corpus humeri

**Axial CT image of Art.
glenohumeralis dex.**

M. deltoideus

Caput humeri

Fossa glenoidea

Proc. coracoideus

M. supraspinatus

Spina scapulae

ANATOMICAL STRUCTURE	CLINICAL COMMENT	PLATE NUMBERS
Systema Nervosum		
N. thoracicus longus	Injury may produce "winged scapula" caused by denervation of serratus anterior muscle; can be injured with repetitive overhead motion	436, 438
N. axillaris	Position of nerve close to surgical neck of humerus makes it vulnerable to injury with fractures or dislocations of humerus; poorly fitting crutches can also compress axillary nerve	441
N. medianus	Compressed in carpal tunnel syndrome, producing pain and paresthesia in lateral three and one-half digits; major risk factors include obesity, pregnancy, diabetes, and hypothyroidism	470, 486
R. recurrens n. mediani	May be injured in superficial lacerations of palm over thenar eminence	469
N. ulnaris	Vulnerable to compression or injury where it passes posterior to medial epicondyle of humerus, and at wrist in ulnar tunnel (Guyon's canal)	483, 487
N. radialis	Vulnerable to compression or injury where it lies against humerus in radial groove (e.g., with humerus fracture); common symptom is wrist drop due to weakness of wrist extensors; poorly fitting crutches can also compress radial nerve	488, 489
Systema Skeletale		
Clavicula	Most clavicular fractures are caused from fall on outstretched arm or direct trauma delivered to lateral side of shoulder; middle third of clavicle is most commonly fractured; supraclavicular nerve block relieves acute pain associated with fracture	427, 429
Humerus	Proximal humerus, especially surgical neck, is fractured due to low-energy falls in elderly persons and high-energy trauma in young persons; axillary nerve and circumflex humeral arteries can be injured; hematoma from anterior/posterior circumflex humeral artery damage as result of dislocation may complicate reductions; midbody fractures are also relatively common and may affect radial nerve and/or deep brachial artery; distal humerus fractures may affect ulnar nerve medially and radial nerve laterally	427, 428, 430
Ulna	Subcutaneous location of olecranon makes it vulnerable to fracture by direct trauma, especially when elbow is flexed; ulnar styloid process may also be fractured with distal radial fractures	446, 449
Radius	Fractures of distal radius are most common fracture of upper limb (Colles' fracture), typically caused by fall on outstretched hand (FOOSH)	449
Os scaphoideum	Most commonly fractured carpal bone, typically from fall on outstretched hand (FOOSH)	459, 460, 462
Systema Musculare		
Aponeurosis palmaris	Progressive fibrosis may result in nodules and eventually a palpable cord that limits finger extension (Dupuytren's contracture)	469
Mm. cuffiae musculotendineae	Injuries to the rotator cuff muscles can result from acute injury or chronic overuse and are a common cause of shoulder pain and disability	431, 434, 441
Tendo m. supraspinati	Most commonly torn rotator cuff tendon	434–436, 441
Tendo m. bicipitis brachii	Can rupture from sudden load on muscle when contracting; used in flexor compartment reflex assessing C5 and C6 spinal nerves	440, 442
Caput longum m. bicipitis brachii	Tendon of long head of biceps brachii muscle can cause shoulder pain from tendinosis of intraarticular portion and can rupture in elderly persons from falls on outstretched arm; when long head has been ruptured, it usually tears from supraglenoid tubercle and retracts down into arm; muscle commonly bulges (Popeye deformity) at midbody of humerus; spontaneous rupture may occur in amyloidosis, infiltrative disease that also causes cardiomyopathy	440

Table 7.1   **Structures with High Clinical Significance**

ANATOMICAL STRUCTURE	CLINICAL COMMENT	PLATE NUMBERS
Mm. compartimenti posterioris antebrachii	Repetitive use of muscles arising from common extensor origin can damage tendons and produce pain over lateral epicondyle region (epicondylitis); activities such as swinging tennis racquet and poor technique with hammer can result in "tennis elbow"; muscle most likely involved is extensor carpi radialis brevis	451
Mm. compartimenti anterioris antebrachii	Repetitive use of muscles arising from common flexor origin can damage tendons and produce pain over medial epicondyle region (golfer's elbow)	452, 453
Systema Cardiovasculare		
Vena mediana cubiti	Accessed in cubital fossa for venipuncture	424
Aa. suprascapularis, dorsalis scapulae, and circumflexa scapulae	Provide collateral circulation around scapula, allowing blood to reach distal part of upper limb if axillary artery is blocked or compressed	437
A. brachialis	During deflation of sphygmomanometer on upper arm, brachial artery is auscultated for Korotkoff sounds to measure systolic and diastolic blood pressure; identified medial to biceps brachii tendon and deep to bicipital aponeurosis in cubital fossa	442, 443
A. radialis	Palpated at lateral aspect of wrist to assess radial pulse; common site of vascular access for percutaneous cardiac procedures, such as angioplasty, and for sampling of arterial blood	14, 443
A. ulnaris	Provides important collateral circulation to hand via palmar arch during catheterization of radial artery; patency is assessed prior to procedure using Allen test, in which both radial and ulnar arteries are compressed, then pressure over ulnar artery is released; return of color to wrist within a few seconds indicates patent ulnar artery	443, 476

*Selections were based largely on clinical data and commonly discussed clinical correlations in macroscopic ("gross") anatomy courses.

The roots of the brachial plexus are typically the anterior rami of the C5–T1 spinal nerves. Variation in the spinal nerve contributions to the plexus, and the nerves that arise from this plexus, is common, due to prefixed (high) and postfixed (low) plexuses.

NERVE	ORIGIN	COURSE	BRANCHES	MOTOR	CUTANEOUS
N. dorsalis scapulae	R. anterior n. spinalis C5	Pierces scalenus medius muscle to run posteriorly and inferiorly on levator scapulae along vertebral border of scapula		Mm. rhomboidei major and minor; Levator scapulae	
N.thoracicus longus	Rr. anteriores nn. spinalium C5–C7	C5–C6 join within scalenus medius muscle, and at 1st rib are joined by C7; runs inferiorly and posterior to brachial plexus and axillary vessels; follows midaxillary line on surface of serratus anterior muscle		M. serratus anterior	
N. suprascapularis	Truncus superior (C5–C6)	Traverses posterior cervical triangle, coursing posterior to inferior belly of omohyoid muscle and border of trapezius muscle to pass through scapular notch deep to superior transverse scapular ligament; continues laterally and then through spinoglenoid notch into infraspinous fossa		Mm. supraspinatus and infraspinatus	
N. subclavius	Truncus superior (C5–C6)	Runs inferiorly at distal aspect of anterior rami		M. subclavius	
N. pectoralis lateralis	Fasciculus lateralis (C5–C7)	Emerges lateral and superficial to axillary artery and vein, coursing just medial to pectoralis minor muscle		Mm. pectorales major and minor	
N. musculocutaneus	Fasciculus lateralis (C5–C7)	Emerges at inferior border of pectoralis minor muscle, pierces coracobrachialis muscle to run between brachialis and biceps brachii muscles; just proximal to elbow, pierces deep fascia to continue as lateral antebrachial cutaneous nerve	Rr. musculares; N. cutaneus lateralis antebrachii	Compartimentum anterius brachii	See N. cutaneus lateralis antebrachii
N. cutaneus lateralis antebrachii	N. musculocutaneus	Runs posterior to cephalic vein and divides at elbow joint into two branches that travel along lateral surface of forearm	Rr. anterior and posterior		Lateral forearm
Nn. subscapulares	Fasciculus posterior (C5–C6)	Upper and lower subscapular nerves emerge to traverse anterior surface of subscapularis muscle; lower subscapular nerve ends in teres major muscle		Mm. teres major and subscapularis	
N. thoracodorsalis	Fasciculus posterior (C6–C8)	Emerges between upper and lower subscapular nerves, courses with thoracodorsal artery along posterior axillary wall, diving deep to latissimus dorsi muscle		M. latissimus dorsi	

Table 7.3

Nervi Plexus Brachialis

NERVE	ORIGIN	COURSE	BRANCHES	MOTOR	CUTANEOUS
N.radialis	Fasciculus posterior (C5–T1)	Runs anterior to latissimus dorsi muscle to inferior border of teres major muscle, where it accompanies deep brachial artery along radial groove of humerus to course between medial and lateral heads of triceps brachii muscle	Nn. cutanei posterior brachii, lateralis inferior brachii, and posterior antebrachii; Rr. musculares, profundus, and superficialis; N. interosseus posterior antebrachii	Mm. triceps brachii, anconeus, and brachioradialis; Extensores radiales longus carpi and brevis carpi; Supinator (also see N. interosseus posterior antebrachii)	Lateral part of dorsum of hand (also see cutaneous branches)
N. cutaneus posterior brachii	N. radialis	Emerges from radial nerve in medial axilla			Posterior part of medial arm
N. cutaneus lateralis inferior brachii	N. radialis	Perforates lateral head of triceps brachii muscle below deltoid tuberosity, coursing anteriorly with cephalic vein			Distal part of lateral arm
N. cutaneus posterior antebrachii	N. radialis	Emerges from plane between lateral and medial heads of triceps brachii muscle to become cutaneous			Posterior part of lateral forearm
N. interosseus posterior antebrachii	R. profundus n. radialis	Continuation of deep radial nerve courses under cover of supinator distally along posterior surface of interosseous membrane of forearm		Compartimentum posterius antebrachii (some exceptions)	
N. axillaris	Fasciculus posterior (C5–C6)	Passes anterior to subscapularis muscle to exit axilla with posterior circumflex humeral artery through quadrangular space	Rr. musculares; N. cutaneus lateralis superior brachii	Mm. deltoideus and teres minor	See N. cutaneus lateralis superior brachii
N. cutaneus lateralis superior brachii	N. axillaris	Pierces deep fascia at posteroinferior edge of deltoid muscle to become cutaneous			Proximal part of lateral arm
N. pectoralis medialis	Fasciculus medialis (C8–T1)	Emerges and runs between axillary artery and vein to pierce pectoralis minor muscle en route to pectoralis major muscle		Mm. pectorales minor and major	
N. cutaneus medialis brachii	Fasciculus medialis (T1)	Emerges and traverses axilla anterior to latissimus dorsi muscle, running posteromedial with axillary vein, piercing deep fascia to descend with basilic vein	Rr. anterior and posterior		Anterior part of medial arm
N. cutaneus medialis antebrachii	Fasciculus medialis (C8–T1)	Emerges medial to axillary artery, traverses axilla to pierce deep fascia supplying anterior arm, and continues on ulnar side of forearm with basilic vein	Rr. anterior and posterior		Anterior arm, medial part of forearm

NERVE	ORIGIN	COURSE	BRANCHES	MOTOR	CUTANEOUS
N. ulnaris	Fasciculus medialis (C7–T1)	Emerges medial to axillary artery, continuing medial to brachial artery along medial head of triceps brachii muscle in groove for ulnar nerve between olecranon and medial epicondyle; enters forearm between heads of flexor ulnaris carpi; runs distally between flexor ulnaris carpi and flexor profundus digitorum, giving off dorsal branch before entering hand	Rr. musculares, dorsalis, palmaris, superficialis, and profundus	Flexores ulnaris carpi and profundus digitorum (medial half); Adductor pollicis; Mm. hypothenaris, interossei dorsales manus and palmares, and lumbricales manus (medial two)	Medial part of palm and dorsum of hand, 5th finger and part of 4th
N. medianus	Fasciculi medialis and lateralis (C6–T1)	Emerges and runs distally with brachial artery to enter forearm between heads of pronator teres; courses distally on deep surface of flexor superficialis digitorum to become superficial at flexor retinaculum of wrist; traverses carpal tunnel deep to flexor retinaculum of wrist	N. interosseus anterior antebrachii; Rr. musculares, palmaris, recurrens, and digitales palmares communes	Compartimentum anterius antebrachii (some exceptions); Mm. thenaris and lumbricales manus (lateral two) (also see N. interosseus anterior antebrachii)	Lateral part of palm, thumb, 2nd and 3rd fingers, and part of 4th finger
N. interosseus anterior antebrachii	N. medianus	At elbow runs distally with anterior interosseous artery along anterior surface of interosseous membrane of forearm		Flexor longus pollicis; Pronator quadratus; Flexor profundus digitorum (lateral half)	

Table 7.5   **Nervi Plexus Brachialis**

MUSCLE	MUSCLE GROUP	PROXIMAL ATTACHMENT	DISTAL ATTACHMENT	INNERVATION	BLOOD SUPPLY	MAIN ACTIONS
Abductor brevis pollicis	Manus	Retinaculum flexorium carpi; tubercula ossium scaphoidei and trapezii	Basis phalangis proximalis pollicis	N. medianus (r. recurrens)	R. palmaris superficialis a. radialis	Abducts thumb
Abductor digiti minimi manus	Manus	Os pisiforme; tendo flexoris ulnaris carpi	Basis phalangis proximalis digiti minimi (facies medialis)	N. ulnaris (r. profundus)	R. palmaris profundus a. ulnaris	Abducts little finger
Abductor longus pollicis	Compartimentum posterius antebrachii	Facies posteriores ulnae, radii, and membranae interosseae antebrachii	Basis ossis 1 metacarpi	N. interosseus posterior antebrachii	A. interossea posterior	Abducts and extends thumb
Adductor pollicis	Manus	*Caput obliquum*: Bases ossium 2 and 3 metacarpi; os capitatum and adjacent ossa carpi *Caput transversum*: Os 3 metacarpi (anterior surface)	Basis phalangis proximalis pollicis	N. ulnaris (r. profundus)	Arcus palmaris profundus	Adducts thumb
M. anconeus	Compartimentum posterius antebrachii	Epicondylus lateralis humeri (posterior surface)	Olecranon (lateral surface); facies posterior ulnae (proximal part)	N. radialis	A. profunda brachii	Assists m. triceps brachii in extending elbow
M. biceps brachii	Compartimentum anterius brachii	*Caput longum*: Tuberculum supraglenoideum scapulae *Caput breve*: Proc. coracoideus scapulae	Tuberositas radii; fascia antebrachii (via aponeurosis bicipitalis)	N. musculocutaneus	A. brachialis	Flexes and supinates forearm
M. brachialis	Compartimentum anterius brachii	Facies anterior humeri (distal half)	Proc. coronoideus ulnae; tuberositas ulnae	Nn. musculo-cutaneus and radialis	Aa. recurrens radialis and brachialis	Flexes forearm
M. brachioradialis	Compartimentum posterius antebrachii	Crista supracondylaris lateralis humeri (proximal two-thirds)	Facies lateralis radii (distal end)	N. radialis	A. recurrens radialis	Weak flexion of forearm when forearm is in midpronation
M. coracobra-chialis	Compartimentum anterius brachii	Proc. coracoideus scapulae	Facies medialis humeri (middle third)	N. musculocutaneus	A. brachialis	Flexes and adducts arm
M. deltoideus	Mm. scapulohumerales	*Pars clavicularis*: Clavicula (lateral third) *Pars acromialis*: Acromion *Pars spinalis scapularis*: Spina scapulae	Tuberositas deltoidea humeri	N. axillaris	A. circumflexa posterior humeri; R. deltoideus a. thoracoacromialis	*Pars clavicularis*: flexes and medially rotates arm *Pars acromialis*: abducts arm beyond initial 15 degrees done by m. supraspinatus *Pars spinalis scapularis*: extends and laterally rotates arm
Extensor brevis pollicis	Compartimentum posterius antebrachii	Facies posteriores radii and membranae interosseae antebrachii	Basis phalangis proximalis pollicis (dorsal surface)	N. interosseus posterior antebrachii	A. interossea posterior	Extends proximal phalanx of thumb
Extensor digiti minimi	Compartimentum posterius antebrachii	Epicondylus lateralis humeri	Aponeurosis extensoria digiti minimi	N. interosseus posterior antebrachii	A. interossea posterior	Extends 5th digit
Extensor digitorum	Compartimentum posterius antebrachii	Epicondylus lateralis humeri	Aponeuroses extensoriae digitorum 2–5	N. interosseus posterior antebrachii	A. interossea posterior	Extends medial four metacarpophalangeal joints, assists in wrist extension
Extensor indicis	Compartimentum posterius antebrachii	Facies posteriores ulnae and membranae interosseae antebrachii	Aponeurosis extensoria digiti 2	N. interosseus posterior antebrachii	A. interossea posterior	Extends 2nd digit and helps extend hand

MUSCLE	MUSCLE GROUP	PROXIMAL ATTACHMENT	DISTAL ATTACHMENT	INNERVATION	BLOOD SUPPLY	MAIN ACTIONS
Extensor longus pollicis	Compartimentum posterius antebrachii	Facies posteriores (middle third) ulnae and membranae interosseae antebrachii	Basis phalangis distalis pollicis (dorsal surface)	N. interosseus posterior antebrachii	A. interossea posterior	Extends distal phalanx of thumb
Extensor radialis brevis carpi	Compartimentum posterius antebrachii	Epicondylus lateralis humeri	Bases ossium 2 and 3 metacarpi	N. radialis (r. profundus)	Aa. radialis and recurrens radialis	Extends and abducts hand
Extensor radialis longus carpi	Compartimentum posterius antebrachii	Crista supracondylaris lateralis humeri (distal third)	Basis ossis 2 metacarpi	N. radialis	Aa. radialis and recurrens radialis	Extends and abducts hand
Extensor ulnaris carpi	Compartimentum posterius antebrachii	Epicondylus lateralis humeri; margo posterior ulnae	Basis ossis 5 metacarpi	N. interosseus posterior antebrachii	A. interossea posterior	Extends and adducts hand
Flexor brevis pollicis	Manus	*Caput superficiale*: Retinaculum flexorium carpi; tuberculum ossis trapezii *Caput profundum*: Os trapezoideum; os capitatum	Basis phalangis proximalis pollicis (lateral surface)	*Superficial head*: N. medianus (r. recurrens) *Deep head*: N. ulnaris (r. profundus)	R. palmaris superficialis a. radialis	Flexes proximal phalanx of thumb
Flexor digiti minimi manus	Manus	Retinaculum flexorium carpi; hamulus ossis hamati	Basis phalangis proximalis digiti minimi (medial surface)	N. ulnaris (r. profundus)	R. palmaris profundus a. ulnaris	Flexes proximal phalanx of little finger
Flexor longus pollicis	Compartimentum anterius antebrachii	Facies anteriores radii and membranae interosseae	Basis phalangis distalis pollicis (palmar surface)	N. interosseus anterior antebrachii	A. interossea anterior	Flexes thumb
Flexor profundus digitorum	Compartimentum anterius antebrachii	Facies medialis and anterior (proximal three-fourths) ulnae and membranae interosseae antebrachii	Bases phalangium distalium digitorum 2–5 (palmar surfaces)	*Medial part*: N. ulnaris *Lateral part*: N. medianus	Aa. interossea anterior and ulnaris	Flexes distal phalanges of medial four digits, assists with flexion of hand
Flexor radialis carpi	Compartimentum anterius antebrachii	Epicondylus medialis humeri	Basis ossis 2 metacarpi	N. medianus	A. radialis	Flexes and abducts hand
Flexor superficialis digitorum	Compartimentum anterius antebrachii	*Caput humeroulnare*: Epicondylus medialis humeri; proc. coronoideus ulnae; lig. collaterale ulnae cubiti *Caput radiale*: Facies anterior radii (proximal part)	Corpora phalangium mediorum digitorum 2-5	N. medianus	Aa. ulnaris and radialis	Flexes middle and proximal phalanges of medial four digits, flexes hand
Flexor ulnaris carpi	Compartimentum anterius antebrachii	*Caput superficiale*: Epicondylus medialis humeri *Caput profundum*: Olecranon; margo posterior ulnae	Os pisiforme; hamulus ossis hamati; basis ossis 5 metacarpi	N. ulnaris	A. recurrens ulnaris posterior	Flexes and adducts hand
M. infraspinatus	Mm. scapulohumerales	Fossa infraspinata scapulae; fascia infraspinata	Tuberculum majus humeri	N. suprascapularis	A. suprascapularis	Lateral rotation of arm
Mm. interossei dorsales manus	Manus	Facing surfaces of adjacent ossa metacarpi	Bases phalangium proximalium digitorum 2-4; aponeuroses extensoriae digitorum 2–4	N. ulnaris (r. profundus)	Arcus palmaris profundus	Abduct digits; flex digits at metacarpophalangeal joint and extend interphalangeal joints
Mm. interossei palmares	Manus	Ossa 2, 4, and 5 metacarpi (palmar surfaces)	Bases phalangium proximalium digitorum 2, 4 and 5; aponeuroses extensoriae digitorum 2, 4, and 5	N. ulnaris (r. profundus)	Arcus palmaris profundus	Adduct digits; flex digits and extend interphalangeal joints

Table 7.7 **Musculi**

MUSCLE	MUSCLE GROUP	PROXIMAL ATTACHMENT	DISTAL ATTACHMENT	INNERVATION	BLOOD SUPPLY	MAIN ACTIONS
Mm. lumbricales manus	Manus	Tendines flexoris profundi digitorum	Aponeuroses extensoriae (lateral sides) digitorum 2–5	*Lateral two*: N. medianus (rr. digitales) *Medial two*: N. ulnaris (r. profundus)	Arcus palmares superficialis and profundus	Extend digits, flex metacarpophalangeal joints
M. opponens digiti minimi manus	Manus	Retinaculum flexorium carpi; hamulus ossis hamati	Os 5 metacarpi (palmar surface)	N. ulnaris (r. profundus)	R. palmaris profundus a. ulnaris	Draws 5th metacarpal bone anteriorly and rotates it to face thumb
M. opponens pollicis	Manus	Retinaculum flexorium carpi; tuberculum ossis trapezii	Os 1 metacarpi (lateral surface)	N. medianus (r. recurrens)	R. palmaris superficialis a. radialis	Draws 1st metacarpal bone forward and rotates it medially
M. palmaris brevis	Manus	Aponeurosis palmaris; retinaculum flexorium carpi	Cutis marginis medialis palmae	N. ulnaris (r. superficialis)	Arcus palmaris superficialis	Deepens hollow of hand, assists grip
M. palmaris longus	Compartimentum anterius antebrachii	Epicondylus medialis humeri	Retinaculum flexorium carpi (distal half); aponeurosis palmaris	N. medianus	A. recurrens ulnaris posterior	Flexes hand and tenses palmar aponeurosis
Pronator quadratus	Compartimentum anterius antebrachii	Facies anterior ulnae (distal one-fourth)	Facies anterior radii (distal one-fourth)	N. interosseus anterior antebrachii	A. interossea anterior	Pronates forearm
Pronator teres	Compartimentum anterius antebrachii	*Caput humerale*: Epicondylus medialis humeri *Caput ulnare*: Proc. coronoideus ulnae	Facies lateralis radii (middle part)	N. medianus	A. recurrens ulnaris anterior	Pronates forearm and flexes elbow
M. subscapularis	Mm. scapulohumerales	Fossa subscapularis	Tuberculum minus humeri	Nn. subscapulares superior and inferior	Aa. subscapularis and thoracica lateralis	Medially rotates and adducts arm; helps hold humeral head in glenoid fossa
Supinator	Compartimentum posterius antebrachii	Epicondylus lateralis humeri; lig. collaterale radiale cubiti; lig. anulare radii; fossa supinatoria ulnae; crista supinatoria ulnae	Facies lateralis, posterior, and anterior radii (proximal third)	N. radialis	Aa. recurrens radialis and interosseus posterior	Supinates forearm
M. supraspinatus	Mm. scapulohumerales	Fossa supraspinata scapulae; fascia supraspinata	Tuberculum majus humeri	N. suprascapularis	A. suprascapularis	Initiates arm abduction
M. teres major	Mm. scapulohumerales	Angulus inferior scapulae (posterior surface)	Labium mediale sulci intertubercularis humeri	N. subscapularis inferior	A. circumflexa scapulae	Adducts and medially rotates arm
M. teres minor	Mm. scapulohumerales	Margo lateralis scapulae (superior two-thirds of posterior surface)	Tuberculum majus humeri	N. axillaris	A. circumflexa scapulae	Laterally rotates arm
M. triceps brachii	Compartimentum posterius brachii	*Caput longum*: Tuberculum infraglenoideum scapulae *Caput laterale*: Facies posterior humeri (proximal half) *Caput mediale*: Facies medialis and posterior humeri (distal two-thirds)	Olecranon ulnae (posterior surface)	N. radialis	A. profunda brachii	Extends forearm; long head stabilizes head of abducted humerus and extends and adducts arm

Variations in spinal nerve contributions to the innervation of muscles, their arterial supply, their attachments, and their actions are common themes in human anatomy. Therefore, expect differences between texts and realize that anatomical variation is normal.

MEMBRUM INFERIUS 8

Surface Anatomy   491–494
Coxa, Natis, and Femur   495–515
Genu   516–523
Crus   524–534
Talus and Pes   535–549
Nervi   550–554

Regional Imaging   555–556
Structures with High
  Clinical Significance   Tables 8.1–8.2
Nervi Plexus Lumbosacralis   Tables 8.3–8.5
Musculi   Tables 8.6–8.9
Electronic Bonus Plates   BP 103–BP 112

ELECTRONIC BONUS PLATES

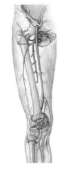
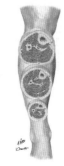

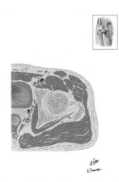

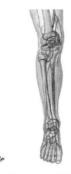

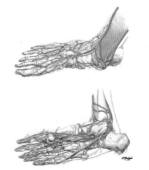

BP 103 Genu and Pes: Arteriae   **BP 104** Coxa: Cross-Sectional Anatomy   **BP 105** Femur and Genu: Arteriae   **BP 106** Crus: Serial Cross Sections

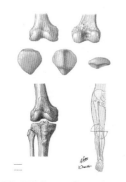

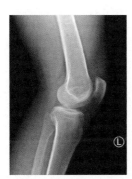

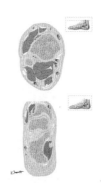

BP 107 Genu: Osteology   **BP 108** Genu: Lateral View Radiograph   **BP 109** Pes: Nervi and Arteriae   **BP 110** Talus and Pes: Cross-Sectional Anatomy

ELECTRONIC BONUS PLATES—*cont'd*

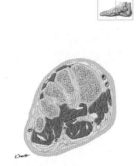

BP 111 Pes: Cross-Sectional
Anatomy

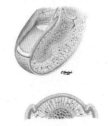

BP 112 Unguis Digiti Pedis:
Anatomy

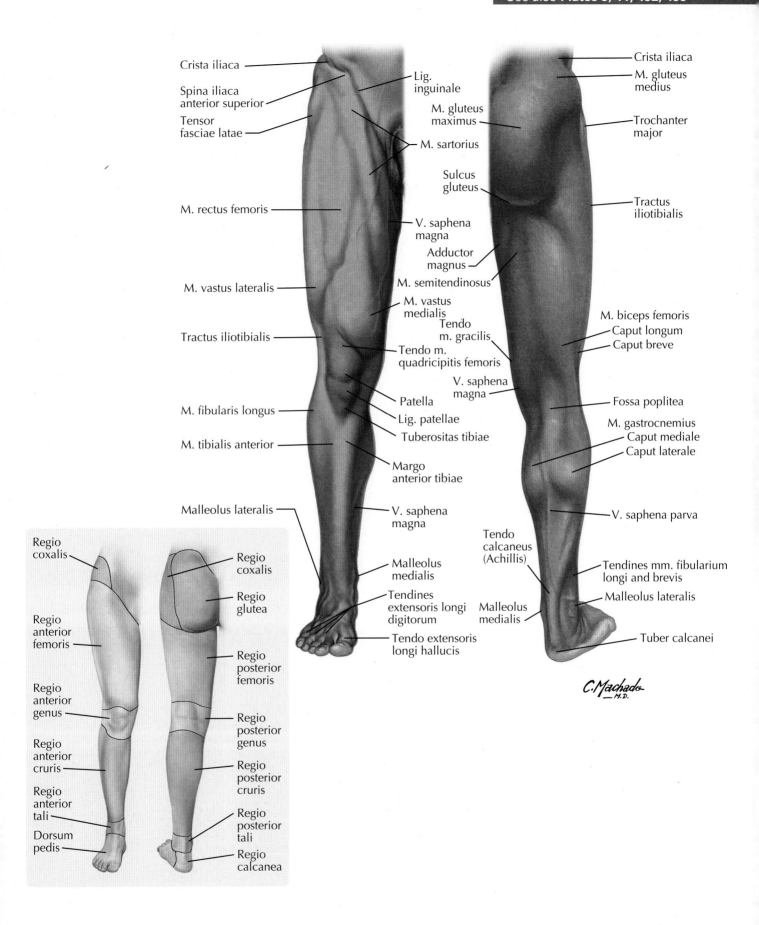

Crista iliaca

Spina iliaca
anterior superior

Tensor
fasciae latae

M. rectus femoris

M. vastus lateralis

Tractus iliotibialis

M. fibularis longus

M. tibialis anterior

Malleolus lateralis

Lig.
inguinale

M. gluteus
maximus

M. sartorius

Sulcus
gluteus

V. saphena
magna

Adductor
magnus

M. semitendinosus

M. vastus
medialis

Tendo
m. gracilis

Tendo m.
quadricipitis femoris

Patella

Lig. patellae

Tuberositas tibiae

Margo
anterior tibiae

V. saphena
magna

Malleolus
medialis

Tendines
extensoris longi
digitorum

Tendo extensoris
longi hallucis

Crista iliaca

M. gluteus
medius

Trochanter
major

Tractus
iliotibialis

M. biceps femoris
Caput longum
Caput breve

V. saphena
magna

Fossa poplitea

M. gastrocnemius
Caput mediale
Caput laterale

V. saphena parva

Tendo
calcaneus
(Achillis)

Malleolus
medialis

Tendines mm. fibularium
longi and brevis

Malleolus lateralis

Tuber calcanei

C.Machado
M.D.

Regio
coxalis

Regio
anterior
femoris

Regio
anterior
genus

Regio
anterior
cruris

Regio
anterior
tali

Dorsum
pedis

Regio
coxalis

Regio
glutea

Regio
posterior
femoris

Regio
posterior
genus

Regio
posterior
cruris

Regio
posterior
tali

Regio
calcanea

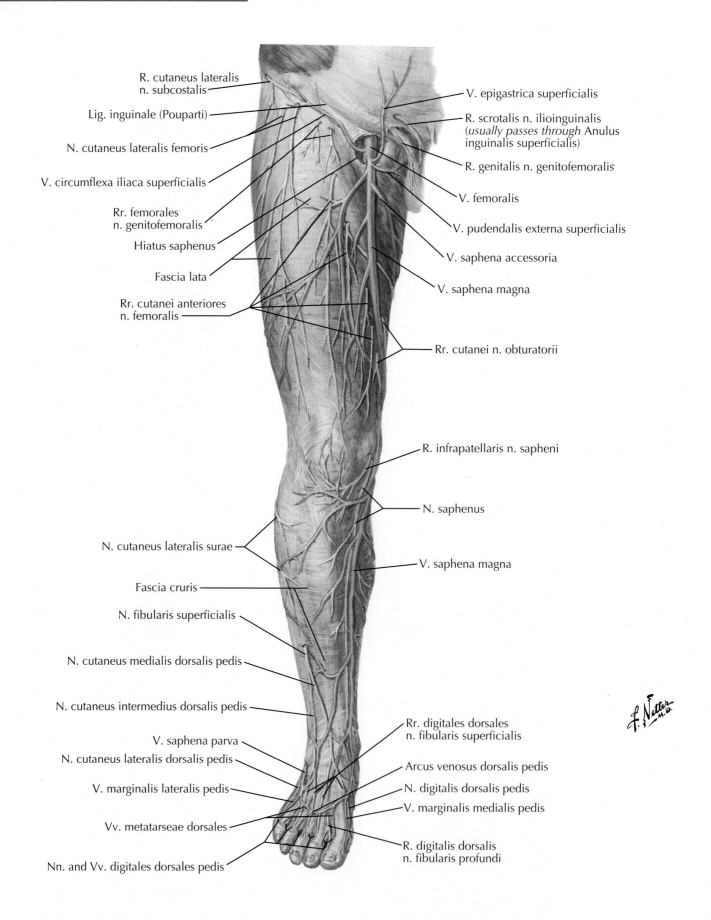

R. cutaneus lateralis
n. subcostalis

Lig. inguinale (Pouparti)

N. cutaneus lateralis femoris

V. circumflexa iliaca superficialis

Rr. femorales
n. genitofemoralis

Hiatus saphenus

Fascia lata

Rr. cutanei anteriores
n. femoralis

N. cutaneus lateralis surae

Fascia cruris

N. fibularis superficialis

N. cutaneus medialis dorsalis pedis

N. cutaneus intermedius dorsalis pedis

V. saphena parva

N. cutaneus lateralis dorsalis pedis

V. marginalis lateralis pedis

Vv. metatarseae dorsales

Nn. and Vv. digitales dorsales pedis

V. epigastrica superficialis

R. scrotalis n. ilioinguinalis
(*usually passes through* Anulus
inguinalis superficialis)

R. genitalis n. genitofemoralis

V. femoralis

V. pudendalis externa superficialis

V. saphena accessoria

V. saphena magna

Rr. cutanei n. obturatorii

R. infrapatellaris n. sapheni

N. saphenus

V. saphena magna

Rr. digitales dorsales
n. fibularis superficialis

Arcus venosus dorsalis pedis

N. digitalis dorsalis pedis

V. marginalis medialis pedis

R. digitalis dorsalis
n. fibularis profundi

Plate 492

Surface Anatomy

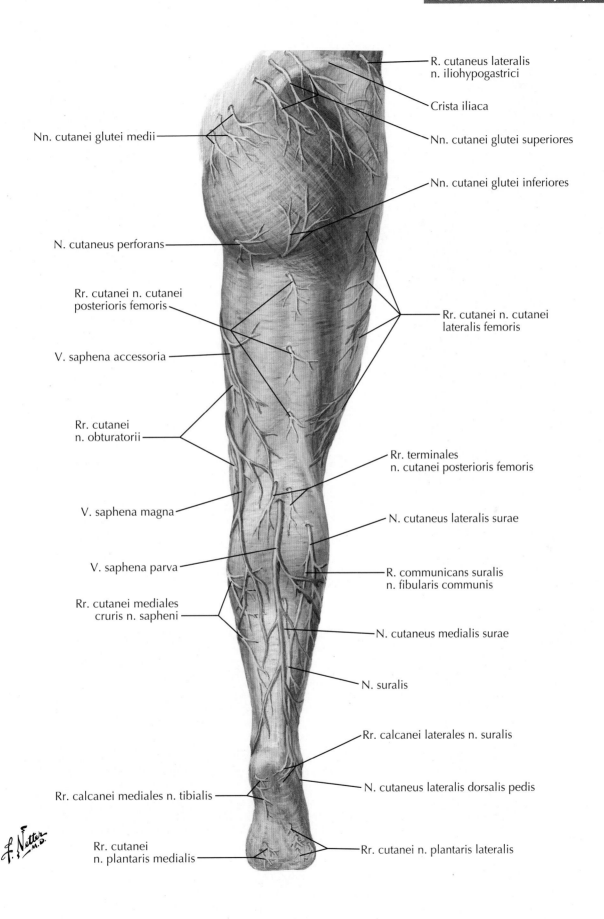

R. cutaneus lateralis
n. iliohypogastrici

Crista iliaca

Nn. cutanei glutei superiores

Nn. cutanei glutei medii

Nn. cutanei glutei inferiores

N. cutaneus perforans

Rr. cutanei n. cutanei
posterioris femoris

Rr. cutanei n. cutanei
lateralis femoris

V. saphena accessoria

Rr. cutanei
n. obturatorii

Rr. terminales
n. cutanei posterioris femoris

V. saphena magna

N. cutaneus lateralis surae

V. saphena parva

R. communicans suralis
n. fibularis communis

Rr. cutanei mediales
cruris n. sapheni

N. cutaneus medialis surae

N. suralis

Rr. calcanei laterales n. suralis

N. cutaneus lateralis dorsalis pedis

Rr. calcanei mediales n. tibialis

Rr. cutanei
n. plantaris medialis

Rr. cutanei n. plantaris lateralis

Surface Anatomy

Plate 493

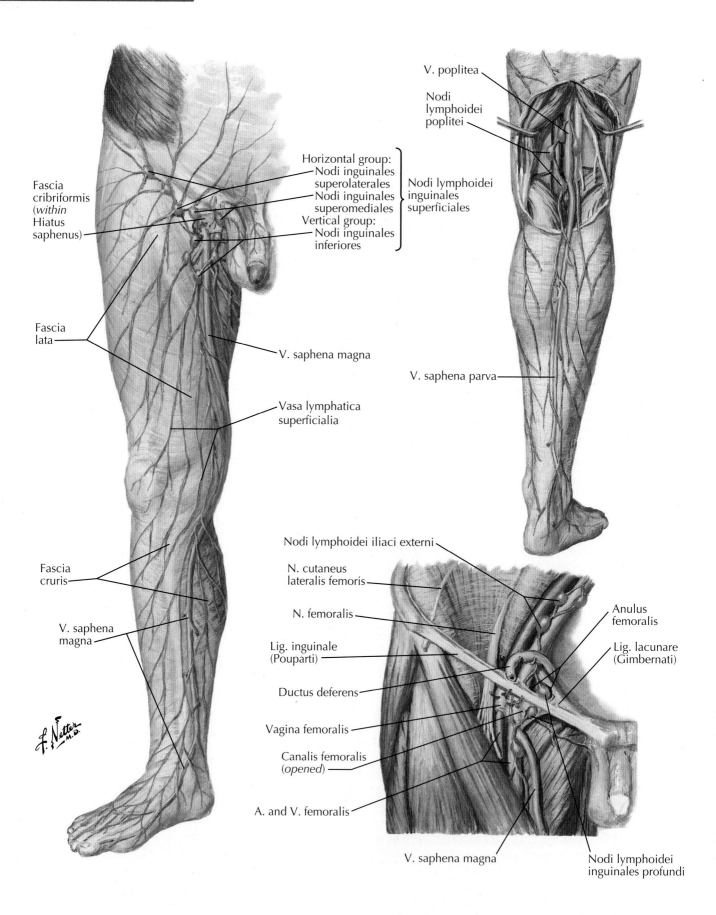

Horizontal group:
Nodi inguinales
superolaterales
Nodi inguinales
superomediales
Vertical group:
Nodi inguinales
inferiores

Nodi lymphoidei
inguinales
superficiales

Fascia
cribriformis
(*within*
Hiatus
saphenus)

Fascia
lata

V. saphena magna

Vasa lymphatica
superficialia

Fascia
cruris

V. saphena
magna

V. poplitea

Nodi
lymphoidei
poplitei

V. saphena parva

Nodi lymphoidei iliaci externi

N. cutaneus
lateralis femoris

N. femoralis

Lig. inguinale
(Pouparti)

Ductus deferens

Vagina femoralis

Canalis femoralis
(*opened*)

A. and V. femoralis

Anulus
femoralis

Lig. lacunare
(Gimbernati)

V. saphena magna

Nodi lymphoidei
inguinales profundi

Plate 494

Surface Anatomy

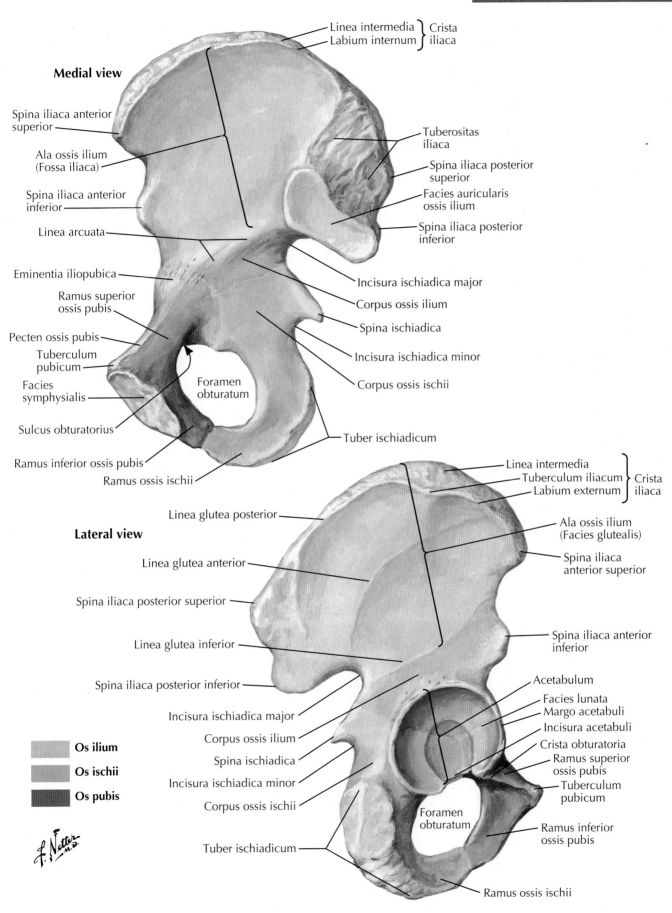

Medial view

Linea intermedia ⎫ Crista
Labium internum ⎭ iliaca

Spina iliaca anterior superior

Ala ossis ilium (Fossa iliaca)

Spina iliaca anterior inferior

Linea arcuata

Eminentia iliopubica

Ramus superior ossis pubis

Pecten ossis pubis

Tuberculum pubicum

Facies symphysialis

Sulcus obturatorius

Ramus inferior ossis pubis

Ramus ossis ischii

Tuberositas iliaca

Spina iliaca posterior superior

Facies auricularis ossis ilium

Spina iliaca posterior inferior

Incisura ischiadica major

Corpus ossis ilium

Spina ischiadica

Incisura ischiadica minor

Corpus ossis ischii

Foramen obturatum

Tuber ischiadicum

Lateral view

Linea glutea posterior

Linea glutea anterior

Spina iliaca posterior superior

Linea glutea inferior

Spina iliaca posterior inferior

Incisura ischiadica major

Corpus ossis ilium

Spina ischiadica

Incisura ischiadica minor

Corpus ossis ischii

Tuber ischiadicum

Linea intermedia ⎫
Tuberculum iliacum ⎬ Crista
Labium externum ⎭ iliaca

Ala ossis ilium (Facies glutealis)

Spina iliaca anterior superior

Spina iliaca anterior inferior

Acetabulum

Facies lunata

Margo acetabuli

Incisura acetabuli

Crista obturatoria

Ramus superior ossis pubis

Tuberculum pubicum

Ramus inferior ossis pubis

Foramen obturatum

Ramus ossis ischii

Os ilium

Os ischii

Os pubis

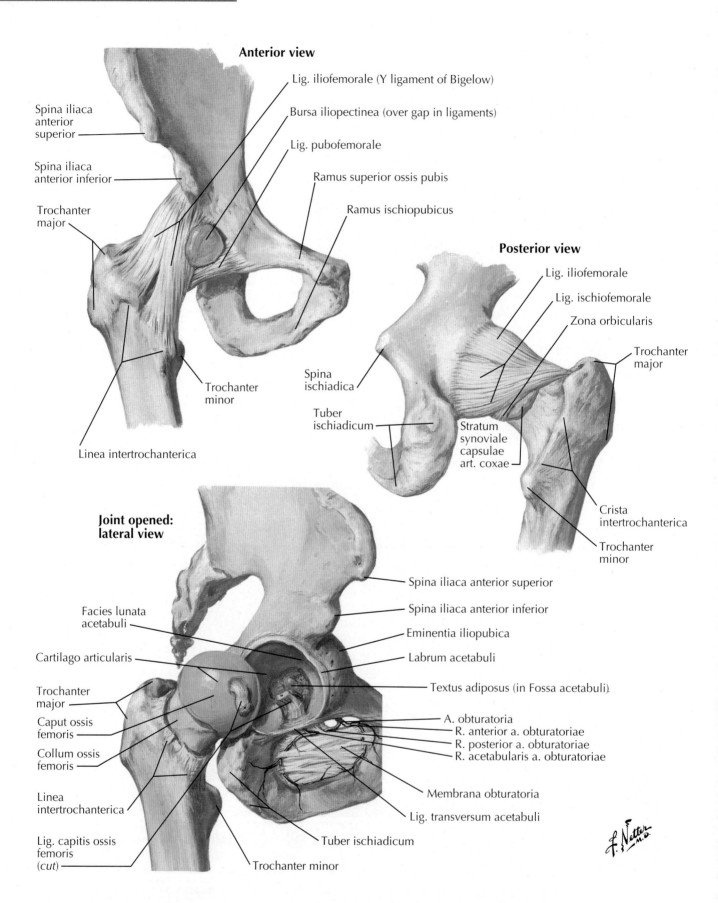

Anterior view

Lig. iliofemorale (Y ligament of Bigelow)

Bursa iliopectinea (over gap in ligaments)

Lig. pubofemorale

Ramus superior ossis pubis

Ramus ischiopubicus

Spina iliaca anterior superior

Spina iliaca anterior inferior

Trochanter major

Trochanter minor

Linea intertrochanterica

Posterior view

Lig. iliofemorale

Lig. ischiofemorale

Zona orbicularis

Trochanter major

Spina ischiadica

Tuber ischiadicum

Stratum synoviale capsulae art. coxae

Crista intertrochanterica

Trochanter minor

Joint opened: lateral view

Facies lunata acetabuli

Cartilago articularis

Trochanter major

Caput ossis femoris

Collum ossis femoris

Linea intertrochanterica

Lig. capitis ossis femoris (*cut*)

Spina iliaca anterior superior

Spina iliaca anterior inferior

Eminentia iliopubica

Labrum acetabuli

Textus adiposus (in Fossa acetabuli)

A. obturatoria

R. anterior a. obturatoriae

R. posterior a. obturatoriae

R. acetabularis a. obturatoriae

Membrana obturatoria

Lig. transversum acetabuli

Tuber ischiadicum

Trochanter minor

Plate 496

Coxa, Natis, and Femur

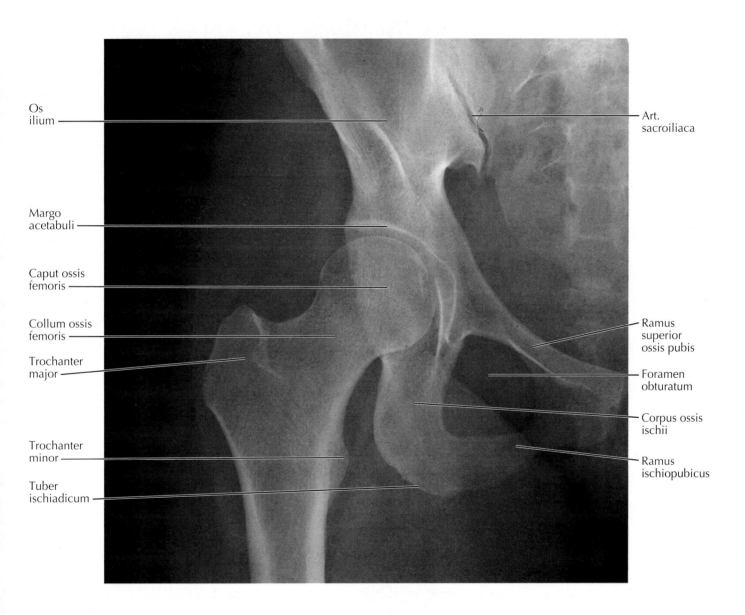

Os
ilium

Margo
acetabuli

Caput ossis
femoris

Collum ossis
femoris

Trochanter
major

Trochanter
minor

Tuber
ischiadicum

Art.
sacroiliaca

Ramus
superior
ossis pubis

Foramen
obturatum

Corpus ossis
ischii

Ramus
ischiopubicus

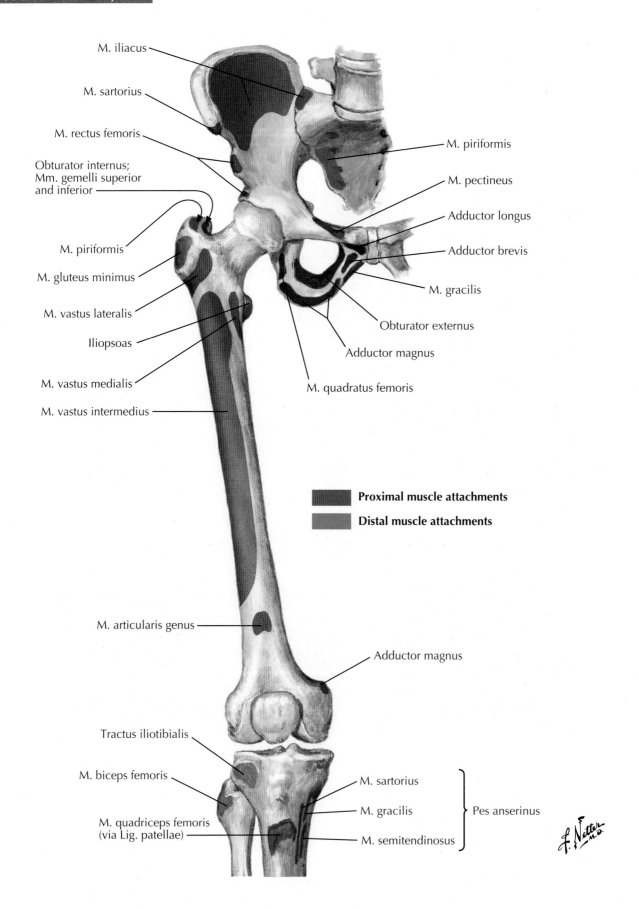

M. iliacus

M. sartorius

M. rectus femoris

Obturator internus;
Mm. gemelli superior
and inferior

M. piriformis

M. gluteus minimus

M. vastus lateralis

Iliopsoas

M. vastus medialis

M. vastus intermedius

M. piriformis

M. pectineus

Adductor longus

Adductor brevis

M. gracilis

Obturator externus

Adductor magnus

M. quadratus femoris

Proximal muscle attachments

Distal muscle attachments

M. articularis genus

Adductor magnus

Tractus iliotibialis

M. biceps femoris

M. quadriceps femoris
(via Lig. patellae)

M. sartorius

M. gracilis

M. semitendinosus

Pes anserinus

Plate 498

Coxa, Natis, and Femur

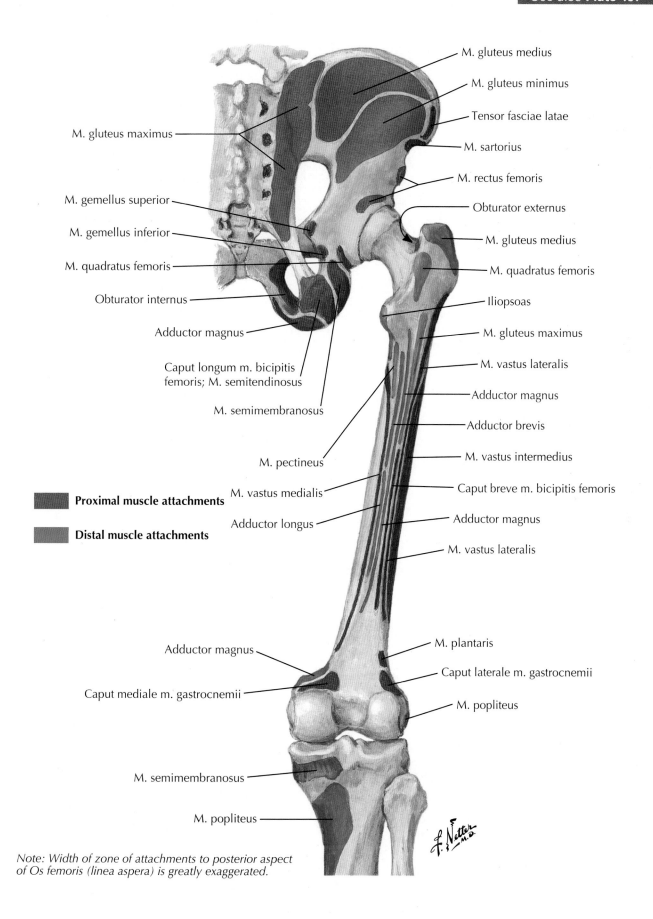

M. gluteus medius

M. gluteus minimus

Tensor fasciae latae

M. gluteus maximus

M. sartorius

M. rectus femoris

Obturator externus

M. gemellus superior

M. gluteus medius

M. gemellus inferior

M. quadratus femoris

M. quadratus femoris

Iliopsoas

Obturator internus

M. gluteus maximus

Adductor magnus

M. vastus lateralis

Caput longum m. bicipitis
femoris; M. semitendinosus

Adductor magnus

Adductor brevis

M. semimembranosus

M. vastus intermedius

Caput breve m. bicipitis femoris

Proximal muscle attachments

M. vastus medialis

Distal muscle attachments

Adductor longus

Adductor magnus

M. pectineus

M. vastus lateralis

M. plantaris

Adductor magnus

Caput laterale m. gastrocnemii

Caput mediale m. gastrocnemii

M. popliteus

M. semimembranosus

M. popliteus

*Note: Width of zone of attachments to posterior aspect
of Os femoris (linea aspera) is greatly exaggerated.*

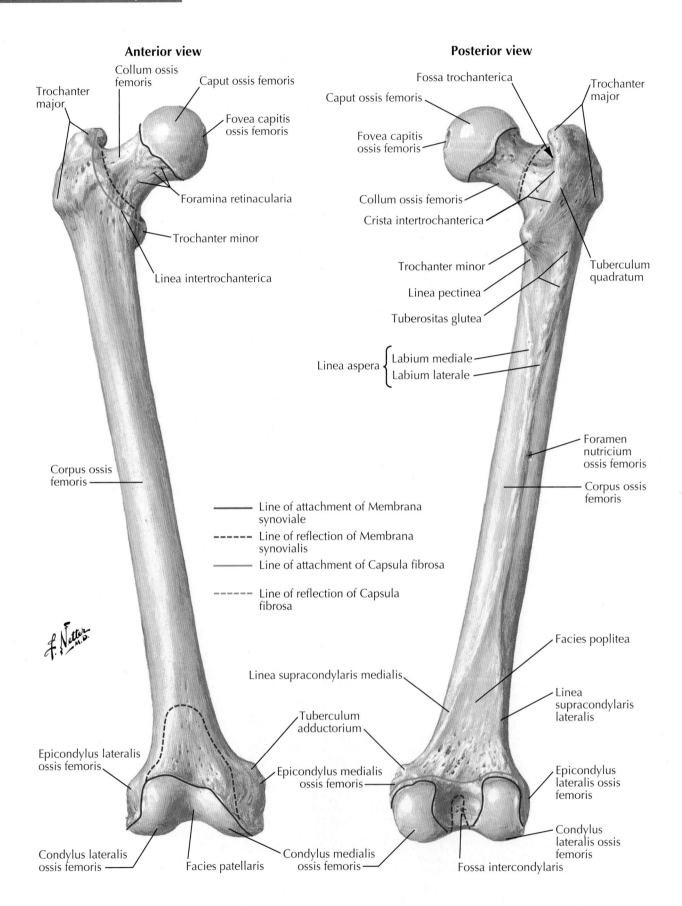

Anterior view

Trochanter major

Collum ossis femoris

Caput ossis femoris

Fovea capitis ossis femoris

Foramina retinacularia

Trochanter minor

Linea intertrochanterica

Corpus ossis femoris

─────── Line of attachment of Membrana synoviale

------- Line of reflection of Membrana synovialis

─────── Line of attachment of Capsula fibrosa

------- Line of reflection of Capsula fibrosa

Linea supracondylaris medialis

Tuberculum adductorium

Epicondylus lateralis ossis femoris

Epicondylus medialis ossis femoris

Condylus lateralis ossis femoris

Facies patellaris

Condylus medialis ossis femoris

Posterior view

Fossa trochanterica

Trochanter major

Caput ossis femoris

Fovea capitis ossis femoris

Collum ossis femoris

Crista intertrochanterica

Trochanter minor

Linea pectinea

Tuberositas glutea

Tuberculum quadratum

Linea aspera { Labium mediale / Labium laterale

Foramen nutricium ossis femoris

Corpus ossis femoris

Facies poplitea

Linea supracondylaris lateralis

Epicondylus lateralis ossis femoris

Condylus lateralis ossis femoris

Fossa intercondylaris

Plate 500

Coxa, Natis, and Femur

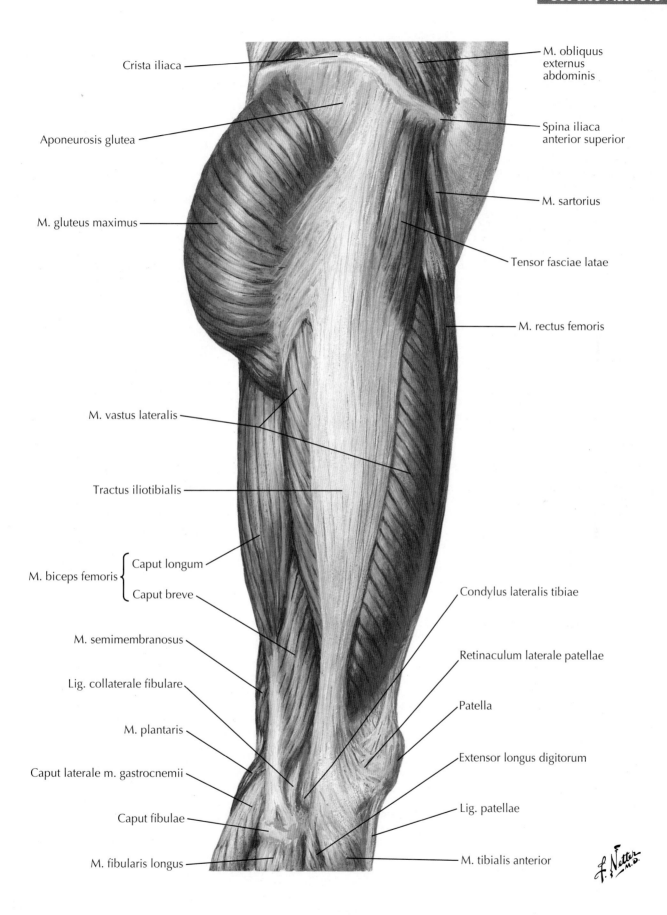

Crista iliaca

M. obliquus externus abdominis

Aponeurosis glutea

Spina iliaca anterior superior

M. gluteus maximus

M. sartorius

Tensor fasciae latae

M. rectus femoris

M. vastus lateralis

Tractus iliotibialis

M. biceps femoris { Caput longum
Caput breve

Condylus lateralis tibiae

Retinaculum laterale patellae

M. semimembranosus

Lig. collaterale fibulare

Patella

M. plantaris

Extensor longus digitorum

Caput laterale m. gastrocnemii

Caput fibulae

Lig. patellae

M. fibularis longus

M. tibialis anterior

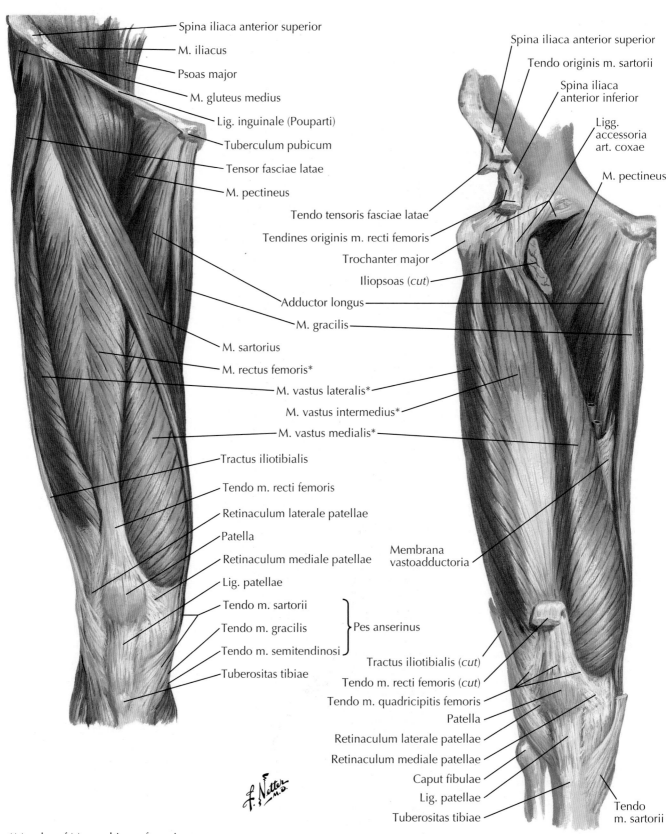

Spina iliaca anterior superior

M. iliacus

Psoas major

M. gluteus medius

Lig. inguinale (Pouparti)

Tuberculum pubicum

Tensor fasciae latae

M. pectineus

Spina iliaca anterior superior

Tendo originis m. sartorii

Spina iliaca anterior inferior

Ligg. accessoria art. coxae

M. pectineus

Tendo tensoris fasciae latae

Tendines originis m. recti femoris

Trochanter major

Iliopsoas (*cut*)

Adductor longus

M. gracilis

M. sartorius

M. rectus femoris*

M. vastus lateralis*

M. vastus intermedius*

M. vastus medialis*

Tractus iliotibialis

Tendo m. recti femoris

Retinaculum laterale patellae

Patella

Retinaculum mediale patellae

Lig. patellae

Tendo m. sartorii

Tendo m. gracilis } Pes anserinus

Tendo m. semitendinosi

Tuberositas tibiae

Membrana vastoadductoria

Tractus iliotibialis (*cut*)

Tendo m. recti femoris (*cut*)

Tendo m. quadricipitis femoris

Patella

Retinaculum laterale patellae

Retinaculum mediale patellae

Caput fibulae

Lig. patellae

Tuberositas tibiae

Tendo m. sartorii

*Muscles of M. quadriceps femoris

Plate 502

Coxa, Natis, and Femur

Deep dissection

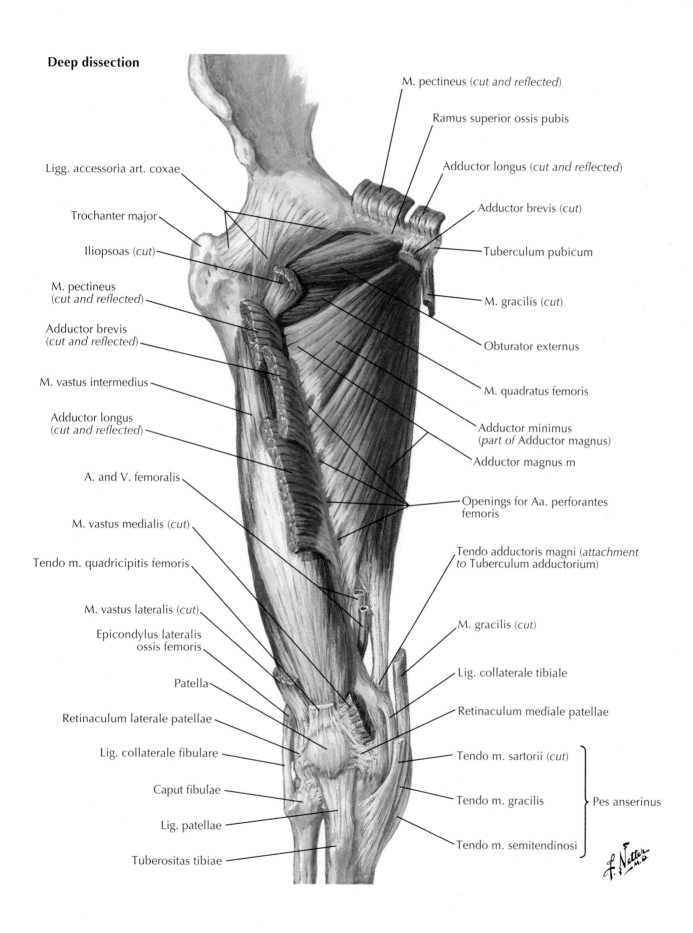

M. pectineus (*cut and reflected*)

Ramus superior ossis pubis

Adductor longus (*cut and reflected*)

Adductor brevis (*cut*)

Tuberculum pubicum

M. gracilis (*cut*)

Obturator externus

M. quadratus femoris

Adductor minimus
(*part of* Adductor magnus)

Adductor magnus m

Openings for Aa. perforantes
femoris

Tendo adductoris magni (*attachment
to* Tuberculum adductorium)

M. gracilis (*cut*)

Lig. collaterale tibiale

Retinaculum mediale patellae

Tendo m. sartorii (*cut*)

Tendo m. gracilis

Pes anserinus

Tendo m. semitendinosi

Ligg. accessoria art. coxae

Trochanter major

Iliopsoas (*cut*)

M. pectineus
(*cut and reflected*)

Adductor brevis
(*cut and reflected*)

M. vastus intermedius

Adductor longus
(*cut and reflected*)

A. and V. femoralis

M. vastus medialis (*cut*)

Tendo m. quadricipitis femoris

M. vastus lateralis (*cut*)

Epicondylus lateralis
ossis femoris

Patella

Retinaculum laterale patellae

Lig. collaterale fibulare

Caput fibulae

Lig. patellae

Tuberositas tibiae

Superficial dissection

Deeper dissection

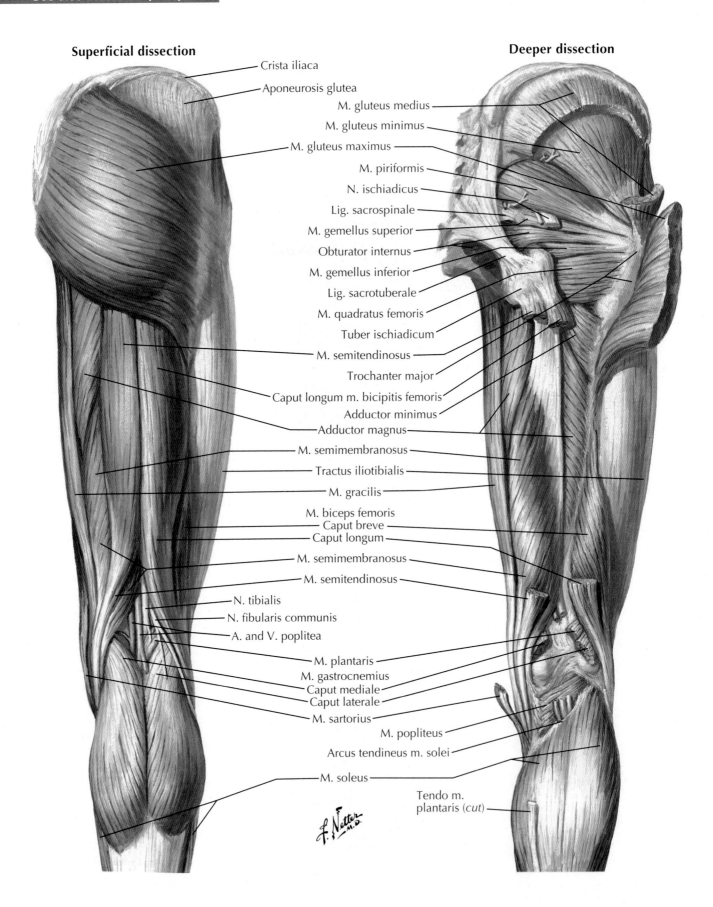

Crista iliaca

Aponeurosis glutea

M. gluteus medius

M. gluteus minimus

M. gluteus maximus

M. piriformis

N. ischiadicus

Lig. sacrospinale

M. gemellus superior

Obturator internus

M. gemellus inferior

Lig. sacrotuberale

M. quadratus femoris

Tuber ischiadicum

M. semitendinosus

Trochanter major

Caput longum m. bicipitis femoris

Adductor minimus

Adductor magnus

M. semimembranosus

Tractus iliotibialis

M. gracilis

M. biceps femoris
Caput breve
Caput longum

M. semimembranosus

M. semitendinosus

N. tibialis

N. fibularis communis

A. and V. poplitea

M. plantaris

M. gastrocnemius
Caput mediale
Caput laterale

M. sartorius

M. popliteus

Arcus tendineus m. solei

M. soleus

Tendo m.
plantaris (*cut*)

Plate 504

Coxa, Natis, and Femur

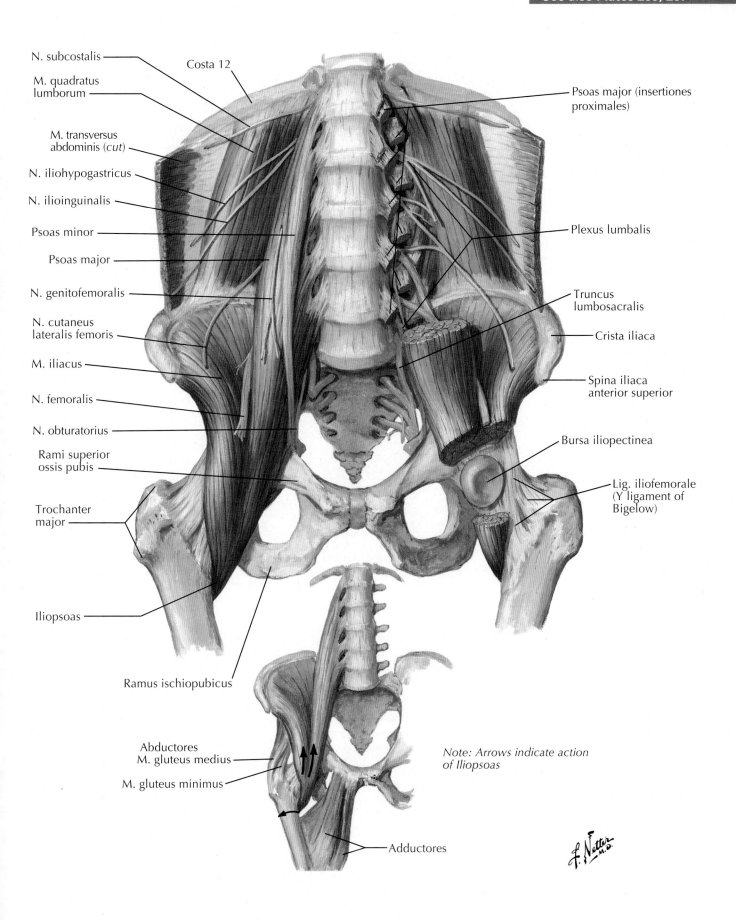

N. subcostalis

M. quadratus lumborum

Costa 12

M. transversus abdominis (*cut*)

N. iliohypogastricus

N. ilioinguinalis

Psoas minor

Psoas major

N. genitofemoralis

N. cutaneus lateralis femoris

M. iliacus

N. femoralis

N. obturatorius

Rami superior ossis pubis

Trochanter major

Iliopsoas

Ramus ischiopubicus

Abductores
M. gluteus medius

M. gluteus minimus

Adductores

Psoas major (insertiones proximales)

Plexus lumbalis

Truncus lumbosacralis

Crista iliaca

Spina iliaca anterior superior

Bursa iliopectinea

Lig. iliofemorale (Y ligament of Bigelow)

Note: Arrows indicate action of Iliopsoas

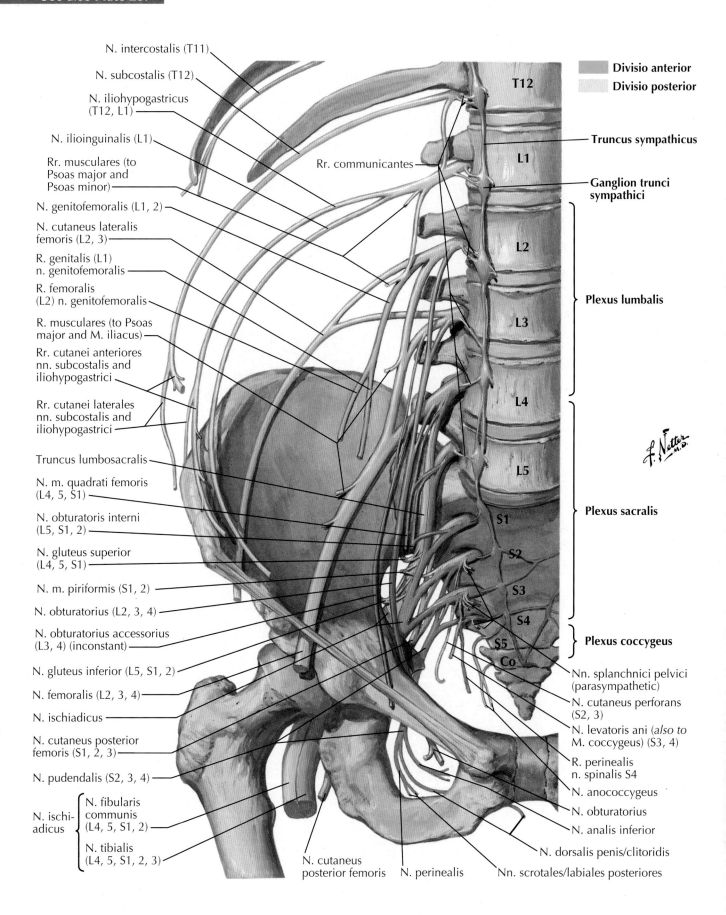

N. intercostalis (T11)

N. subcostalis (T12)

N. iliohypogastricus
(T12, L1)

N. ilioinguinalis (L1)

Rr. musculares (to
Psoas major and
Psoas minor)

N. genitofemoralis (L1, 2)

N. cutaneus lateralis
femoris (L2, 3)

R. genitalis (L1)
n. genitofemoralis

R. femoralis
(L2) n. genitofemoralis

R. musculares (to Psoas
major and M. iliacus)

Rr. cutanei anteriores
nn. subcostalis and
iliohypogastrici

Rr. cutanei laterales
nn. subcostalis and
iliohypogastrici

Truncus lumbosacralis

N. m. quadrati femoris
(L4, 5, S1)

N. obturatoris interni
(L5, S1, 2)

N. gluteus superior
(L4, 5, S1)

N. m. piriformis (S1, 2)

N. obturatorius (L2, 3, 4)

N. obturatorius accessorius
(L3, 4) (inconstant)

N. gluteus inferior (L5, S1, 2)

N. femoralis (L2, 3, 4)

N. ischiadicus

N. cutaneus posterior
femoris (S1, 2, 3)

N. pudendalis (S2, 3, 4)

N. ischi-
adicus { N. fibularis
communis
(L4, 5, S1, 2)

N. tibialis
(L4, 5, S1, 2, 3)

Rr. communicantes

Divisio anterior
Divisio posterior

T12

Truncus sympathicus

L1

Ganglion trunci
sympathici

L2

Plexus lumbalis

L3

L4

L5

Plexus sacralis

S1

S2

S3

S4

S5
Co

Plexus coccygeus

Nn. splanchnici pelvici
(parasympathetic)

N. cutaneus perforans
(S2, 3)

N. levatoris ani (*also to*
M. coccygeus) (S3, 4)

R. perinealis
n. spinalis S4

N. anococcygeus

N. obturatorius

N. analis inferior

N. dorsalis penis/clitoridis

N. cutaneus
posterior femoris

N. perinealis

Nn. scrotales/labiales posteriores

Plate 506

Coxa, Natis, and Femur

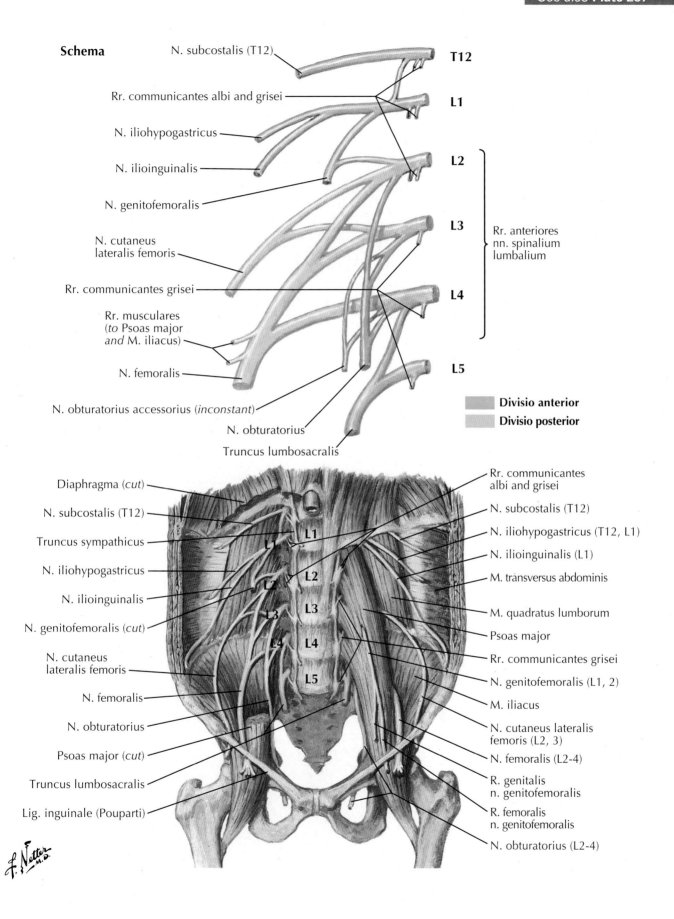

Schema

N. subcostalis (T12)

Rr. communicantes albi and grisei

N. iliohypogastricus

N. ilioinguinalis

N. genitofemoralis

N. cutaneus
lateralis femoris

Rr. communicantes grisei

Rr. musculares
(*to* Psoas major
and M. iliacus)

N. femoralis

N. obturatorius accessorius (*inconstant*)

N. obturatorius

Truncus lumbosacralis

T12

L1

L2

L3

L4

L5

Rr. anteriores
nn. spinalium
lumbalium

Divisio anterior
Divisio posterior

Diaphragma (*cut*)

N. subcostalis (T12)

Truncus sympathicus

N. iliohypogastricus

N. ilioinguinalis

N. genitofemoralis (*cut*)

N. cutaneus
lateralis femoris

N. femoralis

N. obturatorius

Psoas major (*cut*)

Truncus lumbosacralis

Lig. inguinale (Pouparti)

Rr. communicantes
albi and grisei

N. subcostalis (T12)

N. iliohypogastricus (T12, L1)

N. ilioinguinalis (L1)

M. transversus abdominis

M. quadratus lumborum

Psoas major

Rr. communicantes grisei

N. genitofemoralis (L1, 2)

M. iliacus

N. cutaneus lateralis
femoris (L2, 3)

N. femoralis (L2-4)

R. genitalis
n. genitofemoralis

R. femoralis
n. genitofemoralis

N. obturatorius (L2-4)

L1
L2
L3
L4
L5

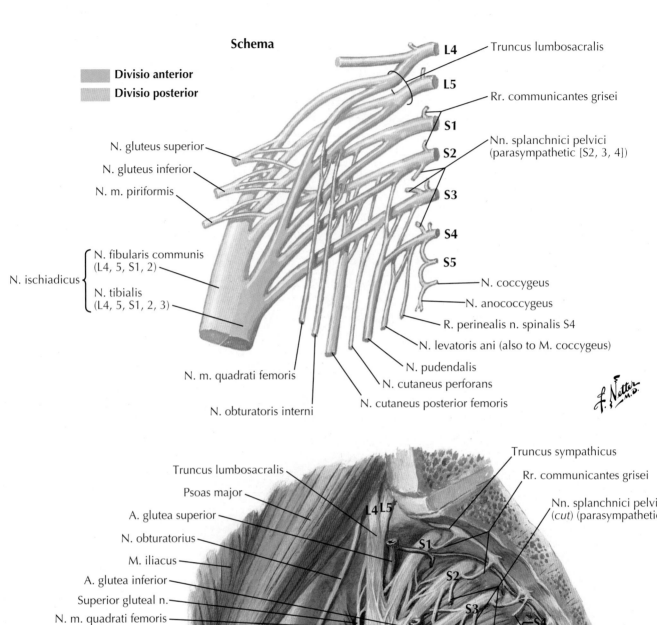

Schema

Divisio anterior
Divisio posterior

L4 — Truncus lumbosacralis
L5
S1 — Rr. communicantes grisei
S2 — Nn. splanchnici pelvici (parasympathetic [S2, 3, 4])
S3
S4
S5

N. gluteus superior
N. gluteus inferior
N. m. piriformis

N. ischiadicus {
N. fibularis communis (L4, 5, S1, 2)
N. tibialis (L4, 5, S1, 2, 3)
}

N. coccygeus
N. anococcygeus
R. perinealis n. spinalis S4
N. levatoris ani (also to M. coccygeus)
N. pudendalis
N. cutaneus perforans
N. cutaneus posterior femoris

N. m. quadrati femoris
N. obturatoris interni

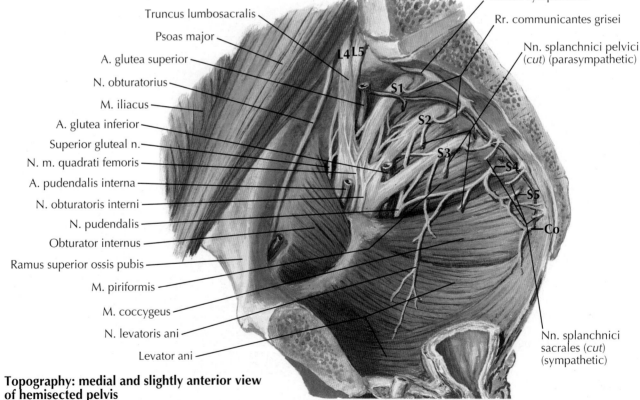

Truncus lumbosacralis
Psoas major
A. glutea superior
N. obturatorius
M. iliacus
A. glutea inferior
Superior gluteal n.
N. m. quadrati femoris
A. pudendalis interna
N. obturatoris interni
N. pudendalis
Obturator internus
Ramus superior ossis pubis
M. piriformis
M. coccygeus
N. levatoris ani
Levator ani

Truncus sympathicus
Rr. communicantes grisei
Nn. splanchnici pelvici (cut) (parasympathetic)

L4 L5
S1
S2
S3
S4
S5
Co

Nn. splanchnici sacrales (cut) (sympathetic)

Topography: medial and slightly anterior view of hemisected pelvis

Plate 508

Coxa, Natis, and Femur

Superficial dissections

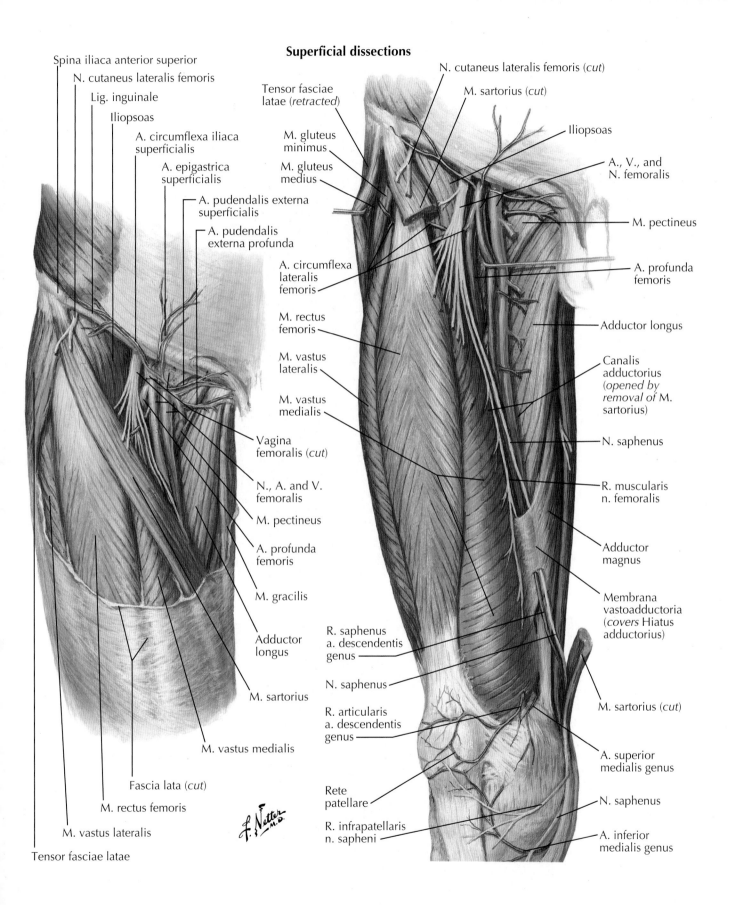

Spina iliaca anterior superior

N. cutaneus lateralis femoris

Lig. inguinale

Iliopsoas

A. circumflexa iliaca superficialis

A. epigastrica superficialis

A. pudendalis externa superficialis

A. pudendalis externa profunda

A. circumflexa lateralis femoris

M. rectus femoris

M. vastus lateralis

M. vastus medialis

Vagina femoralis (*cut*)

N., A. and V. femoralis

M. pectineus

A. profunda femoris

M. gracilis

Adductor longus

M. sartorius

M. vastus medialis

Fascia lata (*cut*)

M. rectus femoris

M. vastus lateralis

Tensor fasciae latae

Tensor fasciae latae (*retracted*)

M. gluteus minimus

M. gluteus medius

N. cutaneus lateralis femoris (*cut*)

M. sartorius (*cut*)

Iliopsoas

A., V., and N. femoralis

M. pectineus

A. profunda femoris

Adductor longus

Canalis adductorius (*opened by removal of M. sartorius*)

N. saphenus

R. muscularis n. femoralis

Adductor magnus

Membrana vastoadductoria (*covers Hiatus adductorius*)

M. sartorius (*cut*)

A. superior medialis genus

N. saphenus

A. inferior medialis genus

R. saphenus a. descendentis genus

N. saphenus

R. articularis a. descendentis genus

Rete patellare

R. infrapatellaris n. sapheni

f. Netter M.D.

Deep dissection

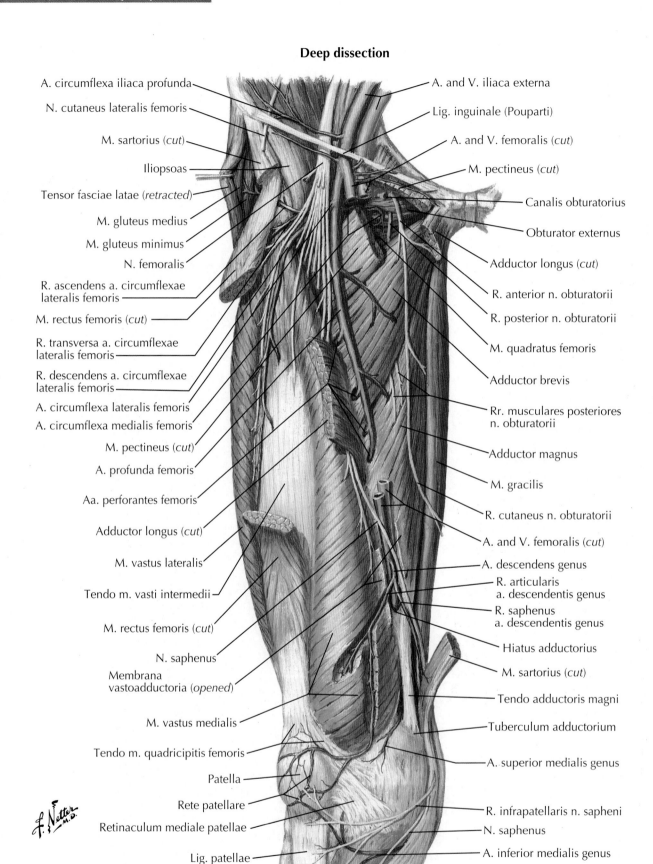

A. circumflexa iliaca profunda

N. cutaneus lateralis femoris

M. sartorius (*cut*)

Iliopsoas

Tensor fasciae latae (*retracted*)

M. gluteus medius

M. gluteus minimus

N. femoralis

R. ascendens a. circumflexae lateralis femoris

M. rectus femoris (*cut*)

R. transversa a. circumflexae lateralis femoris

R. descendens a. circumflexae lateralis femoris

A. circumflexa lateralis femoris

A. circumflexa medialis femoris

M. pectineus (*cut*)

A. profunda femoris

Aa. perforantes femoris

Adductor longus (*cut*)

M. vastus lateralis

Tendo m. vasti intermedii

M. rectus femoris (*cut*)

N. saphenus

Membrana vastoadductoria (*opened*)

M. vastus medialis

Tendo m. quadricipitis femoris

Patella

Rete patellare

Retinaculum mediale patellae

Lig. patellae

A. and V. iliaca externa

Lig. inguinale (Pouparti)

A. and V. femoralis (*cut*)

M. pectineus (*cut*)

Canalis obturatorius

Obturator externus

Adductor longus (*cut*)

R. anterior n. obturatorii

R. posterior n. obturatorii

M. quadratus femoris

Adductor brevis

Rr. musculares posteriores n. obturatorii

Adductor magnus

M. gracilis

R. cutaneus n. obturatorii

A. and V. femoralis (*cut*)

A. descendens genus

R. articularis a. descendentis genus

R. saphenus a. descendentis genus

Hiatus adductorius

M. sartorius (*cut*)

Tendo adductoris magni

Tuberculum adductorium

A. superior medialis genus

R. infrapatellaris n. sapheni

N. saphenus

A. inferior medialis genus

Plate 510

Coxa, Natis, and Femur

Deep dissection

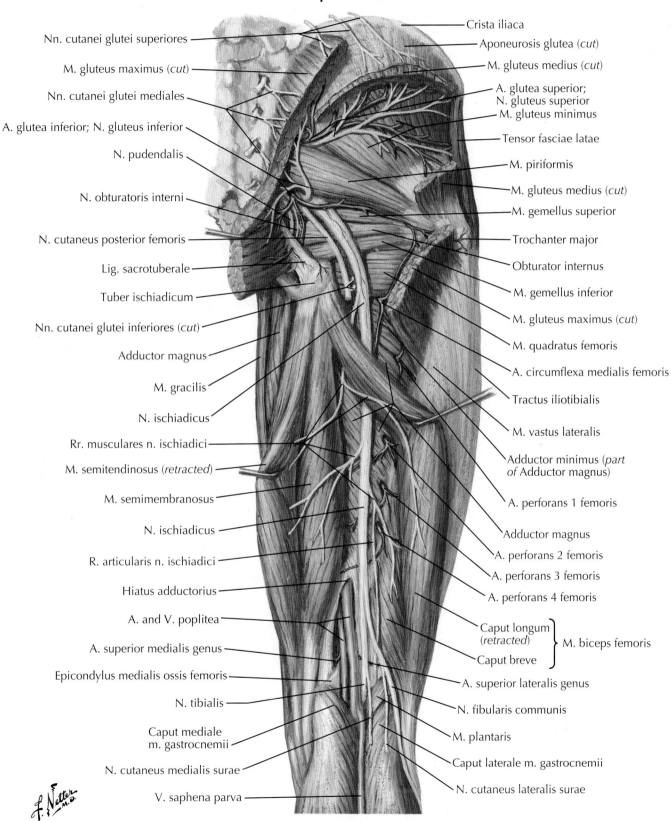

Nn. cutanei glutei superiores

M. gluteus maximus (*cut*)

Nn. cutanei glutei mediales

A. glutea inferior; N. gluteus inferior

N. pudendalis

N. obturatoris interni

N. cutaneus posterior femoris

Lig. sacrotuberale

Tuber ischiadicum

Nn. cutanei glutei inferiores (*cut*)

Adductor magnus

M. gracilis

N. ischiadicus

Rr. musculares n. ischiadici

M. semitendinosus (*retracted*)

M. semimembranosus

N. ischiadicus

R. articularis n. ischiadici

Hiatus adductorius

A. and V. poplitea

A. superior medialis genus

Epicondylus medialis ossis femoris

N. tibialis

Caput mediale m. gastrocnemii

N. cutaneus medialis surae

V. saphena parva

Crista iliaca

Aponeurosis glutea (*cut*)

M. gluteus medius (*cut*)

A. glutea superior; N. gluteus superior

M. gluteus minimus

Tensor fasciae latae

M. piriformis

M. gluteus medius (*cut*)

M. gemellus superior

Trochanter major

Obturator internus

M. gemellus inferior

M. gluteus maximus (*cut*)

M. quadratus femoris

A. circumflexa medialis femoris

Tractus iliotibialis

M. vastus lateralis

Adductor minimus (*part of* Adductor magnus)

A. perforans 1 femoris

Adductor magnus

A. perforans 2 femoris

A. perforans 3 femoris

A. perforans 4 femoris

Caput longum (*retracted*) — Caput breve } M. biceps femoris

A. superior lateralis genus

N. fibularis communis

M. plantaris

Caput laterale m. gastrocnemii

N. cutaneus lateralis surae

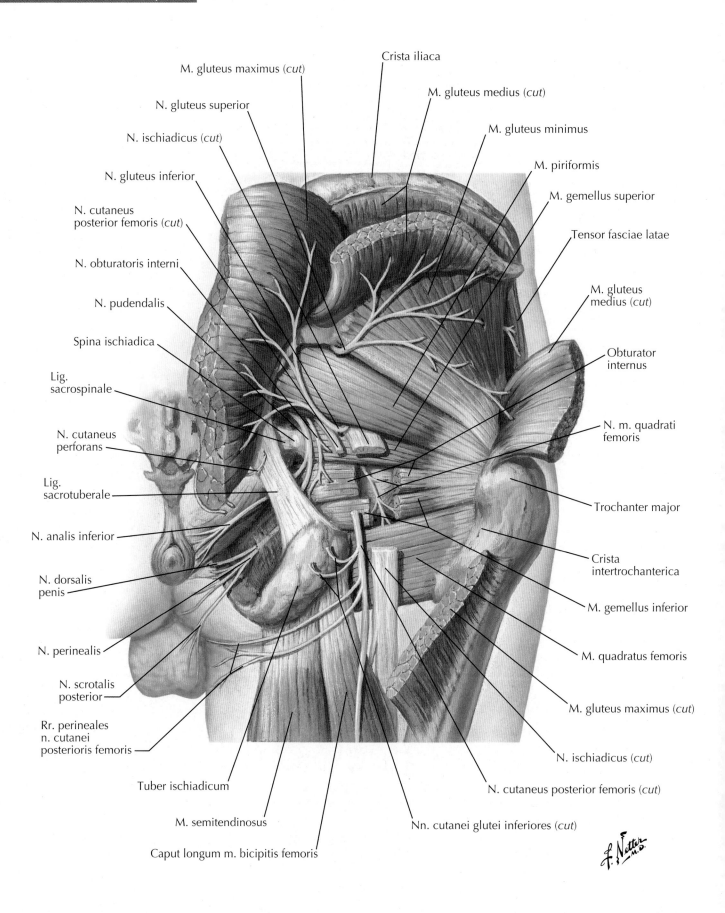

M. gluteus maximus (*cut*)

Crista iliaca

N. gluteus superior

M. gluteus medius (*cut*)

N. ischiadicus (*cut*)

M. gluteus minimus

N. gluteus inferior

M. piriformis

N. cutaneus
posterior femoris (*cut*)

M. gemellus superior

N. obturatoris interni

Tensor fasciae latae

N. pudendalis

M. gluteus
medius (*cut*)

Spina ischiadica

Lig.
sacrospinale

Obturator
internus

N. cutaneus
perforans

N. m. quadrati
femoris

Lig.
sacrotuberale

N. analis inferior

Trochanter major

N. dorsalis
penis

Crista
intertrochanterica

N. perinealis

M. gemellus inferior

N. scrotalis
posterior

M. quadratus femoris

Rr. perineales
n. cutanei
posterioris femoris

M. gluteus maximus (*cut*)

N. ischiadicus (*cut*)

Tuber ischiadicum

N. cutaneus posterior femoris (*cut*)

M. semitendinosus

Nn. cutanei glutei inferiores (*cut*)

Caput longum m. bicipitis femoris

Plate 512

Coxa, Natis, and Femur

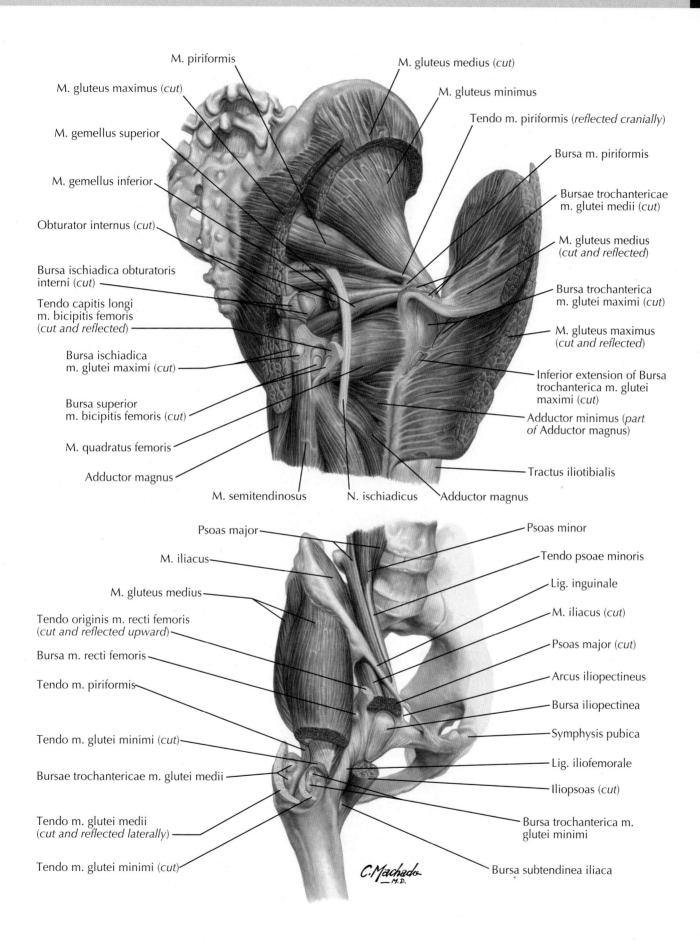

M. piriformis

M. gluteus medius (*cut*)

M. gluteus maximus (*cut*)

M. gluteus minimus

Tendo m. piriformis (*reflected cranially*)

M. gemellus superior

Bursa m. piriformis

M. gemellus inferior

Bursae trochantericae
m. glutei medii (*cut*)

Obturator internus (*cut*)

M. gluteus medius
(*cut and reflected*)

Bursa ischiadica obturatoris
interni (*cut*)

Bursa trochanterica
m. glutei maximi (*cut*)

Tendo capitis longi
m. bicipitis femoris
(*cut and reflected*)

M. gluteus maximus
(*cut and reflected*)

Bursa ischiadica
m. glutei maximi (*cut*)

Inferior extension of Bursa
trochanterica m. glutei
maximi (*cut*)

Bursa superior
m. bicipitis femoris (*cut*)

Adductor minimus (*part
of* Adductor magnus)

M. quadratus femoris

Adductor magnus

Tractus iliotibialis

M. semitendinosus

N. ischiadicus

Adductor magnus

Psoas major

Psoas minor

M. iliacus

Tendo psoae minoris

M. gluteus medius

Lig. inguinale

Tendo originis m. recti femoris
(*cut and reflected upward*)

M. iliacus (*cut*)

Bursa m. recti femoris

Psoas major (*cut*)

Tendo m. piriformis

Arcus iliopectineus

Bursa iliopectinea

Symphysis pubica

Tendo m. glutei minimi (*cut*)

Lig. iliofemorale

Bursae trochantericae m. glutei medii

Iliopsoas (*cut*)

Tendo m. glutei medii
(*cut and reflected laterally*)

Bursa trochanterica m.
glutei minimi

Tendo m. glutei minimi (*cut*)

Bursa subtendinea iliaca

C. Machado
_M.D._

Coxa, Natis, and Femur

Plate 513

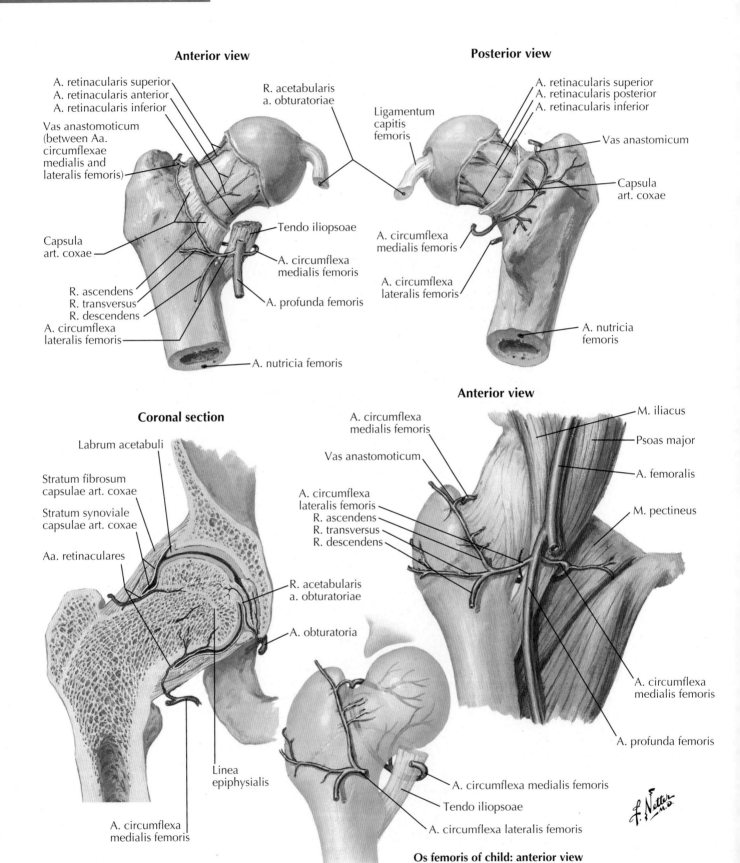

Anterior view

A. retinacularis superior
A. retinacularis anterior
A. retinacularis inferior

Vas anastomoticum
(between Aa.
circumflexae
medialis and
lateralis femoris)

Capsula
art. coxae

R. ascendens
R. transversus
R. descendens
A. circumflexa
lateralis femoris

R. acetabularis
a. obturatoriae

Tendo iliopsoae

A. circumflexa
medialis femoris

A. profunda femoris

A. nutricia femoris

Posterior view

Ligamentum
capitis
femoris

A. retinacularis superior
A. retinacularis posterior
A. retinacularis inferior

Vas anastomicum

Capsula
art. coxae

A. circumflexa
medialis femoris

A. circumflexa
lateralis femoris

A. nutricia
femoris

Coronal section

Labrum acetabuli

Stratum fibrosum
capsulae art. coxae

Stratum synoviale
capsulae art. coxae

Aa. retinaculares

R. acetabularis
a. obturatoriae

A. obturatoria

Linea
epiphysialis

A. circumflexa
medialis femoris

Anterior view

A. circumflexa
medialis femoris

Vas anastomoticum

A. circumflexa
lateralis femoris
R. ascendens
R. transversus
R. descendens

M. iliacus

Psoas major

A. femoralis

M. pectineus

A. circumflexa
medialis femoris

A. profunda femoris

A. circumflexa medialis femoris

Tendo iliopsoae

A. circumflexa lateralis femoris

Os femoris of child: anterior view

Plate 514

Coxa, Natis, and Femur

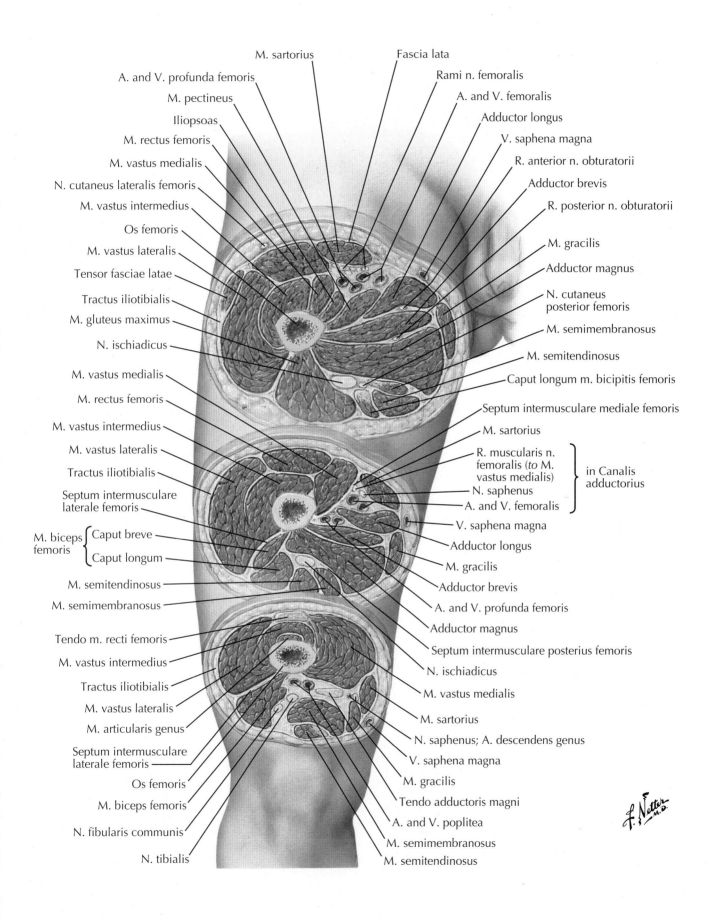

M. sartorius

Fascia lata

A. and V. profunda femoris

Rami n. femoralis

M. pectineus

A. and V. femoralis

Iliopsoas

Adductor longus

M. rectus femoris

V. saphena magna

M. vastus medialis

R. anterior n. obturatorii

N. cutaneus lateralis femoris

Adductor brevis

M. vastus intermedius

R. posterior n. obturatorii

Os femoris

M. vastus lateralis

M. gracilis

Tensor fasciae latae

Adductor magnus

Tractus iliotibialis

N. cutaneus
posterior femoris

M. gluteus maximus

M. semimembranosus

N. ischiadicus

M. semitendinosus

M. vastus medialis

Caput longum m. bicipitis femoris

M. rectus femoris

Septum intermusculare mediale femoris

M. vastus intermedius

M. sartorius

M. vastus lateralis

R. muscularis n.
femoralis (*to* M.
vastus medialis)

Tractus iliotibialis

in Canalis
adductorius

Septum intermusculare
laterale femoris

N. saphenus

A. and V. femoralis

M. biceps
femoris { Caput breve

V. saphena magna

Caput longum

Adductor longus

M. semitendinosus

M. gracilis

M. semimembranosus

Adductor brevis

A. and V. profunda femoris

Tendo m. recti femoris

Adductor magnus

M. vastus intermedius

Septum intermusculare posterius femoris

Tractus iliotibialis

N. ischiadicus

M. vastus lateralis

M. vastus medialis

M. articularis genus

M. sartorius

Septum intermusculare
laterale femoris

N. saphenus; A. descendens genus

Os femoris

V. saphena magna

M. biceps femoris

M. gracilis

N. fibularis communis

Tendo adductoris magni

N. tibialis

A. and V. poplitea

M. semimembranosus

M. semitendinosus

Medial view

M. vastus medialis

Tendo m. quadricipitis femoris

Epicondylus medialis ossis femoris

Patella

Retinaculum mediale patellae

Capsula art. genus

Lig. patellae

Tuberositas tibiae

M. sartorius (*cut*)

M. gracilis (*cut*)

Tendo m. semitendinosi (*cut*)

M. semimembranosus; Tendo

Tendo adductoris magni

Lig. collaterale tibiale

Bursa m. semimembranosi

Bursa anserina

Tendo m. semitendinosi
Tendo m. gracilis
Tendo m. sartorii } Pes anserinus

M. gastrocnemius

M. soleus

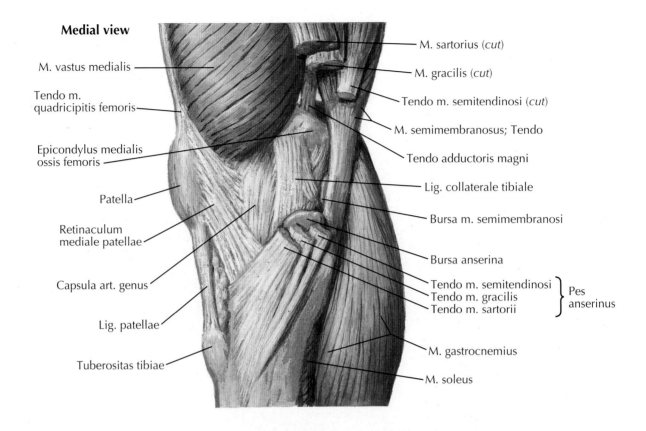

Lateral view

Tractus iliotibialis (*cut*)

M. biceps femoris (*cut*) { Caput longum
Caput breve

Bursa tractus iliotibialis

Lig. collaterale fibulare

Bursa lig. collateralis fibularis

M. plantaris

Bursa subtendinea inferior m. bicipitis femoris

Tendo m. bicipitis femoris

N. fibularis communis

Caput fibulae

M. gastrocnemius

M. soleus

M. fibularis longus

M. vastus lateralis

Tendo m. quadricipitis femoris

Patella

Retinaculum laterale patellae

Capsula art. genus

Lig. patellae

Tuberositas tibiae

M. tibialis anterior

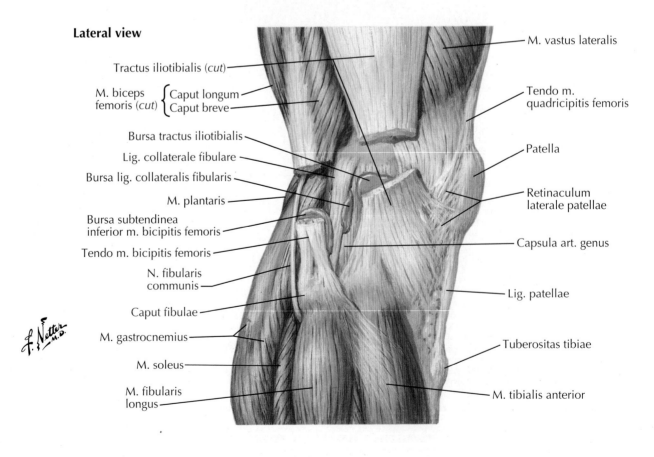

Plate 516   **Genu**

Right knee in extension

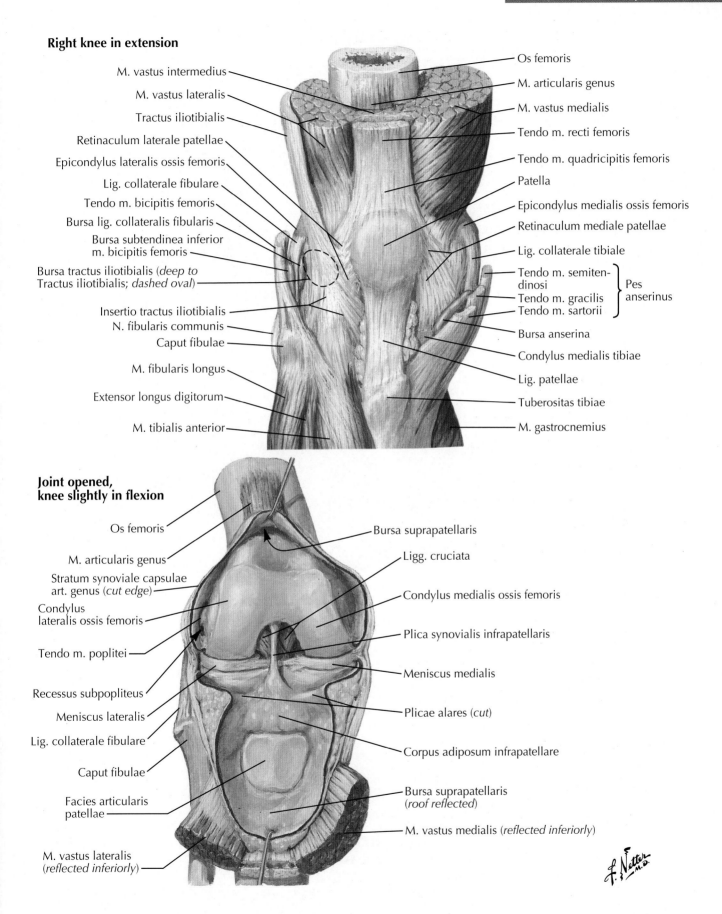

M. vastus intermedius

M. vastus lateralis

Tractus iliotibialis

Retinaculum laterale patellae

Epicondylus lateralis ossis femoris

Lig. collaterale fibulare

Tendo m. bicipitis femoris

Bursa lig. collateralis fibularis

Bursa subtendinea inferior m. bicipitis femoris

Bursa tractus iliotibialis (*deep to* Tractus iliotibialis; *dashed oval*)

Insertio tractus iliotibialis

N. fibularis communis

Caput fibulae

M. fibularis longus

Extensor longus digitorum

M. tibialis anterior

Os femoris

M. articularis genus

M. vastus medialis

Tendo m. recti femoris

Tendo m. quadricipitis femoris

Patella

Epicondylus medialis ossis femoris

Retinaculum mediale patellae

Lig. collaterale tibiale

Tendo m. semiten-dinosi } Pes
Tendo m. gracilis anserinus
Tendo m. sartorii

Bursa anserina

Condylus medialis tibiae

Lig. patellae

Tuberositas tibiae

M. gastrocnemius

Joint opened, knee slightly in flexion

Os femoris

M. articularis genus

Stratum synoviale capsulae art. genus (*cut edge*)

Condylus lateralis ossis femoris

Tendo m. poplitei

Recessus subpopliteus

Meniscus lateralis

Lig. collaterale fibulare

Caput fibulae

Facies articularis patellae

M. vastus lateralis (*reflected inferiorly*)

Bursa suprapatellaris

Ligg. cruciata

Condylus medialis ossis femoris

Plica synovialis infrapatellaris

Meniscus medialis

Plicae alares (*cut*)

Corpus adiposum infrapatellare

Bursa suprapatellaris (*roof reflected*)

M. vastus medialis (*reflected inferiorly*)

Inferior view

Tractus iliotibialis

Bursa tractus iliotibialis

Recessus subpopliteus

Tendo m. poplitei

Lig. collaterale fibulare

Bursa lig. collateralis fibularis

Condylus lateralis ossis femoris

Lig. cruciatum anterius

Lig. popliteum arcuatum

Lig. patellae

Retinaculum mediale patellae

Bursa suprapatellaris

Stratum synoviale capsulae art. genus (*cut edge*)

Plica synovialis infrapatellaris

Lig. cruciatum posterius

Lig. collaterale tibiale (Partes superficialis and profunda)

Condylus medialis ossis femoris

Lig. popliteum obliquum

Tendo m. semimembranosi

Posterior aspect

Superior view

Lig. meniscofemorale posterius

Lig. popliteum arcuatum

Lig. collaterale fibulare

Bursa lig. collateralis fibularis

Tendo m. poplitei

Recessus subpopliteus

Meniscus lateralis

Facies articularis superior condyli lateralis tibiae

Tractus iliotibialis

Corpus adiposum infrapatellare

Tendo m. semimembranosi

Lig. popliteum obliquum

Lig. cruciatum posterius

Lig. collaterale tibiale (Pars profunda *bound to* Meniscus medialis)

Meniscus medialis

Stratum synoviale capsulae art. genus

Facies articularis condyli medialis tibiae

Stratum fibrosum capsulae art. genus

Lig. cruciatum anterius

Lig. patellae

Anterior aspect ↑

Superior view: ligaments and cartilage removed

Attachment of Lig. cruciatum posterius

Attachment of Stratum synoviale capsulae art. genus

Facies articularis superior condyli lateralis tibiae

Attachments of Meniscus lateralis

Attachments of Meniscus medialis

Eminentia intercondylaris

Attachment of Stratum synoviale capsulae art. genus

Facies articularis condyli medialis tibiae

Attachment of Lig. cruciatum anterius

Tuberositas tibiae

Anterior aspect ↑

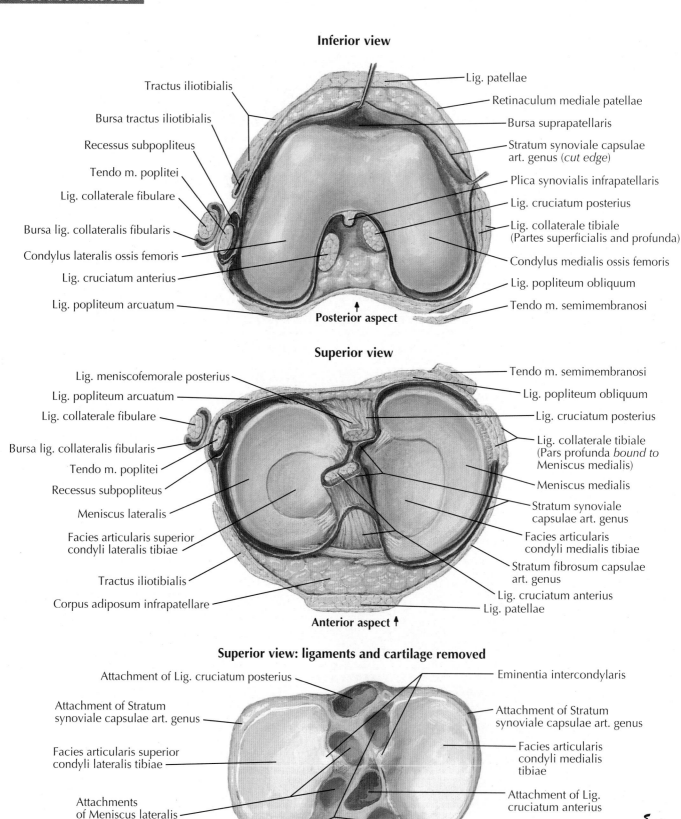

Plate 518

Genu

Right knee in flexion: anterior view

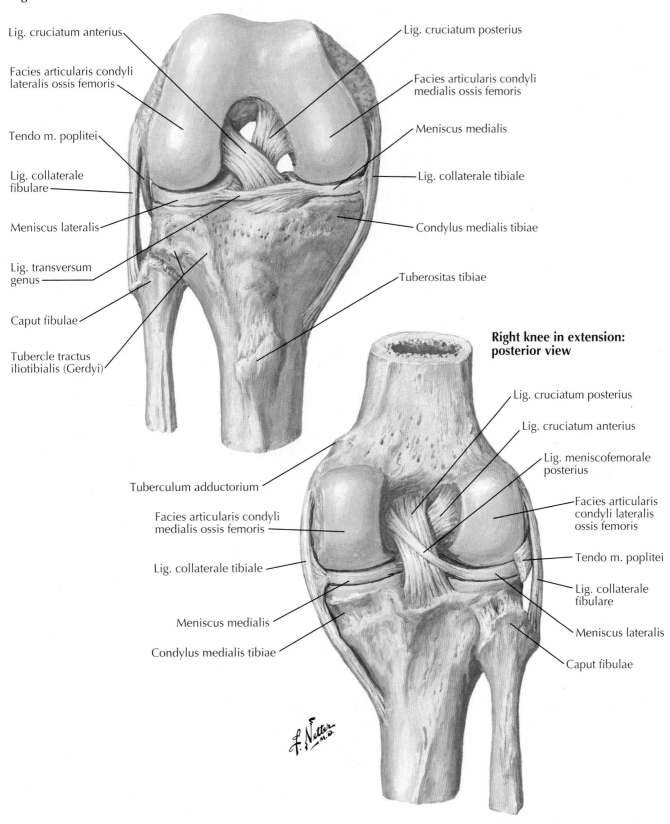

Lig. cruciatum anterius

Facies articularis condyli lateralis ossis femoris

Tendo m. poplitei

Lig. collaterale fibulare

Meniscus lateralis

Lig. transversum genus

Caput fibulae

Tubercle tractus iliotibialis (Gerdyi)

Lig. cruciatum posterius

Facies articularis condyli medialis ossis femoris

Meniscus medialis

Lig. collaterale tibiale

Condylus medialis tibiae

Tuberositas tibiae

Right knee in extension: posterior view

Tuberculum adductorium

Facies articularis condyli medialis ossis femoris

Lig. collaterale tibiale

Meniscus medialis

Condylus medialis tibiae

Lig. cruciatum posterius

Lig. cruciatum anterius

Lig. meniscofemorale posterius

Facies articularis condyli lateralis ossis femoris

Tendo m. poplitei

Lig. collaterale fibulare

Meniscus lateralis

Caput fibulae

f. Netter M.D.

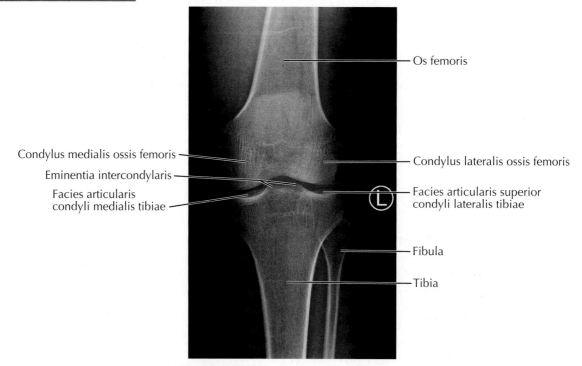

Os femoris

Condylus medialis ossis femoris

Eminentia intercondylaris

Facies articularis condyli medialis tibiae

Condylus lateralis ossis femoris

Facies articularis superior condyli lateralis tibiae

Fibula

Tibia

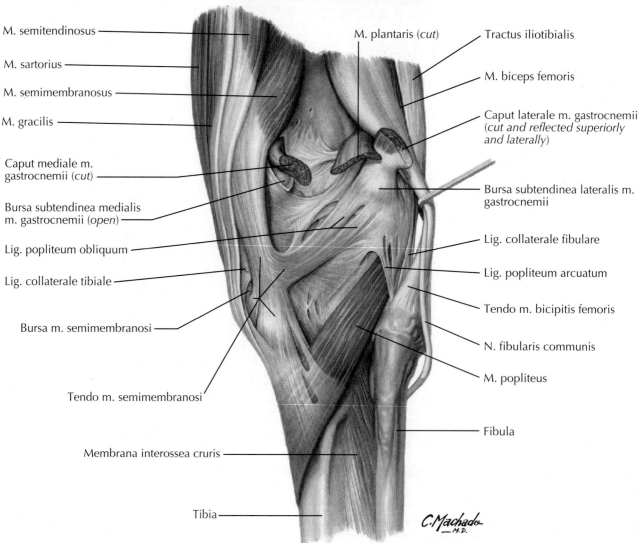

M. semitendinosus

M. sartorius

M. semimembranosus

M. gracilis

Caput mediale m. gastrocnemii (cut)

Bursa subtendinea medialis m. gastrocnemii (open)

Lig. popliteum obliquum

Lig. collaterale tibiale

Bursa m. semimembranosi

Tendo m. semimembranosi

Membrana interossea cruris

Tibia

M. plantaris (cut)

Tractus iliotibialis

M. biceps femoris

Caput laterale m. gastrocnemii (cut and reflected superiorly and laterally)

Bursa subtendinea lateralis m. gastrocnemii

Lig. collaterale fibulare

Lig. popliteum arcuatum

Tendo m. bicipitis femoris

N. fibularis communis

M. popliteus

Fibula

Plate 520

Genu

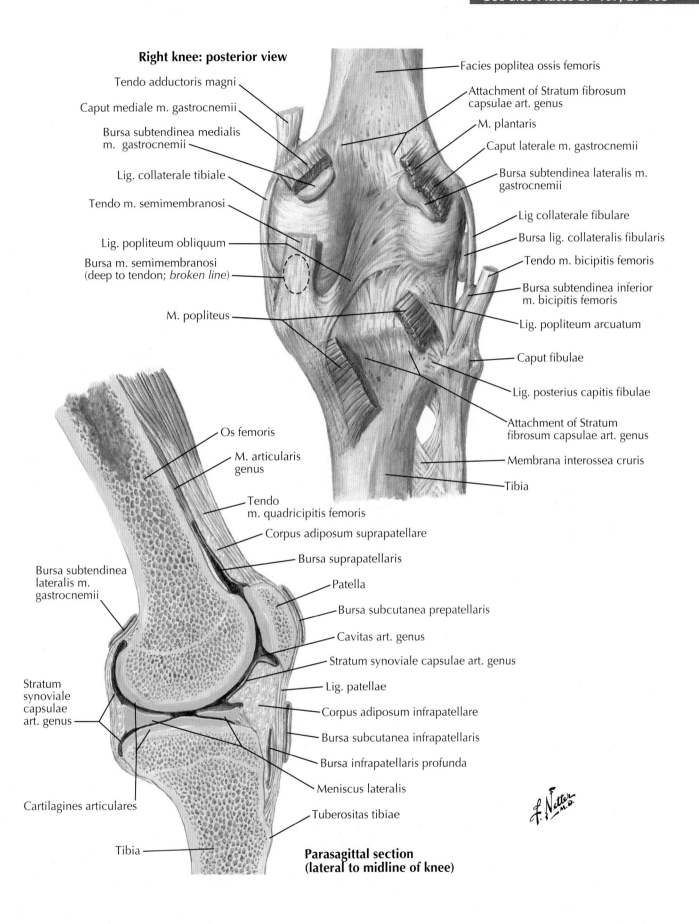

Right knee: posterior view

Tendo adductoris magni

Caput mediale m. gastrocnemii

Bursa subtendinea medialis m. gastrocnemii

Lig. collaterale tibiale

Tendo m. semimembranosi

Lig. popliteum obliquum

Bursa m. semimembranosi (deep to tendon; *broken line*)

M. popliteus

Facies poplitea ossis femoris

Attachment of Stratum fibrosum capsulae art. genus

M. plantaris

Caput laterale m. gastrocnemii

Bursa subtendinea lateralis m. gastrocnemii

Lig collaterale fibulare

Bursa lig. collateralis fibularis

Tendo m. bicipitis femoris

Bursa subtendinea inferior m. bicipitis femoris

Lig. popliteum arcuatum

Caput fibulae

Lig. posterius capitis fibulae

Attachment of Stratum fibrosum capsulae art. genus

Membrana interossea cruris

Tibia

Bursa subtendinea lateralis m. gastrocnemii

Stratum synoviale capsulae art. genus

Cartilagines articulares

Tibia

Os femoris

M. articularis genus

Tendo m. quadricipitis femoris

Corpus adiposum suprapatellare

Bursa suprapatellaris

Patella

Bursa subcutanea prepatellaris

Cavitas art. genus

Stratum synoviale capsulae art. genus

Lig. patellae

Corpus adiposum infrapatellare

Bursa subcutanea infrapatellaris

Bursa infrapatellaris profunda

Meniscus lateralis

Tuberositas tibiae

Parasagittal section (lateral to midline of knee)

f. Netter M.D.

A. circumflexa iliaca profunda

A. circumflexa iliaca superficialis

A. femoralis

R. ascendens a. circumflexae
lateralis femoris

R. transversus a. circumflexae
lateralis femoris

R. descendens a. circumflexae
lateralis femoris

A. circumflexa
lateralis femoris

A. profunda femoris

Aa. perforantes femoris

A. femoralis
(*in* Hiatus adductorius)

A. superior lateralis genus

Rete patellare

A. inferior lateralis genus
(*partially in phantom*)

A. recurrens tibialis
posterior (*phantom*)

A. circumflexa fibularis

A. tibialis anterior

Membrana interossea cruris

A. fibularis (*phantom*)

R. perforans a. fibularis

A. malleolaris anterior lateralis

A. tarsea lateralis

Rr. perforantes aa.
metatarsearum plantarium

Arcus plantaris

A. iliaca externa

A. epigastrica inferior

A. epigastrica superficialis

A. pudendalis externa superficialis

A. obturatoria

A. pudendalis externa profunda

A. circumflexa medialis femoris

A. femoralis

Rr. musculares
a. profundae femoris

Rr. musculares a. femoralis

A. descendens genus

R. articularis a. descendentis genus

R. saphenus a. descendentis genus

A. superior medialis genus

A. poplitea (*phantom*)

A. media genus (*phantom*)

A. inferior medialis genus
(*partially in phantom*)

A. recurrens tibialis anterior

A. tibialis posterior (*phantom*)

A. fibularis (*phantom*)

A. tibialis anterior

A. malleolaris anterior medialis

A. tarsea medialis

A. arcuata

A. dorsalis pedis

A. plantaris profunda

Aa. digitales dorsales pedis

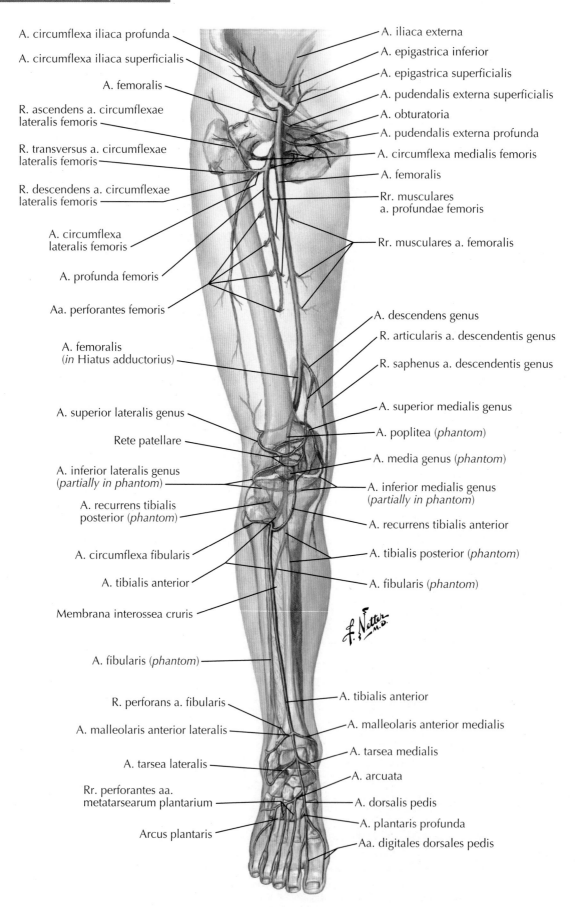

Plate 522

Genu

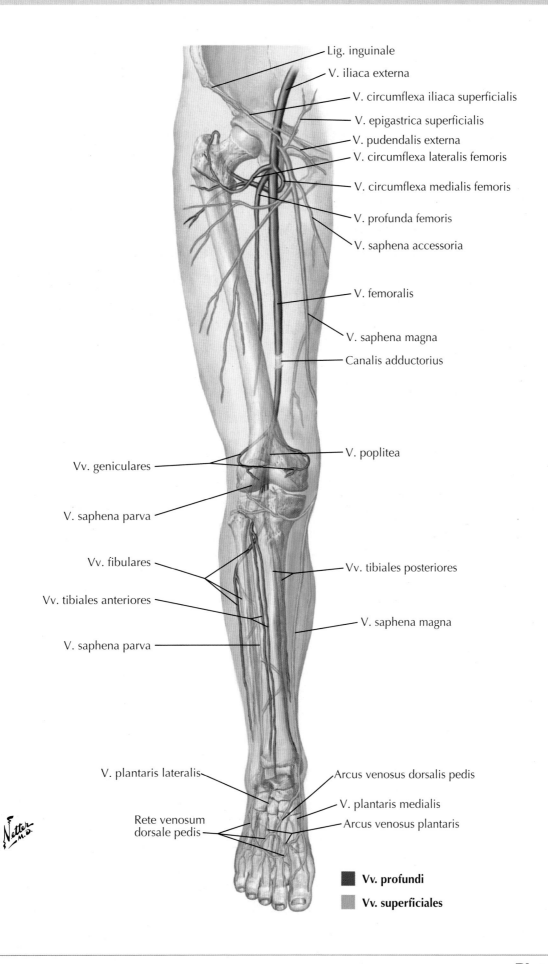

Lig. inguinale

V. iliaca externa

V. circumflexa iliaca superficialis

V. epigastrica superficialis

V. pudendalis externa

V. circumflexa lateralis femoris

V. circumflexa medialis femoris

V. profunda femoris

V. saphena accessoria

V. femoralis

V. saphena magna

Canalis adductorius

V. poplitea

Vv. geniculares

V. saphena parva

Vv. fibulares

Vv. tibiales anteriores

V. saphena parva

Vv. tibiales posteriores

V. saphena magna

V. plantaris lateralis

Arcus venosus dorsalis pedis

V. plantaris medialis

Rete venosum dorsale pedis

Arcus venosus plantaris

Vv. profundi

Vv. superficiales

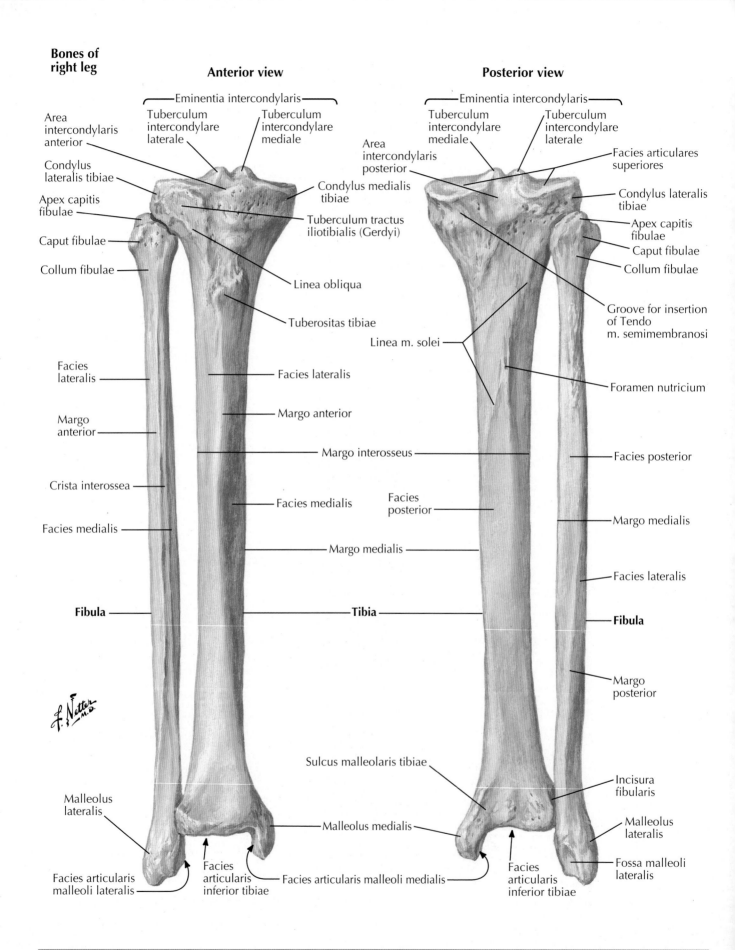

Bones of right leg

Anterior view

Posterior view

Area intercondylaris anterior

Condylus lateralis tibiae

Apex capitis fibulae

Caput fibulae

Collum fibulae

Eminentia intercondylaris

Tuberculum intercondylare laterale

Tuberculum intercondylare mediale

Condylus medialis tibiae

Tuberculum tractus iliotibialis (Gerdyi)

Linea obliqua

Tuberositas tibiae

Facies lateralis

Margo anterior

Crista interossea

Facies medialis

Facies lateralis

Margo anterior

Margo interosseus

Facies medialis

Margo medialis

Fibula

Tibia

Facies posterior

Malleolus lateralis

Facies articularis malleoli lateralis

Facies articularis inferior tibiae

Facies articularis malleoli medialis

Sulcus malleolaris tibiae

Malleolus medialis

Eminentia intercondylaris

Tuberculum intercondylare mediale

Tuberculum intercondylare laterale

Area intercondylaris posterior

Facies articulares superiores

Condylus lateralis tibiae

Apex capitis fibulae

Caput fibulae

Collum fibulae

Groove for insertion of Tendo m. semimembranosi

Linea m. solei

Foramen nutricium

Facies posterior

Margo medialis

Facies lateralis

Fibula

Margo posterior

Incisura fibularis

Malleolus lateralis

Fossa malleoli lateralis

Facies articularis inferior tibiae

Plate 524

Crus

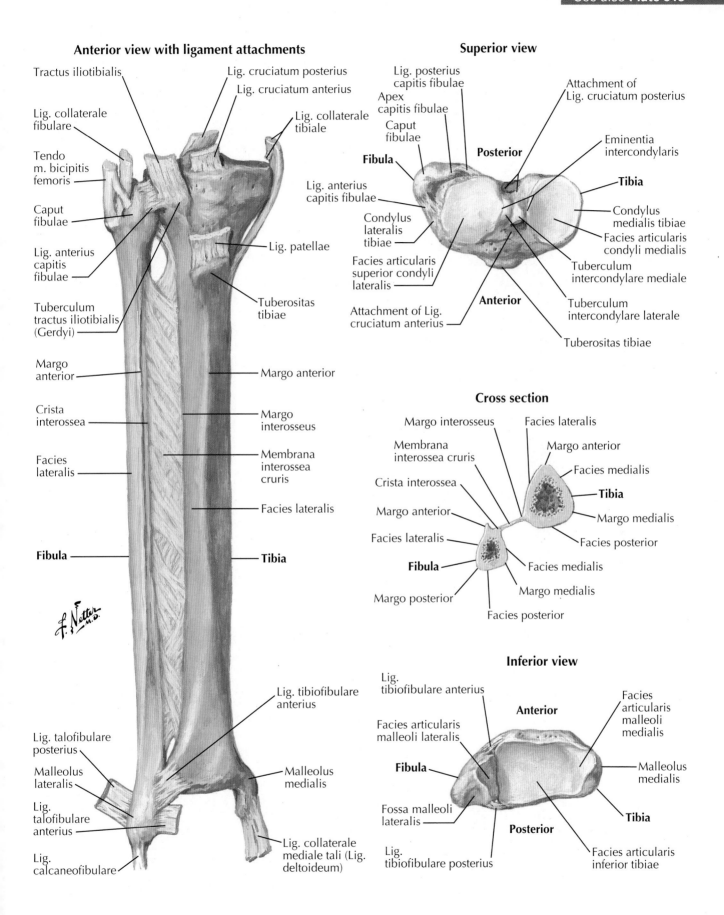

Anterior view with ligament attachments

Tractus iliotibialis

Lig. cruciatum posterius

Lig. cruciatum anterius

Lig. collaterale fibulare

Lig. collaterale tibiale

Tendo m. bicipitis femoris

Lig. anterius capitis fibulae

Caput fibulae

Lig. patellae

Lig. anterius capitis fibulae

Tuberositas tibiae

Tuberculum tractus iliotibialis (Gerdyi)

Margo anterior

Margo anterior

Crista interossea

Margo interosseus

Facies lateralis

Membrana interossea cruris

Facies lateralis

Fibula

Tibia

Lig. talofibulare posterius

Lig. tibiofibulare anterius

Malleolus lateralis

Lig. talofibulare anterius

Malleolus medialis

Lig. calcaneofibulare

Lig. collaterale mediale tali (Lig. deltoideum)

Superior view

Lig. posterius capitis fibulae

Apex capitis fibulae

Caput fibulae

Fibula

Posterior

Attachment of Lig. cruciatum posterius

Eminentia intercondylaris

Tibia

Lig. anterius capitis fibulae

Condylus lateralis tibiae

Condylus medialis tibiae

Facies articularis condyli medialis

Facies articularis superior condyli lateralis

Tuberculum intercondylare mediale

Tuberculum intercondylare laterale

Anterior

Attachment of Lig. cruciatum anterius

Tuberositas tibiae

Cross section

Margo interosseus

Facies lateralis

Membrana interossea cruris

Margo anterior

Facies medialis

Crista interossea

Tibia

Margo anterior

Margo medialis

Facies lateralis

Facies posterior

Fibula

Facies medialis

Margo posterior

Margo medialis

Facies posterior

Inferior view

Lig. tibiofibulare anterius

Anterior

Facies articularis malleoli medialis

Facies articularis malleoli lateralis

Fibula

Malleolus medialis

Fossa malleoli lateralis

Tibia

Posterior

Lig. tibiofibulare posterius

Facies articularis inferior tibiae

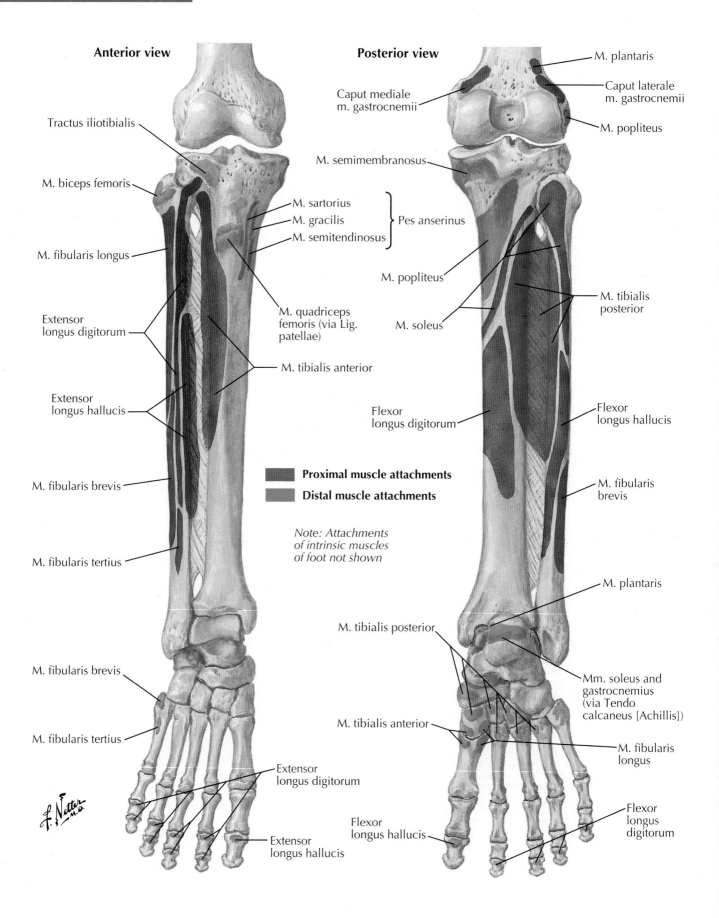

Anterior view

Tractus iliotibialis

M. biceps femoris

M. fibularis longus

Extensor longus digitorum

Extensor longus hallucis

M. fibularis brevis

M. fibularis tertius

M. fibularis brevis

M. fibularis tertius

Extensor longus digitorum

Extensor longus hallucis

M. sartorius
M. gracilis } Pes anserinus
M. semitendinosus

M. quadriceps femoris (via Lig. patellae)

M. tibialis anterior

Posterior view

Caput mediale m. gastrocnemii

M. semimembranosus

M. popliteus

M. soleus

M. plantaris

Caput laterale m. gastrocnemii

M. popliteus

M. tibialis posterior

Flexor longus digitorum

Flexor longus hallucis

M. fibularis brevis

M. plantaris

M. tibialis posterior

Mm. soleus and gastrocnemius (via Tendo calcaneus [Achillis])

M. tibialis anterior

M. fibularis longus

Flexor longus hallucis

Flexor longus digitorum

■ **Proximal muscle attachments**

■ **Distal muscle attachments**

Note: Attachments of intrinsic muscles of foot not shown

Plate 526

Crus

Crus dextrum

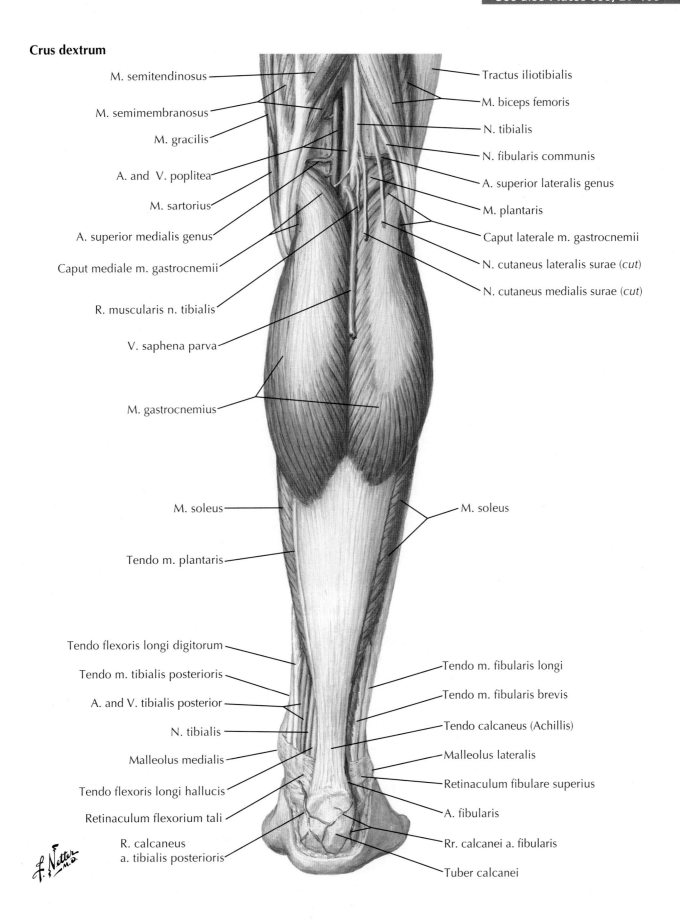

M. semitendinosus

M. semimembranosus

M. gracilis

A. and V. poplitea

M. sartorius

A. superior medialis genus

Caput mediale m. gastrocnemii

R. muscularis n. tibialis

V. saphena parva

M. gastrocnemius

M. soleus

Tendo m. plantaris

Tendo flexoris longi digitorum

Tendo m. tibialis posterioris

A. and V. tibialis posterior

N. tibialis

Malleolus medialis

Tendo flexoris longi hallucis

Retinaculum flexorium tali

R. calcaneus
a. tibialis posterioris

Tractus iliotibialis

M. biceps femoris

N. tibialis

N. fibularis communis

A. superior lateralis genus

M. plantaris

Caput laterale m. gastrocnemii

N. cutaneus lateralis surae (cut)

N. cutaneus medialis surae (cut)

M. soleus

Tendo m. fibularis longi

Tendo m. fibularis brevis

Tendo calcaneus (Achillis)

Malleolus lateralis

Retinaculum fibulare superius

A. fibularis

Rr. calcanei a. fibularis

Tuber calcanei

Crus dextrum

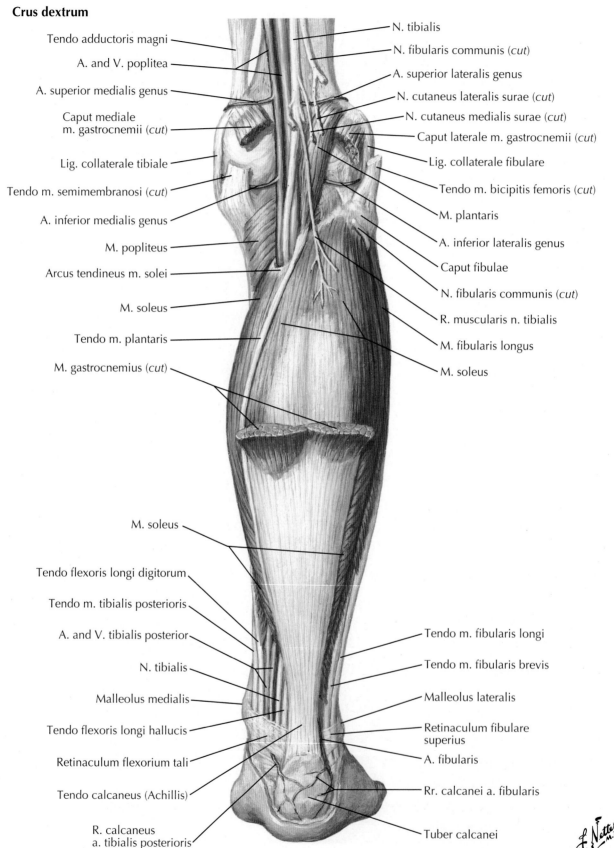

Tendo adductoris magni

A. and V. poplitea

A. superior medialis genus

Caput mediale
m. gastrocnemii (cut)

Lig. collaterale tibiale

Tendo m. semimembranosi (cut)

A. inferior medialis genus

M. popliteus

Arcus tendineus m. solei

M. soleus

Tendo m. plantaris

M. gastrocnemius (cut)

M. soleus

Tendo flexoris longi digitorum

Tendo m. tibialis posterioris

A. and V. tibialis posterior

N. tibialis

Malleolus medialis

Tendo flexoris longi hallucis

Retinaculum flexorium tali

Tendo calcaneus (Achillis)

R. calcaneus
a. tibialis posterioris

N. tibialis

N. fibularis communis (cut)

A. superior lateralis genus

N. cutaneus lateralis surae (cut)

N. cutaneus medialis surae (cut)

Caput laterale m. gastrocnemii (cut)

Lig. collaterale fibulare

Tendo m. bicipitis femoris (cut)

M. plantaris

A. inferior lateralis genus

Caput fibulae

N. fibularis communis (cut)

R. muscularis n. tibialis

M. fibularis longus

M. soleus

Tendo m. fibularis longi

Tendo m. fibularis brevis

Malleolus lateralis

Retinaculum fibulare
superius

A. fibularis

Rr. calcanei a. fibularis

Tuber calcanei

Plate 528

Crus

Crus dextrum

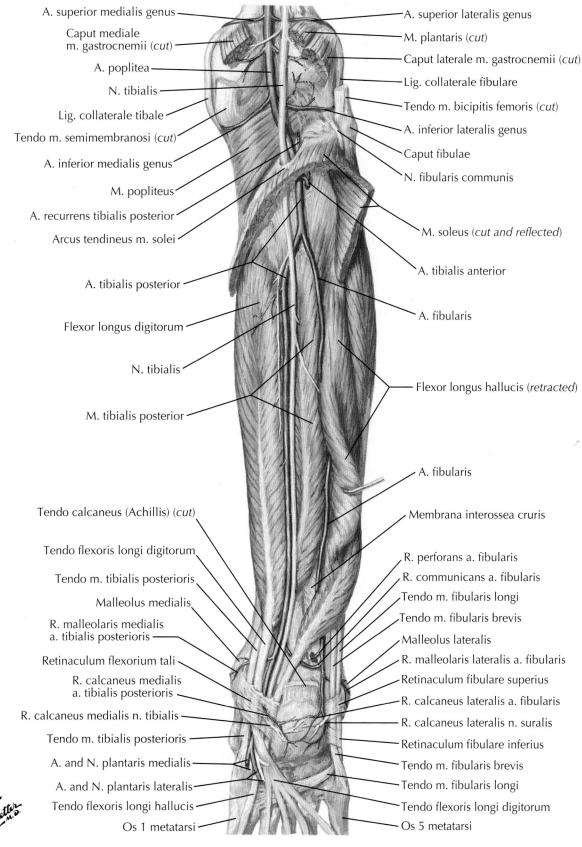

A. superior medialis genus

Caput mediale m. gastrocnemii (*cut*)

A. poplitea

N. tibialis

Lig. collaterale tibale

Tendo m. semimembranosi (*cut*)

A. inferior medialis genus

M. popliteus

A. recurrens tibialis posterior

Arcus tendineus m. solei

A. tibialis posterior

Flexor longus digitorum

N. tibialis

M. tibialis posterior

Tendo calcaneus (Achillis) (*cut*)

Tendo flexoris longi digitorum

Tendo m. tibialis posterioris

Malleolus medialis

R. malleolaris medialis a. tibialis posterioris

Retinaculum flexorium tali

R. calcaneus medialis a. tibialis posterioris

R. calcaneus medialis n. tibialis

Tendo m. tibialis posterioris

A. and N. plantaris medialis

A. and N. plantaris lateralis

Tendo flexoris longi hallucis

Os 1 metatarsi

A. superior lateralis genus

M. plantaris (*cut*)

Caput laterale m. gastrocnemii (*cut*)

Lig. collaterale fibulare

Tendo m. bicipitis femoris (*cut*)

A. inferior lateralis genus

Caput fibulae

N. fibularis communis

M. soleus (*cut and reflected*)

A. tibialis anterior

A. fibularis

A. fibularis

Membrana interossea cruris

R. perforans a. fibularis

R. communicans a. fibularis

Tendo m. fibularis longi

Tendo m. fibularis brevis

Malleolus lateralis

R. malleolaris lateralis a. fibularis

Retinaculum fibulare superius

R. calcaneus lateralis a. fibularis

R. calcaneus lateralis n. suralis

Retinaculum fibulare inferius

Tendo m. fibularis brevis

Tendo m. fibularis longi

Tendo flexoris longi digitorum

Os 5 metatarsi

Flexor longus hallucis (*retracted*)

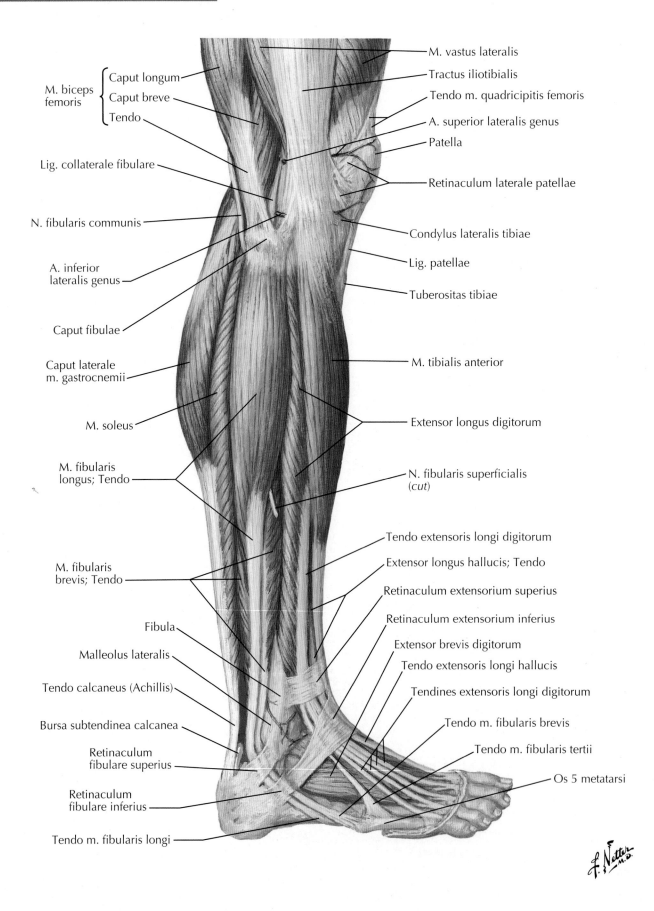

M. vastus lateralis

Tractus iliotibialis

Tendo m. quadricipitis femoris

A. superior lateralis genus

Patella

Retinaculum laterale patellae

Condylus lateralis tibiae

Lig. patellae

Tuberositas tibiae

M. tibialis anterior

Extensor longus digitorum

N. fibularis superficialis (*cut*)

Tendo extensoris longi digitorum

Extensor longus hallucis; Tendo

Retinaculum extensorium superius

Retinaculum extensorium inferius

Extensor brevis digitorum

Tendo extensoris longi hallucis

Tendines extensoris longi digitorum

Tendo m. fibularis brevis

Tendo m. fibularis tertii

Os 5 metatarsi

M. biceps femoris

Caput longum

Caput breve

Tendo

Lig. collaterale fibulare

N. fibularis communis

A. inferior lateralis genus

Caput fibulae

Caput laterale m. gastrocnemii

M. soleus

M. fibularis longus; Tendo

M. fibularis brevis; Tendo

Fibula

Malleolus lateralis

Tendo calcaneus (Achillis)

Bursa subtendinea calcanea

Retinaculum fibulare superius

Retinaculum fibulare inferius

Tendo m. fibularis longi

Plate 530

Crus

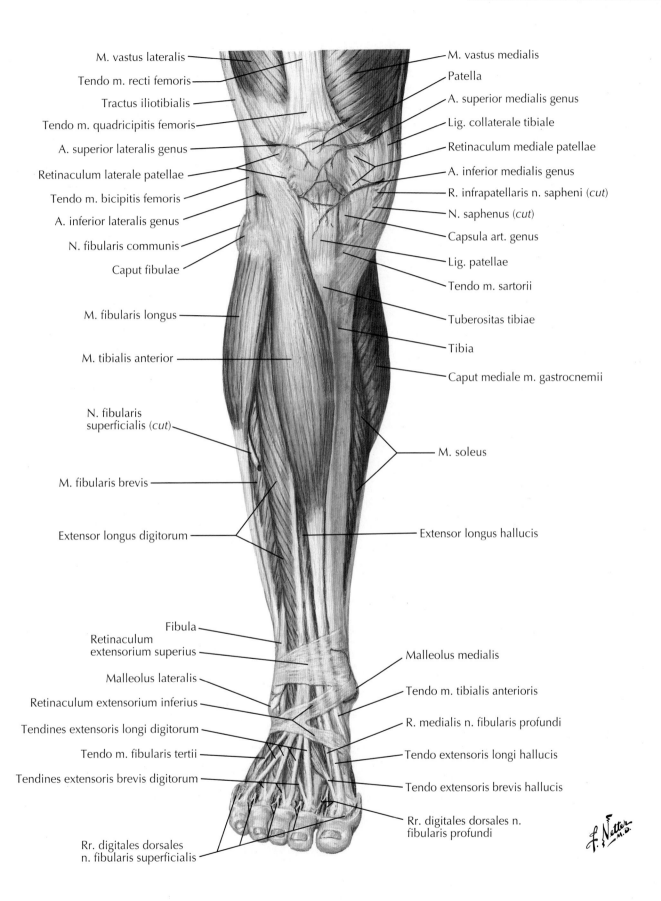

M. vastus lateralis

Tendo m. recti femoris

Tractus iliotibialis

Tendo m. quadricipitis femoris

A. superior lateralis genus

Retinaculum laterale patellae

Tendo m. bicipitis femoris

A. inferior lateralis genus

N. fibularis communis

Caput fibulae

M. fibularis longus

M. tibialis anterior

N. fibularis superficialis (cut)

M. fibularis brevis

Extensor longus digitorum

Fibula

Retinaculum extensorium superius

Malleolus lateralis

Retinaculum extensorium inferius

Tendines extensoris longi digitorum

Tendo m. fibularis tertii

Tendines extensoris brevis digitorum

Rr. digitales dorsales n. fibularis superficialis

M. vastus medialis

Patella

A. superior medialis genus

Lig. collaterale tibiale

Retinaculum mediale patellae

A. inferior medialis genus

R. infrapatellaris n. sapheni (cut)

N. saphenus (cut)

Capsula art. genus

Lig. patellae

Tendo m. sartorii

Tuberositas tibiae

Tibia

Caput mediale m. gastrocnemii

M. soleus

Extensor longus hallucis

Malleolus medialis

Tendo m. tibialis anterioris

R. medialis n. fibularis profundi

Tendo extensoris longi hallucis

Tendo extensoris brevis hallucis

Rr. digitales dorsales n. fibularis profundi

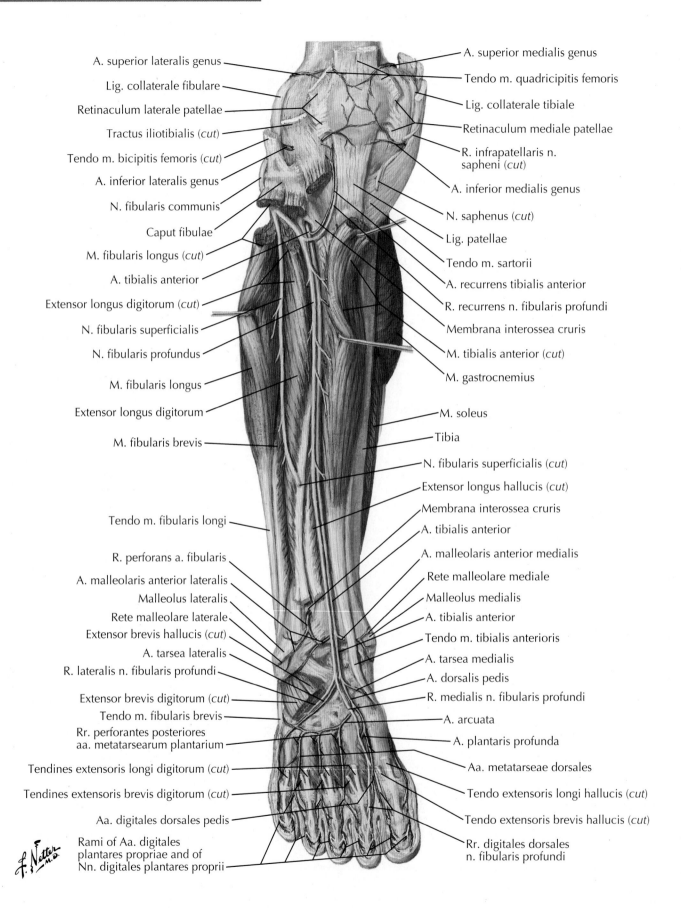

A. superior lateralis genus

Lig. collaterale fibulare

Retinaculum laterale patellae

Tractus iliotibialis (*cut*)

Tendo m. bicipitis femoris (*cut*)

A. inferior lateralis genus

N. fibularis communis

Caput fibulae

M. fibularis longus (*cut*)

A. tibialis anterior

Extensor longus digitorum (*cut*)

N. fibularis superficialis

N. fibularis profundus

M. fibularis longus

Extensor longus digitorum

M. fibularis brevis

Tendo m. fibularis longi

R. perforans a. fibularis

A. malleolaris anterior lateralis

Malleolus lateralis

Rete malleolare laterale

Extensor brevis hallucis (*cut*)

A. tarsea lateralis

R. lateralis n. fibularis profundi

Extensor brevis digitorum (*cut*)

Tendo m. fibularis brevis

Rr. perforantes posteriores
aa. metatarsearum plantarium

Tendines extensoris longi digitorum (*cut*)

Tendines extensoris brevis digitorum (*cut*)

Aa. digitales dorsales pedis

Rami of Aa. digitales
plantares propriae and of
Nn. digitales plantares proprii

A. superior medialis genus

Tendo m. quadricipitis femoris

Lig. collaterale tibiale

Retinaculum mediale patellae

R. infrapatellaris n.
sapheni (*cut*)

A. inferior medialis genus

N. saphenus (*cut*)

Lig. patellae

Tendo m. sartorii

A. recurrens tibialis anterior

R. recurrens n. fibularis profundi

Membrana interossea cruris

M. tibialis anterior (*cut*)

M. gastrocnemius

M. soleus

Tibia

N. fibularis superficialis (*cut*)

Extensor longus hallucis (*cut*)

Membrana interossea cruris

A. tibialis anterior

A. malleolaris anterior medialis

Rete malleolare mediale

Malleolus medialis

A. tibialis anterior

Tendo m. tibialis anterioris

A. tarsea medialis

A. dorsalis pedis

R. medialis n. fibularis profundi

A. arcuata

A. plantaris profunda

Aa. metatarseae dorsales

Tendo extensoris longi hallucis (*cut*)

Tendo extensoris brevis hallucis (*cut*)

Rr. digitales dorsales
n. fibularis profundi

Plate 532

Crus

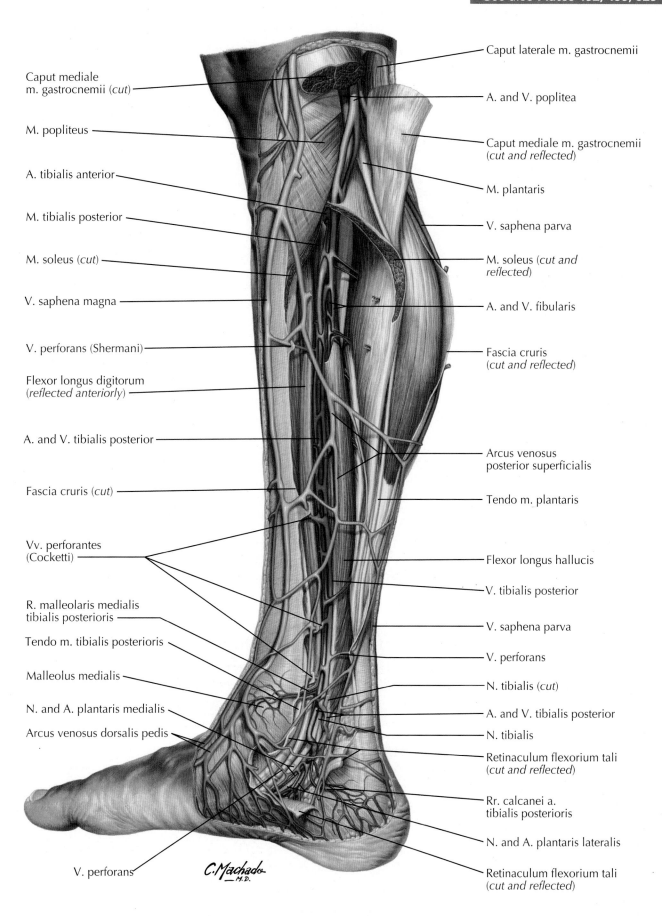

Caput mediale
m. gastrocnemii (*cut*)

M. popliteus

A. tibialis anterior

M. tibialis posterior

M. soleus (*cut*)

V. saphena magna

V. perforans (Shermani)

Flexor longus digitorum
(*reflected anteriorly*)

A. and V. tibialis posterior

Fascia cruris (*cut*)

Vv. perforantes
(Cocketti)

R. malleolaris medialis
tibialis posterioris

Tendo m. tibialis posterioris

Malleolus medialis

N. and A. plantaris medialis

Arcus venosus dorsalis pedis

V. perforans

Caput laterale m. gastrocnemii

A. and V. poplitea

Caput mediale m. gastrocnemii
(*cut and reflected*)

M. plantaris

V. saphena parva

M. soleus (*cut and
reflected*)

A. and V. fibularis

Fascia cruris
(*cut and reflected*)

Arcus venosus
posterior superficialis

Tendo m. plantaris

Flexor longus hallucis

V. tibialis posterior

V. saphena parva

V. perforans

N. tibialis (*cut*)

A. and V. tibialis posterior

N. tibialis

Retinaculum flexorium tali
(*cut and reflected*)

Rr. calcanei a.
tibialis posterioris

N. and A. plantaris lateralis

Retinaculum flexorium tali
(*cut and reflected*)

*C.Machado
—M.D.*

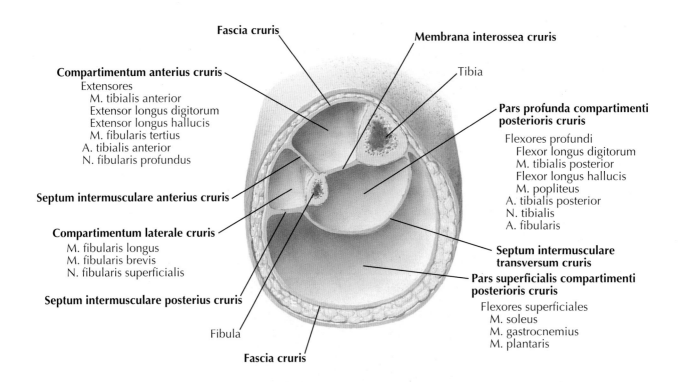

Fascia cruris

Membrana interossea cruris

Compartimentum anterius cruris
Extensores
M. tibialis anterior
Extensor longus digitorum
Extensor longus hallucis
M. fibularis tertius
A. tibialis anterior
N. fibularis profundus

Tibia

Pars profunda compartimenti posterioris cruris

Flexores profundi
Flexor longus digitorum
M. tibialis posterior
Flexor longus hallucis
M. popliteus
A. tibialis posterior
N. tibialis
A. fibularis

Septum intermusculare anterius cruris

Compartimentum laterale cruris
M. fibularis longus
M. fibularis brevis
N. fibularis superficialis

Septum intermusculare transversum cruris

Pars superficialis compartimenti posterioris cruris

Flexores superficiales
M. soleus
M. gastrocnemius
M. plantaris

Septum intermusculare posterius cruris

Fibula

Fascia cruris

Cross section just above middle of leg

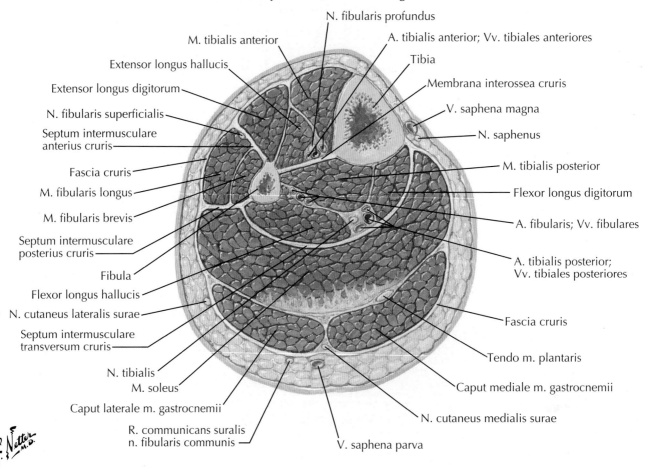

N. fibularis profundus

M. tibialis anterior

A. tibialis anterior; Vv. tibiales anteriores

Extensor longus hallucis

Tibia

Extensor longus digitorum

Membrana interossea cruris

N. fibularis superficialis

V. saphena magna

Septum intermusculare anterius cruris

N. saphenus

Fascia cruris

M. tibialis posterior

M. fibularis longus

Flexor longus digitorum

M. fibularis brevis

A. fibularis; Vv. fibulares

Septum intermusculare posterius cruris

A. tibialis posterior; Vv. tibiales posteriores

Fibula

Flexor longus hallucis

N. cutaneus lateralis surae

Septum intermusculare transversum cruris

Fascia cruris

Tendo m. plantaris

N. tibialis

Caput mediale m. gastrocnemii

M. soleus

Caput laterale m. gastrocnemii

N. cutaneus medialis surae

R. communicans suralis n. fibularis communis

V. saphena parva

Plate 534

Crus

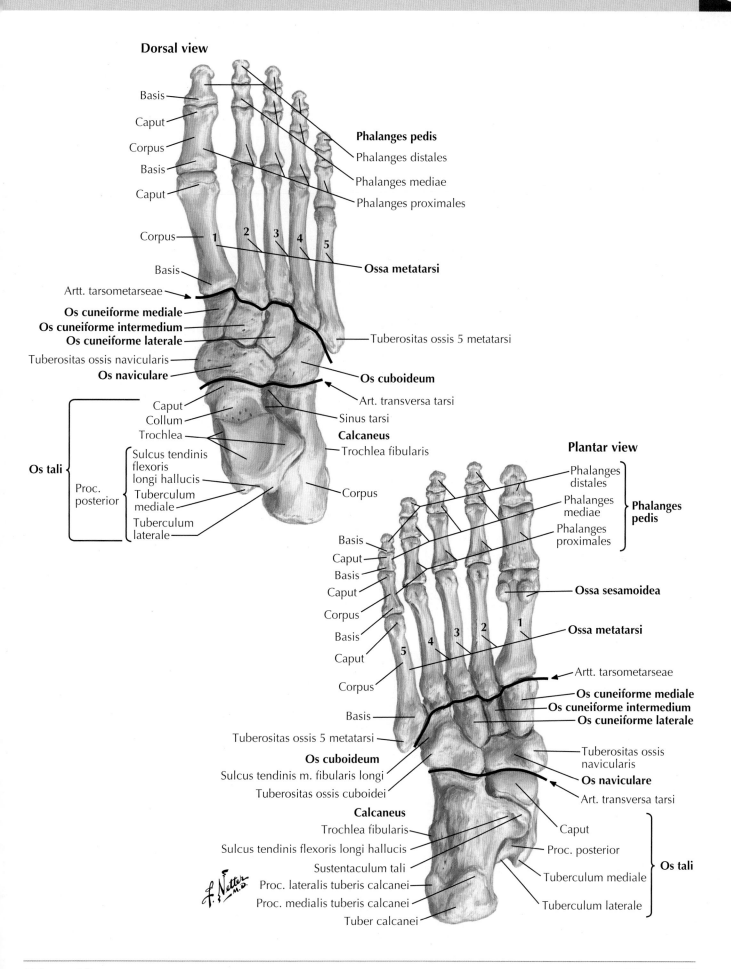

Dorsal view

Basis
Caput
Corpus
Basis
Caput

Phalanges pedis
Phalanges distales
Phalanges mediae
Phalanges proximales

Corpus
1 2 3 4 5

Basis
Ossa metatarsi

Artt. tarsometarseae
Os cuneiforme mediale
Os cuneiforme intermedium
Os cuneiforme laterale
Tuberositas ossis navicularis
Os naviculare

Tuberositas ossis 5 metatarsi

Os cuboideum
Art. transversa tarsi

Caput
Collum
Trochlea

Sinus tarsi
Calcaneus
Trochlea fibularis

Os tali
Proc. posterior
Sulcus tendinis flexoris longi hallucis
Tuberculum mediale
Tuberculum laterale

Corpus

Plantar view

Phalanges distales
Phalanges mediae
Phalanges proximales

Phalanges pedis

Basis
Caput
Basis
Caput
Corpus
Basis
Caput
Corpus

5 4 3 2 1

Ossa sesamoidea

Ossa metatarsi

Artt. tarsometarseae
Os cuneiforme mediale
Os cuneiforme intermedium
Os cuneiforme laterale

Basis

Tuberositas ossis navicularis

Tuberositas ossis 5 metatarsi
Os cuboideum
Sulcus tendinis m. fibularis longi
Tuberositas ossis cuboidei

Os naviculare
Art. transversa tarsi

Calcaneus
Trochlea fibularis
Sulcus tendinis flexoris longi hallucis
Sustentaculum tali
Proc. lateralis tuberis calcanei
Proc. medialis tuberis calcanei
Tuber calcanei

Caput
Proc. posterior

Tuberculum mediale

Tuberculum laterale

Os tali

F. Netter M.D.

Talus and Pes

Plate 535

Lateral view

Caput

Art. transversa tarsi

Os naviculare

Collum

Os tali

Trochlea

Os cuneiforme intermedium
Os cuneiforme laterale

Proc. lateralis

Artt. tarsometarseae

Proc. posterior

Ossa metatarsi

Sinus tarsi

Phalanges pedis

Corpus

2

Trochlea fibularis

3

4

Tuber calcanei

5

Calcaneus

Sulcus tendinis m. fibularis longi

Os cuboideum

Tuberositas ossis 5 metatarsi

Tuberositas ossis cuboidei

Sulcus tendinis m. fibularis longi

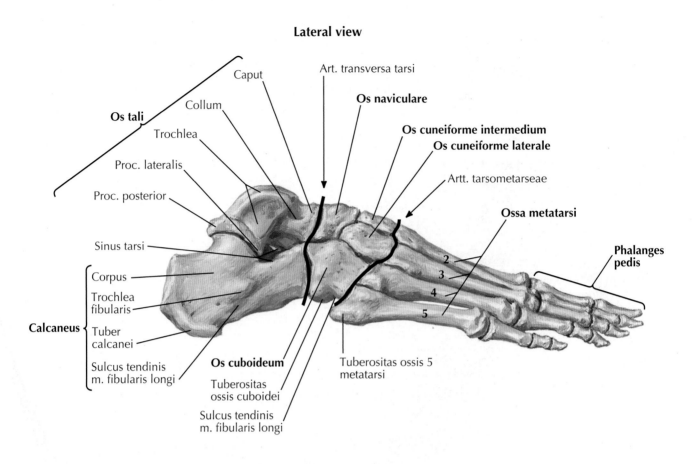

Medial view

Art. transversa tarsi

Os naviculare

Tuberositas ossis navicularis

Collum

Os tali

Caput

Os cuneiforme intermedium

Trochlea

Os cuneiforme mediale

Proc. posterior

Artt. tarsometatarseae

Ossa metatarsi

Phalanges pedis

2

1

Tuber calcanei

Tuberositas ossis 1 metatarsi

Calcaneus

Sulcus tendinis flexoris longi hallucis

Os sesamoideum

Sustentaculum tali

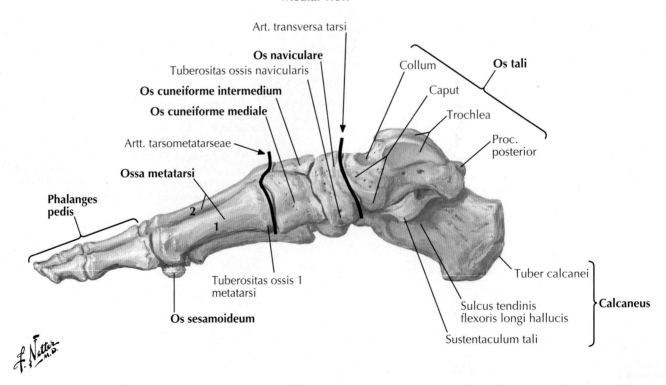

Plate 536

Talus and Pes

Pes dexter

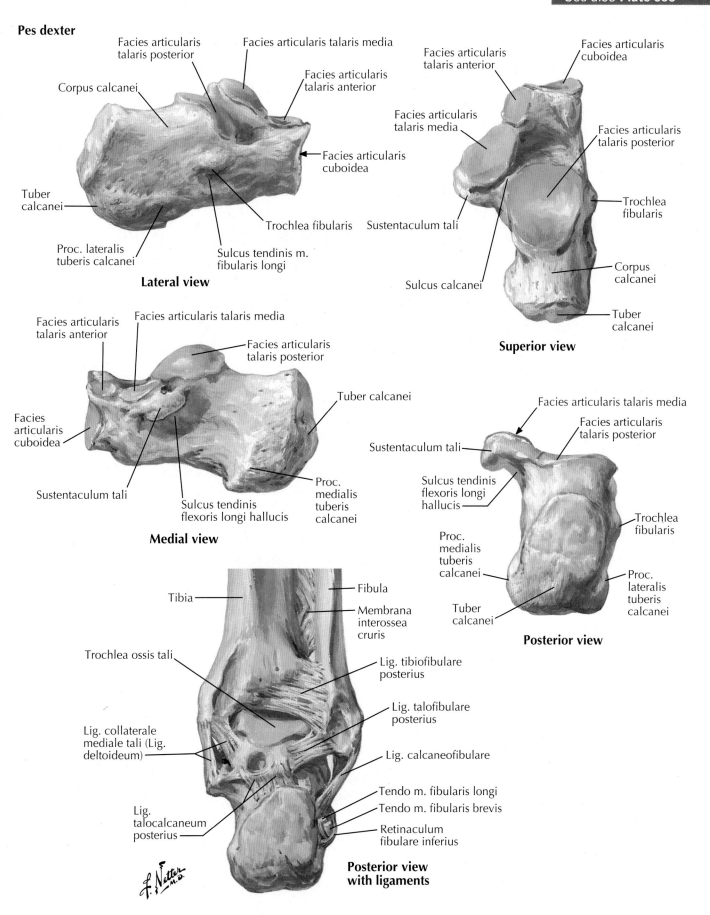

Facies articularis
talaris posterior

Corpus calcanei

Facies articularis talaris media

Facies articularis
talaris anterior

Facies articularis
cuboidea

Tuber
calcanei

Proc. lateralis
tuberis calcanei

Sulcus tendinis m.
fibularis longi

Trochlea fibularis

Lateral view

Facies articularis
talaris anterior

Facies articularis
talaris media

Sustentaculum tali

Sulcus calcanei

Facies articularis
cuboidea

Facies articularis
talaris posterior

Trochlea
fibularis

Corpus
calcanei

Tuber
calcanei

Superior view

Facies articularis
talaris anterior

Facies articularis talaris media

Facies articularis
talaris posterior

Facies
articularis
cuboidea

Tuber calcanei

Sustentaculum tali

Sulcus tendinis
flexoris longi hallucis

Proc.
medialis
tuberis
calcanei

Medial view

Facies articularis talaris media

Facies articularis
talaris posterior

Sustentaculum tali

Sulcus tendinis
flexoris longi
hallucis

Proc.
medialis
tuberis
calcanei

Tuber
calcanei

Trochlea
fibularis

Proc.
lateralis
tuberis
calcanei

Posterior view

Tibia

Fibula

Membrana
interossea
cruris

Trochlea ossis tali

Lig. tibiofibulare
posterius

Lig. talofibulare
posterius

Lig. collaterale
mediale tali (Lig.
deltoideum)

Lig. calcaneofibulare

Tendo m. fibularis longi

Tendo m. fibularis brevis

Retinaculum
fibulare inferius

Lig.
talocalcaneum
posterius

**Posterior view
with ligaments**

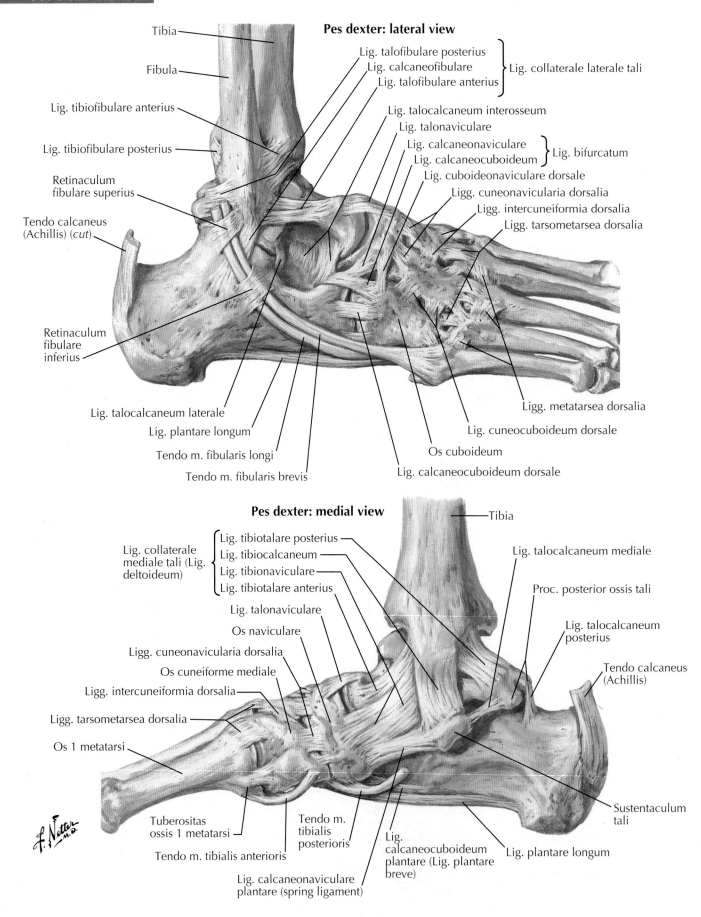

Pes dexter: lateral view

Tibia

Fibula

Lig. tibiofibulare anterius

Lig. tibiofibulare posterius

Retinaculum
fibulare superius

Tendo calcaneus
(Achillis) (cut)

Retinaculum
fibulare
inferius

Lig. talofibulare posterius
Lig. calcaneofibulare   Lig. collaterale laterale tali
Lig. talofibulare anterius

Lig. talocalcaneum interosseum
Lig. talonaviculare
Lig. calcaneonaviculare   Lig. bifurcatum
Lig. calcaneocuboideum
Lig. cuboideonaviculare dorsale
Ligg. cuneonavicularia dorsalia
Ligg. intercuneiformia dorsalia
Ligg. tarsometarsea dorsalia

Lig. talocalcaneum laterale

Lig. plantare longum

Tendo m. fibularis longi

Tendo m. fibularis brevis

Ligg. metatarsea dorsalia

Lig. cuneocuboideum dorsale

Os cuboideum

Lig. calcaneocuboideum dorsale

Pes dexter: medial view

Tibia

Lig. collaterale
mediale tali (Lig.
deltoideum)
{
Lig. tibiotalare posterius
Lig. tibiocalcaneum
Lig. tibionaviculare
Lig. tibiotalare anterius
}

Lig. talonaviculare

Os naviculare

Ligg. cuneonavicularia dorsalia

Os cuneiforme mediale

Ligg. intercuneiformia dorsalia

Ligg. tarsometarsea dorsalia

Os 1 metatarsi

Lig. talocalcaneum mediale

Proc. posterior ossis tali

Lig. talocalcaneum
posterius

Tendo calcaneus
(Achillis)

Sustentaculum
tali

Lig. plantare longum

Tuberositas
ossis 1 metatarsi

Tendo m. tibialis anterioris

Tendo m.
tibialis
posterioris

Lig.
calcaneocuboideum
plantare (Lig. plantare
breve)

Lig. calcaneonaviculare
plantare (spring ligament)

Plate 538

Talus and Pes

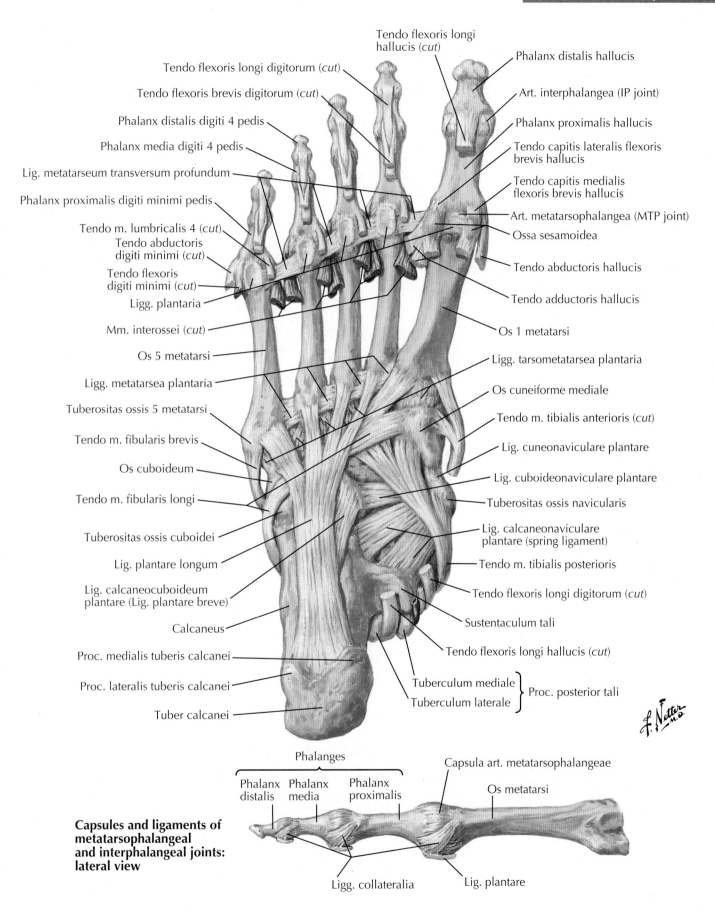

Tendo flexoris longi hallucis (*cut*)

Tendo flexoris longi digitorum (*cut*)

Tendo flexoris brevis digitorum (*cut*)

Phalanx distalis digiti 4 pedis

Phalanx media digiti 4 pedis

Lig. metatarseum transversum profundum

Phalanx proximalis digiti minimi pedis

Tendo m. lumbricalis 4 (*cut*)

Tendo abductoris digiti minimi (*cut*)

Tendo flexoris digiti minimi (*cut*)

Ligg. plantaria

Mm. interossei (*cut*)

Os 5 metatarsi

Ligg. metatarsea plantaria

Tuberositas ossis 5 metatarsi

Tendo m. fibularis brevis

Os cuboideum

Tendo m. fibularis longi

Tuberositas ossis cuboidei

Lig. plantare longum

Lig. calcaneocuboideum plantare (Lig. plantare breve)

Calcaneus

Proc. medialis tuberis calcanei

Proc. lateralis tuberis calcanei

Tuber calcanei

Phalanx distalis hallucis

Art. interphalangea (IP joint)

Phalanx proximalis hallucis

Tendo capitis lateralis flexoris brevis hallucis

Tendo capitis medialis flexoris brevis hallucis

Art. metatarsophalangea (MTP joint)

Ossa sesamoidea

Tendo abductoris hallucis

Tendo adductoris hallucis

Os 1 metatarsi

Ligg. tarsometatarsea plantaria

Os cuneiforme mediale

Tendo m. tibialis anterioris (*cut*)

Lig. cuneonaviculare plantare

Lig. cuboideonaviculare plantare

Tuberositas ossis navicularis

Lig. calcaneonaviculare plantare (spring ligament)

Tendo m. tibialis posterioris

Tendo flexoris longi digitorum (*cut*)

Sustentaculum tali

Tendo flexoris longi hallucis (*cut*)

Tuberculum mediale
Tuberculum laterale } Proc. posterior tali

f. Netter m.d.

Phalanges

Phalanx distalis   Phalanx media   Phalanx proximalis

Capsula art. metatarsophalangeae

Os metatarsi

Capsules and ligaments of metatarsophalangeal and interphalangeal joints: lateral view

Ligg. collateralia

Lig. plantare

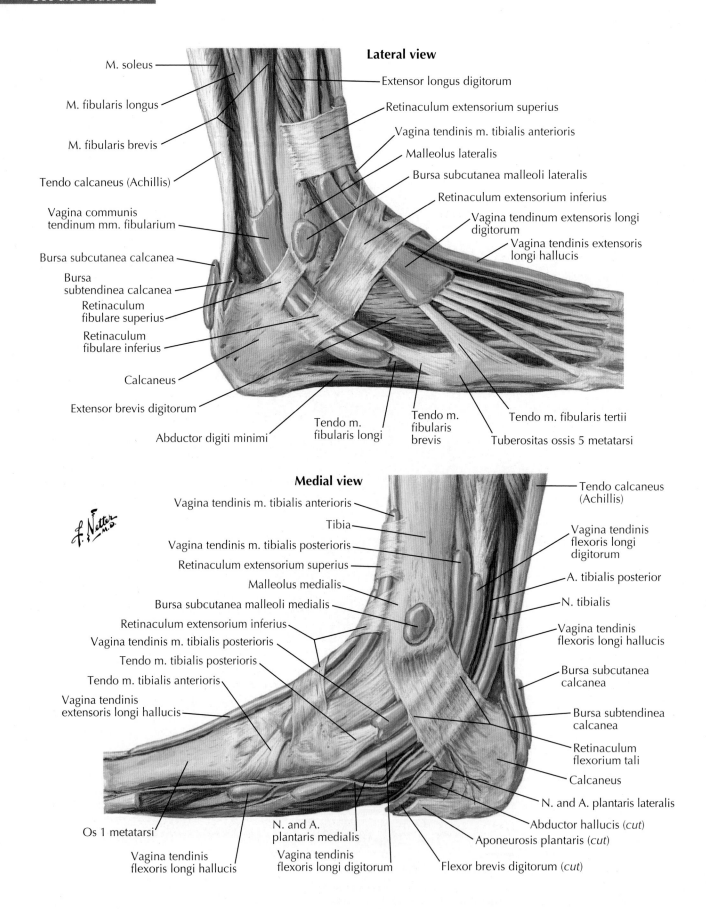

Lateral view

M. soleus

Extensor longus digitorum

M. fibularis longus

Retinaculum extensorium superius

M. fibularis brevis

Vagina tendinis m. tibialis anterioris

Malleolus lateralis

Tendo calcaneus (Achillis)

Bursa subcutanea malleoli lateralis

Retinaculum extensorium inferius

Vagina communis tendinum mm. fibularium

Vagina tendinum extensoris longi digitorum

Vagina tendinis extensoris longi hallucis

Bursa subcutanea calcanea

Bursa subtendinea calcanea

Retinaculum fibulare superius

Retinaculum fibulare inferius

Calcaneus

Extensor brevis digitorum

Abductor digiti minimi

Tendo m. fibularis longi

Tendo m. fibularis brevis

Tendo m. fibularis tertii

Tuberositas ossis 5 metatarsi

Medial view

Vagina tendinis m. tibialis anterioris

Tendo calcaneus (Achillis)

Tibia

Vagina tendinis m. tibialis posterioris

Vagina tendinis flexoris longi digitorum

Retinaculum extensorium superius

Malleolus medialis

A. tibialis posterior

Bursa subcutanea malleoli medialis

N. tibialis

Retinaculum extensorium inferius

Vagina tendinis m. tibialis posterioris

Vagina tendinis flexoris longi hallucis

Tendo m. tibialis posterioris

Bursa subcutanea calcanea

Tendo m. tibialis anterioris

Vagina tendinis extensoris longi hallucis

Bursa subtendinea calcanea

Retinaculum flexorium tali

Calcaneus

N. and A. plantaris lateralis

Os 1 metatarsi

N. and A. plantaris medialis

Abductor hallucis (*cut*)

Aponeurosis plantaris (*cut*)

Vagina tendinis flexoris longi hallucis

Vagina tendinis flexoris longi digitorum

Flexor brevis digitorum (*cut*)

Plate 540

Talus and Pes

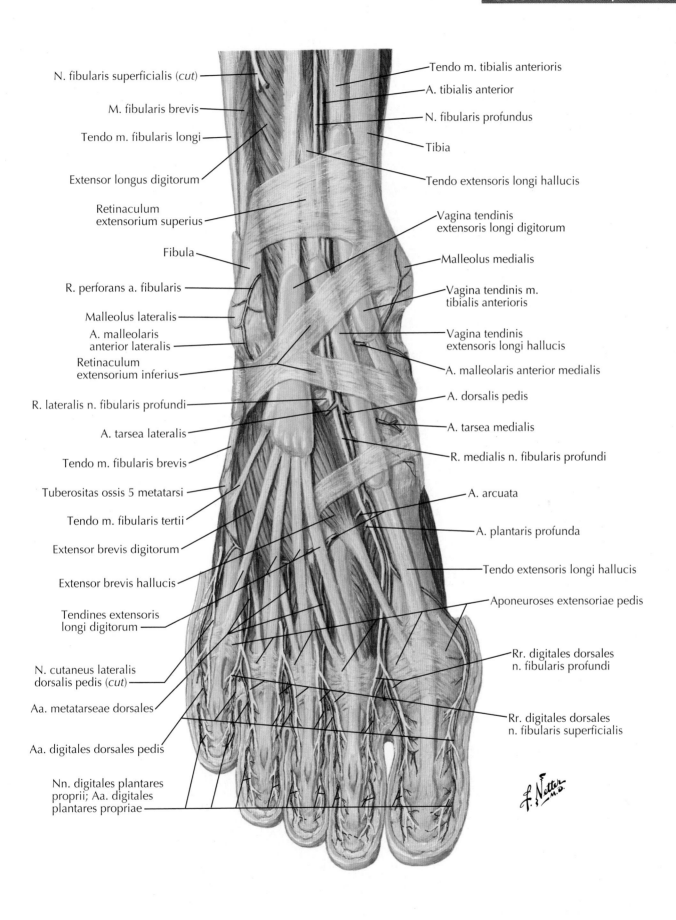

N. fibularis superficialis (*cut*)

M. fibularis brevis

Tendo m. fibularis longi

Extensor longus digitorum

Retinaculum extensorium superius

Fibula

R. perforans a. fibularis

Malleolus lateralis

A. malleolaris anterior lateralis

Retinaculum extensorium inferius

R. lateralis n. fibularis profundi

A. tarsea lateralis

Tendo m. fibularis brevis

Tuberositas ossis 5 metatarsi

Tendo m. fibularis tertii

Extensor brevis digitorum

Extensor brevis hallucis

Tendines extensoris longi digitorum

N. cutaneus lateralis dorsalis pedis (*cut*)

Aa. metatarseae dorsales

Aa. digitales dorsales pedis

Nn. digitales plantares proprii; Aa. digitales plantares propriae

Tendo m. tibialis anterioris

A. tibialis anterior

N. fibularis profundus

Tibia

Tendo extensoris longi hallucis

Vagina tendinis extensoris longi digitorum

Malleolus medialis

Vagina tendinis m. tibialis anterioris

Vagina tendinis extensoris longi hallucis

A. malleolaris anterior medialis

A. dorsalis pedis

A. tarsea medialis

R. medialis n. fibularis profundi

A. arcuata

A. plantaris profunda

Tendo extensoris longi hallucis

Aponeuroses extensoriae pedis

Rr. digitales dorsales n. fibularis profundi

Rr. digitales dorsales n. fibularis superficialis

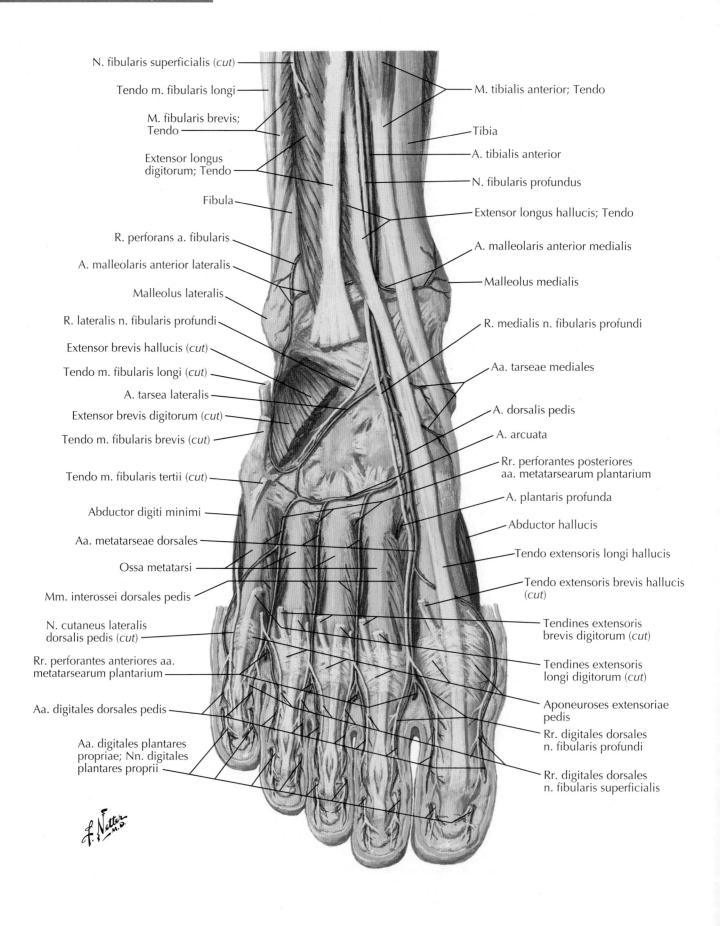

N. fibularis superficialis (*cut*)

Tendo m. fibularis longi

M. fibularis brevis; Tendo

Extensor longus digitorum; Tendo

Fibula

R. perforans a. fibularis

A. malleolaris anterior lateralis

Malleolus lateralis

R. lateralis n. fibularis profundi

Extensor brevis hallucis (*cut*)

Tendo m. fibularis longi (*cut*)

A. tarsea lateralis

Extensor brevis digitorum (*cut*)

Tendo m. fibularis brevis (*cut*)

Tendo m. fibularis tertii (*cut*)

Abductor digiti minimi

Aa. metatarseae dorsales

Ossa metatarsi

Mm. interossei dorsales pedis

N. cutaneus lateralis dorsalis pedis (*cut*)

Rr. perforantes anteriores aa. metatarsearum plantarium

Aa. digitales dorsales pedis

Aa. digitales plantares propriae; Nn. digitales plantares proprii

M. tibialis anterior; Tendo

Tibia

A. tibialis anterior

N. fibularis profundus

Extensor longus hallucis; Tendo

A. malleolaris anterior medialis

Malleolus medialis

R. medialis n. fibularis profundi

Aa. tarseae mediales

A. dorsalis pedis

A. arcuata

Rr. perforantes posteriores aa. metatarsearum plantarium

A. plantaris profunda

Abductor hallucis

Tendo extensoris longi hallucis

Tendo extensoris brevis hallucis (*cut*)

Tendines extensoris brevis digitorum (*cut*)

Tendines extensoris longi digitorum (*cut*)

Aponeuroses extensoriae pedis

Rr. digitales dorsales n. fibularis profundi

Rr. digitales dorsales n. fibularis superficialis

Plate 542

Talus and Pes

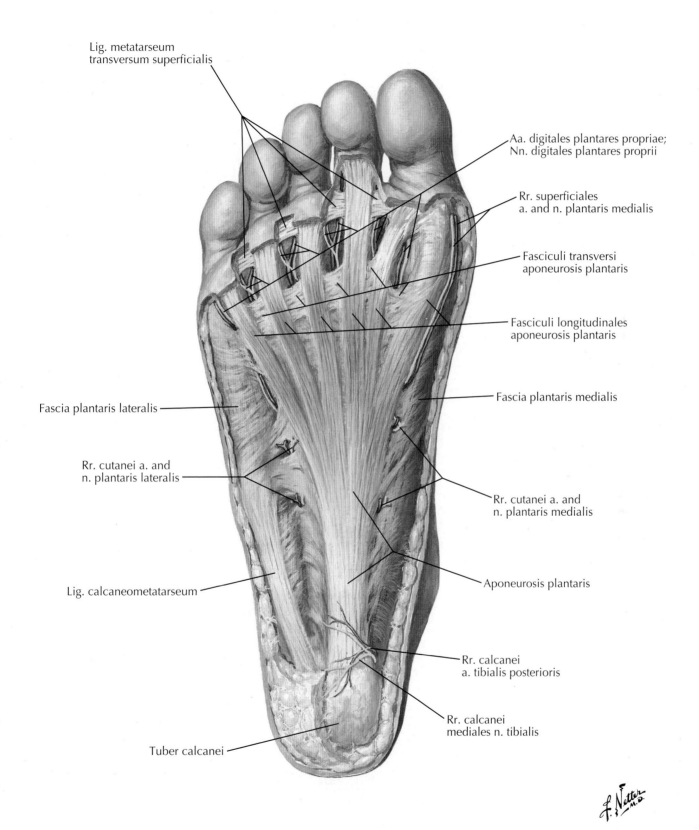

Lig. metatarseum
transversum superficialis

Aa. digitales plantares propriae;
Nn. digitales plantares proprii

Rr. superficiales
a. and n. plantaris medialis

Fasciculi transversi
aponeurosis plantaris

Fasciculi longitudinales
aponeurosis plantaris

Fascia plantaris medialis

Fascia plantaris lateralis

Rr. cutanei a. and
n. plantaris lateralis

Rr. cutanei a. and
n. plantaris medialis

Aponeurosis plantaris

Lig. calcaneometatarseum

Rr. calcanei
a. tibialis posterioris

Rr. calcanei
mediales n. tibialis

Tuber calcanei

First layer muscles in bold

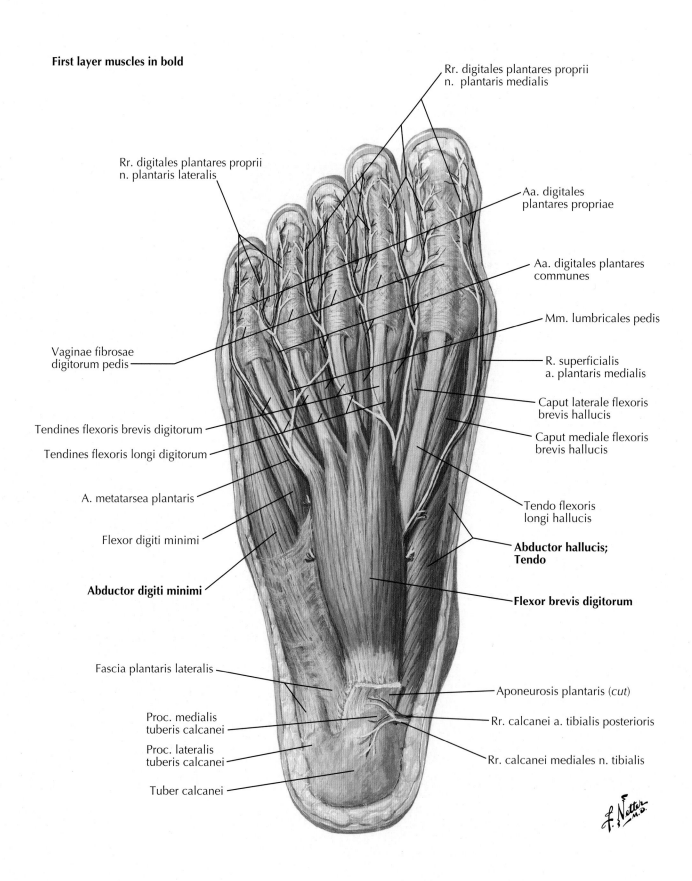

Rr. digitales plantares proprii
n. plantaris medialis

Rr. digitales plantares proprii
n. plantaris lateralis

Aa. digitales
plantares propriae

Aa. digitales plantares
communes

Mm. lumbricales pedis

Vaginae fibrosae
digitorum pedis

R. superficialis
a. plantaris medialis

Caput laterale flexoris
brevis hallucis

Tendines flexoris brevis digitorum

Caput mediale flexoris
brevis hallucis

Tendines flexoris longi digitorum

A. metatarsea plantaris

Tendo flexoris
longi hallucis

Flexor digiti minimi

**Abductor hallucis;
Tendo**

Abductor digiti minimi

Flexor brevis digitorum

Fascia plantaris lateralis

Aponeurosis plantaris *(cut)*

Proc. medialis
tuberis calcanei

Rr. calcanei a. tibialis posterioris

Proc. lateralis
tuberis calcanei

Rr. calcanei mediales n. tibialis

Tuber calcanei

Plate 544

Talus and Pes

Second layer tendons and muscles in bold

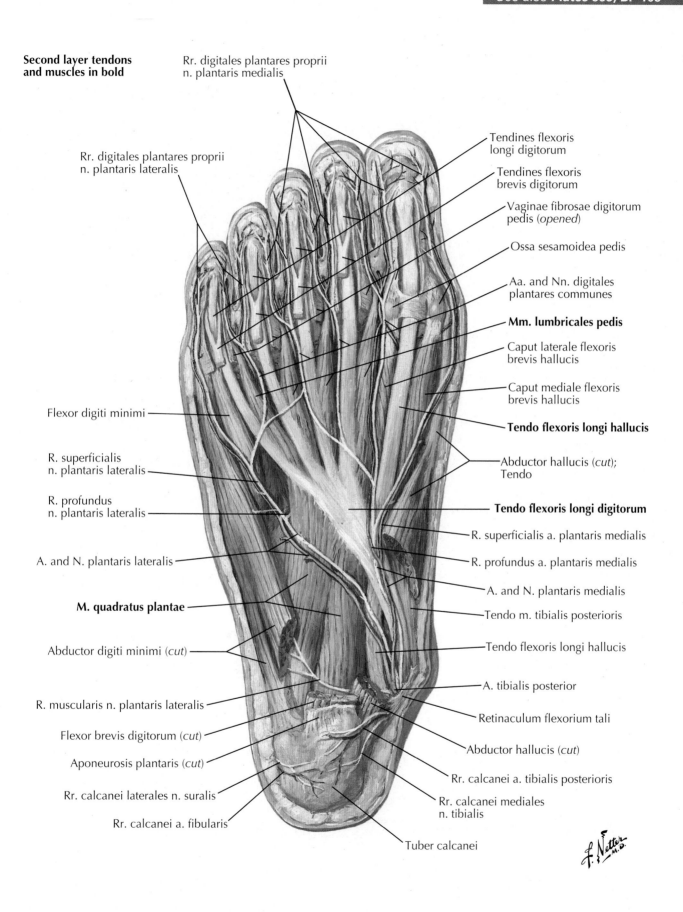

Rr. digitales plantares proprii n. plantaris medialis

Rr. digitales plantares proprii n. plantaris lateralis

Tendines flexoris longi digitorum

Tendines flexoris brevis digitorum

Vaginae fibrosae digitorum pedis (*opened*)

Ossa sesamoidea pedis

Aa. and Nn. digitales plantares communes

Mm. lumbricales pedis

Caput laterale flexoris brevis hallucis

Caput mediale flexoris brevis hallucis

Tendo flexoris longi hallucis

Abductor hallucis (*cut*); Tendo

Flexor digiti minimi

R. superficialis n. plantaris lateralis

R. profundus n. plantaris lateralis

Tendo flexoris longi digitorum

R. superficialis a. plantaris medialis

R. profundus a. plantaris medialis

A. and N. plantaris lateralis

A. and N. plantaris medialis

Tendo m. tibialis posterioris

M. quadratus plantae

Tendo flexoris longi hallucis

Abductor digiti minimi (*cut*)

A. tibialis posterior

R. muscularis n. plantaris lateralis

Retinaculum flexorium tali

Flexor brevis digitorum (*cut*)

Abductor hallucis (*cut*)

Aponeurosis plantaris (*cut*)

Rr. calcanei a. tibialis posterioris

Rr. calcanei laterales n. suralis

Rr. calcanei mediales n. tibialis

Rr. calcanei a. fibularis

Tuber calcanei

Third layer muscles in bold

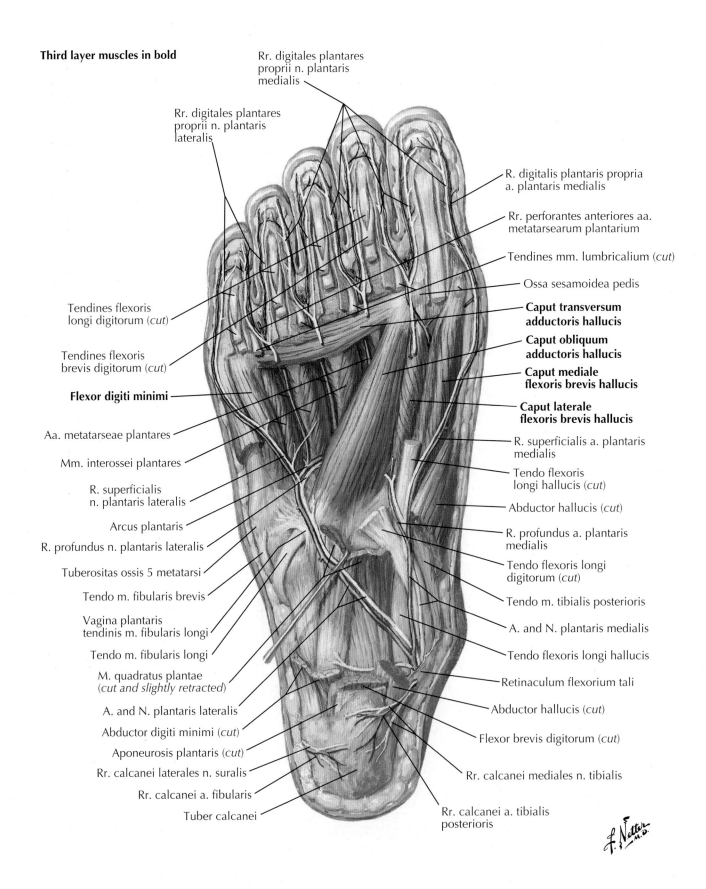

Rr. digitales plantares proprii n. plantaris medialis

Rr. digitales plantares proprii n. plantaris lateralis

R. digitalis plantaris propria a. plantaris medialis

Rr. perforantes anteriores aa. metatarsearum plantarium

Tendines mm. lumbricalium (*cut*)

Ossa sesamoidea pedis

Caput transversum adductoris hallucis

Caput obliquum adductoris hallucis

Caput mediale flexoris brevis hallucis

Caput laterale flexoris brevis hallucis

R. superficialis a. plantaris medialis

Tendo flexoris longi hallucis (*cut*)

Abductor hallucis (*cut*)

R. profundus a. plantaris medialis

Tendo flexoris longi digitorum (*cut*)

Tendo m. tibialis posterioris

A. and N. plantaris medialis

Tendo flexoris longi hallucis

Retinaculum flexorium tali

Abductor hallucis (*cut*)

Flexor brevis digitorum (*cut*)

Rr. calcanei mediales n. tibialis

Rr. calcanei a. tibialis posterioris

Tendines flexoris longi digitorum (*cut*)

Tendines flexoris brevis digitorum (*cut*)

Flexor digiti minimi

Aa. metatarseae plantares

Mm. interossei plantares

R. superficialis n. plantaris lateralis

Arcus plantaris

R. profundus n. plantaris lateralis

Tuberositas ossis 5 metatarsi

Tendo m. fibularis brevis

Vagina plantaris tendinis m. fibularis longi

Tendo m. fibularis longi

M. quadratus plantae (*cut and slightly retracted*)

A. and N. plantaris lateralis

Abductor digiti minimi (*cut*)

Aponeurosis plantaris (*cut*)

Rr. calcanei laterales n. suralis

Rr. calcanei a. fibularis

Tuber calcanei

Plate 546

Talus and Pes

Dorsal view

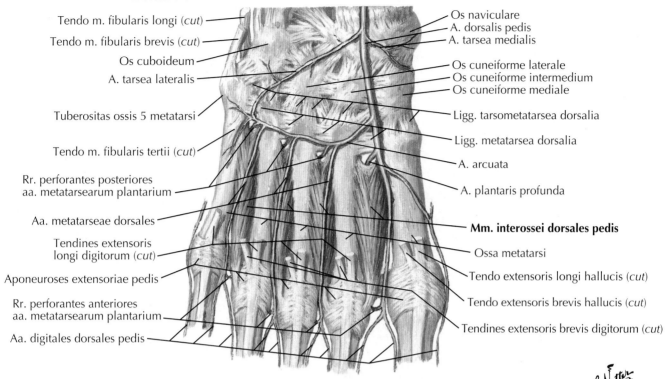

Tendo m. fibularis longi (*cut*)
Tendo m. fibularis brevis (*cut*)
Os cuboideum
A. tarsea lateralis
Tuberositas ossis 5 metatarsi
Tendo m. fibularis tertii (*cut*)
Rr. perforantes posteriores aa. metatarsearum plantarium
Aa. metatarseae dorsales
Tendines extensoris longi digitorum (*cut*)
Aponeuroses extensoriae pedis
Rr. perforantes anteriores aa. metatarsearum plantarium
Aa. digitales dorsales pedis

Os naviculare
A. dorsalis pedis
A. tarsea medialis
Os cuneiforme laterale
Os cuneiforme intermedium
Os cuneiforme mediale
Ligg. tarsometatarsea dorsalia
Ligg. metatarsea dorsalia
A. arcuata
A. plantaris profunda
Mm. interossei dorsales pedis
Ossa metatarsi
Tendo extensoris longi hallucis (*cut*)
Tendo extensoris brevis hallucis (*cut*)
Tendines extensoris brevis digitorum (*cut*)

Plantar view

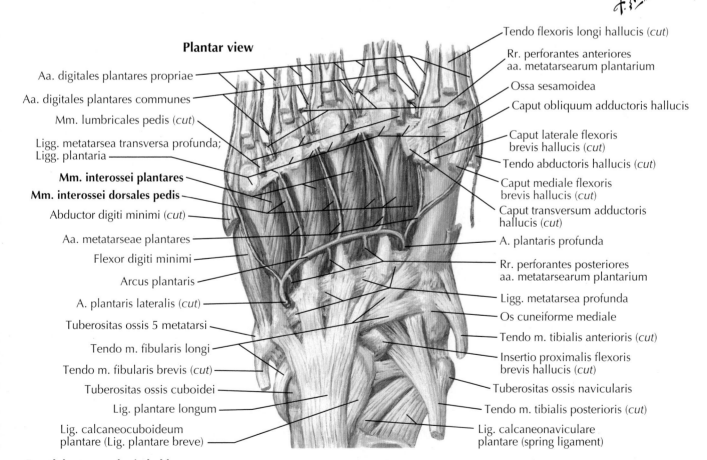

Aa. digitales plantares propriae
Aa. digitales plantares communes
Mm. lumbricales pedis (*cut*)
Ligg. metatarsea transversa profunda; Ligg. plantaria
Mm. interossei plantares
Mm. interossei dorsales pedis
Abductor digiti minimi (*cut*)
Aa. metatarseae plantares
Flexor digiti minimi
Arcus plantaris
A. plantaris lateralis (*cut*)
Tuberositas ossis 5 metatarsi
Tendo m. fibularis longi
Tendo m. fibularis brevis (*cut*)
Tuberositas ossis cuboidei
Lig. plantare longum
Lig. calcaneocuboideum plantare (Lig. plantare breve)

Tendo flexoris longi hallucis (*cut*)
Rr. perforantes anteriores aa. metatarsearum plantarium
Ossa sesamoidea
Caput obliquum adductoris hallucis
Caput laterale flexoris brevis hallucis (*cut*)
Tendo abductoris hallucis (*cut*)
Caput mediale flexoris brevis hallucis (*cut*)
Caput transversum adductoris hallucis (*cut*)
A. plantaris profunda
Rr. perforantes posteriores aa. metatarsearum plantarium
Ligg. metatarsea profunda
Os cuneiforme mediale
Tendo m. tibialis anterioris (*cut*)
Insertio proximalis flexoris brevis hallucis (*cut*)
Tuberositas ossis navicularis
Tendo m. tibialis posterioris (*cut*)
Lig. calcaneonaviculare plantare (spring ligament)

Fourth layer muscles in bold

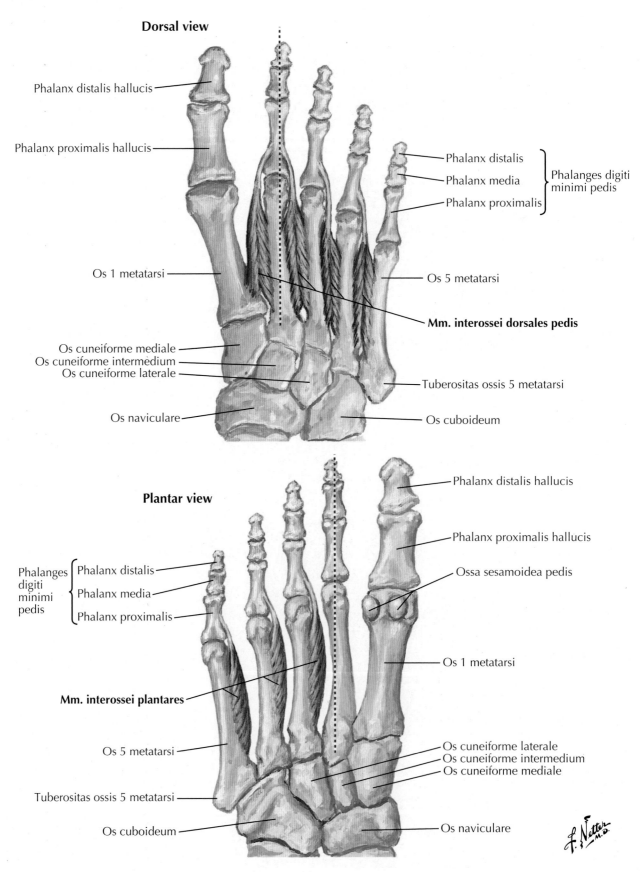

Dorsal view

Phalanx distalis hallucis

Phalanx proximalis hallucis

Phalanx distalis
Phalanx media
Phalanx proximalis
Phalanges digiti minimi pedis

Os 1 metatarsi

Os 5 metatarsi

Mm. interossei dorsales pedis

Os cuneiforme mediale
Os cuneiforme intermedium
Os cuneiforme laterale

Tuberositas ossis 5 metatarsi

Os naviculare

Os cuboideum

Plantar view

Phalanx distalis hallucis

Phalanx proximalis hallucis

Phalanges digiti minimi pedis
Phalanx distalis
Phalanx media
Phalanx proximalis

Ossa sesamoidea pedis

Os 1 metatarsi

Mm. interossei plantares

Os 5 metatarsi

Os cuneiforme laterale
Os cuneiforme intermedium
Os cuneiforme mediale

Tuberositas ossis 5 metatarsi

Os cuboideum

Os naviculare

Note: dashed line is the line of reference for abduction and adduction of the toes.

Plate 548

Talus and Pes

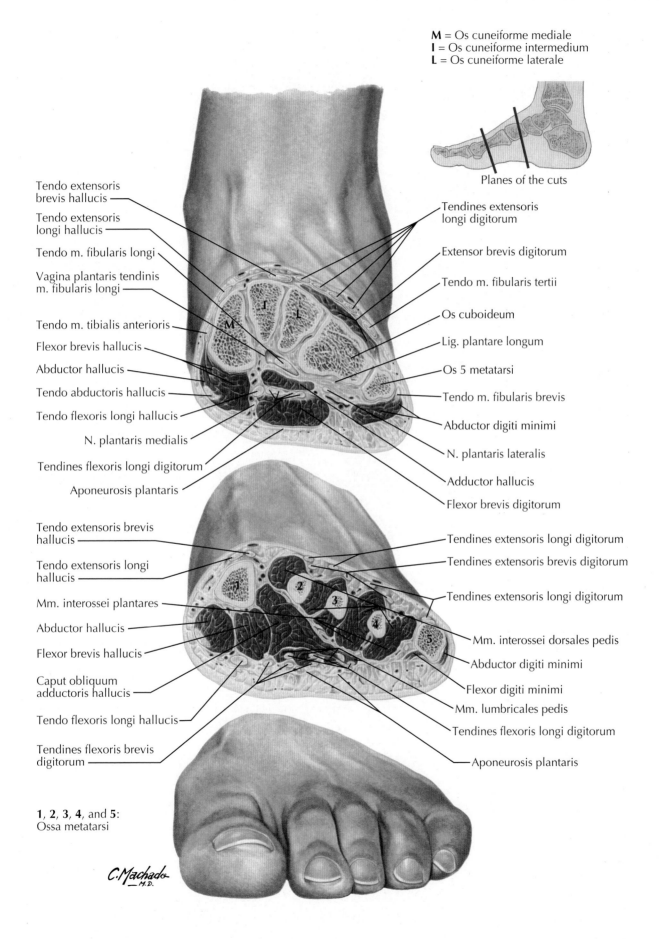

M = Os cuneiforme mediale
I = Os cuneiforme intermedium
L = Os cuneiforme laterale

Planes of the cuts

Tendo extensoris
brevis hallucis

Tendo extensoris
longi hallucis

Tendo m. fibularis longi

Vagina plantaris tendinis
m. fibularis longi

Tendo m. tibialis anterioris

Flexor brevis hallucis

Abductor hallucis

Tendo abductoris hallucis

Tendo flexoris longi hallucis

N. plantaris medialis

Tendines flexoris longi digitorum

Aponeurosis plantaris

Tendines extensoris
longi digitorum

Extensor brevis digitorum

Tendo m. fibularis tertii

Os cuboideum

Lig. plantare longum

Os 5 metatarsi

Tendo m. fibularis brevis

Abductor digiti minimi

N. plantaris lateralis

Adductor hallucis

Flexor brevis digitorum

Tendo extensoris brevis
hallucis

Tendo extensoris longi
hallucis

Mm. interossei plantares

Abductor hallucis

Flexor brevis hallucis

Caput obliquum
adductoris hallucis

Tendo flexoris longi hallucis

Tendines flexoris brevis
digitorum

Tendines extensoris longi digitorum

Tendines extensoris brevis digitorum

Tendines extensoris longi digitorum

Mm. interossei dorsales pedis

Abductor digiti minimi

Flexor digiti minimi

Mm. lumbricales pedis

Tendines flexoris longi digitorum

Aponeurosis plantaris

1, 2, 3, 4, and 5:
Ossa metatarsi

C. Machado
_M.D._

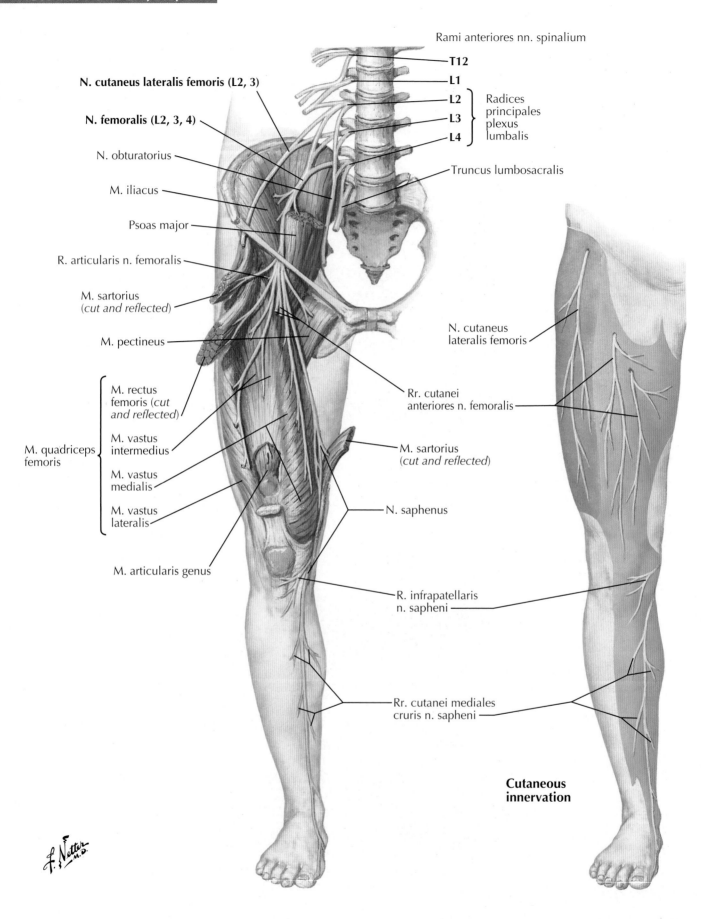

Rami anteriores nn. spinalium

T12

L1

N. cutaneus lateralis femoris (L2, 3)

L2

L3
Radices principales plexus lumbalis

N. femoralis (L2, 3, 4)

L4

N. obturatorius

Truncus lumbosacralis

M. iliacus

Psoas major

R. articularis n. femoralis

M. sartorius
(*cut and reflected*)

M. pectineus

N. cutaneus lateralis femoris

Rr. cutanei anteriores n. femoralis

M. rectus femoris (*cut and reflected*)

M. vastus intermedius

M. quadriceps femoris

M. vastus medialis

M. sartorius
(*cut and reflected*)

N. saphenus

M. vastus lateralis

M. articularis genus

R. infrapatellaris n. sapheni

Rr. cutanei mediales cruris n. sapheni

Cutaneous innervation

Plate 550

Nervi

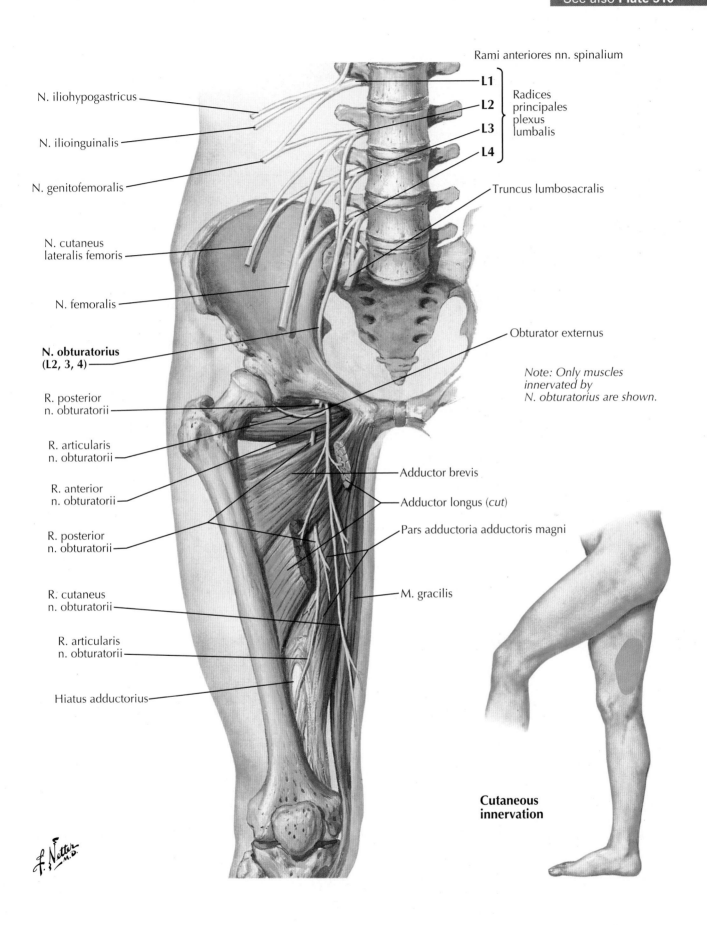

Rami anteriores nn. spinalium

L1
L2   Radices
L3   principales
L4   plexus
      lumbalis

N. iliohypogastricus

N. ilioinguinalis

N. genitofemoralis

Truncus lumbosacralis

N. cutaneus
lateralis femoris

N. femoralis

Obturator externus

**N. obturatorius
(L2, 3, 4)**

*Note: Only muscles
innervated by
N. obturatorius are shown.*

R. posterior
n. obturatorii

R. articularis
n. obturatorii

Adductor brevis

R. anterior
n. obturatorii

Adductor longus (*cut*)

R. posterior
n. obturatorii

Pars adductoria adductoris magni

R. cutaneus
n. obturatorii

M. gracilis

R. articularis
n. obturatorii

Hiatus adductorius

**Cutaneous
innervation**

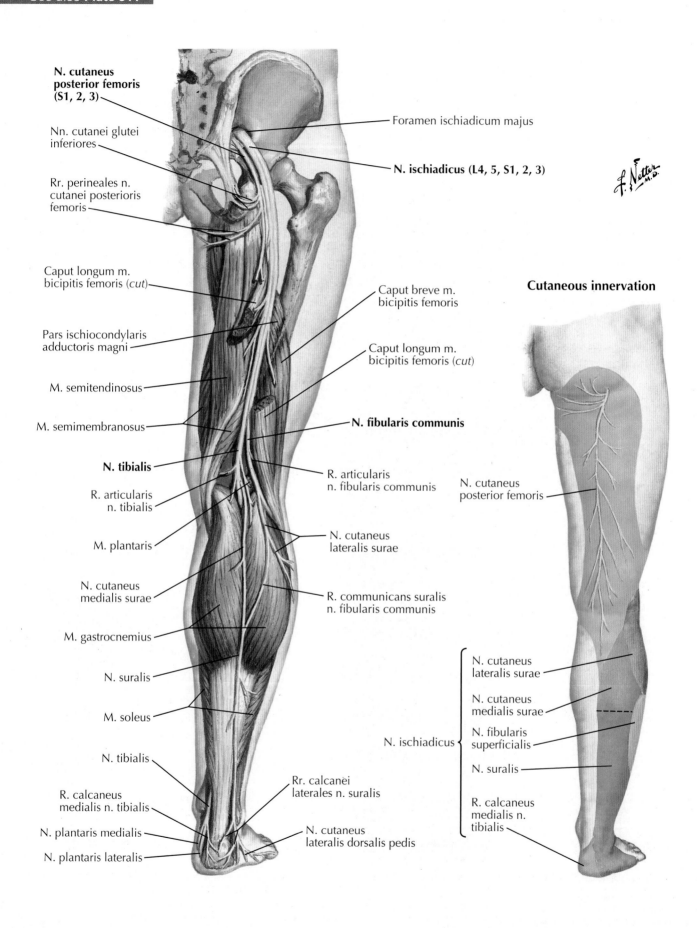

N. cutaneus
posterior femoris
(S1, 2, 3)

Nn. cutanei glutei
inferiores

Rr. perineales n.
cutanei posterioris
femoris

Caput longum m.
bicipitis femoris (cut)

Pars ischiocondylaris
adductoris magni

M. semitendinosus

M. semimembranosus

N. tibialis

R. articularis
n. tibialis

M. plantaris

N. cutaneus
medialis surae

M. gastrocnemius

N. suralis

M. soleus

N. tibialis

R. calcaneus
medialis n. tibialis

N. plantaris medialis

N. plantaris lateralis

Foramen ischiadicum majus

N. ischiadicus (L4, 5, S1, 2, 3)

Caput breve m.
bicipitis femoris

Caput longum m.
bicipitis femoris (cut)

N. fibularis communis

R. articularis
n. fibularis communis

N. cutaneus
lateralis surae

R. communicans suralis
n. fibularis communis

Rr. calcanei
laterales n. suralis

N. cutaneus
lateralis dorsalis pedis

Cutaneous innervation

N. cutaneus
posterior femoris

N. cutaneus
lateralis surae

N. cutaneus
medialis surae

N. fibularis
superficialis

N. suralis

R. calcaneus
medialis n.
tibialis

N. ischiadicus

Plate 552

Nervi

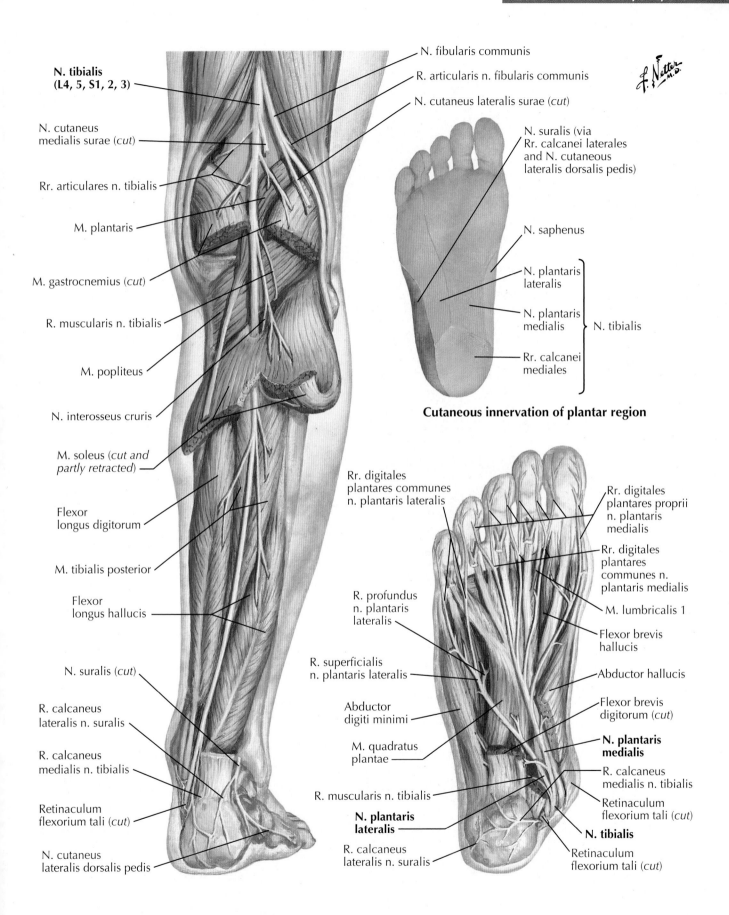

N. fibularis communis

R. articularis n. fibularis communis

N. cutaneus lateralis surae (*cut*)

N. tibialis
(L4, 5, S1, 2, 3)

N. cutaneus medialis surae (*cut*)

Rr. articulares n. tibialis

M. plantaris

M. gastrocnemius (*cut*)

R. muscularis n. tibialis

M. popliteus

N. interosseus cruris

M. soleus (*cut and partly retracted*)

Flexor longus digitorum

M. tibialis posterior

Flexor longus hallucis

N. suralis (*cut*)

R. calcaneus lateralis n. suralis

R. calcaneus medialis n. tibialis

Retinaculum flexorium tali (*cut*)

N. cutaneus lateralis dorsalis pedis

N. suralis (via Rr. calcanei laterales and N. cutaneous lateralis dorsalis pedis)

N. saphenus

N. plantaris lateralis

N. plantaris medialis

Rr. calcanei mediales

N. tibialis

Cutaneous innervation of plantar region

Rr. digitales plantares communes n. plantaris lateralis

Rr. digitales plantares proprii n. plantaris medialis

Rr. digitales plantares communes n. plantaris medialis

M. lumbricalis 1

Flexor brevis hallucis

Abductor hallucis

Flexor brevis digitorum (*cut*)

N. plantaris medialis

R. calcaneus medialis n. tibialis

Retinaculum flexorium tali (*cut*)

N. tibialis

Retinaculum flexorium tali (*cut*)

R. profundus n. plantaris lateralis

R. superficialis n. plantaris lateralis

Abductor digiti minimi

M. quadratus plantae

R. muscularis n. tibialis

N. plantaris lateralis

R. calcaneus lateralis n. suralis

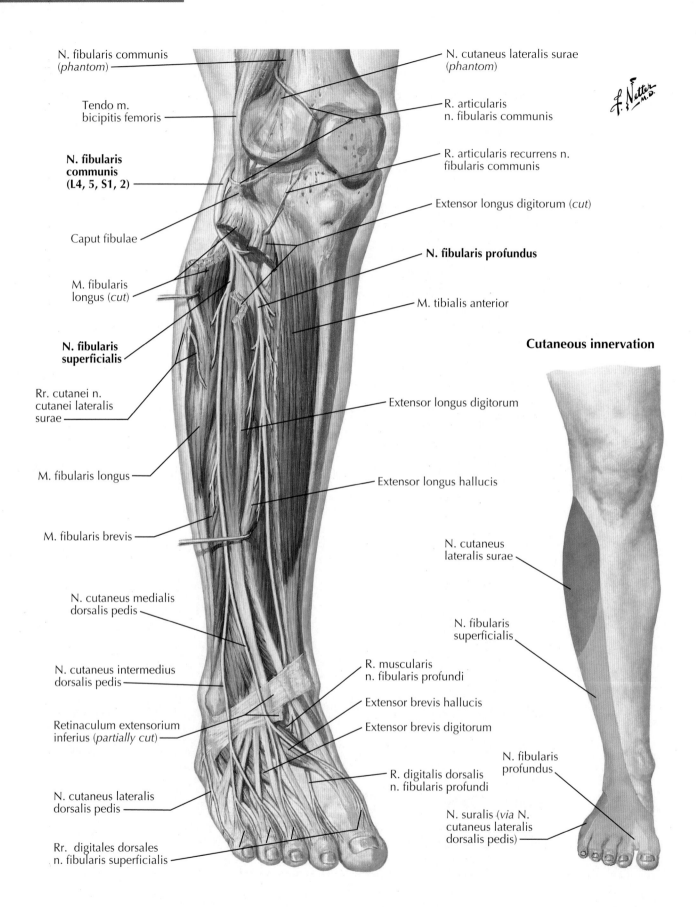

N. fibularis communis
(*phantom*)

Tendo m.
bicipitis femoris

**N. fibularis
communis
(L4, 5, S1, 2)**

Caput fibulae

M. fibularis
longus (*cut*)

**N. fibularis
superficialis**

Rr. cutanei n.
cutanei lateralis
surae

M. fibularis longus

M. fibularis brevis

N. cutaneus medialis
dorsalis pedis

N. cutaneus intermedius
dorsalis pedis

Retinaculum extensorium
inferius (*partially cut*)

N. cutaneus lateralis
dorsalis pedis

Rr. digitales dorsales
n. fibularis superficialis

N. cutaneus lateralis surae
(*phantom*)

R. articularis
n. fibularis communis

R. articularis recurrens n.
fibularis communis

Extensor longus digitorum (*cut*)

N. fibularis profundus

M. tibialis anterior

Extensor longus digitorum

Extensor longus hallucis

R. muscularis
n. fibularis profundi

Extensor brevis hallucis

Extensor brevis digitorum

R. digitalis dorsalis
n. fibularis profundi

Cutaneous innervation

N. cutaneus
lateralis surae

N. fibularis
superficialis

N. fibularis
profundus

N. suralis (*via* N.
cutaneus lateralis
dorsalis pedis)

Plate 554

Nervi

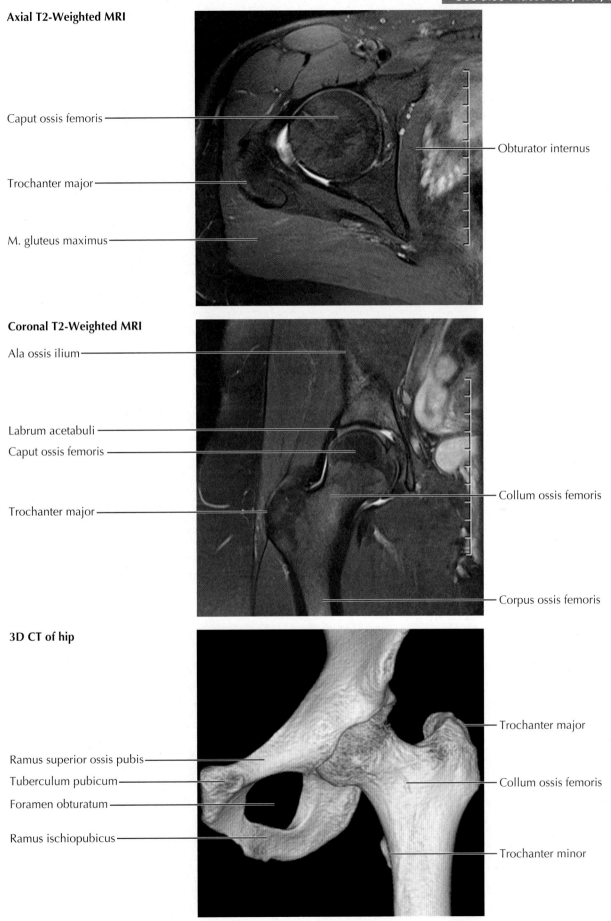

Axial T2-Weighted MRI

Caput ossis femoris

Obturator internus

Trochanter major

M. gluteus maximus

Coronal T2-Weighted MRI

Ala ossis ilium

Labrum acetabuli

Caput ossis femoris

Collum ossis femoris

Trochanter major

Corpus ossis femoris

3D CT of hip

Trochanter major

Ramus superior ossis pubis

Tuberculum pubicum

Collum ossis femoris

Foramen obturatum

Ramus ischiopubicus

Trochanter minor

See also **Plates 530, 537, 538**

Lateral view

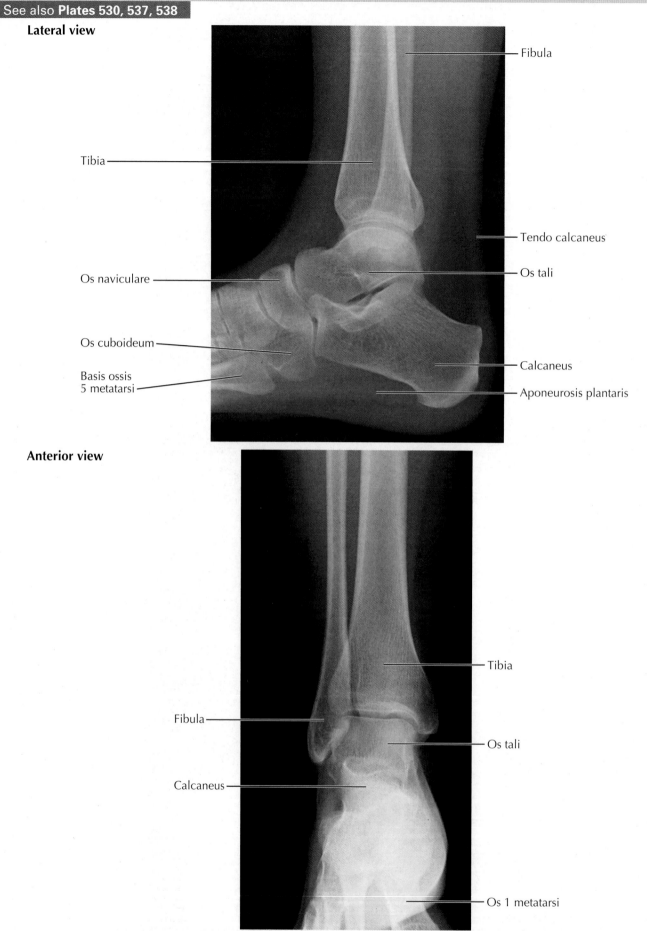

Fibula

Tibia

Tendo calcaneus

Os tali

Os naviculare

Os cuboideum

Calcaneus

Basis ossis
5 metatarsi

Aponeurosis plantaris

Anterior view

Tibia

Fibula

Os tali

Calcaneus

Os 1 metatarsi

Plate 556

Regional Imaging

ANATOMICAL STRUCTURE	CLINICAL COMMENT	PLATE NUMBERS
Systema Nervosum		
N. suralis	Nerve is commonly biopsied for peripheral neuropathies and commonly used as donor graft in neurotization procedures	493, 552
N. fibularis communis	Injury to this nerve from blunt trauma or compression by leg cast weakens dorsiflexion and results in foot drop	550, 552, 554
N. obturatorius	Nerve is blocked or transected for adductor muscle spasticity in cerebral palsy; may be injured during pelvic fractures or pelvic surgical procedures such as lymphadenectomy	551
N. femoralis	Can be compressed from femoral artery hematoma and can be anesthetized for procedures of lower limb just below inguinal ligament	507, 509, 550
N. saphenus	Can be anesthetized in adductor canal to provide pain relief after knee replacement surgery	492, 509, 550
N. cutaneus lateralis femoris	Compression at inguinal ligament leads to meralgia paresthetica, a pain and paresthesia syndrome of anterolateral thigh; risk factors include obesity, pregnancy, and tight-fitting waistbands	509, 550
Systema Skeletale		
Collum ossis femoris	Common fracture in elderly persons from falls; can lead to avascular necrosis of head of femur because of disrupted blood supply	497, 500, 514
Corpus ossis femoris	Midbody is common fracture site in high-energy trauma (motor vehicle collisions)	500
Articulatio coxae	Potential for avascular necrosis of head of femur in hip dislocations or fractures	496, 514
Lig. cruciatum anterius	Most commonly injured knee ligament, typically from sudden pivot of knee causing excessive valgus stress coupled with medial rotation of tibia	517-519
Ligg. collaterale tibiale and cruciatum anterius; Meniscus medialis	"Unhappy triad of the knee"; damage to these structures can result from blow to lateral aspect of joint in extension	517-519
Tibia; fibula	High-energy fractures of body (boot-top skiing fracture) from falling forward at high speed	524
Articulatio metatarsophalangea 1	Joint misalignment leads to hallux valgus (bunion); wearing narrow shoes can contribute, though there is also a strong genetic component	535
Calcaneus	Most common tarsal bone fracture, usually caused by landing forcefully on heel after falling from height	537
Articulatio talocruralis	Most sprains are inversion injuries that occur when foot is plantar flexed, placing stress on lateral collateral ligaments of ankle; fractures often occur to lateral malleolus of fibula and inferior articular surface of tibia	538
Systema Musculare		
Mm. compartimenti medialis femoris	Excessive stretching or tearing of adductor and gracilis muscles is common in sports that require repeated sprints or quick changes in direction (e.g., soccer, hockey)	502, 503
Lig. patellae	Striking patellar ligament with reflex hammer elicits patellar (knee jerk) reflex to test L3 to L4 spinal cord levels (innervation of quadriceps femoris muscle by femoral nerve)	502, 517
Tractus iliotibialis	Can cause lateral knee pain in runners when tight iliotibial tract rubs repetitively across lateral epicondyle of femur (iliotibial band syndrome)	501, 516
Mm. semitendinosus and semimembranosus; Caput longum m. bicipitis femoris	Excessive stretching or tearing of hamstring muscles occurs most often during high-speed running or activities with high kicks	504

Structures with High Clinical Significance

Table 8.1

ANATOMICAL STRUCTURE	CLINICAL COMMENT	PLATE NUMBERS
Systema Musculare—Continued		
M. piriformis	Piriformis muscle strain or structural variations (e.g., split piriformis muscle) may produce compression of sciatic nerve	511
Mm. glutei medius and minimus	Paralysis results in contralateral pelvic dip due to weakened hip abduction when standing on affected limb (Trendelenburg sign or gait)	512
Tendo calcaneus (Achillis)	Inflammation results from repetitive stress on tendon, often from running on uneven surfaces; extreme stress may cause tendon to rupture; striking calcaneal tendon with reflex hammer elicits ankle (ankle jerk) reflex to test S1–S2 spinal cord levels (innervation of superficial calf muscles by tibial nerve)	527, 528, 538
Compartimenta cruris	Acute compartment syndrome may occur after trauma, such as long bone fracture, that increases compartment pressure and thereby compromises vascular flow; symptoms include pain, paresthesias, pallor, pulselessness, and paralysis (five P's); fasciotomy often required to relieve pressure	534
Aponeurosis plantaris	Inflammation results from increased tension, weight, or overuse, causing heel and foot pain (plantar fasciitis)	543
Systema Cardiovasculare		
Vena femoralis	Common site of vascular access for central venous catheters; however, risk of catheter infection is greater than with jugular or subclavian vein access	509
Venae profundae membri inferioris	Venous thrombosis of deep leg veins is due to venous stasis, vessel injury, and/or coagulation disorders (Virchow's triad); can lead to thrombus formation and thromboemboli, such as to the lungs	533
Vena saphena magna	Often used as graft in coronary artery bypass surgery	492
Venae superficiales membri inferioris	Varicose veins are dilated, tortuous superficial veins, often associated with reflux of superficial and/or deep veins; progressive venous disease may cause edema, pain, and ulceration	492, 533
A. femoralis	Common site of vascular access for percutaneous cardiac and vascular procedures; target is segment between origins of inferior epigastric and deep femoral arteries, generally identified using fluoroscopy by its location alongside the femoral head; "high stick" (too cephalad) may result in retroperitoneal hemorrhage	522
Aa. femoralis, poplitea, tibiales, and fibularis	Peripheral arterial disease due to atherosclerosis may occur in major arteries of lower limb, resulting in reduced blood flow; patients experience claudication (cramping pain in thigh or calf) upon exertion	522
Arteriae membri inferioris	Pulse points: femoral artery in femoral triangle, popliteal artery in deep popliteal region of knee, anterior tibial artery between extensor hallucis longus and extensor digitorum longus at ankle joint, dorsalis pedis artery on dorsum of foot, and posterior tibial artery in tarsal tunnel posterior to medial malleolus	14, 509, 527, 540, 541
Vasa Lymphatica and Organa Lymphoidea		
Nodi lymphoidei inguinales superficiales	Superficial inguinal nodes drain lower limb, gluteal region, lower abdominal region, and perineum; are palpable when enlarged	494
Vasa lymphatica membri inferioris	Lymphedema (stasis of lymph flow in lymph vessels obstructed by inflammation, fibrosis, tumor, or abnormally small diameter)	494

*Selections were based largely on clinical data and commonly discussed clinical correlations in macroscopic ("gross") anatomy courses.

The lumbosacral plexus includes the lumbar, sacral, and coccygeal plexuses, whose roots are the anterior rami of spinal nerves (lumbar plexus: typically L2–L4 with a small contribution from L1; sacral plexus: L4–S4; coccygeal plexus: S4–Co). Variation in the spinal nerve contributions to the plexuses, and the nerves that arise from these plexuses, is common and can be due to a prefixed (high) or postfixed (low) plexus.

NERVE	ORIGIN	COURSE	BRANCHES	MOTOR	CUTANEOUS
N. cutaneus lateralis femoris	Divisiones posteriores plexus lumbalis (L2–L3)	Courses posterior to or through inguinal ligament medial to anterior superior iliac spine, then travels superficially in lateral thigh			Lateral thigh
N. femoralis	Divisiones posteriores plexus lumbalis (L2–L4)	Passes posterior to inguinal ligament to lie on iliacus muscle in femoral triangle	Rr. musculares and cutanei anteriores; N. saphenus	Compartimentum anterius femoris; Mm. iliacus and pectineus	Anterior thigh (also see N. saphenus)
N. saphenus	N. femoralis	Leaves femoral nerve in adductor canal, pierces fascia lata to travel superficially with great saphenous vein	Rr. infrapatellaris and cutanei mediales cruris		Medial knee, leg, ankle, and foot
N. genitofemoralis	Divisiones anteriores plexus lumbalis (L1–L2)	Runs on anterior surface of psoas major; genital branch traverses inguinal canal; femoral branch courses into femoral triangle by passing deep to inguinal ligament	Rr. genitalis and femoralis	Cremaster	Lateral part of femoral triangle, anterior scrotum/vulva
N. obturatorius	Divisiones anteriores plexus lumbalis (L2–L4)	At L5 vertebra passes deep to common iliac vessels, enters medial thigh via obturator foramen	Rr. anterior and posterior	Compartimentum mediale femoris	Medial thigh
N. gluteus superior	Divisiones posteriores plexus sacralis (L4–S1)	Exits pelvis via greater sciatic foramen superior to piriformis muscle		Mm. glutei medius and minimus; Tensor fasciae latae	
N. gluteus inferior	Divisiones posteriores plexus sacralis (L5–S2)	Exits pelvis via greater sciatic foramen inferior to piriformis muscle		M. gluteus maximus	
N. musculi piriformis	Divisiones posteriores plexus sacralis (S1–S2)	Innervates piriformis muscle near where it exits pelvis via greater sciatic foramen		M. piriformis	
N. cutaneus perforans	Divisiones posteriores plexus sacralis (S2–S3)	Exits pelvis and pierces sacrotuberous ligament			Inferomedial gluteal region
N. obturatoris interni	Divisiones anteriores plexus sacralis (L5–S2)	Exits pelvis via greater sciatic foramen, inferior to piriformis muscle; re-enters pelvis via lesser sciatic foramen to innervate obturator internus		Obturator internus; M. gemellus superior	
N. musculi quadrati femoris	Divisiones anteriores plexus sacralis (L4–S1)	Exits pelvis via greater sciatic foramen inferior to piriformis muscle		Mm. quadratus femoris and gemellus inferior	
N. levatoris ani	Divisiones anteriores plexus sacralis (S3–S4)	From its source, travels on superior surface of levator ani		Mm. iliococcygeus and pubococcygeus	
N. musculi coccygei	Divisiones anteriores plexus sacralis (S3–S4)	From its source, travels on superior surface of coccygeus muscle		M. coccygeus (ischiococcygeus)	

NERVE	ORIGIN	COURSE	BRANCHES	MOTOR	CUTANEOUS
N. pudendalis	Divisiones anteriores plexus sacralis (S2–S4)	Exits pelvis via greater sciatic foramen inferior to piriformis muscle; enters perineum via lesser sciatic foramen, coursing through ischioanal fossa and pudendal (Alcock's) canal	Nn. analis inferior, perinealis, and clitoridis/dorsalis penis	Mm. perinei; Sphincter externus ani; M. pubococcygeus	Posterior scrotum/vulva, clitoris/penis
N. cutaneus posterior femoris	Divisiones anteriores and posteriores plexus sacralis (S1–S3)	Exits pelvis via greater sciatic foramen inferior to piriformis muscle; runs inferiorly to gluteus maximus muscle and continues distally to popliteal fossa	Nn. cutanei glutei inferiores; Rr. perineales		Inferior gluteal region, posterior thigh, popliteal region
N. ischiadicus	Divisiones anteriores and posteriores plexus sacralis (L4–S3)	Exits pelvis via greater sciatic foramen inferior to piriformis muscle, passing superficial to lateral rotators and deep to gluteus medius muscle to access thigh between greater trochanter of femur and ischial tuberosity	Rr. musculares; Nn. tibialis and fibularis communis	Compartimentum posterius femoris (also see branches)	See branches
N. tibialis	N. ischiadicus	Courses through popliteal fossa and sural region deep to soleus muscle, traversing tarsal tunnel posterior to medial malleolus	Rr. musculares and calcanei mediales; Nn. interosseus cruris, cutaneus medialis surae, and plantares medialis and lateralis	Compartimentum posterius cruris (also see branches)	Heel (also see branches)
N. fibularis communis	N. ischiadicus	Courses medial to biceps femoris muscle and lateral to lateral head of gastrocnemius muscle and neck of fibula	Nn. fibulares superficialis and profundus, and cutaneus lateralis surae; R. communicans suralis	See branches	See branches
N. fibularis profundus	N. fibularis communis	Courses deep to fibularis longus muscle and extensor longus digitorum on surface of interosseous membrane of leg deep to extensor retinaculum	Rr. musculares and digitales dorsales	Compartimentum anterius cruris	Dorsal aspect of adjacent parts of toes 1 and 2
N. fibularis superficialis	N. fibularis communis	Courses between fibularis longus and brevis muscles in lateral compartment of leg, piercing crural fascia distally	Rr. musculares; Nn. cutanei medialis dorsalis pedis and intermedius dorsalis pedis	Compartimentum laterale cruris	Inferior part of anterior leg, dorsum of foot and toes
N. cutaneus lateralis surae	N. fibularis communis	Branches from common fibular nerve just proximal to plantaris muscle			Lateral leg
N. cutaneus medialis surae	N. tibialis	Branches from tibial nerve just proximal to plantaris muscle, runs between both heads of gastrocnemius muscle, pierces crural fascia	N. suralis		Proximal posterolateral leg (also see N. suralis)

Table 8.4

Nervi Plexus Lumbrosacralis

NERVE	ORIGIN	COURSE	BRANCHES	MOTOR	CUTANEOUS
N. suralis	Union of N. cutaneus medialis surae and R. communicans suralis n. fibularis communis	Descends sural region along lateral calcaneal tendon and into foot between lateral malleolus and calcaneus	N. cutaneus lateralis dorsalis pedis		Distal posterolateral leg, lateral foot
N. plantaris lateralis	N. tibialis	Passes deep to abductor brevis hallucis and travels between flexor brevis digitorum and quadratus plantae muscle	Rr. superficialis and profundus	Abductor digiti minimi; Adductor hallucis; Flexor digiti minimi; Mm. quadratus plantae, interossei dorsales pedis and plantares, and lumbricales pedis (lateral three)	Lateral sole, plantar aspect of 5th toe and part of 4th toe
N. plantaris medialis	N. tibialis	Passes deep to abductor brevis hallucis and runs anteriorly along medial border of flexor brevis digitorum	Rr. musculares and digitales plantares communes	Abductor hallucis; Flexores breves digitorum and hallucis; Mm. lumbricales pedis (most medial one)	Medial sole, plantar aspect of toes 1–3, and part of 4th toe

Musculi

MUSCLE	MUSCLE GROUP	PROXIMAL ATTACHMENT	DISTAL ATTACHMENT	INNERVATION	BLOOD SUPPLY	MAIN ACTIONS
Abductor digiti minimi pedis	Mm. pedis	Procc. medialis and lateralis tuberis calcanei; aponeurosis plantaris; septum intermusculare	Basis phalangis proximalis digiti minimi (lateral surface)	N. plantaris lateralis	A. plantaris lateralis; Aa. metatarsea plantaris and digitalis plantaris to digitus minimus	Abducts and flexes 5th digit
Abductor hallucis	Mm. pedis	Proc. medialis tuberis calcanei; retinaculum flexorium tali; aponeurosis plantaris	Basis phalangis proximalis hallucis (medial surface)	N. plantaris medialis	Aa. plantaris medialis and metatarsea plantaris 1	Abducts and flexes 1st digit
Adductor brevis	Compartimentum mediale femoris	Corpus ossis pubis; ramus inferior ossis pubis	Linea pectinea ossis femoris; linea aspera (proximal part)	N. obturatorius	Aa. profunda femoris, circumflexa medialis femoris, and obturatoria	Adducts thigh at hip, weak hip flexor
Adductor hallucis	Mm. pedis	*Caput obliquum*: Bases ossium 2-4 metatarsi *Caput transversum*: Ligg. articulationum metatarsophalangearum digitorum 3–5	Basis phalangis proximalis hallucis (lateral surface)	N. plantaris lateralis	Aa. plantares medialis and lateralis; Arcus plantaris; Aa. metatarseae plantares	Adducts 1st digit, maintains transverse arch of foot
Adductor longus	Compartimentum mediale femoris	Corpus ossis pubis (inferior to crista pubica)	Linea aspera ossis femoris (middle third)	N. obturatorius	Aa. profunda femoris and circumflexa medialis femoris	Adducts thigh at hip
Adductor magnus	Compartimentum mediale femoris	*Pars adductoria*: Ramus ischiopubicus *Pars ischiocondylaris*: Tuber ischiadicum	*Pars adductoria*: Tuberositas glutea; linea aspera; linea supracondylaris medialis *Pars ischiocondylaris*: Tuberculum adductorium ossis femoris	*Pars adductoria*: N. obturatorius *Pars ischiocondylaris*: N. ischiadicus (divisio tibialis)	Aa. femoralis, profunda femoris, and obturatoria	*Adductor part*: adducts and flexes thigh *Hamstring part*: extends thigh
M. articularis genus	Compartimentum anterius femoris	Facies anterior ossis femoris (distal part)	Bursa suprapatellaris	N. femoralis	A. femoralis	Pulls suprapatellar bursa superiorly with extension of knee
M. biceps femoris	Compartimentum posterius femoris	*Caput longum*: Tuber ischiadicum *Caput breve*: Linea aspera; linea supracondylaris lateralis ossis femoris	Caput fibulae (lateral surface)	*Caput longum*: N. ischiadicus (diviso tibialis) *Caput breve*: N. ischiadicus (divisio fibularis)	Aa. perforantes femoris, glutea inferior, and circumflexa medialis femoris	Flexes and laterally rotates leg, extends thigh
Extensor brevis digitorum	Mm. pedis	Calcaneus (superolateral surface); lig. talocalcaneum laterale; retinaculum extensorium inferius (deep surface)	Tendines extensoris longi digitorum 2–4 (lateral sides)	N. fibularis profundus	Aa. dorsalis pedis, tarsea lateralis, arcuata, and fibularis	Extends 2nd through 4th digits at metatarsophalangeal and interphalangeal joints
Extensor brevis hallucis	Mm. pedis	Calcaneus (superolateral surface)	Phalanx proximalis hallucis (dorsal surface)	N. fibularis profundus	Aa. dorsalis pedis, tarsea lateralis, arcuata, and fibularis	Extends great toe at metatarsophalangeal and interphalangeal joints
Extensor longus digitorum	Compartimentum anterius cruris	Condylus lateralis tibiae; facies anteriores membranae interosseae and fibulae (proximal three-fourths)	Phalanges mediae and distales digitorum 2–5	N. fibularis profundus	A. tibialis anterior	Extends lateral four digits and dorsiflexes foot
Extensor longus hallucis	Compartimentum anterius cruris	Facies anteriores fibulae and membranae interosseae cruris (middle part)	Basis phalangis distalis hallucis (dorsal surface)	N. fibularis profundus	A. tibialis anterior	Extends great toe, dorsiflexes foot
M. fibularis brevis	Compartimentum laterale cruris	Facies lateralis fibulae (distal two-thirds)	Tuberositas ossis 5 metatarsi (dorsal surface)	N. fibularis superficialis	Aa. tibialis anterior and fibularis	Everts and plantar flexes foot

Table 8.6   **Musculi**

MUSCLE	MUSCLE GROUP	PROXIMAL ATTACHMENT	DISTAL ATTACHMENT	INNERVATION	BLOOD SUPPLY	MAIN ACTIONS
M. fibularis longus	Compartimentum laterale cruris	Caput fibulae; facies lateralis fibulae (proximal two-thirds)	Basis ossis 1 metatarsi (plantar surface); os cuneiforme mediale (plantar surface)	N. fibularis superficialis	Aa. tibialis anterior and fibularis	Everts and plantar flexes foot
M. fibularis tertius	Compartimentum anterius cruris	Facies anteriores fibulae and membranae interosseae cruris (distal third)	Basis ossis 5 metatarsi (dorsal surface)	N. fibularis profundus	A. tibialis anterior	Dorsiflexes and everts foot
Flexor brevis digitorum	Mm. pedis	Proc. medialis tuberis calcanei; aponeurosis plantaris; septum intermusculare	Phalanges mediae digitorum 2–5 (both sides)	N. plantaris medialis	Aa. plantares medialis and lateralis; Arcus plantaris; Aa. metatarseae plantares and digitales plantares	Flexes lateral four digits
Flexor brevis hallucis	Mm. pedis	Ossa cuboideum and cuneiforme laterale (plantar surfaces)	Basis phalangis proximalis hallucis (both sides)	N. plantaris medialis	Aa. plantaris medialis and metatarsea plantaris 1	Flexes proximal phalanx of 1st digit
Flexor digiti minimi pedis	Mm. pedis	Basis ossis 5 metatarsi	Basis phalangis proximalis digiti minimi (lateral surface)	N. plantaris lateralis	Aa. plantaris lateralis, arcuata, and digitalis plantaris to digitus minimus	Flexes proximal phalanx of 5th digit
Flexor longus digitorum	Compartimentum posterius cruris	Facies posterior tibiae (medial part, inferior to linea musculi solei)	Bases phalangium distalium digitorum 2-5 (plantar surfaces)	N. tibialis	A. tibialis posterior	Flexes lateral four digits and plantar flexes foot; supports longitudinal arches of foot
Flexor longus hallucis	Compartimentum posterius cruris	Facies posteriores fibulae and membranae interosseae cruris (distal two-thirds)	Basis phalangis distalis hallucis	N. tibialis	A. fibularis	Flexes all joints of great toe, plantar flexes foot
M. gastrocnemius	Compartimentum posterius cruris	*Caput laterale*: Condylus lateralis ossis femoris (lateral surface) *Caput mediale*: Facies poplitea ossis femoris (above Condylus medialis)	Facies posterior calcanei (via tendo calcaneus)	N. tibialis	Aa. poplitea and tibialis posterior	Plantar flexes foot, assists in flexion of knee
M. gemellus inferior	Mm. glutei profundi	Tuber ischiadicum	Trochanter major ossis femoris	N. musculi quadrati femoris	A. circumflexa medialis femoris	Laterally rotates extended thigh and abducts flexed thigh
M. gemellus superior	Mm. glutei profundi	Spina ischiadica (external surface)	Trochanter major ossis femoris (medial surface)	N. obturatoris interni	Aa. glutea inferior and pudendalis interna	Laterally rotates extended thigh and abducts flexed thigh
M. gluteus maximus	Mm. glutei superficiales	Os ilium (posterior to linea glutea posterior); facies dorsales ossium sacri and coccygis; lig. sacrotuberale	Condylus lateralis tibiae (via tractus iliotibialis); tuberositas glutea ossis femoris	N. gluteus inferior	Aa. gluteae inferior and superior	Extends flexed thigh, assists in lateral rotation, and abducts thigh
M. gluteus medius	Mm. glutei superficiales	Facies glutea ossis ilium (between lineae gluteae anterior and posterior)	Trochanter major ossis femoris (lateral surface)	N. gluteus superior	A. glutea superior	Abducts and medially rotates thigh
M. gluteus minimus	Mm. glutei superficiales	Facies glutea ossis ilium (between lineae gluteae anterior and inferior	Trochanter major ossis femoris (anterior surface)	N. gluteus superior	A. glutea superior	Abducts and medially rotates thigh
M. gracilis	Compartimentum mediale femoris	Corpus ossis pubis; ramus inferior ossis pubis	Facies medialis tibiae (superior part)	N. obturatorius	Aa. profunda femoris and circumflexa medialis femoris	Adducts thigh, flexes and medially rotates leg

MUSCLE	MUSCLE GROUP	PROXIMAL ATTACHMENT	DISTAL ATTACHMENT	INNERVATION	BLOOD SUPPLY	MAIN ACTIONS
M. ilacus	Iliopsoas	Fossa iliaca (superior two-thirds); crista iliaca; ala ossis sacri; lig. sacroiliacum anterius	Trochanter minor; corpus ossis femoris	N. femoralis	R. iliacus a. iliolumbalis	Flexes thigh
Mm. interossei dorsales pedis	Mm. pedis	Ossa 1-5 metatarsi (adjacent surfaces)	*Medial one*: Phalanx proximalis digiti 2 (medial surface) *Lateral three*: Phalanges proximales digitorum 2-4 (lateral surfaces)	N. plantaris lateralis	Aa. arcuata, and metatarseae dorsales and plantares	Abduct 2nd through 4th digits of foot, flex metatarsophalangeal joints, and extend phalanges
M. interossei plantares	Mm. pedis	Bases and facies mediales ossium 3-5 metatarsi	Bases phalangium proximalium digitorum 3-5 (medial surfaces)	N. plantaris lateralis	A. plantaris lateralis; Arcus plantaris; Aa. metatarseae plantares and digitales plantares	Adduct digits (3–5), flex metatarsophalangeal joint, and extend phalanges
Mm. lumbricales pedis	Mm. pedis	Tendines flexoris longi digitorum	Aponeuroses extensoriae digitorum 2–5 (medial side)	*Medial one*: N. plantaris medialis *Lateral three*: N. plantaris lateralis	Aa. plantaris lateralis and metatarseae plantares	Flex proximal phalanges at metatarsophalangeal joint, extend phalanges at proximal and distal interphalangeal joints
Obturator externus	Compartimentum mediale femoris	Foramen obturatum (margins); membrana obturatoria (external surface)	Fossa trochanterica ossis femoris	N. obturatorius	Aa. circumflexa medialis femoris and obturatoria	Laterally rotates thigh
Obturator internus	Mm. glutei profundi	Membrana obturatoria (pelvic surface); foramen obturatum (margins)	Trochanter major ossis femoris	N. obturatoris interni	Aa. pudendalis interna and obturatoria	Laterally rotates extended thigh, abducts flexed thigh
M. pectineus	Compartimentum mediale femoris	Ramus superior ossis pubis	Linea pectinea ossis femoris	N. femoralis (sometimes also N. obturatorius)	Aa. circumflexa medialis femoris and obturatoria	Adducts and flexes thigh
M. piriformis	Mm. glutei profundi	Segmenta 2–4 ossis sacri (anterior surface); lig. sacrotuberale (inconstant)	Trochanter major ossis femoris (superior border)	N. musculi piriformis	Aa. gluteae superior and inferior, and pudendalis interna	Laterally rotates extended thigh, abducts flexed thigh
M. plantaris	Compartimentum posterius cruris	Linea supracondylaris lateralis ossis femoris (inferior end); lig. popliteum obliquum	Facies posterior calcanei (via Tendo calcaneus)	N. tibialis	A. poplitea	Weakly assists gastrocnemius
M. popliteus	Compartimentum posterius cruris	Condylus lateralis ossis femoris (lateral surface); meniscus lateralis	Facies posterior tibiae (superior to linea musculi solei)	N. tibialis	Aa. inferior lateralis genus and inferior medialis genus	Flexes knee
Psoas major	Iliopsoas	Procc. transversi vertebrarum lumbalium; corpora vertebrarum T12–L5 (lateral surfaces); intervening disci intervertebrales	Trochanter minor ossis femoris	Rr. anteriores nn. spinalium L1–L3	R. lumbalis a. iliolumbalis	Acting superiorly with iliacus, flexes hip; acting inferiorly, flexes vertebral column laterally; used to balance trunk in sitting position; acting inferiorly with iliacus, flexes trunk
Psoas minor	Iliopsoas	Corpora vertebrarum T12 and L1 (lateral surfaces); discus intervertebralis T12/L1	Linea pectinea; Eminentia iliopubica	R. anterior n. spinalis L1	R. lumbalis a. iliolumbalis	Flexes pelvis on vertebral column
M. quadratus femoris	Mm. glutei profundi	Tuber ischiadicum (lateral margin)	Tuberculum quadratum	N. musculi quadrati femoris	A. circumflexa medialis femoris	Laterally rotates thigh
M. quadratus plantae	Mm. pedis	Facies plantaris calcanei (medial and lateral margins)	Tendo flexoris longi digitorum (posterolateral edge)	N. plantaris lateralis	Aa. plantares medialis and lateralis; Arcus plantaris	Corrects for oblique pull of flexor longus digitorum tendon, thus assisting in flexion of digits of foot

Table 8.8   **Musculi**

MUSCLE	MUSCLE GROUP	PROXIMAL ATTACHMENT	DISTAL ATTACHMENT	INNERVATION	BLOOD SUPPLY	MAIN ACTIONS
M. rectus femoris	Compartimentum anterius femoris (m. quadriceps femoris)	Spina iliaca anterior inferior; os ilium (superior to acetabulum)	Tuberositas tibiae (via lig. patellae)	N. femoralis	Aa. profunda femoris and circumflexa lateralis femoris	Extends leg and flexes thigh
M. sartorius	Compartimentum anterius femoris	Spina iliaca anterior superior; os ilium (inferior to that spine)	Facies medialis tibiae (superior part)	N. femoralis	A. femoralis	Abducts, laterally rotates, and flexes thigh; flexes knee
M. semimembranosus	Compartimentum posterius femoris	Tuber ischiadicum	Condylus medialis tibiae (posterior part)	N. ischiadicus (divisio tibialis)	Aa. perforantes femoris and circumflexa medialis femoris	Flexes leg, extends thigh
M. semitendinosus	Compartimentum posterius femoris	Tuber ischiadicum	Facies medialis tibiae (superior part)	N. ischiadicus (divisio tibialis)	Aa. perforantes femoris and circumflexa medialis femoris	Flexes leg, extends thigh
M. soleus	Compartimentum posterius cruris	Caput fibulae (posterior surface); facies posterior fibulae (proximal one-fourth); linea musculi solei tibiae	Facies posterior calcanei (via tendo calcaneus)	N. tibialis	Aa. poplitea, tibialis posterior, and fibularis	Plantar flexes foot
Tensor fasciae latae	Mm. glutei superficiales	Spina iliaca anterior superior; crista iliaca (anterior part)	Condylus lateralis tibiae (via tractus iliotibialis)	N. gluteus superior	R. ascendens a. circumflexae lateralis femoris	Abducts, medially rotates, and flexes thigh; helps to keep knee extended
M. tibialis anterior	Compartimentum anterius femoris	Condylus lateralis tibiae; facies lateralis tibiae (proximal half); membrana interossea cruris	Os cuneiforme mediale; basis ossis 1 metatarsi	N. fibularis profundus	A. tibialis anterior	Dorsiflexes foot and inverts foot
M. tibialis posterior	Compartimentum posterius cruris	Facies posterior tibiae (below linea musculi solei); membrana interossea; facies posterior fibulae (proximal half)	Tuberositas ossis navicularis; ossa cuneiformia (all); os cuboideum; bases ossium 2-4 metatarsi	N. tibialis	A. fibularis	Plantar flexes foot and inverts foot
M. vastus intermedius	Compartimentum anterius femoris (m. quadriceps femoris)	Facies anterior and lateralis corporis ossis femoris	Tuberositas tibiae (via lig. patellae)	N. femoralis	Aa. circumflexa lateralis femoris and profunda femoris	Extends leg
M. vastus lateralis	Compartimentum anterius femoris (m. quadriceps femoris)	Trochanter major; tuberositas glutea; Labium laterale lineae asperae	Tuberositas tibiae (via lig. patellae)	N. femoralis	Aa. circumflexa lateralis femoris and profunda femoris	Extends leg
M. vastus medialis	Compartimentum anterius femoris (m. quadriceps femoris)	Linea intertrochanterica; trochanter major; tuberositas glutea; labium laterale lineae asperae	Tuberositas tibiae (via lig. patellae)	N. femoralis	Aa. femoralis and profunda femoris	Extends leg

Variations in spinal nerve contributions to the innervation of muscles, their arterial supply, their attachments, and their actions are common themes in human anatomy. Therefore, expect differences between texts and realize that anatomical variation is normal.

REFERENCES

Plates 5, 188
Lee MWL, McPhee RW, Stringer MD. An evidence-based approach to human dermatomes. *Clin Anat.* 2008;21(5): 363–373.

Plates 29, 61–63, 67–69
Lang J. *Clinical Anatomy of the Nose, Nasal Cavity, and Paranasal Sinuses.* Thieme; 1989.

Plates 40, 85
Benninger B, Andrews K, Carter W. Clinical measurements of hard palate and implications for subepithelial connective tissue grafts with suggestions for palatal nomenclature. *J Oral Maxillofac Surg.* 2012;70(1):149–153.

Plates 43–45
Baccetti T, Franchi L, McNamara Jr J. The cervical vertebral maturation (CVM) method for the assessment of optimal treatment timing in dentofacial orthopedics. *Semin Orthod.* 2005;11(3):119–129.

San Roman P, Palma JC, Oteo MD, Nevado E. Skeletal maturation determined by cervical vertebrae development. *Eur J Orthod.* 2002;24(3):303–311.

Plate 47
Tubbs RS, Kelly DR, Humphrey ER, et al. The tectorial membrane: anatomical, biomechanical, and histological analysis. *Clin Anat.* 2007;20(4):382–386.

Plates 48, 49, 51–54
Noden DM, Francis-West P. The differentiation and morphogenesis of craniofacial muscles. *Dev Dyn.* 2006;235(5): 1194–1218.

Plate 52
Feigl G. Fascia and spaces on the neck: myths and reality. *Medicina Fluminensis.* 2015;51(4):430–439.

Jain M, Dhall U. Morphometry of the thyroid and cricoid cartilages in adults. *J Anat Soc India.* 2008;57(2):119–123.

Plates 56, 58, 152–158
Chang KV, Lin CP, Hung CY, et al. Sonographic nerve tracking in the cervical region: a pictorial essay and video demonstration. *Am J Phys Med Rehabil.* 2016;95(11):862–870.

Tubbs RS, Salter EG, Oakes WJ. Anatomic landmarks for nerves of the neck: a vade mecum for neurosurgeons. *Neurosurgery.* 2005;56(2 suppl):256–260.

Plate 69
de Miranda CMNR, Maranhão CPM, Padilha IG, et al. Anatomical variations of paranasal sinuses at multislice computed tomography: what to look for. *Radiol Bras.* 2011;44(4): 256–262.

Souza SA, Idagawa M, Wolosker AMB, et al. Computed tomography assessment of the ethmoid roof: a relevant region at risk in endoscopic sinus surgery. *Radiol Bras.* 2008; 41(3):143–147.

Plate 72
Benninger B, Lee BI. Clinical importance of morphology and nomenclature of distal attachment of temporalis tendon. *J Oral Maxillofac Surg.* 2012;70(3):557–561.

Plate 76
Alomar X, Medrano J, Cabratosa J, et al. Anatomy of the temporomandibular joint. *Semin Ultrasound CT MRI.* 2007; 28(3):170–183.

Campos PSF, Reis FP, Aragão JA. Morphofunctional features of the temporomandibular joint. *Int J Morphol.* 2011; 29(4):1394–1397.

Cristo JA, Bennett S, Wilkinson TM, Townsend GC. Discal attachments of the human temporomandibular joint. *Aust Dent J.* 2005;50(3):152–160.

Cuccia AM, Caradonna C, Caradonna D, et al. The arterial blood supply of the temporomandibular joint: an anatomical study and clinical implications. *Imaging Sci Dent.* 2013; 43(1):37–44.

Langdon JD, Berkovitz BKV, Moxham BJ, eds. *Surgical Anatomy of the Infratemporal Fossa.* Martin Dunitz; 2003.

Schmolke C. The relationship between the temporomandibular joint capsule, articular disc and jaw muscles. *J Anat.* 1994;184(Pt 2):335–345.

Siéssere S, Vitti M, de Sousa LG, et al. Bilaminar zone: anatomical aspects, irrigation, and innervation. *Braz J Morphol Sci.* 2004;21(4):217–220.

Plates 77, 87
Benninger B, Kloenne J, Horn JL. Clinical anatomy of the lingual nerve and identification with ultrasonography. *Br J Oral Maxillofac Surg.* 2013;51(6):541–544.

Plate 78
Joo W, Yoshioka F, Funaki T, et al. Microsurgical anatomy of the trigeminal nerve. *Clin Anat.* 2014;27(1):61–88.

Joo W, Funaki T, Yoshioka F, Rhoton Jr AL. Microsurgical anatomy of the infratemporal fossa. *Clin Anat.* 2013;26(4): 455–469.

Plate 84
Fawcett E. The structure of the inferior maxilla, with special reference to the position of the inferior dental canal. *J Anat Physiol.* 1895;29(Pt 3):355–366.

He P, Truong MK, Adeeb N, et al. Clinical anatomy and surgical significance of the lingual foramina and their canals. *Clin Anat.* 2017;30(2):194–204.

Iwanaga J. The clinical view for dissection of the lingual nerve with application to minimizing iatrogenic injury. *Clin Anat.* 2017;30(4):467–469.

Otake I, Kageyama I, Mataga I. Clinical anatomy of the maxillary artery. *Okajimas Folia Anat Jpn.* 2011;87(4):155–164.

Atlas of Human Anatomy

Siéssere S, Vitti M, de Souza LG, et al. Anatomic variation of cranial parasympathetic ganglia. *Braz Oral Res*. 2008; 22(2):101–105.

Plates 96, 122, 123
Kierner AC, Mayer R, v Kirschhofer K. Do the tensor tympani and tensor veli palatini muscles of man form a functional unit? A histochemical investigation of their putative connections. *Hear Res*. 2002;165(1–2):48–52.

Plates 101, 102
Benninger B, Barrett R. A head and neck lymph node classification using an anatomical grid system while maintaining clinical relevance. *J Oral Maxillofac Surg*. 2011;69(10):2670–2673.

Plates 107–109
Ludlow CL. Central nervous system control of the laryngeal muscles in humans. *Respir Physiol Neurobiol*. 2005;147(2–3): 205–222.

Plate 114
Cornelius CP, Mayer P, Ehrenfeld M, Metzger MC. The orbits—anatomical features in view of innovative surgical methods. *Facial Plast Surg*. 2014;30(5):487–508.

Sherman DD, Burkat CN, Lemke BN. Orbital anatomy and its clinical applications. In: Tasman W, Jaeger EA, eds. *Duane's Ophthalmology*. Lippincott Williams & Wilkins; 2006.

Plates 128–141
Rhoton Jr AL. *Congress of Neurological Surgeons. Cranial Anatomy and Surgical Approaches*. Lippincott Williams & Wilkins; 2003.

Plates 131, 167
Tubbs RS, Hansasuta A, Loukas M, et al. Branches of the petrous and cavernous segments of the internal carotid artery. *Clin Anat*. 2007;20(6):596–601.

Plates 143–145, 151
Schrott-Fischer A, Kammen-Jolly K, Scholtz AW, et al. Patterns of GABA-like immunoreactivity in efferent fibers of the human cochlea. *Hear Res*. 2002;174(1–2):75–85.

Plates 186, 199
Tubbs RS, Loukas M, Slappey JB, et al. Clinical anatomy of the C1 dorsal root, ganglion, and ramus: a review and anatomical study. *Clin Anat*. 2007;20(6):624–627.

Plate 192
Bosmia AN, Hogan E, Loukas M, et al. Blood supply to the human spinal cord: part I. Anatomy and hemodynamics. *Clin Anat*. 2015;28(1):52–64.

Plate 193
Stringer MD, Restieaux M, Fisher AL, Crosado B. The vertebral venous plexuses: the internal veins are muscular and external veins have valves. *Clin Anat*. 2012;25(5):609–618.

Plates 198, 199
Tubbs RS, Mortazavi MM, Loukas M, et al. Anatomical study of the third occipital nerve and its potential role in occipital headache/neck pain following midline dissections of the craniocervical junction. *J Neurosurg Spine*. 2011;15(1):71–75.

Vanderhoek MD, Hoang HT, Goff B. Ultrasound-guided greater occipital nerve blocks and pulsed radiofrequency ablation for diagnosis and treatment of occipital neuralgia. *Anesth Pain Med*. 2013;3(2):256–259.

Plates 205–207
Hassiotou F, Geddes D. Anatomy of the human mammary gland: current status of knowledge. *Clin Anat*. 2013;26(1): 29–48.

Plate 223, 224
Hyde DM, Hamid Q, Irvin CG. Anatomy, pathology, and physiology of the tracheobronchial tree: emphasis on the distal airways. *J Allergy Clin Immunol*. 2009;124(6 suppl):S72–S77.

Plate 226
Ikeda S, Ono Y, Miyazawa S, et al. Flexible bronchofiberscope. *Otolaryngology (Tokyo)*. 1970;42(10):855–861.

Plate 239
Angelini P, Velasco JA, Flamm S. Coronary anomalies: incidence, pathophysiology, and clinical relevance. *Circulation*. 2002;105(20):2449–2454.

Plates 239, 240
Chiu IS, Anderson RH. Can we better understand the known variations in coronary arterial anatomy? *Ann Thorac Surg*. 2012;94(5):1751–1760.

Plate 248
James TN. The internodal pathways of the human heart. *Prog Cardiovasc Dis*. 2001;43(6):495–535.

Plates 248–250
Hildreth V, Anderson RH, Henderson DJ. Autonomic innervation of the developing heart: origins and function. *Clin Anat*. 2009;22(1):36–46.

Plate 261
Yang HJ, Gil YC, Lee WJ, et al. Anatomy of thoracic splanchnic nerves for surgical resection. *Clin Anat*. 2008;21(2):171–177.

Plate 304
MacSween RNM, Burt AD, Portmann BC, et al., eds. *Pathology of the Liver*. Churchill Livingstone; 2002.

Robinson PJA, Ward J. *MRI of the Liver: A Practical Guide*. CRC Press; 2006.

Plates 308, 310
Odze RD, Goldblum JR, Crawford JM. *Surgical Pathology of the GI Tract, Liver, Biliary Tract, and Pancreas*. Saunders-Elsevier; 2004.

Plate 327
Thomas MD. *The Ciba Collection of Medical Illustrations.* Vol. 3, Part 2: *Digestive System: Lower* Digestive *Tract.* CIBA; 1970:78.

Plates 343, 368, 385, 398, 416
Stormont TJ, Cahill DR, King BF, Myers RP. Fascias of the male external genitalia and perineum. *Clin Anat.* 1994;7(3):115–124.

Plates 358, 364, 369, 372, 379
Oelrich TM. The striated urogenital sphincter muscle in the female. *Anat Rec.* 1983;205:223–232.

Plochocki JH, Rodriguez-Sosa JR, Adrian B, et al. A functional and clinical reinterpretation of human perineal neuromuscular anatomy: application to sexual function and continence. *Clin Anat.* 2016;29(8):1053–1058.

Plates 362, 368
Myers RP, Goellner JR, Cahill DR. Prostate shape, external striated urethral sphincter and radical prostatectomy: the apical dissection. *J Urol.* 1987;138(3):543–550.

Plates 362, 368, 384, 385
Oelrich TM. The urethral sphincter muscle in the male. *Am J Anat.* 1980;158(2):229–246.

Plate 375
Feil P, Sora MC. A 3D reconstruction model of the female pelvic floor by using plastinated cross sections. *Austin J Anat.* 2014;1(5):1022.

Shin DS, Jang HG, Hwang SB, et al. Two-dimensional sectioned images and three-dimensional surface models for learning the anatomy of the female pelvis. *Anat Sci Educ.* 2013;6(5):316–323.

Plate 405
Nathoo N, Caris EC, Wiener JA, Mendel E. History of the vertebral venous plexus and the significant contributions of Breschet and Batson. *Neurosurgery.* 2011;69(5):1007–1014.

Pai MM, Krishnamurthy A, Prabhu LV, et al. Variability in the origin of the obturator artery. *Clinics (Sao Paulo).* 2009; 64(9):897–901.

Park YH, Jeong CW. Lee SEA comprehensive review of neuroanatomy of the prostate. *Prostate Int.* 2013;1(4):139–145.

Raychaudhuri B, Cahill D. Pelvic fasciae in urology. *Ann R Coll Surg Engl.* 2008;90(8):633–637.

Stoney RA. The anatomy of the visceral pelvic fascia. *J Anat Physiol.* 1904;38(Pt 4):438–447.

Walz J, Burnett AL, Costello AJ, et al. A critical analysis of the current knowledge of surgical anatomy related to optimization of cancer control and preservation of continence and erection in candidates for radical prostatectomy. *Eur Urol.* 2010;57(2):179–192.

Plate 513
Beck M, Sledge JB, Gautier E, et al. The anatomy and function of the gluteus minimus muscle. *J Bone Joint Surg Br.* 2000;82(3):358–363.

Woodley SJ, Mercer SR, Nicholson HD. Morphology of the bursae associated with the greater trochanter of the femur. *J Bone Joint Surg Am.* 2008;90(2):284–294.

Plate 533
Aragão JA, Reis FP, de Figueiredo LFP, et al. The anatomy of the gastrocnemius veins and trunks in adult human cadavers. *J Vasc Br.* 2004;3(4):297–303.

Plate 537
Lee MWL, McPhee RW, Stringer MD. An evidence-based approach to human dermatomes. *Clin Anat.* 2008;21(5): 363–373.

INDEX

References are to plate numbers

A

Abdomen, 2
 bony framework, 268
 L1/L2 disc level, 350
 L3/L4 disc level, 351
 L5 vertebral level, near planum
  intertuberculare, BP80
 paramedian section, 343
 regiones, plana, and lineae, 269
 schema of lymphatic drainage, 344
 surface anatomy, 267
 S1 vertebral level, near spina iliaca anterior
  superior, BP81
 T12/L1 disc level, 349
 T12 vertebral level, BP79
 T12 vertebral level, inferior to processus
  xiphoideus, 348
 T10 vertebral level, through junctio
  oesophagogastrica, 347
Abdominal scans, 345–346
Abductor brevis pollicis, 472, 475, 476, T7.6
Abductor digiti minimi manus, 472, 475, 489,
 T7.6
Abductor digiti minimi pedis, 533, 540, 542,
 544, 545, 546, 547, 549, T8.7
Abductor hallucis, 540, 542, 544, 545, 546, 549,
 BP111, T8.7
Abductor longus pollicis, 451, 454, 455, 458,
 459, 460, 461, 489, T7.6
Acetabulum, 354, 357, 495, BP104
Acinus pulmonis, 226, BP44
Acne appears, BP95
Acromion, 203, 209, 422, 427, 430, 431, 432,
 434, 436, 437, 438, 440, 490
Adductor brevis, 503, 510, 515, 551, T8.7
Adductor hallucis, T8.7
Adductor longus, 502, 509, 510, 515, 551,
 BP104, T8.7
Adductor magnus, 415, 491, 498, 499, 504, 510,
 511, 513, 515, T8.7
Adductor minimus, 415, 504, 513
Adductor pollicis, 473, 475, 476, 487, BP100,
 BP101, T7.6
Adhaesio interthalamica, 138, 174
Adipocytia, BP11
Aditus laryngis, 93
Adnexa uteri, 374
Adrenal cortices, BP95
Affluens acromialis v. thoracoacromialis, 424
Affluens oesophageus v. gastricae sinistrae,
 315
Affluentes pubicus v. epigastricae inferioris,
 280
Affluentes v. anorectalis superioris, 317
Agger nasi, 61
Ala major ossis sphenoidei, 25, 28
Ala minor ossis sphenoidei, 25, 26
Ala nasi, 22
Ala ossis ilium, 268, 353, 361, 495, 555
Ala ossis sacri, 354, BP81
Alveoli pulmonis, BP44
Ampulla ductus deferentis, 385, 391
Ampulla hepatopancreatica, 305
Ampulla tubae uterinae, 374, 376
Ampullae membranaceae, 125
Anastomosis aa. gastroomentalium, 291
Angulus acromii, 427
Angulus inferior scapulae, 178, 427
Angulus mandibulae, 22, 26, 39, 93
Angulus sterni (Louisi), T4.1
Angulus subpubicus, 354
Angulus superior scapulae, 427
Annular hymen, BP91

Ansa cervicalis, 57
Ansa nephri, BP72, BP73
Ansa pectoralis, 438
Ansa subclavia, 229, 249, 250
Antebrachium
 arteriae, BP97
 serial cross sections, 461
 venae superficiales, 425
Anterior tributaries of V. vorticosa, 120
 anterior views, 509
 anterior view of deeper dissection, 510
Anterolateral fasciculus, BP40
Antihelix, 22, 122
Antitragus, 22, 122
Antrum folliculare, BP90
Anulus femoralis, 280, 363, 366, 367, 494, T5.1
Anulus fibrosus dexter, 248
Anulus fibrosus, 181
Anulus inguinalis profundus, 272, 274, 280,
 363, 365, 366, 367, 387, BP53, T5.1
Anulus inguinalis superficialis, 270, 280, 281,
 378, 387, 388, BP53, BP54, T5.1
Anulus lymphaticus cardiae, BP74
Anus, 360, 364, 377, 389, 397
Aorta, 190, 247, 283, 328, 344
Aorta abdominalis, 200, 216, 284, 289, 292,
 293, 294, 296, 308, 310, 324, 332, 336, 337,
 341, 343, 345, 346, 349, 350, 351, 363, 365,
 367, 400, 402, 403, 405, 414, BP50, BP79,
 BP82, BP93, T5.2
Aorta ascendens, 238, 241, 244, 245, 248, 262
Aorta descendens, 14, 215, 227, 258, 345, 347,
 348
Aorta thoracica, 192, 212, T4.3
Apertura ductus nasofrontalis, 67
Apertura externa canaliculi vestibuli, 34
Apertura lateralis, 136
Apertura mediana ventriculi quarti, 135
Apertura sinus maxillaris, 62, 67
Apertura sinus sphenoidei, 61, 67
Apertura superior thoracis, 213, T4.1
Apex, 221, 369
Apex capitis fibulae, 524
Apex ossis coccygis, 352, 355, 360, 362, 381,
 383, 397
Apex patellae, BP107
Apex prostatae, 385
Apex pulmonis, 217, 218, 234, T4.3
Aponeuroses extensoriae manus, BP102
Aponeuroses extensoriae pedis, 542, 547
Aponeurosis bicipitalis, 440, 442, 456
Aponeurosis epicranialis, 199, BP19
Aponeurosis glutea, 275, 501, 504
Aponeurosis m. obliqui externi abdominis,
 271, 272, 273, 282, 378, BP53
Aponeurosis m. obliqui interni abdominis,
 272, 273, 278, 351
Aponeurosis m. transversi abdominis, 273,
 275, 331, 351
Aponeurosis palmaris, 425, 452, 456, 464, 469,
 473, T7.1
Aponeurosis plantaris, 540, 543, 544, 545, 546,
 549, 556, T8.2
Apparatus lacrimalis, 111
Apparatus pilosebaceus, BP1
Appendices omentales, 290, 301, 351
Appendix epididymidis, 388, 390
Appendix testis, 388, 390, 391, 392
Appendix vermiformis, 290, 298, 299, 300, 301,
 BP57, BP81, T5.2
 coronal CT image, MRCP, BP57
Appendix vesiculosa, 374, 390
Aquaeductus mesencephali (Sylvii), 136, 177,
 T2.1
Arachnoidea cranialis, 127, 136
Arachnoidea spinalis, 189, 190

Arbor tracheobronchialis, 226, 230
Arcus anterior atlantis, 28, 45, 177, BP34,
 BP35, BP39
Arcus aortae, 14, 17, 103, 217, 232, 233, 234,
 235, 242, 253, 258
Arcus arteriosi ileales, 297, 313
Arcus arteriosi jejunales, 313
Arcus arteriosus jejunalis, 297
Arcus arteriosus omentalis, BP83
Arcus costalis, 288
Arcus ductus thoracici, 220
Arcus palatoglossus, 83, 89
Arcus palatopharyngeus, 83, 89, 93
Arcus palmaris profundus, 443, 475, BP97
Arcus palmaris superficialis, 443, 470, 472,
 476, 483, BP97
Arcus plantaris, 14, 522, 546, 547, BP105
Arcus posterior atlantis, BP18, BP35
Arcus pubicus, 353, 355
Arcus superciliaris, 22
Arcus tendineus fasciae pelvis, 366, 369, 371,
 373
Arcus tendineus levatoris ani, 283, 358, 359,
 360, 361, 362, 366, 369, 371, 372, 373, 379,
 394
Arcus tendineus m. solei, 528, 529
Arcus v. azygae, BP50
Arcus venosi ileales, 316
Arcus venosi jejunales, 316
Arcus venosus dorsalis pedis, 15, 492, 533
Arcus venosus palmaris profundus, 444
Arcus venosus palmaris superficialis, 15, 444
Arcus vertebrarum, 185
Arcus zygomaticus, 26, 36, 38
Areola mammae, 205
Arrector pili, 12, BP1
Arteria, BP13
 zonula avascularis, BP13
 zonula vascularis, BP13
A. anastomotica intercolica, BP68
A. angularis, 60
A. anorectalis inferior, 314, 400, 404, 405, 406,
 407, BP93
A. anorectalis media, 314, 366, 400, 402, 404,
 405, BP93
A. anorectalis superior, 314, 400, 402
A. anterior cerebri, 163, BP31
A. appendicularis, 298, 313, 314, BP60
A. arcuata, 522, 532, 541, 542, 547, BP105
A. auricularis posterior, 163, 199
A. axillaris, 14, 206, 276, 435, 437, 442, 443,
 BP96
A. basilaris, 163, 166, 176, 177, 191, BP31, BP32
A. brachialis, 206, 437, 440, 442, 443, 445, 456,
 457, 458, 483, BP96, BP97, T7.2
A. bronchialis inferior, 222
A. bronchialis, 221, 222
A. bulbi penis, 384, 407
A. bulbi vestibuli, 372, 406
A. caecalis anterior, 313, 314
A. caecalis posterior, 298, 313, 314
A. caudae pancreatis, 309, 310
A. cervicalis ascendens, 57, 103, 191, 437
A. cervicalis profunda, 163, 191
A. chorioidea anterior, 164, 166
A. ciliaris posterior longa, 120
A. circumflexa anterior humeri, 438, 440, 442,
 443, BP96
A. circumflexa fibularis, 522, BP103
A. circumflexa iliaca profunda, 510, 522, BP103
A. circumflexa iliaca superficialis, 272, 509,
 522, BP103
A. circumflexa lateralis femoris, 510, 514, 522,
 BP103
A. circumflexa medialis femoris, 510, 511, 514,
 522, BP103

A. circumflexa posterior humeri, 437, 438, 441, 442, 443, BP96
A. circumflexa profunda ilium, 274
A. circumflexa scapulae, 437, 438, 440, 443, BP96
A. circumflexa superficialis ilium, 276, 284
A. colica dextra, 313, 314, BP68
  aberrant, BP69
A. colica media, 309, 310, 313, 314, 343, BP68, BP69
A. colica sinistra, 284, 314, 400, BP68
A. colicae sinistrae, 314
A. collateralis media, 441, 443, 445, 455, BP96
A. collateralis radialis, 441, 443, 445, BP96
A. collateralis ulnaris inferior, 442, 443, 455, BP96, BP97
A. collateralis ulnaris superior, 442, 443, 445, 454, 455, BP96, BP97
A. communicans anterior, 163, 166, 176, BP31
A. communicans posterior, 163, 164, 166
A. coronaria dextra, 239, 240, 243, BP46
A. coronaria sinistra, BP46
A. cremasterica, 272, 274, 282, 284, 403
A. cystica, 305, 308, 310, BP64, BP83, T5.2
  variations, BP64
A. descendens genus, 510, 515, 522, BP103, BP105
A. digitalis dorsalis, 481
A. digitalis palmaris communis, 470, 473
A. digitalis palmaris propria, 470, 481
A. digitalis palmaris, 443, BP97
A. dorsalis clitoridis, 377, 406
A. dorsalis nasi, 60
A. dorsalis pedis, 14, 522, 532, 542, 547, BP105, BP111
A. dorsalis penis, 382, 403, 405, 407, BP93
A. dorsalis scapulae, 57, 194, 437, 438
A. ductus deferentis, 388, 400, 403, 405, BP93
A. epigastrica inferior, 272, 274, 276, 280, 284, 336, 363, 366, 373, 375, 402, 403, 405, 522, BP93, BP103
A. epigastrica superficialis, 272, 276, 284, 509, 522, BP53, BP103
A. epigastrica superior, 272
A. facialis, 14, 60
A. femoralis, 14, 276, 284, 403, 409, 420, 421, 514, 515, 522, BP94, BP103, BP105, T8.2
A. fibularis, 14, 522, 528, 529, 533, BP103, BP105, BP106
A. gastrica dextra, 297, 305, 308, 309, 310, 325, BP64, BP83
A. gastrica sinistra, 258, 291, 308, 309, 310, 311, 325, BP65, BP79, BP83
A. gastroduodenalis, 297, 305, 308, 309, 310, 311, 312, 313, 325, BP64, BP65, BP83
A. gastroomentalis, 291, 308, 309, 310, 312, 313, 325, BP83
A. glutea inferior, 284, 336, 400, 404, 405, 420, 511, BP93
A. glutea superior, 284, 336, 400, 404, 405, BP93
A. hepatica communis, 291, 297, 305, 308, 309, 310, 311, 312, 313, 325, 328, BP64, BP79, BP83
A. hepatica dextra, 305, 308, 310, BP64, BP65
A. hepatica propria, 292, 293, 296, 297, 302, 303, 305, 306, 308, 309, 310, 311, 312, 343, 348, BP64
A. hepatica sinistra, 305, 308, 310, BP64, BP65
A. hypophysialis inferior, 164
A. hypophysialis superior, 164
A. ileocolica, 313, 314, BP60, BP68, BP69
A. iliaca communis, 14, 293, 330, 335, 336, 373, 400, 402, 403, 414, BP93
A. iliaca externa sin., 405
A. iliaca externa, 14, 284, 293, 317, 330, 335, 364, 365, 368, 376, 400, 402, 403, 405, 522, BP81, BP90, BP93, BP103

A. iliaca interna, 14, 284, 314, 330, 335, 336, 373, 375, 400, 402, 403, 405, BP81, BP93
A. iliolumbalis, 284, 336, 404, 405, BP93
A. inferior anterior cerebelli, 163, 166, 191
A. inferior lateralis genus, 528, 529, 531, BP103
A. inferior medialis genus, 509, 510, 528, 529, 531, 532, BP103, BP105
A. inferior posterior cerebelli, 166
A. intercostalis posterior, 191, 192, 212, 436
A. intercostalis suprema, 163
A. intercostalis, 205
A. interlobularis, 304
A. interossea anterior, 443, 455, 457, 458, BP96, BP97
A. interossea communis, 443, 457, 458, 461, BP96, BP97
A. interossea posterior, 443, 455, 458, BP96, BP97
A. interossea recurrens, 443, 455, BP96, BP97
A. labialis posterior, 406
A. labyrinthi, 166
A. laryngea superior, 103, 163
A. lingualis, 163
A. lumbalis, 191
A. malleolaris anterior lateralis, 542, BP105
A. malleolaris anterior medialis, 522, 532, 542, BP105
A. marginalis coli, 314, 400, BP69, T5.2
A. masseterica, 73
A. media cerebri, 163, 176, BP31, BP32
A. media genus, 522, BP103, BP105
A. medullaris segmentalis, 191, 192
A. meningea media, 42, 73, 74, T2.4
A. meningea posterior, 163
A. mesenterica inferior, 14, 284, 289, 296, 314, 332, 336, 400, 402, 403, BP68
A. mesenterica superior, 14, 200, 247, 284, 289, 294, 309, 310, 311, 312, 313, 314, 316, 325, 329, 332, 343, 350, BP64, BP65, BP68, BP69, T5.2
A. metatarsea plantaris, 544
A. musculophrenica, 219, 231
A. nutricia femoris, 514
A. nutricia, 481
A. obturatoria accessoria, 400
A. obturatoria, 280, 284, 336, 366, 373, 400, 402, 404, 405, 412, 496, 514, 522, BP90, BP93, BP94, BP103
A. occipitalis, 163, 199
A. ophthalmica, 163, T2.4
A. ovarica, 336, 366, 402, 406
A. pancreatica dorsalis, 308, 309, 310, 312, 313, BP69
A. pancreatica inferior, 309, 310, 312, 313, BP83
A. pancreatica magna, 309, 310, 312
A. pancreaticoduodenalis, 291
A. pancreaticoduodenalis inferior, 309, 310, 312, 313, 314, BP83
A. pancreaticoduodenalis inferior anterior, 310, 312, 313, 325
A. pancreaticoduodenalis inferior posterior, 310, 312, 313, 325
A. pancreaticoduodenalis superior anterior, 309, 310, 312, 313, 325, BP83
A. pancreaticoduodenalis superior posterior, 309, 310, 312, 313, BP83
A. perforans 1 femoris, 511
A. perforans 2 femoris, 511
A. perforans 3 femoris, 511
A. perforans 4 femoris, 511
A. pericardiacophrenica, 276
A. perinealis, 372, 384, 405, 406, 407, BP93
A. pharyngea ascendens, 163
A. phrenica inferior, 216, 291, 293, 332, BP83
A. plantaris lateralis, 529, 545, 546, 547
A. plantaris medialis, 529, 546
A. plantaris profunda, 522, 532, 541, 542, 547, BP105

A. poplitea, 14, 522, 529, BP103, BP105
A. posterior cerebri, 163, 191, BP31
A. prepancreatica, 310, 312
A. princeps pollicis, 443, BP97
A. profunda brachii, 438, 441, 442, 443, 445, BP96
A. profunda clitoridis, 377, 406
A. profunda femoris, 14, 421, 509, 510, 514, 522, BP103
A. profunda penis, 382, 384, 386, 407
A. pudendalis externa profunda, 276, 284, 509, 522, BP103
A. pudendalis externa superficialis, 272, 276, 284, 509, BP103
A. pudendalis interna, 284, 336, 384, 400, 404, 405, 406, 407, 420, 421, BP93, BP94
A. pudendalis, 405
A. pulmonalis dextra, 235, 241, 242, 247
A. pulmonalis sinistra, 232, 233, 235, 242, 247
A. radialis indicis, 443, BP97
A. radialis, 442, 443, 455, 456, 457, 458, 461, 464, 472, 475, 476, 477, 479, 483, BP96, BP97, T7.2
A. radicularis anterior, 192
A. radicularis posterior, 192
A. rectalis media, 284
A. rectalis superior, 284
A. recurrens radialis, 443, 457, 458, BP96, BP97
A. recurrens tibialis anterior, 532, BP103, BP105
A. recurrens tibialis posterior, 522, 529, BP103, BP105
A. recurrens ulnaris anterior, 443, 457, 458, BP96, BP97
A. recurrens ulnaris posterior, 443, 455, BP96, BP97
A. renalis, 14, 284, 311, 325, 332, 333, 334, 350, 402, 403, 419, BP70, T5.2
A. retinacularis anterior, 514
A. retinacularis inferior, 514
A. retinacularis superior, 514
A. sacralis lateralis, 336, 405, BP93
A. sacralis mediana, 284, 314, 336, 365, 366, 400, 402, 404, 405, BP93
A. scrotales anteriores, 405
A. segmenti anterioris inferioris renis, 334
A. segmenti inferioris renis, 334
A. segmenti posterioris renis, 334
A. segmenti superioris renis, 334
A. spinalis anterior, 166, 191, 192
A. spinalis posterior, 166
A. splenica, 293, 307, 308, 309, 310, 311, 312, 313, 325, 328, 329, BP65, BP83
A. striata longa, 166
A. subclavia, 14, 163, 191, 206, 258, 276, 437, BP24
A. subcostalis, 284
A. subscapularis, 437, 438, 443, BP96
A. subcutanea, 12
A. superior cerebelli, 163, 166, 176, 191
A. superior lateralis genus, 511, 522, 527, 528, 529, 530, 531, 532, BP103, BP105
A. superior medialis genus, 509, 510, 511, 522, 527, 528, 529, 531, 532, BP103, BP105
A. supraduodenalis, 308, 309, 310, 312, 313
A. supraorbitalis, 24, 60
A. suprarenalis inferior, 284, 332, 342
A. suprarenalis media, 284, 332, 342
A. suprarenalis superior, 216
A. suprascapularis, 57, 103, 436, 437, 438, T7.2
A. supratrochlearis, 24, 60
A. tarsea lateralis, 522, 532, 541, 547, BP105
A. tarsea medialis, 522, 532, 541, 547, BP105
A. temporalis media, 24
A. temporalis superficialis, 60, 76
A. testicularis, 280, 282, 284, 293, 388, 405, BP93, BP104
A. thoracica interna, 206, 212, 215, 231, 437, T4.2

Atlas of Human Anatomy

A. thoracica lateralis, 206, 209, 276, 436, 437, 438, 443, BP96
A. thoracica superior, 436, 437, 438, 443, BP96
A. thoracoacromialis, 435, 437, 443
A. thoracodorsalis, 437, 438, 443, BP96
A. thyreoidea inferior, 57, 103, 105, 163, 249, 258, 437, T2.4
A. thyreoidea superior, 163
A. tibialis anterior, 14, 522, 532, 533, 541, 542, BP103, BP105, BP106, BP109, BP110
A. tibialis posterior, 14, 527, 528, 529, 533, 545, BP103, BP105, BP106, BP110
A. transversa colli, 57, 103, 437, 438
A. transversa faciei, 24, 60
A. transversa perinei, 407
A. ulnaris, 442, 443, 456, 457, 458, 461, 464, 469, 470, 472, 475, 476, 483, BP96, BP97, T7.2
A. umbilicalis, 274, 336, 373, 400, BP93
A. urethralis, 384, 407
A. uterina, 336, 366, 375, 376, 402, 404, 406, T6.2
A. vaginalis, 335, 366, 369, 372, 375, 376, 402, 404, 406
A. vertebralis, 57, 166, 191, 194, 249, BP18, BP31, BP39, BP50
A. vesicalis inferior, 284, 366, 369, 400, 402, 403, 405, BP93
A. vesicalis superior, 274, 366, 400, 404, 405, BP93
A. zygomaticoorbitalis, 24
Arteriae, 60, 163, 165
Aa. anastomoticae scapulae, 437
Aa. arcuatae, 334
Aa. bronchiales, 222
Aa. centrales anterolaterales, 164, 166
Aa. ciliares anteriores, 120
Aa. colicae, BP68, BP69
Aa. coronariae, 239, BP47, T4.2
  imaging, 240
  right anterolateral views with arteriograms, BP46
Aa. digitales dorsales manus, 479
Aa. digitales dorsales pedis, 522, 541, 542, 547, BP105
Aa. digitales palmares, 469
Aa. digitales palmares communes, 443, 475, 476, BP97
Aa. digitales palmares propriae, 443, 470, 543, 544, 547, BP97
Aa. encephali, 168
Aa. epicraniales, T2.4
Aa. epigastricae superiores, 276
Aa. femoralis, T8.2
Aa. gastricae breves, 308, 309, 325, BP83
Aa. hepaticae, BP65
Aa. hepaticae dextra, BP83
Aa. hepaticae media, BP83
Aa. hepaticae sinistra, BP83
Aa. ileales, 313, 314, 316
Aa. iliacae communes, 284, 405, BP38
Aa. intercostales, 212, BP83
Aa. intercostales anteriores, 276
Aa. intercostales posteriores, 212
Aa. interlobares, 334
Aa. interlobulares, 334
Aa. intestinales, T5.2
Aa. intrarenales, 334
Aa. jejunales, 313, 314, 316
Aa. labiales inferior, 60
Aa. labiales superior, 60
Aa. majores, 14
Aa. manus, 476
Aa. medullae spinalis, T3.1
Aa. medullares segmentales, 191
Aa. membri inferioris, 522, T8.2
Aa. meningeae, 128
Aa. metacarpeae dorsales, 479

Aa. metacarpeae palmares, 443, 475, BP97
Aa. metatarseae dorsales, 532, 547, BP105
Aa. metatarseae plantares, 546, 547
Aa. musculophrenicae, 276
Aa. nutriciae, 481
Aa. omentales, BP83
Aa. perforantes femoris, 510, 522, BP103
Aa. phrenicae inferiores, 258, 308, 309
Aa. pontis, 166
Aa. profundae pedis, 547
Aa. pulmonales, T4.2
Aa. rectae, 297, 313, 314
Aa. retinaculares, 514
Aa. sacrales laterales, 404
Aa. scrotales posteriores, 405, 407, BP93
Aa. sigmoideae, 284, 314, 400
Aa. spinales posteriores, 192
Aa. suprarenales superiores, 284, 332
Aa. tarseae mediales, 542
Aa. testiculares, 284
Aa. thoracicae internae, 276, BP83
Aa. umblicales, 247
Aa. vesicales superiores, 336, 402
Aa .vertebrales, 194
Arteriola glomerularis afferens, BP71, BP72
Arteriola glomerularis efferens, BP71, BP72, BP73
Arteriola intralobularis hepatis, 304
Arteriola periportalis hepatis, 304
Arteriola portalis hepatis, 304
Arteriolae, 481
Articulatio acromioclavicularis, 431, 434
Articulatio atlantoaxialis lateralis, 45, 46, BP34
Articulatio atlantoaxialis mediana, 45
Articulatio atlantooccipitalis, BP18
Articulatio carpometacarpea, 463
Articulatio carpometacarpea pollicis, BP98
Articulatio costotransversaria, 263
Articulatio coxae, 496, T8.1
  anteroposterior radiograph, 497
Articulatio interphalangea, 539
Articulatio interphalangea distalis, 422, 467, 468
Articulatio interphalangea proximalis, 422, 467, 468
Articulatio mediocarpea, 463, 465
Articulatio metacarpophalangea, 422, 467, 468
Articulatio metatarsophalangea, 539, T8.1
Articulatio radiocarpea, 463, 465
Articulatio radioulnaris distalis, 465
Articulatio sacroiliaca, 354, 355, 361, T6.1
Articulatio sternochondralis, 429
Articulatio sternoclavicularis, 217
Articulatio talocruralis, T8.1
Articulatio temporomandibularis, 42, T2.2
Articulatio uncovertebralis, BP34
Articulationes carpometacarpeae, 465
Articulationes intermetacarpeae, 465
Articulationes uncovertebrales, 44, 45
Asterion, T2.2
Atonic stomach, BP55
Atria, 245
Atrium dextrum, 233, 234, 235, 238, 241, BP50
Atrium meatus medii nasi, 61
Atrium sinistrum, 234, 235, 241, 242
Auricula, 28
Auricula dextra cordis, 241, 245
Auricula sinistra cordis, 233, 239
Auris, 121, BP29
Auris externa, 122
Auris interna, 124
  labyrinths orientation, 126
Axilla
  anterior view, 438
  posterior wall, 433
Axillary hair appears, BP95
Axolemma, BP3
Axon, BP3

Axoplasma, BP3
  deeper dissection, 510
  frontal view and section, 168
  imaging, 240
  inferior views, 166
  intrinsic distribution, 192
  lateral and medial views, 169
  posterior view, 511
  rami of arteria vertebralis and arteria basilaris, 170
  right anterolateral views with arteriograms, BP46
  schema, 191

B

Ball-and socket joint, 9
Basis cordis, 235
Basis cranii
  foramina and canales (inferior view), 33
  foramina and canales (superior view), 34
  inferior view, 31
  nervi and vasa sanguinea, 82
  superior view, 32
Basis mandibulae, 39
Basis ossis 5 metatarsi, 556
Basis patellae, BP107
Basis prostatae, 385
Basis pyramidis renalis, 333
Basis stapedis, 121, 125
Bifurcatio tracheae, BP36, T4.3
Blood clot, 365
Body contours rounded, BP95
Brachial plexus, T7.3–T7.4
Brachium
  arteriae, BP96
  serial cross sections, 445
Bregma, 30
Bridging vein, 127, 136, BP31
Bronchi, 7, 226
Bronchi intrapulmonales, 225
Bronchi majores, 225
Bronchi segmentales
  lingulae, 225
  lobi inferioris, 225
  lobi medii, 225
  lobi superioris, 225
Bronchioli, 226
Bronchioli respiratorii, 227
Bronchiolus terminalis, 227, BP44
Bronchus intermedius, 221
Bronchus principalis, 222, 253
Bucinator, 48, 73, BP19, T2.14
Bulbi olfactorii, 69
Bulbus inferior v. jugularis internae, 194
Bulbus oculi, 6, 7, 117, BP27
  transverse section, 116
  vasa sanguinea externa, 120
  vasa sanguinea interna, 119
Bulbus penis, 383, 384, 386
Bulbus pili, BP1
Bulbus superior v. jugularis internae, 194
Bulbus v. vorticosae, 120
Bulbus vestibuli, 371, 372, 379, 406, BP86
Bursa anserina, 517
Bursa iliopectinea, 496
Bursa infrapatellaris profunda, 521
Bursa intermedia manus, 471
Bursa ischiadica m. glutei maximi, 513
Bursa ischiadica obturatoris interni, 513
Bursa lig. collateralis fibularis, 516, 518, 521
Bursa m. piriformis, 513
Bursa m. semimembranosi, 516, 520
Bursa omentalis, 292, 302, 343, BP79
  cross section, 292
  gaster reflected, 291
Bursa subacromialis, 440

Bursa subcutanea infrapatellaris, 521
Bursa subcutanea malleoli lateralis, 540
Bursa subcutanea malleoli medialis, 540
Bursa subcutanea olecrani, 448
Bursa subcutanea prepatellaris, 521
Bursa subdeltoidea, 431
Bursa subtendinea calcanea, 530, 540
Bursa superior m. bicipitis femoris, 513
Bursa suprapatellaris, 517, 518, 521
Bursa tractus iliotibialis, 518
Bursa trochanterica m. glutei maximi, 513
Bursae coxae, 513

C

Caecum, 288, 298, 299, 300, 301, 363, 367,
    BP57, BP80, BP81
    arterial supply and posterior peritoneal
        attachment variations, BP61
    as site of referred visceral pain, BP5
Calcaneus, 535, 536, 537, 540, 556, BP110,
    T8.1
Calcar avis, 139
Calices renales majores, 333
Calices renales minores, 333
Calix renalis major, 350
Calvaria, 30
Calyculi gustatorii, 89
Camera anterior, 118
Camera posterior, 118
Canales radicum dentis, 41
Canaliculi biliferi, 304
Canaliculus cochleae, 125
Canaliculus mastoideus, 33
Canaliculus tympanicus, 33
Canalis adductorius, 515, 523
Canalis analis, 395, T6.2
    arteriae of, 400
    female, 401
    male, 400
    venae of, 401
Canalis carotidis, 33, 34
Canalis carpi release, BP100
Canalis cervicis uteri, 374
Canalis condylaris, 34
Canalis digestorius, 21
Canalis incisivus, 61
Canalis inguinalis, 281, 282, BP104
Canalis n. hypoglossi, 34
Canalis obturatorius, 357, 358, 359, 361, 366,
    369, 510, BP90
Canalis opticus, 25, 34
Canalis pudendalis, 400, 407, 413
Canalis pyloricus, 348
Canalis sacralis, 361
Canalis semicircularis anterior, 125
Canalis semicircularis lateralis, 125
Canalis semicircularis posterior, 125
Canalis vertebralis, 180, 181, 345
Capitulum humeri, 427, 446, 447
Capsula adiposa perirenalis, 337, 350
Capsula art. atlantooccipitalis, 46
Capsula art. coxae, 514
Capsula art. cubiti, 448
Capsula art. genus, 516, 531
Capsula art. glenohumeralis, 441
Capsula art. metatarsophalangeae, 539
Capsula art. radiocarpeae, BP98
Capsula art. temporomandibularis, 42
Capsula articularis, 468
Capsula fibrosa perivascularis, 303, 304
Capsula fibrosa renis, 333, 337, BP72
Capsula fibrosa splenis, 307
Capsula glomerularis, BP71
Capsula prostatae, 371
Capsula prostatae, BP92
Capsulae articulares, BP111

Caput, 2–3, 22
    arteriae, 99
    nervi autonomici, 158
    nodi lymphoidei, 101
    skeleton, 36
    venae, 100
Caput breve m. bicipitis brachii, 433
Caput breve m. bicipitis femoris, 415, 552
Caput claviculare m. sternocleidomastoidei,
    22, 49, 202
Caput costae, BP42
Caput epididymidis, 388
Caput fibulae, 501, 502, 503, 516, 517, 519, 521,
    524, 525, 528, 529, 530, 531, 554
Caput humerale flexoris ulnaris carpi, 460
Caput humeri, 427, 430, 490
Caput laterale cremasteris, 271, 280, BP53
Caput laterale flexoris brevis hallucis, 544, 546
Caput laterale m. gastrocnemii, 491, 501, 511,
    526, 527, 528, 529, 533
Caput laterale m. tricipitis brachii, 432, 436,
    437, 441
Caput longum m. bicipitis, T8.2
Caput longum m. bicipitis brachii, 432, 433,
    436, T7.1
Caput longum m. bicipitis femoris, 415, 512,
    515, 552
Caput longum m. tricipitis brachii, 178, 422,
    432, 433, 436, 437, 441
Caput mandibulae, 39
Caput mediale cremasteris, 271, 280, BP53
Caput mediale flexoris brevis hallucis, 544, 546
Caput mediale m. gastrocnemii, 491, 521, 527,
    529, 531, 533
Caput mediale m. tricipitis brachii, 433, 441, 460
Caput nuclei caudati, 139
Caput obliquum adductoris hallucis, 546, 547,
    BP111
Caput ossis 2 metacarpi, BP101
Caput ossis 3 metacarpi, BP102
Caput ossis 5 metacarpi, 467, BP101
Caput ossis femoris, 354, 420, 496, 497, 500,
    514, 555, BP94, BP104
Caput pancreatis, 291, 294, 296, 297, 305, 312,
    345, 349
Caput profundum flexoris brevis pollicis, 487
Caput profundum pronatoris teretis, 450, 458,
    486
Caput radiale flexoris superficialis digitorum,
    457, 461
Caput radii, 440, 446, 447, 449
Caput sternale m. sternocleidomastoidei, 22,
    49, 202
Caput superficiale pronatoris teretis, 458, 459, 486
Caput transversum adductoris hallucis, 546
Caput ulnae, 453
Caput ulnare flexoris ulnaris carpi, 460
Cardia, 295
Carina tracheae, BP50
Carotides, 58
Carotis communis, 14, 24, 57, 103, 162, 211, 214,
    219, 220, 231, 232, 235, 238, 254, 258, T2.4
Carotis externa, 24, 103
Carotis interna, 24, 33, 103, 163, 166, 176, 177,
    BP31, BP32, T2.4
Carpi, BP100
Carpus
    arteriae, 472
    cutaneous innervation, 482
    deeper palmar dissections, 470
    nervi, 472
    radiographs, 467
    superficial dorsal dissection, 478
    superficial lateral dissection, 477
    superficial palmar dissections, 469
    tendines extensoris, 480
    tendines flexoris, 472

Cartilagines articulares, 448, 521
Cartilagines costales, 203, 268, 347, 429
Cartilagines laryngeae, T2.2
Cartilagines laryngis, 106
Cartilagines tracheales, 225
Cartilago articularis, 481, 496, BP102
Cartilago arytenoidea, 106
Cartilago corniculata, 106
Cartilago costalis, 1, 7, 215, 237, 429, 432,
    BP79
Cartilago cricoidea, 36, 49, 103, 106, 217,
    220
Cartilago epiglottica, 36, 106
Cartilago thyreoidea, 22, 36, 49, 50, 217, 220,
    225
Cartilago trachealis, 36
Cartilago triticea, 106
Caruncula hymenalis, 372, 377
Caruncula lacrimalis, 110
Caruncula sublingualis, 83
Cauda equina, 182, 186, BP38, T3.1
Cauda nuclei caudati, 139
Cauda pancreatis, 291, 307, 330, BP82
Caudalis, as term of relationship, 1
Cavitas abdominis, BP2
Cavitas articularis, 481
Cavitas cranii, BP2
Cavitas nasalis cranii, 37
    arteriae (septum nasalis turned up), BP21
    nervi (septum nasalis turned up), 66
Cavitas nasi, 65, 68
    autonomic innervation, 80
    nervi, 64
    vasa saguinea, 65
Cavitas oris, 18, 65, 84, BP26
    inspection, 83
Cavitas pelvis, BP2
    female, 363
    male, 367
Cavitas pericardiaca, 236
Cavitas pleuralis, 237, BP2
Cavitas thoracis, BP2
Cavitas tunicae vaginalis testis, 387
Cavitas tympani, 122, 123, 125
    medial and lateral views, BP28
Cavitas vertebralis, BP2
Cavitates art. sternoclavicularis, 429
Cavitates articulares, BP33
Cavitates majores corporis humani, BP2
Cavum septi pellucidi, 139
Celiac arteriogram, 311
Cellulae ethmoideae, 26, 67, 69
Cellulae mastoideae, 26
Centrum tendineum diaphragmatis, 215, 216,
    253, 283, 343
Cerebellum, 141–142, 177, BP35
Cervix uteri, 364, 365, 366, 372, 373, 374, 375,
    BP90, T6.3
Cervix vesicae, 369, 371, 373, BP86
Chiasma opticum, 164, 174, 177
Choana, 61
Choana cranii, 38
Choanae, 93
Chorda folliculogenica, 365
Chorda genitalis, 390
Chorda obliqua, 449
Chordae tendineae, 244, 246
Chorioidea, 116, 118
Cilia, 110
Cingulum pectorale, 8
Circulus arteriosus cerebri (Willisi), 167, T2.4
Cisterna chiasmatica, 136
Cisterna chyli, 16, 286, 344, BP76
Cisterna interpeduncularis, 136
Cisterna lumbalis spatii subarachnoidalis
    spinalis, BP80
Cisterna prepontis, 136

Clavicula, 48, 49, 202, 203, 204, 205, 238, 422, 427, 428, 429, 430, 432, 433, 435, 437, 490, BP34, T7.1
Claviculae, 429, T4.1
Clitoris, 379, 380, 397
Clivus, 177, BP35
CM joint radial styloid process, BP99
Cochleocyte internum, 125
Cochleocytia externa, 125
Colliculus axonalis, BP3
Colliculus seminalis, 371, 385, BP92
Colliculus superior, 143
Collum, 2–3, 22
    arteriae, 99
    nervi autonomici, 157
    nodi lymphoidei, 101
    skeleton, 36
    venae, 100
Collum anatomicum humeri, 427
Collum chirurgicum humeri, 263, 427, 490
Collum costae, 203, BP42
Collum fibulae, 524, BP107
Collum glandis penis, 383
Collum mandibulae, 39
Collum ossis femoris, 354, 420, 421, 496, 497, 500, 555, BP94, T8.1
Collum radii, 446, 447, 449
Collum scapulae, 203, 427, 430
Colon, T5.3
Colon ascendens, 288, 290, 296, 301, 331, 350, 351, 363, 367
Colon descendens, 6, 7, 290, 296, 301, 337, 346, 350, 363, BP80, BP81
Colon sigmoideum, 6, 7, 288, 290, 301, 363, 365, 367, 375, 393, 394, 395, 396, 414
    as site of referred visceral pain, BP5
    variations in position, BP60
Colon transversum, 288, 289, 290, 292, 296, 301, 305, 307, 316, 343, 348, 349, 350, 351
Columna renalis, 333, BP73
Columna vertebralis, 8, 179
Columnae anales, 395
Columnae fornicis, 139
Commissura alba anterior, BP40
Commissura anterior labiorum vulvae, 377
Commissura anterior prostatae, 385
Commissura anterior, 174
Commissura hippocampi, 139
Commissura labiorum, 22
Commissura posterior labiorum vulvae, 377, 389
Commissura valvularum semilunarium, 244
Compartimenta cruris, T8.2
Compartimentum anterius cruris, 534
Compartimentum anterius femoris, 502
Compartimentum laterale cruris, 534
Compartimentum mediale femoris, 503
Complexus stimulans cordis, 248
Complexus valvularis cordis, 243–244
Compressor urethrae, 358, 372, 379, 406, T6.4
Concha auriculae, 122
Concha inferior nasi, 61, 67, 68, 93
Concha media nasi, 61, 67, 68
Concha nasalis inferior, 25, 26, 38
Concha nasalis media, 25
Concha superior nasi, 61
Condyloid joint, 9
Condylus lateralis ossis femoris, 500, 517, 518, 520, BP107
Condylus lateralis tibiae, 501, 524, 530, BP107
Condylus mandibulae, 26
Condylus medialis ossis femoris, 500, 517, 518, 520, BP107
Condylus medialis tibiae, 517, 519, 524, BP107
Conjugata diagonalis, 355
Conjugata recta, 355
Connexus intertendinei, 480

Constrictor medius pharyngis, T2.17
Constrictor superior pharyngis, 73, T2.21
Conus arteriosus, 241, 242, 243
Conus medullaris, 182, 186, 350, T3.1
Cor, 7, 21
    anterior exposure, 232
    basis cordis, 235
    innervation of, schema of, 250
    radiographs and ct angiogram, 234
    regiones precordiales auscultationis, 233
    in situ, 231
Cornu Ammonis, 139
Cornu anterius medullae spinalis, 189
Cornu frontale ventriculi lateralis, 177
Cornu inferius cartilaginis thyreoideae, 106
Cornu laterale medullae spinalis, 189, BP40
Cornu majus ossis hyoidei, 93
Cornu occipitale ventriculi lateralis, 139, 177
Cornu posterius medullae spinalis, 189
Cornu superius cartilaginis thyreoideae, 93, 106
Corona radiata, BP90
Corpora cavernosa penis, 383
Corpora vertebrarum, BP33
Corpus adiposum fossae ischioanalis, 378, 394, 420, BP94
Corpus adiposum infrapatellare, 517, 518, 521
Corpus adiposum pararenale, 200, 350
Corpus adiposum suprapatellare, 521
Corpus adiposum cubiti, 448
Corpus albicans, 365
Corpus axis, 26, 177
Corpus calcanei, 537
Corpus cavernosum clitoridis, 377
Corpus cavernosum penis, 368, 382, 386, 391
Corpus ciliare, 118
Corpus claviculae, 429
Corpus clitoridis, 364, 389
Corpus epididymidis, 388
Corpus fornicis, 139
Corpus gastris, 295
Corpus geniculatum laterale, 143
Corpus haemorrhagicum, 365
Corpus humeri, 430, 490
Corpus luteum, 365, 374
Corpus luteum graviditatis, 365
Corpus mamillare, 177
Corpus mandibulae, 25, 39
Corpus ossis 1 metacarpi, 467
Corpus ossis 3 metacarpi, 467
Corpus ossis femoris, 354, 500, 555, T8.1
Corpus ossis ilium, 357, 495
Corpus ossis ischii, 495, 497
Corpus ossis pubis, 420, BP94
Corpus pancreatis, 291, 294, 345
Corpus penis, 267, 389
Corpus perineale, 362, 368, 370, 378, 379, 383, 384, 385, 393, 397, 407, BP84, T6.1
Corpus phallicum, 389
Corpus polare primum, BP87
Corpus polare secundum, BP87
Corpus radii, 447, 453
Corpus residuale, 391
Corpus spongiosum penis, 368, 371, 382, 383, 386, 391
Corpus sterni, 202, 203, 213, 267, 268
Corpus ulnae, 447
Corpus uteri, 364, 365, 374
Corpus vertebrae lumbalis, 185
Corpus vertebrae, 45, 180, 181, 182, 184, 190, 263, 292, 345, 347, 357, 399, BP36, BP37, BP38, BP79, BP80
Corpus vitreum, 119
Corpusculum lamellosum (Pacinii), 12
Corpusculum renale corticale, BP72
Corpusculum renale juxtamedullare, BP72
Corpusculum renale, BP71

Corpusculum tactile (Meissneri), 12
Corrugator cutis ani, 395, 396
Corrugator supercilii, 48, 60, BP19, T2.14
Cortex corticis renis, BP73
Cortex glandulae suprarenalis, 341
Cortex pili, BP1
Cortex renis, 296, 333
Costae, 204, T4.1
    muscle attachments, BP42
Costae cervicales, BP41
Costae fluctuantes, 203
Costae spuriae, 203
Costae verae, 203
Coxa
    cross-sectional anatomy, BP104
    3D CT, 555
    MRI, 555
Cranial imaging, 176, BP31
Cranialis, as term of relationship, 1
Cranium, 8
    anterior view, 25
    lateral radiograph, 28
    lateral view of, 27
    median section, 29
    newborn, 35
    posterior and lateral views, 38
    radiographs, 26
Cremaster, 271, 272, 278, 280, 281, 388, BP54, T6.4
Crena interglutea, 178
Cribriform hymen, BP91
Crista frontalis, 30
Crista galli, 37, 177
Crista iliaca, 178, 195, 198, 267, 268, 275, 330, 331, 352, 353, 356, 357, 491, 493, 501, 504, 511, 512, BP80
Crista interossea, 524, 525
Crista intertrochanterica, 512
Crista obturatoria, 357
Crista occipitalis externa, 38
Crista pubica, 280, 361
Crista sacralis mediana, 357, 358
Crista supracondylaris lateralis, 446
Crista supracondylaris medialis, 427, 446
Crista terminalis, 241, 248
Crista tuberculi majoris, 427
Crista tuberculi minoris, 427
Crista urethralis, 385, 386
Crura antihelicis, 122
Crura diaphragmatis, 200
Crura fornicis, 139
Crus
    compartimenta, 534
    cross sections, 534
    serial cross sections, BP106
Crus ascendens, BP72
Crus clitoridis, 364, 371, 372, 375, 379
Crus descendens, BP72
Crus dextrum diaphragmatis, 216, 253, 283, 289, 348, BP78, BP79
Crus laterale anuli inguinalis superficialis, 280
Crus mediale anuli inguinalis superficialis, 280
Crus membranaceum commune, 125
Crus osseum commune, 125
Crus penis, 371, 383, 386
Crus sinistrum diaphragmatis, 216, 253, 283, 289, 345, 347, 348, 349, 350
Crypta tonsillae lingualis, 89
Cryptae intestinales, BP57
CT angiogram, 311
Cubitus
    ligamenta, 448
    ligamenta radiographs, 447
    ossa, 446
Cucullus extensorius, 474
Cumulus oophorus, BP90

Cupula pleurae, 103, 217, 251, T4.3
Cuspis anterior, 244
Cuspis inferior, 243, 245
Cuspis posterior, 244
Cuspis septalis, 243, 245
Cuspis superior, 243, 245
Cuticula pili, 12, BP1
Cutis, 6, 12, 48, 182, 273
Cutis penis, 382, 383, 388
Cutis scroti, 388, 392
Cystourethrograms
   female, BP85
   male, BP85

D

Deep inguinal ring, 281
Dendrita, BP3
Dentes, 18, 40
Depressor anguli oris, 48, BP19, T2.14
Depressor labii inferioris, 48, BP19, T2.14
Depressor septi nasi, 48, 60, BP19, T2.15
Dermatomata, 188
   membra superius and inferius, 5
Desmosoma, BP13
Detrusor vesicae, BP86
Dexter, as term of relationship, 1
Diametri pelvis, 355
Diaphragma, 211, 234, 257, 274, 276, 283, 285,
   291, 292, 294, 302, 307, 328, 330, 331, 344,
   347, 412, 507, BP36, BP58, BP79, T4.2, T4.4
   facies inferior, 216
   facies superior, 215
   as site of referred visceral pain, BP5
Diaphragma pelvis, 368, T6.1
   female, 358
   inferior view, 360, 362
   medial and superior views, 359
   superior view, 361
Digiti manus, 481
   tendines extensoris, 474
   tendines flexoris, 474
Digitus anularis, 467
Digitus medius, 467
Digitus minimus manus, 467
Dilatator pupillae, T2.3, T2.15
Diploe, 30
Disci intervertebrales, 184
Discus art. radiocarpeae, 463, 465, BP98
Discus art. sternoclavicularis, 204, 263, 429
Discus art. temporomandibularis, 42, 73
Discus intervertebralis, 45, 182, 185, 351, 399,
   BP33, T3.1
Distal forearm, BP99
Distal nail groove, BP112
Distalis, as term of relationship, 1
Divisio autonomica, 4
Divisio mandibularis n. trigemini, 23
Divisio maxillaris n. trigemini, 23
Divisio ophthalmica n. trigemini, 23
Dorsum, 3, 200
   surface anatomy of, 178
Dorsum linguae, 89
Dorsum manus, 463
   arteriae, 479
   nervi, 479
Dorsum pedis, 491
Dorsum penis, 352
Ductuli biliferi intralobulares, 304
Ductuli biliferi periportales, 304
Ductuli efferentes testis appendix testis, 390
Ductulus aberrans, 392
Ductulus bilifer periportalis, 304
Ductus (Vas) deferens, 274, 280, 281, 282, 284,
   367, 368, 371, 385, 387, 388, 390, 391, 392,
   393, 405, 411, 412, 418, 494, BP93, BP104,
   T6.3

Ductus alveolares, BP44
Ductus biliares extrahepatici, 305
Ductus biliares, 6
Ductus biliaris, 292, 293, 296, 297, 305, 306,
   308, 310, 312, 348, BP57, BP63, BP64,
   BP82, T5.3
Ductus bilifer interlobularis, 304
Ductus biliferi interlobulares, 304
Ductus cochlearis, 125
Ductus colligens, BP72
Ductus colligentes, BP73
Ductus cysticus, 302, 305, 306, 308, 310
   Variations, BP63
Ductus deferens vestigialis, 390
Ductus ejaculatorii, BP92
Ductus ejaculatorius, 385
Ductus endolymphaticus, 125
Ductus epididymidis, 392
Ductus glandulae bulbourethralis, 384
Ductus glandulae salivariae, 89
Ductus glandulae sebaceae, BP1
Ductus hepaticus communis, 303, 310, BP57
Ductus hepaticus dexter, 305, 306
Ductus hepaticus sinister, 305
Ductus lactiferi, 205
Ductus longitudinalis, 390
Ductus lymphaticus dexter, 16, 208
Ductus mesonephricus, 387, 390
Ductus pancreaticus, 297, 305, 306, BP57,
   BP62, BP63, BP82
   Variations, BP62, BP63
Ductus pancreaticus accessorius, 306
Ductus papillaris, BP73
Ductus paramesonephricus, 390
Ductus paraurethralis, BP86
Ductus parotideus (Stenonis), 71, 73
Ductus reuniens, 125
Ductus semicirculares, 121
Ductus semicircularis anterior, 125
Ductus semicircularis lateralis, 125
Ductus semicircularis posterior, 125
Ductus submandibularis (Whartoni), 83
Ductus thoracicus, 16, 219, 228, 229, 231, 254,
   259, 283, 286, 319, 344, 347, BP50, BP76,
   BP79, T2.5
Ductus venosus, 247
Duodenum, 292, 293, 294, 302, 306, 330, 337,
   341, 345, 350, BP57, T5.2
   arteriae, 310, 312
   autonomic innervation, 320–321
   in situ, 296
   laminae, BP56
   schema of autonomic innervation, 325
   as site of referred visceral pain, BP5
   venae, 315
Dura cranialis, 122, 125, 136
Dura spinalis, 136, 182, 189, 190, 194, BP35

E

Eminentia hypothenaris, 422
Eminentia iliopubica, 268, 353, 356, 357, 361,
   495, 496
Eminentia intercondylaris, 518, 520, 524, 525
Eminentia thenaris, 422
Emissaria, T2.4
Emissarium condylare, 194
Emissarium mastoideum, 194
Emissarium parietale, 24
Encephalon, 4, 69
   axial and coronal MRIS, BP32
   inferior view, 134
   lateral views, 132
   medial views, 133
Endocrine glands, BP95
Endometrium, 374, 399
Endotheliocyte, BP11

Endothelium fenestratum, BP71
Endothelium, BP13, BP71
Epicondylus lateralis humeri, 440, 446, 447,
   448, 450, 451, 452, 453, 455, 458, 489
Epicondylus lateralis ossis femoris, 500, 503,
   517, BP107
Epicondylus medialis humeri, 427, 441, 442,
   446, 447, 448, 450, 451, 452, 453, 454, 455,
   456, 457, 458, 487, 488
Epicondylus medialis ossis femoris, 500, 511,
   516, BP107
Epicranium (calva), 24, 48
Epidermis, BP1
Epididymis, 20, 387, 388, 390, 391, 392, 418
Epiglottis, 89, 93, T2.5
Epiphysial union hastened, BP95
Epiphysis phalangis distalis, 481
Epithelial tag, 389
Epitheliocytia pilae, 125
Epithelium spermatogenicum, 391
Eponychium, 481, BP112
Erector spinae, 178, 195, 200, 201, 212, 279,
   331, 347, 351, BP79, BP80
Erythrocyte, BP11
Excavatio rectouterina, 364, 365, 374, 375, 393,
   BP90, T6.3
Excavatio rectovesicalis, 343, 367, 368, 393
Excavatio vesicouterina, 364, 365, 369, 375,
   376, 393
Exocrinocyte G, BP55
Exocrinocyte cervicale, BP55
Exocrinocyte parietale, BP55
Exocrinocyte principale, BP55
Extensor brevis digitorum, 530, 532, 540, 542,
   549, 554, BP111, T8.7
Extensor brevis hallucis, 532, 554, BP111, T8.7
Extensor brevis pollicis, 451, 454, 455, 460,
   489, T7.7
Extensor digiti minimi, 451, 454, 460, 461, 489,
   T7.7
Extensor digitorum, 441, 451, 454, 461, 488,
   489, T7.7
Extensor indicis, 451, 455, 460, 461, 489, T7.7
Extensor longus digitorum, 501, 517, 526, 531,
   532, 534, 540, 541, 542, 554, BP106, BP110,
   T8.7
Extensor longus hallucis, 526, 529, 531, 534,
   542, 554, BP106, BP110, T8.7
Extensor longus pollicis, 451, 455, 460, 461,
   489, T7.7
Extensor radialis brevis carpi, 422, 441, 451,
   454, 455, 460, 461, 488, 489, T7.6
Extensor radialis longus carpi, 422, 441, 445,
   451, 454, 455, 459, 460, 461, 488, 489, T7.6
Extensor retinaculum of wrist, BP99
Extensor ulnaris carpi, 422, 441, 451, 454, 459,
   460, 461, 488, 489, T7.6
Extremitas acromialis, 429
Extremitas anterior splenis, 307
Extremitas posterior splenis, 307
Extremitas sternalis, 429

F

Facial hair appears, BP95
Facies anterior patellae, BP107
Facies anterior radii, 449
Facies anterior renis sinistri, 334
Facies articularis acromialis, 429
Facies articularis condyli medialis ossis
   femoris, 519
Facies articularis condyli medialis tibiae, 518
Facies articularis cuboidea, 537
Facies articularis inferior atlantis, BP35
Facies articularis inferior vertebrae, 180, 181,
   185
Facies articularis lateralis patellae, BP107

Facies articularis medialis patellae, BP107
Facies articularis patellae, 517, BP107
Facies articularis radii, 467
Facies articularis sternalis, 429
Facies articularis superior atlantis, BP35
Facies articularis superior capitis costae, BP33
Facies articularis superior condyli lateralis tibiae, 518
Facies articularis superior vertebrae, 180
Facies articularis talaris media, 537
Facies articularis talaris posterior, 537
Facies diaphragmatica cordis, 221, 235, 307
Facies dorsalis ossos metacarpi, 468
Facies lateralis radii, 449
Facies lateralis tibiae, 524, 525, BP107
Facies lunata acetabuli, 357, 420, 496, BP94
Facies medialis tibiae, 524, 525
Facies orbitalis alae majoris ossis sphenoidei, 25
Facies orbitalis maxillae, 25
Facies orbitalis ossis frontalis, 25
Facies orbitalis ossis zygomatici, 25
Facies palmaris ossis metacarpi, 468
Facies patellaris, 500, BP107
Facies poplitea, 500
Facies posterior radii, 449
Facies posterior renis sinistri, 334
Facies posterior tibiae, 524, 525
Facies symphysialis, 357, 495
Falx cerebelli, 130
Falx cerebri, 69, 130
Falx inguinalis, 271, 272, 274, 280, 281, BP53
Fascia adductoris pollicis, 470
Fascia axillaris, 435
Fascia brachii, 435, 445
Fascia clavipectoralis, 435
Fascia clitoridis, 377
Fascia cremasterica, 392
Fascia cribriformis, 494, BP53
Fascia cribrosa, 277
Fascia cruris, 492, 494, 533, 534
Fascia darta scroti, 381
Fascia diaphragmatica, 257
Fascia dorsalis manus, 473
Fascia extraperitonealis, 272, 414, BP54
Fascia iliaca, 282, 366, 394
Fascia inferior diaphragmatis pelvis, 378, 379, 394, 396, 398, 407
Fascia infraspinata, 198, 275, 432
Fascia investiens abdominis, 381
Fascia investiens superficialis colli, 48, 49
Fascia lata, 270, 271, 372, 378, 381, 409, 492, 494, 509, 515
Fascia masseterica, 48
Fascia mm. profundorum perinei, 359
Fascia musculorum infrahyoideorum, 49
Fascia obturatoria, 358, 359, 361, 366, 369, 372, 373, 379, 394, 404, 413, BP90
Fascia over M. interosseus dorsalis 1, 477
Fascia parotidea, 48
Fascia pectinea, 272
Fascia pectoralis, 435
Fascia penis, 270, 272, 343, 368, 382, 383, 384, 388, 397, 398, 407, BP84, BP93
Fascia perinei, 368, 371, 372, 378, 379, 383, 384, 393, 398, BP86
Fascia phrenicopleuralis, 257
Fascia plantaris lateralis, 543, 544
Fascia plantaris medialis, 543
Fascia presacralis, 366, 398
Fascia pretrachealis, 49
Fascia psoae, 200
Fascia rectalis, 366, 378, 385, 393, 394, 395, 396, 398, BP84, BP90
Fascia rectoprostatica, 362, 368, 385, 393, 398
Fascia rectovaginalis, 366
Fascia renalis, 337, 342

Fascia spermatica externa, 270, 271, 272, 278, 281, 368, 381, 383, 388, 392, 407, BP54
Fascia spermatica interna, 272, 282, 388, 392, BP54
Fascia superior diaphragmatis pelvis, 369, 373, 378, 394, 396, 398
Fascia thoracolumbalis, 198, 351
Fascia transversalis, 272, 273, 274, 280, 281, 282, 284, 337, 343, 351, 363, 366, 367, 368, 369, BP54
Fascia umbilicalis prevesicalis, 274, 281, 366
Fascia umbilicalis, 368, 369
Fascia uterovaginalis, 372, 378, BP84, BP90
Fascia vesicalis, 371, 378, 393, 398, BP84, BP90
Fasciae cervicales, 51, 52
Fasciae endopelvicae, 366
Fasciae extraperitoneales pelvis, T6.1
Fasciculi centrales extensoris digitorum, 460
Fasciculi collaterales aponeurosis extensoriae, 474
Fasciculi collaterales extensoris digitorum, 460
Fasciculi longitudinales aponeurosis plantaris, 543
Fasciculi longitudinales mediales, BP40
Fasciculi proprii, BP40
Fasciculi transversi, 469
Fasciculi transversi aponeurosis plantaris, 543
Fasciculus centralis aponeurosis extensoriae, 474
Fasciculus collateralis aponeurosis extensoriae, 474
Fasciculus interfascicularis, BP40
Fasciculus lateralis plexus brachialis, 238, 442
Fasciculus medialis plexus brachialis, 442
Fasciculus posterior plexus brachialis, 433
Fasciculus posterolateralis, BP40
Fasciculus septomarginalis, BP40
Fauces, 90
Femoral mechanical axis, BP107
Femur
  arteriae, BP105
  serial cross sections, 515
Fenestra cochleae, 35
Fenestra vestibuli, 35, 121
Fibrae afferentes, 146
Fibrae ascendentes, 340, 419
Fibrae collagenosae, BP11, BP13
Fibrae descendentes, 340, 419
Fibrae efferentes, 146
Fibrae elasticae, 12, 225, BP11, BP44
Fibrae intercrurales, 270, 280, 281, BP53
Fibrae obliquae tunicae muscularis gastris, 257
Fibrae postganglionicae, 7
Fibrae preganglionicae, 7
Fibrae reticulares, BP11
Fibrae zonulares, 118
Fibrin, 365
Fibroblastus, BP11, BP13
Fibula, 520, 524, 525, 530, 531, 534, 537, 556, BP106, BP108, BP110, T8.1
Filum terminale externum, 186, 187
Filum terminale internum, 186, 187
Fimbria hippocampi, 139
Fimbriae tubae uterinae, 374, 376
Fissura horizontalis, 221
Fissura horizontalis pulmonis dextri, 221, BP50
Fissura lig. teretis, 302
Fissura lig. venosi, 302
Fissura longitudinalis cerebri, 177
Fissura mediana anterior, BP40
Fissura nasalis, 34
Fissura obliqua pulmonis, 217, 218, 219, 221, BP50
Fissura orbitalis inferior, 25, 37, 38
Fissura orbitalis superior, 25, 26, 34, 37
Fissura petrosquamosa, 35
Fissura petrotympanica, 33

Fissura synaptica, BP3
Fixed retrocecal appendix vermiformis, 300
Flexor brevis digitorum, 540, 544, 545, 546, T8.8
Flexor brevis hallucis, 549, T8.8
Flexor brevis pollicis, 472, 475, 476, T7.7
Flexor digiti minimi manus, 472, 475, T7.7
Flexor digiti minimi pedis, 544, 545, 546, 549, T8.8
Flexor longus digitorum, 529, 533, 534, 553, BP106, T8.8
Flexor longus hallucis, 526, 529, 533, 534, 553, BP106, BP110, T8.8
Flexor longus pollicis, 428, 453, 458, 459, 461, 483, 486, T7.7
Flexor profundus digitorum, 453, 458, 459, 460, 461, 483, 486, 488, T7.7
Flexor radialis carpi, 440, 442, 452, 456, 458, 459, 461, 486, T7.7
Flexor superficialis digitorum, 453, 456, 459, 461, T7.7
Flexor ulnaris carpi, 422, 441, 452, 454, 455, 456, 457, 458, 459, 461, 483, 487, 488, T7.7
Flexura dextra coli, 288, 290, 291, 294, 296, 301, 337, 345, 346, 348, 349
Flexura duodenojejunalis, 289, 296, 297, 306, 337, 342
Flexura inferior duodeni, 297
Flexura sinistra coli, 288, 289, 290, 291, 294, 300, 301, 303, 345
Flexura superior duodeni, 297
Folliculi ovarici, BP90
Folliculi ovarici maturantes, 365
Folliculi ovarici tertiarii, 365
Folliculus ovaricus maturus, 365
Folliculus ovaricus primarius, 365
Folliculus ovaricus secundarius, 365
Folliculus pili, 12
Fonticulus anterior, 35
Fonticulus posterior, 35
Fonticulus sphenoideus, 35
Foramen alveolare inferius, 39
Foramen caecum linguae, 89
Foramen caecum ossis frontalis, 34
Foramen ethmoideum anterius, 25, 34, 35
Foramen ethmoideum posterius, 25, 34
Foramen infraorbitale, 25, 26, 35
Foramen interventriculare (Monroi), 136, 177
Foramen intervertebrale, 45, 181, 184, 185, BP34, BP36, BP37, BP81, T3.1
Foramen ischiadicum majus, 184, 356, 357, 358, 552
Foramen ischiadicum minus, 184, 356, 357
Foramen jugulare, 34
Foramen lacerum, 33, 34
Foramen magnum, 34, 38
Foramen mastoideum, 34
Foramen mentale, 25, 39
Foramen nutricium, 524
Foramen obturatum, 268, 353, 354, 497, 555
Foramen omentale, 292, 294, 343, BP79
Foramen ovale, 33, 34
Foramen ovale cordis, 247, T4.2
Foramen palatinum majus, 33
Foramen parietale, 30
Foramen rotundum, 26, 34, 79
Foramen sacrale posterius, BP81
Foramen spinosum, 33, 34
Foramen stylomastoideum, 33
Foramen supraorbitale, 25
Foramen transversarium, 45
Foramen v. cavae, 216, 283, BP78
Foramen venosum (Vesalii), 34
Foramen vertebrale, 180, 181, T3.1
Foramen zygomaticofaciale, 25, 35
Foramina apicum dentis, 41
Foramina cribrosa, 34

Foramina palatina minora, 33
Foramina retinacularia, 500
Foramina sacralia anteriora, 354, 356, 361
Foramina sacralia posteriora, 356
Fornix, 139, 174
Fornix inferior tunicae conjunctivae, 110
Fornix superior tunicae conjunctivae, 110
Fornix vaginae, 374
Fossa acetabuli, 420, BP94
Fossa anterior cranii, 37
Fossa axillaris, 202
Fossa coronoidea, 427, 446
Fossa cubitalis, 422
Fossa glenoidea, 430, 431, 490
Fossa hypophysialis, 63
Fossa iliaca, 357, 363
Fossa incisiva, 31, 33, 38
Fossa infratemporalis, 27, 75, 78
Fossa intercondylaris, BP107
Fossa ischioanalis, 379
Fossa malleoli lateralis, 524, 525
Fossa mandibularis, 35, 42
Fossa navicularis, 386
Fossa olecrani, 447
Fossa ovalis, 238, 247
Fossa pararectalis, 363, 365, 367
Fossa paravesicalis, 365
Fossa poplitea, 491
Fossa posterior cranii, 171
Fossa pterygoidea, 38
Fossa pterygopalatina, 67
Fossa radialis, 427, 446
Fossa retromolaris, 39, T2.3
Fossa sacci lacrimalis, 25
Fossa sublingualis, 39
Fossa submandibularis, 39
Fossa subscapularis, 203, 427
Fossa supravesicalis, 274
Fossa temporalis, 36, 75
Fossa triangularis, 122
Fossa trochanterica, 500
Fossa vestibuli vaginae, 377
Fossae ischioanales, 394
Fovea analis, 389
Fovea capitis ossis femoris, 500
Fovea centralis, 116, T2.1
Fovea costalis inferior, 180, 204
Fovea costalis superior, 180
Fovea costalis, 180
Fovea pterygoidea, 39
Foveola radialis, 422, 454
Foveolae granulares, 30
Frenulum clitoridis, 377
Frenulum labii inferioris, 83
Frenulum labii superioris, 83
Frenulum labiorum vulvae, 377
Frenulum linguae, 83
Frenulum ostii ilealis, 299
Frenulum preputii penis, 383
Fundus gastris, 234, 294, 295, 347
Fundus uteri, 363, 364, 365, 369, 374, 399
Fundus vesicae, 371
Funiculus posterior medullae spinalis, BP40
Funiculus spermaticus, 274, 281, 420, BP53,
  BP94

G

Galea aponeurotica, 48, 199
Ganglia aorticorenalia, 321, 322, 341, 411, 417
Ganglia autonomica abdominis, 319
Ganglia coeliaca, 319, 320, 321, 322, 323, 324,
  325, 328, 329, 339, 340, 341, 411, 412, 417,
  418, 419
Ganglia inferiora, 230
Ganglia lumbalia trunci sympathici, 319, 411,
  412

Ganglia sacralia trunci sympathici, 319, 414
Ganglia spinalia, 419
Ganglia thoracica trunci sympathici, 416
Ganglia trunci sympathici, 340
Ganglion aorticorenale, 6, 287, 319, 321, 323,
  324, 339, 340, 412, 416, 418, 419, BP6
Ganglion cervicale medium, 57, 249, 250, BP6
Ganglion cervicale superius, 6, 249, 250, BP6
Ganglion cervicothoracicum, 229, 249, 250,
  BP6
Ganglion ciliare, 7, 79, BP7
  schema, 159
Ganglion coeliacum, 6, 7, 326, 341, 416, BP6,
  BP79, T5.1
Ganglion geniculi, 143
Ganglion inferius n. vagi, 153
Ganglion lumbale primum trunci sympathici, 6
Ganglion lumbale trunci sympathici, 319, 414
Ganglion mesentericum inferius, 6, 323, 324,
  339, 411, 412, 416, 417, 419, BP6
Ganglion mesentericum superius, 6, 7, 321,
  322, 325, 326, 339, 340, 411, 412, 417, 418,
  419, BP6
Ganglion oticum, 7, 42, 161
Ganglion phrenicum, 216, 321
Ganglion pterygopalatinum, 7, 79, 149, 160,
  BP7
Ganglion renale, 339, 341, 418
Ganglion sacrale primum trunci sympathici, 6
Ganglion spinale, 189, 201, 212, 279, 324, 325,
  328, 329, 340, BP81, T4.1
Ganglion spirale, 125
Ganglion submandibulare, 7, 160, BP7
Ganglion thoracicum primum trunci
  sympathici, 6
Ganglion thoracicum trunci sympathici, 249,
  417, 418
Ganglion trigeminale, 79, 84, 143
Ganglion trunci sympathici, 190, 212, 326, 328,
  329
Ganglion vertebrale, 249, 250
Gaster, 6, 18, 258, 288, 291, 292, 302, 303, 305,
  307, 343, 345, 348, BP79, BP82, T5.2
  arteriae, 308
  autonomic innervation, 320–321
  body habitus, position and contour
    variations, BP55
  in situ, 294
  schema of autonomic innervation, 325
  as site of referred visceral pain, BP5
  vasa lymphatica and nodi lymphoidei, BP74
  venae, 315
Genetics of reproduction, BP87
Genu, 3
  anterioposterior radiograph, 520
  anterior views, 517
  arteriae, BP103, BP105
  interior views, 518
  lateral view radiograph, BP108
  medial and lateral views, 516
  osteology, BP107
  posterior and sagittal views, 521
  posterior view, 520
Genu corpus callosi, 139, 177
Glabella, 22, 25
Glandula bulbourethralis, 20, 274, 343, 371,
  384, 385, 386, 390, 391
Glandula lacrimalis, 6, 7, BP7
Glandula lingualis, 83
Glandula mammaria, 205, T4.3
Glandula parotidea, 6, 7, 49, 71, 93, BP7, T2.5
Glandula pinealis, 21
Glandula pituitaria, 21, 61, 177
Glandula sebacea, 12, BP1
Glandula seminalis, 274, 367, 368, 385, 390,
  391, 393, 405
Glandula sublingualis, 6, 7, 83, BP7

Glandula submandibularis, 6, 7, 22, 93, BP7
Glandula sudorifera, 12
Glandula suprarenalis, 6, 291, 293, 296, 306,
  307, 330, 332, 341, 345, 348, 387, BP50,
  BP82, T5.3
Glandula thyreoidea, 21, 50, 57, 105, 217, 219,
  220, 238, T2.5
  anterior view, 103
  posterior view, 104
Glandula trachealis, 225
Glandula vestibularis major, 379, 390, 406
Glandulae anales, 395
Glandulae bulbourethrales, 385
Glandulae endocrinae, T5.3
Glandulae gastricae propriae, BP55
Glandulae gustatoriae, 89
Glandulae molares, 85
Glandulae mucosae, 7, 89
Glandulae parathyreoideae, 21, 105
Glandulae paraurethrales, 390, BP86
Glandulae prostatae, BP92
Glandulae pyloricae, BP55
Glandulae salivariae, 70–71, 83, 86
Glandulae sebaceae, 110
Glandulae submucosae, 327
Glandulae suprarenales, 19, 21, 332
  dissection, 341
  in situ, 342
  schema of autonomic innervation, 341
Glandulae tarsales (Meibomii), 110
Glandulae urethrales, BP86
Glans clitoridis, 377, 389
Glans penis, 267, 352, 383, 386, 389
Glomerulus intermedius, BP73
Glomerulus superficialis, BP73
Glomus caroticum, 163
Gonadae, 387, 390
Gonadotropic hormone levels, BP88
Granulatio arachnoideae, 127, 129
Granulationes arachnoideae, 136
Granulocyte eosinophilum, BP11
Gubernaculum testis, 387
Gyrus dentatus, 139

H

Hair shaft. See Stipes pili
Hamulus ossis hamati, 452, 458, 462, 464, 467,
  468, BP98
Hamulus pterygoideus, 36, 38, 73
Haustra coli, 298, 301
Helicotrema cochleae, 125
Helix, 22, 122
Hemidiaphragma, 217, 218
Hepar, 6, 18, 217, 247, 291, 296, 305, 337, 341,
  343, 345, 347, 348, 350, BP38, BP58, BP79,
  T5.2
  arteriae, 308, 310
  arterial blood supply variations in, BP83
  in situ, 303
  schema of autonomic innervation, 328
  schema of structure, 304
  as site of referred visceral pain, BP5
  surfaces and Bed, 302
  topography, BP58
  variations in form, BP59
  vasa lymphatica and nodi lymphoidei, BP78
Hernia sac, BP54
Hiatus adductorius, 510, 511, 551
Hiatus anorectalis, 361
Hiatus aorticus, 216, 253
Hiatus canalis n. petrosi majoris, 34
Hiatus canalis n. petrosi minoris, 34
Hiatus for V. dorsalis profunda penis, 361
Hiatus oesophageus diaphragmatis, 216, 253,
  287, T5.1
Hiatus sacralis, T3.1

Hiatus saphenus, 271, 277, 378, 492
Hiatus semilunaris, 67
Hiatus urogenitalis, 361, 370
Hilum pulmonis, 221, 232
Hilum renis, 333
Hilum splenis, 307
Hinge joint, 9
Hippocampus, 139
Hormones, BP95
Humerus, 427, 428, 442, 445, 447, T7.1
Hydrocele, 388
Hymen, BP91
Hypertonic stomach, BP55
Hyponychium, BP112
Hypophysis, 174, 175
Hypothalamus, 21, 174, 175
Hypotonic stomach, BP55

I

Ileum, 316, 350, 351, BP80, BP81
Iliopsoas, 274, 420, 421, 498, 502, 503, 509,
    510, 515, BP94, BP104
Impressio colica hepatis, 302
Impressio colica splenis, 307
Impressio duodenalis hepatis, 302
Impressio gastrica hepatis, 302
Impressio gastrica splenis, 307
Impressio mediastinalis anterior pulmonis,
    221
Impressio oesophagea, 221, 302
Impressio oesophagea hepatis, 302
Impressio renalis hepatis, 302
Impressio trachealis pulmonis, 221
Impressiones costales hepatis, 302
Incisura acetabuli, 357
Incisura cardiaca pulmonis, 217
Incisura cardialis, 294
Incisura fibularis, 524
Incisura inferior vertebrae, 180, 181
Incisura interarytenoidea, 93
Incisura intertragica, 122
Incisura ischiadica major, 268, 353, 495
Incisura ischiadica minor, 268, 353, 495
Incisura jugularis, 22, 49, 202, 203, 217
Incisura lig. teretis, 288
Incisura mandibulae, 36, 39
Incisura pancreatis, 306
Incisura radialis ulnae, 446, 449
Incisura scapulae, 203, 427, 436, 437
Incisura splenica, 307
Incisura superior vertebrae, 180, 181
Incisura supraorbitalis, 22, 25, 35
Incisura thyreoidea superior, 106
Incisura trochlearis, 446, 449
Incisura trochlearisa, 447
Indirect Inguinal Hernia, BP54
Inferior, as term of relationship, 1
Infundibulum hypothalami, 174
Infundibulum tubae uterinae, 374, 376
Insertio m. brachialis, 448
Insertio tendinis flexoris profundi digitorum,
    470
Insertio tendinis flexoris superficialis
    digitorum, 470
Insertiones superiores m. scaleni anterioris,
    55
Insertiones superiores m. scaleni posterioris,
    55
Insulae pancreaticae, 21
Intersectio tendinea, 202, 267, 271
Intestina, 6, 7, 324
Intestinum, 247, 327
Intestinum crassum, 18, 301
    arteriae, 314
    vasa lymphatica and nodi lymphoidei, BP77
    venae, 317

Intestinum tenue, 18, 288, 297, 300, 343
    arteriae, 313
    autonomic innervation, 322
    as site of referred visceral pain, BP5
    vasa lymphatica and nodi lymphoidei, BP76
    venae, 316
Intumescentia cervicalis, 187
Intumescentia lumbosacralis, 187
IP joint, BP99
Iris, 110
Isthmus grandulae thyreoideae, 103
Isthmus uteri, 374

J

Jejunum, 289, 290, 296, 297, 306, 316, 348,
    349, 350, 351
Junctio anorectalis, 420, BP94
Junctio duodenojejunalis, 200
Junctio ileocaecalis, 298, BP80
Junctio oesophagogastrica, 253, 257, 295, 347,
    T5.2
Junctio pharyngooesophagea, 94
Junctio rectosigmoidea, 393, 395, 396
Junctio vesicoprostatica, 420
Juncturae, BP11
Juncturae columnae vertebralis, 185
Juncturae synoviales
    structure of, 9
    types, 9
Juncturae thoracicae, 204
Juxtaglomerulocytia, BP71

K

Kyphosis sacralis, 179
Kyphosis thoracica, 179

L

Labia minora, 364, 375
Labium externum cristae iliacae, 268
Labium internum cristae iliacae, 268
Labium majus, 364, 369, 372, 377, 389, BP86
Labium minus, 364, 369, 372, 377, 380, 389,
    BP86
Labrum acetabuli, 357, 496, 514, 555, BP104
Labrum glenoideum, 431, 490
Labrum ileocaecale, 299
Labrum ileocolicum, 299
Labyrinthus membranaceus, 125
Labyrinthus osseus, 125
Lacuna magna, 386
Lacuna vasorum, 283
Lacus lacrimalis, 110
Lamellae circumferentiales externae, BP9
Lamellae circumferentiales internae, BP9
Lamellae concentricae, BP9
Lamina anterior fasciae renalis, 200, 337
Lamina anterior fasciae thoracolumbalis, 200
Lamina anterior omenti minoris, 320
Lamina anterior vaginae m. recti abdominis,
    271, 272, 273, 280, 378, BP53
Lamina arcus vertebrae, 180, 181, 184, 185,
    T3.1
Lamina cartilaginis cricoideae, 93
Lamina cartilaginis thyreoideae, 103, 106
Lamina cribrosa, 37
Lamina hepatica limitans, 304
Lamina horizontalis ossis palatini, 38, 61
Lamina lateralis proc. pterygoidei, 29, 36
Lamina media fasciae thoracolumbalis, 197,
    200
Lamina medialis proc. pterygoidei, 29, 73
Lamina muscularis mucosae canalis analis,
    395, 396
Lamina muscularis mucosae recti, 395, 396

Lamina muscularis mucosae, 327, BP55
Lamina orbitalis ossis ethmoidei, 25, 35
Lamina orbitalis ossis frontalis, 25
Lamina parietalis tunicae vaginalis testis, 388,
    392
Lamina perpendicularis ossis ethmoidei, 25
Lamina posterior fasciae renalis, 200, 337
Lamina posterior fasciae thoracolumbalis, 200,
    275
Lamina posterior omenti minoris, 320
Lamina posterior vaginae m. recti abdominis,
    272, 278, 280
Lamina profunda fasciae pectoralis, 435
Lamina spiralis ossea, 125
Lamina terminalis, 174
Lamina unguis, 481, BP112
Lamina visceralis tunicae vaginalis testis, 392
Laminae anteriores lig. gastrocolici, 291
Laminae mesosalpingis, 376
Laminae mesovarii, 376
Laminae posteriores lig. gastrocolici, 291
Larynx, 7, BP34, BP95
    intrinsic muscles of, 109
    nervi and coronal section, 108
Lateral nail fold, BP112
Lateral nail groove, BP112
Lateralis, as term of relationship, 1
Lectulus, 481, BP112
Lens, 118, T2.1
Leptomeninges, 190
Levator anguli oris, BP19, T2.16
Levator ani, 274, 283, 301, 318, 324, 343, 358,
    361, 364, 370, 371, 372, 373, 378, 379, 383,
    393, 394, 395, 396, 397, 398, 400, 404, 405,
    406, 412, 413, BP86, BP104, T6.4
Levator labii superioris, 48, BP19, T2.16
Levator nasolabialis, 48, T2.16
Levator palpebrae superioris, 110, 113, T2.3,
    T2.16
Levator scapulae, 195, 198, 432, 436, 437, 488,
    T3.2
Levator veli palatini, 73, T2.3, T2.16
Levatores costarum, T4.4
Lien. See Splen
Ligg. accessoria art. coxae, 503
Ligg. anularia tracheae, 225
Ligg. carpi
    anterior view, 464
    posterior and anterior views, BP98
    posterior view, 465
Ligg. carpometacarpea dorsalia, BP98
Ligg. carpometacarpea palmaria, 468, BP98
Ligg. columnae vertebralis, 184, BP33
Ligg. craniocervicalia, 47
Ligg. craniocervicalia externa, 46
Ligg. intercarpea dorsalia, 465
Ligg. intercarpea interossea, 465
Ligg. interphalangea, 468
Ligg. interphalangea collateralia manus, 468,
    474
Ligg. interphalangia collateralia pedis, 468,
    469, 539
Ligg. interphalangea palmaria, 468, 471
Ligg. lectuli, BP112
Ligg. metacarpea dorsalia, BP98
Ligg. metacarpea palmaria, 468, BP98
Ligg. metacarpea transversa profunda, 468,
    475, BP102
Ligg. metacarpea transversa superficialia, 469
Ligg. metacarpophalangea, 468
Ligg. metacarpophalangea collateralia, 468,
    BP102
Ligg. metacarpophalangea palmaria, 471,
    BP102
Ligg. metatarsea dorsalia, 547
Ligg. pedis, 538, 539
Ligg. pelvis, 376

Ligg. sacrococcygea anteriora, 356
Ligg. sacrococcygea posteriora, 357
Ligg. sacroiliaca posteriora, 184
Ligg. suspensoria mammaria (Cooperi), 205
Ligg. tali, 538
Ligg. tarsometatarsea dorsalia, 547
Ligg. tarsometatarsea plantaria, 539
Ligg. umbilicalia medialia, 247
Lig. anococcygeum, 360, 378, 379, 383, 397, 398
Lig. anulare radii, 448
Lig. apicis dentis, BP18
Lig. arcuatum laterale, 283
Lig. arcuatum mediale, 283
Lig. arcuatum medianum, 216, 283
Lig. arteriosum, 232, 233, 242, T4.2
Lig. bifurcatum, 538
Lig. calcaneofibulare, 525
Lig. calcaneometatarseum, 543
Lig. calcaneonaviculare plantare, 539
Lig. capitis femoris, 514, BP104
Lig. capitohamatum, 464, 465
Lig. capsulare, 431
Lig. cardinale, 366, 372, 374, BP90
Lig. collaterale fibulare, 501, 503, 517, 518, 519, 521, 525, 528, 529, 530, 532
Lig. collaterale laterale tali, 538
Lig. collaterale mediale tali, 537, 538
Lig. collaterale radiale carpi, BP98
Lig. collaterale radiale cubiti, 448
Lig. collaterale tibiale, 503, 516, 517, 518, 519, 520, 521, 528, 529, 531, 532, T8.1
Lig. collaterale ulnare carpi, BP98
Lig. collaterale ulnare cubiti, 448
Lig. coracoacromiale, 431, 434, 440
Lig. coracoclaviculare, 434
Lig. coracohumerale, 431
Lig. coronarium hepatis, 293, 302, 343
Lig. costoclaviculare, 429, 435
Lig. costocoracoideum, 435
Lig. cricothyroideum medianum, 103, 106, 225, T4.1
Lig. cruciatum anterius, 518, 519, T8.1
Lig. cruciatum posterius, 518, 519
Lig. cuboideonaviculare plantare, 539
Lig. cuneonaviculare plantare, 539
Lig. denticulatum, 189, 190
Lig. falciforme, 274, 288, 293, 318, 345
Lig. flavum, 185, 351, BP18
Lig. fundiforme penis, 270, 280, 368
Lig. gastrophrenicum, 291, 293, 330
Lig. gastrosplenicum, 291, 292, 307
Lig. glenohumerale inferius, 431
Lig. glenohumerale medium, 431
Lig. glenohumerale superius, 431
Lig. hepatoduodenale, 291, 294, 296, 297, 348
Lig. hepatogastricum, 294
Lig. hyoepiglotticum, 106
Lig. iliofemorale, BP104
Lig. iliolumbale, 331, 356
Lig. inguinale, 267, 270, 271, 272, 280, 281, 282, 283, 352, 373, 375, 378, 409, 491, 492, 502, 507, 509, 510, 523, BP53, T5.1
Lig. inguinale reflexum, 271, 280
Lig. interclaviculare, 204, 429
Lig. interfoveolare, 274
Lig. interphalangeum collaterale accessorium manus, 468
Lig. interphalangeum collaterale manus, 468
Lig. interphalangeum palmare, 474, 481, BP102
Lig. interspinale, 184, 185
Lig. intraarticulare capitis costae, 204, BP33
Lig. ischiofemorale, BP104
Lig. lacunare, 271, 272, 274, 280, 282, 283
Lig. laterale articulationis temporomandibularis, 42

Lig. laterale pubovesicale, 366
Lig. laterale vesicae, 366
Lig. latum uteri, 363, 364, 365, 372, 373, 390
Lig. lectuli, BP112
Lig. longitudinale anterius, 46, 184, 185, 200, 204, 351, 356, BP35, BP79
Lig. longitudinale posterius, 185, BP33
Lig. lumbocostale, 331
Lig. lunotriquetrum, 464
Lig. mediale pubovesicale, 366
Lig. meniscofemorale posterius, 518, 519
Lig. metacarpeum transversum superficiale, 425
Lig. metacarpophalangeum collaterale, 474
Lig. metacarpophalangeum palmare, 468
Lig. metatarseum transversum profundum, 539
Lig. metatarseum transversum superficiale, 543
Lig. metatarsophalangeum plantare, 539
Lig. nuchae, 178, BP18
Lig. palmare carpi, 425, 456, 457, 464, 469, 470, 472, 476, 487, 488
Lig. patellae, 491, 501, 502, 503, 510, 516, 517, 518, 531, 532, BP106, BP108, T8.2
Lig. pectineum, 271, 272, 274, 280, 282, 283
Lig. phrenicocolicum, 291, 293
Lig. phrenicoesophageum superius, 257
Lig. pisohamatum, 464, BP98
Lig. pisometacarpeum, 464, BP98
Lig. plantare longum, 547
Lig. popliteum arcuatum, 518, 521
Lig. popliteum obliquum, 518, 520, 521
Lig. posterius capitis fibulae, 521
Lig. proprium ovarii, 363, 364, 365, 372, 373, 374, 375, 390
Lig. pubicum inferius, 353, 359, 360, 361, 362, 366, 369, 378
Lig. pubocervicale, 366, 373
Lig. pubofemorale, 496, BP104
Lig. pubovesicale laterale, 369
Lig. pubovesicale mediale, 369
Lig. pubovesicale, 373
Lig. pulmonale, 221
Lig. quadratum, 448
Lig. radiatum capitis costae, BP33
Lig. radiatum carpi, BP98
Lig. radiocapitatum, BP98
Lig. radiocarpeum dorsale, 465
Lig. radiocarpeum dorsale, BP98
Lig. radiolunatum breve, 464
Lig. radiolunatum longum, 464
Lig. radioscaphocapitatum, 464
Lig. radioscapholunatum, BP98
Lig. radioulnare dorsale, 465, BP98
Lig. radioulnare palmare, 464, BP98
Lig. rectovesicale, 293
Lig. sacrococcygeum anterius, 361, 366
Lig. sacrococcygeum laterale, 357
Lig. sacroiliacum anterius, 356
Lig. sacroiliacum interosseum, BP81
Lig. sacroiliacum posterius, 356, 357
Lig. sacrospinale, 184, 356, 357, 358, 360, 412, 415, 504, 512
Lig. sacrotuberale, 184, 356, 357, 358, 360, 362, 379, 397, 398, 404, 412, 413, 415, 504, 511, 512, BP94, BP104
Lig. scaphocapitatum, 464
Lig. scapholunatum, 465
Lig. scaphotrapeziotrapezoideum, 464
Lig. scrotale, 390
Lig. sphenomandibulare, 42, 73
Lig. splenorenale, 291, 293, 307, 330, BP79
Lig. sternochondrale radiatum, 429
Lig. sternoclaviculare anterius, 429
Lig. stylohyoideum, 36
Lig. stylomandibulare, 42

Lig. supraspinale, 182, 184, 185, 200, 356, 357
Lig. suspensorium axillae, 435
Lig. suspensorium clitoridis, 378, 379, 380
Lig. suspensorium ovarii, 363, 364, 365, 373, 374, 375, 376, 390, 402
Lig. suspensorium penis, 271, 368, BP53
Lig. talocalcaneum posterius, BP110
Lig. talofibulare anterius, BP110
Lig. talofibulare posterius, 525
Lig. teres hepatis, 247, 288, 294, 302, 318, 351, BP83
Lig. teres uteri, 285, 363, 364, 365, 372, 373, 375, 376, 378, 390, 402, BP86
Lig. tibiocalcaneum, BP110
Lig. tibiofibulare posterius, 537
Lig. transversum acetabuli, 357, 496, BP104
Lig. transversum humeri, 431
Lig. transversum inferius scapulae, BP24
Lig. transversum perinei, 359, 361, 366, 369, 378, 384, 407
Lig. transversum superius scapulae, 433, 437, BP24
Lig. trapeziotrapezoideum, 464, 465
Lig. trapezoideocapitatum, 464, 465
Lig. triangulare dextrum hepatis, 293, 302
Lig. triangulare sinistrum hepatis, 302
Lig. triquetrocapitatum, 464
Lig. triquetrohamatum, 464, 465
Lig. ulnocarpeum dorsale, BP98
Lig. ulnocarpeum palmare, BP98
Lig. ulnotriquetrum, 465
Lig. umbilicale mediale, 272, 274, 280, 282, 336, 363, 366, 367, 375, 376
Lig. umbilicale medianum, 273, 274, 281, 282, 343, 363, 366, 369, 375, 378, 402
Lig. uterosacrale, 364, 366, 373, 374, BP90
Lig. venosum, 247
Lig. vocale, 106
Limbus corneae, 110
Limbus fossae ovalis, 241
Limen nasi, 61
Linea alba, 202, 267, 270, 271, 272, 273, 280, 351, 363, 367, BP53, BP79, BP81, T5.1
Linea anocutanea, 394, 395, 396
Linea anorectalis, 395
Linea arcuata ossis ilium, 268, 353, 357, 358, 359, 361, 495
Linea arcuata vaginae m. recti, 272, 274, 276, 280
Linea epiphysialis, 514
Linea glutea anterior, 357, 495
Linea glutea inferior, 357, 495
Linea glutea posterior, 357, 495
Linea intermedia, 268, 495
Linea intertrochanterica, 496, 500
Linea mylohyoidea, 39
Linea nuchalis inferior, 38
Linea nuchalis superior, 38, 195, 196
Linea obliqua mandibulae, 39, 524, BP107
Linea obliqua tibiae, 524, BP107
Linea pectinata, 395
Linea semilunaris, 267, 269
Linea supracondylaris medialis, 500
Linea terminalis, 366, 367, 372, 394
Linea trapezoidea, 429
Lineae semilunares, BP58
Lineae transversae, 183
Lingua, 18, 84, 86, 88, 177, BP35
   nodi lymphoidei, 102
Lingula mandibulae, 39
Lingula pulmonis, 219
Liquor cerebrospinalis, 136, 182
Lobuli glandulae mammariae, 205
Lobuli testis, 392
Lobulus auriculae, 22, 122
Lobulus pulmonis, 226, 227
Lobus caudatus hepatis, 291, 294, 302

Atlas of Human Anatomy

Lobus dexter glandulae thyreoideae, 103
Lobus dexter hepatis, 288, 294, 302, 345, 346, BP82
Lobus inferior pulmonis dextri, 347
Lobus inferior pulmonis sinistri, 347
Lobus lateralis prostatae, BP93
Lobus medius prostatae, BP93
Lobus quadratus, 302
Lobus sinister glandulae thyreoideae, 103
Lobus sinister hepatis, 288, 294
  complete atrophy, BP59
Locus lambda, 30
Loop of bowel entering hernia sac, BP54
Lower limb, 11
Lower pelvis, BP94
Lumbosacral plexus, T8.4–T8.6, T8.4–T8.7
Lumen, 327
Lunula, 481, BP112
Luteocytia, 365
Lymphocyte, BP11

M

Macrophagocyte, BP11
Malleolus lateralis, 491, 524, 525, 528, 529, 530, 531, 540
Malleolus medialis, 491, 524, 525, 527, 529, 531, 532, 533, 540, 542, BP110
Malleus, 125
Mamma
  arteriae, 206
  lymphatic drainage, 208
  nodi lymphoidei, 207
  vasa lymphatica, 207
Mandibula, 25, 26, 27, 28, 36, 39
Manubrium sterni, 49, 203, 204, 211, 219, 263, 429, BP34, BP35
Manus
  axial view, BP101–BP102
  spatia, 471, 473
  vaginae tendinum, 471, 473
Margo acetabuli, 356, 357, 361, 497
Margo anterior claviculae, 429
Margo anterior pulmonis, 221
Margo anterior radii, 449
Margo anterior tibiae, 491, 524, 525
Margo dexter cordis, 217
Margo falciformis hiatus sapheni, 282
Margo inferior hepatis, 288, 294, BP58
Margo inferior pulmonis, 217, 221
Margo inferior splenis, 307
Margo infraorbitalis, 22
Margo interosseus radii, 449, 524, 525
Margo interosseus tibiae, 524, 525
Margo lateralis renis, 333
Margo lateralis scapulae, 427
Margo liber unguis, BP112
Margo medialis levatoris ani, 362
Margo medialis scapulae, 178, 427
Margo medialis tibiae, 524, 525
Margo posterior claviculae, 429
Margo posterior fibulae, 524
Margo posterior radii, 449
Margo sinister cordis, 217
Margo superior scapulae, 427
Margo superior splenis, 307
Margo supraorbitalis, 26
Massa lateralis atlantis, 26
Masseter, 72, T2.17
Mastocyte, BP11
Matrix epithelialis, 12
Matrix mesangialis, BP71
Matrix unguis, 481, BP112
Maxilla, 25, 27, 31, 35
Meatus acusticus externus cranii, 36
Meatus acusticus externus, 125, T2.1

Meatus acusticus internus, 34
Meatus inferior nasi, 61
Meatus superior nasi, 61
Medialis, as term of relationship, 1
Mediastinum, 220
  cross section, 237
  left lateral view, 252
  right lateral view, 251
Mediastinum anterius, 215
Mediastinum inferior, BP2
Mediastinum superius, BP2
Mediastinum testis, 388
Medulla glandulae suprarenalis, 341
Medulla oblongata, 7, 177, 324, 340, BP8, BP35
Medulla pili, BP1
Medulla renis, 349
Medulla rubra ossis, 16
Medulla spinalis, 4, 186, 263, 328, 329, 340, 341, BP38
  fiber tracts cross sections, BP40
Melanocyte, 12
Membrana atlantoaxialis posterior, BP18
Membrana atlantooccipitalis anterior, 46
Membrana atlantooccipitalis posterior, 46, BP18
Membrana basalis endothelii, BP71
Membrana basalis glomeruli, BP71
Membrana basalis, 391, BP13
Membrana costocoracoidea, 435
Membrana intercostalis externa, 201, 279, 436
Membrana intercostalis interna, 201, 212
Membrana interossea antebrachii, 449, 451, 453, 461, 464, BP98
Membrana interossea cruris, 520, 521, 529, 532, 534, 537, BP103, BP105, BP106, BP110
Membrana obturatoria, 357, 372, 496
Membrana perinei, 274, 283, 343, 358, 361, 362, 364, 369, 371, 372, 378, 379, 380, 383, 384, 385, 397, 398, 406, 407, 413, 419, BP84, BP86
Membrana postsynaptica, BP3
Membrana presynaptica, BP3
Membrana suprapleuralis, 251
Membrana thyreohyoidea, 103, 106
Membrana tympanica secundaria, 125
Membrana tympanica, 125, T2.1
Membrum inferius, 2–3
  anterior view, 492
  nodi lymphoidei, 494
  posterior view, 493
  structures with high clinical significance, T8.1–T8.3
  surface anatomy, 491
  vasa lymphatica, 494
  vena superficiales, 492, 493
Membrum superius, 2–3
  arteriae, 443, 483
  cutaneous innervation, 423
  nervi, 483, 484
  structures with high clinical significance, T7.1–T7.2
  surface anatomy, 422
  vasa lymphatica and nodi lymphoidei, 426
  venae, 444
Meninges craniales, 127, 129
Meninges spinales, 189, T3.1
Meniscus art. radiocarpeae, 465
Meniscus lateralis, 518, 519, 521
Meniscus medialis, 517, 518, 519, T8.1
Menstrual cycle, BP88
Menstruation begins, BP95
Mesangiocyte, BP71
Mesencephalon, 177

Mesenteria, 289
Mesenterium, 200, 290, 297, 327, 343, 351
Mesenterium urogenitale, 387, 390
Mesoappendix, 298, 322, BP57
Mesocolon sigmoideum, 290, 301, 314, 393
Mesocolon transversum, 288, 289, 290, 291, 292, 293, 296, 301, 314, 316, 330, 343
Mesometrium, 374
Mesosalpinx, 365, 374
Mesovarium, 372, 374
Metacarpal bone, BP99
Mid and proximal forearm, BP99
Middle phalanx, BP99
Mitochondria, BP3
Modiolus anguli oris, 48, T2.3
Modiolus cochleae, 125
Monocyte, BP11
Mons pubis, 377
Mouth, opening of, BP25
MP joint, BP99
Mucocyte superficiale, BP55
Musculature develops, BP95
Musculi, T2.14–T2.22, T5.4, T6.4, T7.5–T7.8, T8.7–T8.10, T8.8–T8.10
Musculi suprahyoidei, 53
Mm. anorectales, 396
Mm. antebrachii
  attachments (anterior view), 459
  attachments (posterior view), 460
  compartimentum anterius, 457
  flexores carpi, 452
  flexores digitorum, 453
  pars profunda compartimenti anterioris, 458
  pars profunda compartimenti posterioris, 455
  pars superficialis compartimenti anterioris, 456
  pars superficialis compartimenti posterioris, 454
Mm. anteriores antebrachii, 10
Mm. anteriores brachii, 10
Mm. anteriores cruris, 10
Mm. anteriores femoris, 10
Mm. arytenoidei obliqui, 107
Mm. brachii
  compartimentum anterius, 440
  compartimentum posterius, 441
Mm. colli, 10
  anteriores and laterales, 55
  anterior view, 49
  lateral view, 54
Mm. compartimenti anterioris antebrachii, T7.2
Mm. compartimenti medialis femoris, T8.2
Mm. compartimenti posterioris antebrachii, T7.2
Mm. cricothyreoidei, 103
Mm. cruris
  attachments, 526
  compartimentum anterius, 531, 532
  compartimentum laterale, 530
  pars profunda compartimenti posterioris, 529
  pars superficialis compartimenti posterioris, 527, 528
Mm. cuffiae musculotendineae, 434, T7.1
Mm. dorsales pedis
  deep dissection, 542
  superficial dissection, 541
Mm. dorsi, 196
Mm. epaxiales, T3.1
Mm. externi bulbi oculi, 112, T2.3
Mm. faciales, 10, 150, BP20
  anterior view, BP19

Mm. femoris
  anterior view, 498
  attachments (anterior view), 498
  attachments (posterior view), 499
  compartimentum anterius, 502
  compartimentum mediale, 503
  lateral view, 501
  posterior view, 499, 504
Mm. glutei
  anterior view, 498
  attachments (anterior view), 498
  attachments (posterior view), 499
  lateral view, 501
  posterior view, 499
  posterior views, 504
Mm. glutei medius, T8.2
Mm. glutei minimus, T8.2
Mm. glutei superficiales, 10
Mm. hypothenaris, 469, 470, 473, 487, BP100, BP101
Mm. iliocostales, T3.2
Mm. infrahyoidei, 53, 219
Mm. intercostales, 219, 238, 263
  externi, 197, 271, T4.4
  interni, T4.4
  intimi, 253, T4.4
Mm. interni laryngis, 107
Mm. interossei dorsales
  manus, 473, 474, 475, 480, BP100, T7.6
  pedis, 547, 548, 549, T8.7
Mm. interossei palmares, 473, 475, 487, BP100, T7.7
Mm. interossei pedis, 547, 548
Mm. interossei plantares, 546, 547, 548, T8.9
Mm. interspinales, T3.2
Mm. intertransversarii, T3.2
Mm. laterales cruris, 10
Mm. latissimus dorsi, T3.2
Mm. longissimi, T3.3
Mm. lumbricales manus, 470, 471, 472, 473, 486, 487, T7.7
Mm. lumbricales pedis, 545, 549, T8.9
Mm. manus, 10, 475
Mm. masticatorii, 72, 73
Mm. mediales femoris, 10
Mm. multifidus, 200, T3.3
Mm. obliquus externus, BP104
Mm. pectorales, 10
Mm. pedis, 10
Mm. perinei, 10
Mm. pharyngis
  lateral view, 97
  medial view, 96
  partially opened posterior view, 92
Mm. plantares pedis
  first layer, 544
  second layer, 545
  third layer, 546
Mm. posteriores
  antebrachii, 10
  brachii, 10
  cruris, 10
  femoris, 10
Mm. profundi dorsi, 197
Mm. respiratorii, BP43
Mm. scapulohumerales, 10
Mm. semimembranosus, T8.2
Mm. semispinales, T3.3
Mm. semitendinosus, T8.2
Mm. spinales, T3.4
Mm. subcostales, 279, T4.4
Mm. superficiales capitis, T2.2
  lateral view, 48
Mm. superficiales dorsi, 10, 195
Mm. suprahyoidei, 87
Mm. thenaris, 467, 469, 470, 486, BP100
Musculus, structure of, BP10

M. anconeus, 428, 441, 454, 455, 460, 461, 488, 489, T7.6
M. articularis genus, 498, 515, 517, 521, 550, T8.7
M. arytenoideus obliquus, T2.18
M. arytenoideus transversus, T2.22
M. auricularis anterior, 48, BP19, T2.14
M. auricularis posterior, 48, T2.14
M. auricularis superior, 48, T2.14
M. biceps brachii, 202, 422, 428, 435, 438, 440, 442, 445, 457, 459, 460, 483, 485, T7.6
M. biceps femoris, 498, 501, 504, 515, 526, 527, 529, 530, T8.7
M. brachialis, 428, 438, 440, 442, 445, 456, 457, 458, 459, 483, 485, T7.6
M. brachioradialis, 422, 428, 440, 441, 442, 454, 455, 456, 457, 458, 459, 460, 461, 483, 488, 489, T7.6
M. bulbospongiosus, 343, 371, 375, 378, 379, 380, 384, 397, 398, 406, 407, 419, BP86, T6.4
M. ciliaris, T2.14
M. coccygeus, 283, 358, 359, 360, 361, 404, 405, 412, 413, 414, T6.4
M. coracobrachialis, 428, 433, 438, 440, 442, 445, 483, 485, T7.6
M. cricoarytenoideus lateralis, T2.16
M. cricoarytenoideus posterior, T2.19
M. cricothyreoideus, 103, T2.14
M. deltoideus, 49, 178, 202, 238, 263, 422, 428, 431, 432, 433, 435, 436, 440, 441, 442, 445, 483, 488, 490, T7.6
M. digastricus, T2.15
M. fibularis brevis, 526, 531, 532, 534, 540, 541, 542, 554, BP106, BP110, T8.8
M. fibularis longus, 491, 501, 516, 517, 526, 528, 531, 532, 534, 540, 554, BP106, T8.8
M. fibularis tertius, 526, T8.8
M. frontalis, 48, T2.15
M. gastrocnemius, 516, 517, 527, 528, 532, 552, 553, BP106, T8.8
M. gemellus inferior, 415, 420, 421, 499, 504, 511, 512, 513, T8.9
M. gemellus superior, 415, 499, 504, 511, 512, 513, BP104, T8.10
M. genioglossus, T2.3, T2.15
M. geniohyoideus, 57, T2.15
M. gluteus maximus, 178, 195, 198, 275, 331, 362, 379, 397, 398, 412, 413, 415, 420, 421, 491, 499, 501, 504, 511, 512, 513, 515, 555, BP81, BP104, T8.8
M. gluteus medius, 178, 415, 420, 421, 491, 502, 504, 505, 510, 512, 513, BP81, BP94, BP104, T8.8
M. gluteus minimus, 498, 504, 505, 510, 512, 513, BP81, BP104, T8.8
M. gracilis, 415, 498, 502, 509, 510, 511, 515, 516, 520, 527, 551, T8.8
M. hyoglossus, T2.15
M. iliacus, 280, 283, 330, 366, 394, 420, 498, 502, 505, 507, 514, 550, BP80, BP81, BP94, T8.9
M. iliococcygeus, 358, 359, 360, 362
M. iliocostalis colli, 196
M. iliocostalis lumborum, 196
M. iliocostalis thoracis, 196
M. infraspinatus, 178, 201, 212, 428, 432, 434, 435, 436, 441, 488, T7.7
M. intercostalis externus, 201, 212, 279, 436
M. intercostalis internus, 201, 212, 279
M. intercostalis intimus, 201, 212, 251, 279
M. interosseus dorsalis manus, 455, 470, 474, 475, 477, 487, BP101, BP102
M. interosseus palmaris, 474, BP101
M. interosseus pedis, BP111
M. ischiocavernosus, 364, 371, 372, 378, 379, 380, 383, 384, 393, 397, 405, 406, 407, T6.4

M. latissimus dorsi, 178, 195, 198, 200, 209, 270, 271, 275, 278, 279, 331, 347, 351, 428, 432, 433, 435, 438, 440, 442, BP79
M. levis, BP71
M. longissimus capitis, 196, 199
M. longissimus colli, 196
M. longissimus thoracis, 196
M. longitudinalis inferior linguae, T2.15
M. longitudinalis superficialis linguae, 89
M. longitudinalis superior linguae, T2.21
M. longus capitis, 253, T2.16
M. longus colli, 253, T2.17
M. lumbricalis, 473, 474, BP101, BP102
M. mentalis, 48, BP19, T2.17
M. mylohyoideus, T2.18
M. nasalis, 48, T2.18
M. nonstriatus, BP44
M. obliquus externus abdominis, 198, 202, 205, 267, 271, 272, 273, 275, 276, 278, 279, 280, 281, 283, 331, 351, 363, 432, 433, 501, BP53, BP79, T5.4
M. obliquus inferior capitis, 196, T3.3
M. obliquus inferior, T2.15
M. obliquus internus abdominis, 195, 271, 272, 273, 275, 276, 278, 280, 281, 283, 351, 363, BP53, T5.4
M. obliquus superior capitis, 196, T3.3
M. obliquus superior, 113, T2.21
M. occipitalis, 48, 199, T2.18
M. oliquus externus abdominis, 270
M. opponens digiti minimi, 472, 475, T7.7
M. opponens pollicis, 472, 475, 476, T7.7
M. orbicularis oculi, 48, T2.18
M. orbicularis oris, 48, 60, BP19, T2.18
M. palatoglossus, 89, T2.19
M. palatopharyngeus, 89, T2.19
M. palmaris brevis, 469, T7.7
M. palmaris longus, 452, 456, 461, 486, T7.7
M. papillaris anterior, 248
M. papillaris superior, 244
M. pectineus, 420, 421, 499, 502, 503, 509, 510, 514, 515, BP94, BP104, T8.9
M. pectoralis major, 49, 202, 205, 208, 209, 219, 238, 262, 263, 267, 270, 271, 422, 428, 432, 433, 435, 438, 440, 445, T4.4
M. pectoralis minor, 208, 219, 238, 433, 435, 442, T4.4
M. piriformis, 283, 358, 359, 360, 361, 404, 405, 412, 413, 414, 415, 498, 504, 511, 512, 513, T8.2, T8.9
M. plantaris, 501, 511, 516, 520, 526, 527, 528, 529, 533, 552, 553, T8.9
M. popliteus, 521, 526, 529, 533, 553, BP106, T8.9
M. procerus, 48, 60, BP19, T2.19
M. pterygoideus lateralis, 73, T2.16
M. pterygoideus medialis, 73, T2.17
M. puboanalis, 343, 358, 360, 362, 393, 420, 421, BP94
M. pubococcygeus, 358, 359, 360, 362
M. pyramidalis, 271, 281, BP104, T5.4
M. quadratus femoris, 415, 498, 499, 504, 510, 511, 512, 513, T8.9
M. quadratus lumborum, 200, 283, 284, 285, 287, 363, 505, T5.4
M. quadratus plantae, 545, BP111, T8.9
M. quadriceps femoris, 498, 550
M. rectococcygeus, 283
M. rectoperinealis, 362
M. rectus abdominis, 202, 267, 271, 272, 273, 274, 276, 278, 280, 281, 343, 347, 351, 363, 366, 367, 368, 399, 420, BP79, BP80, BP81, BP94, BP104, T5.1, T5.4
M. rectus anterior capitis, T2.19
M. rectus femoris, 421, 491, 498, 501, 502, 509, 510, 515, BP94, BP104, T8.10
M. rectus inferior, T2.16

Atlas of Human Anatomy

M. rectus lateralis, T2.16, T2.19
M. rectus medialis, T2.17, BP27
M. rectus posterior major capitis, 196, 199, T3.3
M. rectus posterior minor capitis, 196, 199
M. rectus superior, 113, T2.21
M. rhomboideus major, 198, 201, 212, 263, 275, 432, 488
M. rhomboideus minor, 195, 198, 432, 488, T3.3
M. risorius, 48, BP19, T2.19
M. salpingopharyngeus, T2.19
M. sartorius, 420, 421, 491, 498, 501, 502, 509, 510, 515, 516, 520, 527, 550, BP94, BP104, T8.10
M. scalenus anterior, 57, 103, 211, 219, 220, 231, 238, 251, 252, 253, 254, 436, 437, 438, BP42, T2.19
M. scalenus medius, 49, 51, 253, 436, T2.20
M. scalenus posterior, 49, 51, 253, 254, BP42, T2.20
M. semimembranosus, 415, 499, 501, 504, 511, 515, 516, 520, 526, 527, 552, T8.10
M. semispinalis capitis, 195, 196, 199
M. semispinalis colli, 199
M. semitendinosus, 415, 491, 498, 504, 512, 515, 520, 527, 552, T8.10
M. serratus anterior, 195, 202, 205, 209, 212, 267, 270, 271, 275, 278, 279, 347, 422, 432, 433, 435, 436, 438, BP42, T4.4
M. serratus posterior inferior, 195, 200, 275, 331, T3.4
M. serratus posterior superior, 196, T3.4
M. soleus, 516, 527, 528, 529, 530, 531, 532, 533, 534, 540, 552, BP106, T8.10
M. spinalis colli, 196
M. spinalis thoracis, 196
M. splenius capitis, 195, 196, 199, T3.4
M. splenius colli, 195, 196, 199, T3.4
M. stapedius, T2.3, T2.20
M. sternocleidomastoideus, 49, 199, 202, 209, 219, 432, 438, T2.2, T2.20
M. sternohyoideus, 49, 53, 211, T2.20
M. sternothyreoideus, 49, 211, T2.20
M. styloglossus, T2.3, T2.20
M. stylohyoideus, T2.21
M. stylopharyngeus, T2.21
M. subclavius, 205, 238, 429, 433, 435, BP42, T4.4
M. subscapularis, 212, 263, 428, 433, 435, 436, 440, 442, BP50, T7.7
M. supraspinatus, 195, 198, 428, 432, 433, 434, 435, 436, 437, 441, 488, 490, BP50, T7.7
M. suspensorius duodeni, 289
M. tarsalis superior, 110, T2.3
M. temporalis, 72, T2.21
M. teres major, 178, 428, 432, 433, 435, 436, 438, 440, 442, 445, 488, T7.7
M. teres minor, 212, 428, 432, 433, 435, 436, 441, 488, T7.7
M. thyreoarytenoideus, T2.22
M. thyreohyoideus, 49, 57, T2.22
M. tibialis anterior, 491, 501, 516, 517, 530, 531, 532, 534, 542, 554, BP106, BP110, T8.10
M. tibialis posterior, 526, 529, 533, 553, BP106, T8.10
M. transversus abdominis, 196, 200, 211, 272, 273, 276, 278, 280, 281, 283, 287, 351, 363, 505, BP80, T5.4
M. transversus linguae, T2.22
M. transversus profundus perinei, 343, 364, 379, 385, 393, 398, 405, 406, T6.4
M. transversus superficialis perinei, 343, 378, 379, 380, 383, 384, 393, 397, 398, 406, 407, T6.4
M. transversus thoracis, 201, 212, T4.4

M. trapezius, 22, 49, 178, 198, 199, 209, 212, 263, 275, 422, 428, 432, 433, 435, BP50, T3.1, T3.4
M. triceps brachii, 178, 202, 428, 438, 441, 442, 445, 447, 460, T7.7
M. umbricalis, 474
M. uvulae, T2.3, T2.18
M. vastus intermedius, 498, 502, 503, 515, 517, T8.10
M. vastus lateralis, 421, 491, 498, 501, 502, 509, 510, 511, 515, 516, 517, 530, 531, T8.10
M. vastus medialis, 491, 498, 499, 502, 503, 509, 515, 516, 517, 531, T8.10
M. verticalis linguae, T2.22
M. vocalis, T2.22
M. zygomaticus major, 48, BP19, T2.22
M. zygomaticus minor, 48, BP19, T2.22
Myocyte leve, BP13
Myometrium, 374, 399

N

Nares, 22
Naris, 61
Nasion, 25
Neck of hernia sac, BP54
Nephron, schema, BP72
Nervi, 60
    autonomici, 319
    cervicales, 57
    colli, 56
    cutanei, 23
    dorsales colli, 199
    dorsi, 198
    glutei, 512
    intercostales, 212, 279
    spinales, 186, 190
Nervi craniales, T2.6–T2.11
Nn. alveolares superiores posteriores, 149
Nn. anales inferiores, 415
Nn. anococcygei, 415
Nn. cardiaci, 6
    cervicales, 229, BP6
    thoracici, 249, T4.1
Nn. cavernosi penis, 412, BP7, T6.1
Nn. ciliares breves, 79
Nn. ciliares longi, 79
Nn. craniales, 4, 86, 145
Nn. cutanei glutei
    inferiores, 198, 413, 415, 493, 511, 512, 552
    mediales, 511
    medii, 198, 493
    superiores, 198, 493, 511
Nn. digitales, 476
    dorsales manus, 425, 478
    dorsales pedis, 492
    palmares, 469
    plantares proprii, 543
Nn. dorsales penis, 411, 418
Nn. fibulares superficialis and profundus, BP109
Nn. hypogastrici, 339, 411, 412, 414, 416, 417, 418, 419
Nn. intercostales, 186, 212, 279, T5.1
Nn. labiales anteriores, 415
Nn. labiales posteriores, 415, 416
Nn. oculomotorius, T2.1
Nn. palatini minores, 81, 149
Nn. scrotales anteriores, 411
Nn. scrotales posteriores, 412, 413
Nn. spinales, 4, 186, 190
Nn. splanchnici lumbales, 6, 319, 411, 412, 414, 416, 417, 418, BP6
Nn. splanchnici pelvici, 7, 323, 324, 339, 412, 416, 417, 418, 419, 508, BP7
Nn. splanchnici sacrales, 339, 412, 414, BP6

Nn. splanchnici thoracici, 326
    lumbales, T5.1
Nn. subscapulares, T7.3
Nn. superiores clunium, 275
Nn. supraclaviculares, 423
Nn. temporales profundi, 149
Nn. viscerales thoracici, BP6
N. abducens (CN VI), 148, T2.7
N. accessorius (CN XI), 131, 143, 154, T2.11
N. accessorius spinalis, 33, 34, 198, 436, T2.1
N. alveolaris inferior, 42, 73, 84
N. alveolaris superior anterior, 84, 149
N. alveolaris superior medius, 84
N. alveolaris superior posterior, 84
N. analis inferior, 324, 412, 413, 415, 416, 512, T6.1
N. anococcygeus, 413, 508
N. auricularis magnus, 50, 198, 199, T2.13
N. auricularis posterior, 71
N. auriculotemporalis, 23, 42, 73, 75
N. autonomicus, BP13
N. axillaris, 434, 438, 439, 441, 484, 485, 486, 488, 489, T7.1, T7.4
N. buccalis, 23, 84, 149
N. canalis pterygoidei (Vidii), 79
N. cardiacus cervicalis medius, 249, 250
N. cardiacus cervicalis superior, 249, 250
N. caroticus externus, 6, BP6
N. caroticus internus, 6, BP6
N. coccygeus, 187, 508
N. cochlearis, 125, T2.8
N. cutaneus, 12
N. cutaneus intermedius dorsalis pedis, 492, 554, BP109
N. cutaneus lateralis antebrachii, 423, 424, 425, 440, 445, 456, 457, 458, 479, 483, 485, T7.3
N. cutaneus lateralis dorsalis pedis, 492, 493, 542, 552, 553, 554, BP109
N. cutaneus lateralis femoris, 278, 282, 287, 411, 492, 494, 505, 507, 509, 510, 515, 550, 551, T8.1, T8.4
N. cutaneus lateralis inferior brachii, 423, 441, 488, T7.4
N. cutaneus lateralis superior brachii, 423, 424, 441, 488, T7.4
N. cutaneus lateralis surae, 492, 493, 511, 527, 528, 534, 553, 554, T8.6
N. cutaneus medialis antebrachii, 439, 442, 445, 479, 482, 484, 485, 486, T7.4
N. cutaneus medialis brachii, 278, 424, 439, 442, 445, 483, 484, 485, 486, T7.4
N. cutaneus medialis dorsalis pedis, 492, 554, BP109
N. cutaneus medialis surae, 493, 527, 528, 534, 553, BP106, T8.6
N. cutaneus perforans, 413, 415, 493, 508, T8.4
N. cutaneus posterior antebrachii, 423, 424, 425, 441, 445, 478, 479, 488, T7.4
N. cutaneus posterior brachii, 423, 424, T7.4
N. cutaneus posterior femoris, 186, 413, 415, 420, 508, 511, 512, 515, 552, T8.5
N. digitalis dorsalis manus, 481
N. digitalis dorsalis pedis, 492
N. digitalis palmaris communis, 473
N. digitalis palmaris proprius, 481
N. dorsalis clitoridis, 415, 416
N. dorsalis penis, 382, 384, 407, 412, 413, 512
N. dorsalis scapulae, 438, 439, 488, T7.3
N. ethmoideus anterior, 79
N. ethmoideus posterior, 79
N. facialis (CN VII), 7, 71, 121, 143, 150, BP7, BP26, BP32, T2.1, T2.7
N. femoralis, 186, 274, 280, 282, 287, 409, 411, 420, 494, 505, 507, 510, 550, 551, BP81, BP94, BP104, T8.1, T8.4
N. fibularis communis, 504, 511, 515, 516, 517, 527, 528, 529, 530, 552, 553, 554, BP106, T8.1, T8.5

N. fibularis profundus, 534, 541, 542, 554, BP106, BP109, BP110, T8.5
N. fibularis superficialis, 492, 534, 541, 542, 554, BP106, BP109, T8.5
N. frontalis, 79
N. genitofemoralis, 287, 351, 411, 505, 507, 551, T5.1, T8.4
N. glossopharyngeus (CN IX), 7, 143, 152, BP7, T2.8
N. gluteus inferior, 186, 508, 512, T8.4
N. gluteus superior, 186, 508, 512, T8.4
N. hypogastricus, 340, 414, BP6
N. hypoglossus (CN XII), 155, T2.11
N. iliohypogastricus, 198, 351, 411, 416, 505, 506, 507, 551, T5.1
N. ilioinguinalis, 186, 278, 287, 351, 411, 416, 505, 506, 507, 551, T5.1
N. infraorbitalis, 23, 79, 84, 149
N. infratrochlearis, 23, 60, 79
N. intercostalis, 205, 211, 251, 340, 439, 506, T4.1
N. intercostobrachialis, 278, 424, 436, 438, 483, 484
N. interosseus anterior antebrachii, 458, 486, T7.5
N. interosseus cruris, 553
N. interosseus posterior, 489, T7.4
   antebrachii, 455, 489
N. ischiadicus, 186, 415, 420, 421, 504, 508, 511, 512, 515, 552, BP94, BP104, T8.5
N. lacrimalis, 79
N. laryngeus recurrens, 57, 103, 229, T2.1, T2.10, T4.1
N. laryngeus superior, T2.10
N. levatoris ani, T8.5
N. lingualis, 42, 73, 84, 149
N. mandibularis, 23, 42, 77, 84, T2.7
N. massetericus, 73, 149
N. maxillaris, 23, 79, 84, T2.7
N. medianus, 423, 439, 440, 442, 445, 456, 457, 458, 461, 464, 470, 472, 475, 476, 482, 483, 484, 485, 486, BP100, T7.1, T7.5
N. mentalis, 23, 149
N. musculi coccygei, T8.5
N. musculi piriformis, T8.4
N. musculi quadrati femoris, T8.5
N. musculocutaneus, 423, 438, 439, 440, 442, 445, 458, 482, 483, 484, 485, 486, T7.3
N. mylohyoideus, 42, 73
N. nasociliaris, 79
N. nasopalatinus, 33, 84, 149
N. obturatorius, 287, 402, 412, 420, 505, 507, 550, 551, BP81, BP94, T8.1, T8.4
   accessorius, 507
N. occipitalis major, 198, 199
N. occipitalis minor, 198, 199, T2.12
N. occipitalis tertius, 198, 199
N. oculomotorius (CN III), 7, 143, 148, BP7, T2.6
N. olfactorius (CN I), 46, T2.1, T2.6
N. ophthalmicus, 23, 79, 84, T2.7
N. opticus (CN II), 147, 164, T2.1, T2.6
N. palatinus major, 82, 149
N. pectoralis lateralis, 435, 438, 439, T7.3
N. pectoralis medialis, 435, 438, 439, T7.4
N. perinealis, 412, 413, 415, 512
N. periphericus, BP4
N. pharyngeus, 149
N. phrenicus, 50, 57, 103, 211, 214, 215, 216, 219, 220, 231, 249, 251, 253, 263, 276, 319, 341, 436, 438, T2.12, T4.1
N. plantaris lateralis, 529, 533, 540, 552, BP109, T8.6
N. plantaris medialis, 529, 533, 549, 552, 553, BP109, T8.6
N. pterygoideus lateralis, 149
N. pterygoideus medialis, 73, 98, 149
N. pudendalis, 186, 287, 324, 407, 412, 413, 414, 415, 416, 417, 418, 420, 421, 508, 511, 512, BP94, T6.1, T7.4, T8.5

N. radialis, 423, 433, 438, 439, 441, 445, 457, 458, 482, 483, 484, 485, 486, 488, 489, T7.1, T7.4
N. saphenus, 492, 509, 510, 515, 531, 532, 534, 550, BP106, BP109, T8.1, T8.4
N. scrotalis anterior, 278
Nervus spinalis, 190, 326, 414
   L4, 415
   L5, 415
   lumbalis, 200
   S1, 415
   S2, 415
   S3, 415
   S4, 415
   thoracicus, 201
N. splanchnicus lumbalis, 340, 341
N. splanchnicus thoracicus
   major, BP6
   minor, BP6
N. splanchnicus thoracicus imus, 6, 216, 287, 321, 325, 339, 340, 411, 416, 417, 418
N. splanchnicus thoracicus major, 6, 216, 287, 320, 321, 339, 411, 412, 416, 417, 418
N. splanchnicus thoracicus minor, 6, 216, 229, 287, 321, 325, 339, 411, 412, 416, 417, 418
N. subclavius, T7.3
N. subcostalis, 287, 330, 331, 411, 416, 505, 506, 507
N. suboccipitalis, 199
N. subscapularis inferior, 433, 438, 439
N. subscapularis superior, 433, 438, 439
N. supraclavicularis, T2.13
   intermedius, 424
   lateralis, 424
   medialis, 424
N. supraorbitalis, 23, 60, 79
N. suprascapularis, 436, 439, 488, T7.3
N. supratrochlearis, 23, 60, 79
N. suralis, 493, 552, 553, 554, BP106, BP109, BP110, T8.1, T8.6
N. tensoris veli palatin, 149
N. thoracicus longus, 206, 209, 278, 436, 438, 439, T4.1, T7.1, T7.3
N. thoracodorsalis, 433, 438, 439, T7.3
N. tibialis, 504, 511, 515, 527, 528, 529, 533, 534, 552, 553, BP106, BP109, BP110, T8.5
N. transversus colli, 57, T2.13
N. trigeminus (CN V), 84, 143, 149, 177, BP26, T2.1, T2.6
N. trochlearis (CN IV), 143, 148, T2.6
N. ulnaris, 423, 438, 439, 441, 442, 445, 454, 455, 456, 457, 458, 461, 470, 475, 476, 482, 483, 484, 485, 486, 487, T7.1, T7.5
N. vagus (CN X), 7, 99, 103, 143, 153, 249, 263, 326, 340, BP7, T2.9
N. vestibularis, T2.8
N. vestibulocochlearis (CN VIII), 151, T2.7
N. zygomaticofacialis, 23, 79, 98, 149
N. zygomaticotemporalis, 23, 79, 149
N. zygomaticus, 79, 149
Neurocranium, 8
Neurofibrae, 125
Neurofilamentum, BP3
Neurons, BP3
Neuron postsynapticum, BP3
Neurotubulus, BP3
No communication between ducts, BP62
Nodi anorectales
   medii, BP77
   superiores, BP77
Nodi axillares, 16
   anteriores, 207, 208
   apicales, 207, 208
   centrales, 207, 208
   laterales, 207, 208, 426
   posteriores, 207, 208
Nodi cervicales, 16
   laterales profundi inferiores, 260

Nodi coeliaci, 260, BP74, BP75, BP76, BP78
Nodi cubitales, 16
Nodi gastrici sinistri, BP74
Nodi gastroomentales dextri, BP74
Nodi hepatici, BP74, BP75, BP78
Nodi iliaci, 16
   communes, 286, 338, 408, 410, BP77
   externi, 286, 338, 410, BP77
   interni, 286, 338, 408, 410, BP77
Nodi inguinales, 16, BP77
   profundi, 286, 408, 410
   superficiales, 408, 410
   superficiales inferiores, 409
   superficiales superolaterales, 409
   superficiales superomediales, 409
Nodi intercostales, 260
Nodi interpectorales (Rotteri), 207
Nodi juxtaoesophagei, 260
Nodi lumbales.
   dextri, 286
   sinistri, 286
Nodi lymphoidei, 207, 228, 260, 494
   axillares, T4.3
   coeliaci, BP74
   iliaci externi, 494
   inguinales profundi, 409
   inguinales superficiales, T8.3
   lumbales, T6.2
   lumbales dextri, 408, 410
   lumbales intermedii, 408
   lumbales sinistri, 408
   lumbalis intermedii, 410
   parasternales, 207
   paratracheales, 260
   pelvis, T6.2
   poplitei, 494
   pretracheales, 103
   tracheobronchiales, 286
Nodi mediastinales, 16
   posteriores, 260
Nodi mesenterici
   juxtaintestinales, BP76
   superiores, BP74
   superiores centrales, BP75, BP76
Nodi pancreaticoduodenales, BP75
Nodi paracolici, BP77
Nodi paramammarii, 208
Nodi parasternales, 208
Nodi paratracheales, 228
Nodi phrenici inferiores, 286
Nodi phrenici superiores, 260, BP78
Nodi poplitei, 16
Nodi prevesicales, 338
Nodi pylorici, BP78
Nodi sacrales, 410
   laterales, 286
   mediani, 286, 408, 410
Nodi sigmoidei, BP77
Nodi splenici, BP74
Nodi subpylorici, BP74
Nodi supratrochleares, 426
Nodi tracheobronchiales
   inferiores, 260
   superiores, 228, 260
Nodi vesicales laterales, 338
Noduli lymphoidei, 89
   aggregati appendicis vermiformis, BP57
   aggregati intestini (Peyeri), 16, 297
   solitarii intestini, 297
Nodulus lymphoideus solitarius, 297, BP55
Nodus atrioventricularis, T4.2
Nodus cervicalis lateralis profundus inferior, 228
Nodus cysticus, BP74
Nodus epigastricus inferior, 286
Nodus iliacus
   communis, 410
   externus lateralis, 408

Nodus infraclavicularis, 426
Nodus inguinalis profundus proximalis, 408, 409, 410
Nodus lymphoideus, 282
  inguinalis, 421
  lumbalis intermedius, 351
  mediastinalis, 263
Nodus obturatorius, 408
Nodus pancreaticus superior, BP74
Nodus preaorticus, 410
Nodus sacralis
  lateralis, 408, 410
  medianus, 338, 410
Nodus sinuatrialis, 248, T4.2
Nuclei basales, corpus striatum, 137
Nuclei cochleares
  anterior, 143
  posterior, 143
Nuclei mamillares, 174
Nuclei nervorum cranialium
  medial view, 144
  posterior view, 143
Nucleus accessorius n. oculomotorii, 143
Nucleus ambiguus, 143
Nucleus mesencephalicus n. trigemini, 143
Nucleus motorius n. trigemini, 143
Nucleus n. abducentis, 143
Nucleus n. facialis, 143
Nucleus n. hypoglossi, 143
Nucleus n. oculomotorii, 143
Nucleus n. trochlearis, 143
Nucleus paraventricularis hypothalami, 174
Nucleus posterior n. vagi, 143, 250, 324
Nucleus principalis n. trigemini, 143
Nucleus pulposus, 181
Nucleus ruber, 143
Nucleus salivatorius superior, 143
Nucleus salivatorius inferior, 161
Nucleus spinalis n. trigemini, 143
Nucleus supraopticus, 174
Nucleus tractus solitarii, 143, 144, 150, 152, 153, 340

O

Obturator externus, 421, 510, 551, T8.9
Obturator internus, 274, 283, 358, 359, 360, 361, 362, 371, 372, 373, 384, 394, 400, 413, 415, 420, 421, 498, 499, 504, 511, 512, 513, 555, BP104, T8.9
Oesophagus, 18, 93, 215, 238, 251, 263, 283, 285, 286, 289, 293, 323, 330, 332, 343, BP36, BP50
  arteriae, 258
  arterial variations, BP49
  constrictions and relations, 255
  intrinsic nerves and variations, BP48
  musculi, 256
  nervi, 261
  nodi lymphoidei, 260
  schema of autonomic innervation, 325
  in situ, 254
  vasa lymphatica, 260
  venae, 259
Olecranon, 422, 441, 446, 447, 449, 451, 454, 455, 488
Olfactory pathways, 146
Omentum majus, 288, 290, 292, 294, 301, 343, 350, 351
Omentum minus, 293, 306, 343, BP79
Omos
  anteroposterior radiograph, 430
  CT, 490
  juncturae, 431
  MRI, 490
  musculi, 432, 436
  tendines, 436
  venae superficiales, 424

Oocyte
  primarium, BP87, BP90
  secundarium, BP87
Oocytia, BP90
Oogonium, BP87
Ootidium, BP87
Opisthion, BP18
Ora serrata, 118
Orbiculus ciliaris, 118
Orbita, 37, 67, BP27, T2.2
  arteriae and venae, 115
  nervi, 113
  superior and anterior views, 114
Organa endocrina, T2.5
Organa genitalia externa
  female, 377, 415
  homologues of, 389
  male, 381, 382, 383, 386, 388
  nervi of, 6, 7, 411, 413, 415
Organa genitalia interna
  feminina, 363, 364, 365
  homologues of, 390
  musculina, 368, 385, 391, 392
  nervi of, 417, 418
Organa lymphoidea, 16, T2.5, T4.3, T5.2, T6.2, T8.3
Organa sensuum, T2.1
Orthotonic stomach, BP55
Os, architecture of, BP9
Os 1 metacarpi, 455, 458, 467, 472, 477
Os 1 metatarsi, 529, 539, 540, 548, 556
Os 2 metacarpi, 455, BP102
Os 3 metacarpi, 463, BP101
Os 4 metacarpi, BP101
Os 4 metatarsi, BP111
Os 5 metacarpi, 454, 455, 458
Os 5 metatarsi, 529, 530, 548, BP111
Os capitatum, 462, 463, 465, 467, 472, BP98
Os coccygis, 179, 183, 186, 354, 356, 358, 359, 379, 393, 420, BP94, BP104
Os coxae, 495
  ligamenta of, 357
Os cuboideum, 535, 536, 539, 547, 548, 549, 556
Os cuneiforme
  intermedium, 547, 548
  laterale, 547, 548
  mediale, 539, 547, 548, BP111
Os ethmoideum, 25, 27, 32, 35
Os femoris, 500, 515, 517, 520, 521, BP108
Os frontale, 22, 25, 27, 28, 30, 31, 32, 35, 110
Os hamatum, 462, 463, 465, 472, BP98
Os hyoideum, 36, 49, 50, 103, 106, BP34, T2.2
Os ilium, 354, 497
Os ischii, 354, 420, 421
Os lacrimale, 25, 27, 35
Os lunatum, 462, 463, 465, 467, BP98
Os metacarpi, 468, 474
Os nasale, 22, 25, 26, 27, 35
Os naviculare, 535, 536, 547, 548, 556
Os occipitale, 27, 30, 32, 35, 186, 187
Os palatinum, 31, 35
Os parietale, 25, 27, 28, 30, 32, 35
Os pisiforme, 452, 456, 457, 458, 462, 463, 464, 465, 467, 468, 469, 470, 472, 475, BP98
Os pubis, 343, 354, 358, 359, 370, 384, 399, 414, 421
Os sacrum, 178, 179, 183, 361, 399
Os scaphoideum, 462, 463, 465, 467, 477, BP98, T7.1
Os sesamoideum pedis, 536
Os sphenoideum, 25, 27, 29, 31, 32, 36
Os suturale, 27, 30
Os tali, 535, 536, 556, BP110
Os temporale, 25, 27, 31, 32, 35, 36
Os trapezium, 462, 463, 465, 467, 468, 472, 477, BP98
Os trapezoideum, 462, 463, 465, 467, 472, BP98

Os triquetrum, 463, 465, 467, BP98
Os zygomaticum, 22, 25, 26, 27, 31, 35, 110
Ossa antebrachii, 449
Ossa capitis, 8
Ossa carpi, 462, 466
  movements, 463
Ossa faciei, 8
Ossa manus, 466
Ossa metacarpi, 463, 466, BP98
  cross sections through, BP100
Ossa metatarsi, 535, 536, 547, 549
Ossa pedis
  lateral and medial views, 536
  superior and inferior views, 535
Ossa sesamoidea
  manus, 463
  pedis, 535, 539, 545, 546, 547, 548
Ossicula auditus, 122, T2.2
Osteoblasti, BP9
Ostia aa. coronariarum, 245
Ostia ductulorum prostaticorum, 386
Ostia ductuum ejaculatoriorum, 386, BP94
Ostia ductuum glandularum bulbourethralium, 386
Ostia ductuum paraurethalium, 377, BP86
Ostia ductuum sublingualium, 87
Ostia glandularum ductus biliaris, 305
Ostia glandularum tarsalium, 110
Ostia ureterum, 375
Ostium a. coronariae dextrae, 244
Ostium abdominale tubae uterinae, 374
Ostium cardiale gastris, 238, 295
Ostium ductus
  alveolaris, BP44
  ejaculatorii, 385, 390
  glandulae bulbourethralis, 385
  glandulae vestibularis majoris, 377
  paraurethralis, BP86
Ostium externum urethrae
  femininae, 364, 377, 380, 389, 397, BP86
  masculinae, 267, 352, 383, 386, 389
Ostium externum uteri, 374
Ostium glandulae preputialis, 383
Ostium ileale, 299, 301
Ostium internum urethrae, BP94
Ostium internum uteri, 374
Ostium pharyngeum tubae auditivae, 61, 93
Ostium pyloricum, 297
Ostium ureteris, 369, 371, 385, BP86, T6.3
Ostium uterinum tubae uterinae, 374
Ostium vaginae, 364, 377, 380, 389, BP86
Ovaria, 21
Ovarian hormone levels, BP88
Ovarium, 363, 364, 365, 372, 373, 374, 375, 376, 390, 402, 414, 417, BP90, T6.3
Ovulatio, 365

P

Pain, referred visceral, sites of, BP5
Palatum, 68
  durum, 177
  molle, 61, 83, 93, 145, 177
  paries superior cavitatis oris, 85
Palma, 463
Palpebrae, 110, 115
Pancreas, 6, 18, 200, 292, 293, 343, 348, 350, BP50, T5.3
  arteriae, 310
  schema of autonomic innervation, 329
  in situ, 306
  vasa lymphatica and nodi lymphoidei, BP75
  venae, 315
Panniculus adiposus telae subcutaneae abdominis, 182, 270, 273, BP84
Papilla dermalis pili, 12, BP1
Papilla ductus parotidei, 83
Papilla fungiformis, 89

Papilla lacrimalis
  inferior, 110
  superior, 110
Papilla major duodeni, 297, 305, BP62, T5.2
Papilla mammaria, 202, 205
Papilla minor duodeni, 297, 305, BP62
Papilla renalis, 333
Papilla vallata, 89
Papillae filiformes, 89
Papillae foliatae, 89
Papillae vallatae, 89
Paradidymis, 390
Parasympathetic fibers, BP8
Paries anterior abdominis, 10, 285, 336
  deep dissection, 272
  intermediate dissection, 271
  internal view, 274
  nervi, 278
  superficial dissection, 270
  venae, 277
Paries anterior thoracis
  deeper dissection, 210
  internal view, 211
  superficial dissection, 209
Paries lateralis cavitatis
  nasalis cranii, 62
  nasi, 61
Paries posterior abdominis
  arteriae, 284
  internal view, 283
  nervi, 287
  peritoneum, 293
  vasa lymphatica and nodei lymphoidei, 286
  venae, 285
Paries posterior oropharyngis, 83
Paries posterolateralis abdominis, 275
  arteriae, 276
Paries thoracis venae, 213
Paries vaginae, 372
Parous introitus, BP91
Pars abdominalis oesophagi, 258, 294
Pars abdominalis ureteris, autonomic
  innervation, 340
Pars adductoria adductoris magni, 551
Pars alaris m. nasalis, 60
Pars alveolaris mandibulae, 39
Pars anterior fornicis vaginae, 364
Pars anularis vaginae fibrosae digiti manus,
  470, 473
Pars ascendens duodeni, 289, 296, 297
Pars basilaris ossis occipitalis, 46, 61, 93
Pars cardialis gastris, 257
Pars cartilaginea tubae auditavae, BP30
Pars cervicalis a. vertebralis, 163
Pars cerebralis carotidis internae, 164
Pars cervicalis columnae vertebralis, 45
  Mri and radiograph, BP35
Pars cervicalis medullae spinalis, 177, BP35
Pars cervicalis oesophagi, 254
Pars clavicularis m. pectoralis majoris, 202
Pars convoluta tubuli
  distalis, BP72
  proximalis, BP71, BP72
Pars costalis diaphragmatis, 211, 216
Pars costalis pleurae, 215, 231, 331
Pars cruciformis vaginae fibrosae digiti
  manus, 470, 473
Pars descendens duodeni, 200, 289, 291, 296,
  297, 305
Pars diaphragmatica pleurae, 231
Pars horizontalis duodeni, 289, 297, 343
Pars inferior duodeni, 296
Pars ischiocondylaris adductoris magni, 552
Pars laryngea pharyngis, 93
Pars lumbalis columnae vertebralis
  Mris, BP38
Pars lumbalis medullae spinalis, 419

Pars lumbalis superior medullae spinalis, BP8
Pars media faciei, nervi and arteriae, 81
Pars mediastinalis pleurae, 231
Pars membranacea
  septi interventricularis, 242, 244
  urethrae, 391, BP85
Pars meningea durae cranialis, 127
Pars muscularis septi interventricularis, 244
Pars nasalis pharyngis, 93
Pars occlusa a. umbilicalis, 402, 404, 405, BP93
Pars optica retinae, 116, 118
Pars oralis pharyngis, 93
Pars ossea septi nasi, 38
Pars palpebralis m. orbicularis oculi, 110
Pars parasympathica systematis nervosi, BP7
Pars patens a. umbilicalis, 402, 404, BP93
Pars pelvica peritonei, 368, 371, 394, 398, 417,
  418
Pars periostea durae cranialis, 127
Pars petrosa
  carotidis internae, 164
  ossis temporalis, 26, 35
Pars posterior fornicis vaginae, 364, 375
Pars prerectalis spatii rectovesicalis, 398
Pars profunda
  compartimenti posterioris cruris, 534
  sphincteris externi ani, 343, 393, 395, 396
Pars prostatica urethrae, 385, 386, 391, BP85,
  BP92
Pars pylorica gastris, 295
Pars retroprostaticus spatii rectovesicalis, 398
Pars retrovesicalis spatii rectovesicalis, 398
Pars sacralis medullae spinalis, 419, BP8
Pars spongiosa urethrae, 371, 382, 386, 391
Pars squamosa ossis frontalis, 35
Pars sternalis diaphragmatis, 211, 216
Pars sternocostalis, 202
Pars subcutanea sphincteris externi ani, 393,
  395, 396
Pars superficialis
  compartimenti posterioris cruris, 534
  sphincteris externi ani, 343, 393, 396
Pars superior duodeni, 295, 296, 297, 305, 348
Pars sympathica systematis nervosi, BP6
  schema of, 6–7
Pars synovialis articulationis sacroiliacae,
  BP81
Pars terminalis ilei, 298, 299, 363, 367
Pars thoracica
  medullae spinalis, BP8
  oesophagi, 258
Pars thoracolumbalis columnae vertebralis,
  lateral radiograph, BP36
Pars thyreopharyngea constrictoris inferioris,
  92, 96, 97, 104, 105, 108, T2.15
Pars transversa m. nasalis, 60
Partes corporis human
  anterior view of female, 2
  posterior view of male, 3
Parturition, neuropathways in, 416
Patella, 491, 501, 503, 510, 516, 517, 521, 530,
  531, BP108
Pecten analis, 395
Pecten ossis pubis, 268, 353, 357, 361, 495
Pediculus arcus vertebrae, 180, 181, 184, BP33,
  BP36
Pedunculi arcus vertebrae, BP37
Pelvic scans, 399
  sagittal T2-weighted mris, 399
Pelvis
  arteriae, 404, 405, BP93
  bony framework, 353
  fasciae of, BP84
  female, 404
  male, 405
  nodi lymphoidei, 408
  radiographs of, 354

Pelvis (Continued)
  structures with high* clinical significance,
    T6.1–T6.3
  surface anatomy, 352
  through prostata, BP92
  vasa lymphatica and nodi lymphoidei, 408,
    410
  venae, 405, BP93
Pelvis feminina, 421
Pelvis masculina, 420
Pelvis ossea
  ligamenta of, 356
  measurements, 355
  sex differences of, 355
Pelvis renalis, 333, 350, T5.3
Penis, 383, 399
Pericardium, 214, 215, T4.2
  fibrosum, 231
Pericyte, BP11
Perineum, 2
  arteriae and venae of, 406, 407
  deeper dissection, 379, 382
  fasciae of, BP84
  female, 377, 378, 379, 415
  male, 381, 382, 407, 413
  nervi of, 413, 415
  superficial dissection, 378, 381
  vasa lymphatica of, 409
Peritoneum, 200, 273, 274, 281, 301, 402, 414,
  T6.2
  mesentericum, 322
  parietale, 282, 292, 293, 337, 341, 342, 343,
    351, 363, 367, 368, 369, 371, 372, 373,
    378, BP54, BP84
  urogenitale, 417, 418
  viscerale, 292, 398
Pes
  anserinus, 516, 517, 526
  arteriae, BP103, BP109
  cross section, 549
  cross-sectional anatomy, BP111
    lateral view, 538
    medial view, 538
  hippocampi, 139
  nervi, BP109
Phalanges
  manus, 466
  pedis, 535, 536, 539, 548
Phalanx distalis
  manus, 467, 468, 481, 539
  pedis, 539, 548, BP112
Phalanx media
  manus pedis, 467, 468, 481, 539
Phalanx proximalis
  manus, 467, 468, BP102
  pedis, 539, 548
Pharynx, 98, BP26
  medial view, 95
  muscles, 18
  nervi and vasa sanguinea (posterior view),
    91
  nodi lymphoidei, 102
  opened posterior view, 93
Philtrum, 22, 83
Pia cranialis, 127, 135
Pia spinalis, 189, 190
Pip joint, BP99
Pivot joint, 9
Plana referentiae, 1
Plane joint, 9
Planta, superficial dissection, 543
Planum coronale, 1
Planum interspinale, 269
Planum intertuberculare, 269
Planum sagittale, 1
Planum subcostale, 269
Planum transpyloricum, 269, BP58

Planum transversum, 1
Plasma
  composition of, BP12
  proteins, BP12
Plasmocyte, BP11
Platelets, BP12
Platysma, 48, 49, BP19, T2.19
Pleura parietalis, 190, BP79
Pleura visceralis, 190
Pleura, T4.3
Plexus, 277, 403, BP93
  aganglionicus externus tunicae muscularis, 327
  aganglionicus internus tunicae muscularis, 327
  aganglionicus tunicae serosae, 327
  anorectalis medius, 323
  anorectalis superior, 324, 412
  aorticus abdominalis, 367
  aorticus thoracicus, 325
  arteriosus pialis, 191
  brachialis, 22, 57, 186, 206, 214, 219, 220, 231, 435, 439, 484, 486
  caecales, 323
  capillaris corticalis renis, BP73
  capillaris medullaris renis, BP73
  cardiacus, 249, 250, BP6, BP7
Plexus caroticus externus, 6
Plexus caroticus internus, 6, 82, BP6
Plexus cervicalis, 57, 156, 186, T2.1
Plexus chorioideus
  ventriculi lateralis, 136, 139
  ventriculi quarti, 136
  ventriculi tertii, 136
Plexus coccygeus, 508
Plexus coeliacus, 320, 321, 322, 339, 340, 341, 412, BP6, BP7
Plexus colicus
  dexter, 322, 323
  medius, 323
  sinister, 319, 323
Plexus deferentialis, 411, 412, 418
Plexus dentalis inferior, 149
Plexus enterici, 326, 327
Plexus gastricus, 412
  dexter, 320, 321
  sinister, 319, 320, 321
Plexus gastroduodenalis, 321, 322, 328
Plexus gastroomentalis
  dexter, 320
  sinister, 320, 321
Plexus hepaticus, 319, 320, 321, 322, 328
Plexus hypogastricus
  inferior, 6, 324, 339, 340, 411, 412, 414, 416, 417, 418, 419, BP6, BP7
  superior, 6, 323, 324, 339, 363, 411, 412, 414, 416, 417, 418, 419, BP6
Plexus ileocolicus, 322, 323
Plexus iliacus
  communis, 414
  externus, 319, 414
  internus, 319, 414
Plexus intermesentericus, 287, 319, 322, 323, 324, 339, 340, 351, 412, 414, 416, 417, 418, 419
Plexus lumbalis, 186, 507, BP80
Plexus lumbosacralis, 506
Plexus marginalis coli, 323
Plexus mesentericus
  inferior, 323, 412, BP6
  superior, 320, 321, 322, 329, 412, BP6, BP7
Plexus myentericus, 327
Plexus oesophageus, 229, 325, BP6, BP7
Plexus ovaricus, 414, 417
Plexus pampiniformis, 388, T6.2
Plexus pancreaticoduodenalis, 320, 321, 322

Plexus phrenici, 320, 412
Plexus phrenicus, 319, 321, 341
Plexus prostaticus, 339, 412, 418, 419, T6.1
Plexus pulmonalis, BP6, BP7
  posterior, 229
Plexus rectalis, 323, 324, 339, 412, 414
Plexus renalis, 319, 323, 339, 412
Plexus sacralis, 186, 287, 323, 339, 412, 417, 418, 419, 508
Plexus sigmoidei, 323
Plexus splenicus, 319, 320, 321
Plexus submucosus, 327
Plexus suprarenalis, 323
Plexus testicularis, 319, 411, 418
Plexus uretericus, 319, 412
Plexus uterovaginalis, 414, 416
Plexus venosus, 194, BP39
  anorectalis, 285, 394
  anorectalis externus, 317, 394, 395, 396, 401
  anorectalis internus, 395, 396, 401
  anorectalis perimuscularis, 317, 401
  areolaris, 277
  basilaris, 130
  prostaticus, 405, BP93
  pterygoideus, T2.4
  urethrae, BP86
  uterinus, 376
  uterovaginalis, 285
  vaginalis, 421
  vertebralis externus anterior, 193, 194
  vertebralis internus anterior, 130, 193, 194
  vertebralis internus posterior, 193
  vesicalis, 285, 368, 369, 371, 405, BP93
Plexus vesicalis, 323, 339, 412, 414, 416, 418, 419
Plica aryepiglottica, 93
Plica axillaris
  anterior, 202
  posterior, 202
Plica caecalis vascularis, 298
Plica duodenojejunalis, 289
Plica duodenomesocolica, 289, 296
Plica fimbriata, 83
Plica glandulopreputialis glandis, 389
Plica glossoepiglottica lateralis, 89
Plica glossoepiglottica mediana, 89
Plica ileocaecalis, 298
Plica inguinalis, 390
Plica interureterica, 371
Plica longitudinalis duodeni, 305
Plica n. laryngei superioris, 93
Plica rectouterina, 363, 365
Plica rectovesicalis, 367, 394
Plica salpingopharyngea, 93
Plica semilunaris, 110
Plica sublingualis, 83
Plica synovialis infrapatellaris, 517, 518
Plica umbilicalis lateralis, 274, 293, 363, 367
Plica umbilicalis medialis, 274, 293, 363, 375, 402, BP81
Plica umbilicalis mediana, 273, 363
Plica urethralis primaria, 389
Plica urethralis secundaria, 389
Plica uterosacralis dex., 375
Plica vesicalis transversa, 274, 363, 367, 375, 376
Plicae alares, 517
Plicae caecales, 298, 363, 367
Plicae circulares, 297, 305
Plicae gastricae, 295, 347
Plicae longitudinales canalis gastrici, 295
Plicae mucosae, 374
Plicae transversae recti, 395
Polus inferior renis, 333
Polus superior renis, 296, 333, 348
Pons, 177, BP32, BP35
Porta hepatis, 302
Portio bulbaris urethrae, 386

Portio pendula urethrae, 386
Porus sudorifer, 12
Postnatal circulation, 247
Prenatal circulation, 247
Preputium clitoridis, 375, 377, 389
Preputium penis, 389
Processus accessorius, 181
Processus alveolaris maxillae, 38
Processus articularis inferior vertebrae, 45, 180, 181, 184, 185, BP37
Processus articularis superior vertebrae, 45, 180, 181, 183, 184, 185, BP37
Processus axillaris glandulae mammariae, 206
Processus mamillaris, 181
Processus ciliaris, 118
Processus clinoideus anterior, 28
Processus condylaris mandibulae, 36, 39
Processus coracoideus, 203, 427, 430, 431, 433, 434, 435, 437, 438, 440, 442, 490
Processus coronoideus mandibulae, 28, 36, 39
Processus coronoideus ulnae, 446, 449, 453
Processus gliocytis, BP3
Processus mastoideus, 36, 38, 49
Processus orbitalis ossis palatini, 25
Processus palatinus maxillae, 28, 31
Processus pyramidalis ossis palatini, 35, 38
Processus spinosus vertebrae, 178, 180, 181, 184, 185, 195, 200, 218, 351, 354, 432, BP18, BP37, T3.1
Processus styloideus
  ossis temporalis, 35, 38, 42, 93
  radii, 453, 462, 467, 477
  ulnae, 462, 467
Processus transversi vertebrarum lumbalium, 268
Processus transversus vertebrae, 163, 181, 184, 185, 200, 216, 253, 354, BP37
  lumbalis, 353
Processus uncinati, 45
Processus uncinatus, 45, 67
Processus vaginalis, 387
Processus xiphoideus, 202, 203, 211, 267, 268, 270, 347, T5.1
Processus zygomaticus, 31, 35
Promontorium ossis sacri, 353, 355, 356, 359, 364, 365, 367, 414, BP81, BP90
Pronator quadratus, 450, 458, 459, 461, 473, 475, 486, T7.7
Pronator teres, 440, 442, 450, 455, 456, 457, 458, 459, 460, 461, 483, T7.7
Prostata, 6, 274, 368, 371, 384, 385, 386, 390, 391, 393, 399, 405, 420, BP94, BP104, T6.3
  seminalis, 385
Protuberantia
  mentalis, 22, 25, 39
  occipitalis externa, 38
Proximal nail fold, BP112
Proximal phalanx, BP99
Proximalis, as term of relationship, 1
Psoas
  major, 200, 216, 280, 283, 284, 285, 287, 296, 330, 331, 350, 351, 363, 366, 367, 402, 420, 502, 505, 507, 514, 550, BP38, BP80, BP81, BP94, T8.9
  minor, 283, 351, 363, 367, 505, T8.9
Pterion, T2.2
Puberty, BP89, BP95
Pubic hair appears, BP95
Pulmo, 190, 205
  dexter, 231, 238, 263, 337
  sinister, 231
Pulmonary trunk, 246
Pulmones, 7
  medial views, 221
  in situ, anterior view, 219
Pulpa digiti manus, 481
Pulpa rubra splenis, 307

Punctum lacrimale
  inferius, 110
  superius, 110
Pupilla, 110
Purulence in fossa ischioanalis, 398
Pylorus, 294, 295, 296, T5.2
Pyramidal system, BP15

R

Radices
  dentium, 67
  nervorum spinalium, 187, 189, 190
  principales plexus lumbalis, 550, 551
Radiculae anteriores, 189
Radiculae posteriores, 189
Radius, 446, 450, 451, 452, 455, 458, 461, 462, 463, 465, 467, 475, BP98, T7.1
Radix anterior
  n. spinalis, 189, 190, 212, 279, 326
  n. spinalis L1, 419
Radix inferior ansae cervicalis, T2.12
Radix mesenterii, 293, 306, 335, 363, 367
Radix posterior (N. spinalis), 189, 279, 419
Rami
  a. suprarenalis mediae, 342
  nervi, 481
  n. facialis, 71
  n. femoralis, 515
  n. transversi colli, 50
Rami anteriores nn. spinalium, 190, 253, 550, 551
Rr. articulares n. tibialis, 553
Rr. buccales n. facialis, 71
Rr. calcanei
  a. tibialis posterioris, 533, 545
  a fibularis, 528, 545, 546
  laterales n. suralis, 493, 545, 552
  mediales n. tibialis, 493, 545, 546
Rr. capsulares n. vesicalis inferioris, BP93
Rr. communicantes, 416
  albi, 507
  grisei, 6, 319, 412, 414, 507, 508, BP6
Rr. cutanei
  a. plantaris lateralis, 543
  anteriores n. femoralis, 411, 492
  anteriores pectorales nn. intercostalium, 209
  laterales nn. spinalium thoracicorum, 198
  mediales cruris n. sapheni, 493
  n. cutanei lateralis femoris, 493
  n. cutanei posterioris femoris, 493
  n. obturatorii, 492, 493
  n. plantaris lateralis, 493, 543
  n. plantaris medialis, 493
  posteriores nn. spinalium, 199
Rr. dentales anteriores n. alveolaris inferioris, 84
Rr. digitales
  dorsales n. fibularis superficialis, 554
  dorsales n. radialis, 477, 489
  dorsales n. ulnaris, 479
  palmares communes n. mediani, 483, 486
  palmares communes n. ulnaris, 470
  palmares proprii n. mediani, 470, 483, 486
  palmares proprii n. ulnaris, 483, 487
  plantares proprii n. plantaris medialis, 544
Rr. dorsales nn. digitalium palmarium propriorum, 478
Rr. femorales n. genitofemoralis, 278, 411, 492
Rr. ganglionares pterygopalatini, 79
Rr. interventriculares septales, 239
Rr. mammarii laterales
  aa. intercostalium posteriorum, 206
  a. thoracicae lateralis, 206
Rr. musculares, 507
  a. femoralis, 522, BP103
  a. profundae femoris, BP103
  n. ischiadici, 511
  plexus cervicalis, T2.12

Rr. nasales
  externi a. ethmoideae anterioris, 60
  externi n. ethmoidei anterioris, 60
  laterales posteriores a. sphenopalatinae, 81
  posteriores superiores n. maxillaris, 149
Rr. oesophagei aortae thoracicae, 258
Rr. perforantes a. thoracicae internae, 206, 209
Rr. perforantes posteriores aa. metatarsearum plantarium, BP105
Rr. posteriores mediales nn. cervicalium, 23
Rr. sensorii n. cutanei, 12
Rr. septales (aa. nasi), 65
Rr. splenici a. splenicae, 308
Rr. subendocardiales (Purkinje fibers), 248
Rr. superficiales
  a. and n. plantaris medialis, 543
  plexus cervicalis, 23
Rr. temporales, 71
Rr. tubarii a. ovaricae, 406
Rr. urethrales n. vesicalis inferioris, BP93
Rr. vaginales a. uterinae, 406
Rr. zygomatici n. facialis, 71
R. accessorius a. meningeae mediae, 33, 34, 74, 78, 123, 128
R. acetabularis a. obturatoriae, 496, 514
R. acromialis a. thoracoacromialis, 437, 443, BP96
R. anterior
  a. obturatoriae, 496
  n. cutanei lateralis antebrachii, 485
  n. cutanei medialis antebrachii, 425
  n. obturatorii, 510, 515, 551
  n. spinalis, 184, 189, 190, 214, 279, 325, 412, 416, 417, 419, BP81
R. articularis
  a. descendentis genus, 510, BP103, BP105
  n. femoralis, 550
  n. fibularis communis, 553, 554
  n. ischiadici, 511
  n. mediani, 486
  n. musculocutanei, 485
  n. obturatorii, 551
  n. tibialis, 552
  n. ulnaris, 487, 488
R. ascendens
  a. circumflexae illiacae profundae, 276, 284
  a. circumflexae lateralis femoris, 510, BP103
  a. colicae sinistrae, 314, 400
R. bronchialis inferior, 222
R. bronchialis superior, 222
R. calcaneus
  a. tibialis posterioris, 527, 528
  lateralis a. fibularis, 529
  lateralis n. suralis, 529, 553
  medialis a. tibialis posterioris, 529
  medialis n. tibialis, 529
R. capsularis a. perforantis radiatae, 334
R. capsularis hepatis, BP83
R. cardiacus cervicalis inferior n. vagi, 249
R. cardiacus cervicalis n. vagi, 229, BP7
R. cardiacus thoracicus n. vagi, 157, 229
R. carpeus dorsalis
  a. radialis, 477
  a. ulnaris, 443, 479, BP97
R. carpeus palmaris
  a. radialis, 458, 475
  a. ulnaris, 458, 475
R. clavicularis a. thoracoacromialis, 437, 443, BP96
R. coeliacus
  trunci vagalis anterioris, 153, 320, 321
  trunci vagalis posterioris, 153, 320, 321, 322, 412
R. colicus a. ileocolicae, 314, BP60
R. collateralis n. intercostalis, 279
R. communicans
  albus, 6, 189, 212, 229, 250, 319, 325, 326, 340, 412, 414, 417, 418, 419, BP6

R. communicans (Continued)
  griseus, 6, 189, 229, 250, 319, 325, 326, 339, 340, 412, 417, 418, 419, BP6
  hypoglossus n. spinalis, T2.12
  lacrimalis n. zygomaticotemporalis, 79
  n. radialis, 478
  n. ulnaris, 476, 478, 483, 486, 487, 488
  suralis n. fibularis communis, 493
R. cutaneus anterior
  n. iliohypogastrici, 278, 411
  n. intercostalis, 279, 436
  n. subcostalis, 278
R. cutaneus lateralis
  a. intercostalis posterioris, 209
  n. iliohypogastrici, 275, 278
  n. intercostalis, 209, 279
  n. subcostalis, 275, 278, 492
R. cutaneus n. obturatorii, 510, 551
R. deltoideus a. thoracoacromialis, 432, 437, 443, BP96
R. descendens
  a. circumflexae lateralis femoris, BP103
  a. colicae sinistrae, 314, 400
R. digastricus n. facialis, 71
R. digitalis dorsalis n. fibularis profundi, 492, 554
R. digitalis palmaris
  communis n. ulnaris, 483, 487
  proprius n. mediani, 470
R. dorsalis
  a. intercostalis posterioris, 192, 212
  n. ulnaris, 425, 454, 457, 458, 461, 478, 479, 483, 487, 488
R. femoralis, n. genitofemoralis, 282, 287, 507
R. frontalis a. temporalis superficialis, 24
R. gastricus posterior trunci vagalis posterioris, 321
R. genitalis n. genitofemoralis, 278, 281, 282, 287, 388, 411, 492
R. hepaticus trunci vagalis anterioris, 320, 323
R. ilealis a. ileocolicae, BP60
R. inferior ossis pubis, 268, 360, 364, 495
R. inferior n. vestibularis, 124, 126
R. infrahyoideus a. thyreoideae superioris, 103
R. infrapatellaris n. sapheni, 492, 509, 510, 531, 550
R. intermedius a. hepaticae sinistrae, 310, BP64
R. ischiopubicus, 352, 353, 354, 356, 357, 362, 368, 371, 372, 378, 379, 381, 383, 384, 385, 397, 496, 497, 505, 555
R. lateralis
  nasi a. facialis, 60
  n. fibularis profundi, 541
R. malleolaris
  lateralis a. fibularis, 529
  medialis a. tibialis posterioris, 533
R. mandibulae, 25, 39
R. marginalis
  dexter a. coronariae dextrae, 240
  mandibularis n. facialis, 71
  sinister a. circumflexae cordis, 239
R. mastoideus a. occipitalis, 163
R. medialis n. fibularis profundi, 279, 531, 532, 541, 542, BP111
R. meningeus
  anterior a. vertebralis, 163
  n. maxillaris, 149
  n. spinalis posterior a. vertebralis, 163
R. meningeus n. spinalis, 190
R. muscularis
  a. brachialis, 442
  n. fibularis profundi, 554
  n. plantaris lateralis, 545
  n. tibialis, 527, 528, 553

R. nasalis externus n. ethmoidei anterioris, 23, 79
R. nodi sinuatrialis a. coronariae dextrae, 239, 240, 248
R. oesophageus
   a. gastricae sinistrae, 258, 308, 309
   aortae thoracicae, 222, 258
   n. splanchnici thoracici majoris, 229
R. orbitofrontalis
   lateralis a. mediae cerebri, 166
   medialis a. anterioris cerebri, 166
R. ossis ischii, 495
R. ovaricus a. uterinae, 376
R. palmaris
   n. mediani, 425, 456, 457, 469, 486
   n. ulnaris, 425, 457, 469, 487, 488
   profundus a. ulnaris, 443, 457, 458, 464, 469, 470, 475, 476, 483, BP97
   superficialis a. radialis, 443, 457, 458, 464, 470, 475, 476, BP97
R. palpebralis n. lacrimalis, 23, 79
R. parietalis a. temporalis superficialis, 24
R. pectoralis a. thoracoacromialis, 437, 443, BP96
R. pelvicus a. renalis, 334
R. perforans
   a. fibularis, 522, 529, 532, 541, 542, BP105
   a. thoracicae internae, 436
R. perinealis
   n. cutanei posterioris femoris, 415
   n. spinalis, 508
R. pharyngeus n. vagi, 82, 8
R. posterior, 425
   a. obturatoriae, 496
   n. cutanei lateralis antebrachii, 425, 485
   n. cutanei medialis antebrachii, 425
   n. obturatorii, 510, 515, 551
   n. spinalis, 189, 279
R. posterior lateralis n. spinalis, 279
R. posterior medialis n. spinalis, 279
R. posterioris n. spinalis T7, 275
R. prefrontalis a. mediae cerebri, 166
R. profundus
   n. perinealis, 413
   n. plantaris lateralis, 546, 553
   n. radialis, 457, 461, 489
   n. ulnaris, 457, 458, 464, 469, 470, 475, 476, 483, 487, 488
R. prostaticus a. vesicalis inferioris, BP93
R. pubici a. epigastricae inferioris, 280
R. pubicus a. epigastricae inferioris, 272, 366
R. recurrens
   oesophageus a. phrenicae inferioris, 216
   n. fibularis profundi, 532
   n. mediani, 469, 470, 476, 483, 486, T7.1
R. saphenus a. descendentis genus, 509, 510, 522, BP103, BP105
R. spinalis a. intercostalis posterioris, 192, 212
R. stylohyoideus n. facialis, 71
R. superficialis
   a. transversae colli, 198
   n. perinealis, 413
   n. plantaris lateralis, 553
   n. radialis, 423, 425, 454, 457, 461, 477, 478, 479, 483, 489
   n. ulnaris, 457, 469, 470, 476, 483, 487, 488
R. superior ossis pubis, 268, 353, 354, 356, 357, 361, 364, 383, 495, 496, 555, T6.1
R. superior n. vestibularis, 124, 126
R. uretericus
   a. renalis, 332, 334, 336
   a. vaginalis, 336
Raphe diaphragmatis pelvis, 359, 360
Raphe penis, 389
Raphe perinei, 377, 389
Raphe pharyngis, 61
Raphe pterygomandibularis, 36, 73, T2.3

Raphe urethralis, 389
Recessus anterior fossae ischioanalis, 274, 371, 372, 398
Recessus costomediastinalis cavitatis pleuralis, 215, 217
Recessus duodenalis
   inferior, 289, 296
   superior, 289
Recessus hepatorenalis, 296
Recessus ileocaecalis
   inferior, 298
   superior, 298
Recessus paracolicus, 363, 367
Recessus paraduodenalis, 289
Recessus pharyngeus, 61, 93
Recessus piriformis, 93
Recessus posterior fossae ischioanalis, 398
Recessus retrocaecalis, 290, 298
Recessus sphenoethmoideus, 61
Recessus subpopliteus, 518
Recessus superior bursae omentalis, 293, 343
Rectum, 6, 182, 283, 290, 301, 330, 343, 358, 359, 360, 363, 364, 366, 367, 368, 373, 375, 385, 393, 399, 402, 414, 421, BP84, BP104, T6.2
   arteriae of, 400
   female, 393, 401
   male, 393, 400
   venae of, 401
Referred pain, visceral, sites of, BP5
Reflectio pericardii, 235
Reflectio peritonealis, 393, 395
Reflectio pleurae parietalis, 217, 218
Regio anterior
   cruris, 491
   femoris, 491
   genus, 491
   tali, 491
Regio calcanea, 491
Regio coxalis, 491
Regio epigastrica, 267, 269
Regio glutea, 491
Regio hypochondriaca, 267, 269
Regio hypogastrica, 267, 269
Regio infrascapularis, 178
Regio inguinalis, 267, 269, BP53
   dissections, 280
Regio lateralis abdominis, 267, 269
Regio lateralis colli, 209
Regio lateralis thoracis, 202
Regio lumbalis, 178, 200
Regio pectoralis, 202
Regio posterior cruris, 491
Regio posterior femoris, 491
Regio posterior genus, 491
Regio posterior tali, 491
Regio presternalis, 202
Regio sacralis, 178
Regio scapularis, 178
Regio umbilicalis, 267, 269
Regio vertebralis, 178
Ren, 6, 21, 247, 291, 292, 293, 294, 296, 302, 306, 307, 330, 331, 337, 342, 345, 346, 350, 387, 402, BP79, BP82, T5.3
   gross structure, 333
   schema of vasa sanguinea intrarenalia, BP73
   as site of referred visceral pain, BP5
Renes, 19
   nervi autonomici, 339
   schema of autonomic innervation, 340
   in situ, anterior views, 330
   in situ, posterior views, 331
   vasa lymphatica and nodi lymphoidei, 338
Respiration, anatomy of, BP45
Rete acromiale, 437
Rete carpeum
   dorsale, 479
   palmare, 475

Rete malleolare
   laterale, 532
   mediale, 532
Rete patellare, 509, 510, BP103, BP105
Rete testis, 391, 392
Rete venosum dorsale manus, 444, 478
Retinacula cutis, 12
Retinaculum extensorium
   carpi, 425, 477, 478, 479, 480
   inferius, 529, 531, 540
   superius, 529, 531, 540, BP110
Retinaculum fibulare
   inferius, 529, 530, 537
   superius, 528, 529, 530
Retinaculum flexorium tali, 527, 529, 533, 540, 545, 546, 553, BP110
Retinaculum flexorium
   carpi, 457, 464, 472, 473, 475, 476, 483, BP100
   tali, 553
Retinaculum laterale patellae, 501, 502, 503, 516, 517, 530, 531
Retinaculum mediale patellae, 502, 510, 516, 518, 531, 532
Rima vulvae, 377
Rostrum corporis callosi, 177
Rotatores, T3.3
Ruga palmaris proximalis, 422

S

Sacculi alveolares, BP44
Sacculus, 125
Saccus endolymphaticus, 125
Saccus pericardiacus, 214, 215, 219, 236
Saddle joint, 9
Satellite cells, BP3
Scala tympani, 125
Scala vestibuli, 125
Scapha, 122
Scapula, 203, 212, 427, 428, 436
Sclera, 116, 118
Scrotum, 267, 352, 387, 389
   contents, 388
Segmenta A_2 aa. anteriorum cerebri, 164
Segmenta bronchopulmonalia, 226
   anterior view, 223
   lateral view, 224
   medial view, 224
   posterior view, 223
Segmentum anterius
   bulbi oculi, T2.1
   inferius renis, 334
   pulmonis (S3), 223, 224
   superius renis, 334
Segmentum apicale (S1), 223–224
Segmentum apicoposterius (S1+2), 223–224
Segmentum basale anterius (S8), 223–224
Segmentum basale anteromediale (S7+8), 223–224
Segmentum basale laterale (S9), 223–224
Segmentum basale mediale (S7), 223–224
Segmentum basale posteriusl (S10), 223–224
Segmentum inferius renis, 334
Segmentum initiale, BP3
Segmentum laterale (S4), 223–224
Segmentum mediale (S5), 223–224
Segmentum P2 a. posterioris cerebri, 164
Segmentum posterius
   pulmonis (S2), 223, 224
   renis, 334
Segmentum superius
   pulmonis (S6), 223, 224
   renis, 334
Sella turcica, 28, BP34
Septa
   interalveolaria, 39
   pulpae cutis, 481

Septate hymen, BP91
Septula testis, 392
Septum atrioventriculare, 241, 242, 243, 244
Septum interatriale, 241
Septum intercavernosum fasciae penis, 382, 383, 386
Septum interlobulare pulmonis, 227
Septum intermusculare
    anterius cruris, 534
    laterale brachii, 440, 445, 455, 458, 488
    laterale femoris, 515
Septum intermusculare mediale
    brachii, 440, 442, 445, 455, 457, 458
    femoris, 515
Septum intermusculare posterius
    cruris, 534
    femoris, 515
Septum intermusculare transversum cruris, 534
Septum interventriculare, 245, T4.2
Septum nasi, 26, 68, 69, 93, T2.5
Septum orbitale, 110, T2.1
Septum pellucidum, 139, 174
Septum scroti, 388, 392, 397, 407
Sinister, as term of relationship, 1
Sinus analis, 395
Sinus aortae (Valsalvae), 244
Sinus carotidis, 163, T2.4
Sinus cavernosus, 163, T2.4
Sinus coronarius, 242
Sinus epididymidis, 392
Sinus frontalis, 26, 28, 61, 67, 68, 69
Sinus intercavernosus anterior, 130
Sinus intercavernosus posterior, 130
Sinus lactifer, 205
Sinus maxillaris, 26, 28, 67, 68, BP32
Sinus occipitalis, 130
Sinus ossis sphenoidei, 29
Sinus paranasales, 37, BP23, T2.5
    changes with age, 68
    coronal and transverse sections, 69
    paramedian views, 67
Sinus petrosus
    inferior, 130
    superior, 130
Sinus prostatici, 386
Sinus prostaticus, BP92
Sinus rectus, BP31
Sinus renalis, 333
Sinus sagittalis
    inferior, 130
    superior, 130, 136, BP31
Sinus sigmoideus, 130, BP31
Sinus sphenoideus, 61, 67, 95, 177, BP34
Sinus sphenoparietalis, 130
Sinus transversus, 130, BP31
    pericardii, 232, 233, 242
Sinus urogenitalis, 390
Sinus venosi durales, T2.4
    basis cranii, 131
    sagittal section, 130
Skeleton appendiculare, 8
Skeleton axiale, 8
Skeleton nasi, 37
    anterolateral view, 59
    inferior view, 59
Skeleton thoracis, 8
Somatic fibers, BP8
Somatosensory system, BP14
Spatia extraperitonealia pelvis, 398
Spatia intercostalia, T4.1
Spatia manus, 473
Spatia perinei, 398
    female, 380
    male, 384
Spatia perisinusoidea, 304
Spatium episclerale, 116

Spatium infraperitoneale, 394
Spatium intervaginale subarachnoideum, 116
Spatium palmare medium, 470, 471, 473
Spatium perianale, 398
Spatium perichorioideum, 116
Spatium periportale, 304, BP78
Spatium perisinusoideum, BP78
Spatium postanale
    profundum, 398
    superficiale, 398
Spatium presacrale, 398
Spatium profundum perinei, BP84
Spatium rectovesicale, 398
Spatium retropubicum, 343, 366, 398
Spatium subarachnoidale, 127, 136, 190
Spatium submucosum, 398
Spatium superficiale perinei, 372, 378, 379, 398, 406, 407, BP84
Spatium suprasternale (of burns), 49
Spatium thenaris, 471
Spermatidia, 391, BP87
Spermatocyte primarium, 391, BP87
Spermatocyte secundarium, 391
Spermatocytia primaria, 391
Spermatocytia secundaria, 391, BP87
Spermatogonium, 391, BP87
Spermatozoa, 391, BP87
Sphincter ampullae hepatopancreaticae, 305, 328
Sphincter ductus
    biliaris, 305
    pancreatici, 305
Sphincter externus ani
    female, 358, 364, 369, 371, 378, 379, 398, BP84, BP86, T6.4
    male, 274, 362, 371, 384, 385, 386, 419, BP84, BP93, T6.4
Sphincter externus urethrae, 274, 362, 364, 369, 371, 378, 379, 384, 385, 386, 398, 419, BP84, BP86, BP93, T6.4
Sphincter internus ani, 394, 395, 396
Sphincter internus urethrae
    female, 370, 371
    male, 371, 385
Sphincter pupillae, T2.3, T2.20
Sphincter pyloricus, 295
Sphincter urethrovaginalis, 358, 369, 372, 378, 379, T6.4
Sphincteres urethrae, female, 370
Spina iliaca anterior inferior, 268, 283, 353, 356, 357, 361, 495, 496
Spina iliaca anterior superior, 267, 268, 270, 271, 280, 281, 283, 300, 352, 353, 356, 357, 378, 381, 491, 495, 496, 501, 502, 509, BP53, T5.1
Spina iliaca posterior inferior, 357, 495
Spina iliaca posterior superior, 178, 356, 357, 495
Spina ischiadica, 184, 268, 283, 353, 354, 355, 356, 357, 358, 359, 360, 361, 400, 413, 415, 495, 512, T6.1
Spina scapulae, 178, 198, 432, 434, 436, 490
Splen, 218, 291, 292, 294, 303, 307, 345, 347, 348, BP79, BP82, T5.2
    arteriae, 308, 310
    as site of referred visceral pain, BP5
    venae, 315
Splenium corporis callosi, 139, 177
Squama frontalis, 35
Sternum, 48, 203, 215, 237, 262, 432
Stipes pili, 12, BP1
Stoma, 98
Stratum basale, 12
Stratum corneum, 12
Stratum externum (Henle), BP1
Stratum fibrosum capsulae art. genus, 518
Stratum granulosum, 12

Stratum internum (Huxley), BP1
Stratum lucidum, 12
Stratum membranosum
    telae subcutaneae abdominis, 270, 273
    telae subcutaneae perinei, 368, 371, 378, 379, 380, 383, 384, 393, 397, 398, 406, 407, BP84
Stratum musculare
    circulare coli, 299
    circulare duodeni, 295, 305, BP56
    circulare gastris, 257, 295
    circulare ilei, 299
    circulare oesophagi, 94, 257
    circulare recti, 362, 395, 396
    longitudinale canalis analis, 394, 396
    longitudinale duodeni, 295, 305, BP56
    longitudinale gastris, 257, 295
    longitudinale ilei, 297, 299
    longitudinale intestini tenuis, 327
    longitudinale jejuni, 295
    longitudinale oesophagi, 257, 295
    longitudinale recti, 362, 396
    longitudinale tracheae, 225
Stratum myelini, BP3
Stratum papillare, 12
Stratum preosseum, BP9
Stratum reticulare, 12
Stratum spinosum, 12
Stratum synoviale capsulae art. glenohumeralis, 431
Stratum synoviale capsulae art. coxae, 496
Stratum synoviale capsulae art. genus, 518
Stratum synoviale capsulae articularis, 481
Stratum synoviale capsulae art. cubiti, 448
Stria terminalis, 139
Stroma fibromusculare prostatae, BP92
Stroma intermusculare, 327
Substantia alba, 189, BP40
Substantia fundamentalis, BP11, BP13
Substantia grisea, 189
Sulci diaphragmatici, BP59
Sulci ramorum a. meningeae mediae, 30
Sulcus a. subclaviae, 221, BP42
Sulcus calcanei, 537
Sulcus coronarius, 389
Sulcus deltopectoralis, 422
Sulcus gluteus, 178, 491
Sulcus hypothalamicus, 174
Sulcus infraorbitalis, 25
Sulcus intermedius posterior, BP40
Sulcus intertubercularis, 427
Sulcus lateralis anterior, BP40
Sulcus m. subclavii, 429
Sulcus medianus linguae, 89
Sulcus medianus posterior, BP40
Sulcus mylohyoideus, 39
Sulcus n. radialis, 427
Sulcus n. spinalis, 45
Sulcus n. ulnaris, 427
Sulcus nasolabialis, 22
Sulcus obturatorius, 495
Sulcus oesophageus, 221
Sulcus papillae, 89
Sulcus paracolicus, 290, 298, 351
Sulcus posterolateralis, BP40
Sulcus sinus sagittalis superioris, 30
Sulcus terminalis linguae, 89
Sulcus urethralis
    primarius, 389
    secondarius, 389
Sulcus v. azygae, 221
Sulcus v. brachiocephalicae, 221
Sulcus v. cavae inferioris, 221
Sulcus v. cavae superioris, 221
Sulcus v. subclaviae, BP42
Supinator, 428, 450, 455, 457, 458, 459, 460, 483, 489, T7.7

Sustenocyte, 391
Sustentaculum tali, 537, 539
Sutura coronalis, 25, 26, 28, 30, 35
Sutura frontozygomatica, 26
Sutura intermaxillaris, 31
Sutura lambdoidea, 26, 28, 30, 35
Sutura metopica, 35
Sutura sagittalis, 26, 30, 35
Suturae cranii, T2.2
Sympathetic fibers, BP8
Symphysis pubica, 267, 268, 280, 283, 352,
    353, 354, 355, 356, 360, 361, 362, 364, 366,
    369, 375, 378, 380, 381, 384, 420, 421,
    BP94, T5.1, T6.1
Synapses adrenergicae, BP8
Synapses cholinergicae, BP8
Synapsis, BP3
Synchondrosis manubriosternalis, 429
Systema cardiovasculare, 13, BP12, T2.4, T3.1,
    T4.2, T5.2, T6.2, T8.2
    composition of blood, BP12
    venae systematicae majores, 15
Systema digestorium, T2.5, T5.2, T6.2
Systema endocrinum, 21
Systema genitale masculinum, 391
Systema musculare, 10, T3.1, T4.2, T5.1, T7.1,
    T8.2
Systema nervosum, 4, T2.1, T3.1, T4.1, T5.1,
    T6.1, T7.1, T8.1
    centrale, 4
    periphericum, 4
    segmental motor function, 11
Systema respiratorium, 17, T2.5, T4.3
Systema skeletale, 8, T2.2, T3.1, T4.1, T6.1,
    T7.1, T8.1
Systema urinarium, 19, T6.3
Systemata genitalia, 20, T4.3–T4.4, T6.3

T

Taenia libera, 290, 298, 299, 393, 396
Taenia mesocolica, 298, 299
Taenia omentalis, 298, 301
Talus
    cross-sectional anatomy, BP110
    radiographs, 556
Taste pathways, schema, 162
Tectum mesencephali, 177
Tela subcutanea
    abdominis, 270, 368, 378, BP84
    epicranii, 48
    penis, 270, 271, 272, 368, 381, 382, 383, 388,
        BP84
    perinei, 378
Tela submucosa, 297, BP55, BP56, BP57
    appendix vermiformis, BP57
    duodeni, BP56
    esophagi, 257
    gastris, BP55
    intestini tenuis, 297
Tela subserosa intestini tenuis, 327
Tendines capitum flexoris superficialis
    digitorum, 453
Tendines extensoris
    brevis digitorum, 531, 532, 542, 547
    digitorum, 422, 451, 454, 455, 461, 473, 479,
        480, BP102
    longi digitorum, 491, 530, 531, 532, 541, 549
Tendines flexoris brevis digitorum, 544, 545,
    546
Tendines flexoris longi digitorum, 545, 546,
    549
Tendines flexoris profundi digitorum, 453, 468,
    471, 473, BP101, BP102
Tendines flexoris superficialis digitorum, 422,
    456, 468, 471, 472, 483, BP101, BP102
Tendines mm. lumbricalium, 471, 546

Tendines originis m. recti femoris, 502
Tendinous slips to aponeuroses extensoriae,
    475
Tendo abductoris
    hallucis, 539, 547
    longi pollicis, 454, 458, 461, 477, 479, 480
Tendo adductoris
    hallucis, 539
    magni, 510, 515, 516, 521, 528
Tendo calcaneus, 528, 529, 530, 540, 556,
    BP106, T8.2
Tendo capitis lateralis flexoris brevis hallucis,
    539
Tendo capitis longi m. bicipitis brachii, 431
Tendo capitis longi m. bicipitis femoris, 513
Tendo capitis medialis flexoris brevis hallucis,
    539
Tendo extensoris
    brevis digitorum, BP111
    brevis hallucis, 531, 532, 547, 549, BP111
    brevis pollicis, 454, 458, 477, 479, 480
    digiti minimi, 451, 454, 455, 461, 479, 480
    digitorum, 474, BP101, BP102
    indicis, 422, 454, 479, 480, BP101, BP102
    longi digitorum, 529, BP111
    longi hallucis, 491, 530, 531, 532, 541, 542,
        547, 549, BP111
    longi pollicis, 422, 454, 461, 473, 477, 479,
        480
    radialis brevis carpi, 454, 455, 461, 477, 479,
        480
    radialis longi carpi, 454, 455, 479, 480
    ulnaris carpi, 454, 455, 461, 479, 480
Tendo extensorius communis, 428, 451, 454,
    455
Tendo flexoris
    brevis digitorum, 539
    longi digitorum, 527, 528, 529, 539, 545,
        BP110
    longi hallucis, 527, 529, 539, 544, 545, 546,
        547, 549
    longi pollicis, 458, 464, 472, 473, BP101,
        BP102
    profundi digitorum, 471, 473, 474, 481
    radialis carpi, 422, 457, 458, 461, 464, 470,
        472, 473, 483
    superficialis digitorum, 471, 473, 474
    ulnaris carpi, 422, 458, 464, 470, 472, 475,
        BP98
Tendo flexorius communis, 428, 452, 453, 456
Tendo iliopsoae, 514
Tendo m.
    bicipitis brachii, 440, 442, 448, 456, 457, 458,
        T7.1
    bicipitis femoris, 516, 525, 528, 531, 554
    brachioradialis, 458
    fibularis brevis, 528, 529, 530, 537, 540, 542,
        546, 547, BP110
    fibularis longi, 528, 529, 530, 532, 537, 540,
        541, 544, 546, 547, 549, BP110, BP111
    fibularis tertii, 530, 531, 540, 541, 542, 547,
        549, BP110
    gastrocnemii, BP110
    gracilis, 491, 502, 503
    infraspinati, 434, 436, 441
    latissimi dorsi, 445
    palmaris longi, 422, 456, 457, 458, 461, 464,
        469, 470, 472
    pectoralis majoris, 445
    pectoralis minoris, 433, 438, 440
    piriformis, 513
    plantaris, 527, 528, 533, 534, BP106, BP110
    poplitei, 517, 518, 519
    quadricipitis femoris, 491, 503, 516, 521, 531,
        532, BP108
    recti femoris, 502, 515, 517, 531
    recti superioris, 120

Tendo m. *(Continued)*
    sartorii, 502, 531, 532, BP106
    semimembranosi, 518, 520, 521, 529
    semitendinosi, 502, 503
    subscapularis, 431, 434
    supraspinati, 431, 434, 441, 490, T7.1
    teretis minoris, 434
    tibialis anterioris, 531, 532, 539, 540, 541,
        549, BP110, BP111
    tibialis posterioris, 527, 528, 529, 533, 540,
        546, BP110
    transversi abdominis, 351
    tricipitis brachii, 454, 455, 488
Tendo m. fibularis brevis, 491
Tendo m. fibularis longi, 491
Tendo obturatoris interni, 360, 362
Tendo psoae majoris, BP94
Tendo psoae minoris, 283
Tendo tensoris fasciae latae, 502
Tendo, 516, 544, 545, BP104, BP110, BP111
Tensor fasciae latae, 421, 491, 501, 502, 509,
    510, 511, 512, 515, BP94, T8.10
Tensor tympani, T2.21
Tensor veli palatini, 73, T2.22
Tentorium cerebelli, 130
Terminationes neurales liberae, 12
Termini generales, 1
Terminus durae spinalis, 182, 186
Testes, 21, 387, 391
Testis, 343, 387, 388, 390, 391, 392, 418, T6.3
    anterior view, 403
    arteriae, 403
    descent of, 387
    venae of, 403
Textus adiposus, 21
    epiduralis, 182, 190, BP39
    extraperitonealis, 273, 281, 282
    fossae acetabula, 496
    gluteus, 420, 421
    mammae, 205
    spatium retropubicum, 272, 362
Textus connectivus
    hepatis, BP78
    prevertebralis, BP34
Textus perianales, 389
Thalami, 139
Thalamus, 138, 324
Theca externa, BP90
Theca interna, BP90
Thorax, 2
    axial ct images, 262
    bony framework, 203
    cor, coronal section of, 238
    coronal cts, BP51
    coronal sections, BP50
    cross section at T3/T4 disc level, 264
    cross section at T4/T5 disc level, 265
    cross section at T3 vertebral level, 263
    cross section at T7 vertebral level, 266
    nervi, 249
    nervi autonomici of, 229
    nodi lymphoidei, 228
    pulmones in
        anterior view, 217
        posterior view, 218
    surface anatomy, 202
    vasa lymphatica, 228
Thymus, 16, 21, 219, 231
Tibia, 520, 521, 524, 531, 532, 534, 541, 542,
    556, BP106, BP108, BP110, T8.1
    additional views and cross section, 525
    anterior and posterior views, 524
Tibial mechanical axis, BP107
Toenail growth, BP112
Tonguelike process, BP59
Tonsilla lingualis, 89, 93
Tonsilla palatina, 83, 89, 93

Tonsilla pharyngea, 61, 93, 177, BP34, BP35
Tonsillae, 16
Tortuosity of ducts, BP62
Torus levatorius, 93
Torus tubarius, 61, 93
Trabecula septomarginalis, 248
Trabeculae splenis, 307
Trachea, 7, 93, 103, 217, 220, 222, 225, 231, 238, 251, 263, BP34, BP36
Tractus corticospinalis anterior, BP40
Tractus descendentes medullae, 230
Tractus hypothalamohypophysial, 174
Tractus iliopubicus, 280, 363, 366, 367
Tractus iliotibialis, 415, 491, 498, 501, 502, 511, 513, 515, 517, 518, 525, 526, 527, 531, T8.2
Tractus opticus, 139
Tractus paraventriculohypophysial is, 174
Tractus portales, 303
Tractus portalis, 303
Tractus reticulospinalis lateralis, BP40
Tractus reticulospinalis medialis, BP40
Tractus rubrospinalis, BP40
Tractus spinalis, 143
Tractus spinocerebellaris anterior, BP40
Tractus spinocerebellaris posterior, BP40
Tractus spinoolivaris, BP40
Tractus supraopticohypophysialis, 174
Tractus tectospinalis, BP40
Tractus tuberohypophysialis, 174
Tractus vestibulospinalis lateralis, BP40
Tragus, 22, 122
Trias portae hepatis, 296, 303
Trigonum, 369
    anale, 352, 381
    auscultationis, 178, 275, 432
    cystohepaticum, 305, 310
    deltopectorale, 432
    femorale, BP53
    fibrosum sinistrum, 243
    inguinale, 274, 280, T5.1
    lumbale (Petiti), 178, 275
    lumbocostale, 283
    urogenitale, 352, 381
    vesicae, 371, 375, 385, 386, BP86
Trochanter major, 178, 268, 353, 354, 420, 491, 496, 497, 500, 502, 503, 504, 505, 511, 512, 555, BP104
Trochanter minor, 268, 283, 353, 354, 496, 497, 500, 555
Trochlea fibularis, 537
Trochlea humeri, 427, 446
Trochlea m. digastrici, 49, 53
Trochlea ossis tali, 537
Trunci lumbosacrales, 287
Trunci lymphatici lumbales, 338, BP76
Trunci vagales, 283
Truncus brachiocephalicus, 57, 103, 163, 211, 220, 230, 231, 232, 233, 234, 238, 263
Truncus coeliacus, 14, 216, 247, 258, 284, 289, 293, 306, 308, 309, 310, 311, 312, 313, 325, 330, 332, 343, 349, BP64, BP67, BP69, BP83
    variations, BP67
Truncus corporis callosi, 177
Truncus costocervicalis, 57, 163, 194
Truncus encephali, 140, 143, 144
Truncus hepatomesentericus, BP67
Truncus inferior plexus brachialis, 433
Truncus lumbosacralis, 287, 339, 412, 507, 508, 551, BP81
Truncus lymphaticus bronchomediastinalis, 228
Truncus lymphaticus dexter, BP76
Truncus lymphaticus intestinalis, 286, BP76
Truncus lymphaticus jugularis, 228, BP76
Truncus lymphaticus lumbalis, 286

Truncus lymphaticus subclavius, 228, 286, BP76
Truncus medius plexus brachialis, 433
Truncus n. spinalis, 279
Truncus pulmonalis, 232, 233, 234, 241, 245, 247
Truncus sympathicus, 6, 215, 216, 229, 249, 250, 251, 283, 319, 323, 324, 325, 328, 329, 339, 341, 351, 411, 412, 414, 417, 418, 419, 507, BP6, BP79
Truncus thyreocervicalis, 57, 103, 163, 194
Truncus vagalis anterior, 229, 319, 320, 321, 322, 323, 325, 328, 329, 339, 412, BP7
Truncus vagalis posterior, 319, 321, 322, 323, 325, 339, 341, 412, BP7
Tuba auditiva (Eustachii), 125, BP30
Tuba uterina, 363, 364, 365, 372, 373, 374, 375, 390, 402, 414, 417, T6.3
Tuber calcanei, 491, 528, 537, 543, 544, 545, 546
Tuber ischiadicum, 268, 352, 353, 354, 355, 356, 357, 360, 362, 378, 379, 381, 383, 384, 394, 397, 495, 496, 497, 504, 511, 512, T6.1
Tuber maxillae, 38
Tuberculum, 268
    adductorium, 500, 510, 519, BP107
    anale, 389
    anterius atlantis, 43, 45
    articulare, 42
    auriculare (tubercule of Darwin), 122
    caroticum (of Chassaignac), 45
    conoideum, 429
    corniculatum, 93
    costae, BP42
    cuneiforme, 93
    dorsale radii, 462
    genitale, 389
    iliacum, 356
    infraglenoideum, 427
    intercondylare laterale, 525, BP107
    intercondylare mediale, 525, BP107
    labii superioris, 22, 83
    labioscrotale, 389
    majus, 427, 430, 431, 440
    mentale, 25, 39
    minus, 427, 430, 440
    ossis scaphoidei, 462, 464, BP98
    ossis trapezii, 462, 464, BP98
    pharyngeum, 46
    posterius atlantis, 43, 45, 196
    pubicum, 267, 268, 271, 272, 281, 283, 352, 353, 356, 357, 361, 362, 378, 383, 495, 502, 555
    supraglenoideum, 427
    tractus iliotibialis, 524, BP107
Tuberositas, 466
    deltoidea, 427
    iliaca, 268, 353, 495
    ossis 5 metatarsi, 540, 541, 546, 547, 548
    ossis navicularis, 539
    radii, 440, 446, 447, 449
    tibiae, 491, 502, 503, 516, 517, 518, 519, 524, 525, 530, 531, BP107
    ulnae, 440, 446, 449
Tubuli
    mesonephrici, 390
    reunientes, BP72
    seminiferi contorti, 391, 392
Tubulus colligens, BP72
Tunica adventitia arteriae, BP13
Tunica adventitia tracheae, 225
Tunica albuginea corporis cavernosi, 382, 386
Tunica albuginea corporis spongiosi, 382, 386
Tunica albuginea testis, 392
Tunica conjunctiva bulbi oculi, 110, BP27
Tunica conjunctiva palpebrae inferiori, 110

Tunica conjunctiva palpebrae superioris, 110
Tunica darta scroti, 270, 271, 272, 368, 388, 392, 397, 407, BP84
Tunica intima arteriae, BP13
Tunica mucosa
    intestini crassi, 301
    intestini tenuis, 297, 327
    gastris, 295
    oesophagi, 94, 257
    parietis posterioris trachea, 225
Tunica muscularis intestini crassi, 301
Tunica muscularis intestini tenuis, 297
Tunica serosa appendicis vermiformis, BP57
Tunica serosa intestini tenuis, 297, 327
Tunica submucosa intestini tenuis, 327
Tunica vaginalis testis, 343

U

Ulna, 446, 450, 451, 452, 455, 462, 463, 465, 467, BP98, T7.1
Umbilicus, 267, 274, 318, 399, BP80, BP83, T5.3
Umbo membranae tympanicae, 125
Unguis digiti manus, 481
Unguis digiti pedis, BP112
Upper limb, segmental innervation of, 11
Ureter, 19, 274, 285, 293, 330, 333, 335, 336, 350, 351, 363, 364, 365, 366, 367, 368, 369, 372, 373, 374, 375, 376, 385, 393, 394, 402, 403, 405, 406, 412, 414, BP80, BP81, BP90, BP93, T6.3
    arteriae, 336
    nervi autonomici, 339
Urethra
    feminina, 19, 358, 359, 360, 364, 369, 370, 371, 373, 375, 379, 390, 421, BP85, BP86
    musculina, 19, 283, 362, 371, 386, 390, BP85
Uterus, 372, 375, 390, 393, 402, 414, BP84, T6.3
    arteriae and venae of, 406
    development of, BP89
    enlarges, BP95
    ligamenta, 373, 374
    supporting structures, 372, 373, 374
Utriculus, 125
    prostaticus, 371, 385, 386, 390, BP92
Uvula
    palatina, 83, 93
    vesicae, 371, 385, 386

V

Vagina, 358, 359, 360, 364, 369, 370, 372, 373, 375, 379, 390, 393, 397, 399, 402, 417, 421, BP86, T6.3
    bulbi, 116
    carotidis, 49
    communis tendinum flexorum, 470, 471, 472, 476
    externa n. optici, 116
    femoralis, 272, 274, 282, 494, 509
    fibrosa digiti manus, 473, 481
    m. recti abdominis, 270, 271, 351
    radicularis epithelialis externa, BP1
    radicularis epithelialis interna, BP1
    synovialis digiti manus, 471, 473, 481
    synovialis digiti minimi, 470
    tendinis extensoris longi hallucis, 540, 541
    tendinis flexoris longi pollicis, 470, 471, 472, 473
    tendinis flexoris radialis carpi, 472
    tendinis intertubercularis, 431, 440
    tendinis m. tibialis anterioris, 540
    tendinis m. tibialis posterioris, 540
Vaginae synoviales digitorum manus, 470, 471

Vaginae tendinum manus, 471, 473
Vaginae tendinum tali, 540
Vaginal epithelium partially cornifies, BP95
Vallecula epiglottica, 89
Valva aortae, 238, 245, T4.2
Valva atrioventricularis dextra, 237, 246
Valva atrioventricularis sinistra (Valva mitralis), 237, 245
Valva trunci pulmonalis, 243, 248
Valvae cordis, 246, T4.2
Valvula analis, 395
Valvula coronaria
    dextra, 242, 244
    sinistra, 242, 244
Valvula noncoronaria, 242, 244
Valvula semilunaris anterior, 243
Valvula semilunaris dextra, 243
Valvula semilunaris sinistra, 243
Vas anastomicum, 514
Vas capillare, BP11
Vas lymphaticum, 304
Vas sinusoideum, 304, BP78
Vasa anastomotica paravertebralia, 192
Vasa anastomotica prevertebralia, 192
Vasa lymphatica, 16, T2.4, T4.3, T5.2, T6.2, T8.3
Vasa lymphatica mammae, 16, 207, T4.3
Vasa lymphatica membri inferioris, 16, 494, T8.3
Vasa lymphatica membri superioris, 426
Vasa lymphatica oesophagi, 260
Vasa lymphatica perinealia, BP77
Vasa lymphatica superficialia membri inferioris, 494
Vasa lymphatica thoracis, 228
Vasa recta spuria, BP73
Vasa recta vera, BP73
Vasa sanguinea, innervation, schema of, BP52
Vasa sinusoidea, 303, 304
Vasa vasis, BP13
V. anastomotica, 50, 401
V. anorectalis inferior, 317, 401
V. anorectalis media, 285, 317
V. anorectalis superior, 317, T5.2
V. appendicularis, 317, 318
V. axillaris, 15, 277, 435, 444
V. azyga, 15, 213, 229, 347, BP79, T4.3
V. basilica, 15, 422, 424, 425, 426, 444, 445, 461, 478
V. basivertebralis, 193, BP39
V. brachiocephalica dextra, 15, 194, 211, 213, 228, 233, 259
V. brachiocephalica sinistra, 15, 194, 211, 213, 228, 233
V. caecalis anterior, 317, 318
V. caecalis posterior, 317, 318
V. capsularis renis, BP73
V. cardiaca magna, 239
V. cardiaca parva, 239
V. cava inferior, 15, 200, 229, 234, 241, 242, 246, 247, 248, 253, 285, 291, 292, 293, 294, 296, 302, 306, 312, 315, 330, 332, 341, 345, 346, 347, 348, 350, 351, 363, 367, 400, 401, 402, 403, 414, BP38, BP79, BP82, BP93
V. cava superior, 15, 103, 213, 234, 241, 246, 247, 248, 253, 259, 262, 344
V. cavernosa, 405
V. centralis, 303, 304
V. cephalica accessoria, 424, 425
V. cephalica, 15, 202, 209, 238, 277, 422, 424, 425, 426, 432, 435, 438, 444, 445, 461, 478
V. cervicalis profunda, 194, BP39
V. circumflexa iliaca profunda, 274, 285

V. circumflexa iliaca superficialis, 267, 277, 492, 523
V. circumflexa lateralis femoris, 523
V. circumflexa medialis femoris, 523
V. circumflexa posterior humeri, 424
V. colica dextra, 316, 317, 318
V. colica media, 316, 317, 318
V. colica sinistra, 317, 318
V. communicans, BP39
V. cremasterica, 403
V. dorsalis
    profunda clitoridis, 358, 359, 360, 364, 366, 369, 377, 380
    profunda penis, 270, 362, 368, 382, 403, 405, 407, BP93
    superficialis clitoridis, 377
    superficialis penis, 267, 277, 352, 382, 405, BP93
V. epigastrica inferior, 272, 274, 280, 285, 363
V. epigastrica superficialis, 267, 277, 285, 492, 523, BP53
V. epigastrica superior, 272
V. episcleralis, 120
V. facialis profunda, 24, 100, 115
V. femoralis, 15, 277, 285, 403, 420, 421, 523, BP53, BP94, T8.2
V. fibularis, 533
V. gastrica dextra, 315, 316, 318
V. gastrica sinistra, 315, 316, 317, 318, BP79
V. gastroomentalis dextra, 315, 317, 318
V. gastroomentalis sinistra, 315
V. glutea inferior, 285, 420
V. glutea superior, 285, 317
V. hemiazyga accessoria, 259
V. hemiazyga, 213, 259
V. hepatica, 13, 247, 303
V. ileocolica, 316, 317, 318
V. iliaca communis, 15, 285, 373, BP81
V. iliaca externa, 15, 285, 317, 405, 523
V. iliaca interna, 15, 285, 317, 373, 405
V. iliolumbalis, 285
V. intercostalis, 205
    anterior, 213
    posterior, 213
    superior dextra, 213, 251
V. interlobularis, 304
V. interna cerebri, BP31
V. intervertebralis, 193, BP39
V. jugularis anterior, 50, 103
V. jugularis externa, 15, 22, 50, 103, 220, 231, 238, 259, T2.4
    dextra, T2.4
V. jugularis interna, 15, 49, 50, 57, 208, 211, 219, 220, 228, 231, 238, 259, BP31, T2.4
V. lateralis superficialis penis, 382
V. lumbalis, 332
V. magna cerebri (Galeni), 130, BP31
V. marginalis medialis pedis, 492
V. mediana antebrachii, 422, 424, 425, 444, 461
V. mediana basilica, 425, 444
V. mediana cephalica, 425
V. mediana cubiti, 424, 426, 444, T7.2
V. medullaris
    segmentalis anterior, 193
    segmentalis posterior, 193
V. mesenterica
    inferior, 289, 315, 317, 401
    superior, 200, 315, 316, 317, 318, 345, 350
V. musculophrenica, 277
V. nasofrontalis, 24
V. obturatoria, 280, 285, 317, 373
V. ophthalmica superior, 120
V. ovarica, 285, 402
V. pancreatica magna, 315
V. pancreaticoduodenalis inferior anterior, 315

V. pancreaticoduodenalis inferior posterior, 315
V. pancreaticoduodenalis superior anterior, 315, 317
V. pancreaticoduodenalis superior posterior, 315
V. perforans radiata, BP73
V. perforans, 444, 533
V. phrenica inferior, 332
V. poplitea, 15, 494, 523
V. portae hepatis, 247, 292, 294, 296, 297, 302, 303, 305, 306, 308, 310, 315, 316, 317, 318, 343, 345, 348, 349, BP74, BP75, BP79, T5.2
    affluentes, 318
    anastomoses portocavales, 318
    anomalies, BP66
    variations, BP66
V. prepylorica, 315, 317
V. profunda femoris, 15, 523
V. pubica, 285
V. pudendalis externa superficialis, 492
V. pudendalis externa, 277, 285, 523
V. pudendalis interna, 285, 407
V. pulmonalis dextra, 247
    inferior, 241
    superior, 241
V. pulmonalis sinistra, 247
V. pulmonalis, 227
V. renalis, 15, 285, 332, 346, 350, 402
    variations, BP70
V. retromandibularis, 50
V. sacralis mediana, 285, 365, 401
V. saphena accessoria, 492, 493, 523
V. saphena magna, 15, 270, 271, 277, 285, 381, 421, 491, 492, 493, 494, 515, 523, 533, 534, BP53, BP106, BP110, BP111, T8.2
V. saphena parva, 491, 492, 493, 494, 511, 527, 533, 534, BP110
V. spinalis anterior, 193
V. spinalis posterior, 193
V. splenica, 292, 293, 307, 315, 316, 317, 318, 341, 345, 349
V. subclavia, 15, 259, 277, T2.4
V. subcostalis, 285
V. subcutanea, 12
V. sublobularis, 303, 304
V. submentalis, 50
V. supraorbitalis, 24
V. suprarenalis
    dextra, 285, 332, 341, 342
    inferior dex, 285
    sinistra, 332, 341, 342
V. supratrochlearis, 24
V. temporalis media, 24
V. testicularis, 280, 282, 293
V. thoracica interna, 277
V. thoracica lateralis, 277
V. thoracodorsalis, 444
V. thoracoepigastrica, 270, 277
V. thyreoidea inferior, 219, 259
V. tibialis posterior, 527, 533
V. transversa faciei, 24
V. ulnaris, 444
V. umblicalis, 247
V. uterina, 285
V. vertebralis accessoria, 194
V. vertebralis, 194, 259
V. vesicalis superior, 285
V. vorticosa, 120
Vv. anorectales, T6.2
Vv. anorectales inferiores, 318
Vv. anorectales mediae, 318
Vv. brachiales, 15, 438, 444, 445
Vv. brachiocephalicae, 103, 253
Vv. bronchiales, 222

Atlas of Human Anatomy

Vv. cardiacae, 239, BP47
Vv. ciliares anteriores, 120
Vv. columnae vertebralis, 193
   venae vertebrales, 194
   venous communications, BP39
Vv. comitantes, 470
Vv. communicantes, 194
Vv. cruris, 533
Vv. digitales palmares, 15, 444
Vv. epigastricae inferiores, 277
Vv. epigastricae superiores, 213, 277
Vv. gastricae breves, 315
Vv. hepaticae, 253, 285, 315
Vv. ileales, 316, 317
Vv. iliacae communes, 401
Vv. iliacae internae, T6.2
Vv. intercapitulares, 425, 444, 478
Vv. intercostales anteriores, 277
Vv. intercostales, 15
Vv. interosseae anteriores, 444
Vv. jejunales, 316, 317
Vv. lumbales, 285
Vv. medullae spinalis, 193
Vv. membri inferioris, 523
Vv. metacarpeae dorsales, 425, 478
Vv. metacarpeae palmares, 444
Vv. metatarseae dorsales, 492
Vv. oesophageae, 259, 318, T5.2
Vv. pancreaticae, 317
Vv. paraumbilicales, 277, 318, T5.2
Vv. perforantes anteriores, 213
Vv. perforantes, 424, 425, 533
Vv. phrenicae inferiores, 285
Vv. profundae, 15
Vv. profundae encephali, 172
Vv. profundae membri inferioris, T8.2
Vv. pulmonales, T4.2
Vv. pulmonales dextrae, 242
Vv. pulmonales sinistrae, 242
Vv. radiales, 15, 444
Vv. rectae, 316
Vv. sacrales laterales, 285
Vv. scrotales anteriores, 277
Vv. sigmoideae, 317

Vv. subependymales encephali, 173
Vv. sublobulares, 303
Vv. superficiales, 15
   antebrachium and manus, 425
   cerebri, 129
   colli, 50
   membri inferioris, T8.2
   omos and brachium, 424
Venae superficiales membri inferioris
   anterior view, 492
   posterior view, 493
Vv. superiores cerebri, T2.4
Vv. suprarenales sin, 285
Vv. thoracicae internae, 213, 215
Vv. thyreoideae inferiores, 103, 231
Vv. tibiales anteriores, 15
Vv. tibiales posteriores, 15, 523
Vv. ulnares, 15
Vv. vertebrales anteriores, 194, BP39
Venter frontalis m. occipitofrontalis, 60, BP19
Venter inferior m. omohyoidei, 22, 49, 432,
   435, 438, T7.12
Venter posterior m. digastrici, 58
Venter superior m. omohyoidei, 49, 58
Ventilation, anatomy of, BP45
Ventriculi, 245
   encephali, 135, 141
Ventriculus dexter, 235, 237, 241, 245
Ventriculus lateralis, 139
Ventriculus quartus, 177
Ventriculus sinister, 234, 238, 242
Ventriculus tertius, 177
Venulae rectae, BP73
Venulae stellatae, BP73
Vertebrae, 187
   cervicales, 44, 179, BP17, T2.2
     atlas and axis, 43
   lumbales, 179, 181, 399, T3.1
   radiograph and MRI of, 182
   thoracicae, 179, 180
Vertebrae cervicales, 45
Vesica biliaris, 6, 18, 217, 288, 291, 294, 302, 305,
   306, 310, 345, 348, BP57, BP58, BP82, T5.3
   as site of referred visceral pain, BP5

Vesica urinaria, 6, 7, 19, 182, 274, 281, 282,
   288, 300, 323, 330, 335, 343, 363, 364,
   365, 366, 367, 368, 369, 370, 375, 384,
   385, 387, 393, 399, 402, 405, 414, 419,
   420, BP84, BP85, BP90, BP94, BP104,
   T6.3
   arteriae, 336
   female, 371
   innervation of, 419
   male, 371
   nervi autonomici, 339
   orientation, 369
   schema, 419
   supports, 369
   vasa lymphatica and nodi lymphoidei, 338
vesicae urinariae, 369
Vesiculae synapticae, BP3
Vestibulum vaginae, 372, 377, 390
Vestibulum, 121, 125
Vestibulum nasi, 61
Vincula longa tendinum, 474
Vinculum breve tendinis, 474
Viscera abdominis, 288
Viscera pelvis
   anterior view, 402
   arteriae, 402
   female, 364, 375, 402, 414
   male, 368, 412
   nervi of, 412, 414
   venae of, 402
Visual pathway, 147
Voluntary urethral sphincters, 370
Vomer, 25, 31

W

White blood cells, BP12

Z

Zona centralis prostatae, 385
Zona peripherica prostatae, 385
Zona squamosa analis, 395
Zona transitionalis prostatae, 385